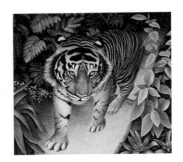

The Nightingale Research Foundation Review of

The Clinical and Scientific Basis of Myalgic Encephalomyelitis/ Chronic Fatigue Syndrome*

Byron M. Hyde, M.D.
Medical and Scientific Editor

◆

Jay Goldstein, M.D.
Director, Chronic Fatigue Syndrome Institute, Anaheim, California, USA
Intellectual and Conceptual Advice

◆

Paul Levine, M.D.
NIH, Bethesda, Maryland, USA
Editorial Advice

* Also known as Post-Viral Fatigue Syndrome and Chronic Fatigue and Immune Dysfunction Syndrome

The Nightingale Research Foundation

Front Cover Illustration: The boy whose portrait is on the cover comes from a province in Canada where none of the demonstrated physiological brain scanning techniques is accessible. The brain images represented are from different patients and simply illustrate different investigative techniques.

Back Cover Illustration: The Nightingale Research Foundation symbol is "Tiger in Kew Gardens" by Beryl Cook. Reproduced from the original painting, courtesy of Beryl Cook and with the assistance of Portal Gallery, London, England.

For Nightingale Research Foundation:
Production Editor: Bonnie Cameron
Copy Editor: Anne Duncker
Communications: Lydia Neilson
Project Administrator: Laurie Wilson
Assistant Editor: Glenn Sheskay

Published by The Nightingale Research Foundation simultaneously in Ottawa, Ontario, Canada and Ogdensburg, New York State, USA

Library of Congress Catalog Card Number 92-064489

Canadian Cataloguing in Publication Data

Main entry under title:

The Nightingale Research Foundation review of the clinical and scientific basis of myalgic encephalo-myelitis/chronic fatigue syndrome

"...proceedings of the Cambridge Easter Symposium on Myalgic Encephalomyelitis/Chronic Fatigue Syndrome."-Foreword.
"Also known as post-viral fatigue syndrome and chronic fatigue and immune dysfunction syndrome".
Includes indexes.

ISBN 0-9695662-0-4

     1. Myalgic encephalomyelitis--Congresses. 2. Chronic fatigue syndrome--Congresses. I. Hyde, Byron M. II. Goldstein, Jay A. III. Levine, P.H. (Paul H.) IV. Nightingale Research Foundation. V. Cambridge Easter Symposium on Myalgic Encephalomyelitis/Chronic Fatigue Syndrome (1990: Cambridge University). VI. Title. VII. Title: The Clinical and scientific basis of myalgic encephalomyelitis/chronic fatigue syndrome.

RB150.F37N44 1992   616.7 ' 4   C92-090416-5   75617

Printed and bound in Canada

This text is printed on acid free paper manufactured by an environmentally friendly process.

This book was created on a Macintosh IIci, donated by Apple Canada, assembled in Microsoft Word donated by Microsoft Corporation and was formatted in Aldus PageMaker, donated by Aldus Canada.

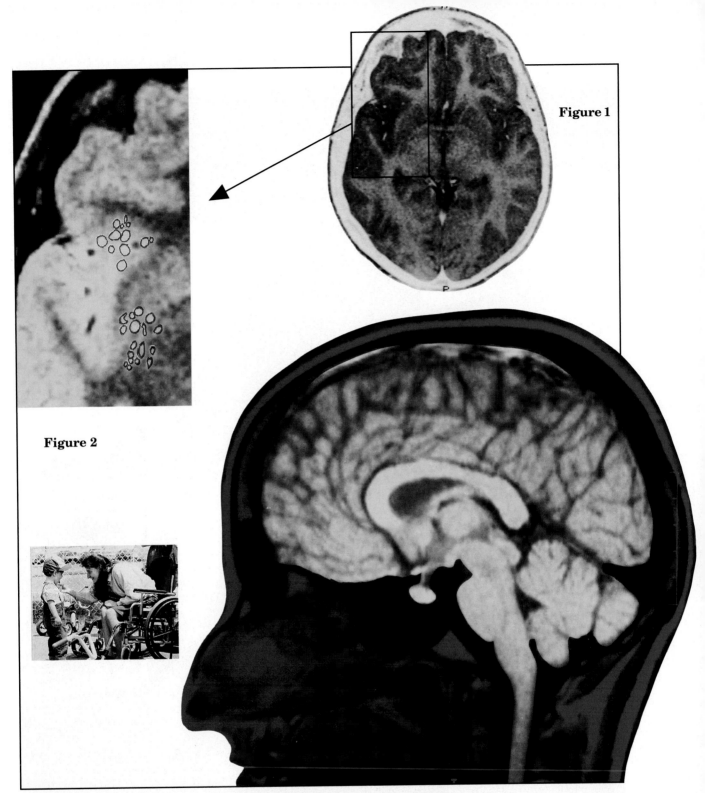

Figure 1

Figure 2

Magnetic Resonance Imaging (MRI)

This large colour accentuated sagittal MRI brain scan is that of a 17 year-old girl who was a top academic student in grade 8 when she was involved in an apparently minor MVA that was followed by contact with an infectious mono-like illness. She then developed a typical severe M.E./CFS-like clinical picture. Six years later, she still suffers from significant CNS dysfunction with intellectual and physical abilities far below her previous norm.

A cluster of UBOs or punctuate anomalies can just be seen in the transverse (horizontal) cut (Figure 1) of the same girl's brain. These anomalies are located in the posterior part of the left anterior lobe. Figure 2 represents an enlargement of the pathological area, clearly demonstrating two clusters of UBOs. These lesions appear to be in the pre-motor cortex or in the somato-motor cortex, the area responsible, in part, for muscle control. This girl has been confined to a wheelchair for much of the past several years. The QEEG scan indicated contre coup type injury.

i

Dr. John Richardson M.B., B.S.

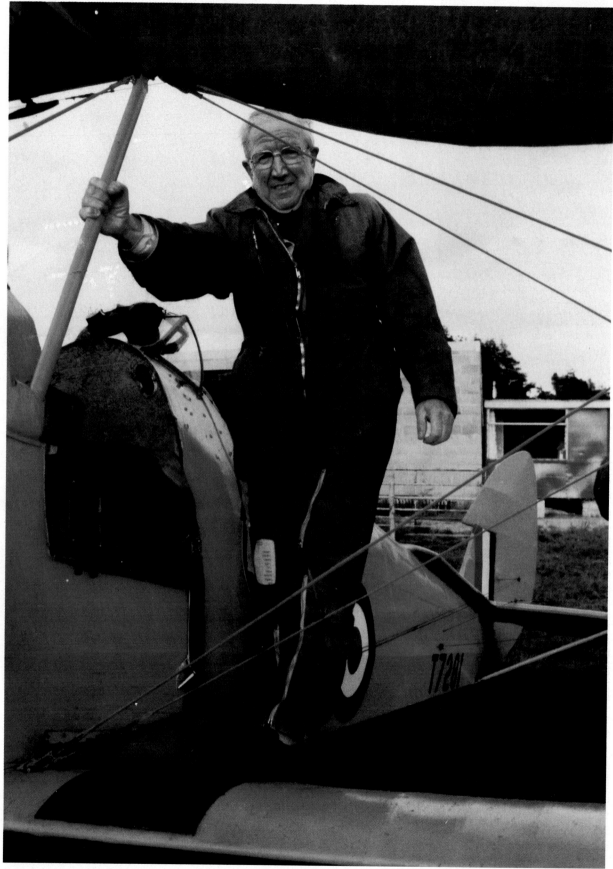

Reproduction by Golden Lang Colour Laboratories, photo retouching by John Evans Photography Ltd.

Dr. John Richardson M.B., B.S.

This book is not only dedicated to my friend and mentor, Dr. John Richardson, but it owes its very existence to him.

John Richardson was born in Shildon, County Durham, England in 1915. His was a talented musical family and, like his parents, he obtained an excellent musical education. His grandfather was a renowned violinist, his father an equally accomplished organist and his mother a gifted soprano. When John was a boy, he was taught the elements of music and, by the age of 14, he had become the local church organist. He learned the art of organ building from Edwin Taylor, organist and choirmaster for St Mary's in Darlington, Yorkshire and went on to build five pipe organs. He could easily have made his living as a professional musician. He has composed symphonies and played for the Princess of Wales in Balmoral Castle. An avid horticulturist, he grows semi-tropical fruits in his large greenhouse beside his home, Belle Vue House in Ryton, overlooking Hadrian's Wall and the River Tyne.

John Richardson's medical career started prior to the second world war when he decided to study physical medicine and attended the University of Edinburgh. When the war broke out in 1939, he joined the Royal Air Force and saw service in Germany. In 1941, he married Margaret Naseby. They have four children, David, Margaret, June and Gillian. Dr. Richardson remained in the services until after the war when he attended Newcastle University and obtained his M.B.

Dr. Richardson, a very young energetic 75 year-old, still practises full-time medicine. His wife Margaret would prefer that he not fly around over the moors in the WWI Tiger Moth.

As part of his general practice, he started to see patients with M.E./CFS in 1953. Since then, he has been compassionately examining, diagnosing and treating M.E./CFS patients on a continual basis for longer than any physician alive today.

This book is dedicated to Dr. John Richardson for the following three reasons:

(1) When I first hammered on the doors of the Faculty of Medicine at the University of Toronto, I did not know Dr. John Richardson, but had I, he would have been my physician role model. He has the most ceaselessly inquisitive and scientific mind, but he takes care of his patients like the good Samaritan.

Over the years he has listened to them, learned from them and done his best to help them during the long period when many physicians were simply dismissing these patients' problems as conversion hysteria or anxiety neurosis.

(2) When I started my study of M.E./CFS in 1985, I was assisted by many kind, notable and brilliant physicians and researchers in Australia, Britain, Canada, Japan, Iceland, New Zealand, and the United States of America. Many took me into their homes and gave me not only an understanding of the disease process of M.E./CFS but also kindness and friendship. John Richardson, over several visits, spent days with me, going minutely over his research, his correspondence and intellectual storehouse of knowledge. As in all things, John Richardson went far beyond the expected. I was a poor Telemachus but he was a unique Mentor.

(3) This book and the Cambridge Symposium were to be the joint work of an informal association of British physicians who meet under the title of the EME or the Epidemic Myalgic Encephalomyelitis Study Group. However, death and illness struck down many of the notables in their group and the enormous necessary work in England was not done. Up to the day of the symposium, we were led to believe that significant fund raising, delegates and staffing would be forthcoming from the second group of British organizers who took up the task from the EME. In the end, none of this anticipated assistance arrived, only unpaid accounts. In the midst of this trying and difficult experience, John Richardson and his Newcastle Research Group rose to the challenge, and helped fund some of the costs. John Richardson insisted that the show should go on and it did. Without John Richardson's determination and equitable personality, there would not have been a Cambridge Symposium. Without that Symposium this book would never have been written.

At 10 p.m., on one of my last visits to his home, and after listening to him discuss the cardiac findings in M.E./CFS patients for several hours, Dr. Richardson turned to me and asked if I was up to doing one or two house calls. With the top of his BMW down, we sped off into the night, over the moors and dodging wandering sheep to visit some of his bedridden M.E./CFS patients. He reminded me of a unique person in a series of books that I had read as a child. The books were based upon The Flying Yorkshireman, a country man who did not resemble a hero but who always came through when the going was difficult.

Adult QEEG/BEAM Scan, QSI Medical Corporation

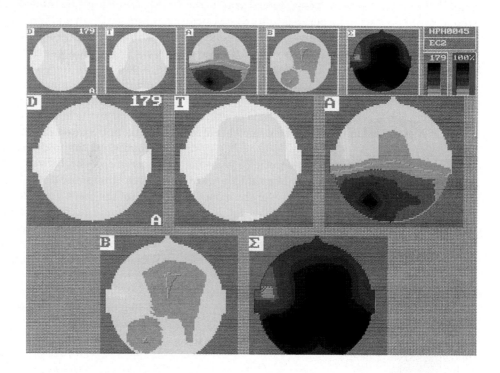

The QEEG, **Q**uantitative **E**lectro-**E**ncephalo-**G**ram, is a computer driven EEG that produces an easily read two dimensional colour coded print of electrical brain activity. The above QEEG scan was performed at the QSI Medical Corporation headquarters in Toronto. The patient is a 42 year-old respiratory technologist who has been house-bound and severely disabled for over six years.

This high quality inexpensive QEEG scanner offers several benefits in brain imaging. It is painless and non-invasive. It provides considerably more information than a classical EEG yet is easily read by any trained technologist or physician.

The electrical asymmetry of the above scan immediately suggests the underlying pathology; the abnormal activity in the Σ view indicates both left and right abnormalities in the motor cortex. The electrical abnormality in the **A** view is situated in the left posterior parietal area of auditory and visual comprehension, consistent with this patient's clinical pathology.

Photon Emission Tomography - PET Scan

These PET scan images of a 34 year-old patient of Dr. Byron Hyde were provided by Dr. Stephen Lottenberg, University of California at Irvine.

These images demonstrate significant mid-brain changes. This young lawyer has never returned to work during the past ten years after becoming brain disabled with CFS following an incapacitating viral infection. To date, the PET scan is the only brain imaging tool that has been shown to demonstrate adequately sub-cortical physiological injury.

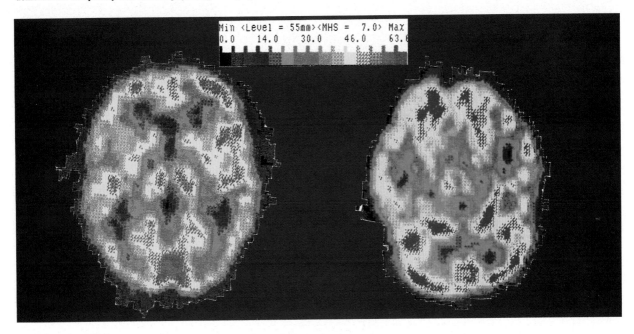

Child SPECT Scan

In the horizontal SPECT brain images in this section, we have adhered to the illogical but standard protocol that the right side of the SPECT image represents the left side of the brain and vice versa. The upper part of the SPECT scan logically represents the frontal (anterior) part of the brain. Except for the MRI pages, the coloured brain imaging techniques in this text represent physiological brain function rather than anatomical features.

This HMPAO SPECT scan was provided by Dr. Michael Goldberg of Tarzana, California. The scan was performed by Dr. Ismael Mena with a Shimadzu brain dedicated SPECT unit at UCLA Harbor, California.

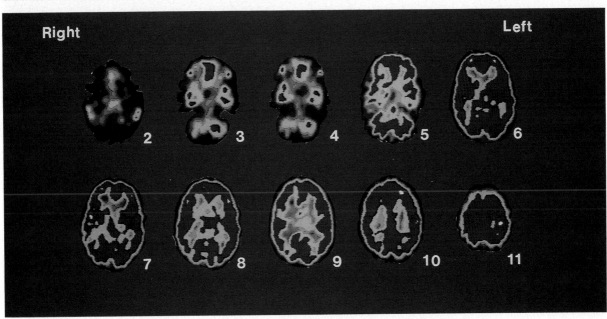

These scans are of an 8 year-old boy with M.E./CFS. There is a marked decreased perfusion in the left posterior parietal lobe, the area of the angular gyrus and the area responsible for visual and auditory comprehension. The right cerebellum is also deficient. This quiet, withdrawn child has developed considerable learning difficulty as well as balance problems and nystagmus.

Child SPECT Scan

These Xenon-133 and HMPAO SPECT scans of a 10 year-old M.E./CFS girl patient were provided by Dr. Michael Goldberg of Tarzana, California. The scan was performed by Dr. Ismael Mena with a Shimadzu brain dedicated SPECT unit at UCLA Harbor, California.

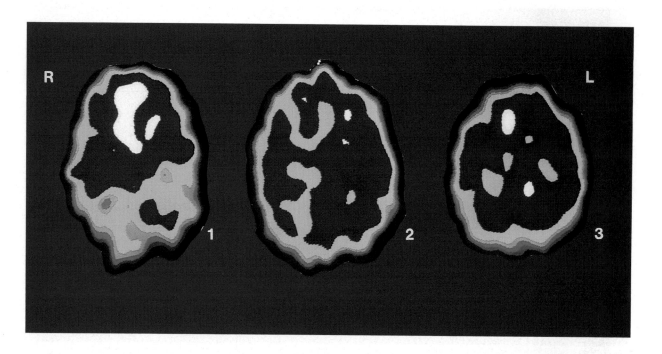

The three Xenon scans demonstrate marked decreased perfusion in the right frontal and right posterior parietal lobes. This decreased cerebral blood flow was found to fluctuate around 50 ml/min/100g or approximately half of the normal expected blood flow. There is also a marked decrease in perfusion of the cerebellar region.

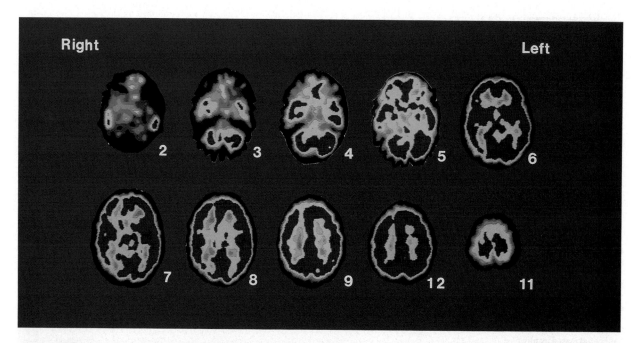

The ten HMPAO scans reveal the details of bilateral decreased frontal perfusion, more extreme on the right, as well as a bilateral temporal hypoperfusion. There is a decrease in both posterior parietal lobes, more extreme in the right lobe. There is hypoperfusion of the right medial lobe of the cerebellum. There may also be decreased perfusion of the basal ganglia.

It is possible that this child may have multiple problems including marked emotional volatility under stress, ataxia or nystagmus problems and a learning disability for comprehending both visual and auditory information.

The Negative Effects of Exercise on an M.E./CFS Dysfunctional Brain

These Xenon SPECT scans of a 37 year-old female M.E./CFS patient and the concept were provided by Dr. Jay Goldstein of Anaheim, California. The technical expertise is that of Dr. Ismael Mena, UCLA Harbor, California.

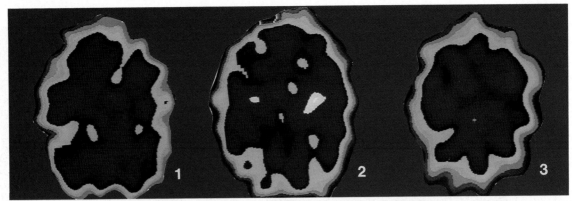

Resting

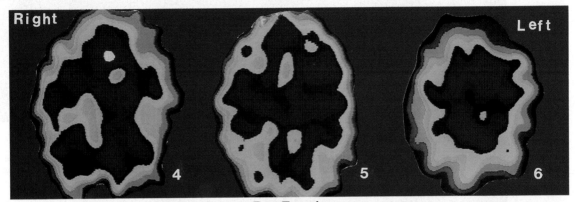

Post-Exercise

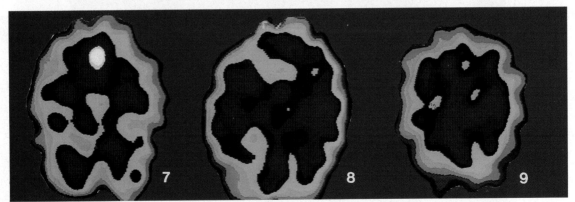

24 Hours Post-Exercise

Resting State **Images 1, 2 and 3,** represent the abnormal resting state of an M.E/CFS brain. There is a perfusion defect in the left inferior frontal lobe as well as the right and left posterior parietal lobes.

Immediate Post-Exercise State **Images 4, 5 and 6** represent the immediate post-exercise function of the brain of the same patient. There is a significant decrease in perfusion of the right and left frontal lobes and the right and left posterior parietal lobes. An occipital perfusion defect is starting to appear. The functional resting defects noted in images 1, 2 and 3 have become aggravated.

24 Hours Post-Exercise State **Images 7, 8 and 9** illustrate the severely decreased brain perfusion of the same patient 24 hours after the brain has been stressed by physical exercise. This 24 hour delayed effect may explain much of the M.E./CFS dysfunction that occurs the day after exercise or other stress factors.

The pathological brain changes demonstrated in 1, 2 and 3 were exaggerated by normal physical activity. Similar dysfunctional images could probably be produced in an M.E./CFS patient as a result of sleep deprivation, a secondary infectious state, cognitive, sensory or emotional factors. A normal healthy patient will probably exhibit increased brain perfusion after similar modest exercise. See Dr. Goldstein, Addendum I, showing common stress pathway.

Adult SPECT Scan

These HMPAO SPECT scans of a 35 year-old pilot were provided by Dr. Byron Hyde. This scan was performed by Dr. Jean Léveillé at Hôtel Dieu Hospital in Montreal, employing a SX300 Picker.

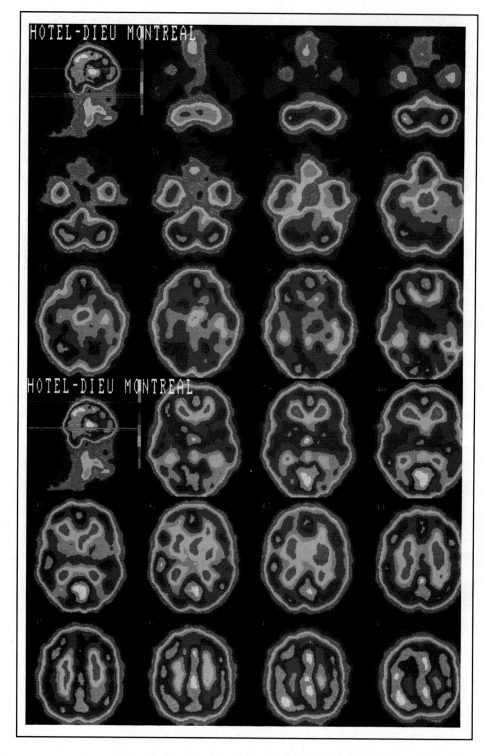

After a significant febrile illness in June 1990, this 35 year-old pilot developed chronic headaches, difficulty in concentration, a marked loss of energy and inability to exercise. He has developed nystagmus. His reading skills have markedly decreased and he has developed emotional lability that occurs after any physical, cognitive or emotional stress factors. He had no significant disability or illness before falling ill in June 1990.

SPECT scans performed at Hôtel Dieu in Montreal demonstrate marked abnormalities of perfusion in the left posterior parietal lobe, together with decreased perfusion of the left frontal region. He also has a decreased perfusion in the area of the right motor cortex. These SPECT findings are consistent with the clinical description.

Foreword

This text is the work of The Nightingale Research Foundation, a charitable foundation located in Ottawa, Canada and incorporated in 1988 to conduct and assist research into the cause and cure of Myalgic Encephalomyelitis / Chronic Fatigue Syndrome (M.E./CFS) and to serve as an educational institution, for the Canadian public, physicians, nurses, teachers and their professional societies.

Our Foundation is named after Florence Nightingale, who fell ill with an infectious disease during her service in the Crimean War. She then developed a disease process that was indistinguishable from M.E./CFS. Despite her severe disability, she went on to reform both public health and health care, helping to bring medicine and particularly the care and treatment of the ill patient into the twentieth century.

This text that provides a basis of general information for clinicians and researchers interested in M.E./CFS was initiated by the Cambridge Easter Symposium on Myalgic Encephalomyelitis/Chronic Fatigue Syndrome. The Symposium was held at Cambridge University, England in April 1990. The Symposium was international in scope and brought together, for the first time, researchers from around the world who were contributing to the growing body of scientific information regarding this disease process.

Had it not been for the efforts of Dr. John Richardson, his Newcastle Research Group and Nightingale staff, the Symposium would have never been held. Without the constant confidence of our supporters and the rugged and continued determination of Nightingale's staff, this text could never have been completed.

We have attempted to obtain material in every area of M.E./CFS knowledge, but we have not always been successful. Some information is under copyright and could not be released. Some promised material just never arrived. Scientific knowledge of M.E./CFS is growing so rapidly that we were not always able to keep up with all of the explosive changes in information. To compensate for some of the omissions, Nightingale staff have written review chapters only when an appropriate contributor was not available or the chapter was delayed. These review chapters represent Nightingale's opinions and are not necessarily those of the clinicians and researchers mentioned.

Furthermore, in a few cases, we have requested and obtained permission from certain prestigious journals to reproduce works of historical significance. Due to the sheer length of some of the original manuscripts, it was necessary for us to reproduce some of the authors' work in abstract form.

For historical purposes, we have attempted to obtain photographs of all of the leading M.E./CFS experts, past and present, who have contributed so much to our knowledge of this disease process. The dimensions and quality of the photographs received were not always uniform. Consequently, the size and the quality of the photographic reproduction is in no way related to the importance of the paper or the author. Some photographs were obtained through the kind assistance of the authors' friends, colleagues and secretaries, as well as medical and newspaper archives to whom we extend our appreciation.

This text has come to represent much of our historical, clinical and scientific knowledge of M.E./CFS. We believe that this reference work will provide a welcome and exciting addition to our knowledge of a most fascinating disease process.

The Board of Directors
The Nightingale Research Foundation
June 1992

Preface

Unravelling the Enigma

This book attempts to outline, with broad strokes of the brush, the extent of an infectious illness, which affects both the immune and central nervous systems. This infectious illness has occurred in numerous well documented epidemics since the 1934 epidemic in the Los Angeles County General Hospital, magnificently described by Gilliam[1] in 1938.

Since that date, well over 50 similar clusters or epidemics[2] have appeared in the medical literature under a plethora of names. David Bell was right to title his book about this disease process "The Disease of a Thousand Names[3]". For the purpose of this book I will refer to the disease as M.E./CFS, a fence-sitting title for Myalgic Encephalomyelitis / Chronic Fatigue Syndrome. It is not our intention to suggest M.E./CFS as yet another name. We could have equally tacked on the term PVFS or Post Viral Fatigue Syndrome, a term that, in England, has now partially replaced CFS as a generic term, or CFIDS, a term coined by the epidemiologist, Dr. Seymour Grufferman, and used by many of the U.S. patient groups. At The Nightingale Research Foundation in Ottawa, Canada, we have stuck with the name Myalgic Encephalomyelitis because there have been at least 10 names used in the literature since we started looking at this disease process in 1984 and we are simply tired of trying to keep up with the name changes. We have also tried to avoid the term "fatigue". Fatigue is immeasurable and largely indefinable. Fatigue is a normal phenomenon as well as being associated with almost all chronic disease states. Fatigue, which is simply one of the common features of healthy life and disease, neither defines M.E./CFS nor clarifies the illness. The term "fatigue" **does** cause disparagement to those who study this serious debilitating illness and those who suffer from it. It is an error to name a disease after just one of its many symptoms.

It has always been known by investigators that these epidemics of M.E./CFS tended merely to highlight the same disease activity in the general public in the epidemic area. At first, these epidemics tended to occur in hospitals and residential schools. In the hospitals, there has been a predilection for the disease to attack chiefly the staff[1,4,5] rather than the patients. In residential schools, the illness seems to have attacked both staff and students.[6]

From the very first well-documented 1934 epidemic[1], the question has arisen concerning the relationship of both an infective agent and immunization as a cause of this illness. Unfortunately, immunization has become one of the holy of holies and it is almost totally excluded from discussion in the literature as a cause of disease. Part of this may well be the close association of governments to immunization. It is my understanding that part of the problem that Assistant Surgeon General Gilliam of the United States faced in the publication of his report, and the reason for the four-year delay in publication, was the fact that the authorities were not willing to let it be known that this epidemic may have been spread to the staff by the use of human serum in immunization procedures.[7]

It takes no great leap of imagination to note that hospital staff continue to be significantly more immunized than their patients and that both teachers and students enjoy a much higher immunization rate than the general public. It is these very groups that are most numerically afflicted by M.E./CFS. It is not my intention to attack immunization. I would not live happily in a world without immunization. Immunization, as a public health benefit, has not only saved countless millions from death and chronic disability, but has also saved governments fortunes and allowed armies to be assembled in vast numbers. One does not suggest with impunity that immunization is a cause of disease. Yet I am strongly suggesting that governments spend more money on research relating to immunization and its consequences than they are presently doing. Immunization is a two edged sword and the relationship between M.E./CFS, infection and immunization has never been seriously studied.

Since 1979, there has been an enormous but poorly

Incidence of new cases of M.E. / CFS per year[20]

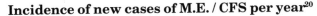
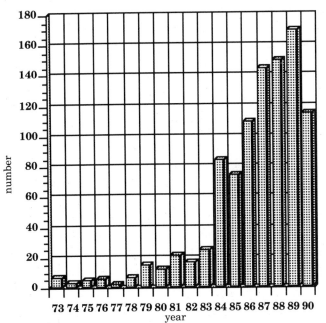

documented increase in cases of M.E./CFS amongst the general public[8]. These increases compounded slowly until the late Summer of 1984 when it appears that a critical mass was reached and a veritable explosion of M.E./CFS occurred. Numbers, however, did not drop as one would expect after an epidemic period, but rather appear to have continued to rise in ever-increasing numbers.

Although one of the infectious causes may represent a newly discovered virus, the illness that we are describing is not new. Thomas Sydenham, the father of English medicine, described a similar disease spectrum as Muscular Rheumatism in 1681[14]. But from 1681 to the present time, what has been described is always the same. This disease has usually closely followed the patient's contact with an environmental stimulus and usually this stimulus has been an infectious disease.

A Loss of Homeostasis

In terms of its major dysfunction, M.E./CFS represents an acute change in the balance of neuropeptide messengers, and due to this, a resulting loss in the ability of the central nervous system (CNS) to adequately receive, interpret, store and recover information. This dysfunction also results in the inability of the CNS to consistently programme and achieve normal, smooth end organ response. The problem is one of maintaining systemic functioning within nor-

mal limits in the face of a chronic infectious stress. The resulting loss of normal internal homeostasis arises from the fact that a chronic viral infection provokes reactive changes in these peptides with a consequent pathophysiological changes and autonomic dysregulation.

These powerful excitatory and inhibitory mechanisms for rapid physiological adjustment work well with short term stressors. Frequently, these mechanisms shut down the biological system allowing for compensatory adjustments of the homeostatic mechanisms. When the stressor is an infectious agent, the messenger mechanisms stimulate compensating immune reactions to rid the body of this infectious stressor and ultimately return the individual to a normal homeostasis.

By definition, chronic infections have managed to escape these initial compensatory immune mechanisms. However, the neurochemical homeostatic events continue to be employed uselessly and to the detriment of the organism. This modulatory biochemical complex, biologically derived over the millenium to assist the organism, destabilizes the autonomic neuronal outflow and the individual can no longer function systemically within normal limits. Two theories of viral cause have been proposed.

The Retrovirus Concept

Dr. Paul Cheney believes that the present epidemic[9], starting in 1979, represents a new disease process caused by the emergence of an entirely new retroviral infection. His views should be taken seriously, for, if he is correct, the new retrovirus, first noted by Dr. Michael Holmes in New Zealand on July 23rd 1986[10], isolated and further clarified by Drs Paul Cheney and Elaine DeFreitas at the Wistar Institute in 1990[11] may be pivotal in our understanding of M.E./CFS. Is it the same as the second retrovirus successfully grown and whose structure was further elucidated by Dr. John Martin in The Los Angeles County Hospital?[12] If so, it will bring us full circle to that first epidemic in 1934.

The Enterovirus Concept

In 1958, it was pointed out by Dr. Björn Sigurdsson[15] that both the patients who had fallen ill with Akureyri disease in 1948, (another synonym for M.E./ CFS.), and also the healthy population from the same area, failed to succumb to a paralytic poliomyelitis epidemic that swept Iceland during that period. Later, when the same Akureyri population were first immunized against poliomyelitis, it was observed that this population responded with a much higher seroconversion than the non-Akureyri population of Iceland. This is one of the reasons why many researchers feel that there is a cross-over effect between M.E./CFS and the closely related poliomyelitis-enterovirus family and, indeed, that M.E./CFS is caused by an enteroviral infection.

One personal observation that I can make is that, since the introduction of poliomyelitis immunization in 1954-56, and until 1979, there appears to have been a decrease both in poliomyelitis and M.E./CFS epidemics reported. This is only a cursory observation since no funding has been available to investigate these occurrences.

It is not generally realized, but in the 1954-56 period, M.E./CFS itself changed abruptly. I have made the point of examining many patients who were affected with M.E./CFS prior to 1956 and who suffered a paralytic association along with the typical symptom picture of M.E. / CFS. For all purposes, post-1956 M.E./CFS patients have been spared overt paralysis. One can only conclude that poliomyelitis immunization may have somehow spared many subsequent M.E./CFS patients the paralytic features common in earlier epidemics.

Again, one has to question the rise of Post-Polio Syndrome. Since 1881, when the first paralytic poliomyelitis epidemic was described, occurring on the north central Swedish/Norwegian border[16], there has been no clearly described body of information that discusses Post-Polio Syndrome. Post-Polio Syndrome began clearly to surface around 1979 and only received its name during the same period[17] when M.E./ CFS also catapulted into public attention. Lauro Halstead writes that *"...prior to 1980 the name (post-polio syndrome) did not exist and without a name it was not possible to talk or write about it."* It is most curious for an epidemic disease such as paralytic poliomyelitis, that had been around since 1881, to suddenly spawn a major new manifestation. There is no difference in the clinical picture between these two disease syndromes except that in Post-Polio Syndrome there has been a clear observation of an earlier paralytic poliomyelitis illness. Yet, when we at Nightingale question patients with M.E./CFS who were born prior to 1955, we find that over a third of them had a parent, sibling or house resident who was paralysed with poliomyelitis. Poliomyelitis was a scourge, but it was just not that common. Are many M.E./CFS patients simply post-polio patients who had contracted a subclinical case of poliomyelitis years earlier? Is M.E./CFS in part simply a poliomyelitis variant?

Physicians do not understand paralytic poliomyelitis as well as they should, nor as well as they think they do. We do not know why, when a poliovirus epidemic swept through a town, infecting and immunizing the vast majority of the population without even giving them a minor cold, only a few in that same population with the same virus fell ill, died or were paralysed. Did some of those individuals who fell ill and died with poliomyelitis have an immune dysfunction problem? Did some of them harbour a subclinical chronic virus infection that had previously injured their immune system?

We still do not understand the cause of Encephalitica Lethargica[18] or of the major changes in that disease from the time it appeared in 1915 until 1934, when for all intents and purposes it disappeared[19], curiously in the same year that M.E./CFS appeared. One cannot but be impressed by the similarity of the sleep dysfunctions and associated pain syndromes and the inability, until now, to isolate a causative agent in both M.E./CFS and Encephalitica Lethargica.

Who is right about the cause of M.E./CFS, the British researchers who believe we are dealing with a persisting enteroviral infection or the American and New Zealand scientists who believe they have found a new and explosive retrovirus that has provoked such severe disability in so many hundreds of thousands of children and adults in the world today? The clinicians and scientists in this book may not yet have all of the answers, but like the discoverers of the New World, they have mapped out the bold features of the terrain.

Byron Hyde, M.D., Editor
The Nightingale Research Foundation,
Ottawa, Canada

References

1. Gilliam A.G. **Epidemiological Study of an Epidemic, Diagnosed as Poliomyelitis, Occurring Among the Personnel of The Los Angeles County General Hospital During The Summer of 1934,** Public Health Bulletin No. 240, April 1938, The United States Public Health Service.

2. see this book, Review of Epidemics.

3. Bell D. **The Disease of a Thousand Names,** First Edition, Possard Publications, Lyndonville, New York.

4. The medical staff of the Royal Free Hospital, An Outbreak of Encephalomyelitis in the Royal Free Hospital Group, London, in 1955, Br. Med. J., 1957; 2:895-904.

5. Shelokov A., Havel K., Verder E., Welsh W. Epidemic Neuromyasthenia, An outbreak of poliomyelitis-like illness in student nurses. N.E.J.M., 1957; 257:345-55.

6. Hyde B., Bergmann S. Akureyri Disease, Forty Years Later. Lancet, 1988;1191-2.

7. Conversation between A. Gilliam and Alexis Shelokov reported to B. Hyde by A. Shelokov, 1988, 1991.

8. Cheney P. Kalamazoo Symposium, Oct 19, 1991.

9. Cheney P. Kalamazoo Symposium, Oct. 19, 1991.

10. Holmes M. The Cambridge Symposium on Myalgic Encephalomyelitis (M.E.), Lady Mitchell Hall, Cambridge University, England, April 9-12, 1990.

11. DeFreitas E., Hilliard B., Cheney P., Bell D. et al. Evidence of Retrovirus in Patients With Chronic Fatigue Immune Dysfunction Syndrome, Presented at the 11th International Congress of Neuropathology, Kyoto, Japan, September 4, 1990. (see CFIDS Chronicle, September 1990).

12. Personal communication with Dr. John Martin, November 1991 concerning further decoding of virus structure.

13. Personal communication Dec 1991 with co-worker, Dr. David Bell.

14. Sydenham, T. **The Works of Thomas Sydenham, M.D.** (translation from the Latin edition of Dr Greenhill by R.G. Latham M.D.), Vol 1, London, Sydenham Society (1847).

15. Sigurdsson B., Gudnadottir M., Petursson, G. Response to Poliomyelitis Vaccination, The Lancet, 1,370-371, Feb. 1958.

16. Bergenholtz, noted in Wickman, Ivan, (translation Maloney, W.) **Acute Poliomyelitis** (Heine-Medin's Disease), The Journal of Nervous and Mental Disease Publishing Company, (1913).

17. Munsat, T. **Post-Polio Syndrome**; Butterworth-Heinemann, Halstead, Lauro, Chapter 3, pg 24, (1991).

18. Von Economo C. (translation.Newman, K.O.) **Encephalitis Lethargica**; its sequelae and treatment. London (1931).

19. Brain W. Russell. **Diseases of the Nervous System**, pg. 428-438, Oxford Medical Publications, Second Edition, (1940).

20. Nightingale Research Foundation, unpublished figures

In Appreciation

This text would not have been possible without the financial help, support and services of the following individuals, associations and corporations. Nor could we have succeeded without our staff, the majority whom have donated their time and talents without any thought of financial remuneration, and others who have worked long hours for very modest wages.

I would like to single out three of our staff. First, **Lydia Neilson** who, despite her illness, and in addition to being our principal fund raiser, has always been there to help those who despaired of life. Somehow, in her weakness she found strength and was able to use this strength to help others.

Also this book would never have been completed were it not for the tireless efforts of our Production Editor, **Bonnie Cameron**, whose organizational abilities and technical ingenuity made this book possible. Attempts to coordinate the work of so many clinicians and researchers scattered across the globe has been daunting.

The administrative excellence of **Laurie Wilson** has been invaluable during the preparation of this text.

I would like in particular to acknowledge one individual, **Kim Bechthold**, whose companies and Principal Patrons, Genmark Corporation of San Francisco and BioCapital Corporation of Toronto, came to the rescue of both the Symposium and this book, ensuring their success. This was and is equally true of **an anonymous Alberta family** whose son and brother was ill and the Hobin family of **Barry Hobin and Associates**, Architects of Ottawa. Without their considerable and timely financial assistance we would not have succeeded in this venture.

I would also like to thank and acknowledge, Dr. Henry Eisenberg from Syracuse, New York, Dr. Charles Poser, Beth Israel Hospital, Harvard, and Sandra Gwyn who were responsible for my taking up this challenge, Dr. Jay Goldstein in California, Dr. John Richardson in England and Dr. Peter O. Behan in Glasgow, whose ideas have greatly influenced this work, and my wife, Maureen O'Neil and my private secretary, Margaret O'Neill, who put up with me throughout this period.

My thanks also go out to those thousands who are not mentioned here, whose modest donations and letters of encouragement have inspired us to complete our mission and make this publication available to all who might benefit from its existence.

Byron Hyde M.D.

Principal Patrons

BioCapital Corporation, Ontario
An Anonymous Alberta Family
Province of Ontario
Royal Canadian Legion, Montgomery Branch
Apple Canada
Bell Northern Research
Newcastle Research Group, G.B.
Department of Health and Welfare, Canada
G.W. Cadbury Trust, Great Britain
Corel Systems Corporation
Royal Bank of Canada
Barry Hobin and Associates, Architects
G. & P. Chilton & clients of Midland Walwyn
Genmark Corporation, California

Patrons

The Hon. H. Perrin Beatty
Canadian Life and Health Insurance Ass.
Clare Francis, Great Britain
Goldberg, Shinder, Gardner & Kronick
Miriam Gallacher, Ontario
Brian and Donna Haley, BC
Kim Harvey, BC
IBM Canada
Adrienne Kowalski, BC
John and Pauline Perry
Power Corporation, Quebec
Richard & Donald Purcell, Ontario
Dr. Gérald Séguin, Ontario
Donna Sinclair, BC

M.E./CFS Associations & Support Groups

I would like to laud **Marc Iverson**, President of the CFIDS Association and Publisher of the CFIDS Chronicle in Charlotte, North Carolina, who without any prior medical training, and although desperately ill, has managed to produce the best continuous source of medical information on M.E./CFS anywhere in the world. The efforts of Marc Iverson and his staff must truly be one of the most remarkable contributions to modern American medical history.

The following support groups or their members have been instrumental in the success of this book. Many of them also raised considerable funds that enabled us to stay solvent during this period.

Alberta M.E./CFS Associations, including Calgary, Edmonton, High Prairie, Lethbridge, Peace River & Red Deer Associations; **British Columbia** M.E. Society, and, Victoria, Comox, Vernon, Kelowna support groups; **Ontario** M.E. Support groups in Burlington, Chatham, Collingwood, Hamilton-Wentworth, Kitchener-Waterloo, London, Orillia, Oshawa, Ottawa, Quinte-Bellville, St. Catharines

Australia New South Wales M.E. Association; **Great Britain**, M.E. Action Campaign; **New Zealand**, ANZYMES Association; **South Africa** South Africa M.E. Association; **USA**, CFIDS Association, North Carolina Association, Massachusetts Association and their members

Principal Benefactors

Air Canada; Bell Canada; Canadian Airlines; Cybermedix Laboratories, Ontario; Miss Patricia Hession; Janet & Golden Lang Of **Golden Colour Laboratories**, Ontario; the Crout Family; **National Printers**, Ontario; Margaret Siebrasse, Quebec; **Taggart Family Trust**, Ontario; Phyllis & Cyril Putt, BC; Paul and Sue-Ellen Roache, Australia

Benefactors
If not otherwise mentioned, those following are from Ontario:

An Anonymous Ontario Family; Paul Beatty; Milus Bollenberghe Topps Watchorn, Ontario; **Burroughs Welcome Pharmaceuticals**, Canada; **Bristol Myers Pharmaceuticals**, Canada; **CUPE Canadian Union of Postal Workers; Dan Can Electric**, Terry Deutscher, Robert Dingman, Alberta; **Ferano Construction**; André Gagnon, **General Scrap Iron**, Alberta **HEM Pharmaceuticals**, Philadelphia, Louise Matte-Lewis and Family and Friends, Patricia Muster, BC; Sean O'Sullivan, **Reliable Services, Scotia Pharmaceuticals**, Nova Scotia; **Smith Kline and French Pharmaceuticals**, Canada **Sun Life of Canada,** William & Irene Turriff, BC, Essence Vida, BC

Significant Assistance

Mary Pamela Allen, BC.; Walter Bick, **Bicks Pickles**; Barbara & Peter Burke, Dr. Song Yin Cai, Philippe Cassidy, Omelan Chabursky, Brian Child, Joan Cotsworth, BC; Warren Foster, BC; Ron & Marie Foxcroft, Deirdre Franklin, **Les Filles de la Sagesse D'Ottawa**, Gwendolyn Hancock, Mr. & Mrs. Houghton, Elizabeth Howson, Dorothy Jackson, BC Beverley & Peter Jones, **Kelowna Elks Club, BC**; Joyce Lang, BC; J.R. MacDonald, Que; **McAlpine & Hordo**, B.C Beatrice McPhatter, BC W.H. Merril, Mrs. C. Palumbo, Lucielle Parizeau, **Pfizer Canada Inc.**, Roy Postlewhite, Sarah Pouliot, Christie Richards, Washington D.C.; H.A. Schnurr, BC Lily Smith, Dr. Graeme Taylor, Earl Trouten, **Troco Limited**, Ontario; Pamela Turriff, BC; Robert & Susan Vadeboncoeur, Quebec; George D. Willits, Miriam Wright, The Estate of Evelyn F. Wright, Dr. Lydia Wu, Max Wyman, BC

Financial Assistance

Sylvia Abbott, BC; Hazel Bain; Jean Baird; Collins Barrow, Alberta; Peter Bell, BC; E.G. Bernard, BC; Susan Best; Paul Bilodgau; **Blackburn Properties**; Brian Blackwell, BC; Chad Blackwood, BC Arthur Blair; Sylvia Boivin, BC; Jean Booth,

BC; Elizabeth Borek; Susan Botting; Alice Brodie; George Bruce; **Butler Research**; Gillian Canning, Quebec Larry Corless, AB; W.E. Couling, BC; Sally Coulter; Cathy Clemens; George W. Clemens; Dr. R. J. Conklin, BC; René Desormeaux; Dr. Larry Dobson; Beryl Farr, Nancy Finn, AB; Barbara Fitzgerald; Bozena Frydova, B.C.M. Garamszeghy; John & Mildred Garlick; Dr. Lorna Guiou; Dr. David Gotlib, Drs Eva & Paul Groff; Dan and Shirley Gilbert, Alberta; Robert and Mary Gilhuly; Novella Gouldsborough, MB **Grief Containers**, Niagara Falls; Kenneth Gross; Ross Hall; Theresa Iverson, BC; Mabel Kung, Mr & Mrs Guy Launay, **Leduc Cleaners, Alberta Loeb Inc., Luxors Gifts Ltd., BC**; Jennifer Lynch, Judge W.E. MacLatchy, Maureen Madigan, Anita Manstan, Al Martin, Carolyn Matthews, Mary Percival Maxwell, Mr & Mrs J. Mendel, Quebec; **Merck Sharp & Dohme Research**, Terling Park, Great Britain; Susan Mertens, BC; **Metropolitan Toronto Police**; R.E. Miller; **Mollenhayer Construction Ltd**; Lorraine Molloy; **MDS Laboratories**, Canada; Frank Mrack, Saskatchewan; Betty Miller; Dr. Brian Myhill-Jones, B.C.; Brian Newby, Alberta; Jack Newby, Alberta; John H. Newton, BC Marion Oades; **Ontario Secondary School Teachers' Federation**, Brian Orshinsky, Saskatchewan Frank Palumbo; G.R. Pauling, Alberta M.Petre Family; Raymond & Margaret Philips, BC; Rebecca Pratt; Darlene Quartermain; Lorna Quion; Dr. R.J. Richards; B.G. Robertson; **Royal Canadian Legion, Strathcona Branch**; **Roussel Canada**, Barbara Russell, BC; Mrs. J.M. Samuel, New Mexico; Richard Sandborn; Lois Schneider, AB; Alan Shiff; Margaret Shouldice; Lloyd Singer; **Sino Acupuncture Clinic**, Marcia Smith; Robert McCallum, **Stiefel Canada Inc,** Frank Stoelzle, BC; **Syntex Inc. Canada**, Susan Tarras, BC; Dr. Lary Turner; **UpJohn Pharmaceuticals Canada**, Nico Van Duyvenbode; Jean and Rick Van Loon; Miroslava Vintor, BC; Jane Wallace, Saskatchewan Esther Wallner BC, David Ward, BC Dan Watts; H.O Westra, BC, Ruby Wilkins; Joan Wright; Sarah Wright; **Wyeth Limited, Canada**

Principal Nightingale Staff

Bonnie Cameron, Anne Duncker, Ratna Kanagaretnam, Lydia Neilson, Margaret O'Neill, Kathrine Tatsis, Laurie Wilson

Cambridge Symposium Support Staff

We would particularly mention **Valerie Oades Gamache** who was the principal individual responsible for bringing the Symposium together and for all of the final detailed organization. I would also like to mention **Ann Frampton** who was able to recover a part of the funds held by the British organizers and ensure that they were paid to the British creditors.

Jim Brook, Claire Comeau, Borys Chabursky, Marc Chuma, Anne Duncker, Ann Frampton, Valerie Gamache, Toni Jeffreys, Abdul Khan Grimshaw, Raymonde Guilbault, the late Martin Lev, Margaret O'Neill, Joan Rothery, Helen Urwin

Specialist and Associate Nightingale Staff

Matthew Allen, Brenda Barsellotti, Ikbal Boga, Judy Cameron, Borys Chabursky, Dianne Delaney, Denise Dinsley, Valerie Gamache, Armett E. Hill, P. Kanagaretnam, Peggy Kitcher, Jill Peters, Sharyn Robertson, Michel Rochon, Glenn Sheskay, Robert Towsley

Finally, I should like to mention and thank our honorable board, past and present, who supported us in this work.

Past and Present Honorary Board

The Hon. Monique Bégin, P.C.
The Hon. Guy Charbonneau
The Hon. David Crombie, P.C.
Dr. Josephine Flaherty
Arnell Goldberg, Q.C.
Dr. Gilles Hurteau
Dr. Antoine D'Iorio
Dr. John Last
The Hon. Martin O'Connell, P.C.
Joan Pennefather

Since we have so many people to thank, we may have inadvertently omitted some names. Naturally our thanks also go out to these people.

Byron Marshall Hyde, Chairman
Danielle Dougall, Vice President

The Clinical and Scientific Basis of Myalgic Encephalomyelitis / Chronic Fatigue Syndrome

Contents

A Road Map to M.E. / CFS /
PVFS / CFIDS

Chapter 1

The Disease of a Thousand Names

The following descriptive names have been compiled from the work of Dr. Gordon Parish, Dr. David S. Bell, Dr. Henri Rubinstein and Dr. Byron Hyde. The following represent just a few of the names that have been given to this protean illness:

The Poliomyelitis Names:

A disease resembling or simulating poliomyelitis; atypical poliomyelitis; abortive poliomyelitis, encephalitis simulating poliomyelitis; encephalitis resembling poliomyelitis; postpolio syndrome; posterior poliomyelitis, sensory poliomyelitis.

Postpolio syndrome is considered by the medical community to be an indisputable entity. Unlike M.E./CFS there is no physician who doubts its existence. However, postpolio syndrome symptomology is identical to that of M.E./CFS. The only difference is that, in postpolio syndrome, there is clear evidence of paralytic poliomyelitis in the patient concerned. Curiously, no note was ever made of postpolio syndrome except in the recent medical literature, despite the fact that poliomyelitis has been in existence as an epidemic disease since 1881 when the first epidemic of poliomyelitis occurred in Sweden. The rise in postpolio syndrome closely parallels the increasing incidence of M.E./CFS observed since 1979. It is our opinion at Nightingale that postpolio syndrome is no more than M.E./CFS [in an individual with previous history of clinical poliomyelitis.]

Names based upon location:
Iceland disease, Akureyri disease, Coventry disease, Tapanui flu, Otago mystery disease. Royal Free disease, Lake Tahoe mystery disease, Lyndonville chronic mononucleosis, the English disease;

Neuromyasthenia-names:
Neuromyasthenia, Neurasthenia, Epidemic neuromyasthenia, Epidemic pseudo myasthenia, Sporadic postinfectious neuromyasthenia, Neurocirculatory asthenia;

Myalgic Encephalomyelitis names:
Myalgic encephalomyelitis, benign encephalomyelitis, benign myalgic encephalomyelitis, benign subacute encephalomyelitis, epidemic myalgic encephalomyelitis or encephalomyelopathy, acute infective encephalomyelitis, epidemic diencephalomyelitis, lymphoreticular encephalomyelopathy;

Myalgia type names:
Epidemic malaise, persistent myalgia following sore throat. Damadian's ache, Myofascial syndrome, Muscular rheumatism, Fibromyalgia syndrome, Fibromyositis, Fibrositis, Epidemic myositis, Lymphocytic meningo encephalitis with myalgia and rash, Syndrome polyalgique idiopathique diffus (S.P.I.D.);
(The Fibromyalgia names are based upon a symptom complex seen in M.E., Lupus, Rheumatoid arthritis and several other non-associated illnesses.)

Personal names:
Da Costa's Syndrome, Beard's disease;

Symptom based names:
Chronic fatigue syndrome, CFS, La Spasmophilie, (France), Raggedy Ann Syndrome, the English sweats, Effort syndrome, Tétanie chronique idiopathique;

Bacterial names:
Chronic brucellosis, Chronic lyme disease;

Combined virus/symptom names:
Post-viral fatigue syndrome, PVFS, Persistent viral fatigue syndrome;

Immune based names:
Chronic immune activation syndrome, CIAS, Chronic immune dysfunction syndrome, CIDS, Low natural killer cell syndrome (Japan), Multiple chemical sensitivity syndrome, Ecological disease, Allergic fatigue syndrome, Antibody negative lupus, Antibody negative lyme disease, Chronic activated immune dysfunction syndrome, CAIDS, Chronic fatigue and immune dysfunction syndrome, CFIDS, Naxalone-reversible monocyte dysfunction syndrome (NRMDS);

Epstein-Barr Virus based names:
Chronic Epstein-Barr virus syndrome, CEBV, Chronic active Epstein-Barr virus infection, CAEBV, Virus epidemic in recurrent waves, Chronic mononucleosis, Familial chronic mononucleosis, Chronic infectious mononucleosis, Chronic active Epstein-Barr virus infection, Chronic mononucleosis-like syndrome;

Hypothalamic Names:
Epidemic vegetative neuritis, Neurocirculatory asthenia, vasoregulatory asthenia, vasomotor instability, vasomotor neurosis, Habitual chronic hyperventilation syndrome;

The Atypical Names:
Atypical multiple sclerosis, Atypical migraine;

Media names:
Yuppie flu, Yuppie plague;

Miscellaneous names:
Soldier's heart, Epidemic vasculitis syndrome.

Myalgic Encephalomyelitis (M.E.)

Many readers may not understand the significance of the above term that has been used in Great Britain for many years to describe this disease process. **My** refers to muscle and **algic** to pain. **Encephalo** refers to brain, **myel** to spinal cord and **itis** denotes inflammation. The name Myalgic Encephalomyelitis is consistent with our knowledge of the disease process except for the suffix **itis**; there is no evidence of active inflammation. A pathologically more appropriate name would be Myalgic Encephalomyelopathy - **opathy** simply referring to the fact that there is pathology.

Chapter 2

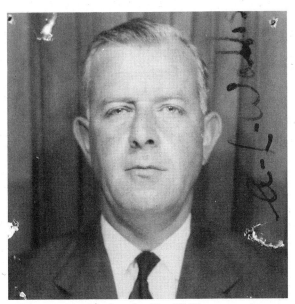

Andrew Lachlan Wallis

This damaged photograph of Dr. Andrew Lachlan Wallis was sent to us by the N.S.W. Australia, Medical Board. It is the sole photograph that we have been able to recover of Dr. Wallis, who registered in N.S.W. in 1958 and then appears to have disappeared. Dr. Wallis' thesis outlines guidelines for the diagnosis of adults that have not been improved upon. Dr. Wallis was the first to describe M.E./CFS in large numbers of children and was the first to define the illness in children. He was the first to describe the microscopic brain pathology in M.E./CFS.

The Definitions of M.E./CFS, A Review

B. Hyde, M.D.

(Please see Chapter 5 for Dr. Hyde's photograph and curriculum vitae.)

*Under **"define"**, two of the examples given in the Third Edition of the Shorter Oxford English Dictionary are: (a) **To determine the boundary or limits of.** (b) To set forth the essential nature of.*

Yet one of the problems facing physicians and researchers interested in M.E./CFS, is that the perception of the limits and boundaries of the disease varies greatly in relation to the prejudices of those who describe the disease.

Some apparently reasonable physicians insist that no children are affected by M.E./CFS, that no infectious agent is apparent, and that there are no physical signs. I hope that this text will put an end to such naive objections.

The Clan War

M.E./CFS finds itself in a fierce clan war between biochemical, subcellular, brain imaging and virological scientists who are challenging the centuries-old imaginative world of psychiatry. Frequently the psychiatric theory proponents are not even psychiatrists but traditionalists who have learned their subject well and have lost their ability to look again. Many skins will be bruised before this conflict has ended.

An Adequate Definition

The formation of an adequate definition of a disease appears to be an easy task. It is not. Rheumatoid arthritis has been redefined every few years for most of this century and still researchers are far from satisfied. The problem is simply that if you know the exact cause, the method of acquiring and the pathophysiology of a disease, one does not need a definition.

If we have a definitive test for a specific disease, there is little need for definition, only the need of a good historian or a good checklist. One of the biggest problems with M.E./CFS is that researchers are so much at each other's throats that an excellent definition is beyond reasonable consensus. But from what we do know, we should be able to build a reasonable working definition.

Early attempts to define M.E./CFS consisted of simple symptom check lists, sometimes mixed in with insights from the particular epidemic under examination. One such check list stands out above all others and that is the working definition of A.L.Wallis of the epidemic M.E./CFS illness that occurred in 1955 in Cumberland in England It is particularly useful as it is also the first definition to demonstrate some of the specifics of M.E./CFS in children.

The Wallis Descriptive Definition for Adults

(1) A systemic illness with relatively low fever or subnormal temperatures.

(2) Marked muscle fatigability.

(3) Mental changes with impairment of memory, changes in mood, sleep disorders and irritability or depression.

(4) Involvement of the autonomic nervous system resulting in orthostatic tachycardia, coldness of the extremities, episodes of sweating or profound pallor, sluggish pupils, bowel changes and frequency of micturition, possibly as a result of a lesion of the hypothalamus.

(5) Diffuse and variable involvement of the central nervous system, leading to ataxia, weakness and/or sensory changes in a limb, nerve root or a peripheral nerve.

(6) Muscular pain, tenderness and myalgia, and

(7) Recurrence in some patients over a period of several years.

Wallis' Variations Seen in Children

(1) **Depression:** This often occurred with weeping tendencies, and appeared early. There were four cases severe enough to warrant psychiatric inpatient treatment.

(2) **Loss of energy:** This occurred in all but the mildest cases and frequently persisted.

(3) **Retardation of thought process:** Work involving abstract thought was difficult to perform in all with protracted illness or recurrences. Serial seven test was poorly performed, often with errors, often starting the test well and then getting bogged down.

(4) **Impairment of thought process:** This was a common feature, and the contents of papers or magazines read only a few minutes earlier could not be recollected.

(5) **Impairment of memory:** Recent retention and recall: Items of work to be done or purchases to be made had to be listed as memorising proved unreliable.

(6) **Disorders of sleep:** Inversion of sleep rhythm was common with nightmares in children. Hallucinations on waking occurred in 6 cases.

(7) **Behaviour disorders:** Temper tantrums were frequent in young children. In older children unsociability and lack of attention and effort on return to school was frequent. If behaviour was checked, children tended to weep.

Persistent Traits in Children

(1) Nocturnal enuresis
(2) Disobedience at school and at home
(3) Unmotivated acts of aggression
(4) Facile lying in normally truthful children
(5) Rapid changes in mood

It is interesting to compare these findings with those quoted by Behan and Behan over 30 years later in children with sporadic M.E./CFS. Apparently the Behans had not seen the manuscript published by

Wallis when they wrote these findings in the CRC Reviews.

Behan and Behan,
Ten Findings in Children with PVFS
(post-viral fatigue syndrome)

(1) There is anxiety and clinging dependency.

(2) There is reluctance to attend school.

(3) There is lack of interest in playing games with other children.

(4) There is lassitude.

(5) Sleep pattern is disturbed.

(6) Nightmares and irritability are common.

(7) A significant amount of body weight may be lost.

(8) In some cases such severe weakness occurs that the child is confined to a wheel chair for several months.

(9) Nearly all affected children are diagnosed first as hysterical. with depression or "parental over-involvement".

(10) When forced to attend school and take part in physical exercises, this has been followed by disastrous deterioration in the clinical condition, with overwhelming exhaustion and weakness supervening.

Comments:

Wallis studied these M.E./CFS children and adults for a period of approximately two years and then apparently left for Australia; Behan and Behan had the advantage of studying these children for years. These traits may persist chronically.

Wallis points out that this disease in part represents a hypothalamic injury and that the disease is characterized by a subnormal temperature after the prodromal period of three or four days. These findings of subnormal variability are described in every well-documented M.E/CFS epidemic. It is unfortunate that the CDC diagnosis did not benefit from a review of this literature.

In 1959, Henderson and Shelokov, writing in the New England Journal of Medicine, describe a check list of the acute findings of M.E./CFS or what they called Epidemic Neuromyasthenia.

The Henderson and Shelokov Summary

(1) Fatigability, malaise, prodromal sore throat

(2) Muscle weakness, cramps, spasms and twitches

(3) Bursting headache, neck pain, eye pain

(4) Irritability, depression, lack of concentration, emotional instability, impaired mentation

(5) Visual problems, photophobia, diplopia

(6) Dizziness, nausea, cutaneous sensory changes

(7) Urinary, menstrual difficulties

Of the 23 features mentioned in this summary, the vast majority can be attributed to an acute CNS injury and 17 of the features could only be attributed to a CNS or muscle pathology. In the Henderson Shelokov list, fatigue is only one of 27 notations and is not elevated to special status. As with Gilliam and later Wallis, the urinary and menstrual difficulties are mentioned.

The first and only attempt to date to systemize M.E./CFS in the form of a useful working definition was made in 1988 by a United States Government researcher, Dr. Gary Holmes and his learned team. Their definition was a good start. Yet all of these researchers had believed that Epstein-Barr virus was the cause of what they called Chronic Epstein-Barr Syndrome and this was perhaps one of their collective difficulties. However, a review of the literature on M.E./CFS epidemics would have revealed that the epidemic disease they described had an incubation period of as little as 4-5 days and that EBV had an incubation period of 30-50 days. This failure to return to the literature haunts the very basis of their definition.

The CDC Definition

This article is reprinted with the kind permission from Holmes et al, Chronic Fatigue Syndrome: A Working Case Definition. Ann Intern Med. 1988; Vol. 108, Number 3: pages 387-389.

Chronic Fatigue Syndrome: A Working Case Definition

Gary P. Holmes, M.D.; Jonathon E. Kaplan, M.D.; Nelson M. Gantz, M.D.; Anthony L. Komaroff, M.D.; Lawrence B. Schonberger, M.D.; Stephen E. Straus, M.D.; James F. Jones, M.D.; Richard E. Dubois, M.D.; Charlotte Cunningham-Rundles, M.D.; Savita Pahwa, M.D.; Giovanna Tosato, M.D.; Leonard S. Zegans, M.D.; David T. Purtilo, M.D.; Nathaniel Brown, M.D.; Robert T. Schooley, M.D.; and Irena Brus, M.D.; Atlanta, Georgia; Worcester and Boston, Massachusetts, Bethesda, Maryland; Denver, Colorado; New York and Manhasset, New York; San Francisco, California; and Ohama, Nebraska

The chronic Epstein-Barr virus syndrome is a poorly defined symptom complex characterized primarily by chronic or recurrent debilitating fatigue and various combinations of other symptoms, including sore throat, lymph node pain and tenderness, headache, myalgia, and arthralgias. Although the syndrome has received recent attention, and has been diagnosed in many patients, the chronic Epstein-Barr virus syndrome has not been defined consistently. Despite the name of the syndrome, both the diagnostic value of Epstein-Barr virus serologic tests and the proposed causal relationship between Epstein-Barr virus infection and patients who have been diagnosed with the chronic Epstein-Barr virus syndrome remain doubtful. We propose a new name for the chronic Epstein-Barr virus syndrome - the chronic fatigue syndrome - that more accurately describes this symptom complex as a syndrome of unknown cause characterized primarily by chronic fatigue. We also present a working definition for the chronic fatigue syndrome designed to improve the comparability and reproducibility of clinical research and epidemiologic studies, and to provide a rational basis for evaluating patients who have chronic fatigue of undetermined cause.

[MeSH Terms; axilla; chronic disease; depression; Epstein-Barr virus; fatigue; fever; lymph nodes; memory disorders; neck, pharyngitis. Other indexing terms; chronic Epstein-Barr virus syndrome; chronic fatigue syndrome; sore throat]

The Chronic Epstein-Barr virus syndrome, also known as chronic mononucleosis or chronic mononucleosis-like syndrome, is a syndrome of unknown cause that has been the subject of interest in both medical and popular literature, particularly since 1985. As it was described[1-4] in four groups of patients, the syndrome consists of a combination of nonspecific symptoms - severe fatigue, weakness, malaise, subjective fever, sore throat, painful lymph nodes, decreased memory, confusion, depression, decreased ability to concentrate on tasks, and various other complaints - with a remarkable absence of objective physical or laboratory abnormalities. The syndrome was linked in these and other reports to Epstein-Barr virus, because many, but not all, of the patients had Epstein-Barr virus antibody profiles that suggested reactivation of latent infection.

Reference laboratories soon began to advertise Epstein-Barr virus serologic tests for use in the diagno-

From the Division of Viral Disease, Centers for Disease Control, Atlanta, Georgia: Department of Medicine, University of Massachusetts Medical School, Worcester, Massachusetts; Department of Medicine, Brigham and Women's Hospital, Boston, Massachusetts; Laboratory of Clinical Investigation, National Institutes of Health, Bethesda, Maryland: Department of Pediatrics, National Jewish Center for Immunology and Respiratory Medicine, Denver, Colorado: Atlanta Medical Association, Atlanta, Georgia; Department of Medicines, Mount Sinai Medical Center, New York, New York: Department of Pediatrics, North Shore University Hospital, Manhasset, New York; Division of Biochemistry and Biophysics. Food and Drug Administration, Bethesda, Maryland; Department of Psychiatry, University of San Francisco School of Medicine, San Francisco, California, Department of Pathology and Microbiology, University of Nebraska Medical Center, Omaha, Nebraska; Department of Medicine, Massachusetts General Hospital, Boston, Massachusetts, and Department of Medicine, Beth Israel Medical Center, New York, New York.

sis of the chronic Epstein-Barr virus syndrome[5]. Although reliable data are not available, indications are that the syndrome has been diagnosed commonly by physicians, often on the basis of poorly defined diagnostic criteria. Since late 1985, the Division of Viral Diseases, Centers for Disease Control has responded to several thousand telephone and mail requests for information about the chronic Epstein-Barr virus syndrome, both from physicians and from patients in whom the syndrome has been diagnosed. Judging from the inquiries received, many physicians appear to have based their diagnoses on little more than the presence of detectable serum Epstein-Barr virus antibody titers.

More recent studies[6,7] have cast doubt on the diagnostic value of positive Epstein-Barr virus serologic results and on the proposed relationship between Epstein-Barr virus infection and patients who have been diagnosed with the chronic Epstein-Barr virus syndrome. Although some statistically significant associations between positive Epstein-Barr virus serologic tests and illnesses diagnosed as the chronic Epstein-Barr virus syndrome were identified in one study using age-, sex-, and race-matched controls[6], the serologic associations between the syndrome and cytomegalovirus, herpes simplex virus types 1 and 2, and measles virus were as strong as or stronger than the association with Epstein-Barr virus. Epstein-Barr virus serologic results in this study were also found to be poorly reproducible, both within and among laboratories, leading to the conclusion that the results of these tests are not directly comparable unless they have been done in parallel.

With the apparent lack of correlation between serum Epstein-Barr virus titers and the presence of chronic fatigue symptoms, it is premature to focus research and diagnostic efforts on Epstein-Barr virus alone. Many public health officials and clinicians are concerned that a diagnosis of the chronic Epstein-Barr virus syndrome may not be appropriate for persons with chronic fatigue who have positive Epstein-Barr virus serologic tests, and that definable occult diseases may actually be the cause of symptoms such as fatigue, weakness, and fever. It is also inappropriate to use a name for the syndrome that implies a specific causal agent. We, therefore, propose a new name - the chronic fatigue syndrome - that describes the most striking clinical characteristic of the chronic

Epstein-Barr virus syndrome without implying a causal relationship with Epstein-Barr virus.

Because of the nonspecific nature of the symptoms and the lack of a diagnostic test, researchers have had difficulty devising a case definition for the chronic Epstein-Barr virus syndrome. When definitions have been described, they have differed greatly among the various published studies, making direct comparisons of the study results difficult. We have organized an informal working group of public health epidemiologists, academic researchers, and clinicians, to develop a consensus on the salient clinical characteristics of the chronic Epstein-Barr virus syndrome and to devise a definition for the chronic fatigue syndrome that will be the basis for conducting future epidemiologic and clinical studies. Because the syndrome has no diagnostic test, the definition at present is based on signs and symptoms only. This definition is intentionally restrictive, to maximize the chances that research studies will detect significant associations if such associations truly exist. It identifies persons whose illnesses are most compatible with a possibly unique clinical entity; persons who may have less severe forms of the syndrome or who have less characteristic clinical features may be excluded by the new definition.

The chronic fatigue syndrome is currently an operational concept designed for research purposes that physicians must recognize not necessarily as a single disease but as a syndrome - a complex of potentially related symptoms that tend to occur together - that may have several causes. Periodic reconsideration of conditions such as those listed under major criteria, part 2, should be standard practice in the long-term follow-up of these patients.

Case Definition for
The Chronic Fatigue Syndrome

A case of the chronic fatigue syndrome must fulfill major criteria 1 and 2, and the following minor criteria: 6 or more of the 11 symptom criteria and 2 or more of the 3 physical criteria; or 8 or more of the 11 symptom criteria.

Major Criteria

1. New onset of persistent or relapsing, debilitating

fatigue or easy fatigability in a person who has no previous history of similar symptoms, that does not resolve with bedrest, and that is severe enough to reduce or impair average daily activity below 50% of the patient's premorbid activity level for a period of at least 6 months.

2. Other clinical conditions that may produce similar symptoms must be excluded by thorough evaluation, based on history, physical examination, and appropriate laboratory findings. These conditions include malignancy; autoimmune disease; localized infection (such as occult abscess); chronic or subacute bacterial disease (such as endocarditis, Lyme disease, or tuberculosis), fungal disease (such as histoplasmosis, blastomycosis, or coccidioidomycosis), and parasitic disease (such as toxoplasmosis, amebiasis, giardiasis, or helminthic infestation); disease related to human immunodeficiency virus (HIV) infection; chronic psychiatric disease, either newly diagnosed or by history (such as endogenous depression; hysterical personality disorder; anxiety neurosis; schizophrenia; or chronic use of major tranquilizers, lithium, or antidepressive medications); chronic inflammatory disease (such as sarcoidosis, Wegener granulomatosis, or chronic hepatitis); neuromuscular disease (such as multiple sclerosis or myasthenia gravis); endocrine disease (such as hypothyroidism, Addison disease, Cushing syndrome, or diabetes mellitus); drug dependency or abuse (such as alcohol, controlled prescription drugs, or illicit drugs); side effects of a chronic medication or other toxic agent (such as a chemical solvent, pesticide, or heavy metal); or other known or defined chronic pulmonary, cardiac, gastrointestinal, hepatic, renal, or hematologic disease.

Specific laboratory tests or clinical measurements are not required to satisfy the definition of the chronic fatigue syndrome, but the recommended evaluation includes serial weight measurements (weight change of more than 10% in the absence of dieting suggests other diagnoses); serial morning and afternoon temperature measurements; complete blood count and differential; serum electrolytes; glucose; creatinine, blood urea nitrogen, calcium, phosphorus; total bilirubin, alkaline phosphatase, serum aspartate aminotransferase; serum alanine aminotransferase; creatine phosphokinase or aldolase, urinalysis; posteroanterior and lateral chest roentgenograms; detailed personal and family psychiatric history;

erythrocyte sedimentation rate; antinuclear antibody; thyroid-stimulating hormone level; HIV antibody measurement; and intermediate-strength purified protein derivative (PPD) skin test with controls.

If any of the results from these tests are abnormal, the physician should search for other conditions that may cause such a result. If no such conditions are detected by a reasonable evaluation, this criterion is satisfied.

Minor Criteria
Symptom Criteria

To fulfill a symptom criterion, a symptom must have begun at or after the time of onset of increased fatigability, and must have persisted or recurred over a period of at least 6 months (individual symptoms may or may not have occurred simultaneously). Symptoms include:

1. Mild fever - oral temperature between 37.5°C and 38.6°C, if measured by the patient - or chills. (Note: oral temperatures of greater than 38.6°C are less compatible with chronic fatigue syndrome and should prompt studies for other causes of illness.)

2. Sore throat.

3. Painful lymph nodes in the anterior or posterior cervical or axillary distribution.

4. Unexplained generalized muscle weakness.

5. Muscle discomfort or myalgia.

6. Prolonged (24 hours or greater) generalized fatigue after levels of exercise that would have been easily tolerated in the patient's premorbid state.

7. Generalized headaches (of a type, severity, or pattern that is different from headaches the patient may have had in the premorbid state).

8. Migratory arthralgia without joint swelling or redness.

9. Neuropsychologic complaints (one or more of the following: photophobia, transient visual scotomata, forgetfulness, excessive irritability, confusion, difficulty thinking, inability to concentrate, depression).

10. Sleep disturbance (hypersomnia or insomnia).

11. Description of the main symptom complex as initially developing over a few hours to a few days (this is not a true symptom, but may be considered as equivalent to the above symptoms in meeting the requirements of the case definition).

Physical Criteria

Physical criteria must be documented by a physician on at least two occasions, at least 1 month apart.

1. Low-grade fever - oral temperature between 37.6°C and 38.6°C or rectal temperature between 37.8°C and 38.8°C (See note under Symposium Criterion 1.)

2. Nonexudative pharyngitis.

3. Palpable or tender anterior or posterior cervical or axillary lymph nodes. (Note: lymph nodes greater than 2 cm in diameter suggest other causes. Further evaluation is warranted.)

Acknowledgements: The authors thank Mrs. Josephine M. Lister for manuscript preparation.

Requests for reprints should be addressed to Gary P. Holmes, M.D.; Division of Viral Diseases, Center for Infectious Diseases, Centers for Disease Control; Atlanta GA, 30333.

References

1. Tom M, Morag A, Ravid Z, et al. Prolonged atypical illness associated with serological evidence of persistent Epstein-Barr virus infection. *Lancet.* 1982; 1:61-4.

2. DuBois RE, Seeley JK, Brus I, et al. Chronic mononucleosis syndrome. *South Med J.* 1984; 77:1376-82.

3. Jones JF, Ray CG, Minnich LL, et al. Evidence for active Epstein-Barr virus infection in patients with persistent, unexplained illnesses: elevated anti-early antigen antibodies. *Ann Intern Med.* 1985:102:1-7.

4. Straus SE, Tobato G, Armstrong G, et al. Persisting illness and fatigue in adults with evidence of Epstein-Barr virus infection. *Ann Intern Med.* 1985:102:7-16.

5. Merlin TL, Chronic Mononucleosis: pitfalls in the laboratory diagnosis. *Hum Pathol.* 1986:17:2-8.

6. Holmes GP, Kaplan JR, Stewart JA, Hunt B, Pimsey PF, Schonberger LB. A cluster of patients with a chronic mononucleosis-like syndrome: is Epstein-Barr virus the cause? *JAMA.* 1987:287:2297-2302.

7. Buchwald D, Sullivan JL, Komaroff AL. Frequency of "chronic active Epstein-Barr virus infection" in a general medical practice. *JAMA.* 1987:287:2303-7.

end of document

Comments on the above paper

The first criticism of this paper is that it takes one symptom of disease, fatigue, and elevates it to an unrealistic importance. The first sentence states that "The chronic Epstein-Barr syndrome is...characterized primarily by chronic or recurrent debilitating fatigue ...". Yet the problem with fatigue is that it is neither specific, definable nor scientifically measurable. Fatigue is both a normal and a pathological feature of every day life. Every normal person gets fatigued. Fatigue is a common feature of much major psychiatric disease and major medical disease. Since fatigue is such an integral part of many illnesses by calling fatigue the primary characteristic, the authors necessitated the elimination of hundreds of other diseases. To truly follow the criteria set out by the CDC definition probably makes M.E./CFS the most expensive illness to investigate of any known disease. Fatigue is not an object, it is simply a modifier in search of a noun.

Also, taking fatigue as the flagship symptom of a disease not only bestows the disease with a certain Rip Van Winkle humour, but it removes the urgency of the fact that the majority of M.E./CFS symptoms are in effect CNS symptoms. Interestingly, CNS dysfunction was not part of the CDC exclusion list. Was this an oversight or were the authors suggesting that M.E./CFS was a CNS dysfunction? That would have made a lot of sense, since to most physical M.E./CFS scientists and clinicians, M.E./CFS represents a major attack on the CNS by the chronic effects of a viral infection. This relationship of the systemic features of M.E./CFS to CNS dysfunctions are only beginning to be explored in this text.

The second criticism is illustrated in the seven references all of which refer to Epstein-Barr and five of which refer back to the authors of the CDC paper. It is unusual in a scientific paper to attempt to prove one's points by primarily citing oneself. I mentioned earlier that there were many expert American M.E./CFS clinicians and historians that were not called upon or referred to. Had they been heard, many of the following errors would have been avoided.

Low-grade fever: There may be fever in the first few days of the prodromal period but the predominant temperature abnormality is one primarily of subnormal and marked diurnal variability.

Non-exudative pharyngitis: There may be pharyngitis in the first few days of the prodromal period and patients complain of dryness and irritation of the pharynx but there is no publication on consistent cultured bacterial or viral pharyngitis beyond that generally found in a normal population.

Palpable or tender anterior or posterior cervical or axillary lymph nodes. (not to exceed 2 cm.) M.E./CFS: Patients suffer from cutaneous hypersensitivity, they tend to lose weight during the early months of disease making normal lymph nodes more apparent. I know of no M.E./CFS expert who would care to stake his reputation on his ability to distinguish any difference in the lymph nodes of 10 M.E./CFS patients from those of 10 normal controls. These tender points more likely represent fibromyalgia points than sensitive lymph nodes.

These three features are all important in infectious mononucleosis (glandular fever), a disease associated with EBV; they are not important in M.E./CFS. I can only wonder if these authors, all published in the field of this herpes virus, and with the help of their patients, all attempting to prove their illness, did not confuse the two illnesses of mononucleosis and M.E./CFS.

The third criticism is the exclusion of certain diseases. For example, thyroid dysfunction with an early increase of TSH, and ovarian- uterine dysfunction, both related to a primary possible hypothalamic injury are a real part of the inception or consequences of M.E./CFS and should not be excluded. To exclude certain patients with bladder, GIT, cardiac, pulmonary and certain other endocrine dysfunctions that have started after the M.E./CFS illness started, may be equivalent to removing some of the systemic side effects patients with this illness incur.

The Oxford Guidelines

This British paper was developed developed in Oxford England by 21 invited clinical and scientific researchers. Six other individuals were invited but did not attend. Of those present, eight were in psychiatry or psychology as was the Chair, Dr. Sharpe. Another six were research scientists. Non-psychiatric clinicians in attendance, who spend at least half of their working day with M.E./CFS patients were few.

Reprinted with the kind permission of The Journal of the Royal Society of Medicine, MC Sharpe et al, A Report - Chronic Fatigue Syndrome: Guidelines for Research, JRSM Volume 84, February 1991, pp 118-121.

A Report
Chronic Fatigue Syndrome: Guidelines for Research

Keywords: chronic fatigue syndrome; research; definition

Authors

Dr. M.C. Sharpe MRC Psych   Clinical Lecturer, Department of Psychiatry, University of Oxford

Dr. L.C. Archard PhD   Senior Lecturer, Department of Biochemistry, Charing Cross and Westminster Medical School, London

Professor J.E. Banatvala MD   Professor of Virology, Department of Virology , St. Thomas' Hospital Medical School, London

Dr. L.K. Borysiewicz FRCP   Wellcome Trust Senior Lecturer, Department of Medicine, University of Cambridge

Professor A.W. Clare MD.   Clinical Professor of Psychiatry, Trinity College, Dublin

Dr. A. David MRCPsych   MRC Training Fellow, Institute of Psychiatry, London

Professor RHT Edwards FRCP Professor of Medicine , Department of Medicine, University of Liverpool

Dr. KEH Hawton DM Consultant Psychiatrist, Department of Psychiatry, University of Oxford

Professor HP Lambert MD.   Emeritus Professor of Microbial Disease , St. George's Hospital Medical School, London

Dr. RJM Lane MD   Consultant Neurologist, Regional Neurosciences Center, Charing Cross Hospital, London

Dr. EM McDonald MRC Psych   Research Psychiatrist, Institute of Psychiatry, London

Professor JF Mowbray FRCP Immunopathology, Department of Immunopathology, St. Mary's Hospital Medical School, London

Dr. DJ Pearson FRCP   Senior Lecturer, Department of Medicine, University of Manchester

Dr. TEA Peto MRCP   Consultant Physician, Department of Infectious Diseases, John Radcliffe Hospital, Oxford

Dr. VR Preedy PhD   Research Biochemist, Department of Biochemistry, King's College Hospital, London

Dr. AP Smith PhD   Research Psychologist, Department of Psychology, University of Sussex

Dr. DG Smith MB   General Practitioner, Horndon-On- The-Hill, Essex

Dr. DJ Taylor DPhil   MRC Staff Scientist, MRC Biochemical and Clinical Magnetic Resonance Unit, John Radcliffe Hospital, Oxford

Dr. DAJ Tyrrell MD   Director, MRC Common Cold Unit, Harvard Hospital, Salisbury

Dr. S Wessely MRCPsych   Wellcome Training Fellow in Epidemiology, Institute of Psychiatry, London

Dr. PD White MRCPsych   Senior Lecturer, Department of Psychological Medicine, St. Bartholomew's Hospital, London

Other signatories who contributed to the guidelines but who were unable to attend the meeting

Professor PO Behan MD   Professor of Neurology, Department of Neurology, University of Glasgow

Dr. F Clifford Rose FRCP   Director, Academic Unit of Neuroscience, Charing Cross and Westminster Medical School, London

Professor TJ Peters FRCP   Professor of Clinical Biochemistry, Department of Biochemistry, King's College Hospital, London

Dr. PG Wallace MRCGP   Head of Research Unit, Department of General Practice, St. Mary's Hospital Medical School, London

Professor DA Warrell FRCP   Professor of Tropical Medicine and Infectious Diseases, Nuffield Department of Medicine, John Radcliffe Hospital, Oxford

Dr. DJM Wright MD Consultant Microbiologist, Department of Microbiology, Charing Cross Hospital, London

Introduction

Patients who present with a principal complaint of disabling fatigue of uncertain cause have received much attention in recent years. Correspondingly there has been an increasing amount of research into this problem. The findings have however often been contradictory. Resolution of these contradictions depends on the ability to compare research studies, but such constructive comparison has rarely been possible. This is largely because research has been carried out by investigators trained in different disciplines, using different criteria to define the condition. Whilst such an eclectic approach is to be welcomed, agreement on case definition, and assessment methods is necessary if progress is to be made.

The principal lack of agreement concerns definition of the clinical syndrome to be studied. A number of clinical syndromes have been described, all apparently referring to similar groups of patients, but differing sufficiently to preclude comparison of published studies. The various names used include epidemic neuromyasthenia[1], idiopathic chronic fatigue and myalgia syndrome[2], benign myalgic encephalomyelitis[3], chronic infectious mononucleosis[4], Royal Free disease[5], postviral fatigue syndrome[6], fibrositis-fibromyalgia[7,8], and chronic fatigue syndrome[9].

An attempt to address the problem of case definition was made by Holmes and colleagues in 1988[9], who chose the name chronic fatigue syndrome (CFS) because it is descriptive and free from unproven etiological implications. They also proposed an operational definition for the syndrome. Although a welcome advance, this definition proved to be unsatisfactory in practice.[10,11] Other definitions e.g. by Lloyd and colleagues[12] are also unsatisfactory[13], and have not been widely accepted.

Additional sources of difficulty have arisen from inadequate and poorly described sampling procedures, choice of comparison groups, shortcomings in study design and measures of poor or unspecified reliability.[14]

In an attempt to remove these obstacles to progress, a meeting of research workers with a known interest in the field was convened. The format of the meeting was modelled on the MRC (Medical Research Council) workshop on Alzheimer's disease.[15]

Aims

The aim of the meeting was to seek agreement amongst research workers on recommendations for the conduct and reporting of future studies of patients with chronic fatigue. Specifically we set out to agree on which patients should be included, how such studies should be approached, and on the minimal data that should be reported.

Procedure

The meeting (attended by all those listed at the beginning of the paper) was held at Green College, Oxford, on 23 March 1990, and chaired by Professor Anthony Clare. It was restricted to invited research workers, all of whom had studied patients with CFS. The disciplines represented included biochemistry, general medicine, general practice, imaging, immunology, infectious diseases, microbiology, neurology, physiology, psychiatry, and psychology.

Before the meeting all participants (and several others who were unable to attend) were circulated with a questionnaire, and their responses were used to draw up an initial discussion document which formed the basis of discussion during the meeting. Points on which agreement was reached were recorded and a draft of this paper circulated to participants.

The Guidelines

The following guidelines were agreed.

Symptoms

A preliminary research glossary is appended. This comprises definitions for symptoms and suggestions for their description.

Signs

There are no clinical signs characteristic of the condition, but patients should be fully examined, and the presence or absence of signs reported.

Syndromes

Two broad syndromes can be defined:

Chronic fatigue syndrome (CFS)

(a) A syndrome characterized by fatigue as the principal symptom.

(b) A syndrome of definite onset that is not life long.

(c) The fatigue is severe, disabling, and affects physical and mental functioning.

(d) The symptom of fatigue should have been present for a minimum of 6 months during which it was present for more than 50% of the time.

(e) Other symptoms may be present, particularly myalgia, mood and sleep disturbances.

(f) Certain patients should be excluded from the definition. They include:

(i) Patients with established medical conditions known to produce chronic fatigue (e.g. severe anaemia). Such patients should be excluded whether the medical condition is diagnosed at the presentation or only subsequently. All patients should have a history and physical examination performed by a competent physician.

(ii) Patients with a current diagnosis of schizophrenia, manic depressive illness, substance abuse, eating disorder or proven organic brain disease. Other psychiatric disorders (including depressive illness, anxiety disorders and hyperventilation syndrome) are not necessarily reasons for exclusion.

Post-infectious fatigue syndrome (PIFS)

This is a subtype of CFS which either follows an infection or is associated with a current infection (although whether such associated infection is of aetiological significance is a topic for research).

To meet research criteria for PIFS patients must
(i) fulfil criteria for CFS as defined above , and
(ii) should also fulfil the following additional criteria:
(a) There is definite evidence of infection at onset or presentation (a patient's self-report is unlikely to be sufficiently reliable).
(b) The syndrome is present for a minimum of 6 months after onset of infection.
(c) The infection has been corroborated by laboratory evidence.

In reporting studies it should be clearly stated which of these two syndromes is being studied. The degree of disability should be measured and stated. The criteria and method used to exclude subjects from study must be clearly described and the degree of examination and investigation specified. All patients should be assessed for associated psychiatric disorder and the results of this assessment reported.

Sampling

The way in which the patient sample was obtained should be clearly described. In particular it is essential to know whether the sample was recruited from primary care or from secondary referral centres. Because of the risk of introducing bias at this stage the use of random samples or consecutive referrals is preferred.

Comparison Groups

The term comparison group is preferred to control group. The precise choice of comparison groups should be determined by the hypothesis being tested. In the current state of knowledge multiple comparison groups may be required as there are pitfalls in the sole use of 'healthy' or 'normal' selected controls.

Suggested comparison groups include patients with neuromuscular disorder, patients with conditions causing inactivity, and patients with depressive disorder. The method used to obtain the comparison group should be clearly specified.

Study design

The design of studies must be chosen with regard to the hypothesis being tested. Both cross-sectional and longitudinal designs may be useful; the former to establish associations , and the latter to demonstrate temporal sequence (eg of infection and symptoms).

Longitudinal single case designs that examine correlations of relevant variables with fluctuations in symptom severity may be useful.

Measurements

All measures (both clinical and laboratory based) should be reliable, valid and reproducible between centres.

Reliable measures of subjective fatigue and of disability are lacking and require development. When reporting studies the reliability of all measures should be assessed and specified whenever possible.

Glossary

This glossary provides provisional definitions of the principal symptoms and suggests how they may be described. Each symptom is considered as follows:

(i) A description of the symptom (what it is).
(ii) What it is to be distinguished from (what it is not).
(iii) Criteria for rating its presence.
(iv) Additional description.

Fatigue

(i) When used to describe a symptom this is a *subjective* sensation and has a number of synonyms including, tiredness and weariness. A clear description of the relationship of fatigue to activity is preferred to the term fatiguability. Two aspects of fatigue are commonly reported: mental and physical. Mental fatigue is a subjective sensation characterized by lack of motivation and of alertness. Physical fatigue is felt as a lack of energy or strength and is often felt in the muscles.

(ii) Fatigue as a symptom should be distinguished from low mood and from lack of interest. The symptom of fatigue should not be confused with impairment of performance as measured by physiological or psychological testing. The physiological definition of fatigue is of a failure to sustain muscle force or power output.

(iii) To be regarded as a symptom, fatigue must:
(a) be complained of;
(b) significantly affect the person's functioning;
(c) should be disproportionate to exertion;
(d) should represent a clear change from a previous state; and
(e) be persistent or, if intermittent, should be present more than 50% of the time.

(iv) The symptom should be described as follows:
(a) severity: mild, moderate, or severe;
(b) frequency: continuous or intermittent. If intermittent the proportion of the time present;
(c) relation to activity: it should be stated whether the fatigue is greatly increased by minor exertion and whether it occurs at rest.

Disability

(i) This refers to any restriction of lack (resulting from loss of psychological or physiological function) of ability to perform an activity in the manner or within the range considered normal for a human being (i.e. things people cannot do in the areas of occupational, social, and leisure activities because of their illness[16]).

(ii) Disability (e.g. inability to walk) should be distinguished from impairment of function (e.g. weak legs) and from handicap (e.g. unable to work).

(iii) There should be a definite and persistent change from a previous level of functioning and it is desirable to seek supportive evidence from an informant.

(iv) The disability should be described as follows:
(a) area of disability (i.e. occupational, social, leisure, self-care);
(b) degree of disability.

Mood disturbance

(i) The term mood disturbance has been used to include depression, loss of interest and loss of pleasure (anhedonia), anxiety, emotional lability and irritability.

(ii) These phenomena should be distinguished from each other.

(iii) To be regarded as a symptom the mood disturbance should be
(a) complained of;
(b) should represent a significant change from a previous state; and
(c) should be relatively persistent or recurrent. Judgements of the appropriateness of mood disturbance are unreliable and should be avoided.

(iv) The symptoms should be described as follows:
(a) type: depressed mood, anhedonia, anxious mood, emotional lability, irritability;
(b) severity: standard scales are available to assess the severity of depressed mood and anxiety. In addition it should be determined whether the patient's disorder is sufficient to meet operational diagnostic criteria for major depressive disorder, generalized anxiety disorder or panic disorder according to a recognized psychiatric classification, e.g. the current edition of the Diagnostic and Statistical Manual of the American Psychiatric Association, DSM-III-R[17];
(c) duration and frequency of the mood disturbance should be reported.

Myalgia

(i) This refers to the symptom of pain or aching, felt in the muscles.
(ii) It should be distinguished from feelings of weakness and from pain felt in other areas such as joints.

(iii) The myalgia should be
(a) complained of;
(b) be disproportionate to exertion;
(c) be a change from a previous state;
(d) should be persistent or recurrent.

(iv) The symptom should be described as follows:
(a) severity: mild, moderate, or severe;
(b) frequency and duration;
(c) relation to exertion: if after exertion the time of onset relative to the exertion and duration should be described.

Sleep disturbance

(i) The symptom of sleep disturbance refers to a subjective report of a change in the duration or quality of sleep.
(ii) Sleep disturbance should be distinguished from feelings of daytime fatigue or tiredness.
(iii) The sleep disturbance should

(a) be complained of;
(b) not simply be a response to external disturbance;
(c) be a change from a previous state;
(d) be persistent.

(iv) The symptom should be described as follows:
(a) type: hypersomnia or increased sleep; insomnia or reduced sleep (which should be further described as either difficulty getting off to sleep, early waking, or subjectively disturbed or unrefreshing sleep);
(b) severity: the amount of change in duration of sleep should be quantified in hours.

Other symptoms

Many other symptoms may be present and should be recorded as follows:
(i) The definition used.

(ii) Symptoms should be carefully distinguished from one another.

(iii) The criteria for rating its presence.

(iv) Additional information, e.g. severity.

Conclusions

The contributors hope that these guidelines will provide a basis for fruitful research studies, and for inter-disciplinary collaboration essential to this field of research. The guidelines are preliminary and will undoubtedly require further refinement and revision. The authors would welcome comments and suggestions.

M C Sharpe
University Department of Psychiatry
Warneford Hospital, Oxford OX3 7JX

Acknowledgments: *The convenors wish to thank all the participants and Professor Anthony Clare for his chairmanship. They also wish to thank Duphar Pharmaceuticals, Dr. Peter White and Professor Michael Gelder, for financial support.*

References

1. Henderson DA, Shelokov A. Epidemic neuromyasthenia- clinical syndrome? *N Engl J Med* 1959;**260**:757-64.

2. Byrne E. Idiopathic chronic fatigue and myalgia syndrome (myalgic encephalomyelitis); some thoughts on nomenclature and aetiology. *Med J Aust* 1988;**148**:18-82.

3. Galpine JF, Brady C. Benign myalgic encephalomyelitis. *Lancet* 1957;757-8.

4. Isaacs R. Chronic Infectious mononucleosis, *Blood* 1948;**3**:858-61.

5. The medical staff of the Royal Free Hospital. An outbreak of encephalomyelitis in the Royal Free Hospital Group London, in 1955. *BMJ* 1957;**2**:895-904.

6. BehanPO. Behan WMH, Bell EJ. The postviral fatigue syndrome- an analysis of the findings in 50 cases. *J Infect* 1985;**10**:211-22.

7. Pritchard C. Fibrositis and the chronic fatigue syndrome. *Ann Intern Med* 1988; **106**:906.

8. Yunus MB. Fibromyalgia syndrome: new research on an old malady. *BMJ* 1989; **298**:474-5.

9. Holmes GP, Kaplan JE, Gantz NM, *et al.* Chronic fatigue syndrome a working case definition. *Ann Intern Med* 1988; **108**:387-9.

10. Manu P, Lane TJ, Matthews DA. The frequency of the chronic fatigue syndrome in patients with symptoms of persistent fatigue. *Ann Intern Med* 1988; **109**:554-6.

11. Komaroff A, Geiger A. Does the CDC working case definition of chronic fatigue syndrome (CFS) identify a distinct group? *Clin Res* 1989; **37**:778A.

12. Lloyd AR, Wakefield A, Boughton C, Dwyer J. What is myalgic encephalomyelitis? *Lancet* 1988;i:1286-7.

13. David A, Wessely S, Pelosi A. Myalgic encephalomyelitis or what? *Lancet* 1988;ii:100-1.

14. David A, Wessely S, Pelosi A. Post viral fatigue: time for a new approach. *BMJ* 1988;**296**:696-8.

15. Wilcock GK, Hope RA, Brooks DN, *et al.* Recommended minimum data to be collected in research studies on Alzheimer's disease. *J Neurol Neurosurg Psychiatry* 1989;**52**:693-700.

16. World Health Organization. International classification of impairments, disabilities and handicaps. Geneva: WHO, 1980.

17. American Psychiatric Association. *Diagnostic and Statistical Manual of Mental Disorders*, revised 3rd edn. Washington DC: APA, 1987.

end of document

Comments

This Oxford paper appears to me to serve a single purpose and that is to introduce the term, **post-infectious fatigue syndrome** as an acceptable term under which to publish. The term chronic Epstein-Barr disease was rarely used in the United Kingdom and in general they still tend to disdain the "Americanism" Chronic Fatigue Syndrome. In attempting to both rubber-stamp and clarify the term CFS they simply added confusion to the already too complicated CDC definition. It is my opinion that their definition shows no new insight into the disease process.

The authors state that the syndrome is not lifelong. There is no evidence or basis for such a categorical statement. We have seen ample evidence of lifelong CNS dysfunction in M.E./CFS.

Reviewing the many eminent physicians present at this workshop, it is my observation that it includes only two medical participants who routinely may spent up to 50% or more, of their time, investigating M.E./CFS patients.

Since this definition has appeared, the Behan group in Glasgow, certainly the most productive, the best financed and most important M.E./CFS clinical and research group in the U.K., has only published under the term PVFS or post-viral fatigue syndrome, yet another name.

The National Institute of Health Definition

The NIH definition update workshop held in the Spring of 1990 has yet to be published. Certainly improvements have been made in the CDC definition at this workshop. However, those that organized this meeting appear to have made a deliberate attempt to avoid inviting any American scientists who engaged in neuropsychological or physiological brain mapping and evaluation of M.E./CFS patients. A disproportionate part of that meeting was taken up by one physician, who in my recollection, appeared to work as a vociferous lobbyist for the unsupported position that CFS patients get better if you tell them that nothing is wrong with them.

Behan Definition

Please see Chapter 22, Post-Viral Fatigue Syndrome Research in Glasgow.

Conclusion

It is a tragedy that clinicians and scientists who spend the majority of their time studying M.E./CFS patients have not put together a short, usable working definition with subgroups. These would include:

(1) a short working definition for researchers and clinicians

complemented by:

(2) a definition relating to children and adolescents,

(3) an inexpensive epidemiological definition.

Until we have a better understanding of the infectious etiology and the pathophysiology of M.E./CFS or a resolute marker, a perfect definition will elude even the most knowledgable.

In the meanwhile, it is clear that if CNS dysfunction were utilized as the primary feature of the disease, the list of disease exclusions would be considerably and economically shortened. It is hard to avoid the fact, that the majority of symptoms given in each and every one of these definitions, Wallis, Henderson-Shelokov, CDC and Oxford, lean heavily on CNS dysfunction or CNS symptoms as the primary system involved.

> **M.E./CFS is a systemic disease with many systemic features, but it is characterized primarily by CNS dysfunction, of which fatigue is only one of many components.**

Chapter 3

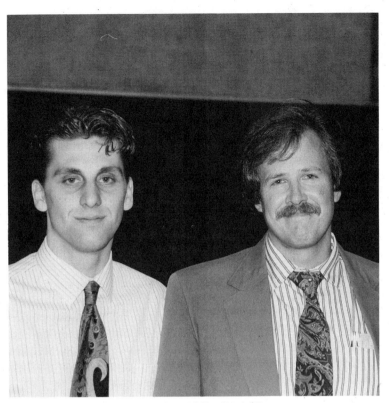

Borys Chabursky with Dr. Daniel Peterson

A Description
of Patients who Present with a Presumed Diagnosis of M.E./CFS

Borys Chabursky, Byron Hyde, MD, Anil Jain, MD

Borys Chabursky is a student at the University of Toronto. He is in the third year of a four year undergraduate specialist programme in Pharmacology and Toxicology. He has worked for the Nightingale Research Foundation as the National Director of Fund Raising and is a member of the media relations team for the National Society for Fund Raising Executives, Toronto chapter. He has also done research work with Dr. Hyde in Ottawa, Dr. Ryll in Sacramento and Dr. Mildon in Toronto. He has published in the CFIDS journal. Additionally, Borys worked for several pharmacies doing marketing, public relations and business development.

(Please see Chapter 5 for Dr. Hyde's photograph and curriculum vitae. Please see Chapter 4 for Dr. Jain's photograph and curriculum vitae.)

Since 1985, we have collectively seen and examined over 6,000 patients who have arrived at The Nightingale Research Foundation, either self -diagnosed or referred as possible M.E./CFS patients. The following represents some of our observations concerning individuals who may or may not actually suffer from M.E./CFS.

It is our belief that M.E./CFS may represent two superimposed disease processes:

(1) a dynamic disease process involving a post-encephalitic viral provoked injury followed by a variable recovery process. It is those patients that do not recover to their previous or adequate level of function that we come to know as suffering from chronic M.E. /CFS disease.

(2) a chronic disease process involving a low-grade encephalopathy resulting from either a persistence of the viral infection or the chronic metabolic effects of the initial destabilizing infection. This process may be the result of one or more infectious agents and involves a primary or secondary immune dysfunction.

It is also our belief that M.E./CFS represents a major acquired CNS dysfunction in which the brain function undergoes a metabolic alteration. We believe that the CNS is diffusely injured at several levels and that these areas include the cortex, the limbic system, the basal ganglia, the hypothalamus and areas of the spinal cord and its appendages. This persisting multilevel CNS dysfunction defines the nature of the disease process.

Most physicians first see M.E./CFS patients once they have become chronic and their disease process relatively static. Although the diversity and extreme nature of the dysfunctions tends to decrease once the patient's disease is chronic, the ongoing disabling features may be sufficient to create persisting major work and school disability.

Techniques of History Taking

One of the first questions that we ask a prospective M.E./CFS patient is: How did your illness begin? and frequently the patient replies, "with a flu-like illness". If you ask the patients what they mean by a flu-like illness, a multitude of descriptions ensue. It is the symptom picture that we wish to discover rather than a name that in itself can suggest different diseases to different people.

We also ask the patient to supply us with a typed, year by year summary of major life events from birth to the present time. Since many M.E./CFS patients will reply with dozens, sometimes hundreds of pages of history, we ask them to limit the description for each year from one to three sentences.

This short summary gives us a checklist of academic attainment, loss of schooling, geographical changes and major illnesses, major family illnesses, immunizations, school and work record. The summary provides us with a useful clothes horse to act as a frame for more precise questions. We also ask for the patient's report cards and work record to assess both lost schooling and academic achievement. The report card often gives a better social and medical understanding than physicians' records.

We place great store in the history of the patient from birth. When we look at the history of the disease we are interested in the type of onset, the environment of the onset of illness and how the disease process unfolds.

Although we, as many physicians, have difficulty with the CDC definition guidelines[1], all physicians should have a CDC checklist as well as their own. The patient's profile should be checked off to conform with legal requirements.

Discussion of these findings

It is most unusual for an acutely ill patient to approach us in an attempt to fraudulently seek compensation. On the contrary, most of these patients want an instant magic pill so that they can return to work immediately and are not happy when we do not have that magic potion. Fraud is not likely to be missed if the physician is knowledgeable of the patient and of

---

Diseases Masquerading as M.E./CFS

We have discovered in those patients who present at our office with a possible diagnosis of M.E./CFS, that the morbidity of perhaps as many as 25% may arise from one of the following illnesses:

Multiple Sclerosis
Thyroid illness
Localized and Metastatic malignancies
Brain tumours, including astrocytomas, gliomas
Transverse Myelitis
Myopathic illnesses, including:
     myasthenia gravis
     mitochondrial myopathies
     post-infectious polymyositis
Vitamin B 12 Deficiency Disorders
     Pernicious aenemia
     Vegetarianism and intentional dietary deprivation
     Intestinal disease associated with or independent of M.E./CFS

Rheumatoid illness or lupus (SLE)
Sarcoma
Renal or Liver disease
Infectious illnesses including:
     Toxoplasmosis
     AIDS
     Lyme Disease (Borrellia burgdorferi)
     Tuberculosis
     Brucellosis
Various psychiatric and social-psychiatric states including:
     Anxiety neurosis
     Uncomplicated Endogenous or Reactive Depression
     Psychopathic Personality Disorder
     Schizophrenia and other psychiatric disease.

the disease process. Almost all acutely ill adult patients suffer from work related deprivation anxiety. In chronically ill patients, other factors come into play.

We have had a small but interesting group of HIV positive patients who do not tell us they are HIV positive and may be even delusional, insisting that they have M.E./CFS. They are often phobic and then never return when told they are HIV positive. All patients should be checked for HIV and questioned as to sexual activity and intravenous drug use.

All patients presenting with M.E./CFS who fit into the guidelines should have the immediate benefit of a MRI. In areas of state supported medicine, this may at times represent a difficulty. These MRI tests should be ordered with specific understanding of localization of M.S., M.E./CFS UBOs (unidentified bright objects) and other space occupying lesions. This may save a later legal action against the attending physician and may, in a few cases, result in the discovery of a treatable lesion.

CT scans are definitely not useful for M.E./CFS patients and sometimes serve little purpose for M.S. patients. If anything, CT scans play a negative role in the investigation of an M.E./CFS patient, since, once the physician finds that it is normal, there is a tendency to tell the patient there is nothing wrong with the brain. The treating physician, as well as the radiologist, should learn to read the MRI.

MRI lesions, called UBO's can often be found in M.E./CFS patients, particularly in the first year of illness. These lesions may be mistaken for early M.S. They are only rarely larger than 1 cm in length and less in width.[2] M.E. patients may also have oligoclonal banding[3] in the spinal fluid in the first six months and thus be misdiagnosed as M.S.

M.E./CFS patients may be misdiagnosed as suffering from rheumatoid disease. This is particularly true in children. The knees, ankles and elbows may be dramatically swollen but are not red or hot or internally ankylosed. A typical M.E./CFS patient will have a classical lupus rash in the submaxillary region, considerable pain and often be incorrectly diagnosed as "a rheumatoid waiting to happen". Frequently the sedimentation rate is 0-5 in this group, unusual for a true rheumatoid.

Few patients with M.E./CFS present or continue as chronic depression. Despite this, we do diagnose severe depression in this group and have investigated patients who have succeeded in committing suicide. We almost always refer the few patients with severe depression for psychiatric assistance. These may be the only M.E./CFS patients that psychiatrists ever see, supporting the belief held by some psychiatrists that M.E./CFS is essentially a depressive illness.

As many as 20% of all women with typical chronic M.E./CFS illness will eventually develop thyroid abnormalities. Thyroid disease is not necessarily an exclusion of M.E./CFS.

M.E./CFS or M.E./CFS-like illnesses

The British and others utilize the name Post-Viral Fatigue Syndrome because, among other reasons, they believe the American term, Chronic Fatigue Syndrome, is too open to misinterpretation. However, it is not just the American name but the definition that may be too unfocused.

The name Post-Viral Fatigue Syndrome would suggest that the triggering illness is the cause of the disease process. That may not be the case.

M.E./CFS can start acutely or insidiously, but, when it starts acutely after an observed triggering infection, it is much easier to diagnose. But the reason that the Acute Onset form is easier to diagnose is not due to the infectious start but rather the explosive symptoms that are more often observed following an Acute Onset form.

Nor are Acute and Insidious Onset M.E./CFS necessarily different diseases. Frequently, in one family an Acute Onset and an Insidious Onset will occur within the same time frame. At times, a patient with an earlier Acute Onset appears to trigger an insidious onset in a new contact.

We recognize several clinical entities within the collectivity of these terms, all obscured by these general diagnostic names. They are as follows:

(1) **Acute Onset M.E./CFS** is characterized by brain and physical dysfunction, immediately after:

(a) an apparent infectious triggering agent,

(b) an infectious disease in close family member or partner,

(c) a specific immunization(s), or transfusion(s),

(d) a traumatic incident, eg: automobile accident, surgery.

The Acute Onset Group can frequently tell you the hour, day and year when the illness started. The onset is frequently dramatic and they can usually be diagnosed within two weeks of the onset of their illness.

The Acute Onset Group frequently contains a sub-group that may represent a significantly delayed reaction and is as follows:

(2) Delayed Acute Onset M.E./CFS

There is no difference from the Acute Onset M.E./CFS in its characteristics, however, M.E./CFS follows:

(a) **Mononucleosis-Like Illness**: Six months to two years earlier, an infectious mononucleosis-like illness occurred that may have persisted with marked prostration for two or more months followed by a complete clinical recovery.

(b) **Encephalitis**: Six months to two years earlier, an encephalitic illness occurred, severe in nature but of very short duration, usually less than one week of prostration, followed by a complete clinical remission without any persisting sequellae.

(c) **Subclinical Poliomyelitis**: Many years earlier, when in childhood, the individual had a parent, sibling or close contact who had paralytic poliomyelitis. The M.E./CFS patient never demonstrated any poliomyelitis-like illness. This Delayed Acute Onset Group may be the same group as the post-polio patients but who had suffered a subclinical case of poliomyelitis. Up to one third of adult M.E./CFS patients may fit into this group.

(3) Insidious Onset M.E./CFS

This group tends to slowly ease themselves into the spectrum of M.E./CFS illness. Clinically they are difficult to diagnose when not associated with an epidemic.

This form of M.E./CFS is often incomplete. The onset symptoms are frequently less dramatic and fewer in number than an Acute Onset Type. They tend to resemble the chronic pattern seen one or more years after the start of an Acute Onset M.E./CFS.

In this group, by definition, an infectious triggering episode is never discovered. Not infrequently, other family members may have or have had M.E./CFS. A detailed history reveals that they frequently have had previous similar episodes that they omitted to discuss. They may well represent recurrent bouts of a previous acute onset illness that started in early childhood and is not remembered. A detailed life history, as noted above, is important to document in this group.

This large insidious group has been poorly investigated and rarely appears in the literature.

(4) **Pure Fatigue Syndrome** without any evidence of brain or physical dysfunction, depression or other psychiatric disturbance.

This fourth group of Pure Fatigue Syndrome is quite curious and appear regularly. They are not M.E./CFS. The patient arrives in our office with the following complaint. "Doctor, I am tired all of the time. I am tired when I wake up. I am tired when I run my 5 or 10 or 20 miles everyday. I don't have any appreciable muscle pain or cognitive problem but just this fatigue."

This group tends to have no obvious psychiatric history.
They tend to have active full-time jobs.
They tend to have normal family lives.
They tend to be fairly positive persons, anxious and concerned with their job and health. The few that have been tested by SPECT have normal brain imaging. We don't know what to make of this patient group.

Although it is most rare to find any pathology in this group, they should not be treated in a cavalier manner since they may represent a single area brain lesion. One such patient that we investigated fell into this group. He was referred to a neurologist who sent the patient home telling him that he simply suffered from depression. He was not depressed. However, the patient died of a brain tumour two years later.

(5) **Pure Muscle or Fibromyalgia Illness** with pain and fatigue but without any evidence of brain exhaustion or dysfunction, depression or psychiatric disturbance.

A recent symposium on CFS at the NIH in 1991[4], concluded that Fibromyalgia was a symptom of several disease processes, and that Fibromyalgia Syndrome was a synonym for CFS.

We believe there is a third process of pure Fibromyalgia Illness without any other apparent attached disease process. This group must be distinguished from Fibromyalgia Syndrome, that is simply a synonym for M.E./CFS. **It must be this group, the Pure Muscle or Fibromyalgia Illness Group, that recover when exercised. In our experience, exercising M.E./CFS or Fibromyalgia Syndrome patients results in an increasing disability of both cognitive and muscular strength.**

(6) Post-Varicella induced Brain Dysfunction

Varicella (chicken pox) is well-known as a cause of brain and systemic injury in prenatal and very early childhood, giving rise to deafness, and other sensory and cardiac defects. Varicella can cause up to 19% death rate in adults over the age of 20[5] or persisting major central nervous and systemic illness in adults. This process should be distinguished from M.E./CFS. To our knowledge, no one has studied and published the post-encephalitic brain injuries in this group of individuals using QEEG, SPECT and PET scanning techniques. Post-Varicella brain and muscle dysfunction, as well as post Herpes Zoster fatigue syndrome, should not be confused with the M.E./CFS group since they probably represent a specific post-encephalitic brain and cellular injury. It cannot be concluded that their brain and muscle defects are the same as those of M.E./CFS patients.

(7) Post-Hepatitis B Fatigue Syndromes

This is a separate disease entity and should not be included as part of M.E./CFS.

(8) Post-Recovery M.E./CFS Group

This group have definitely suffered a moderate or severe case of typical M.E./CFS, and have been considerably disabled for an extended period of time, sometimes in excess of two years. They have, after considerable difficulty, justifiably obtained disability insurance, but now are partially or, in a few cases, completely recovered.

This fairly large subgroup has certain common characteristics. They have largely lost self-confidence both as to their intellectual and physical capacities.

Most of these individuals have, in the past, improved and returned to work or school only to fall ill again with a recurrence of their disease process. Now, seemingly recovered, they wish to return to work but they are frightened to lose their hard-earned disability pension, fall ill again and be left both disabled and without any income.

The Employer's Perspective:

Often their employer does not want them back.

They have been replaced with another employee who is adequately filling their old job and who can be depended upon.

The employer is very concerned that the patient is contagious.

Concerned that the illness is of a psychiatric nature, the employer is frightened and apprehensive about psychiatric patients and possible emotional confrontation. Often this group may have been excellent and productive workers, but, having fallen ill with M.E./CFS, attempted to continue to work with disastrous consequences to the employer and employee. The excellent work is forgotten and the irregular work pattern and productivity are remembered.

The employer is concerned about legal repercussions, filling out forms, accident policies and the views of other employees.

Some employers rehire these M.E./CFS patients simply to fire them, and thus prevent any loss of cost-effective company insurance package.

Many of these patients feel that they are strong enough to return to part-time jobs but, if they do, they will not qualify for long-term disability insurance benefits and they will, in addition, lose their previous insurance benefits or access to them thus losing all access to a disability net.

Summary

We are concerned about the delayed group that may represent a significant number of M.E./CFS patients. Do these cases represent an earlier infection that provokes a chronic immune injury? This could set the individual up for the triggering infection that will eventually result in M.E./CFS.

We are very concerned that some of these M.E./CFS patients may harbour an insidious malignancy. We have seen this occur infrequently but often with disastrous results. Even when a patient has a confirmed diagnosis of M.E./CFS, re-evaluation should be an annual event to rule out such eventualities.

We are concerned with the **Post-Recovery Group**.

They represent a major problem for disability insurance and the government employment offices to solve. However, there is little chance of immediate help from either Government or insurance companies since both have been studiously blind to the reality of M.E./CFS. Physicians, insurance companies and governments have been largely inept in dealing with this sociological work crisis. Why then should an employer take in a potential problem?

It is obvious that the prospective diagnosis of M.E./CFS attracts many individuals who are ill and undiagnosed. In the course of our study of M.E./CFS we have seen innumerable very disabled children with rheumatoid disease and others with disease resembling Encephalitica Lethargica. Because they do not conform to clear-cut diagnostic criteria they have been abandoned in their wheel chairs and forgotten in their homes. To abandon our jurisdiction is neither what physicians were trained to do nor what governments were elected to do.

References

1. Holmes G., Kaplan J., Gantz N. et al. Chronic fatigue syndrome; A working case definition. Annals of Internal Medicine, 108, 387-389.

2. Biddle R. See chapter 48 this text.

3. Poser C. See chapter 43 this text.

4. Schluederberg A. Workshop on the Definition and Medical Outcome Assessment of CFS in Research,. National Institute of Allergy and Infectious Diseases, Bethesda, March 18-19, 1991.

5. Gordon JE. Chicken pox: An epidemiological review. Am. J. Med Sci 1962; 244: 362-389

Chapter 4

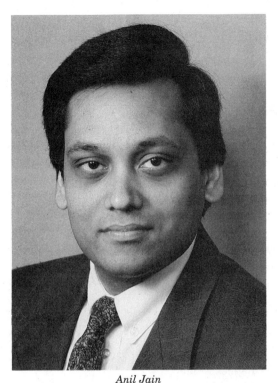

Anil Jain

General Information
Post-Infectious, Acute Onset M.E./CFS
(Post-Viral Fatigue Syndrome)

Byron Hyde, MD, Sheila Bastien, PhD, Anil Jain, MD

Dr. Jain received his Bachelor of Sciences from the University of Ottawa. Subsequently, he graduated in Medicine from the Faculty of Medicine, University of Ottawa in 1985. He then completed his internship from the Ottawa General Hospital. Following this, he worked in Family Practice and in the emergency department at the Springdale Hospital in Springdale, Nfld., Canada for two years. Over the last four years, Dr. Jain has dedicated the majority of his practice for diagnostic evaluation and treatment of thousands of patients suffering from M.E. / CFS in North America. He is presently the clinical Director of the Nightingale Research Foundation (Canada) on M.E.

(Please see Chapter 5 for Dr. Hyde's photograph and curriculum vitae. Please see Chapter 51 for Dr. Bastien's photograph and curriculum vitae.)

In the previous chapter we discussed several of the non-psychiatric disabling syndromes that we have encountered at The Nightingale Research Foundation. This chapter reviews the general information concerning Acute Onset M.E. / CFS and, in particular, the form that is triggered or caused by an apparent infectious illness. This is the same entity as Post-Viral Fatigue Syndrome. As explained in the previous chapter, this is an arbitrary clinical classification based upon the form of onset. This arbitrary classification has been made by researchers in order to narrow the disease range down to a manageable and similar group.

Using the type of onset, i.e. Post-Viral Fatigue Syndrome[1] as a defining technique, is a far from perfect way to subdivide the various forms of M.E./CFS. If we define the disease by symptom picture, some patients seem to start at the beginning of this process, i.e. at the Initial Stage, and some appear to skip this early period and fall ill at the level resembling the Early Chronic Stage where there is a blunting or obscurity of many of the symptoms but not necessarily of the disability.

```
┌─────────────────────────────────────────┐
│            M.E. / CFS Stages             │
│                                          │
│  (1) Initial Stage    (3) Early Chronic Stage │
│  (2) Recuperation Stage (4) Late Chronic Stage│
└─────────────────────────────────────────┘
```

Clinically, there are three forms of this disease. The first is a complete form where the patient runs through the four stages, starting at the Initial Stage. This is the pattern one sees regularly with Post-Infectious, Acute Onset M.E./CFS. It is relatively easy to diagnose and does not require a waiting period of 6 months.[2]

The second is the Insidious Onset M.E./CFS that usually starts with the blunted symptom picture seen in the Chronic Stages and thus represents a more clinically difficult diagnosis.

To make matters worse, as in all diseases, the entire symptom picture is not always present in any one patient, thus making the clinical diagnosis of incomplete forms difficult or clinically impossible to diagnose. A similar problem exists in the diagnosis of rheumatoid disease processes.

Post Infectious, Acute Onset M.E./CFS
Post-Viral Fatigue Syndrome.

This chronic disease process is characterized by the acute onset of:

(1) Obvious central nervous system (CNS) and muscle dysfunction accompanied by a plethora of strange, frightening and unstable symptoms. The CNS symptoms and dysfunctions include:

> cognitive
> sensory
> sleep
> motor
> and frequently pain dysfunction.

(2) Rapid fatigue, shut-down or exhaustion of muscle and CNS functions after no apparent cause or after minor:

> physical
> intellectual
> sensory or
> infectious interaction.

and associated with an unusually slow rate of recov-

ery or rebound to the previous decreased level of function.

(3) Neuropsychological and reactive psychiatric changes.

Variable expression of the above disease pattern exist, are common, and can be explained by injury to different functional areas of the central nervous system. The most common incomplete expression is the non-myalgic form. This symptom variability is quite comprehensible if the physician realizes that M.E./CFS, like paralytic poliomyelitis, can injure certain areas of the CNS while missing others.

Incubation Period 1

The incubation period has been well documented in various epidemics[1] and also in some of the more recent sporadic cases of M.E./CFS. The documented incubation period of the triggering disease is probably about 5-6 days, but varies from 4 to 15[4, 5, 6, 7, 8,9] days. However, the role of the triggering infection is not understood. Are we measuring the incubation period of the triggering disease or of the actual M.E./CFS disease. Are they the same or different diseases?

```
┌────────────────────────────────────────────────┐
│      Known Incubation Period of M.E./CFS.       │
│                                                 │
│  1934 Los Angeles*.....................4-7 days⁴│
│  1948 Akureyri epidemic*..............5-10 days⁵│
│  1955 Royal Free epidemic*............5-6 days⁶ │
│  1955 Cumberland epidemic.............5-7days⁷  │
│  1955 Massachusetts epidemic..........5 days⁸   │
│  1965 Texas epidemic**................21 days⁹  │
│  1984 Labour Day Montreal cluster*....7-10 days¹⁰│
│  1984 Ontario cluster.................5 days¹¹  │
└────────────────────────────────────────────────┘
```

Known Incubation Period of M.E./CFS.	
1934 Los Angeles*	4-7 days[4]
1948 Akureyri epidemic*	5-10 days[5]
1955 Royal Free epidemic*	5-6 days[6]
1955 Cumberland epidemic	5-7days[7]
1955 Massachusetts epidemic	5 days[8]
1965 Texas epidemic**	21 days[9]
1984 Labour Day Montreal cluster*	7-10 days[10]
1984 Ontario cluster	5 days[11]

* *multiple examples documented*
** *This 21 day period is not a true incubation period since Dr. Leon-Sotomayor discounts the prodromal period or triggering infection as being different from the actual disease process. This 21 day period would closely associate with our own observations in which there is the initial infectious incident followed by a pause then the gradual development of the full blown features of the illness. This period can take up to 21 days.*

Incubation Period 2

The incubation period 1, mentioned above, relates to the incubation period of either the epidemic disease or the triggering disease. This does not explain the apparent delayed association that we have documented all too frequently of an infectious mononucleosis-like disease or an encephalitic process that preceded the actual M.E./CFS illness by a variable period, usually from 6-24 months. Nor does it explain the frequent association of an M.E./CFS patient with an earlier close contact with a paralytic poliomyelitis patient[11].

Transmission of Infection

The major mode of infectivity appears to be by airborne or respiratory route[4,13]. There is no evidence in the literature that the infection was waterborne or that potables were the cause of the illness. Bodies of water, or sewage may, however, sustain the causative infectious agent.

It is not known if the triggering or prodromal disease is the cause of M.E./CFS or if the triggering disease is a convenient non-specific destabilizing virus that provides the ultimate injury to a pre-existing destabilized immune system.

It is not known if M.E./CFS in any one individual is caused by:

(a) a single unique virus,
(b) one or more families of viruses
(c) a virus that requires a particular immune window or breakdown in order to create a persisting virus infection
(d) or if M.E./CFS operates in an AIDS-like system with one virus that immobilizes the immune system and another infectious agent that causes the disabling illness.

Although the Lake Tahoe epidemic in 1984 appears to have been first documented in a girls' high school basketball team[14], there is also an anecdotal story from the Lake Tahoe epidemic, that 5 unrelated men all fell ill with M.E./CFS after having slept with the same prostitute[15]. This prostitute was visiting from Africa. There is no mention of sexual transmission of M.E./CFS in the literature. We have countless cases documented in our files where one spouse with M.E./CFS has had long-term repeated sexual contact with an existing or new spouse without transmission of the illness. We have had a few cases of apparent rapid transmission to a new sexual partner. However, it is

most unusual for the two disease processes to display exactly the same clinical spectrum.

At the same time, we have many cases of individuals in the same family who have fallen ill at significantly different time periods. It is not known if this indicates transmission of a chronic infectious illness, if we are observing a latent infection with spurts of infectivity as note by Wallis[16] or if we are merely observing late expression of the disease process in which all parties were infected at the same proximate time. We have a few instances in which several generations in the same family have developed the illness. In the Mercy San Juan Hospital epidemic[17], the illness seems to have been passed down through as many as five related and unrelated non-sexual, casual contacts.

Attack Rate		
Population at risk	No. of Cases	Attack Rate per 100
Los Angeles 1934		
Student Nurses 401	65	16.2
Graduate Nurses 891	73	8.2
Attendants 266	5	1.9
Orderlies 318	5	1.6
Akureyri epidemic[5,21]		
6,887	465	6.75
high school and university students		
ages 10-14 46	9	5.1
ages 15-19 231	66	28.6
ages 20-24 56	11	19.6
Royal Free Hospital[6]		
3,500	292	8.3
Men 950	27	2.8
Women 2,550	265	10.4
Nurses 800	149	18.6
Cumberland epidemic[7]		13.9
Orton region		19.8

*Eventually 1116 case were documented in the Akureyri epidemic giving a considerably larger attack rate for the general population of 6,887 of 16.2 rather than 6.75

Degree of Infectivity

During the first few weeks of the Initial Stage, M.E./CFS appears to be infective but highly selective within clusters and epidemics. During the Recovery and Chronic Stages, M.E./CFS does not appear to present a significant infective risk. Wallis states that *"the level of infectiousness is fairly high as shown by the numbers of families where secondary attacks had occurred subsequent to the primary illness."*[18]

Period of Infectivity

Clinically, it would appear that the main period of infectivity of M.E./CFS occurs in the period preceding the overt illness and during the early days of the Initial Stage. In most cases, the chronic phases of this disease do not appear to be particularly infective.

In a very few clusters and individual cases the disease infectivity appears to continue for many months. e.g. (a) Four individuals in an open lesbian community in Ontario fell ill with both acute onset and insidious onset M.E./CFS. This irregular series of new illness involved new sexual partners and casual dinner contacts in which there was neither kissing nor other sexual contact. Fomites were shared. e.g.(b) In the Mercy San Juan Hospital epidemic[17] infectivity was followed through 5 new generations of contacts. One can only surmise that we may be dealing with two different infectious processes. Wallis states that the time of maximum infectivity appeared to be at or about the time of initial onset of symptoms. Recurrences of symptoms of the disease became a well-marked feature, and, at that time, contacts would develop the typical disease, suggesting, therefore, that the host was again infectious.[19]

Variability of Disease Expression

There is little in the literature of variable expression of illness but there appears to be considerable vari-

ability within the same epidemic both in degree of illness, symptoms, myalgic or non-myalgic forms, chronicity and even form of illness manifested.

In the August 1984 North Carolina orchestra M.E./CFS epidemic[20], it appears that the orchestra broke down into three groups:

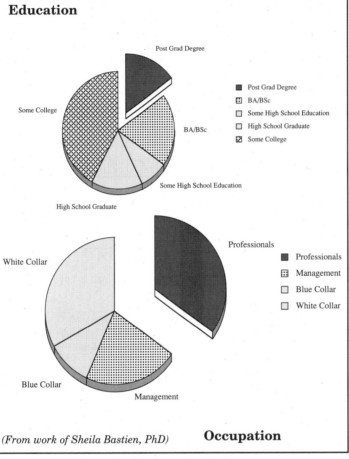

(From work of Sheila Bastien, PhD)

Education

- Post Grad Degree
- BA/BSc
- Some High School Education
- High School Graduate
- Some College

Occupation

- Professionals
- Management
- Blue Collar
- White Collar

(a) one with M.E./CFS
(b) one with an assumed acquired immune dysfunction but no observable disease
(c) and one with no observable disease and no observable immune dysfunction.

The group with no M.E./CFS but observable immune dysfunction, within five years manifested a considerably larger number of malignancies than would be anticipated.

In an August 1984 Ontario cluster[11] seven family members fell ill with presumably the same virus infection.

Five members of the same household came down with a tracheobronchitis and two with Bornholme's disease and no tracheobronchitis. Those that fell ill with Bornholme's disease then developed M.E./CFS. The tracheobronchitis started in mid-August and persisted for up to six weeks and preceded the cases of M.E./CFS by one week.

In this epidemic, one case of M.E./CFS was totally cleared within one year and another has become chronic. Twenty days after falling ill with tracheobronchitis and no M.E./CFS, that individual kissed a non-family member and that outside person fell ill within 5 days with M.E./CFS. This illness was a typical acute onset form but was self-limiting after two months.

During the Akureyri epidemic[5] in northern Iceland, during the same epidemic period, approximately 5 children fell ill with Parkinson's disease[21] as an apparent result of the Akureyri epidemic. These children eventually died of Parkinson's disease.

In any one cluster we have noted some patients with severely disabling disease and some mildly disabling disease, some with pain syndromes and some with no pain syndromes.

Who Falls Ill with M.E./CFS?

In the early epidemics, there was an initial preponderance of disease among health care workers in hospitals and in nursing schools[4,6,17, 22]. There have been several epidemics among schools[5,7,23], that, in the case of the Akureyri and Lake Tahoe epidemics, involved both teachers and students. Historically, there has been a tendency for the staff of institutions to manifest increased disease incidence. There have been several epidemics among military establishments.[24,25,26] Except for the Akureyri and the 1955 Cumberland, England epidemic[7] until 1979, most M.E./CFS disease tended to occur as institutional epidemics. Although there is much early anecdotal talk of M.E./CFS in the community, sporadic M.E./CFS did not become widespread and appear significantly in the literature until after the apparent increase in 1979[27]. From that time on a steady increase among the general public was observed by several clinicians with 1984 marking an apparent major increase in the numbers falling ill with M.E./CFS[28].

We have noted M.E./CFS in children from the age of 3 to adults in their late 60's. In children and in adults, there tends to be a marked increase of reported cases of females, with girls and women representing as many as 65-75% of all of the cases. In children, we have found that there seems to be an increased frequency of M.E./CFS in girls in grades 7 and 8 and again in youths in their last year of high school and first year at University.

We have found a definite occupational bias with teachers, health care workers and social workers significantly affected and to a lesser degree, other professions such as the clergy and lawyers. We have also found that, within the health professions, those

that work in psychiatric institutions and nursing teachers seem to be particularly singled out. In the teaching professions, teachers who work in schools for the disabled appear to be particularly at risk.

It has been suggested that these individuals represent a group of high contact with a potentially ill public and are thus exposed to more infectious illness. This is true. However, these select groups also tend to be the same population that keep their immunizations up to date and, in fact, they may be some of the few adults who routinely receive immunization due to their line of work. Several of the epidemics occurred after the individuals were either exposed to immunization or would have been expected to have been just immunized. These groups that are noted to have a high risk of falling ill with M.E./CFS do not work in occupations where there is higher stress than the average worker. However, they do work in occupations that require higher levels of immunization. This relation to inoculation is also seen in other infectious diseases. It has been observed that there is an increased risk of poliomyelitis occurring after prophylactic inoculation against diphtheria, whooping cough and smallpox. The risk seems greater 8-14 days after the inoculation.[29]

Racial and Working Class Anomalies

Among blue collar workers, we again note the high proportion of individuals who are health care workers. Unlike the consensus in the United States, and despite the relatively low black and native populations in Canada, we have seen several blacks of both African and American origins ill with M.E/CFS. We have seen Mohawk, Woodland Cree and Algonquin native persons with M.E./CFS. Numbers are not large, but consistent with their low relative populations. In Canada there tends to be a much more egalitarian mix of patients with M.E./CFS rather than the higher income, higher educated groups seen in the United States series[30]. We believe this bias is either a sampling error or may simply represent one of access to physicians.

It is of particular interest that Dr. Luis Leon-Sotomayor, a Spanish American, observed a significant number of blacks who fell ill in the Texas epidemic. This was described in his book **Epidemic Diencephalomyelitis**[9]. Also, in the Punta Gorda epidemic in Florida, described by Poskanzer, Henderson et al[37], there were a large number of blacks observed with M.E./CFS. The Punta Gorda epidemic was of particular interest due to the fact that of the some 60 epidemics noted in this book, it was the sole epidemic in which a door-to-door study was involved. The absence of blacks might simply be interpreted as disabled M.E./CFS black patients avoiding a group of white physician researchers. To my knowledge, no black U.S. researcher has been funded to study M.E./CFS by NIH or CDC.

Geographical Distribution

One wonders if, as with M.S., there is not a geographical epicentre of M.E./CFS and if there is not an in creased frequency of M.E./CFS in the northern British Isles, particularly in the area north of Hadrian's wall and extending up to the Glasgow area. We also find it curious that, in the some 26 Canadian physicians with M.E./CFS that we have seen from Ontario and Quebec, twenty-one originally came from or worked in Scotland, England and Ireland and of the remaining five, one was from Denmark, one from Belgium and one from Mexico, but of European origin. Only two were born and raised in Canada and one of those was married to a physician with M.E./CFS who came from Ireland.

Natural History of M.E./CFS

The natural history of post-infectious M.E./CFS resembles that of a single infectious injury with an initial rapid period of symptom and disability improvement from the prodromal infection, after which a new disease process sets in from which the patient either recovers or is left with a chronic illness and a decreased level of performance, frequently in the areas of intellectual, neuropsychological, physical and emotional abilities. This decreased level of performance can stabilize at this new level, slowly improve or deteriorate depending upon many physical and psychosocial aspects of support. This new level of functioning is quite variable and may be dependent upon the site and degree of the initial central nervous system injury. It is rare for a patient who has been ill for one year or more to totally recover. It is also rare for the patient to show a progressive deterioration once the Chronic Stage has been reached. We have observed these few exceptions.

The Natural History of M.E./CFS:

does not resemble Alzheimer's disease with a cumulative increase in disability until the patient succumbs. M.E. is rarely progressive.

does not resemble M.S., although the symptoms may at times be similar, where there tend to be periods of increased activity of the disease process with a stepwise increase in disability.

does resemble that of epidemic paralytic poliomyelitis in that these patients show an initial recovery period after which many are left with permanent disability.

Anterior or Paralytic Poliomyelitis

As with anterior poliomyelitis, the deaths that have been recorded tend to occur early in the first weeks of the disease. There are however, few deaths from M.E./CFS recorded in the literature[7,31].

Repeat infections of paralytic poliovirus were rare and when they did occur, appeared to have been associated with different polio or other enteroviral types. It is not known if the recurrences of M.E./CFS represent a resurgence of a latent and existing disease or a reinfection with a new viral entity.

As with anterior poliomyelitis, M.E./CFS tends to occur as a single isolated event that causes the maximum disability during the first few months and during which period the patients tend to improve. During this early period even patients severely disabled with poliomyelitis or M.E./CFS may significantly recover while some show limited recovery.

As with anterior poliomyelitis, there tends to be continued recovery in most M.E./CFS patients after the first acute episode , but any recovery tends to be marginal after two years. Psychosocial dysfunction may aggravate the physical aspects of what would have been a stabilized moderate to severe illness.

Rehabilitation in paralytic poliomyelitis usually has to take into account only the physical disability. There tends to be little or no brain dysfunction in classical anterior poliomyelitis, while, in M.E./CFS, brain dysfunction is the defining characteristic of the disease.

In poliomyelitis, any physical disability is eventually stabilized and the process of rehabilitation can be affected by modifying the home and work place, structurally assisting the patient with braces, wheel chairs, automobile modifications, and changing the work focus to one more congruent with the physical limitations of the disability.

Stable Chronic Stage of Poliomyelitis

No matter what degree of disability is attained by the paralysed poliomyelitis patient, that patient's condition has one over-riding characteristic, stability. The degree of disability is stable and that stability can be depended upon. It is this expectation and this assurance of stability that allow any serious health, re-education and work planning.

Unstable Chronic Stage of M.E./CFS

One of the diagnostic principals underlying the understanding of M.E./CFS is the chronically unstable nature of the illness. This lack of stability results both in the patient's lack of dependability in the work place and the patient's increasing loss of confidence in her own abilities. A typical example of an M.E./CFS patient is illustrated by a disease process where there is a lack of stability or dependability of:

(a) the central nervous system's functions,
(b) the neuropsychiatric behavioural patterns
(c) the reactive psychiatric patterns
(d) muscle function

Thus, even as the patient's physical and CNS functions improve, she may develop a significant loss of confidence in her own ability to perform. Frequently this psychological loss of confidence or ability becomes one of the dominant forces in perpetuating the patient's disability.

A Description of Prior Illnesses, Triggering Infections, and Stages of M.E./CFS

SIGNS OF PRIOR ILLNESS

We routinely note in our clinic the occurrence of a curious illness that can sometimes be documented three months to two years prior to the prodromal illness. This may present as:

(1) a mononucleosis-like illness that causes a period of chronic illness that may last up to six months, or

(2) It may resemble an acute encephalitic process. When it occurs as an encephalitic process, the illness is usually very short lasting (2-4 days), very severe with at times an almost comatose patient, a rapid and apparent complete recovery and without other apparent lingering sequellae. The patient will usually state that this had been the worst headache of his life.

(3) A third type is that of a minor episode that resembles the main chronic M.E./CFS disease. This minor episode tends to last several weeks or even months. During this time, the person rarely misses school or work but is quite unwell. The patient then usually recovers for a brief period only to fall ill with the full blown features of M.E./CFS. (For further details see Chapter 6, M.E./CFS: The Physical Signs of Disease).

Observed Triggering Infections

The most common presentation is that of a minor non-specific viral-like illness, sore throat, with or without febrile episode. There is frequently diarrhoea and/or gastric pain.

There is nothing in the prodomal disease to forewarn of the impending chronic illness. There is a habit of calling this prodromal infection, a flu-like illness but there is no indication that it is an influenza. "Flu" has entered the public domain as a synonym for any unknown minor infection. However, to our knowledge, despite the tens of thousands of cases of M.E./CFS, only a few physicians have ever attempted to culture, successfully recover this "flu-like" virus and publish their results. Those that have would suggest that influenza is most rare and that enteroviruses may be among the most frequently encountered family of prodromal viruses.

We are not in a known Lyme disease area and perhaps, for this reason, have never seen a case of Lyme disease as an onset although we have demonstrated positive Lyme disease tests in approximately 12 chronic M.E./CFS cases.

Triggering infections include:

(1) Non-specific viral illness
(2) Tracheobronchitis
(3) Encephalitic-like illness
(4) Bornholme's disease
(5) Ménière's syndrome
(6) Epidemic conjunctivitis
(7) Hand, Foot and Mouth disease in children
(8) Undiagnosed forms of hepatitis
(9) Infectious Mononucleosis-like disease
(10) Myocarditis or pericarditis

Half of the above list; (4), (6), (7), (8) & (10) could be potentially classifiable as enteroviral infections and, with the exception of Ménière's disease, whose cause is unknown, and infectious mononucleosis, enterovirus infections are known to give rise to all of the above triggering infections. One cannot, of course, be sure if (1), (2) & (3), in M.E./CFS patients are due to enterovirus or other viruses.

Despite the now almost universal rejection of EBV as a cause of M.E./CFS, clinically an infectious mononucleosis-like illness appears in a modest but significant recent number of M.E./CFS histories. Most frequently this illness occurs 6 months to 2 years prior to the onset of M.E./CFS. Less frequently, it occurs just prior to onset of M.E./CFS.

Initial False Recovery Phase

Many M.E./CFS patients will frequently start to improve from the triggering or presenting illness before demonstrating the full-blown features of M.E./CFS. When it occurs, this recovery phase from the prodromal infection is very short lasting, from a few hours to one or two days, until the actual typical M.E./CFS features become apparent. Drs. Behan make the point that in M.E./CFS *"there is no latent period after the initial disease and before the characteristic M.E./CFS symptoms develop."*[32] They apparently use this argument to separate M.E./CFS from the auto-allergic reaction that follows a wide variety of different viral diseases known as Acute Disseminated Encephalomyelitis or ADEM. Contrarily, we have frequently observed that there is an aborted recovery. This biphasic character of the disease can also be typical of paralytic poliomyelitis[33].

Four Stages of Post-Infectious M.E./CFS

Acute Onset M.E./CFS can be arbitrarily and profitably subdivided into 4 overlapping stages.

Initial Stage:	0-6 months
Recuperation Stage:	2 weeks-24 months
Early Chronic Stage:	1-6 years
Late Chronic Stage:	from 6 years on

The Initial Stage

0-6 months

The Acute Onset M.E./CFS illness frequently declares itself by a dramatic barrage of symptoms following one of several prodromal symptom pictures. These are noted in this chapter as well as by Drs. Behan[32, 34] and Luis Leon Sotomayor[9].

(1) There is usually a significant degree of malaise, or total body discomfort such as one encounters in an acute attack of influenza. This malaise is associated with a rapidly fluctuating temperature change in which the body temperature tends to have a **below normal** temperature variability that may shoot up to modest elevation of temperature. This peak is often associated with episodes of drenching sweats not necessarily associated with any physical or emotional activity.

(2) There is a severe exhaustion or prostration that can assume the proportions of narcolepsy or even Encephalitica Lethargica. The patient can be awoken but soon falls back to sleep. In most patients, this period lasts for a few days to a few months but we have seen cases that have persisted for years. This persistence is particularly noticeable among children and youths.

(3) There may be an exacerbation of the prodromal symptoms.

(4) There is an alarming fluctuation and variability of symptoms.

(5) There is frequently tachycardia with ectopic beats.

(6) There is frequently marked initial anorexia.

(7) The disease process tends to usher in a permanent hypotensive process. However, about 10%, particularly those who had mild hypertension at onset, will react with a malignant type hypertension sometimes resembling a carcinoid syndrome[9].

(8) The patient frequently suffers from irritability, severe anxiety or panic attacks at the start of the disease process. This anxiety is very much related to the great number and inexplicable nature of the symptoms. In some cases this may be associated with hyperventilation. This condition may persist for the duration of the illness.

(9) There is a tendency for the multiple symptoms and signs to come in "storms". In the Initial Stage these storms seem to have a life of their own without any apparent triggering mechanism. In the Recuperation and later stages, the storms may be provoked by unusual but not necessarily excessive activity or association with infectious disease[9].

(10) It may take 3 weeks to 6 months to develop the full symptom picture of M.E./CFS.

Recuperation Stage
2 weeks-24 months, usually 1-12 months

The Recuperation Stage is characterized by a decrease in the number and severity of symptoms and symptom storms. The patient also tends to have an amnesic loss of remembrance of these early symptoms. During this period, some patients will rapidly return to normal and any minor permanent disability will be discounted as they return to a usual level of work and social activity. Others will return to work but will have to discount much of their social life due to the severity of on-going features of their disability. There tends to be an uneven return of abilities.

Some patients may recover most or all of their physical but not their cognitive abilities. This is seen particularly in children. Others may recover their mental abilities but not their physical strengths. Cardiac irregularities, if they occurred, and if they were not associated with myocarditis, tend to return to a normal pattern. Chordae tendinae ruptures that may occur in the Initial Stage and signs of mitral valve prolapse may be erroneously dismissed as pre-existing defects. Even those functions commonly associated with brain function, i.e. memory, emotional control, reading comprehension, aphasia, ataxia and sensory perception will vary as to the degree or completeness of recovery. All this suggests an unequal level of damage, variable location of injury and variable recovery of brain function.

Some patients will start to recover within two weeks while others may show little recovery until five or six months after onset. We have never seen a patient who has not recovered to some degree from this initial bomb blast of symptoms. Symptom decrease should not be confused with decrease of disability.

This period of recovery is variable and is almost always over by one or two years. At that time the patient will either be no longer disabled and back to work, or will be left at various levels of disability according to the variation in the individual disease process. Although most recovered patients will insist that they have completely recovered, on scrutiny many will have returned to work and social activity simply at a reduced level of brain and physical ability.

Physicians who observe the recovery of one M.E./CFS patient, her return to the work-force or to full-time school, sometimes generalize this recovery into the expectation that all ME./CFS patients will recover and that those that do not, have something morally wrong with them.

Early Chronic Stage
1-6 years

The early chronic stage is characterized by the same features as the Inital Stage. However, rapid shut down or exhaustion of muscle and CNS functions is the chief complaint as the patient attempts to return to normal activity. The CNS cognitive, sensory, sleep, motor, gastric and pain dysfunctions still exist, but exist in a more diffuse but not necessarily less disabling pattern. Insidious onset M.E./CFS has a clinical and symptom spectrum that resembels this early chronic stage as do recurrences.

This Early Chronic Stage is when the physical and medical aspects starts to merge with the psychosocial aspects of the disease, sometimes creating a treatment impasse. It is impossible to separate the physical from the psychosocial aspects when rehabilitation is the issue. The social aspects of the disease hinders the improvement of the physical disease and the physical aspects hinder the socio-economic life of the patient. Due to the financial and technical constraints of modern medicine, few general practitioners, internists or psychiatrists are able to cope with the lengthy time involved in the psychosocial aspects of rehabilitation.

This is the stage in which many M.E./CFS speciality physicians first see the M.E./CFS patient. If the patient is unlucky, she will already have been improperly diagnosed by several physicians, may have undergone minor or major surgery or investigative intervention. Marinacci, tongue in cheek, mentions patients from the 1934 epidemic "who had a hysterectomy in 1938, in the hope that the mental symptoms would be relieved, but the procedure was not beneficial."[35] At the Nightingale clinic we have rarely seen an adult female patient who had suffered from M.E./CFS for over five years, who has not had either a pelvic intervention or pelvic surgery.

It is thus understandable that, due to the multiple interpretations and her failure to show significant improvement, the patient may well have lost faith in her physicians and sought out well meaning and perhaps at times fraudulent individuals who practice what is loosely termed "alternative medicine". Humankind is still quite scientifically primitive. Many people still believe in variations of magic, they just don't use the term magic. It is rare to find an M.E./CFS patient who is not on several vitamins, oriental and perhaps other mystical "curative" agents, loosely called, "natural products". Most do no harm except to the pocket book. Some are dangerous. Inquiry should always be made as some of these "natural" products may be life-threatening, e.g. germanium.

The Early Chronic Stage is characterized by a fairly unstable level of dysfunction. During this period, most patients continue to show a very slow and uneven period of recovery and readaption to their altered state of CNS, muscle and social function. Recovery should not be confused with adaption. During this same period some patients will adapt to their altered internal environmental circumstances and others will not be able to make the transition. The

difference in those who adapt and those who do not is not simple. We believe the following factors are important in the individual's success or failure to be rehabilitated.

Some Factors Affecting Rehabilitation

Males with supporting spouse
Women without family obligations
Pre M.E./CFS intellectual assets
Level and type of pre M.E./CFS education
Degree and area of CNS injury
Social and economic support facilities
Family, medical and government support
Access to knowledgeable re-education program

Most of this group will have had a reversal of the initial hypersomnia and will now have a sleep dysfunction that involves non-restorative sleep and features of narcolepsy. To the detriment of earlier phases of sleep pathology, it is this period that sleep pathologists have most investigated. Sleep patterns are interrupted by arousal patterns.

Many patients in this stage of illness will not recover sufficiently to either enjoy work or social activities. This early Chronic Stage is marked by major changes in their life pattern. Unstable marriages will become increasingly destabilized and marriage breakdown and divorce will occur. Money reserves will have been liquidated. Many of the social confines of poverty may have set in and the patients, most of whom will have had life and social expectations set at a higher level, will now see those hopes and expectations destroyed. It is difficult for a physician, in a 15 minute visit, to relate to this change, particularly if the patient is still wearing a snappy, wealthy looking $1000 dollar Kenzo suit she had bought five years previously.

It is the period when students and youths and some adults will be most prone to suicide.

The more dramatic features noted in the Initial Phase will have diminished, but the patient will be left with a chronic brain, muscle and social dysfunction. Depending upon the ability of the patient to adapt to her changed circumstances and the area of most brain dysfunction, she may exhibit various levels of social and psychological impairment.

The Married Male Teacher

It is also the period when different social and financial abilities start to direct the course of the disease process. For instance, a disabled male teacher will often be able to return to work. He will have little or no social life. He will depend upon his wife for preparing course work and for marking exams. He will tend to sleep during the lunch break and return home at 4p.m. to sleep until a late dinner and then return to his bed, to sleep until the next morning. He will tend to spend the weekends in bed or in a state of exhaustion, but he will pick up his cheque. He is usually a total loss as a teacher and his relationship with the students will become trying. He will cease to perform many of his physical, intellectual and social functions as a teacher, parent or spouse.

The Married Female Teacher

A woman teacher at the same level of disability as her male counterpart will **not** be able to return to work or assume any other similar or appropriate work. Unlike her male counterpart, she will not be able to sleep in her car during lunch time in the local shopping centre parking lot. Her husband, who will be working, will rarely prepare her course work or mark her students' papers. She will have to return home at four or five p.m. and prepare supper for her children and husband and help her children with their homework. She will have to do the washing and cleaning. Despite the reputed social revolution, many husbands will not take on their share and certainly not their wife's share of the essential household activities. Some do, but it cannot be counted upon in most families. The net effect is that neither the work, home nor social abilities can be met by a mentally and physically exhausted woman with M.E./CFS.

The Spinster

We find that when a woman can get back to work, she is usually single and does not have children or other obligations.

The Senior Executive

A senior executive with an excellent executive assistant and secretarial staff can also get through with these work support structures. His changes in mental and social abilities are often equated with eccentricity. He can place more of his executive burdens on his senior staff. If his incompetency becomes too painful, he will frequently be bought out with a considerable financial settlement. A labourer with an active physical job will not be able to keep up with the changes in his altered physical condition.

Late Chronic Stage:
from 6 years on.

There has been no publication and to our knowledge, no research done on the chronic features of disease in M.E./CFS.

Without adequate recovery and support, there is an increasing tendency for the patient to become a hermit.

These patients tend to be forgotten. They have adjusted to their altered abilities. They will still show some minor improvements in function, but this is due to their accepting their altered abilities. We rarely see these individuals since they have given up any hope that physicians can be of service to them.

Despite their previous relatively high earning ability, many of these M.E./CFS patients will have become poor, long out of the work force, with no appreciable disability insurance. They frequently have disorganized houses and minds and, unless they have sufficient social structure, can become street people. They tend to no longer be recognized as having a post-infectious disease process.

It is our opinion, that far from M.E./CFS simply being a disease of the upper middle class, many of those that fall ill as children, adolescents and young adults become a significant proportion of the chronic poor.

Dr. John Richardson in the Newcastle-Upon-Tyne area in England has found a higher than usual level of retroperitoneal carcinoma[36] in this group. Retroperitoneal carcinoma is a very rare disease. He has also noted an apparent decrease in breast cancer. We also have noted what appears to be a lower than normal incidence of breast cancer in M.E./CFS patients.

There appears to be a recurrence of irregular cardiac rhythms in chronic illness, particularly after 20 years, but this may simply be a feature of aging.

If M.E./CFS is poorly funded and poorly investigated, this late chronic phase is almost totally devoid of research and is replete with all of the mythologies that occur when scientific scrutiny is absent.

References

1. Sharpe M.C. et al (1991) A report ...chronic fatigue syndrome: guidelines for research. J. Royal Soc Med 84:118-21.

2. Holmes G., Kaplan J., Gantz N. et al. Chronic fatigue syndrome; A working case definition. Annals of Internal Medicine, 1988;108:387-9.

3. See Chapter on Epidemics, this text.

4. Gilliam A.G. **Epidemiological Study of an Epidemic, Diagnosed as Poliomyelitis, Occurring Among the Personnel of The Los Angeles County General Hospital During The Summer of 1934**,Public Health Bulletin No. 240, April 1938, The United States Public Health Service.

5. Sigurdsson B., Sigurjonsson J., Sigurdsson J.H.,Thorkelsson J and Gudmundsson K. (1950) A disease epidemic in Iceland simulating poliomyelitis. American Journal of Hygiene, 1950;52:222-38.

6. The medical staff of the Royal Free Hospital, An Outbreak of Encephalomyelitis in the Royal Free Hospital Group, London, in 1955, Br. Med. J., 1957;2:895-904.

7. Wallis A.L. **An investigation into an unusual disease seen in epidemic and sporadic form in a general practice in Cumberland in 1955 and subsequent years**, Doctoral Thesis submitted to University of Edinburgh (1957), page 18.

8. Pittsfield, Massachusetts Epidemic. Described by Hyde B.Canada Diseases Weekly Report, Proceedings of a Workshop on Chronic Fatigue Syndrome, Jan 1991, Vol. 17S1E, p. 7 also Hyde B. Bergmann S. Chronic Aspects of Akureyri Disease in **Post-Viral Fatigue Syndrome**, Jenkins and Mowbray, John Wiley, p.210, (1991).

9. Leon-Sotomayor Luis. **Epidemic Diencephalomyelitis**, Pageant Press, 1969, page 13.

10. Sean O'Sullivan M.D., Donna Rosenthall, September 1, 1984 Montreal Cluster, personal communication with Byron Hyde.

11. See this chapter.

12. Schluederberg A. Workshop on the Definition and Medical Outcome Assessment of CFS in Research, National Institute of Allergy and Infectious Diseases, Bethesda, March 18-19, 1991.

13. See Chapter 3, this text, Description of Patients.

14. Daniel Peterson, M.D., Girls' highschool basketball team, personal communication with Byron Hyde.

15. Paul Cheney, M.D., African prostitute, personal communication with Byron Hyde, M.D.

16. Wallis A.L. Idem (7) pages 25-26.

17. Ryll Erich, Chabursky B. 1975 Mercy San Juan Hospital epidemic, in preparation.

18. Wallis A.L. Idem (7) pages 25-26.

19. Wallis A.L. Idem (7) page 26.

20. Grufferman S. see abstracts, The Cambridge Symposium on Myalgic Encephalomyelitis (M.E.), The Nightingale Spring 1990;Vol.1,Issue 3:12 16.

21. Bergmann S. Iceland, personal communication in 1988 with B. Hyde.

22. Shelokov A., Havel K., Verder E., Welsh W. Epidemic Neuromyasthenia, An outbreak of poliomyelitis-like illness in student nurses. NEJM, 1957;257:345-55.

23. Parish J.G. Unpublished review of Lake Tahoe Disease.

24. Gsell O. Encephalomyelitis myalgic epidemic eine poliomyelitisahnliche krankheit, Schweiz Med Wochenschr (reviews 3 milirary epidemics)1958;88:488-91.

25. Graybill J., Silva J., O'Brien M., Reinarz J. Epidemic Neuromyasthenia, A Syndrome or a Disease (Lackland Air Force Base, Texas) JAMA 1972; 219:1440-3.

26. Hyde B. M.E. Epidemics in the U.S. Airforce, The Nightingale, The Nightingale Research Foundation 1991; Vol.1 Issue 5, Summer:15-7 .

27. Preface, this text.

28. Cheney P., Goldstein J., Hyde M. Separate papers read at Kalamazoo Michigan Symposium, Oct. 1991.

29. Wilson G.S. Poliomyelitis and prophylactic inoculation against diphtheria, whooping-cough and small pox, Report of the Medical Research Council Committee on inoculation procedures and neurological lesions. The Lancet, 1956;Dec 15;1223-1231.

30. Bastien S. Vancouver Workshop On Research Directions for M.E./CFS, May 1991.

31.   Rose J.R. An outbreak of encephalomyelitis in Sierra Leone, Lancet 1957;2:914-6.

32. Behan P., Behan W. Post-viral fatigue syndrome, a review. CRC Reviews. Cleveland, Ohio:CRC Press, 1988.

33.   Weinstein Louis. Chapter 188, **Principles of Internal Medicine**, Ed. Harrison T.R Fourth Edition, pg 1142.

34. Behan P. Diagnostic and Clinical Guidelines for Doctors, a Publication of the Myalgic Encephalomyelitis Association of Great Britain. 1991.

35. Marinacci Alberto. **Applied Electromyography**, chapter. The Value of the Electromyogram in the Diagnosis of Iceland Didease, page 92, Lea & Febiger, 1968.

36. Richardson J. Workshop on M.E./CFS in Newcastle, 1989.

Chapter 5

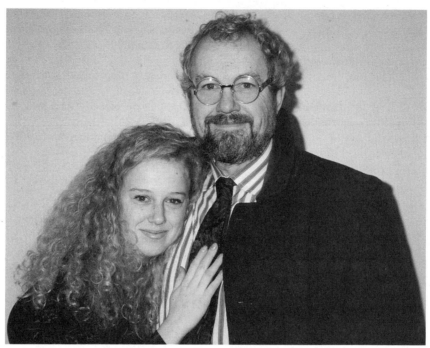

Byron M. Hyde with his daughter Dominique

Clinical Observations of Central Nervous System Dysfunction in Post-Infectious, Acute Onset M.E./CFS

Post-Viral Fatigue Syndrome

Byron Hyde M.D., Anil Jain M.D.

Dr. Hyde attended the Haileybury School of Mines and worked as a geophysicist. He then did premedicine in the Faculty of Medicine and University College, University of Toronto, obtaining a degree in chemistry and nutrition. He graduated in Medicine from the University of Ottawa where he was Director and Chief of the International Exchange Program for the Canadian Association of Medical Students and Interns (CAMSI). Dr. Hyde founded the International Summer School in Tropical Medicine. He interned at Hôtel Dieu in Montreal, was a resident at St. Justine Hospital in Montreal and to the Ottawa Civic Hospital. He also studied in Munich at the University Kinderklinik and in Paris at the Necker Hospital for Children. He was a research chemist at the Roscoe B. Jackson Laboratory at Bar Harbour, Maine, a leading world laboratory in immunological research. Following this, he was Chief Technician in charge of the Electron Microscope Laboratory in Toronto at the Hospital for Sick Children. This was followed by a similar post at the University of British Columbia. Dr. Hyde has authored a book on Electron Microscopy and two non-medical books. Dr. Hyde has been a physician for 20 years and has performed charitable work as a physician in Laos and the Caribbean. He held the position of Chairman of the Ottawa Community Health Services Association, and is presently Chairman of The Nightingale Research Foundation (Canada) and Chairman of the 1990 Cambridge Easter Symposium and the Workshop on Canadian Research Directions for Myalgic Encephalomyelitis / Chronic Fatigue Syndrome in May 1991, at the University of British Columbia. He has worked exclusively with M.E. / CFS patients since 1985.

(Please see Chapter 4 for Dr. Jain's photograph and curriculum vitae.)

Post-Infectious Acute Onset M.E./CFS

Post-Viral Fatigue Syndrome

Post-Infectious, Acute Onset M.E./CFS *is commonly referred to as Post-Viral Fatigue Syndrome. It is our opinion that the primary cause of disability in this disease process is an acquired central nervous system (CNS)* *dysfunction. We believe that M.E./CFS represents an acutely acquired, chronic change in the ability of the central nervous system to process, with any dependability, the functions of reception, interpretation, storage and recovery of information and to programme dependable, normal, smooth end-organ response. Depending upon the patient, we believe a physiological encephalopathy exists in one, but usually several of the cortical areas responsible for motor, sensory, cognitive and emotional function. Those deeper levels of CNS function that are responsible for the coordination of motor, sensory, cognitive, emotional, hormonal and at time rational value judgement may also be physiologically injured. In particular, we believe that there is evidence of subcortical injury to the hypothalamic-pituitary-end organ axis and also to the limbic system, that area responsible for coordination for so many CNS functions. This is not simply theory, but it is based upon an enormous body of clinical information that we discuss in this chapter. Scientific evidence presented in this text is increasingly strengthening this belief. The following clinical observations were made from a review of the literature covering over 6,000 of our patients.*

Few patients have all of the symptoms and complaints described here, but many will have a large number of these problems. We have seen a few patients with almost all of the symptoms described in this chapter.

M.E./CFS, like most diseases, has a considerable variability of expression. However, where some chronic diseases such as paralytic poliomyelitis are known essentially by a variable peripheral neurological dysfunction, M.E./CFS is primarily a disease of variable CNS dysfunction, e.g. motor, cognitive, sensory and emotional dysfunction. Although Jamal[1] has demonstrated that motor dysfunction is discernible in M.E./CFS, it is primarily the patient's subjective complaints of physical dysfunction that have been most evident.

Most cases of M.E./CFS are studied only when they reach the Chronic Stages. This is understandable, but it is a little like studying chicken pox-varicella one year after the spots have disappeared. As in most viral illnesses, the most florid picture occurs early in the disease. In that manner, the disease process of M.E./CFS most similarly imitates a poliomyelitis infection rather than that of a known retrovirus. It is possible that this disease process exists, due to a preceding viral injury of the immune system and what we are describing is the effect of a superimposed acute viral injury that the faulty or damaged immune system has failed to overcome.

CNS Dysfunction in M.E./CFS

Central nervous system dysfunction can be divided into:
    Brain dysfunction
    Spinal cord and root ganglia dysfunction

Anterior Horn Cell Injury

The little that we do know about spinal cord dys-

function in the M.E./CFS patient is from the publications of Alberto Marinacci in the 1950's-1960's[2]. Marinacci demonstrated that anterior horn cell injuries did occur in M.E./CFS patients,[3] but, unlike in anterior poliomyelitis, these cells were injured, not destroyed. Leon-Sotomayor also states, that "Electromyograms done in 20 patients (early in the disease process) showed findings consistent with a patchy denervation-type of polyneuritis most likely caused by a diffuse anterior horn cell injury".[4] The nature of this injury has never, to my knowledge, been investigated further. During the 1950's when Dr. Marinacci examined those recently fallen ill with M.E./CFS, he noted that the spinal cord damage in M.E./CFS was different from that of paralytic poliomyelitis in which there was an **irreversible** injury to the anterior horn cells. Marinacci found that in M.E./CFS there was usually **reversible** damage to these cells. His work suggests that these "recovered" anterior horn cells in some M.E./CFS patients were unstable and could in the future break down as physiological motor units. This is exactly the same concept used to explain post-polio syndrome.

Marinacci notes that on electromyography, during the first two weeks of the acute stage of M.E./CFS, only polyphasic normal amplitude motor units are found. After three weeks one starts to detect scattered fibrillation and positive sharp waves. This is further evidence for the concept of prodromal injury, minor recovery, onset of major illness that we sometimes see in M.E./CFS.

Sporadic Cases

In the **chronic stages** of this 1950's group, high

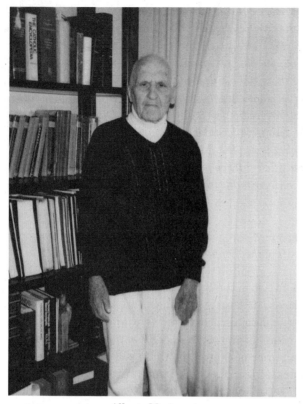

Alberto Marinacci

Hospital, when first examined by electromyogram 14 -18 years later, still demonstrated isolated polyphasic motor units and a few fibrillation potentials denoting mild persistent injury to the lower motor neurons or radiculopathy. This suggests that epidemic cases may be more severe than sporadic cases.

Clinically, we see this motor dysfunction in chronic M.E./CFS patients who are perfectly functional until they shovel snow or do some other exercise that exceeds their normal level of activity. This activity then causes a persistent tremor, fasciculation or twitch in a specific nerve distribution, e.g. ulnar nerve distribution. Duration of this involuntary muscle movement depends upon the individuals limitations and rarely lasts more than a week or two after the provoking incident.

In our experience, sporadic onset M.E./CFS tends to be correlated with and results in more insidious onset patients with less dramatic symptoms and less disability than the acute onset forms of M.E./CFS that we see more frequently in epidemics or epidemic years. This would also conform with Marinacci's differences in sporadic and epidemic cases.

Experimental Support

Transmission of M.E./CFS to monkeys has been successfully demonstrated, producing CNS and PNS injury in at least two separate sets of experiments. The first was in 1934[5] where "cross-sections of the spinal cord demonstrated numerous minute haemorrhages in the grey matter". The second was in the 1949-51 Adelaide, Australia epidemic where a radiculitis of the sciatic nerve was demonstrated with small punctate lesions of the myelin sheath.[6]

Human Pathology

In Canada, during the 1984 North American pandemic, a physician who fell ill with M.E./CFS ordered his own sural nerve biopsy. Observations of his sural nerve biopsy[7] showed inappropriately thin myelin sheaths, loss of large myelinated fibres, mild inflammatory changes and evidence of previous axonal degeneration. Although such lesions would explain some of the acute features such as peripheral muscle spasms, insufficient human biopsy material has been examined to confirm the impression that there is a

polyphasic and some giant motor units developed in a segmental distribution. In mild cases, that accounted for approximately 20% of the patients, these findings rapidly disappeared and there tended to be no reappearance of the M.E./CFS illness. In moderate cases, or approximately 80%, recovery occurred over a period of 18 months. In about 5% of the patients, both the complaints and abnormal electromyographic findings persisted for over 3 years. This more seriously injured group tended to have recurrences of their disability.

Clinically, in accordance with Marinacci's work, we observe a large number of local neuralgias and muscle spasms early in the disease with a tendency to improvement over several months, suggesting possibly spinal cord and peripheral nervous system involvement early in the disease process.

Epidemic Cases

Dr. Marinacci was able to study approximately 20% of the original 1934 epidemic group. It is interesting that the 20% of the patients who fell ill during the 1934 epidemic at the Los Angeles County General conductive defect in specific peripheral nerves of many M.E./CFS patients. Since this clinical finding tends to clear in most patients once the disease has reached a chronic phase, it would not be profitable to look for these lesions except in the Acute Stage. Neither the experimental nor the human pathology case cited are sufficient to generalize the findings, but they do indicate the value of further research in these areas.

Acquired Brain Dysfunction in M.E./CFS

The process can be categorized under:

> Central Endocrine Dysfunction
>> Fluid Balance Dysfunction
>> TSH Dysfunction
>> Temperature Regulation Dysfunction
>> Sexual Dysfunction
> Natural Killer Cell Dysfunction
> Cognitive dysfunction
>> Volition dysfunction
> Sensory dysfunction
>> tactile dysfunction
>> pain dysfunction
>> auditory dysfunction
>> visual dysfunction
>> proprioceptive dysfunction
> Seizure activity
> Hypnagogic dysfunction
> Sleep disorders
> Dream disorders
> Amnesia
> Motor dysfunction
> Emotional dysfunction

Central Endocrine Dysfunction

Dr. John Richardson[8] has noted that M.E./CFS is, in large part, an injury of the endocrine system functions originating in the hypothalamic and pituitary areas of the lower brain. Most of the hormones of the hypothalamus or pituitary gland cannot be measured directly in a normal laboratory and many others can only be measured by indirect methods that rely on target organ response.

The area of the hypothalamic nuclei acts as the master control of much of the endocrine system and, through its actions, the anterior pituitary gland is triggered by the corticotropin releasing hormone

(CRH), to stimulate the thyroid, adrenal and sex organs. The anterior pituitary produces:

Thyroid stimulating hormone (TSH)   , thyroid
Adrenocorticotropin hormone (ACTH) , adrenals
Gonadotrophin hormones   , sex glands

Although most M.E./CFS physicians are increasingly aware of this endocrine problem in M.E./CFS, it is unfortunately one area that research physicians have avoided until the recent published work of Dr. Demitrack and associates.[9]

Fluid Balance Dysfunction

We routinely observe that there is a metabolic fluid imbalance in M.E./CFS. This is also documented by Gilliam[10]. Leon-Sotomayor[11] also notes this oedema and suggests it is due to loss of vasomotor reflexes and venous pooling in the hands with the development of carpal tunnel syndrome that is more pronounced in the night. Although it can be a chronic feature, clinically, we have noted, particularly in the first few months of illness, that patients tend to have puffy hands and wrists as well as puffy lower extremities and joints. Many women, but also men, have at times marked diurnal weight changes. We know clinically that there is an irregular diurnal and nocturnal output of urine. Dr. Peter Behan has discussed his observations of an unusual fluid output related to a hypothalamic injury.[12] It is interesting to note that water excretion can also be influenced by thyroid hormone dysfunction, which increases urine solute by augmenting both catabolism and the oral intake of foodstuffs.[13]

Thyroid Stimulating Hormone (TSH) Dysfunction

One of the most common endocrinological findings we observe in M.E./CFS is thyroid dysfunction and the first thyroid hormone to show an abnormal pattern is TSH. This was first mentioned by Fudenberg[14] and also by Hyde[15] in 1990. All varieties of thyroid disease dysfunction other than malignancy have been observed routinely in M.E./CFS patients at the Nightingale clinic. In our experience, as many as 20% or more of all women who develop M.E./CFS will within five years develop some form of thyroid disease. They should be watched and when indicated, treated for this condition.

Temperature Regulation Dysfunction

Patients routinely complain of dysfunctional temperature regulation in M.E./CFS. We have noted that a marked fluctuation of body temperature with a lower than normal average temperature is pathognomonic of M.E./CFS patients. This is also described by Gilliam[16] who notes that there is "an instability of temperature, with a frequent daily range from 97-99 F. That was much more characteristic of this illness than a real elevation of temperature". We routinely observe patients with severely cold extremities, cyanosis and a visible line demarcating the cold from the area of normal skin temperature. This finding was also illustrated by Dr. Leon-Sotomayor[17] with photographs of patients with cyanotic discoloration of the knee and foot as well as another showing blotchy appearance of the hands with cyanotic changes over the knuckles and nail beds. The fact that this loss of normal blood flow may be persistent has been indicated by Gilliam[18] noting the unequal and slow growth of nails on the hand most affected. M.E./CFS patients frequently develop problems in adapting to both cold and hot weather. They appear unable to regulate their internal thermostats adequately.

Sexual Dysfunction

Much of the sexual dysfunction seen in the early and even chronic stages of M.E./CFS is probably related to the malaise, the pain syndromes and the chronic exhaustion experienced with the onset of the disease process. However, this does not explain the lack of orgasm in women and men that in some cases becomes chronic, the lack of ability to maintain erection early in the disease and the prolactin abnormalities we sometimes see in women. There is hardly any mention of the sexual dysfunction in the literature, except for mention by Dunnet of loss of libido for many months[19] and Ramsay[20] who describing a woman two years after she fell ill during the London Free epidemic, states "excessive frigidity had made sexual intercourse impossible". We routinely record total cessation of menses, irregular menses, many gynaecological pain syndromes, and infrequently, what appears to be an early, reversible softening of testes.

Natural Killer Cell Dysfunction

There appears to be a loss of natural killer cell

activity that is particularly striking in the first year of illness in our M.E./CFS patients. Renoux and Renoux have suggested that a left cortex injury can inhibit T cell and specifically natural killer cell activity and that brain lateralization for cognitive processes should be extended to immune recognition. It is of interest that physiological brain imaging suggests that the left cortex is one of the primary areas of injury in M.E./CFS patients.[21]

Blood Pressure Regulation

M.E./CFS patients routinely suffer from postural hypotension and, in general, their blood pressure measurements tend to be lower than one would expect in the normal public. We believe that this unusually large number of patients with relatively low blood pressures is related to hypothalamic or other changes. Conversely, we have seen a small but significant number of M.E./CFS patients who will develop malignant hypertension with the onset of disease. Some of these will have an almost carcinoid feature with flushing and typical diencephalon seizure state. Others seem to be unable to adjust blood pressure with body activity, resulting in high blood pressure on modest activity and very low pressure when reclining. We believe that, in each of these cases, there may have been an alteration to the hypothalamic nuclei responsible for maintaining normal arterial pressure. Leon-Sotomayor also noted the de nouveau occurrence of hypertension in 10% of his series of 50 patients, "It is conceivable that lesions in the diencephalon could give rise to permanent hypertension, as was observed in five patients reported in the present series".[22]

Acquired Cognitive Dysfunction

Central nervous system dysfunction, and in particular, inconsistent CNS dysfunction is, undoubtedly, both the chief cause of disability in M.E./CFS and the most critical in the definition of the entire disease process. Of the CNS dysfunctions, cognitive dysfunction is one of the most disabling characteristics of M.E./CFS. When this simple fact is understood, it becomes immediately apparent why this is such a devastating disease for children, students and adults, both within and outside the educational system. Today, few adult work situations exist where consistent use of education and developed cognitive skills are not necessary to maintain a place in the work force.

Patients can return to work with pain, with muscle spasm, with fatigue, with motor dysfunction, but when the patient consistently has difficulty in making new memories, recalling old memories and coordinating new and old information he becomes of little use in the modern work force. It is the combination of the chronicity, the dysfunctions, and the instability, the lack of dependability of these dysfunctions, that creates "the most chronic of chronic disabilities[23]." It is these combined acquired, chronic brain and physical dysfunctions that define M.E./CFS.

Some of these acquired cognitive dysfunctions of M.E./CFS are listed in the following table:

Acquired Cognitive Dysfunctions in M.E./CFS

Loss of Verbal and Performance Intelligence Quotient
Dysfunction in Simultaneous Processing
    Easy distraction
    Decreased concentration
Receptive and expressive dysphasia
Reading Comprehension Dysfunction
    Sequencing Dysfunction
Visual Comprehension and Discrimination
Discalculia
Abstract Reasoning Dysfunction
Memory Dysfunction
    Dysfunction in making new memories
    Dysfunction in recalling formed memories
    Immediate and delayed verbal recall
    Visual Recall Dysfunction
    Spacial Perception Dysfunction
Volition Dysfunction

Discussion of Acquired Cognitive Dysfunctions

All of the following acquired dysfunctions can be readily demonstrated by a knowledgeable neuropsychologist. In the case of an insurance or disability claim, the help of a knowledgeable neuropsychologist may be essential. Testing is also useful for treatment research. However, at the time of writing, many physicians will not have access to such expertise, and the patient may not have funds or adequate insurance to cover this type of investigation. If the physician is familiar with some of the defects, he can make a rough assessment from a careful history.

Loss of Verbal and Performance Intelligence Quotient

"Many of these patients behave stupidly"
Marinacci[24]

Patients will freely discuss cognitive dysfunctions but many will be unhappy and unaccepting if they are told that they have lost a significant amount of their verbal and performance I.Q. Admission of I.Q. loss represents a threat to their work and social abilities and to their own sense of identity. Dr. Bastien has observed that the average patient with M.E./CFS may lose approximately 20% of his estimated pre-illness IQ.[25] Some will lose more than this. Past the age of puberty, loss of verbal I.Q. will not be as significant as the loss of performance I.Q. The enquiring observer tends to judge a person's I.Q. not simply by verbal but also by dress and learned cultural responses that tend to blind us from adequately assessing I.Q. It is almost impossible to assess I.Q. loss unless we know the I.Q. of the patient before the illness. After the fact, we must rely on group, academic or professional I.Q. expectations.

We can also roughly assess I.Q. loss if we realize that I.Q. is the sum of all of the more visible individual cognitive losses.

Dysfunction in Simultaneous Processing
    Easy distraction
    Decreased concentration

Early in the disease process, patients may be distracted and unable to concentrate simply due to the severe headaches that frequently are associated with the onset[26]. Others have "noise" in their head that is often described as buzzing and thus mistaken for Ménière's disease or as the sound of the crackle and hissing of a short-wave receiver slightly off of the frequency channel. The symptom storms, the myalgias and the anxieties also make it difficult to concentrate. However, there comes a period in the disease process when these symptom storms settle down and the patient becomes acquainted with his new internal environment and, when that occurs, the primary lack of concentration ability becomes obvious.

Most brain functions do not operate separately but have back-up systems. Thus patients with M.E./CFS may be able to understand a single person speaking directly to them. However, the same patient may not be able to understand the same conversation from the same person on the telephone. If even slightly tired they may become irritable even with telephone conversations from friends. They have difficulty in concentrating and following the conversation even more than with a face to face conversation. Visual or multisensorial cues are important in M.E./CFS.

An M.E./CFS patient may have no difficulty at a dinner party with two or three persons and one table conversation, but with multiple persons and conversations, may not be able to understand a word that is said. In addition she may not even be able to recall the guests and, in extreme cases, may not even recall the dinner party the next day.

The same person may have no difficulty and no anxiety walking in the country, but will experience panic in crowds and even more so in a busy shopping centre where she is deluged with multiple discordant sensory information.

All individuals tend to concentrate better when the input of information is specific and simple, but a normal individual has the ability to block out extraneous and unwanted information or noise. M.E./CFS patients lose the ability to distinguish noise from required information and tend to shut down all intake after simple fatigue or minimal prolongation of the information signal. This receptive shutdown has alarming connotations for making memories and at times can create danger to the M.E./CFS patient.

Receptive and expressive dysphasia

Closely allied to concentration is the difficulty in understanding speech and in speaking. The patients will complain that they were able to hear the spoken words clearly, the words were not garbled, but they made absolutely no sense. These patients had lost the ability to interpret normal language. When the M.E./CFS patient speaks, important elements are frequently left out of the sentence such as the verb or subject. Sometimes the syntax is askew. At times, the patient's reply makes absolutely no sense or does not respond to the question asked. Patients are usually aware of the structural faults in their own conversation and at times become overly conscious of this, but rarely do they tend to be aware of their

totally inappropriate and nonsensical responses that at times can be quite hilarious. This is a most common complaint and tends to improve as the disease progresses unless the patient is fatigued, anxious or experiences sensory storms.[27]

These patients will show faulty testing in immediate and delayed verbal recall dysfunction tests.

Reading Comprehension Dysfunction Sequencing Dysfunction

This dysfunction is closely allied spacially with that of receptive dysphasia, that area is localized in the area of the annular gyrus of the posterior left parietal lobe. The patient can still read, but what she reads is not comprehended nor can it be compared with known information that had previously been stored. This dysfunction is one of the primary cognitive problems encountered by an M.E./CFS patient[28] and plays havoc with any job description or learning ability. Unless she redevelops these skills in a structured retraining programme, even an M.E./CFS patient with a PhD in English can become and remain functionally illiterate. These skills do improve during the recuperation stage but sometimes much is lost.

In **sequencing dysfunction** patients will variously lose the ability to look up phone numbers in a telephone directory or to look for words in a dictionary. They develop problems in retrieving and placing files. Patients not only become confused with restaurant menus, but also find it impossible at times to make any decision. Students tend to have significant troubles with lists of true and false questions.

Visual Comprehension and Discrimination Dysfunction

Patients will complain routinely of going through a red light. They see it is red, but the significance either does not register or is slow to register.

Facial Agnosia

It is not unusual for an M.E./CFS patient to develop facial agnosia. e.g. Teachers fail to recognize and associate children's faces with their name. A patient had a dinner party for a business associate and despite sitting beside his associate's wife all night, failed to recognize the guest the next day when they met by accident. The guest remarked on the wonderful dinner and the patient neither remembered the person nor could figure out what dinner was being discussed.

Such patients can suffer from bouts of "jamais vu". These patients may have difficulty in any manner of visual recall.

Discalculia

Perhaps the one overriding cognitive dysfunction observed in almost all M.E./CFS patients, irrespective of their prior mathematical abilities, is the development of discalculia.[29]

Patients either have difficulty or cannot make small change, add up columns, do serial sevens subtraction. M.E./CFS patients frequently cannot remember even their own phone numbers or combinations although they tend to have less difficulty with touch positions on a touch telephone or touch combination locks.

A few exceptional children are able to overcome this problem with mathematics and discalculia. However, in devising an educational programme for most children with M.E./CFS it may be worthwhile to abandon mathematics and related subjects if any hope of salvaging the child's education is to be considered.

Confusion with timetables is routine, with the patients routinely showing up at the wrong time or on the wrong day.

Abstract Reasoning Dysfunction
Memory Dysfunction
    Dysfunction in making new memories
    Dysfunction in recalling formed memories
    Immediate and delayed verbal recall dysfunction
    Visual Recall Dysfunction

These are well discussed within the text of this book.

Volition Dysfunction

This lack of volition is characteristic of M.E./CFS patients yet we cannot find it mentioned in any of the numerous publications. Volition dysfunction can be initially confused with depression but it is quite different. Patients may relate that they can walk, but they manifest that they are conscious of a dissociation of the mind and the body and that they have to "tell their legs" to walk. This dissociation is not a psychotic manifestation but is akin to the Olympic runner who has to tell her legs, to push, to build up speed, to pass that person a metre ahead in the race. This dissociation of mind and body function is similar to that encountered in the sleep paralysis observed in the hypnapagogic period. This volition form of mind body dissociation is much more common than is sleep paralysis.

If you are walking with an M.E./CFS patient and you stop to observe something in a store window, the M.E./CFS patient will frequently keep on walking. When you ask why they did not stop and wait, they will sometimes tell you that it is just too hard to get their legs moving again. In reality, it may be too hard simply to get their mind to give the command. Stopping, like starting can be a problem for M.E./CFS patients. This stopping and starting problem is a central dysfunction and along with the rigid mask like faces that develop with fatigue, may be similar to that seen in Parkinsonianism. There are other findings similar to those of a physiological Parkinson's disease. Dr. Ichise of the Mount Sinai Hospital in Toronto has observed that SPECT scans routinely show basal ganglia hypoperfusion in M.E./CFS.[30]

In the commencement of movement, all individuals have an initial inertia during which time the muscle mass builds up efficiency. Athletes build up to maximum output rapidly, but even in non-athletes the warm up period is relatively short. In M.E./CFS patients, this muscle warm up period seems significantly longer, but it is the "mental warm up period" that is affected in this volition dysfunction. The brain functions of an M.E./CFS patient are often like that of a locomotive, that does not readily make changes in volicity and can only change tracks with deliberation.

Proprioceptive Dysfunction

The patient in the acute stages often has periods of loss of positional sense of the extremities. In the dark, the patient may walk like a person with tabes dorsalis. The patient develops faulty judgement in the position of curbs and which frequently causes twisted ankles.

Gilliam notes that in case 105, "there was a loss of position sense of the hands and feet".[31]

Amnesia

To our knowledge, long standing amnesia does not occur in M.E./CFS. However, shorter periods do. The patients are regularly lost for seconds, less frequently for minutes and this may provoke panic attacks, particularly if the amnesic attack is associated with disorientation, where the patient, momentarily, neither knows where she is nor who she is. Although it is quite common to lose orientation of place totally, it is extremely rare to lose orientation of person. We have had patients who have lost large parts of the day but this is infrequent. Amnesic patients can, in most cases, be easily cued back to reality. It is extremely rare to observe hallucinations, but these short hallucinogenic bursts tend to be self-limiting occurring at the beginning of the illness and should not necessarily be taken as an indication of a psychotic breakdown.

Patients will regularly tell you that they are amnesic and that they cannot remember major elements of the previous day unless they are cued. This is not really amnesia but rather a difficulty to recall past events. Whole periods of recent history appear to have never been imprinted and even with cues the patient cannot recall major incidences. Often they confabulate to obscure the obvious memory loss.

Absence spells probably account for some of the momentary amnesic losses and failure to make new memories for others.

Sensory Dysfunction

This section is closely associated with the subsection of Cognitive Dysfunction. We have separated it simply due to the occurrence of "**sensory storms**". Sensory storms were first described by Luis Leon-Sotomayor as Diencephalon Seizures, a term no longer in vogue.[32] Sensory storms were an important and astute observation and seem to have been missed by subsequent writers.

The necessity of multiple sensory clues

Sensory dysfunction tends to have cumulative effects. For instance, a normal person performs remembered tasks without the necessity of multiple sensory clues. An M.E./CFS patient may require multiple sensory clues to perform a given task, e.g. the M.E./CFS patient is the principal driver of an automobile that he has had for 6 years. He knows the position of all of the major controls or functions of the automobile. He then falls ill with M.E./CFS and at night can no longer find the switch for the headlights or the door handle unless the interior lights are on. He has not forgotten where the switch is, since as soon as the light is on, his hand instinctively finds the switch, but he needs an external sensory stimulus to recall specifics of gross memory reserves.

Tactile Dysfunction or Apraxia

It is the rule for patients to frequently drop things since they cannot gauge the weight of the object, due to loss of normal tactile recognition. Ramsay states that "Many...tend to drop or fail to grasp articles...and the destruction rate of household crockery has in consequence risen alarmingly".[33] They lose the ability to recognize or locate by touch and require visual confirmation to recognize familiar objects, e.g. cannot locate home light switches in the dark. They tend to have poor position discrimination of their extremities and head.

Pain Dysfunction

In the Royal Free Hospital epidemic, "Spontaneous pain was the commonest sensory manifestation."[34]

The quality of pain reception may be significantly impaired. At disease onset, patients have been known to protest due to the unbearable pain provoked by the weight of the bed sheets. The multiple "hit and run" pain storms that frequently torment M.E./CFS patients are undoubtedly in part seizure phenomena but can more clearly be appreciated as dysfunctional pain receptors in either the peripheral or central pain recognition areas. To our knowledge, other than the work of Leon-Sotomayor[35], there has been no publication devoted to the origins of the jungle of pain syndromes associated with M.E./CFS. The pain symptoms associated with M.E./CFS will be reviewed separately since it is difficult to ascribe all of these pain phenomena to brain dysfunction or even to be exact as to the pain receptor origins in each case.

Auditory Dysfunction

Many different forms of central auditory dysfunction are recognized by patients with M.E./CFS. These include:

(1) inability to comprehend in the presence of multiple auditory signals,

(2) loss of tone perception in which music previously appreciated becomes "flat and boring"

(3) discomfort, pain and "noise" associated with hearing a modest decibel sound signal. Part of the associated pain may be in the outer ear and may be due to spasm of the tympanic muscles, as one of the major characteristics of this disease is muscle spasm.

(4) and finally, a sudden loss of appreciated sound volume.

But perhaps the greatest hearing problem is associated with the difficulty and at times inability to interpret spoken or auditory information. This dysfunction is one of the most central problems of M.E./CFS and represents physiological injury to the area of the angular gyrus in the region of the left posterior parietal lobe. This same area is responsible for visual interpretation, another major problem for M.E./CFS patients.

Interference greatly accentuates this auditory dysfunction, e.g. if two or three people are speaking or if there is a radio turned on, the patient frequently has difficulty in interpreting information.

Auditory comprehension is usually keyed by the initial transmitted information. The initial information asks the question or outlines the area to be comprehended. Frequently the M.E./CFS patient does not register the initial burst of focusing information and thus cannot make sense of the follow-up information. The M.E./CFS patient is frequently heard to ask, "Can you repeat what you were just saying!"

Making sense of new auditory information requires the patient to store short-term information and "to make memories". This simple process often represents a difficulty for the M.E./CFS patient.

Sensory Storms

Sensory storms are a common feature of post-infectious M.E./CFS. It is essential for the physician to understand the terror that they can provoke in a patient, particularly if that patient has little judgement or support. These storms are likely to occur more frequently during the acute stage where they tend to have no particular triggering factor. The fact is that they often have a life of their own and can create a certain amount of terror or panic when they arise unannounced. Not only are the patients struck with an explosion of sensory phenomena, but they almost invariably develop an accompanying malaise. At worst, the patient feels as if she were going to die. It is possible that such storms may precipitate a suicide attempt. It is important to forewarn the patient that these storms may occur, but are generally short lived and tend to decrease significantly in the chronic stages of disease. In chronic stages, storms can be triggered by and occur after physical, intellectual or infectious stress.

Leon-Sotomayor describes these storms as very variable in which one, several or all of the following may predominate.

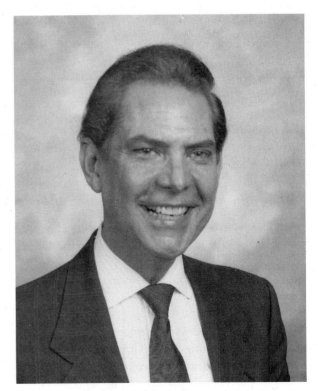

Luis Leon-Sotomayor

Elements of Sensory Storms

(a) emotional disturbance, increased nervousness, aggravation of tremors and blepharospasm

(b) abrupt or insidious onset with subnormal temperature or low-grade fever

(c) pleurodynia

(d) diaphragmatic tendinitis

(e) abdominal pain

(f) spotty myalgia and tendinitis, usually over the calves and pectoralis muscle group

(g) fibrillatory muscle twitching and muscle jerks; jerking of the muscles is usually more severe during sleep, usually awakening the patient

(h) increased bowel movement

(i) episodic weakness, shortness of breath and fainting episodes. Orthostatic hypotension, tachypnea and tachycardia are constant findings in the acute stage of the illness

(j) episodic sympathetic overactivity followed by neuromyasthenia symptoms

(k) abrupt waxing and waning of the symptoms is the most characteristic feature of the illness

(l) episodic nervousness, changes in personality, tendency to depression, tremors, nocturnal paresthesias, insomnia, nightmares and carpopedal tunnel syndrome are also characteristic of this condition

(m) periorbital tenderness, palpebral swelling, burning and dryness of the eyes

(n) abrupt vasomotor changes manifested by conjunctival injection, facial flushing or pallor, acrocyanosis and increased sensitivity to environmental temperatures. Patients can be feeling hot and perspiring one minute and cold and shivering the next. Profuse perspiration can be induced by emotional factors or by minimal physical exertion

The clinical picture was also characterized by a high incidence of relapses during the first six months of the illness. The relapse usually presents the same clinical manifestation as the acute attack usually with less severity. Clinical manifestation during the relapses may present as colitis, rheumatoid-like picture, carcinoid syndrome-like picture. Neuromyasthenia, mental depression, irritability, generalized myositis and tendinitis, and fluid retention with facial puffiness were commonly present during relapses.[32]

Visual Dysfunction:

(Also see Addendum V, Dr. Sadun)

Perhaps one of the most interesting and the most complex of the dysfunctions involves the patients' external and central ophthamological processes. A small number of patients will have no visual complaints but, for the majority who do, there is a considerable collection of visual phenomena. Although most clinicians remark on these findings, there is almost nothing in the literature concerning the opthamological changes.

Pain: The patient complains of pain, usually behind but sometimes above the eye. The posterior fundus at times will demonstrate a large cherry red discoloration.[36] It is most unusual to demonstrate any optic nerve involvement.

Photophobia: Patients often appear with dark sunglasses. When examined, the patient will frequently demonstrate a contradictory cogwheel dilatation of the pupil rather than the normal pupillar contraction when challenged with a light source. The contrary pupillar reflex tends to be one sided. There may be a ptosis over that eye. A few of these patients demonstrate an Adies pupil with loss of patella reflex. This Adies pupil comes and goes.

Latency of Accommodation: The patient will frequently complain of a sluggish or decreased range of accommodation, often described as a slow zoom lens. Patients with previous normal accommodation will, with onset of M.E./CFS, relate that, when changing gaze from near to far objects, their accommodation adjustment is unusually slow to react.

Nystagmus: There is an apparent increased incidence in nystagmus when the patient is asked to look into the upper outer quadrants. Pellew[37] describes the variability of this nystagmus, "A patient examined in the morning might have nystagmus, which would disappear at midday, recur later, disappear later and recur the next day." This waxing and waning, this inconsistency in the same patient in the same day is typical of almost all findings of M.E./CFS.

Double Vision: Patients will complain of double or blurred vision, particularly when tired. This, at times, has been associated with obvious lack of parallelism.

External Ophthalmoplegia: Described in the London Free epidemic as "common, usually affecting one or both sixth nerves and occasionally the third nerve".[38] We frequently observe failure of the two eyes to track together.

Internal Ophthalmoplegia: We regularly observe abnormal contraction and enlargement of the pupil and assume injury of the iris or ciliary muscle (third nerve) dysfunction. It is usually one-sided.

Tearing and Dry Eyes: Patients will complain contrarily of inappropriate and excessive tearing and at the same time of lack of sufficient tear formation or excessively dry, irritated and even painful eyes. The excessive tearing is usually short-lived and is replaced by a dryness of the eyes. In effect, all of the mucous membranes tend to dry, including buccal and vaginal, developing a situation that can be mistaken for Sjögren's syndrome.

Tunnel Vision: At times, an M.S. patient with central optic nerve injury will direct her gaze to the peripheral areas. We see the reverse in M.E./CFS patients. Early in the disease process, we infrequently have patients mention that they are looking at the world "through a tunnel". Because it sounds so bizarre, most patients will not describe this for fear that the physician will believe that they are psychiatric patients. This complaint may be associated in some cases with peripheral scotomas, but the presence of scotoma is not sufficient to explain all of the cases. Many patients without describing tunnel vision will mention loss of peripheral vision. Loss of normal peripheral vision represents a frequent problem for a car driver with M.E./CFS.

Night Vision Loss: Patients frequently complain of night vision loss. They stumble in their own homes and at times have a manner of walking that resembles that of tabes dorsalis patients of another era. As in tabes dorsalis, the normal proprioception cannot come into play without a visual reference.

Colour Vision: We have had patients complain of colour appreciation changes, of a loss of colour intensity. On examination, we have at times noted one-sided and bilateral loss of colour vision. We have had one patient with no history of colour blindness but who developed red green blindness and when verified one year later was normal. We rarely examine patients for colour blindness unless they have a particular complaint. At present, we have no way of telling if this visual variation predated the illness, is a common feature of M.E./CFS or is simply a normal variant.

Palpebral Oedema: This is usually one sided and usually on the left side.[13]

Central Visual Dysfunction

Visual Comprehension Dysfunction: The primary central visual dysfunction is equivalent to the auditory dysfunction mentioned above. The patient fails to integrate and store visual information in a meaningful way. As mentioned, the single area of major cortical damage in M.E./CFS appears to be in the posterior left parietal lobe[20], the area that integrates and interprets visual and auditory sensory information. This dysfunction provokes the following problems:

Reading: Some patients are so damaged that they permanently lose much of their ability to comprehend easily what they read. For most patients, this disability occurs significantly during the initial stage from 0-6 months and then improves to reach a new plateau, subjectively below their previous level. This can be a catastrophe for students or those who depend upon reading for their livelihood.

Writing: To write, one must not only have the ability to recall, but also to read and comprehend what one has written. M.E./CFS patients can make ridiculous spelling and grammar errors and fail to notice these omissions. e.g. leaving out the verb structures in a sentence, difficulties in spelling or comprehending simple words like "and". There appears to be a cross over effect in which patients have improved writing skills with their non-dominant hand compared to healthy controls. Many of these patients develop a deformed handwriting consistent with that of brain damaged patients. Like many of the symptoms of M.E./CFS, this too waxes and wanes. Early in the disease, there is frequently a rapid deterioration in the handwriting ability over the time it takes to write one or two pages.

Distance and Spacial Dysfunction: Human brains interpret distance not only by parallax but by the complex ability to recall, associate and compare appropriate visual and visual memory cues. Perhaps no sensory linked function is so important in the busy urban world. Our depth and speed perception is essential as a guarantee of our safety. These functions, working in tandem, interpret motion, speed and vector. They protect us as much in crossing a road as they protect the integrity of a teacup when we place it upon a shelf. The following problems are frequently mentioned by patients:

(a) **Jay walking:** Inability to jay walk or cross streets without a light, due to loss of ability to judge speed, distance, deceleration and vector. This problem has not only been the cause of patients walking into moving automobiles, fortunately with only their dignity ruffled and a few bruises, but also of the death of one young girl who walked or fell into the path of a train and perished. All of these visual perception problems are aggravated by mind altering medications.

(b) **Traffic motion:** This inability to judge the speed and position of cars coming from the side occurs equally with drivers or passengers. This does not seem to bother drivers as much since they tend to lose their lateral vision and don't even see cars from side roads or passing cars. However, it is difficult for drivers of an M.E./CFS passenger who is vociferously demonstrating his inability to judge the deceleration or acceleration of an approaching automobile.

(c) **Repeating:** Sometime, particularly when descending an escalater or a walled staircase, the last step seems to repeat itself and the patient stumbles. This repetitive visualization of identical steps seems somehow to confuse the individual's perception. It may be related to height sensing mentioned next.

Depth of Field Dysfunction:

(a) **Height Sensing:** Inability to judge the position of the road or floor when either stepping off a curb or descending a stair. Patients have particular problems at the bottom of a moving escalator. Many twisted ankles occur due to this disability. It is common for patients to fall while descending stairs as they not only have problems with distance judgement but also suffer from an associated vertigo.

(b) **Irregular Walking Surface:** Many patients have positional difficulty particularly when walking on fields or unpaved surfaces, since they tend to fatigue particularly easily due to the necessity of concentrating all of their judgement abilities. This problem is exaggerated by lack of adequate light and/or fatigue.

(c) **Wall crashing:** Patients routinely walk into the door jamb or wall rather than walking through the open door.

(d) **Mending:** Inability to judge position of button holes, threading needles and finger position.

(e) **Dishes:** Patients regularly crash dishes into the shelf, misjudging the shelf position and at times breaking the dish.

Reversals:

If this occurs, it happens in the first days of the illness and is most infrequent. We are aware of four patients who complained of such short term reversals of vision. In one case, a respirologist complained of left-right reversal. He had fallen ill with Acute Onset M.E./CFS, and, early in the disease, attempted to continue working. While driving home, his view of the road became reversed. Fortunately he ended up in a snow bank. On SPECT and QEEG he had a lesion in the left visual cortex. He has remained severely ill and bed-ridden for the past 4 years. The others all had vertical reversals lasting less than one hour. One case of Dr. John Richardson was hospitalized for one week with a vertical reversal.

Clouding: This frequently described phenomenon resembles an opaque or milky film or veil sensation bilaterally covering the field of vision. It is as though the individual had a turtle-like opaque film that covered the eye momentarily. This phenomenon lasts seconds and can recur through the various stages of disease.

Visual-Auditory Dysfunction

Television: When most people are ill, they can at least read a book or watch television. In the first few months of disease, M.E./CFS patients have difficulty even watching a T.V. sitcom and following the story line. This combined visual and auditory dysfunction is particularly obvious at this simple level.

Seizure Activity:

Two of Britain's leading M.E./CFS experts take opposing positions regarding seizure activity. We have heard Professor Peter Behan categorically state[39] that there is no seizure activity in M.E/CFS while Dr. John Richardson, who has continually followed M.E./CFS for longer than any living clinician, states that all M.E./CFS patients by definition have seizure activity. We are totally in agreement with John Richardson. It would be worthwhile for a clinician to briefly review a pictorial view of seizure activity such as that of CIBA's Frank Netter, perhaps the world's best known illustrator of the central nervous system, which clearly indicates these seizure forms.[40]

Our conception of CNS seizure activity has been highly modified since the mid-1930's by technology. Up to that time seizures were known by their clinical description or by activity stimulated by implanting electrodes or stimulating certain areas of animal and human brains. In the early 1920's, a German scientist, Hans Berger (1873-1941) discovered that human brains produced an electrical activity that could be recorded and measured by an electroencephalogram, or ECG. At that time, clinicians and scientists in their wisdom rejected the possibility that the brain could have such electrical wave activity[41] and it was not until the late 1930's that this opinion began to change when two British scientists discovered the same principal. By the early 1940's the revolution was so complete that, if a seizure activity could not be documented by EEG, it was considered to be a form of conversion hysteria. It is easy for a physician to forget that the EEG picks up electrical activity only from the outer 1 mm skin of the upper cortex of the brain and that any central or lower brain activity is not readily accessible to EEG identification.

We routinely refer M.E./CFS patients with obvious seizure activity to neurologists, often in very august institutions, and when the EEG is normal, the neurologist frequently acts in a dismissive manner to the patient and to us, suggesting that this patient suffers from coversion hysteria. Sometimes however, we can record these dismissed cases with seizure activity,

utilizing a QEEG scanner i.e. a computer driven EEG.

The appearance of the QEEG (CEEG, BEAM) scan is beginning to modify our concept of seizure activity again. Based upon this new evolving technology, the classification of brain seizures is perhaps about to undergo another revolution. Yet QEEG technology still will not be good enough to measure deep seizure activity. Many of the following clinical seizure observations are still beyond the limit of available technology.

During the Initial Stage from 0-6 months, various seizure manifestations occur. EEG changes were documented in 40 of the 48 cases tested from the Royal Free epidemic and Children's Hospital cases by Pampiglione.[42] Although Pampiglione states that these EEG changes tended to persist for years, we have not been able to duplicate those findings with conventional EEG. From personal experience at our clinic, unless one employs a QEEG, the major EEG changes tend to fall off and are difficult to verify after the patient has been ill for 6 months. Using a QEEG, i.e. a computer driven EEG, these abnormalities can be noted for years or perhaps as long as the illness persists.

It is our observation that all seizure activity is greater in the Initial Stage (0-6 months) of M.E./CFS and decreases considerably in the recuperation stage (2-12 months). In the chronic stages, occasional bursts of increased activity may persist.

We have observed the following seizure activity:

Grand Mal Seizure: This occurs rarely and is usually noticed in epidemic situations. e.g.: In a single Gloucester Ontario primary school, reputedly as many as 7 teachers fell ill with typical M.E./CFS during the fall of 1984. In this cluster, one developed typical grand mal seizure. This seizure activity ceased after one year.

Absence (Petit Mal) Seizures: Probably all M.E./CFS patients experience this form of seizure activity. These seizures usually consist of simple episodes usually lasting less than 10 seconds. We have seen these absence spells extended to longer periods in which **ambulatory automatism** occurs, e.g. A bus driver having left his designated route by several city blocks was awakened by his demonstrative passengers. During this time, the bus driver had unconsciously navigated several busy streets and intersections. We have also noted this behaviour in two cases that extended almost to amnesic lengths, for "several missing hours" in which the patient was not observably "asleep".

Frequently the patient is not aware of the existence of these absence spells and a relative or associate must be questioned concerning the history.

SIMPLE PARTIAL SEIZURES:

These should always be recorded because they may suggest the area of dysfunction. The following seizure activities are routinely recorded. The patient may decline to admit to these if the physician terms them seizures.

Somatosensory Seizures: The patient complains of tingling or pins and needles in the extremities and face. These can be almost continuous during the first few weeks of illness, can frequently be pressure activated and are sometimes associated with focal motor seizures or single muscle spasm e.g.: left side of the face in one of the branches of the trigeminal nerve. These can be primarily one-sided or bilateral. The most common pattern is that the patient reports diffuse bilateral changes with a marked increase in the left side activity.

Autonomic Seizures: Described in detail by Leon-

Sotomayor[35] above, it is the rare M.E./CFS patient that does not experience profuse episodic sweating, flushing or facial pallor. The patient usually complains of the malodorous nature of the sweats. The odour may simply represent a heightened sensitivity with limbic system derangement. The seizure can go beyond this simple description, but when it does, it is seen almost exclusively during the first weeks of the illness. Brain[43] mentions this as a term employed by Penfield, as Diencephalic Autonomic Epilepsy which appears to be due to neural discharge from centres of the hypothalamus. There is flushing of the face, a rise in blood pressure, sweating, dilatation and contraction of the pupils, tachycardia, and retardation of the respiratory rate.

Focal Motor Seizures: as noted above. These are frequently noted in the hypnagogic period but can occur at any time during the initial stage. This can involve involuntary movement of both single muscle and/or muscle groups.

Neck muscles may go into spasm, twisting the head to one side.

Auditory Seizures: These are common and frequently are associated with Ménièrés Syndrome. The patient has ringing or hissing in the head and may also have associated pain. There is no evidence of external or middle ear disease and although hearing comprehension may be markedly decreased, simple auditory tests are not usually affected.

Visual Seizures: These are rare outside of the initial and recuperation stages, i.e. 0-24 months. They should not be confused by the peripheral scotomas or photophobia that occur commonly. They are usually described as lightning-like flashes. Very transient microsecond sectional blindness also occurs.

COMPLEX PARTIAL SEIZURES:

These tend to be episodic, very short-term and frequently dramatic responses.

Olifactory Hallucinations: The patient frequently complains of intense and unusual smells that are not apparent to others. This doubtlessly represents a limbic system derangement.

Episodic Dysphasia/Dyspagia: The patient has episodic difficulty in maintaining volume of speech. The patient may have spasmodic difficulties of the larynx and upper oesophagus with or without activation by swallowing. This can also be easily triggered by certain foods. These findings tend to occur frequently in some patients, can be quite frightening and have caused laryngeal blocking with certain foods and fatigue.

Déjà Vu/Jamais Vu Episodes: Jamais vu episodes are the more frequent with patients getting lost in their own building or lost driving on a road they normally know well.

Uncategorized Seizures:

Tremulous Attacks. The patient has subjective attacks of tremulousness. They last up to one minute. Sometimes these are so pronounced that the patient feels he is in an earthquake. These can happen day or night but appear more pronounced when the patient is lying down. They tend not to be externally visible and are common even in chronic cases.

Psychomotor Attacks: The patient does not lose consciousness but may be amnesic, confused and anxious. This is of short duration, usually persisting for approximately 15 seconds.

Episodic Affective Disorders: Abrupt changes in emotional response frequently triggered by fatigue or multiple sensory input barrages and may consist of inappropriate fear, anxiety, pleasure or happiness.

Sleep Dysfunction

(also see Addendum Harvey Moldofsky)

HYPNAGOGIC & HYPNAPAGOGIC DYSFUNCTION

Sleep dysfunction is the rule in M.E./CFS but we separate this group as it is so dramatic and different from the usually described sleep dysfunction. This normal dreamlike, delusional period through which the mind passes while falling asleep or awaking is characteristic of several abnormal patterns in M.E./CFS. This narcoleptic state is common in M.E./CFS.

Hypnagogic Period

Hypnagogic Myoclonus: Frequent in normal children but rare in adults, these are brusque, sometimes almost violent movements of arms or legs. Sometimes the sleeping partner is kicked or struck while the spouse with M.E./CFS is totally unaware of the incident. They are common in adult M.E./CFS patients.

Hypnapagogic Period

(1) Sleep paralysis: This cataplexy-like state occurs when the patient awakens and is conscious, but there is a total loss of body tone and an inability to move an arm or leg. This results in a frightening paralysis, as though one had been injected with curare that spared the respiratory muscles. This paralysis lasts from several seconds to one or two minutes.

This form of dysfunction occurs when there is a failure of the normal uniform activation or spread of consciousness and function over the nervous system. The levels concerned with consciousness awaken before the levels concerned with motor function.

(2) Waking Dreams: This could be considered to be the reverse of cataplexy where there is a dissociation of consciousness when the subject is partially awake. At times in childhood, the child may rise from sleep with every evidence of being awake but terrified and still living a dreadful nightmare. At times it takes the comforting parent several minutes to convince the child that this very real experience was simply a dream. Such a state is rarely seen in normal adulthood but exists commonly in M.E./CFS adults and children.

Thematic Dreams: Usually these dream-like states persist for only a few minutes. However, we have one Chilean patient who awoke, living a dream in which he was a mediator between the Pope and General

Pinochet who was still then the Dictator of Chile. This dream state persisted through breakfast and lunch during which time the patient was like an automaton living his dream.

Pain Dreams: Another form of hypnapagogic dream is the pain dream. These hypnapagogic dream states are not common, but they are interesting and we have not seen them described in the literature. They occur in the myalgic form of M.E./CFS. The dream is curious in that it is formless and storyless and consists only of terrible pain localized in one part of the body. One actually dreams of pain. Like any dream, it seems to go on for what appears to be an eternity until the patient awakes fully, only to find that the severe pain persists. This pain can endure for most of the day but is usually over within one or two hours.

SLEEP DISORDERS

Post-encephalitic sleep disorders occur frequently but in M.E./CFS they are the rule and few if any M.E./CFS patients with a full blown disease escape sleep dysfunction. These sleep disorders with the associated symptoms at times appear uncannily to be taken from a text on encephalitica lethargica.

Hypersomnia:

The process starts within days of the illness. It commonly resembles an extension of the short duration hypersomnia associated with an acute viral infection such as influenza. However, in many cases the period of hypersomnia extends so that it resembles that sometimes seen in infectious mononucleosis or, in some cases, encephalitica lethargica. This form of encephalitica lethargica sleep pattern is seen in both adults and children. It appears more dramatic and may even be more common in children. It is difficult to be sure. However, one's heart naturally goes out to children and the anxious parent who is very aware of this situation. The adult who sleeps 18 hours a day at home frequently goes unnoticed unless the patient is in a particular research project. The child who sleeps 18 hours a day becomes the focus of concern.

The state of the patient in the hypersomnic state resembles that found in normal sleep. The breathing is normal and does not resemble a comatose state. The patient can always be aroused to some extent, may reply rationally, will take food, but cannot be depended upon to stay awake or finish eating any food offered. As soon as the patient is left alone she tends to fall back to sleep.

The patient tends to lose significant weight rapidly during the initial hypersomnic period.

Russel Brain states that hypersomnia is most frequently caused by a dysfunction of the posterior hypothalamus and upper part of the mid brain[43].

Causes of Insomnia:

There is almost no consistent evaluation of sleep dysfunction in the published medical literature although these themes are a frequent topic of conversation among M.E./CFS clinicians. The following represent our observations. Marked insomnia alternating with episodes of acute narcolepsy is rarely observed in the Initial Stage of the disease process but is the rule in the Recuperation and Chronic Stages of M.E./CFS. Insomnia is a primary central dysregulation. However, we have noted that when a patient is asked why he doesn't sleep, some of the answers and observations are as follows:

(a) **Night Temperature Variation**: During normal sleep, the body temperature may fall as much as 2 degrees.[44] In M.E./CFS the patient's temperature is frequently 2 degrees subnormal while awake and one can only wonder if the drop in sleeping temperature is not additive. These patients experience wide variability of temperature, frequently with pronounced sweats while asleep. This unusual nocturnal rhythm disturbs the normal sleep process.

(b) **Night Extremity Hypothermia**: Perhaps related to the bradycardia, the extremities, fingers, toes and nose become so cold they start to hurt and this pain awakes the patient. This hypothermia of the extremities also occurs frequently during the day with the onset of environmental cold spells. These patients respond poorly to chilling.

(c) **Urine Output**: Healthy patients decrease urine formation at night, M.E./CFS patients, particularly in the first months, appear to increase urine output. Nocturia is frequently reported in patients who never previously had to awaken in the night to relieve themselves. The bladder area becomes overly sensitive in the majority of M.E./CFS patients and this pain or spasm also helps to awaken the patient.

(d) Malodorous Sweats: The patient will often complain of the malodorous night sweats associated with this disease. These sweats are more frequent in the Initial Stage. The smell may be real or it may be related to a hypersensitive limbic system.

(e) Nightmares: These vivid colourful and frightening dreams tend to occur primarily during the Initial Stage. The terrifying nature of these dreams frequently awakens the patient. They are discussed in greater detail in this chapter.

(f) Diurnal Rhythm Inversion: The patient tends to sleep during the day and is unable to sleep during the night.

(g) Seizures, Myoclonus and Fasciculations: The abrupt muscular or limb movements wake the patient or the sleeping companion.

(h) Sleep Palsies and Paresthesias: These sometimes result in uncomfortable cutaneous sensations that awaken the patient.

(i) Fear of Dying: This is just one of many terrifying neuroses that develop due to the initial frightening symptom picture of M.E./CFS. The patients may not have been diagnosed and feel they have some terminal illness. They frequently feel so ill that they assume that this is how one feels just prior to death. This is more than simple malaise and it continues even into the chronic stages of the disease.

(j) Unresolved Conflict or Anger with the Physician: Unresolved conflict is an important component of sleep neurosis. Many patients feel they are abandoned by their physician.

(k) Pain on Movement: Some patients are in severe or persistent pain that is worse during the Initial Stage of the illness. Normal sleep movement triggers these pains and the patient awakens.

(l) Sensory Seizures or Storms: Referred to by Leon-Sotomayor as diencephalon fits or seizures,

these occur day or night but when they occur at night they tend to awaken the patient.

(m) Spasm: M.E./CFS's common name in France is Spasmophilie and for good reason since patients frequently have painful spasms associated with their illness. At night, these spasms tend to awaken the patient. While in bed they tend to occur in the foot, the big toe.

(n) Light Flashes: These light flashes mentioned as a phenomenon that usually occur during the day, also occur when the patient is asleep. They awaken the patient in the same way that a streak of lightning does.

(o) Causalgia: These intense, short-lived, herpes-like pains, can occur anywhere in the body. Usually they occur during the day, particularly involving the left anterior chest and simulating an acute myocardial incident. When they occur during sleep, they always awaken the patient. This kind of pain is particularly frequent after an active day such as getting out of bed for a physician or hospital visit.

(p) Night Headaches: These may be related to cervical spine spasm or can occur as an intense pancephalic exploding headache that occurs during the late night. Frequently these pains awaken the patient at 4 or 5 a.m. Once the patient is out of bed for a few minutes the pain rapidly diminishes and the patient can then fall back to sleep. We have speculated that this may be related to the marked night bradycardia that is known to occur. Holter monitor should be requested.

(q) Hyperacusis: M.E./CFS patients tend to have marked hypersensitivity to sound and so the patient awakens due to sounds that would otherwise not have disturbed sleep.

(r) Remembered Sleep Apnia: We have only recorded this in three patients but the patient is frightened and, unlike in cases of classical sleep apnia, the patient remembers the occurrence. This may occur as a hypnapagogic incident, but it tends to occur during the night and not during the normal hypnapagogic period.

(s) Night Bradycardia and Night Hypotension. Discussed in the following text.

(t) Medication Reactions: Patients frequently have adverse reaction to certain medications. Sometimes it is sufficient to awaken the patients or keep them continuously awake. The reaction seldom lasts longer than 24 hours but can be quite frightening to the patient. We have seen this with H2 blocker medications but any medication can provoke this reaction.

(u) Cardiac Irregularities: Ectopic or irregular rhythm or heart pain awakens the patient. This tends to occur early in the illness.

(v) Ataxia: Patients have awoken due to the sensation that they were in an earthquake. The bed seems to be moving and the patient suffers from marked ataxia. This also occurs less commonly during the day and occurs in short brusque bursts such as an earthquake tremor. At the start of the illness, rarely, these attacks can last for several hours but the episodes rapidly decrease in length as the disease progresses. In recalling this phenomena among the physicians at the Royal Free epidemic, Jane Eden describes these attacks as *"what really shook us was the way our beds seemed to lurch and pitch like a coracle crossing a stormy sea. Morning usually brought a calm somewhat tempered by the thought that one must have been imagining it after all."*[45]

(w) Explosive Stool Loss: Patient awakens having soiled himself and the bedclothes. This occurs only in the Initial Stage.

This alphabet of common causes of M.E./CFS insomnia have all been recorded in numerous of our patients.

Sleep Bradycardia: Similar to sleep apnea in its format except that, instead of a significant decrease of the respiratory rate, in this case it is the significant slowing of the heart below the normal nocturnal decrease. The patient usually awakens during the night due to a significant headache. Once the patient is up for a few minutes, the headache decreases and the patient may return to sleep. These periods are also associated with a marked fall in blood pressure. Holter monitor should be ordered in all M.E./CFS patients.

Narcolepsy: Narcolepsy results from an impaired CNS control of wakefulness and the sleep/wake cycle. To our knowledge, no one has yet published on narcolepsy and the intrusion of REM sleep into the waking state in M.E./CFS but that is simply a question of time and research. Although excellent M.E./CFS sleep dysfunction studies have been published by Moldofsky, he has only looked at patients in later stages of the disease and neither he nor others have to our knowledge published on any of these fascinating epiphenomena or changes occurring in the early disease stages.

Narcolepsy is very common in M.E./CFS. The patient is sleepy much of the day, especially in those periods when normal people also tend to be sleepy, such as after meals. We have noted sleep attacks during the middle of meals, while walking up stairs in an attempt to get to a bed before sleep takes over, where the patient literally lies down and falls asleep at the table or on the stairs. These attacks are usually preceded by an overwhelming desire to sleep.

M.E./CFS patients are unusually subject to narcolepsy, to sleep attacks, sleep paralysis and hypnagogic and hypnapagogic hallucinations.

We have not noted Cataplexy in an M.E./CFS patient.

Dream Disorders

It is perhaps incorrect to speak of dream disorders, but there is certainly a change in content, colour and violence of the dreamscapes of M.E./CFS patients. It is also rare for a non-psychiatric physician to take the time to enquire about dreams, but if the question is asked one is told of:

(a) the intense brightness and colour of dreams;
(b) the violence of these dreams;
(c) the frequent attack nature of dreams;
(d) the frequency of hypnagogic and hypnapagogic dream states;
(e) the pain dreams.

Leon-Sotomayor suggests that sensory seizures originating in the mid-brain may provoke the unusual dream patterns.[32] As early as 1911, Wickman,[46] describing acute poliomyelitis dreams in similar terms and, in 1934, Gilliam,[10] describing the dream states

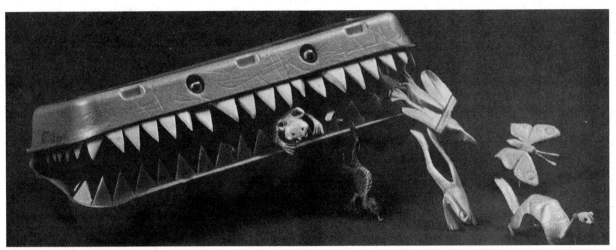

Courtesy of Rudi Haas, The Egg Carton Zoo

during that first M.E./CFS epidemic, mentions the vivid and increased dream activity. Behan and Behan[47] mention that, in their view, sleep disorders are "not accompanied by hypna(pa)gogic hallucinations or sleep paralysis" However, Wallis[48] has noted them in his dissertation, "children continued their dreams on wakening". In our experience, M.E./CFS hypnapagogic dreams are all fairly common features in both children and adults and are worthy of the physician's interest.

The M.E./CFS dream is usually an attack dream in which some unseen assailant or inanimate object persists in attacking the patient. The colours are vivid and they are described as being the most brilliantly coloured, the most intense, the most persistently frightening of dreams. Some of the dreams are violent and work related, some explicitly sexual, but never pleasant in nature.

e.g. Rudi Hass,[49] the Austrian artist-photographer suffered from a severe case of M.E./CFS after falling ill in Africa. This particular case was associated with a triggering attack of what, at the time, was diagnosed as possibly Lhasa Fever or even Apollo fever. He awoke from a dream one morning and, utilising egg cartons, fashioned some of the monsters in his dreams. This is illustrated above.

e.g. An economist would not relate the content of her dreams but to quote her she stated: "My god, they were very ugly, very vivid, very detailed, very coloured, very personal, very oppressive, with dying, death and violence everywhere".

e.g. A male Irish physician had dreams consisting of "murder, bloodshed, mayhem and butchered Caribbean bodies all over the place".

e.g. A female social worker described "decapitated heads with blood streaming from their eyes, ears and nose". Curiously, her triggering onset was with epidemic conjunctivitis.

e.g. Children dreaming of Pac man-like monsters persistently attacking them.

e.g. A secretary in a research laboratory described "My sister had just returned from Africa, thrilled with the boa constrictor she had brought back. However, this large writhing beast, wrapped itself around my neck and arm and threatened to kill me. But I had no sister in reality and I had no knowledge either of anyone coming from Africa or of snakes".

e.g. A woman writer from Radio Canada related, "It was like Clock-Work Orange. There were toughs breaking into the house. I couldn't call the police because they were part of the group. It was rape and pillage in which I was involved. They broke up and smashed the house. There were people in the dream that were acquaintances. It was like Star Wars, with flashing lights. I awoke huddled in a ball, cringing. My husband was sleeping beside me but the dream continued for another ten minutes and I could not stop it although I was wide awake. The visual part of the dream then stopped, but the terror continued for over an hour."

Pain Syndromes Associated With M.E./CFS

Pain syndromes in M.E./CFS can vary from totally disabling, to occurring only after exercise, to non-existent.

When they occur, and that is in over 60% of M.E./CFS patients, the variety of pain syndromes can be legion. The very number of them can cause grave anxiety to the patient and help create skepticism on the part of the physicians who frequently believe that no one in their right mind can have this many symptoms. Physicians have been trained to associate pain with local or referred pathology. They almost never associate or ascribe pain as a central dysfunction. Once they have scrupulously investigated pain for its possible cardiac, surgical or malignant origins they tend to feel impugned if their search has revealed no local pathology and fall back and blame the patient for the pain syndrome by terming it hysteria, conversion hysteria, or somatization . Some of these pain symptoms may result from peripheral nerve and end organ derangement. More likely, the majority of these pain syndromes are manifestations of central pain receptor deregulation or injury. The sheer number of pain syndromes suggest that the amygdala in the limbic system, the right posterior central gyrus of the parietal lobe as well as the posterior tracts of the spinal cord could all be affected.

The very chronicity of these pain syndromes cautions physicians from creating a dependence upon narcotics.

Muscular Rheumatism, T. Sydenham, 1681 [50]

"The pains are sometimes in one part, sometimes in another; they seldom are attended with fevers. They are less fixed to one spot, are more erratic, and more uncertain. At times it afflicts this or that joint; at times the inward parts only. Here it produces suffering, which suffering goes off when the point again transfers itself outwardly, then it harasses the patient in turns, and prolongs itself to the duration of the most chronic amongst the chronic diseases."

The three most important M.E./CFS pain syndromes are the following:

(1) Malaise

"Malaise has probably occurred in every epidemic described in the literature"[51]. Malaise is accentuated in the Initial Stage and it recurs for as long as the disease process exists. Malaise is almost impossible to describe. It is often referred to as the pain and discomfort that one has during the acute phase of an influenza. However, it is not always the same. The patient feels terrible, feels as though he is about to die. There is no fever as in influenza nor dimming of consciousness that, mercifully, usually occurs in the malaise of a febrile influenza attack. The malaise tends to wander, to wax and wane. It particularly injures the sensory and dulls the cognitive abilities of the brain. The pain seems to originate everywhere, both on and within the chest and abdominal areas, head and extremities. The rapid muscle and brain fatigue that is normal in M.E./CFS becomes accentuated.

This malaise is often exaggerated or cumulative in association with specific events. It occurs as a rule after any physical exercise that goes beyond the normal everyday work output. Malaise may occur often in place of what would have been an infectious illness, e.g. all of the family comes down with an influenza or simple sore throat and cough. The M.E./CFS patient may come down with no external symptoms of an infectious illness although one would anticipate such an event since everyone else in the family is ill. The M.E./CFS patient simply develops this terrible malaise. e.g. We see this often when a child in the family falls ill with chicken pox. The healthy adult who is immune, due to an earlier varicella infection, is usually symptom free, - not so the M.E./CFS patient. The M.E./CFS patient develops a severe malaise and not only encounters all of the above problems but often becomes bedridden for no apparent reason unless the physician has seen this varicella effect before.

The patients term these probably infectious equivalents *"crashes"*. Many M.E./CFS patients will inform the physician that since they fell ill with M.E./CFS five years earlier they never once had a typical *"cold"* or external sign of an upper respiratory infection. They most likely will have had many *"crashes"*.

(2) Lower Cervical, Upper Dorsal Pain

It is the most frequently encountered chronic pain and it tends to continue well into the chronic stages. This is discussed in the text and tends not only to be a persistent form of pain but also possibly triggers the chest wall pains and the chronic occipital pain that so frequently occur in M.E./CFS patients.

(3) Bladder, Genitalia Pain and Discomfort in Women

This also is discussed in the text. However it is the singularly most misdiagnosed pain symptom that leads to sometimes drastic and unnecessary intervention. Since nothing is found on these interventions, the patient is usually blamed as being hysteric or seeking surgery, whereas it is really the physician's ignorance of this almost constant pain association in M.E./CFS. Since this pain at times is associated with **interstitial cystitis** where a vein in the wall of the bladder mucosa may rupture, this appearance of blood may be incorrectly interpreted as either infectious or more sinister pathology. Nota Bene.

The following is a review of the common pain syndromes encountered in M.E./CFS patients.

These pain syndromes frequently come in *"storms"* in association with other dysfunctions already noted.

Cephalgias and Other Head Area Pain: It may seem unusual to catalogue pains, but they are a principal part of many patients' disability. These too occur in storms and when that occurs they can lead to a diagnosis of panic attack. These cephalgias tend to be more dramatic during the early part of the illness and the intensity of the pain tends to decay with time. With the exception of the encephalitic pain, all of these pain syndromes are fairly common if the patient is affected with a myalgic form of the disease.

Encephalitic Pain: The earliest type of pain, if it occurs, is one of encephalitic intensity with severe prostration. This occurs in only a small percent of patients.

Most Common Head Pain: The most common and prominent pain complaints are of dull, persistent, moderate to severe bilateral pain in the occiput and in the area *"behind the eyes"*. The patients sometimes describe it as a feeling of having been clubbed.

Expanding Head Pain: Different from the encephalitic-like pain, it lacks the prostration and fever but is nevertheless a total head pain which the patient describes *"as though my head were expanding and blowing up"*.

Ear Pain: This pain is very short lived, lasting at times only for seconds, severe and worse during the Initial Stage. Referred to in England as tensor tympani pain, it consists of a precise needle like pain primarily in one ear. Less frequently, this phenomenon occurs in the nose. The same type of pain occurs very frequently in the bladder area and less frequently in the anus. It occurs as a spasm where there is a potential muscle sphincter.

Ophthalmic Pain: M.E./CFS patients frequently complain of photophobia with eye pain or discomfort. Cursory exam will reveal that these patients' pupils expand rather than contract when a penlight is shone into their eyes. The pupil movement tends to be irregular and cogwheel-like.

Also, frequently due to the decreased tearing usually present, the patient will have irritated his eyes due to excessive rubbing. These dry eyes should be treated with artificial tears.

Tooth Hypersensitivity Pain: This is common and the patient may develop both heat and cold sensitivity.

Spike-like Pain: This is described by Thomas Sydenham[51] in 1681 as Clavicus Hystericus and again by Gilliam in the 1934 epidemic[52]. Sydenham writes, *"Often times, it attacks the exterior of the head, creating intolerable superficial pain; so isolated, however, as for the thumb, laid across, to cover it. Here it keeps fixed. This is the Clavus Hystericus. So boring and so severe as to feel as if an iron nail were being driven in."* In the scalp, this site frequently gives rise to an eliptical bolus that can usually be rolled around under the finger. It may be a fibromyalgia equivalent. This severe pain occurs anywhere on the scalp and sometimes the extremities and is described by the patient as a nail being driven into the body. The pain is of moderate duration and maximum intensity, rarely lasting longer than one hour.

Fibromyalgia Pain: Associated with pain in the typical fibromyalgia sites of the body. The patient can frequently roll a painful, ellipsoid object under the finger, even under the scalp. These are probably not lymph glands. They frequently occur in *"sensory storms"*. They tend to move about the body in any one storm. Both the storm and the pain tends to be wasting.

Formification: Formification means the movement of ants. This is perhaps one of the most frightening of any of the pain syndromes. Fortunately it is not common. It occurs during the Initial Stage only, and patients have described it as the swarming of bees, buzzing and moving within the head and reaching down into the spinal cord. Patients tend to be terrified with this symptom. When it occurs it may last up to a few hours. It rarely repeats itself more than two or three times. It may be a cause of severe panic and possibly suicide.

Cervical Pain: There are few M.E./CFS patients, even when the non-myalgic patients are considered, who do not describe the nagging pain in the cervical spine area. The pain tends to be localized from C4 to T3 and can persist even into the chronic phases of the disease. It is perhaps neuralgia from this area that extends itself up into the occiput and down into the anterior and posterior chest wall.

Sore Throat: Many patients will describe recurrent sore throats with M.E./CFS. This is quite distinct from "bacterial pharyngitis" where an obvious infection can be cultured. The most common cause of this discomfort is the associated Sjögren's-like syndrome. The patient has the typical lupus-like rash, dry eyes with decrease in tearing, and a concomitant dryness in the buccal area caused by an apparent decrease in activity of the buccal glands. They have dry mouths and sore throats. It is usually an error to treat these cases with antibiotics.

"Spasmophilie" Spasm Associated Pain:

It is this symptom that gives rise to the common French name for M.E./CFS, i.e. Spasmophilie, meaning muscle spasm. Localized spasmodic or tetanic muscle spasm is common in this disease. The muscle sphincters are particularly prone to persistent pain of this type. This spasm, in addition to the areas

already noted, may also be associated with spasm in the oesophagus and duodenal sphincter that we frequently record. These stomach area spasms are so common that a good number of our patients arrive with cimetadine or other H2 antagonist treatment, not for their central effect, but for suspected ulcer disease.

Both single muscle and muscle groups may be involved. There is, early in the disease, the cramp like kick in the area of the left diaphragm that is described like a baby kicking in a pregnant woman. This frequently arises immediately after eating and often results in the physician ordering an upper GI series. Nothing is found on X-Ray. The spasm of irritable bowel syndrome is common and is discussed elsewhere.

We see this spasmodic pain in tendons and have recorded a very few tendon ruptures, usually in athletic individuals early in the disease. This spasmodic pain is frequent in the long strap muscles such as the sternocleidomastoid muscle in the anterior triangle of the neck, the sartorus, the calcaneal (Achilles) tendon and gastrocnemius muscle. When the spasm occurs in the neck, the head is usually turned painfully to that side. In the extremities this can be observed as bunching of tissue, pain and sometimes bruising.

A frequent spasm occurs in the foot and great toe. The great toe is dorsiflexed and frequently the whole foot is in spasm. This also occurs when the patient is in bed. It sometimes awakens the patient who has to get out of bed to massage or stand on the foot. The spasm lasts a few minutes only. In the London Free Epidemic, many somewhat humorous photographs appear in one of the publications demonstrating great toe spasm. Both this and carpal spasm are a common feature of M.E./CFS.

Chest and Abdominal Pain

Pain in this area can be easily broken down into:

Fibromyalgia Pain: This is described under Cephalgias. However the prominent area of pain is on or in the chest wall. The sensitive neck and axillary gland pain often described is probably related to fibromyalgia rather than lymph gland pain in most cases. The classical fibromyalgia points are noted although most of the forms are incomplete.

Sentinel Point: A sub-variety of fibromyalgia may be the quixotic fusiform swellings that come and go, usually in the left chest and axilla and less commonly in other locations. These swellings can cause intense local pain, occur in *"attacks"*, can be rolled under the finger, and then, after an hour or two, the swelling decreases and the acute pain with it. Although pain can be raised on palpation of this area at any time, moderate residual pain from the *"attack"* can follow in this area for several days. There is one specific site, usually locate superior and medial to the left nipple, that may occur in patients who have few other fibromyalgia-like points. Early in the disease, frequently the patient will be seen, holding his left chest, often hand under the shirt in a Napoleon fashion. This point is one of the few that has been known to persist for weeks, months and even years. When this point occurs in the designated location in a woman, frequently that woman is biopsied for possible breast malignancy. It occurs less frequently in other areas.

Causalgia and other Neuralgic Pain: This lancing pain is sharp, severe and brief. The patient usually describes it as like a cattle prod or electric shock. They are not uncommon in Myalgic Acute Onset forms of the disease. They are seen frequently in those patients who start their disease with Borneholme's disease, but can occur independently of this syndrome.

Borneholme's Disease

"For this be sure, tonight thou shalt have cramps,
Side stitches that shall pen thy breath up."
                    The Tempest, 1.ii., W. Shakespeare

In addition to those chest pains mentioned, some M.E./CFS patients start their disease as Bornholme's disease, also known as intercostal neuralgia. These patients tend to have a persistence of their chest pain syndrome and the accompanying neuralgia.

Perhaps the most succinct description of this disease as a prelude to M.E./CFS appeared in a letter to the editor by J.A. Cotterill in The Lancet, on June 9, 1973. It is well worth reading.

Some patients have an associated myocarditis. Many patients with M.E./CFS have an associated mitral cusp prolapse. This finding is not taken very seriously in North America but either patients with mitral cusp prolapse are particularly prone to falling ill with M.E./CFS or it comes as part of the disease process. Dr. John Richardson has a film of a patient with acute onset M.E./CFS who did not have prolapse prior to falling ill and on open heart surgery was shown to have freshly ruptured chordae tendinae attached to the mitral valves.

Many patients have left and, less frequently, right diaphragmatic pain with tenderness on palpation.

Abdominal pain: In addition to the diaphragmatic pain, about twenty percent of the patients will have an acute or gradual onset of irritable bowel syndrome with all of the discomfort that this implies.

Urogenital Pain: But by far the most common abdominal pain occurs in the lower abdomen and particularly the urogenital system as described at the onset of the pain section. This symptom is definitely worse in postpubertal females and is associated with any and every form of menstrual irregularity and cessation. Part of the pain in women is in relation to a typical *"perimenstrual"* distress syndrome with all the symptoms and changes that occur with that condition.

So consistent is this pain area that it is rare to find a woman with chronic M.E./CFS that has not had surgery or at least a cystoscopy and multiple genitourinary exams to evaluate the cause of the pain. Almost all of these women will have been placed on antibiotics for suspected urinary tract infections. The principal element is probably severe muscle spasm. A high degree of interstitial cystitis is seen in this group.

Although it occurs considerably less frequently in men, when it does occur it is usually misdiagnosed as prostatism despite the young age of the general population. The patients, both men and women will complain of pain, sometimes excruciating pain, urgency, difficulty in starting and stopping the stream, frequency, incomplete voiding and nocturia. There is also frequently sharp pain in a specific site of the penis. Many males will also describe erectile impotence. When this occurs it is usually only in the early stages of the disease. Women during the same period will describe failure of sensation and orgasm.

Adolescent children will also have urogenital symptoms and they are often associated, even in early teenage, with the onset of bed wetting. It is understandable that physicians will mistake this for urinary tract infection. Serial urinalysis will clarify the non-infective nature of this complaint. Blood should not be considered a necessary sign of infection but of a possible interstitial cystitis or vein rupture in the bladder wall. This symptom will last for weeks to years.

Pain in the Extremities

Hypothalamic Dysfunction Pain: Patients will not only complain of severe episodic sweats but also of severe blanching of their extremities, nose, ears, lower arms and hands as well as lower legs and feet. Observation will often reveal a blanched clearly demarcated line separating warm from icy cold tissue. The whitened extremities may persist for hours and can be extremely painful.

Rarely, this also occurs as isolated spots anywhere on the torso or upper extremities. It is quite curious and again a clearly demarcated line can be drawn around the cold spot. This rarely persists longer than an hour. Infrequently, these cold spots turn brown, or bruised the next day as though the patient had been hit by a Lacrosse ball in full flight.

A variation of this hypothalamic dysfunction occurs with a complete diencephalon seizure discussed earlier.

Periarthritic Pain: This type of pain is sufficiently common to have had several M.E./CFS patients diagnosed as having incipient rheumatoid arthritis. Since M.E./CFS is routinely associated with a lupus like submaxillary rash and elevated rheumatoid or ANA factors, it is an honest mistake. These patients tend to have low sedimentation rates and the swelling in the joint is never red, nor hot, nor is there ankylosis.

The patient routinely indicates the knee and elbow and makes the physician think in terms of an arthritic process, whereas, in most cases, they are dealing with a periarthritis. This is mentioned by

Sigurdsson[53] in which polyarthritis developed after this illness in a number of cases.

Bone Pain: This pain is described in the bones of the extremities. We don't know if it actually originates in the bone. The pain is so intense that frequently the physician sends the patient for an X-Ray and of course nothing is found. The pain tends to persist into the chronic stages of the disease but is worse in the initial stages. This pain is described as bone breaking as in *"break bone fever"* or as one encounters in an expanding bone lesion. As severe as it is, it does not persist, rarely lasting longer than two hours. It then rapidly disappears leaving no pain sequelae.

Muscle Pain: One of the old names of M.E./CFS was **muscular rheumatism**. There are three forms of common muscle pain.

(a) The patient complains of feeling as though he had been beaten with an axe handle. He feels bruised and hurt. This pain lingers for several hours and then departs, usually only after the patient has slept. It is sometimes associated with a dull generalized headache as well as an increased inability to concentrate.

(b) The second pain is very similar to spike-like pain that has been described in the head The patient will describe a severe pain, usually in the main muscle mass in the leg, extensors or flexors. It is described as a nail or as though a knife or arrow had been stuck into the leg although it can occur anywhere. This pain tends to last a few hours and then abate.

(c) The third is associated with particular muscle group use. e.g. When a patient does highway driving for considerable distances, he will frequently develop "foot drop" and associated pain. This usually resolves over a few days. It is also seen in the extensors of the leg and in the shoulder muscles after shopping. Frequently, the painful muscle can be palpated and is hard and swollen.

Emotional Dysfunction

Of the approximately 60 M.E./CFS epidemics noted in the literature there is not one which does not describe the acute onset of emotional dysfunction. In 1951, Pellew in Australia,[54] described two patients hospitalized at the same time in the same hospital.

One had paralytic poliomyelitis and the other M.E./CFS. After two months, the poliomyelitis patient was almost totally paralysed except that he had some movement in his right great toe. He was described as *"the most cheerful patient in the ward"*. Whereas the M.E./CFS patient over two months totally recovered his muscle power *"but was extremely irritable and almost melancholic."*

This abrupt change from a person with a normal emotional control to one of pathological emotional dysfunction is noted in every epidemic. Gilliam, in one of his classical lines, states that *"the emotional upsets - varied in degree from relatively slight displays of irritability and impatience to violent manifestations of dislike for people and things formerly liked...crying spells resulting from no known provocation."* [55] Sigurdsson notes *"complaints of nervous instability, irritability were conspicuously frequent for months after".* [56]

Some physicians have jumped upon this emotional dysfunction as an explanation of the entire disease in the same way that some physicians have looked at muscle dysfunction or loss of respiratory control or hyperventilation. M.E./CFS is a diffuse brain dysfunction. There seems to have been a separation of emotional function from that of all other brain functions as far back as 1900 B.C. (Kahun Medical Papyrus)[57] and 1550 B.C. (Eber's Papyrus).[58] From that period until the time of Augustine the emotions were considered to reside in a woman's uterus (the hysteria). We noted earlier that this mentality persisted until the 1950's when Marinacci observed that *"cases who had a hysterectomy in 1938, in the hope that the mental symptoms would be relieved, but the procedure was not beneficial".* [59]

Injury to the left frontal lobe and at times both lobes is increasingly documented in QEEG, SPECT and PET scans of the M.E./CFS brain. In 1991, we won a Supreme Court decision in Alberta[60] by demonstrating frontal lobe and limbic system damage in an M.E./CFS patient who had lost the ability to make rational decisions. Anatomical and physiological damage to the centres of the brain that affect emotional control should be considered, as injuries to other areas of the brain are considered. One does not have an injury to the motor functions of the brain due to the fact that the patient's mother did not love her or that she had been depressed. One has an injury to the motor functions of the brain due to an infection, or immune injury or other physical and pathological change. Injuries to the areas of the brain affecting emotion are of the same nature as those that affect physical function. It is time for all physicians to put away their emotional copy of the Ebers papyrus and to accept the infectious and immune theory of disease as a cause for much emotional dysfunction.

Summary

This overload of symptoms and complaints follows an infectious disease in a patient with no previous history of similar episodes. These changes not only cause severe and chronic anxiety even in the most phlegmatic of patients, but also tend to be too much for most treating physicians. It is because of all these unmanageable complaints that the patient becomes more persistent of the physicians time and the physician becomes more frustrated and more skeptical.

Passed off for years as hysteria, somatization and anxiety neurosis, this chronic disease state with all of these sensory changes can only be explained in terms of an acute injury to the brain resulting from an infectious or other CNS injury and in a chronic dysfunctional aftermath. We have completed this partial symptom list since, to our knowledge, no such bibliography of M.E./CFS CNS dysfunctions exist in the literature.

Patients with an insidious onset may have this symptom picture as well, but much more frequently they will more closely resemble a more blunted chronic stage of M.E. with disability but little of the extremes of sensory and cognitive derangement described here.

References

1. Jamal G. Hansen S. Journal of Neurology, Neurosurgery and Psychiatry 1985; 48:691-694

2. Marinacci Alberto, **Applied Electromyography**, chapter. The Value of the Electromyogram in the Diagnosis of Iceland Disease, Lea & Febiger, (1968)

3. Marinacci A.A. and Von Hagen K. Bulletin of the Los Angeles Neurological Society, Vol 30, No 4, part 1, December 1965, page 166-7

4. Leon-Sotomayor L., Epidemic Diencephalomyelitis, Pageant Press, 1969, page 85

5. Van Wart, R. Courville C, Hall E. (1934) Epidemic of Poliomyeltis in Los Angeles, American Journal of Public Health, Vol 24, Number 12, Dec 1934, 1207-1209

6. Pellew RAA. Clinical description of disease resembling poliomyelitis, seen in Adelaide, 1949-1951, (1951) Med.J.Australia, I, 944-946

7. During the 1984 pandemic a sural nerve biopsy was taken from a Nova Scotia physician suffering from M.E./CFS in December 13, 1984, reported by Dr King of the Victoria General Hospital, Halifax, Canada. The immuno-fluorescence was reported by Dr T. Ghose

8. Richardson J. The Cambridge Symposium on Myalgic Encephalomyelitis (M.E.) April 9-12, 1990

9. Demitrack M.A. et al. Journal of Clinical Endocrinology and Metabolism, December 1991

10. Gilliam, A.G., **Epidemiological Study of an Epidemic, Diagnosed as Poliomyelitis, Occurring Among the Personnel of The Los Angeles County General Hospital During The Summer of 1934,** Public Health Bulletin No. 240, April 1938, The United States Public Health Service, page 15

11. Leon-Sotomayor L., **Epidemic Diencephalomyelitis,** Pageant Press, 1969, page 10

12. Behan P. Hamilton Ontario Speech, Oct 1991

13. R. Douglas Collins, **Laboratory Diagnosis,** J.B. Lippincott, (1968) page 37

14. Fudenberg H.H. Chronic Fatigue Syndrome and Fibromyalgia Pathogenesis and Treatment, First International Conference, Los Angeles Biltmore, Los Angeles Biltmore, February 1990

15. Hyde B.M. Chronic Fatigue Syndrome and Fibromyalgia Pathogenesis and Treatment, First International Conference, Los Angeles Biltmore, Los Angeles Biltmore, February 1990

16. Gilliam, A.G. idem (10), page 23

17. Leon-Sotomayor L., idem (11), page 119

18. Gilliam idem (11), page 24

19. Dunnet BMJ, 1963,1,1187

20. Ramsay A.M. Encephalomyelitis in North West London, An endemic infection simulating poliomyelitis and hysteria, The Lancet, Dec 14, 1957, page 1197

21. Renoux G. Renoux M. (pg 17-19) **Immune modulation agents and their mechanism,** R.L. Fenichel and M.A. Chirigos, Marcel Dekker Publisher (1984)

22. Leon-Sotomayor L., idem (11), pages 88-89

23. Sydenham, T. The Works of Thomas Sydenham, Latin Edition of Dr Greenhill (translated by R.G. Latham), The Sydenham Society, 1848

24. Marinacci A. Von Hagen K. idem(3) pg 165

25. Bastien S. Loss of verbal and performance I.Q. paper given at Vancouver Workshop on Research Directions, UBC. May 1991,

26. Pellew R.A. A , idem (6) page 944

27. Leon-Sotomayor L. idem (11) page 15

28. Goldstein, J. Chronic Fatigue Syndrome and Fibromyalgia Pathogenesis and Treatment, First International Conference, Los Angeles Biltmore, February 1990

29. Bastien S. idem (25) Discalculia

30. Itchese, paper given at Vancouver Workshop on Research Directions, UBC. May 1991

31. Gilliam A.G. idem (10) page 15

32. Leon-Sotomayor L., **Epidemic Diencephalomyelitis,** Pageant Press, 1969, pages15-17

33. Ramsay A.M. idem (20) page 1199

34. Medical Staff of the Royal Free Hospital, An outbreak of encephalomyelitis in the Royal Free Hospital Group, London in 1955, British Medical Journal(1957) 2: 895-904

35. Leon-Sotomayor L.

36. Richardson J. Newcastle-upon-Tyne Symposium, 1989

37. Pellew R.A.A. A Clinical Description of a Disease resembling Poliomyelitis seen in Adelaide 1949-1951, The Medical Journal of Australia, June 30, 1951 pg 944-946

38. idem (23) page 896

39. Behan P. , Hamilton Ontario Speech, October 1991.

40. Netter F. **The CIBA Collection of Medical Illustrations, Vol 1, Nervous System, Part 11** 1986, pp 43-45

41. Berger Hans 1873-1941, (German inventor of EEG), see Isaac Asimov's Chronology of Science and Discovery, Harper & Row, page 504, (1989)

42. Pampiglione G., Harris R., Kennedy J., Electroencephalographic investigations in myalgic encephalomyelitis Postgraduate Medical Journal (November 1978) 54: 752-754

43. Brain W. Russell, Diseases of the Nervous System, Oxford University Press, second Edition,1942, page 819

44. Brain W. Russell, idem (43) page 831

45. Eden J. We called it the pestilence, World Medicine, June 15, 1977, page 25

46. Wickman I. **Acute Poliomyelitis** (1913) The Journal of nervous and Mental Disease Publishing Company, New York.

47. Behan P. Behan W. Post viral fatigue syndrome, a review. CRC Reviews. Cleveland, Ohio: CRC Press, 1988

48. Wallis A.L. **An investigation into an unusual disease seen in epidemic and sporadic form in a general practice in Cumberland in 1955 and subsequent years,** Doctoral Thesis submitted to University of Edinburgh (1957).

49. Haas R. Blohm H. Suzuki D. **Egg Carton Zoo,** Oxford University Press, (1986)

50. Sydenham, T., The Works of Thomas Sydenham (translated from the Latin edition of Dr Greenhill, London (1848)

51. Medical Staff of the Royal Free, idem (34), page 902

52. Gilliam A.G. idem (8)

53. Sigurdsson Bjorn et al. A disease epidemic in Iceland simulating poliomyelitis, American Journal of Hygiene, vol 52, pp. 222-2238, page 234

54. Pellew R.A.A. idem (37) page 945

55. Gilliam A.G. idem (8) page 24

56. Sigurdsson Bjorn idem (53), page 238

57. Kahun Papyrus, see introduction, The Papyrus Ebers: the greatest Egyptian medical document, Translated by B. Ebbell, Copenhagen: Levin & Munksgaard, 1937:108

58. Ebers Papyrus, idem (57)

59. Marinacci A. idem (3) page 163

60. Transcript of Alberta Supreme Court Judgement, August 1991, Appeal, November 1991

Chapter 6

M.E. / CFS: The Physical Signs of Disease

Byron Hyde, MD, Anil Jain, MD

(Please see Chapter 5 for Dr. Hyde's photograph and curriculum vitae. Please see Chapter 4 for Dr. Jain's photograph and curriculum vitae.)

M.E. / CFS patients may demonstrate a multitude of physical signs both of the prodromal illness and the chronic features of their disease process. Knowledge of these physical signs, along with a good history, often provides sufficient information to make a clinical diagnosis of a complete or classical M.E. / CFS. Increasingly, we are able to support our clinical diagnosis with laboratory tests, brain imaging and neuropsychological testing. When the patient is a poor historian, or if we are dealing with an incomplete form of the disease process, we are increasingly able to lean upon these testing procedures to assist us in making that diagnosis. The problem of supporting a diagnosis with testing procedures is no longer a doubt, it is however often an exercise in access, affordability and frustration for both the patient and physician.

This chapter is divided into the following sections:

*(1) **Prior Illness**: Frequently patients will note an unusual earlier illness that occurs from 3 months to two years prior to the prodromal illness.*

*(2) **Prodromal signs**: The prodromal signs result from an acute interaction of the virus and a host that may be immune compromised. This response usually occurs independently of the host's interaction with his external environment.*

*(3) **Chronic M.E./CFS signs**: These are the characteristic physical signs of M.E. / CFS disease.*

SIGNS OF PRIOR ILLNESS

We routinely note in our clinic the occurrence of a curious illness that can sometimes be documented usually as having occurred three months to two years prior to the prodromal illness. This may present as:

(1) a mononucleosis-like illness that causes a period of chronic illness that may last up to six months, or

(2) It may resemble an acute encephalitic process. When it occurs as an encephalitic process, the illness is usually very short lasting (2-4 days), very severe with at times an almost comatose patient, a rapid and apparent complete recovery and without other apparent lingering sequellae. The patient will usually state that this had been the worst headache he had had in his life.

(3) A third type is that of a minor episode that resembles the main chronic M.E./CFS disease. This minor episode tends to last several weeks or even months. During this time, the person rarely misses school or work but is quite unwell. The patient then usually recovers for a brief period only to fall ill with the full blown features of M.E./CFS.

1934 Los Angeles Epidemic

This prior illness was noted by Gilliam on several occasions. In one of these he recounts in the case history of a social worker. Case #102 fell ill on July 7 with a severe headache, *"never anything like it before"*. She recovered, returned to work, only to fall ill three months later on October 8 with a severe case of atypical poliomyelitis [M.E./CFS].[1]

"The patient recalled a transient illness, for which he did not at the time seek medical care, often several months earlier, which resembled the systemic or meningeal phase of poliomyelitis."[2]

Gilliam notes that in 25 cases, the systemic or meningeal symptoms occurred so far prior to the time the patient reported off duty that there might be considerable error in fixing the dates on which they occurred.[3]

1948 Akureyri Epidemic

In the text, Post-Viral Fatigue Syndrome, Hyde and Bergmann state *"When the ten 1948 Akureyri patients were interviewed in May 1988, it was found that three had first fallen ill in 1947. In each case, the disease was of a similar nature, with burning pain in one or more limbs, severe prostration and profound muscular weakness. The illness was short-lived, lasting about two weeks, followed by an apparent complete recovery. The fact that a similar type of disease occurred in three of the ten patients the year before falling seriously ill in 1948 was quite unanticipated."*[4]

1949-51 Adelaide Australia Epidemic

Pellew notes that *"Many patients said that they had been feeling vaguely off colour for perhaps three months with occasional bouts of headache, associated with lassitude and aches in limbs lasting for two days or so."*[5]

1955 Royal Free Epidemic

Crowley notes that among the late summer Royal Free illness patients *"Between March 1 to July there were four cases of infectious mononucleosis-like illness. One woman had a mild transitory [Royal Free] illness in July 1955 that totally resolved. She returned to work and five months later, in December, she fell ill and was hospitalized with a mononucleosis-like illness. Six days later her fiancé was hospitalized with an encephalitis".*[6]

Eden, a clinical student at Royal Free in 1955 states: *"Since early spring some clinical students at the Royal Free Hospital had been having highly unpleasant symptoms. They started of as a sore throat and rather stiff neck. By the way our necks felt, our cervical lymph nodes should have been enlarged. And so they were, but only to the size of small peas. The shivering, aching limbs, aching back, disturbed sleep suggested a high fever but the thermometer obstinately refused to budge above 99."* She describes the typical but mild M.E./CFS like symptoms in some detail. She continued to work for several months when she notes, *"The bomb didn't go off until July."* She then goes on to describe the start of the severe disabling epidemic.[7] (page 25)

Clearly, some earlier infectious agent had attacked these patients who all later fell ill with M.E./CFS. Perhaps one of the reasons there was such great difficulty in finding the infecting illness was that the prodromal illness that occurred months and even up to two years after their prior illness was not the complete cause of the patient's final M.E./CFS illness. Was this infection the cause of some latent illness? Was this earlier illness due to a retrovirus?

SIGNS OF THE PRODROMAL DISEASE

The prodromal disease of M.E./CFS may have considerable variability. However it is not known if M.E./CFS (a) is caused simply by the prodromal disease virus that contains within its own structure the ability to destabilize the host's immune system and thus create both the acute and chronic illness or (b) the prodromal infection is the final infectious insult, that reaches a destructive disease orbit by riding upon an already destabilized immune system. This earlier immune injury may have, in effect, altered the immune system, thus creating a window though which the prodromal infection, by avoiding the normal immune defenses, could lead to a chronic and possibly hybrid illness.

The possibility of a single virus cause has been suggested by Mowbray[8] who has indicated that potentially any enteroviral persistence may cause M.E./CFS. This echovirus type 30 and coxsackie B viruses persistence is discussed in considerable detail by Schnurr and Schmidt.[9] Yet Bendinelli,[10] who states that, although coxsackievirus suppresses the immune system in mice and in human cells in vitro, *"We know of no evidence that suggest that coxsackievirus (CV) suppresses immunity in humans"*. He then continues that *"There are, however, early observations that concomitant CV infections can lead to unusually severe poliovirus and potentiate certain protozoan and fungal infections"*.

Michael Holmes, Elaine DeFreitas and John Martin,[11] all discoverers of the possible role of a retrovirus in M.E./CFS, appear to assume that this retrovirus may be the unique cause of M.E./CFS. It could also be reasonable to assume that such a retrovirus, if it proven to exist, may cause a primary immune injury, similar in manner to the HIV process, that may precede the triggering infection by a considerable period.

As pointed out by Leon-Sotomayor[12] "The acute state of the illness may have several clinical presentations" Leon-Sotomayor then goes on to list 15 different clinical presentations he has observed. He also makes an important statement that *"The relapse usually presented the same clinical manifestation as the acute attack but less intense."*[13] This point is important since the onset symptoms and physical findings tend to be echoed throughout the disease process. Different onsets frequently cause somewhat different variants of the central disease picture. Behan and Behan[14] also discuss a more limited list of findings that are included in the Leon-Sotomayor review of the various presentations. We concur with both of these authors on the variability of onset disease.

It is important to note that all of the findings in the Leon-Sotomayor list originated in the same epidemic. In any one cluster or epidemic we also have observed this variable onset picture, although different epidemics tend to have their own signature of onset and symptom picture. Undoubtedly, part of the differences in description depends upon the observer and what he believes to be important.

The physical presentations noted by Leon-Sotomayor are listed in the following table. Since these patients all fell ill during the same epidemic and in the same geographical area it is highly unlikely that there were a multitude of viral causes but rather a multitude of host viral responses. Different viral receptors on the same virus may attach to different organ receptors, and even different brain receptors causing hypothalamus, basal ganglia or limbic system injuries.

Clinically, several of the following injuries can occur in any one patient. Many, but not all, of these clinical findings tend to decrease in severity once the disease becomes chronic.

Anterior Poliomyelitis Contact

One of the very early and curious findings that we have repeatedly observed is an early contact with a poliomyelitis patient. In those adult M.E./CFS patients who were born prior to 1955, that is prior to the introduction of generalized polio immunization, we have observed a striking correlation with poliomyelitis.

In excess of 30% of M.E./CFS patients born before 1955 can give a history of living with a parent, sibling, relative or close friend who had been disabled by paralytic poliomyelitis. Poliomyelitis was just not that common. Are these individuals really post-polio syndrome patients, who had subclinical cases of poliomyelitis?

PRODROMAL ILLNESS

Dr. Leon-Sotomayor has listed the following prodromal illnesses associated with M.E./CFS.[12]

CNS Onset

(a) Involuntary muscle jerks, carpopedal spasm, myoclonic episodes that may mimic tetanus or strychnine poisoning.

(b) Psychiatric complaints with hyperventilation syndrome.

(c) Neurovegitative (hypothalamic) episodes with fatigue and abrupt fluctuation of blood pressure (90/60 to 160/110), both orthostatic and hypertension may be present, tachypnea to shallow breathing, bounding pulse, profuse perspiration.

(d) CNS with aseptic meningitis-like picture, Parkinson-like picture, diencephalic fits with chills, cold extremities, pounding of the heart, palpitations, borborygmus, temperature of 96-100, changes of respiratory pattern, sinus arrhythmia, diplopia. This "storm" lasts for a few minutes with components persisting for hours.

(e) Thyrotoxic and thyrotoxic-like picture with staring eyes, irritability, palpitations, tremor, increased perspiration, diarrhoea, leukocytosis, weight loss, vasomotor instability, and elevated BMR.

(f) Postprandial dysporia characterized by palpitations, nausea, perspiration, tremulous feeling mimicking hypoglycemia, carcinoid or dumping syndrome.

(g) Ophthalmological picture with pain, loss of accommodation, both dryness and burning of the eyes in addition to increased lacrimation, photophobia, blepharospasm,

Respiratory System Onset

(h) Upper respiratory infection, with pharyngitis, earache and with or without, Ménière's-like syndrome

(i) Infection-like illness with chills, malaise, leukeoid reaction and fever.

(j) Pulmonary infarction or pneumonia-pleurisy-like symptoms.

Genito-Urinary System Onset

(k) Genito-urinary complaints with puffiness of the face, palpebral oedema, microscopic haematuria, proteinuria, high specific gravity of urine, oligouria, polyuria, orchitis and oophoritis.

Cardiovascular System Onset

(l) Cardiovascular complaints with any of the following C.H.F., pericarditis, myocarditis, cardiovascular collapse, cardiac arrhythmia (PAT or PVC) hypertension, orthostatic hypotension.

Gastroenteric System Onset

(m) Acute abdomen presentation with appendicitis-like picture, diverticulitis-like picture, colitis, pancreatitis or cholecystitis-like picture.

We have seen only one cardiovascular collapse but Dr. John Richardson has had two cases of cardiovascular collapse with death. Autopsy of one of his patients, a professional football player, who died on the playing field, revealed no cardiac infarct.[15] Our single case involved a pulmonary infarction in which the patient had a cardiac arrest and fortunately was resuscitated. We have seen the meningitis-like picture on many occasions but that tends to precede the

M.E./CFS illness by months. We have seen the thyrotoxic picture on several occasions but that tends to occur long after the onset of illness. All of the other forms noted by Leon-Sotomayor and Behan and Behan have been routinely observed by us.

In addition to the above, we have noted the following prodromal onsets:

Paralysis and Paresis

Prior to the mid-1950s and the general introduction of polioimmunization, many of the M.E./CFS cases were permanently paralysed during the initial illness and some recovered from this early paralysis[16]. These paralysed patients were never considered to be poliomyelitis since the persistence of sensory, cognitive and emotional dysfunctions, the waxing and waning of muscle strength and other symptoms were very atypical of classical anterior poliomyelitis. Many M.E./CFS patients were treated as cases of hysterical paralysis[17]. Many M.E./CFS patients were considered to represent a variant of poliomyelitis. With the introduction of immunization and the abrupt cessation of clinical poliomyelitis in the mid-1950s and the continuation of non-paralytic M.E./CFS, few proponents of the infectious origins of M.E./CFS continued to believe that there was any relationship between the two illnesses. One of us (BMH) has personally examined M.E./CFS patients (Akureyri Disease) in Akureyri and in Reykjavik in Iceland, in Canada and the United States, some of whom, despite the passing of almost 50 years, are still paralysed. Except for the paralysis, there is no clinical difference between these two types of patients. It is difficult not to conclude that polioimmunization, which appears to be equally effective against all enteroviral paralysis, may have saved tens of thousands of present day M.E./CFS patients from paralysis. Perhaps "poliomyelitis" epidemics have not stopped, perhaps their cell target has simply changed.

Hand, Foot and Mouth-like Disease (HFM)

We have noted this illness on many occasions in M.E./CFS children and in a significant number of young adults as prodromal illness.

Hand, foot and mouth disease is usually associated with coxsackie A16 and A5, but also A4,7,9 and 10, as well as coxsackie B 2, and 5 and enterovirus 71. Except in the case of enterovirus 71, it is reputedly an illness normally seen in children from 1 to 5 years old[18]. We have never seen this clinical illness associated with M.E./CFS patients under the age of 5. We have documented the illness on several occasions in children usually between the ages of 5 and 14. HFM disease is sometimes misdiagnosed as herpangina. We have also seen HFM disease less frequently in adults as a prodromal or triggering disease of M.E./CFS.

The clinical description is a disease of mild or no fever with sore throat. It is associated with a rash described as small 4 mm macules becoming vesicules in the anterior mouth and lips, located on the palms and fingers, soles and toes and sometimes buttocks. It tends to be associated with malaise, headaches and anorexia. An associated abdominal pain, cough, conjuctivitis, coryza, diarrhoea, pleuritis, nausea/vomiting, pleuritis, carditis or pneumonia have also been described[18].

We refer to this disease as hand, foot and mouth-*like* disease since we usually have only the patient's history to go on and have never had a chance to test the fresh vesicles for viral particles that we have seen. There is another difference with the official description, namely that, in the adults, the rash is in the locations noted but more usually described as starting below the knee and below the elbow.

Acute Hemorrhagic Conjuctivitis-Like Disease[19] (AHC)

This poliomyelitis-like disease is associated with enterovirus 70, coxsackie A24 and hepatitis A (also an enterovirus or enterovirus-like virus). It was pandemic in the tropics in the period 1967-1973 and was associated with paralysis and death[19]. It is reputedly not seen in the temperate regions. However, this may be strictly due to the protective polioimmunization in temperate countries. We have seen AHC in three persons who were in Africa during and after this period. We have documented a similar cluster of physicians and health care workers[20] who fell ill with a clinically identical illness, certain of whom remain considerably ill with M.E./CFS at the time of writing. We have encountered others. It is not a frequent prodromal cause, but the individuals who do fall ill tend to persist in their M.E./CFS illness.

Reticulo Endothelial System Onset[21]

We have rarely seen this form, but it occurred in the 1955 Cumberland, England epidemic described by Wallis[21] and observed on several occasions by Dr. Gordon Parish elsewhere in England.[22] In this form, there is marked enlargement of the lymphatic glands, more so in children. The cervical glands were the most commonly enlarged, followed by the inguinal and axillary glands in that order. The spleen and liver were typically involved, enlarged and painful. Jaundice was also seen in some cases. In the London Free epidemic, 10% of the cases had liver enlargement[23]. Crawley states that *"More than half the cases then showed varying degrees of lympho-reticular disturbance "* [24].

Death

Wallis[25] describes the pathological features of one of the few deaths attributable to M.E./CFS that occurred in a developed country. This death occurred in the Cumberland epidemic. The pathological report is of interest. He describes the report of Dr. R. Klein of the Crichton Royal, Dumfries, Scotland, *"There are in the entire diencephalon, particularly round the third ventricle, numerous small haemorrhages, which extend into the adjacent parts of the mid-brain. Similar haemorrhages can be seen in the corpora mamillare and the supra-mammilary nucleus, the haemorrhages are mostly around small vessels, but some are also to be seen in the free tissue"*[25]. It should be noted that this would correspond in size and location to the UBO's identified by Biddle in the Lake Tahoe epidemic[26]. This patient of Dr. Wallis was an abstainer, so an alcoholic encephalopathy was not part of the differential diagnosis. The many suicide deaths usually occur during the recuperative or chronic stages of the disease.

Delay in Onset of Principal Disease

In the London Free epidemic it was noted that when the primary features of the prodromal illness are over, it may take as long as 3 weeks for most of the features of M.E./CFS to develop[27]. *Pellew*[28] *notes that some patients had no muscular weakness even at two months after onset, then muscular weakness would develop by three months. We concur in this finding and have noted development of certain chronic features of the disease to take up to six months. It is possible that many of the signs and symptoms are present at an earlier date but the patient is often so disabled by exhaustion and bedridden that all of his disease features are not experienced until a certain physical or social activity is reached.*

Henderson and Shelokov, Chapter 15, this text, note that after the prodromal period and "After a period of days to three or four weeks, there is an abrupt exacerbation of symptoms..."

PHYSICAL SIGNS OF CHRONIC DISEASE

Chronic M.E./CFS signs: The chronic signs are manifestations of both specific and ongoing host injury that resulted from the prodromal injury, chronic aspects of the disease process and the lack of internal homeostasis that is characteristic of a M.E./CFS patient. The prominence of the physical signs is often dependent on the host's acute interaction with his environment. This host interaction may be sensory, intellectual, physical or strictly relate to an unstable internal homeostasis. These characteristic physical signs of M.E./CFS disease, and the lack of stability or dependability of the hosts internal homeostasis, become more apparent when the host is challenged by these environmental stimuli.

As noted in the introduction of this chapter, many of these physical signs can be potentiated by environmental interaction. These interactions can be sensory, intellectual, emotional, physical or related to the failure of the host's normal homeostasis that is pathognomic for M.E./CFS. It is an error to believe that the majority of these signs are related to disuse atrophy or lack of conditioning or that they can be improved by forced physical activity.

Inconsistency of Signs: Pellew observed that[29], "*A patient examined in the morning might have nystagmus which would disappear at midday, recur later, disappear later and recur next day.* This on again off again pattern, typical of M.E./CFS, may persist for years although there is a tendency of decrease rather than increase in frequency. Other that this inconsistency, the lack of a normal internal homeostasis, the unusual rapidity of development of cognitive and muscle inconsistency and lack of dependability, the slowness of muscle and cognitive recovery, there are no pathogonomic signs specific to the illness. It is this inconsistency that provokes the major disability of M.E./CFS patients.

These physical signs that we and others note all require a more systematic evaluation. The physical signs of chronic disease will be discussed under the following headings.

Vital signs
Cutaneous
Ophthalmalogic
Neurologic
Genito-urinary
Muscular
Orthopedic
Gastroenteric

Vital Signs

Pulse and Heart Rate: Pulse is frequently irregular and bounding during the course of the early prodromal illness. In the early Initial Stage, many patients will have an unusual decrease in resting rate and an unusual increase in activity rate. A Holter monitor is necessary to document many of these features.

There also tends to be a failure of the heart rate to keep up with the physiological requirements of rapidly changing cardiovascular demands. This has been noted by T. Montague.[30] Clinically this can be documented both in orthostatic hypotension and the inability of the heart rate to keep up with a rapid change in demand, e.g. a patient who tries to bound up 5-6 steps from a resting position will frequently experience an unusually slow speed up of heart rate, chest spasm and shortness of breath.

We have observed nocturnal bradycardia as measured by Holter monitor.

Blood Pressure: The blood pressure may increase or decrease during the first few days of the prodromal period only to fall to a persisting lower than normal blood pressure in chronic patients. As mentioned earlier, some normotensive patients and perhaps more frequently in patients with pre-existing mild hypertensive disease, one can observe the rapid development of malignant hypertension, sometimes with the appearance of carcinoid syndrome. The carcinoid features tend not to continue but the malignant hypertension when it occurs, tends to persist and to be poorly controllable.

Temperature: Temperature is sometimes mildly elevated during the first one to three days of the illness. Pellew notes a typical finding[29] *"The range of temperature was from just above normal to 102 °F, the average being just under 100 °F and the duration of fever, with fall by lysis, was short, about three days being usual"*. This is typical of the prodromal phase.

Once the typical chronic features set in, the normal diurnal temperature changes. First the base temperature is lowered, reaching regularly two degrees below the normal temperature. In addition there is an increase in the normal diurnal variation with swings up to 100°F (37.8°C)[31]. Gilliam[32] states that *" a frequent daily range from 97°- 99°F was much more characteristic of this illness than a real elevation of temperature"*.

Dr. Anne Mildon[33] of Toronto has documented malignant hyperthermia, a very rare condition, in several M.E./CFS patients.

Respiratory Rate: Early in the disease, one may note hyperventilation in M.E./CFS patients. This is not common and is frequently associated with sensory or diencephalonic storms. More frequently we see bouts of shallow breathing after minimal physical activity.

CUTANEOUS SIGNS

Cutaneous changes are common to most M.E./CFS patients but, like many of the symptoms, they are rarely consistent and tend to wax and wane. They tend to be exaggerated with exercise, sensory stimulation, symptom storms and intellectual activity. A patient who arrives at the physician's office rested, will, after a long interview, tend to begin to manifest an increase in visible cutaneous changes. There may be daily drenching sweats early in the disease that decrease in frequency in the chronic stages.

The most common cutaneous changes can be confused with either systemic lupus erythematosus (SLE) or even dermatomyositis (D) but, in our experience, even severe cases of M.E./CFS do not respond to corticosteroids. However, no matter how severe the case of M.E./CFS may be, we have never seen a case that has been progressive or that has lead to death as in the case of SLE and dermatomyositis.

Facial Features: M.E./CFS patients frequently develop what Dr. Ramsay[34] referred to as the ghastly pallor. This sudden blanching of the face with an almost Parkinsonian mask-like appearance is seen more frequently in the first year of illness but commonly can persist for the life of the illness. It is usual for a fatigued M.E./CFS patient to exhibit a mottled malar erythematous discolouration similar or identical to that seen in systemic lupus. This mottled discoloration also occurs in the area of the sternum.

One-sided palpebral oedema in not infrequent and has been described by Leon-Sotomayor[35]. Early in the disease we have observed third nerve injury and mild Horner's syndrome. This does not persist. However misdiagnoses and improper treatment have led to permanent cases of tardif dyskinesia.

What is described as painful shotty glands, frequently in the posterior cervical triangle[36] are described very frequently in the literature. However it is difficult to be too impressed with this finding in chronic cases. In chronic cases, neck sensitivity of this nature probably represents fibromyalgia points.

Hands and Feet: Other common cutaneous signs are cold Raynaud's hands. They are often blotchy with cyanotic nail beds. There are frequently liver palms and an engorged or prominent vein that follows the crease of the flexor pollicis brevis muscle on the palm. This muscle mass on the palm adjacent to the thumb is frequently atrophied in chronic cases. All of these have been pointed out by Dr. Ryll in the Mercy San Juan Hospital epidemic of 1975[37]. In the acute disease, the finger tips may be shiny and smooth, the nail beds cyanotic with an almost sclerodermatous appearance. Paul Cheney has noted that there may be a loss of fingerprints in extreme cases.[38] Wilson and Walker[65] discuss similar findings in the 1934 California epidemic. They note *"Vasomotor and trophic disturbances were almost constant findings among* *the adult patients. In the cases of more extreme involvement exfoliation of the skin of the affected extremities occurred, followed by glossy atrophy of the skin and atrophy of the subcutaneous tissue.*" Rarely, there may be a coarse tremor, particularly after activity. These signs tend to be more common in the left hand. Carpopedal spasm is seen frequently.

Comparison of M.E./CFS and SLE[43,44]		
Sign Primary candidate	M.E./CFS young to middle age women	SLE middle age women
Sedimentation rate elevated in 10%	usually 0-5	high
SLE Cells	never	80%
Rheumatoid factor	in approx. 20%	20%
Migratory polyarthritis	often	often
Arthralgias without objective changes	usual	usual
Deforming arthropathy	never	can occur
Muscle atrophy and weakness	usual	usual
Pericarditis, myocarditis	occurs, early infrequent	occurs late frequent
GIT symptoms	common	common
Sjogren's-like or Sicca Syndrome	common	common
Thyroid disease	common in women	common
Exacerbation triggered by surgery, trauma, emotional stress, sunlight, non-essential drugs	common	common
Mottled erythematous maculopapular eruption Malar butterfly	common	common
Upper chest and neck	common	common
Telangiectases and ecchymotic spots on hands and feet	occurs	occurs
Thinning and atrophy of skin of finger tips with loss of fingerprints	common	common
Raynaud's disease	common	common
Alopecia	occurs	common
Patchy oedema	common	common
Erythema nodosum	occurs	common
Purpura	occurs	common
Oedematous swelling of face and extremities	occurs	occurs
Response to steroids ASA, NSAIDS	poor	good

Vein Engorgement: Dr. Erich Ryll[66] noted engorgement of veins in the Mercy San Juan Hospital epidemic in 1975. He states that these are some-

times quite painful. Similar features were also noted by Leon-Sotomayor.[39] We have seen this primarily in the neck and hand. We have observed this frequently but not noted associated pain. Carpopedal spasm was noted in the London Free epidemic[40] and is a frequent complaint but rarely observed.

Raynaud's Disease: This is common in M.E./CFS but we have never seen it go on to ulceration or gangrene. We have seen this involving the fingers, toes, hands and sometimes the ears and nose with pallor and both pain and loss of sensation. It sometimes can involve well circumscribed spots on the extremities or body. The line demarcating normal from pathologically cold skin is often so distinct that it is visible with the eyes and apparent with touch. It can form visible glove and stocking distribution that may lack normal sensation. Acrocyanosis is illustrated by Leon-Sotomayor[41]. However, the cyanotic colour alterations in the hands and feet and the white and numb fingers and toes described by Fog[42] are a more frequent observation. These acute Raynaud's disease changes are visible and appear sometimes without expectation. The patient may complain of severe localized pain in the area.

Alopecia: This is not a common finding but we see from time to time patchy loss of hair. It occurs in the pubic area and also involves body, facial and scalp area hair. Alopecia totalis is very rare.

Ophthalmalogic Signs

We routinely find ophthalmalogical signs. These include;
-Conjunctival injection is frequent[45]
-Palpebral swelling, usually left sided[33]
-Sicca Syndrome or pseudo-Sjogren's syndrome with excess tearing and excess drying of the tear and buccal glands is a common chronic feature
-Patients regularly complain of photophobia and we regularly note unequal and contrary pupillar reaction to light in chronic patients.[46] During the acute stage of the London epidemic they observed that "the pupils were sometimes unequal, and might be defective in reactions to light and accommodation[46]. External ophthalmoplegia was common."
-Movement of the pupil may be irregular or cogwheel
-We have seen cases of Adies' pupil with loss of patellar reflex

-Rapid variation of visual accommodation within one day and with fatigue. Also sluggish accommodation is very common. Both of these tend to settle down in the chronic stages.

-A variable and increase in nystagmus is routinely observed

-Cherry red posterior fundus early in the disease process that tends to persist for weeks[47]

-Loss of night vision

-Possible loss of colour vision

-External ophthalmoplegia

-Diplopia is mentioned in Fog's description of the 1952 Danish epidemic,[42] and in the South African epidemic in 1959[48] as it is in almost all epidemics.

Neurologic Signs

Modified Romberg test (with eyes closed) is usually always positive (eyes closed). Hand tremor can occur. Loss of equilibrium and motor weakness are common.

Neck stiffness, increased and decreased tendon reflexes have been described in the Initial Stage but are infrequent in chronic illness. Loss of abdominal reflexes is sometimes noted in the early disease.

Abnormal EEG was noted by Pampiglione in the London Free[49] epidemic and Leon-Sotomayor noted 7 out of 25 abnormal EEGs early in the disease.[50] Although Grand Mal epilepsy is rare, seizure activity is the rule in M.E./CFS. This is discussed in detail in this text in the chapter on CNS dysfunction.

Involuntary muscle movement is common in the early stages and tremor in later stages. In acute and chronic patients with straight leg raising we frequently note cogwheel movement of the leg. This was observed in the South African epidemic described by Hill[48] who notes *"When these muscles were tested against resistance, they contracted in a curious interrupted or cog-like fashion"*. In the London Free epidemic[51] they observed *"a peculiar jerking in a limb on voluntary movement - that was distinctive and characteristic - of this encephalitis., "one nurse developed cogwheel rigidity in the right arm"*. The Medical Staff of the Royal Free[23].

Hypoalgesia, and hyperesthesia were observed in the acute stages of the Los Angeles[52], Akureyri[53], Adelaide[54] and London[55] epidemics. Sometimes simply the weight of the sheets creates excessive pain. We have found this common in the Initial Stages but only cutaneous and muscular hyperesthesia are routinely observed in the chronic stages.

The nerve distribution most frequently observed in the Akureyri[56] epidemic were the ulnar, axillary, lateral femoral cutaneus, first sacral, fifth lumbar and first thoracic nerves. We also find in both acute and chronic patients these same nerves involved except the area of the first thoracic extends up to the fourth cervical.

Fasciculations, tremors and even short spasms of tetanic contraction are common but rarely documented by the physician.

Spinal Fluid Pressure

Gilliam notes[57] that *"Nearly all cases in which the spinal fluid pressure was recorded showed the fluid to be under increased pressure."* This is important since, possibly due to rapid draining of spinal fluid, we have seen at least three iatrogenic cases of brain stem hernia, one in a child, all resulting in permanent injury considerably worse that the original illness.

Cardiovascular Signs

Early in the disease there tends to be sinus arrhythmia, PVCs, tachycardia. Leon-Sotomayor[58] and Richardson[59] have noted an associated myocarditis and friction rub early in the disease and muffled heart sounds. There appears to be an increased incidence of mitral valve prolapse. Dr. John Richardson[59] has documented sudden cardiac death in the absence of coronary occlusion in athletes early in the disease. This is very rare. Many patients have unrecognized myocarditis and pericarditis early in the disease that one cursory examination may fail to reveal. Dr. Richardson has also commented on the increased incidence of mitral valve prolapse in M.E./CFS[59].

Dr. Leon-Sotomayor is perhaps the lone cardiologist to comment extensively on this illness.

On ECG, Leon-Sotomayor noted[58]:

sinus tachycardia except when recumbent
sinus arrhythmia

PVC or PAC
non-specific unstable ST-T wave changes
other supraventricular arrhythmias
elevation of ST-segments
peaking of T waves
prominent U waves
TU- segment depression
High incidence of post-exercise ST segment and T wave abnormalities.

Leon-Sotomayor attributes many of these changes to an unstable autonomic influence.

Genito-urinary Signs

Although chronic exhaustion is probably the leading cause of sexual dysfunction, patients frequently complain of dysparunia and impotence. Frequently, there is a distinct vaginal dryness as there tends to be in all mucous membranes. Pudental pain syndromes are common but rarely any physical signs are seen except for interstitial cystitis with an engorged bladder wall vein or ecchymosis. Genital complaints are less common in men. Early in the disease process nocturia, difficulty in starting and stopping stream, and pain are common. Orchiditis is seen rarely and usually in association with a Bornholme's-like onset. Even quite young male patients may have pseudoprostatitis.

Marked menstrual changes are common.

MUSCULAR-ORTHOPEDIC SIGNS

Muscle Strength

A few patients will have such profound muscle weakness that they will be confined to a wheel chair or almost permanently in bed. This degree of disability is more common in children than in adults. These adults fortunately are the exception. A very few of these disabled patients will react to weight bearing by convulsive, tetanic convulsions. These sorry patients are usually dismissed as cases of somatization. We believe this may represent a limbic dysfunction.

Most patients will usually relate to the physician that their muscles are weak. Yet, although electrophysiological and microscopic work reveals changes, there is little to account for the profound muscle weakness described by most patients. To compound matters still further, most M.E./CFS patients can lift a weight equivalent to what any similar non-M.E./CFS underconditioned person can lift. Are these patients simply unreliable witnesses?

How can this conundrum be logically answered?

Pain: The first point to note is that non-myalgic M.E./CFS patients generally appear to have much less muscle weakness. Many M.E./CFS patients have inhibition of muscle strength by pain. This pain can either be immediate such that running up six steps or running across an 18 foot road allowance will bring them to a grinding stop. The second is the delayed pain reaction. Particularly in the first months or even years of illness, any modestly prolonged muscle activity may result in a delayed pain syndrome of considerable intensity that may persist for days. This pain may be specific to a particular muscle group and also generalized as a malaise and tends to prevent muscle activity.

Specific Muscle Group Weakness: The patient may tell the physician that **all** of his muscles are weak. This is not often true. A review of the epidemics will usually point out that the authors state that only specific muscle groups are affected. Usually these specific muscle groups persist in weakness, although this pain and weakness may wander over time to another group. What the patient is complaining of is more likely heaviness and the feeling of exhaustion and malaise in the muscles.

Loss of Dependability: Another problem that M.E./CFS patients experience is the increased speed with which some muscles loose their strength and coordination and the slowness of recovery to a comfortable ability. With activity, the patient tends to lose proprioception and position sense, the ability to estimate the position of his limb. He becomes clumsy and incoordinated.

Incoordination: We see this loss of fine muscle coordination frequently described by patients who have difficulty maintaining legible writing. This is mentioned by Innes[60] "His handwriting became less legible".

Much of the weakness that the patient describes is

really rapidly developing incoordination. There is a lack of smoothness of muscle movement, particularly for complex muscle tasks and this is most likely a central control fault. This has also been noted by Dr. Bastien in this text. Antagonists and agonist muscle groups may contract at the same time. A patient without pain will have less problem lifting up a child than she will have with small rapid movements of drying many dishes. Place the same patient in the dark and she will frequently lose the ability to coordinate even simple muscle movements. Walking around a mile on a sidewalk may be difficult, but not as difficult as trying to walk 500 feet on uneven ground. The problem is not one of distance but one of poor central coordination, positional dysfunction, poor balance and loss of smooth muscle action.

Gilliam[61] states that *"Muscle weakness tends to be confined to localized muscle groups and not to the general distribution that would be expected if due to immobilization alone."* We too have tended to find specific muscle groups weaker than others. If this is true, then it may not be relevant to test, as is usually done, the same muscle group in every patient for cellular and neuromuscular dysfunction.

Thus, testing a single muscle group such as the flexors of the left forearm with a simple muscle task and finding it to have normal function and strength may be akin to testing a poliomyelitis patient, paralyzed from the waist down. No matter how good the researcher's technique may be, the patient will be found to be in perfectly normal muscular strength and health.

Shortness of Breath: This is frequently related to diaphragmatic incoordination, pain, or weakness or pain in the chest wall muscles. Some of the exhaustion and weakness experienced by the patient may be due to decrease in function of these muscle groups in which the patient is unable to respond to increased oxygen needs with increased activity.

Fibromyalgia Points: Fibromyalgia points are commonly tender. Insertions of major tendons are often tender and activity has resulted in infrequent rupture of tendon. These ruptures usually occur in the lower posterior leg. Muscle bunching or spasm can frequently be palpated after minor activity. A stiff painful neck may be common in the Initial Stages.

Polyarthritis: Sigurdsson[62] notes that *"polyarthritis developed after this illness in a number of instances".* We also find this, but the arthritic involvement is particularly apparent in children and adolescents in the Chronic Stages of M.E./CFS. These cases are frequently misdiagnosed as rheumatoid disease despite lack of supportive rheumatoid tests. This is also discussed by Wilson, Walker[65] in the 1934 epidemic, where they observe, *"A unique feature of this (1934 California) epidemic was the occurrence of inflammatory changes in and about the joints, which was observed in 34% of the adult patients in the present series. In 10% there were merely transitory but sharply localized pain and tenderness in the joints."* It should be noted that Wilson, Walker were orthopedists, the number of arthritic patients were twelve, and that their series were referred for these specific complaints and did not represent the epidemic as a whole. We routinely see a small number of these cases at Nightingale.

Anaerobic Activity: Patients tend to utilise anaerobic muscle activity rather than aerobic activity. This can be readily measured if the correct apparatus is available. Measurement of these features proide a useful diagnostic tool.

Gastroenteric Signs

Abdominal distress is frequent with pain and appropriate guarding that mimics cholecystitis, gastric and duodenal ulcer and acute appendicitis. We usually note diaphragmatic sensitivity, generally left-sided, early in the disease. Liver and spleen enlargement have been noted.[63] The staff of the London Free also noted that *"there was extreme tenderness of the subcostal regions, and attempts at palpation might evoke resentment due to pain."* These acute abdomen situations tend to occur early in the disease.

There is also a tendency early in the disease for weight loss with anorexia and constipation, whereas in the later stages there is a tendency for weight gain, dietary fanaticism, loose stools and irritable bowel syndrome. The typical irritable bowel syndrome with bloating, rapid diurnal fluid and weight change, colic, heightened gastrocolic reflex or dumping syndrome and severe bowel urgency or even bowel incontinence develops in about 20% of M.E./CFS patients. Some of this is related to the development of acquired food sensitivities. Food neurosis is a common finding in this group and it becomes difficult to separate true food sensitivities to the almost religious zeal of dietary mania.

Our most difficult patients have been those with explosive retroperistalsis. Fortunately this is not a common feature of the disease. Hardtke[64] points out a much more common problem is the incoordination of the larynx and the oesophagus and it is a frequent complaint of the *"need to swallow carefully to avoid choking on liquids"*. We regularly note this problem with liquids and solids. It is a wonder that some of our

patients have not suffocated to death by the temporary blocking of the larynx by certain foods.

Summary

It is frequently stated that there are no physical signs in M.E./CFS. Yet it is rare that we do not encounter numerous physical signs although these are more apparent in the Initial Stage of the disease. In the chronic stages there are also less dramatic persisting physical signs. Brain imaging, nerve conduction and neuropsychological techniques discussed in this book continue to amplify the physical changes apparent to the careful and learned observer.

References

1. Gilliam A.G. (1938) **Epidemiological study of an epidemic, diagnosed as poliomyelitis, occurring among the personnel of the Los Angeles County General Hospital during the summer of 1934,** United States Public Heath Bulletin No. 240, pages 1-90, page 18.

2. Gilliam A.G. idem (1) page 9.

3. Gilliam A.G. idem (1) page 11.

4. Hyde B., Bergmann S. Chronic Aspects of Akureyri Disease, page 214, chapter on **Post-viral Fatigue Syndrome,** Jenkins and Mowbray, John Wiley & Sons, (1991) page 211.

5. Pellew R.A. (1951) A clinical description of a disease resembling poliomyelitis seen in Adelaide, The Medical Journal of Australia, 1, 944 page 944.

6. Crowley N., Nelson M., Stovin S. Epidemiological aspects of an outbreak of encephalomyelitis at the Royal Free Hospital, London, in the Summer of 1955, Journal of Hygiene[Camb] 1957;55;102-122, page 117-118.

7. Eden, J. We called it the pestilence, World Medicine, June 15, 1977, page 25.

8. Yousef G. E., Bell E.J., Mann G.F. and Mowbray J.F. (1988) Chronic enterovirus infection in patients with postviral fatigue syndrome. Lancet, i, 146-150.

9. Schnurr D., Schmidt N., Persistent Infections, Chapter 11, pages 181-201, Bendinelli & Friedman, **Coxsackieviruses, A General Update,** Plenum Press (1988).

10. Bendinelli M. Interactions with the Immune System, pg 95, idem (2).

11. Holmes, DeFreitis and Martin See this text.

12. Leon-Sotomayor L., **Epidemic Diencephalomyelitis,** Pageant Press, 1969, pages 13-15.

13. Leon-Sotomayor L., idem(12) page 17, see also this text, Clinical Observations.

14. Behan P., Behan W. Post viral fatigue syndrome, a review. CRC Reviews. Cleveland, Ohio: CRC Press, pages 12-13, 1988.

15. Personal communication with Dr. John Richardson of Ryton, England.

16. Gilliam A.G. (1938) **Epidemiological study of an epidemic, diagnosed as poliomyelitis, occurring among the personnel of the Los Angeles County General Hospital during the summer of 1934,** United States Public Heath Bulletin No. 240, pages 1-90.

17. Hyde B., Bergmann S. Chronic Aspects of Akureyri Disease, page 214, chapter on **Post-viral Fatigue Syndrome,** Jenkins and Mowbray, John Wiley & Sons, (1991).

18. Moore M., Morens D. Enteroviruses, including polioviruses, Chapter 17, pages 447-449, Belshe R. **Textbook of Human Virology,** PSG Publishing Company, Littleton, Massachusetts 1985.

19. Moore M. idem 11, page 451.

20. Labor-day 1984 Montreal cluster, Sean O'Sullivan M.D, Tilsonburg Ontario. In publication.

21. Wallis A.L. An **Investigation into an unusual disease seen in epidemic and sporadic form in a general practice in Cumberland in 1955 and subsequent years,** Doctoral Thesis, University of Edinburgh pages 16-17(1957).

22. Parish J. G., personal communications.

23. The medical staff of the Royal Free Hospital, An Outbreak of Encephalomyelitis in the Royal Free Hospital Group, London, in 1955, Br. Med. J., 1957; 2:896.

24. Crowley N., Nelson M., Stovin S. Epidemiological Aspects of an Outbreak of Encephalomyelitis at the Royal Free Hospital, London, in the Summer of 1955. Journal of Hygiene (Cambridge) 1957: 55: 102-122.

25. Wallis A.L. idem(21) pages 46-48.

26. Biddle R. Lake Tahoe epidemic MRI findings in publication.

27. The medical staff of the Royal Free Hospital, idem(23) pages 896.

28. Pellew R.A. (1951) A clinical description of a disease resembling poliomyelitis seen in Adelaide, The Medical Journal of Australia, 1, 944 page 946.

29. Pellew R.A. idem (28), page 945.

30. Montague T., Marrie T., Klassen G., Bewick D., Horacek B.M. Cardiac Function at Rest and with Exercise in the Chronic Fatigue Syndrome, Chest, Vol 95, p779-784, April 1989.

31. The Medical Staff of the Royal Free, idem (23) page 899.

32. Gilliam A.G. idem (16) page 23.

33. Mildon A. Canada Diseases Weekly Report, Supplement, Jan 1991 Vol 17S1E, page 18.

34. Ramsay A. Melvin, Dr. Ramsay used this term, ghastly pallor frequently when speaking at EME meetings in London.

35. Leon-Sotomayor L.idem(12) palpebral oedema, page 121.

36. Galpine J., Brady C. Benign Mylagic Encephalomyelitis, The Lancet Aril 13, 1957, pages 757-758, page 758.

37. Ryll E. 1975 Mercy San Juan Hospital Epidemic in Sacramento, California, work in preparation.

38. Cheney P. San Francisco Conference, SanFrancisco Hilton, 1989.

39. Leon-Sotomayor L. idem(12)vein engorgement page 121.

40. The Medical Staff of the Royal Free idem (23), toe spasm, page 899.

41. Leon-Sotomayor L. idem, (12) acrocyanosis, page 119.

42. Fog T. (Danish)Ugeskrift for Laeger, Vol 115, July-Sept 1953, pages 1244-1250.

43. Harrison T.R. **Principals of Internal Medicine,** fourth Edition, 1962, Tumulty P., SLE 1892-96.

44. Andrews G., Domonkos A. **Disease of the Skin,**Fifth Edition, Saunders, 1966, SLE 129-133.

45. Leon-Sotomayor L. ,idem(12) Conjuctival injection, page 119.

46. The Medical Staff of the Royal Free idem (23), page 896.

47. John Richardson Cherry Red Fundus, Workshop Newcastle upon Tyne, 1989.

48. Hill R., Cheetham R., Wallace H. Epidemic Myalgic Encephalomyelopathy, The Lancet, Saturday 4 April 1959, 689-693.

49. Pampiglione G., Harris R., Kennedy J. Electro-encehpalographic investigations in myalgic encephalomyelitis, Postgraduate Medical Journal November 1978, 54, 752-754.

50. Leon-Sotomayor idem (12) abnormal ECG page 20.

51. The Medical Staff of the Royal Free idem (23), page 898.

52. Gilliam A.G. idem (16) page 21 hypalgesia, hyperesthesia.

53. Sigurdsson B. Sigurjonsson J. Sigurdsson J.H.J., Thorkelsson J & Gudmundsson K.R. (1950) A disease epidemic in Iceland simulating poliomyelitis, American Journal of Hygiene, 52, 222, page 227.

54. Pellew R.A. idem (28) page 945.

55. The Medical Staff of the Royal Free idem (23), page 897.

56. Sigurdsson B. idem (53) page 231.

57. Gilliam A.G. idem (16)page 33.

58. Leon-Sotomayor, idem (12) page 18.

59. Richardson J., Workshop Newcastle upon Tyne, 1989.

60. Innes S. Encephalomyelitis resembling benign myalgic encephalomyelitis, The Lancet, May 9, 1970 969-971, page 970.

61. Gilliam A.G. idem (16), page 26.

62. Sigurdsson B. idem (53), page 234.

63. The Medical Staff of the Royal Free idem (23), page 897.

64. Hardtke E. Iceland Disease in Indiana, Journal of the Indiana State Medical Association Vol 48, March 1955, number 3, page 248.

65. Wilson J, Walker P. Acute Anterior Poliomyelitis, (Aspects of 1934 California Epidemic), Archives of Internal Medicine, (1936), Vol. 57, No.3, March.

66. Ryll E., Chabursky B. Mercy San Juan Hospital Epidemic, California, in preparation.

Opening Remarks of the Honorary Chairmen

Chapter 7

Symposium Speaker and Honorary Chairman

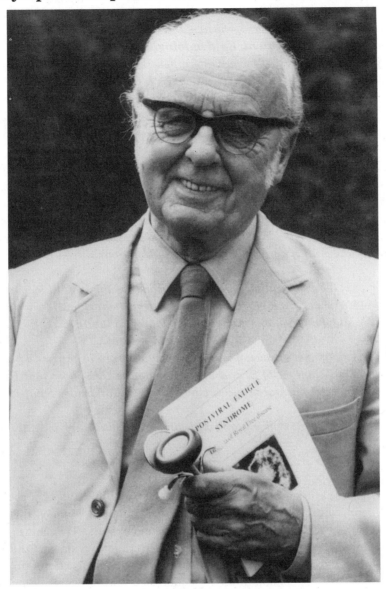

The late A. Melvin Ramsay

Myalgic Encephalomyelitis - Then and Now
An Epidemiological Introduction

A. M. Ramsay, MB, Ch.B
Hon. Consultant Physician, Royal Free Hospital, London

E. G. Dowsett, MB
Hon. Consultant Microbiologist, Basildon\Thurrock Health Authority, Essex

Dr. Ramsay was born in Preston, Lancashire, in 1901. He was educated at the Mackie Academy, Stonehaven, and proceeded to Aberdeen University where he graduated MA in 1923 and MB, ChB in 1926. From 1926 to 1935 he was in general practice in South Africa and then returned to the United Kingdom to enter hospital practice *at Fulham Hospital. He was transferred to the North Western Fevers Hospital in 1937 and went on to become Deputy Medical Superintendent. He was involved in the instruction of nurses and undergraduate medical students in the practical principles of the management of infectious diseases. In 1939, he received the degree of MD (Aberdeen) with a thesis on the **Clinical, Epidemiological and Bacteriological Findings in 1205 cases of Puerperal Sepsis**. In 1947, the North Western Fevers Hospital was taken over by the Royal Free Hospital and Dr. Ramsay became consultant Physician to the Infectious Diseases Department. He was also consultant in smallpox to the Ministry of Health and Lecturer in infectious diseases to the University of London. He later became Lecturer and Examiner in infectious diseases for postgraduates who were training for the Diploma of Public Health. He has written extensively on infectious disease and was co-author of a textbook on the subject.*

The earliest cases of a new and extremely puzzling type of infection were admitted to the Infectious Diseases Department at Hampstead in the Spring of 1955. In July, this outbreak spread to the main body of the Royal Free Hospital and was responsible for around 300 cases before terminating in November. The infection became known as "Royal Free Disease". Dr. Ramsay presented papers on the subject at international conferences in Madrid (1958) and Vienna (1965). Between 1971 and 1974, he was President of the Association for the Study of Infectious Diseases (now the British Society for the Study of Infection).

Dr. Ramsay was very active in the organization of a symposium on the subject of "Epidemic Neuromyasthenia" held at the Royal Society of Medicine in April 1978 and shared the chairmanship. He was a member of the Study Group on the subject of "Myalgic Encephalomyelitis" since its inception in 1978.

Dr. Ramsay, much loved by patient or physician and all who had the privilege to meet him, died a few weeks prior to the First World Symposium on M.E. and the production of this paper that he was to present at Cambridge. Dr. Ramsay was instrumental in encouraging the 1990 Cambridge Symposium.

(Please see Chapter 28 for Dr. Dowsett's photograph and curriculum vitae.)

History

This survey is based on 35 years experience of Myalgic Encephalomyelitis, beginning with the dramatic epidemic which affected the Royal Free Hospital in July 1955. In May of the same year, sporadic cases of a new and puzzling illness began to be admitted from the local community in North West London to the Infectious Diseases Unit at Hampstead and to other hospitals in the area. On July 13th, a ward sister and a resident doctor at the Royal Free Hospital in Grays Inn Road fell ill with the same infection, and, by July 25th, 70 similar cases had occurred. The hospital was closed until October 29th, by which time 290 cases had been identified in hospital staff of all grades (predominantly nurses) though only 12 patients were affected. This epidemic ceased on November 24th although smaller outbreaks occurred in associated units the following Spring.[1]

Nomenclature

The illness, though similar to non-paralytic poliomy-

elitis in many clinical aspects, could clearly be distinguished and was diagnosed as Benign Myalgic Encephalomyelitis. This name gives a clearer clinical description than many of the eponyms used previously. (Iceland Disease, Akureyri's Disease, Epidemic Neuromyasthenia)[2] or invented subsequently (Post viral syndrome, Chronic Fatigue, Immune Dysfunction Syndrome). These share the common disadvantage of obscuring the world-wide incidence or of trivialising the clinical severity of the illness.

Diagnosis

Three factors have done much to cause the obscurity surrounding the aetiology, pathogenesis and prognosis of myalgic encephalomyelitis.

First, there has been an absence of objective evidence of organic disease from laboratory and other studies, often leading to an inappropriate diagnosis of psychiatric or behavioural disturbance. Fortunately, recent advances in molecular biology and in neurophysiological techniques will now enable us to rewrite that history.

Second, the failure to distinguish the characteristic fatigue of myalgic encephalomyelitis from other more short lived post infective debility (e.g. following Influenza or Infectious mononucleosis) or from other causes of fatigue has led to unrealistic estimates of recovery.

Third, the failure to agree on firm diagnostic criteria has distorted the data base for epidemiological and other research, thus denying recognition of the unique epidemiological pattern of myalgic encephalomyelitis.

We adopted the following diagnostic criteria:

A syndrome initiated by a viral infection commonly described as a respiratory/gastro intestinal illness but a gradual or more dramatic onset following neurological, cardiac or endocrine disability is recognised.

The cardinal features, in a patient who has previously been physically and mentally fit, with a good work record are:

1. Generalised or localised muscle fatigue after minimal exertion with **prolonged** recovery time.

2. Neurological disturbance, especially of cognitive, autonomic and sensory functions, often accompanied by marked emotional lability and sleep reversal.

3. Variable involvement of cardiac and other bodily systems.

4. An extended relapsing course with a tendency to chronicity.

5. Marked variability of symptoms both within and between episodes.

Epidemiology

We base our epidemiological experience on 700 patients seen in clinic, some 50% of whom have evidence of enteroviral infection,[5] and 2,000 postal questionnaires (including 420 from patients ill for more than 10 years).

Prevalence

Myalgic encephalomyelitis is an endemic illness with epidemic periodicity. It is a common disability in the UK, based on evidence from GP referrals to clinics. In the sporadic form, it appears to be at least three times as common as multiple sclerosis in South East England. Epidemic myalgic encephalomyelitis is said to affect between 3 and 7% of the exposed population in the UK and USA[4], suggesting an infecting agent not previously encountered in childhood.

Age/Sex

The peak age at onset in both sexes lies in the mid thirties, with a smaller peak between 15 and 20 years in females only. Females of all ages suffer more severely than males and the F/M ratio of 3:1 in the acute stage rises to 9:1 after 10 years illness. Myalgic encephalomyelitis is rare under the age of 15 (less than 10% of total) and less common after 45 (20% of the total).

Season/Geography

As in poliomyelitis, the seasonal and geographical distribution of myalgic encephalomyelitis reflects the interaction of hygiene and climate. The prodromal illness is more common in Summer and Autumn in the UK and commonly affects the whole community. It is not invariably followed by myalgic encephalomyelitis but secondary cases arising after days or weeks in family or social contacts are reported by 25% of patients.

Social Groupings

There is a marked ethnic and sociological divide in this country with professional classes (predominantly teachers and health care workers) most commonly affected.

Prognosis

Myalgic encephalomyelitis is an illness with high morbidity and low mortality (if cardiac complications and suicide can be excepted). Complete recovery, however, appears to be confined to one third of cases, predominantly young people who have been able to rest from onset of the illness. A tendency to relapse spontaneously or under stress (physical/mental exertion, hormonal disturbance, secondary infection, and other factors commonly noted in poliomyelitis) remains for many years. The remaining two thirds of patients are equally divided between those who pursue a fluctuating course initially and then stabilise at a lowered energy level and those who have a severe and debilitating downhill course. Stabilisation often permits limited work and socialisation.

Economic Outcome

A study of our patients who have been ill for more than 10 years indicates a disastrous economic outcome. Over 80% of professional and technical workers suffering chronic disease have been obliged to retire early or work part time. The peak incidence of myalgic encephalomyelitis in the third decade has led to serious family disruption in 70% of patients in all occupational groups. The potential financial loss to the community (based on a comparison with multiple sclerosis) suggests £300 million annually in lost earnings, to say nothing of lost skill and lost parental care and education. If we must add to this, the distress caused by misdiagnosis or disbelief, myalgic encephalomyelitis remains an illness with a tragic aftermath which still presents a challenge to the skill of the medical profession.

References:

1. Ramsay, A. M. Post viral fatigue syndrome - The saga of the Royal Free Disease. Gower Medical Publishing London (1986)

2. Acheson, E. D. The syndrome variously called Benign Myalgic Encephalomyelitis, Iceland Disease and Epidemic Neuromyasthenia. Am J. Med (1959) 26 569-595

3. Dowsett, E. G. Human Enteroviral infections J. Hosp: Infect (1988) 11 103-115

4. Behan, P. O. Behan, W. M. H. Post viral fatigue syndrome. C. R. C. Critical Reviews in Neurobiology (1988) 4 157-178

5. Dowsett, E. G.; Ramsay, A. M.; Bell, E. J.; McCartney, R. A. Myalgic Encephalomyelitis - a persistent enteroviral infection? Post grad med. J. (in press)

Chapter 8

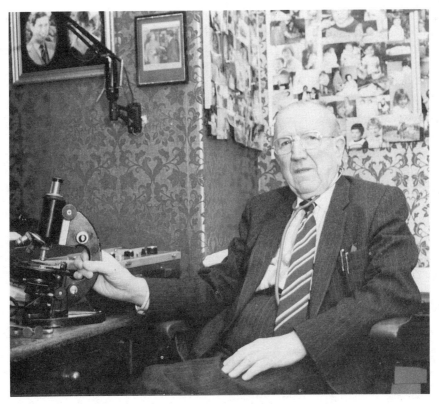

J. Richardson

M.E., The Epidemiological and Clinical Observations of a Rural Practitioner

Dr. J. Richardson MB BS, Belle Vue, Grange Road, Ryton, Tyne & Wear NE40 3LU England

Dr. John Richardson was a founding member of the Department of Family and Community Medicine at the University of Newcastle-upon-Tyne, England. He has had extensive experience in Physical Medicine, Cardiology, Neurology, and Histopathology as well as Obstetrics. He has delivered more than 5 600 babies in his own practice. Dr. Richardson has been examining and treating M.E. patients on a continual basis for the last 37 years, longer than any physician alive today. He has carried out four decades of research into the effects of viruses and subsequent organ pathology.

Polio and M.E.

In the days when polio regularly occurred, the following terms were used :	
Polioencephalitis	inflammatory disease of the grey matter of the brain.
Polio haemorrhagica superior	a haemorrhagic type of above. (Oxley)
Polio acuta infantum	encephalitis with fits, fever etc. and paralysis.

Acute bulbar polio Posterior polio	affecting grey matter of posterior part of the 4th ventricle.
Acute anterior polio or paralytic polio	the one we remember and easy to "see".
Posterior spinal polio or sensory polio	in the posterior grey horns of the spinal cord.
Ascending polio	which we now define as Guillain-Barré syndrome.

Thus polio itself was a pleomorphic entity. Moreover, 20% of cases had a concomitant myocarditis from which 20% succumbed.

The Role of Immunization in M.E.

I suggest that we are dealing with something similar to the posterior polio variety now in some of those with Coxsackie and enteroviral infections. Moreover, this has followed in the wake of the international immunisation for the anterior polio variety. Historically, it can be seen from the literature that the varying national programmes of immunisation for smallpox, polio, rubella and pertussis resulted in a number of cases of encephalitis which was not due to the vaccine used. The evidence is that immunisation in some, could result in activation of a dormant virus of another species; it is well known that a viral illness can activate another dormant virus, e.g. herpes.

We must recall also that rarely was there more than one member in a family who succumbed to polio, though it was shown that the virus could be cultured from the stools of other members of the family. I have recently cultured live virus from the mother whose baby was immunised against polio, the mother having developed a transient facial palsy.

This does not make it easy to specify in time when infection actually occurs. The first titre we do may be high but I have shown in many a persisting high titre month after month, for several years. In retrospect, it may have been high before the first blood was taken.

Related Cardiac Pathology

This raises the question of host reaction and mutation and my family studies confirm that this does take place. "Resistance de passage" makes the virus lethal to the host and innocuous to a foreign or subsequent host. This is seen in family studies such as the W family, where the mother had Coxsackie infection with viral meningitis and was in the last trimester of pregnancy. The baby had endocardial fibroelastosis and died before it was one year of age. I titred the other members of the family and they had significant high titres to the same group. Recently the eldest son of 17 years of age succumbed with viral myocarditis and had to have a heart transplant. That this is not a complete cure is shown by the fact that

his VP1 titre has risen from 25% to 375% and his CMV titre to 1/300.

Pathological Aetiology

I suggest that it is too complex to define simplistically. The reason?

1. Some suggest that a persisting viral infection may be the cause. This can be so, as shown by my family studies, but without any illness. Thus, this on its own is too simplistic.

2. Some say autoimmune dysfunction may be the cause. This may be so, but it begs the question of how, and also does not answer precisely the following questions :

(A)   Is it failure to eradicate the virus before end organ effect?

(B)   Is it failure to prevent cells decoating virus and allowing replication in cells?

(C)   Is it failure in NK cell mechanisms to eradicate cells already infected?

(D)   Is it indiscriminate autoimmune reaction attacking all host tissue, irrespective of infection? This may be evidence of molecular mimicry.

(E)   Is it purely cellular pathology, as collagen and CNS white matter is also affected?

In the light of this, and from my studies, I submit the following as a guide-line, maybe for future channels of research :

Group 1   Comprises those who have a viral illness, most of whom recover without sequelae. Is this purely a blood stream infection?

Group 2   Comprises about 20% who have had a second illness with the same virus. Does this suggest that the virus remained hidden and, due to some stimulus or co-factor, was again stimulated? Is it reinfection?

Group 3   Comprises those where there is definitive end organ effects - be it CVS, CNS, gland, white matter, collagen etc etc.

Group 4 Comprises those with multi-organ effect as in diabetes etc.

Group 5 Alas this is the death column.

From this I deduce the following :

Group 1: There is evidence for complete recovery and possible immunity.

Group 2: There is evidence for reinfection or reactivation of persisting virus.

Group 3&4: There is evidence for tissue tropism which accepts the virus may be previously hidden (self-host) or acquired (family mutation).

To return to the previous hypothesis :

Cellular access

I now believe that it is the host and not the virus which has tropism. Is this because the previous host has mutated the virus? This would explain family sequential illness, where one member "mutated" the virus and made it more acceptable to another family host of similar genetic structure.

Decoating and replication

I now accept this as a step following access and again due to family mutation or failure of interferon activity, only more sinister.

NK activity

Is the lack of this due to the host treating the "sick cell" as an embryonic tissue (coating some with protective CGT) and thus not lysing the cells? In my series in a sinister number this can go on to a state of malignancy.

Results can be :

Group 1 Complete recovery.

Group 2 Recrudescence with or without complete recovery.

Group 3 Organo-tropism and organ pathology. In the series presented it is useful to break it down to ectoderm, mesoderm or endoderm derived organs. In some, eg muscle, repair can occur and be more or less complete. In some, eg CNS, this may not be so and we

must be careful. It raises the query, is it myelin, is it cellular, or is it vasonervorum, i.e. vascular?

Group 4 Is it inordinate immunological activity, i.e. truly auto-immune? If so, then why?:

I might be criticised for presenting alarming material but I have tried to present the truth and this in perspective. The slides which follow will demonstrate the truth as all the patients are well known to me and have been followed up for years, together with the family members. Hence, it is not merely a matter of figures, for the truth is much more dramatic than the slides and statistics.

This bears on the symptomatology, for the symptoms vary. In muscle, it is healthy fatigue which results in the marathon runners holding their arms high in ecstasy, but in the M.E. victim is it gross fatigue even before the exercise commences? In the CNS it is not the tiredness which results in happy deep sleep and awakening refreshment, but in disturbed rest and awakening tiredness. Lastly, it is not "depression" but "oppression".

Investigations

Clinical Examination

Skeletal Muscle: The muscles of the limbs, back and abdomen, should be palpated for softened, tender areas and measured for loss of bulk. Fasiculation at rest is rare but on raising and lowering the legs, peculiar jerking muscle movements are to be found in some cases; this is the visual evidence of the 'jitter' which is found on myographic studies. Raising the arms above the head tends to show flail-like movements in more severe cases and a tendency for the palmar surface to be turned outwards - the so called pronator sign. Some of these I have recorded on video tape.

Neurology: In the long tracts, overt signs are often not remarkable, save perhaps for cord involvement when temperature and touch sensation are sometimes abnormal.

Facial Nerve Involvement: In the face, it is not unusual to find loss of sensation in a 5th nerve segment and audiometry often confirms the tensor-tympani syndrome, i.e. intolerance of high frequencies, which are often painful. Lack of sensation of one side of the tongue or mouth was not an uncommon finding if sought for and the patient would admit having had a scald from time to time.

Bladder dysfunction: It is routinely seen early in M.E. and may persist for several months, very similar to what used to be seen in poliomyelitis. This tends to be seen more frequently in women, and may consist of nocturia, frequent dribbling, pain and less frequently interstitial cystitis. In men, these same symptoms may present as an apparent or pseudo-prostatitis. Frequently, this symptom is misdiagnosed as a bladder or urinary tract infection. The bladder dysfunction may represent a hypothalamic disorder and is referred to in the Purves-Stewart book of Neurology.

Akinetic lapses: This can be observed at any time of day, but is more frequently noted during the hypnogogic period, either when waking or falling asleep. The patients are aware of their surroundings and can hear conversation but are unable to respond or to move. This may last from one to ten minutes and then remit.

Seizure activity: Seizure activity of various types is a common finding in the first year of M.E. but is rarely recognized. Absence spells, noted by family, are an almost universal finding in M.E., though rarely noted by patient or physician. Frank Grand Mal or Jacksonian type seizures do occur but much less frequently and usually remit.

Cogwheel-like rigidity: In some 10% of cases, chiefly those who complain of considerable muscle fatigue etc., there is a sign which should be looked for. This is to grasp the leg above the knee whilst the patient sits on the examination couch and raises and lowers the leg slowly. The observer will find in some, an odd jerking somewhat different from cogwheel rigidity in that it occurs with the patients voluntary movement and cannot be mimicked. It may have some origin in the response of the myofibrils themselves as we know there is a change in the relationship of type 1 and type 2 fibres. Reflexes are usually normal in these cases but sometimes can be accentuated and then the difficulty arises as to whether this phenomenon may have its origin in the spinal reflex arc and not in the muscle itself.

Modified Romberg Abnormality: This is a common feature and may persist years after all other symptoms disappear. The patient may be able to stand well with eyes closed and feet together, but the patient finds it difficult or impossible to do toe heel walking.

Opthamology

Nystagmus, does occur, sometimes only in the abducting eye, but this is not common. However, if one observes M.E. patients in the "CNS group", up to 15% of these have nystagmus.

This failure to focus completely can be shown by computerised testing to be due to saccadic movements of the eye similar to the 'jitter' shown in the limbs and like the limbs, when it is more marked can be seen as nystagmus.

Fundoscopy was performed in every case and not infrequently hyperaemic fundi were observed that may involve the whole of the posterior fundus, or to appear early, as a "cherry red spot".

One notable feature in a number of cases was the inability to focus.

Trying to read resulted in nausea and giddiness in some and in children can be overlooked and put down to school or lesson avoidance. This was observed significantly in many in the acute stage but can persist rather relentlessly.

ENT

Hyperacusis: The tuning fork test is useful for picking up the acute case who finds sounds above the 6.000 range to be very painful. This may be of hyperthalamic origin or be a sign of the tensor tympani syndrome. In the latter there is pain behind the ear apart from sound, but augmented by the tuning fork test. In the hypothalamic disorder the pain only occurs with the TF test and is a spontaneous pain *not* generated in the end organ.

Dermatological

Facial pallor can frequently be observed and this is a feature noted by relatives as usually preceding an exacerbation of symptoms. Relatives note facial pallor when the patient is experiencing a 'bad patch' which may not be a full blown relapse. Sometimes, however, an erythema occurs almost of the 'butterfly' type. This may also involve the 'necklace area' of the chest - similar to that seen in the acute flushing of embarrassment, only in these cases the patient is not embarrassed. These signs appear to be of autonomic CNS origin.

Head, Foot and Mouth Disease: Other changes occur and may be of acute origin as with the hand, foot and mouth disease, usually of Coxsackie A or ECHO virus origin and these have been photographed also.

Liver Palms: Late signs sometimes are the so called liver palms and I have seen two cases where as a late sequel dermatomyositis developed with pulmonary symptoms also. However, one case had diabetes of Coxsackie origin and a liver biopsy showed only a vasculitis of the liver. Thus the liver palm is not definitive of one single syndrome.

The M.E. scoring chart and Hamilton chart should be answered in every case. Typical findings would be about 15 in the former and only 2 in the latter. (The M.E. score chart was formed by the author from symptoms which were annotated as occurring in at least 80% of the hundreds of cases which were carefully recorded). The score chart delineates some of the features mentioned above.

MRI of brain was also undertaken in selected cases but it is not proposed to discuss this here.

Cardiovascular

A routine careful examination is essential, also a pericardial friction rub should be carefully listened for in each case. This is more often elicited at the lower sternal area with the breath held in expiration. Many complain of discomfort in bed when lying in a particular position, no doubt due to a possible mediastinal inflammation, which may be the basis of the pericarditis.

In my 4 decade study, mitral valve disease per se is not occurring as frequently as it did nor is it due to streptococcus infection. The viral disease produces pericarditis, myocarditis and sometimes endocarditis.

It is often not easy to define. In the case of some for whom we have performed open heart surgery, interesting things come to light. One male of middle age developed a systolic mitral murmur suddenly and it was obvious to me that he had ruptured one of his chordae tendinae. This was proved at operation which again I recorded on video. He had to have a valve prosthesis and did well afterwards. In another who had a six vessel coronary grafting performed, the histology showed stenosis **without atheroma**. In my humble opinion, this is similar to the old mitral stenosis in that it is collagen which is involved and occurred in a man who had had a longish history of viral pericarditis with friction rubs appearing and disappearing for months at a time. Two other cases with myocarditis came to transplant surgery and one died. In one youth in whom it was touch and go for a transplant, I gave him gammaglobulin in high doses and he is currently well. It should be emphasised that only a minority developed these serious sequelae.

Dysrythmias, however, are not at all uncommon and occur in the acute stage and can remit. It must not be assumed that this is always so, as some tend to relapse as we have seen and in one where the medication was withdrawn by a hospital department a sudden recurrence occurred and he collapsed and died. They should be followed up for long periods of time. However, sadly in some cases, a fatal collapse occurs. This has happened recently in a 31 year old who collapsed suddenly whilst walking to work. It is also a matter of public knowledge that athletes have died thus when they should have been resting. Also in mutant mice, this can be proven, in that mice, which are forced to swim after virus infection developed a cardiomyopathy whereas resting mice do not. It is not surprising that this should be, as it is well known that patients who were incubating polio and exercised were much more severely affected.

Malignancy

Although malignancy is not a common finding in M.E., certain unusual malignant features have stood out over the last 37 years.

(A) **Retroperitoneal Undifferentiated Carcinoma.** This is an extremely rare malignancy and almost never encountered in general practice. However, over the past 37 years, I have documented close to 10 such malignancies. This appears to occur 15 to 25 years after the patient first falls ill with M.E. Some of these malignancies may be of pancreatic origin.

(B) **Increased Incidence of gliomas, astrocytomas and lymphomas**. These number 16 over the years in patients who had evidence of CNS involvement. Sadly another patient, a man in his 40s has developed a similar lesion and will not survive.

(C) **There appears to be an unusual decrease in the expected finding of breast carcinoma** when the M.E. patient group is compared to the non M.E. patient group. In all my years of practice, I have had only one case of carcinoma of the breast in female patients.

Electrocardiography

If there is any doubt whatsoever this should be done and repeated if need be for the ECG can vary from day to day in some cases. One feature found over the years was the tendency on exercise tolerance testing, using the Tenturi treadmill, for tachycardia to occur without pain, rising from a resting rate of say 70 to a rate of 160 per minute, but without ischaemic changes occurring. This again is not the M.E. syndrome itself but can occur with it as shown.

The usual criteria for myocarditis or pericarditis will apply. I have examined many cases where cardiac involvement has been found, and in fact several died suddenly of dysrythmias. This does not exclude M.E. and in fact, if the cardiac symptoms abate and the patient still complains of feeling very ill, the physician may become very frustrated, not realising that the patient also has M.E. which is the main cause of the distress.

These are the minimal clinical examination requirements.

Investigations

Muscle biopsy studies have been carried out and viral protein has been isolated in peripheral muscle similar to isolation in a viral myocarditis, but this would not be feasible at the moment for all routine examinations.

Serological Studies

A full viral antibody screen is wise, especially for the enteroviruses, but a note of caution, do not assume that the first titre is the highest and a serial repetition is wise to determine any tendency for rise or fall in titre.

Immunoglobulin estimations using the ELISA technique is helpful. This defines the specific IgM and IgG in these cases. IgM was positive in 78% and may signify recent infection. IgG was positive in 21% and may signify prolonged or previous infection. Complement tended to be depleted initially in about 50% with a rise above normal after the acute phase. ESR is not usually raised but can be if auto-immune inflammatory disease is a sequel.

In 76% of this series where auto-antibodies have developed, a leucopenia has been observed with an aplastic type of anemia in the rare case (one required transfusion and it is of interest that after this she recovered - another, a boy, had a RBC count less than 2,000,000). This is due no doubt to a hypothalamic lack of control of absolute RBC numbers. There is evidence that the hypothalamus does control the RBC population at its fairly steady level of around 5,000,000 per cu mm and whilst not frequent nevertheless an erythropenia has been observed in some cases.

VP1 TEST

Recently developed in the Department of Immunology in St. Mary's Hospital, London by Professor James Mowbray.

This defines the presence of persisting viral protein of enteroviral origin. It is helpful, providing it is construed correctly, but it is not a test for M.E. per se. It will be equally positive in myocarditis of enteroviral origin as well as negative if adenovirus is the agent. If it is negative it therefore should be taken to indicate either a non-entero viral infection or if enteroviral, that viral protein is not being replicated and released by infected cells. I have found the VP1 highly positive and the ordinary serological antibodies of the Coxsackie only 1.8.

Interpretation

It is important to realise that these tests all point to an assumed aetiological agent but do not define the severity of the ensuing illness. Not only so but it is possible that other co-factors may be responsible for the incompetent immune response and host vulnerability.

However, it should be reiterated that the height of the titre bears little relationship to the severity of the illness. I have titred family contacts in over 400 families and many have had titres as high as the patient but without illness, albeit some succumbed at a later date.

Autosomal Antibody Tests

Thyroid antibodies are found in my series in about 50% as well as other mitochondrial antibodies. This links with other immune changes.

LFTs are sometimes abnormal and signify sometimes a vasculitis of the liver.

C.P.K. in some is raised at rest and with mild effort can rise to fairly high levels. In my experience this coincides with tender and often palpably softened areas of muscles and, as is found with cardiac tissue, does not correlate with pain per se but rather with muscle fibre necrosis.

Discussion

Aetiology and Relationship to Sequelae

In differentiating between sequelae and concomitant illness it is well to consider aetiology. It is obvious to me that this is not simple for, as shown, a high titre does not signify illness. This is seen with the Mantoux test. Not only so but a family contact with a high titre may not be ill until some years later and may then succumb with a serious illness which could have been justifiably expected with the first contact.

Final Remarks

Myalgic encephalomyelitis has been an elusive as well as a provocative subject and much has been written both by antagonists and protagonists alike, often treating it in isolation, either as a myth or as a separate entity unrelated to other pathology of the same aetiology. This has resulted in a combination of misconceptions as follows :

1. Any concomitant illness of the same aetiology, e.g. myocardial, glandular, thyroid, pancreatic, renal etc., is assumed to be the reason for the malaise. The reasoning is then, that when this is corrected, the patient should be better. In these patients, it is not so.

2. The corollary to 1, that if there is no concomitant illness definable by the doctor, then it must all be in the mind. Varying hypotheses have been put forward to explain this. None of these is really convincing to those of us who have worked in the field for many years and, indeed, cause us considerable distress. This must be minimal compared to the distress felt by the patient when the effects of the illness are compounded by a negative approach, sometimes amounting to a denial of the illness itself.

This has resulted in suicides in some cases and the very act itself is then seen as verification of the original "all in the mind" diagnosis. There is conclusive evidence of the viral aetiology in myocarditis by Archard et al. and also in pancreatitis and diabetes by Professor J. Banatvala, who is also interested in the genetic HLA typing in these cases. I have also documented these.

There is also abundant evidence showing the effects of a virus in the CNS and I have documented a case of M.E. whose serology was positive and sadly, after suicide, the enterovirus was detected in the brain by hybridisation probe analysis. Moreover, the postmortem isolation in this case is of importance as it supported the previous serological evidence of viral infection.

Historical

Finally, it may be well to consider that we do not have poliomyelitis in this part of the world, as least not in the way in which it was remembered. For those who can remember, the diagnosis was obvious and the results long lasting, but that was the anterior variety. Yet, here again, many will not be aware that up to 20% with the virus of anterior poliomyelitis had also a viral myocarditis and the death rate was about

20%. Many have forgotten posterior poliomyelitis was also a defined entity, "affecting the posterior grey horns of the spinal cord". (Dorland American Illustrated Medical Dictionary). This was not so obvious to the beholder but was just as real to the victim as the anterior variety; the aetiological agent was of the same order. After immunisation the scene changed and it is probable that the word "changed" is the correct definition, for this did not eradicate the virus but changed or modified the host response.

In the literature, polioencephalitis is described as seen as well as the spinal and bulbar syndrome. Harrison makes mention of one epidemic where "most patients had this type of disease. The diffuse form is characterised by confusion, agitation, coma, anxiety with a feeling of impending doom, or somnolence. Quivering or jerking of the facial muscles or extremities, flushing of the face, tremor of the hands and restless movements occur. Insomnia may be severe.

In fatal cases, confusion is marked and progressive to lethargy and death. In focal polioencephalitis, there may be clinical evidence of brain damage, or the lesions may be silent and demonstrable only at necropsy. Visual-verbal agnosia, myoclonic jerks, grand-mal convulsions, which occasionally persist for a long while after recovery, spastic hemiparesis, ataxia of one arm or leg, - all were observed. If the medullary respiratory centre was involved, then the rhythm, rate and depth of breathing was affected and the cold, mottled, clammy skin was seen." (Harrison text book of Medicine.)

This is so reminiscent of the process involved in M.E. that we should perhaps begin to consider and take the matter seriously.

> *"To suggest that the diagnosis of M.E. is covered by the term "fatigue of mind and muscle" is equivalent to defining diabetes as merely polydipsia and polyuria and ignoring the eye, the renal, the CNS and arterial consequences which may ensue."* J. Richardson

Opening Remarks of Some
of the Chairmen

Chapter 9

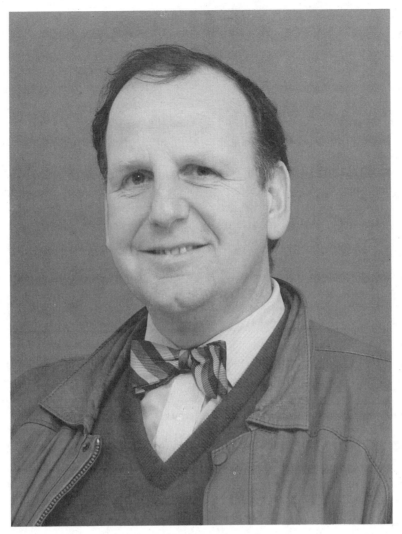

John Campbell Murdoch

This article is reprinted with the kind permission of The New Zealand Medical Journal.

The Myalgic Encephalomyelitis Syndrome

John Campbell Murdoch, MD, PhD, FRCGP, MRNZCGP
General Practitioner, Mornington Health Centre / Elaine Gurr Professor of General Practice
Department of General Practice, Otago Medical School, University of Otago
P.O. Box 913, Dunedin, New Zealand

Dr. Murdoch graduated MBChB from the University of Glasgow and held several positions, mainly in the field of General Practice, in Glasgow, Scotland. While working at the University of Dundee from 1977 to 1983, Dr. Murdoch graduated MD and practised as Senior Lecturer in General Practice, Community and Occupational Medicine and as Principal in General Practice at West Gate Health Centre. Once Dr. Murdoch had completed his PhD at the University of Dundee, he accepted his present appointments in New Zealand. Dr. Murdoch has extensive publications to his credit in M.E. Dr. Murdoch was one of the Chairmen at the First World Symposium at Cambridge University.

Over the past five years in New Zealand, there has been debate concerning the clinical validity of a syndrome, the main features of which have been relapsing fatigue, muscle pain and muscle weakness, particularly on exercise. Other features have included neuropsychological symptoms such as irritability, memory impairment and depression. The illness has affected females more than males and is most common between the ages of 20-40 years. The term "Tapanui flu" has commonly been used in this country, largely due to the fact that the first description of the syndrome here was from West Otago[1]. Since that original description, there have been two further clinical accounts from New Zealand[2,3] and two other studies looking at a possible aetiology for the syndrome[4,5]. In contrast to this paucity of both clinical description and research, there has been much media coverage of the subject and the correspondence columns of these journals have contained beliefs aplenty from both doctors and sufferers, but there has been little informed debate on the facts of the matter, particularly with regard to recent research.

The medical literature has contained frequent reports of patients experiencing similar symptoms since 1934 when, during a polio epidemic, members of the medical and nursing staff of the Los Angeles County Hospital became ill with muscle pain and paresis[6]. Since then, there have been numerous reports of outbreaks in various parts of the world, referred to as benign myalgic encephalomyelitis - a term first suggested for this "new clinical entity" in a Lancet editorial in 1956[7]. The history of the published work on this clinical entity seems to fall into three main phases. The early reports coincided usually with poliomyelitis epidemics and the underlying theme was the desire to connect these with a similar virus[8]. The publication of the papers by McEvedy and Beard in 1970[9,10] claimed that mass hysteria was the cause, but recent studies have suggested a viral and immunological aetiology for the syndrome.

The clinical features of the syndrome have been remarkably consistent over the years during which it has been described, with the main features being extreme fatigue, myalgia, distressing psychological symptoms and a tendency for the illness to relapse after apparent recovery. Many of the earlier reports were of outbreaks of the illness in closed institutions amongst nursing staff, soldiers, nuns and schoolgirls

and the illness seems to have been milder and of shorter duration in these groups[8,11]. It is possible that the reason for this was that the opportunities for observing and recording were greater in these situations where access to medical observation was easier. In the community based outbreaks, eg. in Iceland[12], Adelaide[13], Florida[14], Cumbria[15], and recent case descriptions in Scotland[16-18] the symptoms appear to have been similar to those described in New Zealand. The most recent descriptions of the syndrome have come from the United States where large numbers of people have been diagnosed as suffering from "chronic mononucleosis syndrome"[19-22] and the United Kingdom where the preferred pathogen has been the Coxsackie virus, and where the membership of the Myalgic Encephalomyelitis Society has recently passed the 10,000 mark. Even on purely phenomenological grounds it would seem necessary to take this problem seriously.

The first essential step seems to be to agree on a definition for the syndrome, whatever we wish to call it. A recent list of the criteria for chronic fatigue syndrome by Holmes and his colleagues seems to provide the basis for consensus on the syndrome.[23] A patient is deemed to have the syndrome, if, in addition to two major criteria, eight or more of eleven symptom criteria or six or more of symptom criteria and two or more of physical criteria, are present. A similar list of criteria was suggested by a Working Group of physicians, researchers and patients convened by the Roy McKenzie Foundation in 1987[24]. This suggested that four key features should be present at some time during the course of the illness. These were (a) a relapsing or intermittent course, (b) exhaustion, (c) muscle pain or tenderness and (d) unusual muscle fatigue. There will continue to be dispute over nomenclature. In the view of those who attended the Working Group, the term "M.E. syndrome" seemed to be an acceptable compromise between the doctors who deny any inflammatory process in the nervous system, the patients who have come to accept the term and the long history of the name in the medical literature. The name given to the syndrome is, however, relatively unimportant compared to the need to ensure that a common definition is being used.

Having first agreed what we are describing there seems to be three urgent tasks which will use up all the available energy at present being expended in the controversy surrounding this syndrome. The first is to establish the epidemiology of the syndrome. There is undoubtedly a "halo effect" associated with any outbreak of illness, as was found by Holmes and his colleagues when investigating the epidemic in Nevada[25]. In that case, fifteen out of 134 cases were found to have severe persistent fatigue of undetermined etiology lasting more than two months. However, using the same stringent definition, a study in a Boston general medical practice found that 215 of 500 unselected patients, aged 17 to 50 years, seeking primary care for any reason, were suffering from a chronic fatigue syndrome[26]. They had been experiencing severe fatigue, usually cyclic, for a median of 16 months (range 6-458 months), associated with sore throat, myalgias, or headache. Using the definitions given above, there is a need to carry out periodic community surveys to establish whether such a prevalence exists in this country and whether this prevalence is growing. Murdoch has estimated that the prevalence of M.E. syndrome in the greater Dunedin area in 1985-6 was 127 per 100, 000, but this figure assumes that he had seen all the cases in the area in those two years and is certainly an underestimate[2].

The second issue concerns the management of the patients presently enduring these symptoms. While it is true that we do not fully understand why patients have such problems, it is important that a scientific assessment of the value of various general approaches to management be undertaken. Vallings[3] has demonstrated what can be achieved by a family physician by analysing the response to a whole range of therapies and found that group support was the most effective. The real problem in our dealing with this syndrome is our approach to the patient rather than our differences with regard to aetiology. Werry[27], in stating his belief that many of these patients suffer from depression, has made a plea for diagnostic probing which "should be made clear to the patient for what it really is - our acceptance that something is wrong and that this is our fumbling for a diagnosis, not the assignment of one." It is the relief from the burden of illness, or healing, which patients seek in their encounters with physicians and this healing cannot occur where the physician fails to recognise that the patient is ill or fails to give any meaningful explanation for the illness. Doctors schooled in scientific medicine have a problem where the patient's illness cannot yet be described in these terms. Perhaps in these cases we need to develop an understanding of the philosophic discipline of phenomenology which could be used, according to Baron[28] to bridge the gap between the way we think about disease as physicians and the way we experience illnesses as people.

Finally we need to apply ourselves to research into the possible etiologies of this most interesting clinical condition. Because of the nature of the illness occurring in outbreaks over the past 50 years, effort has been concentrated on finding a viral cause for the syndrome. In the United Kingdom the favoured virus has been Coxsackie B (CBV) and serological studies have suggested higher titres of neutralising antibodies to CBV in sufferers than controls[29]. Enterovirus-specific probes have detected the presence of virus-specific RNA in muscle biopsies from 20 of 96 patients with postviral fatigue syndrome[30]. Positive cultures of enteroviruses were obtained from the faeces of 22% of 76 patients and from 7% of controls in another study[31]. In the United States, the Epstein Barr Virus (EBV) has been associated with chronic fatigue syndrome in several studies[19, 20]. There is a problem, however, in incriminating EBV in the etiology of fatigue states because the virus is a ubiquitous pathogen which infects virtually everyone by early adulthood[21] and because capsid IgG titres may persist at high levels for up to 10 years after infection[32]. The role of EBV in chronic fatigue states has been reviewed recently by Straus[21, 33] and his conclusion is that, while there is evidence to suggest a pathogenic role for EBV in some patients, it is by no means the universal cause. Another virus which has been suggested to have a role is the Human Herpesvirus Type 6 (HHV6) which has been recovered from the peripheral blood mononuclear cells of some patients from the Lake Tahoe outbreak[21].

The problem with the interpretation of these studies is that no one virus can be demonstrated to be present in all cases, in the same way that AIDS patients are all HIV positive. A possible hypothesis is that such patients are immunosuppressed by an unknown retrovirus or herpes virus and that they then become infected by other viruses such as CBV or EBV. Behan et al.[34] demonstrated in an uncontrolled study that 35 of 50 patients with acute or chronic fatigue had altered lymphocyte function in vitro. The acute group showed a reduction in the numbers of suppressor / cytotoxic (T8) lymphocytes and the chronic group showed a highly significant reduction in helper cells (T4) and a reversed T4 / T8 ratio. In fatigue states associated with EBV, the results with respect to lymphocyte function have been mixed with one study showing increased[20] and another decreased helper to suppressor ratios[35]. Two studies[36, 37] have shown decreased natural killer cell activity in patients with chronic fatigue syndrome.

Since the publications of McEvedy and Beard in 1970 which suggested that the cause of M. E. syndrome was mass hysteria, there has been debate on the role of psychological factors in its etiology. David et al.[38] in an important review of this topic, have drawn attention to the fact that hysteria is an outmoded diagnosis which is, in any case, inappropriate to patients seen sporadically in primary care presenting with unexplained fatigue and emotional upset. "Abnormal illness behaviour[39]" is their preferred term for the psychological aspects of the problem and they point out that this may co-exist with a physical etiology. This view is reinforced by Straus[21] who reports that a very high proportion of patients with chronic fatigue syndrome have a history of depression, phobias and anxiety, and that over half of his patients score as being depressed on a Beck's Depression Scale. Taerk et al[40] have reported that 67% of a sample of 24 patients with neuromyasthenia met criteria for major depression and that 50% had a major depressive episode prior to the development of neuromyasthenia. They suggest that the syndrome may be the result of an organic illness in psychologically susceptible individuals. It is important, therefore, that psychological factors, particularly depressive illness, be assessed in the groups of patients to be studied. The presence of such findings may not necessarily deny the validity of the immunological research described above, since there is now growing evidence that psychological factors have a profound effect on immune function[41-42].

Fatigue, pain and emotional upset are the most common problems affecting humanity, and yet we understand little about their causation. While the physical characteristics of fatigue within skeletal muscle can be expounded[43], the distinction between psychological and physiological aspects is so unclear that one reviewer has concluded that experiments could not be done in this field[44]. It is perhaps not surprising therefore that the study of a phenomenon producing all three of these most common symptoms should generate so much heat and so little light. Much more research needs to be done on this most difficult subject before any of us can have the privilege of being dogmatic.

References

1. Poore M, Snow P, Paul C. An unexplained illness in West Otago. NZ Med J 1984; 97:351-4.

2. Murdoch JC. Myalgic encephalomyelitis (ME) syndrome - an analysis of the clinical findings in 200 cases. NZ Family Physician 1987; 14:51-4.

3. Vallings R. Myalgic encephalomyelitis - a consideration of treatment. NZ Family Physician 1989; 16:9-13.

4. Murdoch JC. Cell-mediated immunity in myalgic encephalomyelitis syndrome. NZ Med J 1988; 101:511-2.

5. Simpson LO, Shand BI, Olds RJ. Blood rheology and myalgic encephalomyelitis: a pilot study. Pathology 1986; 18:190-2.

6. Hart TM, Luck JV. Orthopedic aspect of the Los Angeles County poliomyelitis epidemic. Amer J Public Health 1935; 24:1224-8.

7. Editorial. A new clinical entity? Lancet 1956; 1:789-90.

8. Acheson ED. The clinical syndrome variously called benign myalgic encephalomyelitis, Iceland disease and epidemic neuromyasthenia. Amer J Med 1959; 26:569-95.

9. McEvedy CP, Beard AW. Royal Free epidemic of 1955: a reconsideration. Brit Med J 1970; 1:7-11.

10. McEvedy CP, Beard AW. Concept of benign myalgic encephalomyelitis. Brit Med J 1970; 1:11-15.

11. Henderson DA, Shekelov A. Epidemic neuromyasthenia - clinical syndrome? N Eng J Med 1959; 260:757-64, 814-18.

12. Sigurdsson B, Sigurjonsson J, Sigurdsson J et al. A disease epidemic in Iceland simulating poliomyelitis. Amer J Hygiene 1950; 52:222-38.

13. Pellew RAA. A clinical description of a disease resembling poliomyelitis in Adelaide 1949-1951. Med J Aust 1951; 1:944-8.

14. Poskanzer DC, Henderson DA, Kunkle EC et al. Epidemic neuromyasthenia. An outbreak in Punta Gorda, Florida. N Eng J Med 1957; 257:356-64.

15. Wallis AL. An unusual epidemic. Lancet 1955; 2:1091.

16. Fegan KG, Behan PO, Bell EJ. Myalgic encephalomyelitis - report of an epidemic. J Roy Coll Gen Practit 1983; 33:339-41.

17. Keighly BD, Bell EJ. Sporadic myalgic encephalomyelitis in a rural general practice. J Roy Coll Gen Practit 1983; 33:335-7.

18. Calder BD, Warnock PJ. Coxsackie B infection in a Scottish general practice. J Roy Coll Gen Practit 1984; 77:1376-81.

19. Dubois RE, Seeley JK, Brus I et al. Chronic mononucleosis sydrome. Southern Med J 1984; 77:1376-81.

20. Jones JF, Ray CG, Minnich LL et al. Evidence for active Epstein Barr virus infection in patients with persisting unexplained illnesses. Ann Int Med 1985; 102:1-6.

21. Straus SE, Tosato G, Armstrong G et al. Persisting illness and fatigue in adults with evidence of Epstein Barr virus infection. Ann Int Med 1985; 102:1-6.

22. Straus SE. The chronic mononucleosis syndrome. J Infect Dis 1988; 157:405-12.

23. Holmes, GP, Kaplan JE, Gantz NM et al. Chronic fatigue syndrome: a working case definition. Ann Int Med 1988; 108:387-9.

24. Murdoch JC. ME Syndrome. Therapeutic Notes No. 205 Dept of Health, Wellington 1988.

25. Holmes GP, Kaplan JE, Stewart JA et al. A cluster of patients with a chronic mononucleosis syndrome. JAMA 1987; 257:2297-2302.

26. Buchwald D, Sullivan JL, Komaroff AL. Frequency of chronic active Epstein Barr virus infection in a general medical practice. JAMA 1987; 257:2303-7.

27. Werry JS. The ME Syndrome. NZ Med J 1988; 101:642.

28. Baron RJ. An introduction to medical phenomenology: I can't hear you while I'm listening. Ann Int Med 1985; 103:606-611.

29. Calder BD, Warnock PJ, McCartney RA et al. Coxsackie B virus and the postviral syndrome - a prospective study in general practice. J Roy Coll Gen Practit 1987; 37:11-14.

30. Bowles NE, Archard LC, Behan WMH et al. Detection of Coxsackie B virus specific RNA sequences in skeletal muscle biopsies of patients with the postviral fatigue syndrome. Ann Neurol 1987; 22:126.

31. Yousef GE, Bell EJ, Mann GF et al. Chronic enterovirus infection in patients with postviral fatigue syndrome. Lancet 1988; 1:146-150.

32. Horwitz CA, Henle W, Henle G et al. Long term serologic follow-up of patients for Epstein Barr virus after recovery from infectious mononucleosis. J Infect Dis 1985; 151:1150-53.

33. Straus SE. EB or not EB - that is the question. JAMA 1987; 257:2335-36.

34. Behan PO, Behan WMH, Bell EJ. The postviral fatigue syndrome - an enalysis of the findings in 50 cases. J Infection 1985; 10:211-22.

35. Hamblin TJ, Hussain J, Akbar AN et al. Immunological reason for chronic ill health after infectious mononucleosis. Brit Med J 1983; 287:85-7.

36. Kibler R, Lucas Do, Hicks MJ et al. Immune function in chronic Epstein Barr virus infection. J Clin Immunol 1985; 5:46-54.

37. Caligiuri M, Murray C, Buchwald D et al. Phenotypic and functional deficiency of natural killer cells in patients with chronic fatigue syndrome. J Immunol 1987; 139:3306-13.

38. David AS, Wessely S, Pelosi AJ. Postviral fatigue syndrome: time for a new approach. Brit Med J 1988; 296:696-99.

39. Pilowsky I. Abnormal illness behaviour. Brit J Med Psychol 1969; 42:347-51.

40. Taerk GS, Toner BB, Salit I et al. Depression in patients with neuromyasthenia. Psychosomatic Med 1987; 49:214.

41. Baker GHB. Psychological factors and immunity. J Psychosomat Res 1987; 31:1-10.

42. Locke SE, Kraus L, Leserman J et al. Life change stress, psychiatric symptoms and natural killer cell activity. Psychosomatic Med 1984; 46:441-53.

43. Editorial. Fatigue. Lancet 1988; 2:546-8.

44. Kennedy HG. Fatigue and fatigability. Brit J Psychiat 1988; 153:1-5.

Chapter 10

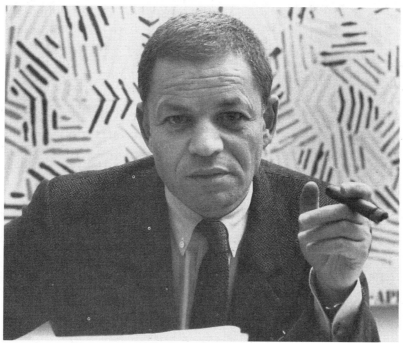

Henri Rubinstein

"Spasmophilia" and/or "Myalgic Encephalomyelitis" ?

Henri Rubinstein, MD
Neurology (EMG) Consultant, Hopital St-Joseph, 11, rue Franklin 75116 Paris, France

Dr. Rubinstein studied medicine in Paris, France, specializing in Neurology at Salpetrière and Sainte-Anne Hospitals. He currently operates a private practice and also practices in the Neurology Department at the St-Joseph Hospital. Dr. Rubinstein has published numerous books and articles, more recently Spasmophilie and L'Equation du Bonheur. Dr. Rubinstein is France's best-known expert in Spasmophilie, or M.E.

Dr. Rubinstein was one of the Chairmen at the First World Symposium on Myalgic Encephalomyelitis at Cambridge University. This was his address to the delegates.

It is now common knowledge that medical practices vary according to countries and cultures; even within the realms of occidental medicine, where therapeutic results are globally equal.

In Germany, a tired individual will be treated for low blood pressure, in the United States, a patient with constrictive chest pain will have six more chances to get a coronary bypass than in Great Britain. In England, a sick person will often leave his doctor's office without any prescribed drug, while, in Italy, he may get a prescription for more than ten different medicines.

In France, we suffer from "crises de foie", a rare ailment across the Atlantic. Above all, we are spasmophiliac, a specifically French syndrome; in any case an unrecognized syndrome in English-speaking countries, who acknowledge only the "hyper-ventilation syndrome", considered to be a demonstration of anxiety.

What about spasmophilia which has an effect on the health of fifteen to twenty percent of the French population?

We understand spasmophilia as a neuro-muscular hyperexcitability that causes chronic fatigue, anxiety, nervous breakdown, loss of intellectual efficiency, headaches, muscular pain, spasmodic colopathy, chest pains, insomnia ...

The primary causes of this neuro-muscular hyperexcitability syndrome are believed to be found in metabolic disorders related to the metabolism of calcium, magnesium, potassium, phosphorus and others, involving either intake deficiency or perturbed cellular membrane permeability.

Spasmophilia syndrome appears to be triggered by physical and/or psychologic stress and occurs, usually, among healthy people, with no known psychiatric background, leading to chronic illness often diagnosed as psychotic depression or anxiety neuroses.

In 1981, the publication of my book **Do You Have Spasmophilia?** answered to a real need among laypeople and focused on this little known disease. The book heartened a lot of patients who were frightened by the symptoms related to the neuro-muscular hyperexcitability.

To find a clear explanation for their numerous perturbations was a great relief for these people who are often misunderstood by their physicians.

The now classical description of various, but especially agonizing symptoms, crippling chronic fatigue, muscular pain, loss of intellectual efficiency, headaches, digestive and cardio-vascular spasms, sleep disorders, allowed, above all, the recognition of the reality and the genuineness of the spasmophilia syndrome.

This is an authentic disease, radically different from mental pathology. Spasmophilia is neither a kind of hysteria, nor an anxious neurosis or a nervous breakdown, nor an expression of stress.

To give a name to this disorder, to take it out of the field of the imaginary diseases, to codify some easy and harmless therapeutic attitudes was a first step. Listening to the patients and believing what they said was, for them, an intense relief. Their newly found well-being was the best evidence of it.

Most of these patients stated that they did not live in particularly dramatic or distressing situations, either in their jobs or in their families; that they did not feel depressed and had no reason to be depressed. But most of the doctors did not believe them. The patients described simply, sometimes angrily, how one day, they felt ill, they became anxious and tired. They related how, for sometimes many years, they could not return either to their previous state or to their health.

They described the real obstacle course they had to struggle with in the medical world that insisted that they were not sick, or that they had a nervous breakdown, or they had too much stress, or that they needed to relax, or to calm down, or to endure, or to change their way of life, their diet, their habits, to take tranquilizers or anti-depressants, or to go to an analyst ...

For this large number of patients, the discovery of spasmophilia was a real break-through. At last the physicians took into consideration what the patients had lived through, what they had been told. At last the patients no longer felt guilty, because the real reasons for their illness were said to be outside of themselves. Their illness was induced by exterior facts, a lack of minerals triggered by a special kind of background, "terrain" in french.

At last they got a glimpse of a way of recovery, and could hope to go back to their previous health, after having corrected and balanced their metabolic disorders.

This hope has become reality for a majority of people with spasmophilia, 70 to 80% regain their health, more or less quickly, after an episode of unbalanced spasmophilia. Of course, they still have to be careful, like a diabetic person for example who continues to check his blood sugar level, but their pathological symptoms have vanished, they lead a normal life, they feel well.

Today, new and exciting facts make it necessary to take a second look at the spasmophilia problem; not for the description of a list of symptoms but for the mechanisms that cause this illness and for its therapeutic consequences.

As a matter of fact, Anglo-Saxons, who, for a long time, turned down the concept of spasmophilia, now describe "Myalgic Encephalomyelitis", a disease that looks almost exactly like our spasmophilia. British and Canadian physicians who wrote to me about this matter were astonished by the numerous likenesses between their subject and mine. And they willingly acknowledge my clinical description.

These are extremely important facts, "M.E." is supposed to be caused by a virus, to be contagious and widely disseminated. "M.E." is said today to be the biggest single cause of chronic fatigue, anxiety and depression.

Like the 'flu, an acute viral disease, it provokes, for a few days, an intense fatigue, diffuse pains, mind obnubilation. "M.E.", a chronic viral disease, causes these very symptoms for months, even for years. An acute infectious beginning may occur in primary "M.E." but secondary "M.E.", where the signs of an obvious viral infection are missing appear to be more frequent.

This virus, as yet unidentified, is either close to the group of viruses that cause paralytic poliomyelitis or is a retro-virus involved in the creation of an acquired immune dysfunction syndrome.

This virus, as contagious as the ones that cause influenza and poliomyelitis is much more prevalent that the AIDS' virus. But, like the AIDS' virus, "M.E.'s" virus provokes an acquired collapse of immunologic defenses. People no longer have any resistance to ordinary infections like colds or sinusitis often associated with mental and physical chronic fatigue.

To demonstrate a viral cause of the spasmophilia syndrome it would be useful to explain some of its still mysterious characteristic features :

Characteristic Features

sudden onset of the symptoms, often described by the patients.
long duration of the disease.
impossibility for the patient, if not healed, to return to normal mental or physical state.
importance of sleep disturbances.
importance of persistent digestive disorders (because of the intestinal location of the virus).
importance of cerebral dysfunctions and of loss of intellectual efficiency.
resistance to healing in 20% of the patients, even if they receive a correct medical treatment.
absence of significant metabolic disorders seen in some patients.
high frequency of infections among the patients (sinusitis, cold, cystitis ...), related to the decline of immune defences.
high frequency of allergic symptoms.

To say more, if the viral assumption is true, we can better understand some of the classical features of spasmophilia :
- acute and chronic fatigue.
- high prevalence of the disease.
- the metabolic disorders, instead of being the primary causes, could be the result of the infection.
- even the very notion of spasmophiliac background, or "terrain" could be a consequence of the large diffusion of the viral infection.

I am neither a virologist nor a bacteriologist, and I don't state positively that spasmophilia has a viral origin; this fact has to be substantiated by the current research. This is why we are here, to tell what we know, to make new hypotheses, and to exchange information.

But I see disconcerting correspondences that arouse our attention, because they lead us farther from the psychological explanations of these agonizing symptoms. Too many doctors are still using these explanations because they don't know, or forget, what biologists have discovered.

Maybe there are several kind of spasmophilia syndromes, some of them related to a viral origin, and others to metabolic disorders. Maybe it is the virus that make us weaker when under stress. We all live through numerous stressful situations, why do only some of us fall ill ?

In a few years, spasmophilia became a well-known syndrome in France. Now the viral hypothesis gives us a new perspective or point of view. That's the way progress works.

From a therapeutic point of view, "Myalgic Encephalomyelitis" is said to be presently incurable. In my opinion, the viral hypothesis is quite encouraging, because we can use minerals, gamma-globulins and other substances together to stimulate immunity. We can search for the virus in the digestive tract. It makes it possible to consider the use of auto-vaccines development of a vaccine.

If a viral origin appeared to be true for spasmophilia, stress, anxiety, depression, are we no longer responsible for these ailments? Will we no longer be responsible for our laziness, our bad temper, our aggressivity, our sadness? Are we no longer responsible for going over our problems during our sleepless nights?

The guilty party is here, easily perceptible in the electron microscope. It is a new virus that wants to get its freedom in the city, that wants to be known, that wants everybody to realize how important it is in our disinfected brave new world.

But it is a very nice virus, indeed. He does not kill us!! He makes us only more human, more fragile, more anxious, even more creative!

He is also an obliging and civil virus, acting like a scapegoat, the scape-virus assumes our responsibility to evacuate it. We are no longer responsible for our diseases, as the virus has destroyed our immunity processes. But we can decide to react, to fight, to counter-attack, to strengthen our natural defenses to live a fuller life.

It is a habit of our time, to make the patients feel guilty. If we are sick, it is our fault, we eat too much, we smoke too much, we do not engage in enough sports, we live a dangerous sexual life, we do not know how to relax, we do not fight the stress ...

The truth is different. If unfortunately, we become sick, it is not our responsibility. Viruses can be mild, like the one for the 'flu, severe, like the one for "ME" or deadly, like the one for AIDS, but the viruses are the same for all us.

Pathogenic agents, toxic or hazardous products are the same for all of us. Losses of minerals, and stress factors are the same for all of us. Risks and perils are the same for all of us in life's wheel of fortune.

People who advocate an everyday prevention want us to live a tasteless, odourless, smooth, eventless life. I doubt this kind of life is less dangerous, but I am sure it would make us die from boredom.

Unfortunately, any of us, at any moment, may draw an unlucky card and become sick, unintentionally; but we must learn to react, and know how to react in order to be healthy again.

Our organism knows how to recognize the real aggressors, our body knows how to start its defence mechanisms in order to maintain or find again its balance. The physician's task is to "put to work the Doctor inside us" as Albert Schweizer said. A physician has to use his technical knowledge to give us the will to heal.

Guilt destroys the defences. A guilty patient is often unable to find enough energy to defend his body.

French spasmophiliacs have already learned to know themselves better, learned how to choose among the medical technologies the ones they trust. They no longer believe theories which contradict the experience they live. A great number of viruses have appeared during history, which have been swept off by medical science.

If the virus of breakdown wants to have its place in the sun and if there is still no vaccine effective against it, we can, at least, do everything we can to defeat it.

Chapter 11

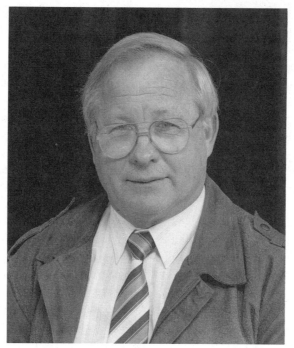

Peter Snow

Tapanui Flu (A quest for a diagnosis)

Peter Snow, MB, ChB, FRNZCSP
Medical Officer
Otago Tapanui Hospital, Suffolk Street, Tapanui, West Otago, New Zealand

Dr. Snow is a solo rural medical practitioner serving a rural community, Tapanui, in the south of the South Island of New Zealand. His research interests include Maori prehistory, Selenium deficiency and Chronic Fatigue Syndrome. Dr. Snow is the describer of the original New Zealand epidemic of Chronic Fatigue Syndrome on "Tapanui Flu".

Dr. Snow was one of the evening chairmen at the 1990 First World Symposium on Myalgic Encephalomyelitis at Cambridge University.

Tapanui is a small rural town in the far south of the south island of New Zealand which services a productive farming forestry district, much like many small towns in New Zealand.

The Condition

Some twelve years ago I became aware of a recurring epidemic of a chronic fatiguing illness associated with lymphadenopathy, myalgia, muscle weakness, hepatomegaly, splenomegaly, arthralgia, myopericarditis, personality changes, headache, vertigo and a multitude of odd neurological symptoms such as parasthesias, dysethesias, shooting pains, dead arm, and dead leg, to name a few.

This illness was noted to appear during the late Winter, peak about late Spring to subside during the Summer months (equivalent to late summer-fall in the North temperate zone). I also noted that this condition was common amongst my farmer clients who experienced a type of contagious abortion in their sheep, cattle, deer or pigs.

The Investigation

During the year of 1983, an investigation of this illness was undertaken which had three aims; to describe the illness, to describe the characteristics of the people affected, and to look for causes. Our conclusions were that a definite disease entity did exist.

We considered a wide range of viral agents: Hepatitis A and B, Infectious Mononucleosis, Coxsackie A and B, ECHO, CMV, Epstein Barr. All investigations proved negative. Non A, B hepatitis remains a possibility.

Associated Animal Illness

Zoonoses were and still are considered, because of the common association with contagious abortion in stock. Most of the abortion cases were undiagnosed but as Toxoplasmosis and Campylobacter abortion, these diseases were considered but proved negative amongst the trial group. Leptospirosis is not a problem in the southern part of the South Island and screening for this disease proved negative.

Selenium

Toxic reaction to farm chemicals was considered but found to be not related. This district is in a very low selenium deficient area. Farm stock require selenium supplementation for good health and some farmers self dose with selenium. No causal relationship to the taking of selenium was found.

The age and sex distribution suggested that it wasn't a disease of psychogenic origin.

The results were published in the N.Z.M.J. The response to the results by the public was intense; they appeared to be aware of the presence of such a disorder throughout New Zealand. The disease was dubbed "Tapanui Flu", much to the displeasure to the residents of our small community!

The Years that Followed

The disease over the years has demonstrated its chronic remitting and relapsing nature. Approximately 15% of sufferers have had a permanent recovery. The rest have demonstrated some degree of impaired health.

The most common complaint has been fatigue of varying degrees exacerbated by effort, recurring lymphadenopathy, hepatomegaly, sore throats, cardiac irregularities resulting in distressing palpitations, arthralgia and arthritis of any joint, but commonly the knees, elbows, temporomandibular joint and shoulders, fibromuscular rheumatism of the neck, buttocks, and intercostals. Cold hands and feet have been a not uncommon finding mainly in the elderly sufferer but not unknown in the young. These were associated with joint destruction, atrophy and pigmentation of the skin. Other skin reactions have been variable. Approximately 50% cannot recall a rash; most cannot recall insect bites, but four of the patients can recall being bitten by insects unknown whilst overseas, resulting in an expanding red rash. The most common rash in New Zealand is a red Tineaform like rash that can recur and come in crops. These are sterile and contain no fungi. They are similar to but not identical with the northern Hemisphere ECM.

I associate this condition with a high incidence of multiple autoimmune diseases such as Thyroiditis, Pernicious Anaemia and Addison's disease.

Finally, the striking long term complications seem to be some degree of neurological involvement. This includes cortical dysfunction such as personality changes, memory loss, impairment of concentration, bizarre visual hallucinations (particularly prior to sleep) vertigo, diploplia, visual loss and impairment, cranial nerve involvement such as Bell's palsy, Horners and Supratrochlear palsy's, paraesthesia's, dysethesia's, loss of power in limb or muscle group, incoordination, ataxia, shooting or lightning pains, sometimes severe, neuritis (intercostal, brachial, sciatic, facial etc.) nerve entrapment syndromes and enthesiopathies, severe headaches often associated with stiff necks and photophobia. All or some of the above can be present in the one patient. Some of the symptomatology is vague and fleeting.

Characteristically, these patients are considered for diseases such as Rheumatoid Arthritis, Multiple Sclerosis, Amytrophic Lateral Sclerosis, Alzheimers, Sciatica, Nerve entrapment syndromes, Myelitis, Cardiopathies of various sorts, and psychiatric disorders. I have been convinced however that the disease process is a multisystem disorder of one aetiology, a view not unreasonably considered with skepticism.

Lyme Borrelosis

Whilst we were describing Tapanui Flu, Steere et al were publishing their works on Lyme Disease, which, in the American model, appeared to be identical to our condition. The Spirochaetal aetiology raised some exciting possibilities, particularly if this Borrelia resembled the Treponemes in its clinical presentation.

It is true that the presentation of the original Tapanui Flu was dominated by fatigue but the syndrome as it progressed seemed the same.

It is also true that New Zealand does not have the Ixodes tick daminni or ricinus of North America and Europe. We do have an Ixodes in some of our sea birds, one of which is a transequatorial migrator, spending a lot of its time feeding off the coast of North America coming to the New Zealand Southern Island groups to breed. This tick is currently under investigation. We do however have a sundry of blood suckers that may be capable of being vectors such as fleas, mosquito's, sandflies and a variety of other non ixodes blood sucking ticks.

The similarities impressed sufficiently for a further trial to be done.

The Borrelia trial

Initial serological investigations on tests performed at C.D.C. Atlanta and then Colorado indicate a positive response to a number of sufferers and some skin specialists indicated they had seen ECM type lesions so a trial was organised by the N.I.H. where Dr. Nick Wilson epidemiologist, Dr. Nigel Dickson, Paediatrician, and members of the Department of Health carried out a sex matched control trial using the flagellar antigen ELIZA test of Dr. Klaus Hansen of the Statenserum Institutes Copenhagen. This test was used because of its greater specificity and a greater claimed accuracy.

Results of this survey indicated only one of the sufferers had a positive titre of 400 OD. All of the others, both sufferers and controls, proved negative to the Hansen test which, incidentally, showed negative results to the positive controls from the United States.

The conclusions were

(1) We do not have Borrelosis in New Zealand.

(2) We may have a strain variation, but according to Dr Klaus Hansen this was unlikely.

(3) Because of the suggestive clinical picture a new spirochaete or Borrelia is feasible.

(4) The result would also question what is happening in the States with regard to Lyme Borrelosis where there is some criticism about the validity of the interpretation of the results. This criticism is centered around the lack of specificity of the test used and the selection of cut off points to indicate a positive result. The other point of interest is that, world wide, it seems as if only about 10% of those tested with the syndrome are positive.

Datwyler has suggested an abrogated immune response because of antibiotic suppression of the immune system.

(5) It could also suggest that the European results should be questioned, which are apparently at variance with the American finding.

(6) The sceptics could be right that the large numbers of so called positives are false, which still leaves the world with what is now a well defined three stage fatiguing syndrome!

Where to From Here

In New Zealand and, indeed, world wide, the condition seems to be occuring at the same rate which, because of its chronicity, means that a large number of sufferers are accumulating. I believe that the effect that the disease has on people's lives is devastating and, coupled with the implied complications using the spirochaetal model, the disease should be viewed with some gravity. I consider that insufficient effort has been put into researching this disorder, particularly in my own country. Finally, I believe the concepts arising out of the Borrelia research in the United States and Europe will have a profound impact on our understanding of the chronic fatigue syndromes being reported from around the world.

Chairman

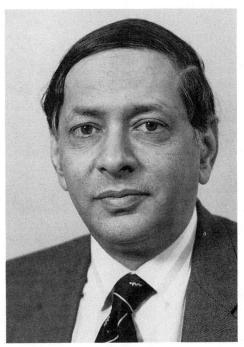

J. E. Banatvala

J.E. Banatvala, MA, MD, MRCP, FRCPath
Professor of Clinical Virology, United Medical and Dental Schools of Guy's and St. Thomas' Hospitals, St. Thomas' Campus, Lambeth Palace Road, London SE1 7EH England

Professor Banatvala has held his present position as Professor of Clinical Virology at St. Thomas' Hospital since 1975 and was previously Reader and Senior Lecturer at the same institution. He is also a past Vice President of The Royal College of Pathologists and a past President of the European Society Against Virus Diseases. Professor Banatvala's interests include intrauterine infections and persistent infections, with particular emphasis on enteroviruses. Dr. Banatvala was one of the Symposium chairmen.

Chairman

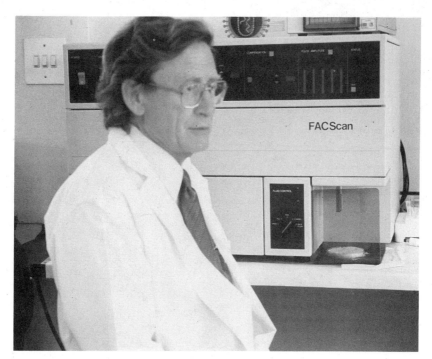

Alan Smith

Alan Smith, MD
Senior Specialist Virologist, Southern Transvaal Health Region
Senior Lecturer, University of the Witwatersrand
Senior Specialist Virologist, National Institute for Virology
Pte Bag X4, Sandringham 2131
Johannesburg, South Africa

Dr. Smith has held his present position as Senior Specialist Virologist at the National Institute for Virology for seven years with a special emphasis on the mechanisms of viral pathogenesis. Previously, he has practised as a Medical Toxicologist (AECI), a Factory Medical Officer (AECI), a General Practitioner in Johannesburg, SAIMR Registrar Haematology, and has also worked at Baragwanath Hospital in both the Medicine and Surgery Departments.

Dr. Smith has a particular interest in computers, whether it be the application of direct interfacing to laboratory equipment, the application of databases for quality control in laboratories, utilizing databases in laboratories for epidemiology research, or LANs (Local Area Networks).

Dr. Smith was one of the Symposium chairmen.

An Historical Review of M.E. / CFS Like Disease

Chapter 12

Myalgic Encephalomyelitis (Chronic Fatigue Syndrome): An Historical Perspective

Byron Hyde, MD, Chairman, The Nightingale Research Foundation, 383 Danforth Ave., Ottawa, ONT K2A 0E1

This article is reprinted with the kind permission of Health and Welfare Canada, Proceedings of a Workshop, January 1991, Vol 17S1E, pages 5-8.

(Please see Chapter 5 for Dr. Hyde's photograph and curriculum vitae.)

Introduction

There have been several viral theories of the cause for myalgic encephalomyelitis (M.E.) postulated over the past 45 years. The principle theories are as follows:

1. Single Enterovirus Theory: one of the following viruses can cause M.E.: poliovirus[1], coxsackie virus[2], and echo group of viruses[3].

2. Multiple Enterovirus Theory: any or all of the above viruses are capable of causing M.E.[4].

3. Precursor + Multiple Enterovirus Theory[5]: an initial immune injury occurs which may be of a temporary or chronic nature and is followed by the causal infection with any of the enteroviruses. This initial immune injury can be due to infection of a different or the same group of viruses or can be due to non-viral immune system injury.

4. Single Herpesvirus Theory: one of the following herpesviruses causes M.E.[6,7,8]:

  Epstein-Barr virus (EBV)
  Cytomegalic virus
  Human herpesvirus 6 or roseola virus 1 (HHV6)
  Inoue-Melnick virus
  Varicella-zoster (chicken-pox) virus.

5. Multiple Herpesvirus Theory: any or all of the herpesviruses (above) are capable of causing M.E.

6. Retrovirus Theory[9,10]: a retrovirus, similar in action but different from the acquired immunodeficiency syndrome (AIDS) and HTLV viruses, can cause M.E.

7. Common Precursor Retrovirus Theory: a common precursor to AIDS and M.E. exists. This may be associated with HHV6 or some other yet unknown virus or viral-like body.

It is the third theory that the Nightingale Research Foundation uses as its working premise. Subjective evidence suggests that there is a lack of significant viral studies funded for M.E. and that this is part of the reason why current information in this area is ambiguous.

This article will discuss the history of M.E.-like disease and the enterovirus or polio-like viruses and their probable role in the cause of M.E. Let us first look at the history.

History

The origins of M.E. are ancient.. A disease complex that may have been M.E. was described in 1900 B.C. and is partially preserved in a papyrus fragment from that date. It is obvious that the origins of this text were considerably older. A complete copy of that information exists in the papyrus Ebers and is dated circa 1400 B.C.[11] Much of the mythology of M.E. was incorporated into western medicine at the time of Hippocrates in the fourth century B.C. and later taken up by Galen in the second century A.D. Galen, in fact, was one of the first to suggest that the disease complex known today as M.E. was related to physical disease and not hysteria. His view was not heeded.

For most of the next 2,000 years there were very few physicians who believed that M.E. or any disease had an infectious cause. The theory of infection, though hinted at by the atomists, was never seriously entertained. The early Egyptian mythology that any unexplained illness is simply due to the gods or hysteria has never died but has simply been clothed in the modern pseudoscientific terminology of the day and has persisted with few critics for most of the last 2,000 years.

The first epidemic of what appears to have been M.E. to strike an English-speaking country arrived in England from Holland at the time of Henry VIII[12]. In fact one of his several wives, Anne Boleyn, fell ill during this epidemic, then called "The English Sweats"[13]. But medical language was rarely written in such a manner that we can be absolutely sure of what they were talking about. This lack of adequate description changed in the 1650s when M.E. was first described by "the English Hippocrates", Thomas Sydenham. Even then, M.E. had several names. It was described by physicians in various ways including "muscular rheumatism", while the common public name at the time was simply "The English Disease"[13]. One of Sydenham's remedies for the many muscle aches of M.E. was Balm of Gilead. It probably was the first symptomatic M.E. medication that actually worked. Let me describe how to compound this first English prescription for M.E.:

Balm of Gilead, The First Treatment

> *Mix one pound of the best bees wax over a moderate fire in a like quantity of canary wine. Add of the best olive oil and Venice turpentine washed to whiteness in rose water, add half a pound. Evaporate the wine by boiling at a gentle heat. Remove the mixture from the fire, and add two ounces of red sandal wood, finely powdered. Stir until cool[13].*

From this preparation one learns why the British were obliged to become a seafaring nation. This exotic balm was applied externally. Not only did this balm assist the muscle aches, it undoubtedly improved many a patient's perfume.

Florence Nightingale

In 1854, the very active Florence Nightingale, while organizing the field services for the British Army, succumbed to an infectious disease in the Crimea. She recovered briefly only to fall ill again. At 35 she had been an extraordinary worker and had worked for years with a diligence that would have exhausted the most hardened general. She became chronically ill with chest pain, headaches, and a rapid muscle fatigue that lasted until she was 60 years of age. She had persistent upper back pain. Numerous heart specialists failed to find any fault with her heart or,

for that matter, any other disease. She would take a short, halting walk in the garden in front of her house but was unable to walk any distance and frequently had to be carried. She was unable to concentrate when more than one person spoke to her and so received only private audiences of one or two persons. Yet, isolated physically from the world in her bed and chambers, she reorganized the British hospital and health services, developed and pushed through the architectural concepts for British hospital construction, started a nursing school, and organized the field services for the Prussian army and the sewer system of Calcutta. We name our Foundation after Nightingale since it is highly likely that she suffered either from M.E. or a disease indistinguishable from it[14].

In 1856, Finsen[15] observed an epidemic of muscle rheumatism and chest pains in Iceland. This was probably the first recorded coxsackie epidemic, later to be called Bornholm disease, and one of the several precursors of M.E. The same epidemic repeated itself in a more serious fashion in Iceland in the district of Ofjord in 1865[15].

The First Therapeutic Regime

In the American Civil War, M.E. surfaced as "Soldiers' Disease" and the neurologist-in-chief for the Union Forces, Silas Weir Mitchell, published a book on this disease. The book was largely concerned with treatment, proposing total bed rest and hypernutrition for a period of several months[16].

The Paralytic Years, 1881-1955

Despite the work of Jenner of smallpox fame and other important scientific workers, until approximately 1880 very few physicians thought in terms of or even believed in infectious diseases or the concept of microbes causing disease. In 1881 this all changed with the first recorded epidemic of paralytic poliomyelitis. This epidemic[17] of 18 cases occurred in northern Sweden. Almost simultaneously another small epidemic of 5 cases appeared in Norway. In 1885 an epidemic of 13 cases occurred in southern France. By 1890[18], when an epidemic of 44 cases of poliomyelitis struck Stockholm, paralytic poliomyelitis was at epidemic proportions as far away as California. In Sweden in 1905, Wickman[19] described the first of the colossal epidemics that were to occur.

In this first macro-epidemic, 1,031 cases were recorded in Stockholm, while a simultaneous and similar epidemic took place in Norway.

Blind to the increasing information indicating that poliomyelitis was due to an infectious process, as late as 1901 Déjerine[20] in France insisted that paralytic poliomyelitis was the result of a psychological predisposition. It is a view proposed by some physicians today when discussing M.E.

The 1934 Epidemic

It was not until the full-blown poliomyelitis epidemic that swept California in the summer of 1934[1] that M.E. was actually recognized as a separate epidemic disease. During that poliomyelitis epidemic another and different type of epidemic occurred among the personnel of the Los Angeles County General Hospital. There were no deaths and 198 or more cases occurred among the nurses, physicians, ambulance drivers, and other medical support staff.

It is important to note that the 1934 epidemic followed as part of a larger California epidemic in which 1,301 cases of paralytic poliomyelitis were hospitalized in the Los Angeles General Hospital alone. Another 1,198 that presented were diagnosed as not having poliomyelitis. What did they have? It is quite probable that many had M.E., but when there were 1,301 paralyzed and dying cases of poliomyelitis, M.E. patients would have been rightly dismissed as unimportant. It is perhaps for this reason that recorded epidemics of M.E. were largely reported among doctors and nurses, individuals who, due to their proximity, could not be ignored.

The investigation of this 1934 epidemic by the Past Assistant Surgeon of the United States Public Health Services, Dr. A. G. Gilliam, was not published until 4 years after the event, in 1938. Dr. Leake, Medical Director, United States Public Health Services, makes a point in the foreword of **Public Health Bulletin, No. 240** of stating that *"none of these cases is definite poliomyelitis."* The report was, nevertheless, published by Gilliam as **An epidemic, diagnosed as poliomyelitis**.

The First Legal Action

Though a lot is known about the epidemic itself, little is known about what happened to the 198 doctors and nurses concerned and, although 54 years later I have been able to track down some of the surviving doctors, I have yet to contact any of the nurses, a few of whom must still be alive. Part of the reason for the lack of published follow-up is the fact that the 198 staff members sued the hospital and eventually settled for $6 million in 1939. Such an amount in 1939, divided among the group, would have purchased 3 houses in the best section of Los Angeles. Contingent on receiving the payment was non-publicity of the epidemic.

Immunization as a Cause

It is apparent from the work of Gilliam[1] that the large majority of the medical staff fell ill with M.E. after being injected with immune prophylactic globulin prepared from the serum of those who had fallen ill during this epidemic. Was this the first recorded clinical transfer of M.E.? The majority of these health-care workers have never fully recovered.

The symptoms of this epidemic were those of M.E. The patients developed relapsing muscle weakness, unusual pain syndromes, personality changes, memory loss, aphasias — all typical M.E. symptoms. Many of the staff doctors never returned to full employment although they were all very young at the time. The nurses in particular were all treated as having hysteria and as late as 1968 Marinacci writes, tongue in cheek, that several of the nurses affected in the 1934 epidemic had been hysterectomized as a technique to treat their hysteria, and that the surgery had not helped[21]. This first, carefully recorded, epidemic disease came to be called atypical poliomyelitis.

The Poliomyelitis Association

Up until 1955, when general poliomyelitis immunization was introduced, many, if not most, of the M.E. epidemics occurred concurrently with or followed epidemics of paralytic poliomyelitis. After the introduction of poliomyelitis immunization, paralytic poliomyelitis stopped but M.E. persisted.

Paralysis

But the nature of M.E. itself also changed. When you

investigate any large numbers of these pre-1955 M.E. patients, as I have done, it is not hard to observe that many are paralyzed and in wheelchairs. When post-1955 M.E. patients are examined, severe muscle failure is common, but paralysis is for all purposes totally lacking. This paralytic facet of M.E. is last described in the M.E. literature by Acheson[22]. This large review of epidemic M.E. is well-worth reading. It describes an epidemic disease process that is identical to endemic M.E. now with one exception: today, in the western world, there are no associated cases of paralysis. Clearly the introduction of poliomyelitis immunization has had an effect on preventing paralysis in M.E. patients. Since 1955 there have been few records of death or paralysis in M.E. epidemics. Clearly this suggests a viral connection between M.E. and poliomyelitis.

The 1936 Wisconsin epidemic of M.E. occurred when a student nun returned to her cloistered school from Brooklyn[22]. Her friend in Brooklyn developed poliomyelitis at the same time as the student nun fell ill with M.E. It appears that the novice from Brooklyn was the source of the epidemic that followed in her dormitory. Up to 1942, 3 epidemics of M.E. in Switzerland were called abortive poliomyelitis[23]. The 1948 epidemic in Iceland started as a poliomyelitis epidemic[24,25] and finished as a major M.E. epidemic involving 1,116 patients. The non-stop 1949-51 M.E. epidemic in Adelaide, South Australia[26,27,28,29], was associated with an epidemic of paralytic poliomyelitis. The 1951 M.E. epidemic in upper New York State, described by Dr. White of Queen's University, Kingston[30], was associated with a poliomyelitis epidemic. In 1953, the M.E. epidemics in both Copenhagen, Denmark[31,32], and Coventry, England[33], were associated with poliomyelitis, as was the Royal Free epidemic[34]. Another name for M.E. was Coventry Disease and it was this name that was used by the M.E. patients in Pittsfield, Massachusetts[35].

The 1956 Pittsfield outbreak combined an M.E. and poliomyelitis epidemic. This reputedly started when an American airman was brought home from Iceland with paralytic poliomyelitis. His arrival in Pittsfield started a mixed polio-M.E. epidemic.

This poliomyelitis-M.E. association is so constant that it becomes boring to even recount the events. Patients with M.E. symptoms were generally abandoned and forgotten in the midst of the epidemic turmoil. There was no time for them. The medical and nursing staff were usually exhausted from caring for the enormous numbers of dying and paralyzed patients.

The Poliovirus Theory of ME is Also Abandoned

After 1955 and the general introduction of polio immunization, people stopped falling ill with both paralytic poliomyelitis and paralytic M.E. but non-paralytic M.E. continued. Since poliomyelitis no longer existed as a major public health problem in the temperate climatic zones, it was only normal to conclude that the continuation of M.E. must have been due to another virus or group of viruses. This conception, of course, was based upon theories of poliovirus immunization.

These theories frame our entire understanding of poliomyelitis and were responsible for M.E. researchers abandoning the polio theory as a cause. For 35 years researchers have looked for another cause. To date, they have met with considerable failure. Before proceeding to discuss other agents, let us make a few final comments on poliomyelitis.

Poliomyelitis is caused by death or injury to the anterior horn cells. These anterior horn cells exist in the anterior part of the spinal cord. Other cells in the lower part of the brain were also attacked in some cases of poliomyelitis. These "motor" cells were responsible for the normal muscle stimulation and function. With the death of these anterior horn cells, innervation to the muscles was interrupted and the muscle "died". But why were these anterior horn cells or other motor cells selectively destroyed or injured in poliomyelitis?

Anterior horn cells have specific receptors for paralytic poliomyelitis viruses. The virus is capable of paralyzing only because it has a specific reciprocal receptor on the motor nerve cell.

Simply stated, polio immunization may work not just by an increase in the antibody response to polioviruses that are capable of causing paralytic poliomyelitis but by a selective blockade by non-virulent poliovirus vaccine strains of the receptors in the anterior horn and other motor cells.

In August of 1989 we received a call at the Nightingale Research Foundation from the Provincial Viral Laboratories. One of our patients had a dangerous rising titre to polio 3 virus. "Is she in the hospital? Is she paralyzed?" "No," I said, "she has simply got M.E." She happened to be one of the few M.E. patients for whom we could tell exactly what virus had caused her illness.

The Immunization Link

At the Nightingale Research Foundation we believe, like Albert Sabin, that many of the enteroviruses cause paralytic "poliomyelitis". We also believe that many of the enteroviruses cause M.E. It is a fact that the majority of M.E. patients today, as well as in the post-1955 period, are not in high-stress occupations as the popular press frequently suggests, but are teachers, nurses, physicians, and other health-care workers. This group represents those most closely related to infectious illness, frequent immunizations, and those most frequently immunized.

Up to 1955, recognized M.E. was clearly previously associated with poliomyelitis. Many of the symptom complexes associated with poliomyelitis epidemics we call M.E. today. In the past we attributed these findings to abortive polio, atypical polio, or posterior polio. The viruses that cause paralytic poliomyelitis are some of the same viruses that cause M.E. But these enteroviruses that are capable of causing paralysis attach to more than one set of tissue receptors. These other receptors are found on different cells in the brain and spine as well as in other body areas. The symptoms described by M.E. sufferers are due to injury to these other cells.

In North America, subjective observations would indicate that very little of the global viral research budget is dedicated to investigation of enteroviruses.

Without heed, we are sitting on the edge of a cliff, waiting for disaster. For many sufferers of M.E. that disaster is already here, and few are listening.

References

1. Gilliam AG. *Epidemiological study of an epidemic, diagnosed as poliomyelitis occurring among the personnel of the Los Angeles County General Hospital during the summer of 1934.* United States Public Health Bulletin No. 240, April 1938: 1-90.

2. Calder BD, Warnock PJ. *Coxsackie B infection in a Scottish general practice.* J R Coll Gen Pract 1984; 34: 15-19.

3. Lyle WH. *An outbreak of disease believed to have been caused by Echo 9 virus.* Ann Intern Med 1959; 51: 248-69.

4. Behan PO, Behan WMH. *Post viral fatigue syndrome, a review.* CRC Reviews. Cleveland, Ohio: CRC Press, 1988.

5. Hyde B. The Nightingale Research Foundation Journal 1989; 1: 16-17.

6. Jones JF, Ray CG, Minnich LL, Hicks MJ, Kibler R, Lucas DO. *Evidence for active Epstein-Barr virus infection in patients with persistent, unexplained illnesses: elevated anti-early antigen antibodies.* Ann Intern Med 1985; 102: 1-7.

7. Tosato G, Straus S, Henle W, Pike SE, Blaese RM. *Characteristic T cell dysfunction in patients with chronic active Epstein-Barr virus infection (chronic infectious mononucleosis).* J Immunol 1985; 134: 3082-88.

8. Straus SE, Tosato G, Armstrong G, et al. *Persisting illness and fatigue in adults with evidence of Epstein-Barr virus infection.* Ann Intern Med 1985; 102: 7-16.

9. Young AJ. *A profile of mononuclear lymphoid cells in patients with chronic fatigue syndrome.* University of Otago Medical School, NZ, 1989.

10. Ablashi D. *Reverse transcriptase recovered in two children with chronic fatigue syndrome.* Presented at the Great Lakes Midwest CFS Conference, October 21-22, 1989

11. *The Papyrus Elbers: the greatest Egyptian medical document.* Translated by B. Ebbell. Copenhagen: Levin & Munksgaard 1937: 108-13.

12. Sylvest E. *History of epidemics, 1933.*

13. Sydenham/Greenhill T. *The works of Thomas Sydemham.* Greenhill translation, bk 1, 1948.

14. Cook ET. *Life of Florence Nightingale.* Vols 1 & 2. MacMillan 1913.

15. Finsen J. **Uagttagekser angaaende Sygdomsforholdene i Island.** Copenhagen 1874: 145.

16. Mitchell SW. *Fat and Blood*. J. B. Lippincott, 1877.

17. Wickman I. *Acute poliomyelitis*. J Nerv Ment Dis 1913: 3.

18. Medin O. ***Uber eine Epidermie von spinaler Kinderlahmung.*** Verhandl. d. x. Internat. Kongr. Berlin 1890.

19. Wickman I. ***Studien uber poliomyelitis acuta.*** Arb. a.d. Path. Inst. d. Universitat Helsingfors. 1, 1905.

20. Déjerine JJ. ***Séminologie du système nerveux.*** Dans: ***Traité de la pathologie générale.*** Paris: Bouchard, 1901.

21. Marinacci A. *Applied electromyography*. Philadelphia: Lea & Febige, 1968: 91.

22. Acheson ED. *The clinical syndrome variously called benign myalgic encephalomyelitis, Iceland disease, and epidemic neuromyasthenia*. Am J Med 1959; 26: 569-95.

23. Gsell O. *Abortive poliomyelitis*. Leipzig: Verlag Thieme, 1938: 20-1.

24. Sigurjonsson J. *Poliomyelitis and the Akureyri disease, mixed epidemics of poliomyelitis and a disease resembling poliomyelitis with the character of the Akureyi disease*. Nord Med 1959; 61: 174-82.

25. Sigurdsson B, et al. *A disease epidemic simulating poliomyelitis*. Am J Hyg 1950; 52: 222-38.

26. Pellew RAA. *A clinical description of a disease resembling poliomyelitis seen in Adelaide, 1949-1951*. Med J Aust 1951; 1: 944-46.

27. Jackson JF. *Monthly incidence of cases*. 14th Annual General Report, South Australia Institute for Medical and Veterinary Science, July 1951-June 1952; 17.

28. Pellew RAA, Miles JAR. *Virus and animal studies. Further investigation on a disease resembling poliomyelitis seen in Adelaide*. Med J Aust 1955; 42: 480-2.

29. Pappenheimer AM, Bailey OT, Cheever FS, Daniels JB. *Experimental polyradiculitis in monkeys*. J Neuropath Clin Neurol 1951; 1: 49-62.

30. White DN, Burtch RB. *Iceland disease - a new infection stimulating acute anterior poliomyelitis*. Neurology 1954; 4: 506-16.

31. Fog AT. ***Neuritis vegitiva epidemica.*** Ugeskr Laeger 1953; 115: 1244-51.

32. Krarup NB. ***Ophobet optraeden of myositer (epidemic of myositis : poliomyelitis).*** Ugeskr Laeger 1952; 114: 1534.

33. Macrae AD, Galpine JF. *An illness resembling poliomyelitis observed in nurses*. Lancet 1954; 2: 350-2.

34. Ramsay AM, O'Sullivan E. *Encephaliomyelitis simulating poliomyelitis*. Lancet 1956; 1: 761-64.

35. Henderson DA, Shelokov A. *Epidemic neuromyasthenia - clinical syndrome?* N Engl J Med 1959; 260: 757-64, 814-8.

The Twentieth Century History of M.E. / CFS

Chapter 13

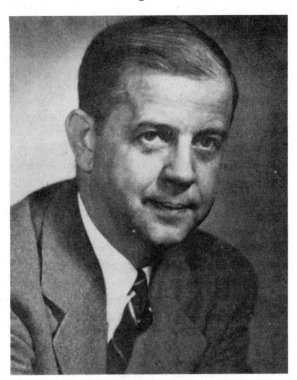

Alexander G. Gilliam

The 1934 Los Angeles County Hospital Epidemic

Review Chapter written by Byron Hyde, M.D., Review of Publication of A.G. Gilliam, M.D.

Taken from:

Epidemiological Study of an Epidemic, Diagnosed as Poliomyelitis, Occurring Among the Personnel of the Los Angeles County General Hospital, During the Summer of 1934

Public Health Bulletin No. 240

Curriculum vitae and photograph courtesy of The Archives of Environmental Health, Vol. 8, Issue 3, pp 761-2, 1964. Reprinted with permission of the Helen Dwight Reid Educational Foundation. Published by Heldref Publications, 1319 13th Street, N.W., Washington, D.C. 20036-1802. Copyright 1992.

Dr. Gilliam was born in Petersburg, Va, and graduated from the University of Virginia and its medical school, after which he took the Doctor of Public Health degree in 1934 at Johns Hopkins University in Epidemiology under Dr. Wade Hampton Frost, whose teaching deeply affected his subsequent career. He was an officer of the United States Public Health Service for 25 years. This period really embraced two careers in epidemiology: first, in the field of infectious diseases, and later in cancer epidemiology. He was the first epidemiologist assigned to the National Cancer Institute, where he worked from 1948 until his retirement from the service in 1960 to become Associate Professor, then Professor of Epidemiology at his alma mater, Johns Hopkins. It was early in this third career that his life was tragically cut off by malignant disease which he bore with great fortitude to the end.

His infectious disease investigations touched upon many problems, of which poliomyelitis was the one to which he devoted most time. He served during World War II with the United States of America typhus commission and while on an over-seas assignment acquired a near-fatal attack of scrub typhus. After the war, he served for two years as the Chief of Epidemiology in the Office of Malaria Control in War Areas, which later became the Communicable Disease Center. His subsequent interest in cancer was broad, but centered upon leukemia, cervical carcinoma, and breast and lung cancer. He was author or co-author of some 45 publications.

While these studies were of uniformly high excellence, an equally important contribution was his introduction of sound epidemiologic methods into new field and his constant insistence of the avoidance of errors of interpretation based on what he so frequently referred to as "jokers" in the data and their methods of analysis. In a kindly way, he was intolerant of shoddy work. His influence as a teacher on his colleagues and students, while difficult to measure, was undoubtedly large.

Those who knew Dr. Gilliam will best remember him for his personal warmth and kindliness. He leaves a very large number of affectionate friends, and a place in epidemiology that will be impossible to fill.

Abstract: *Gilliam describes a disease process, with an acute fulminant onset, related to an infectious disease process that, over a course of six months, generally improves to a level of stability and even one where some of the patients can return to work. For many individuals, the pattern is one of long standing, chronic illness. There is considerable variety in the severity of the disease. It would appear that most individuals described never returned to their original state of health. Since no thorough follow-up examination of these patients was ever conducted, one can only speculate as to the percentages that remained chronically ill. Gilliam also describes the recurrent nature of this disease process. Nevertheless, from the work of Marinacci in the 1950's, one can state that a great many of the women patients who fell ill in the 1934 epidemic never returned to normal work levels or normal health. Although others may have described features of this disease process at earlier dates, this is the first truly excellent scientific examination of an Epidemic of M.E./CFS. Despite the excellent material organized by Dr. Gilliam, it is rarely inspected for the wealth of information it contains. This review also relates Gilliam's work to subsequent findings.*

U.S. Government Resistance to Publication

In April 1938, having overcome the serious obstruction by senior officials in the United States' health bureaucracy[1], Dr. A. G. Gilliam published the first scientific review of an epidemic of what is known today as M. E. or CFS[2]. This small 90 page book should be required reading for any researcher or student of M.E./CFS, for it outlines, for the first time, in clear medical language, many of the largely unresolved problems facing investigators even today.

Was illness provoked by prophylactis?

Not only did Gilliam give the first clear description of the acute and subacute characteristics of M.E./CFS and its epidemiological features, but his book also implicitly posed a question that has been both avoided and unanswered to this day. "(A) Did the 198 health care workers fall ill, or remain ill, solely as a result of the poliomyelitis epidemic of 1934 or (B) did some of the 198 fall ill, or remain ill, as a result of the "prophylactic serum" that Gilliam persistently documents as having been given, often prior to any symptom, to the majority of patients in this epidemic?"

If the first part of the question is true, it would suggest that the viruses causing paralytic poliomyelitis, having sustained one or more passages through a human intestine, a perfect immune modifying system, produced a changed or altered virus capable of acting on different CNS receptors and causing the significantly different disease that Gilliam describes. If the second part of the question was a factor, it is just possible that a new and then unidentified virus, such as the foamy cell retrovirus, was being transmitted into some of these patients with the prophylactic injections. Whatever the process, the second wave of illness appears to have been caused iatrogenically by the injecting of prophylatic serum. Gilliam told Dr. Shelokov that he has been "stymied by his superiors from telling the whole story." For all of these reasons and more, it is worthwhile to go back into source material and take another look at the 1934 Los Angeles Epidemic.

If the question concerning the pooled adult serum and convalescent prophylactic serum as a potential cause of some of the pathology is not clearly stated in the text of his book, there is ample reason for this. We know of the battle that Gilliam fought to even have the epidemic findings published. It was obvious that he was not going to rock any more boats if he was to see the document in print. Today, few know that many of the 198 disabled by the epidemic brought a legal action for compensation against the state and the hospital. The action has never been published but we do know the result. The disabled health care workers were finally compensated in 1938-39, with several millions of dollars[3].

What were the grounds of their victory? Why did the hospital and the state settle? I would be surprised if the role of the pooled human serum given to the majority of these victims was not critical in the final judgement.

Gilliam describes observations lasting from onset to six months after the beginning of the epidemic. Very rarely is the symptom picture described as persisting beyond six months simply because the study did not last longer than that period. This 1934 description is consistent with that found today in early M.E. / CFS patients. Also, as Gilliam points out in his case histories[4], the symptom picture is more pronounced in the first six months and particularly early on in the illness.

> *This observation is the same today: the symptom picture is both more intense and more varied during the first 6 months of illness in the majority of post-infectious M.E./CFS patients.*

Persistence of Illness

The epidemic was studied and graphed from the apparent beginning on the 5th of May until approximately the 16th of November, a period of 28 weeks. Clinical histories were recorded from the beginning of the epidemic in May until mid-December 1934[5]. The longest period of follow-up appears to be 30 weeks[6]. Accordingly, it would be unsubstantiated to assume that those that fell ill in the epidemic were, for the main part, back to work and in reasonably good health, as one would assume from reading some of the case histories.

As far as I am aware, no follow-up study of the chronic features was ever produced. In fact, other than the work of Marinacci, the later literature then forsakes these patients. I assume, correctly or otherwise, that the legal settlement obtained by these patients required total suppression of further medical reporting by the press. Yet it is obvious from the work of Marinacci as late as 1955, that the number of women afflicted in this epidemic was apparently large, many of whom were still ill in 1955[7], 21 years later. This question will be addressed at the end of this document.

In 1989, I was able to speak to two male physicians, one female physician, and to the relatives of one male physician who had recently committed suicide after a long history of unspecified psychiatric illness. All had fallen ill in the 1934 epidemic. The female physician had returned to work shortly after and had worked until retirement in her late 60's. One of the male physicians had never returned to work and another had reputedly had a spotty work history due to chronic illness. There had also been great difficulty in maintaining any long-term marital relationship. However, I was not able to ascertain whether this was due to the illness or other factors. I have no way of knowing if these four cases are representative of the 198 persons who first fell ill. To date, I have totally failed to find any of the women who fell ill. Undoubtedly some are still alive at the time of writing in 1991.

The 1934 Document

It is worthwhile quoting Dr. Gilliam's first paragraph in his report:

"Coincidental with an epidemic of poliomyelitis in the city and county of Los Angeles, CA., in the summer of 1934, there occurred among the employees of the Los Angeles County General Hospital an epidemic of illness diagnosed at the time as poliomyelitis. If this diagnosis may be accepted in any large proportion of the cases, the epidemic is unique in the history of poliomyelitis because of the altogether unusual symptomatology, and the extraordinarily high attack rate in an adult population. If the disease were not poliomyelitis, the epidemic is equally extraordinary in presenting a clinical and epidemiological picture, which, so far as known, is without parallel[8]."

In this epidemic, 198 employees of the Los Angeles County General Hospital fell ill. There were no deaths and the personnel most severely attacked were nurses, technicians and physicians, with an attack rate of 10.7 and 5.4 respectively[9].

It is generally considered today, as it was then, that the major epidemic, starting in May 1934 in the San Francisco[9] area and rapidly engulfing all of southern California, was an epidemic of paralytic poliomyelitis. Yet, by the then considered norms, it was an unusual epidemic.

Gilliam states that, within the hospital epidemic, the 198 adults:

"rarely exhibited the disability that is classically associated with poliomyelitis, namely, paralysis of a kind that might be expected to result from destruction of anterior horn cells."[10]

Gilliam discusses the epidemic figures in Los Angeles City and County. The epidemic was documented for 7 months, from May 6 until December 1, 1934. However the peak period was typical of a poliomyelitis epidemic and lasted 2 months, from May 19 until July 14. He does not give the figures for the state of California or even for the many hospitals in the Los Angeles area, but he does note that 2,499 cases suspected of being poliomyelitis were treated in the General Hospital. Of these, 1,301 cases were reported as poliomyelitis and 1,198 were not commented upon. The median onset of the L.A. epidemic was June 23 and the median onset of the 198 hospital cases was within the following week.[11]

Was the 1934 California epidemic, poliomyelitis or M.E. / CFS? Are they both simply different facets of the same infectious agents?

It was a very large epidemic, but the question arises: was it a bona fide poliomyelitis epidemic or was it an enormous M.E. / CFS epidemic? Were the 1,301 cases that demonstrated primarily muscle weakness, poliomyelitis, and the remaining 1,198 cases part of a giant M.E. / CFS epidemic?

Some of the figures uncharacteristic of a typical poliomyelitis epidemic[12] noted by Gilliam are as follows:

(a) High attack rate: 73.3 per 100,000

(b) Low case fatality rate: 1.39%

(c) High adult age distribution: 29% of all cases were 29 and over but this does not document those 1,198 turned away.

(d) Paralytic cases: Leake and others estimated that the paralytic rate in the Los Angeles area was 50%, but this included any cases that showed slight and often transient localized muscular weakness, only discovered by a careful test of muscle function.

(e) Low residual paralysis rate: Hart and Luck estimated this to be less than 2% of all reported cases.

Experimental Studies[13]:

Rockefeller Institute reference poliomyelitis virus

When this virus was injected into monkeys, it demonstrated a 96.3% complete paralytic rate with only 4.7% recovery.

Los Angeles strains

When this virus was injected into monkeys, it demonstrated a complete paralysis rate of only 22% with 84% recovering. Monkeys infected and recovered from the L.A. virus demonstrated both immunity and higher neutralizing titre when challenged by the Rockefeller strain of virus. This suggested a virus with similar characteristics but a remarkable difference in the severity of the clinical outcome. In other words, the L.A. virus that caused pain, headache, muscle tenderness, muscle weakness, sensory disturbance, cognitive disturbance, irritability, drowsiness, emotional upsets, insomnia, menstrual difficulties, urinary retention and provoked a remitting course with symptoms identical to what we see today in M.E. / CFS, protected the monkeys used in the experiment from more virulent poliomyelitis virus strains.

This experimental model was acted out in real life in Iceland some 20 years later when a poliomyelitis epidemic devastated the population in Iceland, but not where the epidemic of Akureyri Disease had struck in 1947 and 1948[14].

Pathology

In the few human cases coming to autopsy, the lesions were consistent with those regularly found in poliomyelitis. However, "neurophagia was not marked and diffuse and perivascular round cell infiltration was very prominent". Likewise, the monkeys showed "a lesser degree of cell destruction with a comparatively greater amount of diffuse and perivascular infiltration" than seen in monkeys injected with the Rockefeller strain[15].

Acute and Insidious Onset Type Disease

Gilliam is the first to note that the disease process starts in two distinct fashions[6]. He subdivided the 191 cases for which he had good records into the following groupings:

Onset	Category	Percentage
(A) Immediately after an apparent acute infection	poliomyelitis	125/191(65%)
(B) Insidiously or with a gradual onset	missed poliomyelitis	66/191(35%)

The significance of these two names is that he considered both forms as polio variations, but he considers the gradual onset group to be cases of polio in which the initial diagnosis had been missed.

Gilliam goes further than any modern clinician in breaking this Type B, insidious onset group, into three sub-classifications. I have not seen this type of breakdown anywhere else but it is quite informative.

Type one: The patient has earlier hospital admission with another diagnosis, namely bladder infection or enterocolitis. The patient is apparently then discharged and returns at a later unspecified time with what we would recognize today as classical M.E. / CFS symptomology.

Comment: *Type one suggests an initial apparent incitory illness followed with a lacunar period of apparent recovery prior to the onset of M.E./CFS symptomology that many clinicians note.*

Type two: The patient recalls a transient illness, often having occurred several months earlier, (not specified by Gilliam) which resembled systemic poliomyelitis (presumably muscle weakness or fatigue?) or meningeal symptoms.

Comment: *To my knowledge this meningeal type precursor is described nowhere in the subsequent literature but should be. All of us who have seen more than 100 M.E./CFS patients are well aware that many have had a previous unusual illness, either resembling and perhaps erroneously diagnosed as infectious mononucleosis (glandular fever) that may linger for months, following a period of apparent total recovery - or - as a meningeal type illness.*

The meningeal symptoms as a distant precursor are, to my knowledge, mentioned nowhere in the literature except in the London Free epidemic. At Nightingale, we frequently note in both acute and gradual onset patients, a severe meningeal symptom history, usually in the previous 2 year period. The patient will describe an isolated incident in which he / she experienced a severe disabling meningeal type headache "the worst I ever had", "I thought my head was going to explode", "I never get headaches but I remember that one" lasting anywhere from 3-10 days, associated with complete prostration and frequently severe hyperpyrexia. This meningeal episode is usually unique and followed by a complete recovery with no sequellae until 1-2 years later when they fall ill with M.E. / CFS. Approximately 20% of all of our acute or gradual onset M.E./CFS patients will give such a history if questioned. It is my opinion that a similar percentage of non M.E./CFS patients, whether well or with other illness, can rarely recall a similar meningeal episode or do so with such precision.

Type three: No earlier symptom history but a gradual development of illness occurred.

Comment: *This insidious onset with no obvious acute infection stage is regularly described in the literature.*

Temperature:[16]

Gilliam notes the following regarding temperature:

"...fever above 100°F was not a particularly prominent symptom...instability of temperature, with a

frequent daily range from 97-99 °F, was much more characteristic of this illness than a real elevation of temperature..."

In fact, of the hospitalized patients, only 32% of the acute onset group and 16% of the insidious onset group had temperatures confirmed at over 100°F.

> Their charts demonstrated **major temperature fluctuation as the primary finding and the elevation in temperature was the exception.**

Comment: Curiously, the CDC criteria for CFS note elevated temperature as a diagnostic criterion of CFS[17]. In the several thousands of patients we have seen, we have rarely encountered significantly elevated temperature, although patients routinely cite the subjective sensation of feeling hot. When we find an abnormal temperature, we usually register a subnormal temperature. Since we rarely have M.E./CFS patients in hospital, we have never been able to document a fluctuating temperature, although it is reasonable to assume a fluctuation beyond the normal diurnal range. We believe that the CDC criteria may be based upon subjective statements of the patient rather than the nurse taking the temperature.

Age, Occupation and Sex Ratios
Associated with Illness[18]

The attack rate is associated with age, sex and occupation.

Occupation	Cases	Attack Rate
Nurses	138	11.4
Social Service Workers	5	9.6
Laboratory Technicians	3	6.4
Physicians	20	6.2
Maids	6	2.6
Orderlies	6	2.3
Attendants	5	1.8

"...females suffered a greater incidence than males and that among females there was a quite definite selection of the younger age groups below 30..."

"...the epidemic developed more rapidly in the groups

most heavily attacked...earlier and in...higher (numbers) in the communicable disease wards and in the main admitting office..."

The employees of the hospital comprised both residents who lived in the hospital and non-residents. Residents were seven times more likely to fall ill than non-residents.

The epidemic developed in residents working on the communicable diseases wards or in the main admitting office and somewhat later in non-residents at the stations of duty.

Gilliam is not precise in subgrouping the lab technicians as the group with the third highest attack rate. Lab technicians have many different functions. In our experience, the only lab technicians that we have seen who have fallen ill with M.E./CFS are those who draw blood. It is possible that they fall ill due to the fact of constant exposure to a wide variety of patient's blood. However, a more likely explanation is that every coughing patient sent for a blood or urine sample, coughs all over these technicians. If the disease is spread primarily by cough or close contact as Gilliam suggests, then these lab technicians at the front line of drawing blood are the ideal candidates to fall ill with M.E./CFS.

Incubation Period

Gilliam notes that the minimum incubation period was 4 days[18]. This was inferred from workers who came to work at the hospital for the first time and either started to work on the contagious ward or started to work on non-contagious wards. None of the new workers who went to work on the non-contagious stations fell ill, however 6 workers who went to work on the contagious wards fell ill starting on the 4th day. Noting nurses who moved from a non-contagious to a contagious nursing station, it was again on the 4th day that these nurses started to fall ill.

Gilliam's tabulations bring to six, the number of persons in whom the apparent incubation period was 4 days. There is a second peak on their graph at 7 days. It therefore appears possible that the incubation period in this illness is as short as 4 days. But Gilliam, in noting the high attack rates on the

Signs and Symptoms Noted by 1934 Patients

(extrapolated from throughout the 90 pages)

General

easy fatigue on slight exertion
malaise
lethargy, drowsiness
loss of appetite, sometimes to the point of anorexia
diarrhea
constipation
inflamed and/or infected throat
nausea was common and vomiting rare
mild oedema of extremities
negatively affected by cold weather
restlessness
relapses without any obvious precipitating causes
recurrences in some cases were more disabling than the
    original attack
pain in the epigastrium aggravated by eating

Dermatological

one handed failure of nails to grow
rare intense itching
both hypertrichosis and hair loss

Bladder and Uterine Dysfunction

difficulty in voiding, rarely with obstruction
painful burning urination
dismenorrhea
menstrual disturbance in at least 14 patients who had
    previously had no difficulty with increase, decreases
    in flow and change of cycle.

Neurological

photophobia sometimes associated with severe ocular
pain
diplopia
loss of or disturbance of position sense in hands and feet
ataxia

Hypothalamic

unusual sweating
chills

Neuromuscular

stiffness of the neck, back
unsteady gait
fibrillary twitching and spasms
easy fatigue in specific muscle groups
persistent paralysis was quite rare but difficulty in
    lifting against gravity common

difficulty with fine muscle coordination
respiratory difficulties
weakness out of proportion to the muscle atrophy
wandering muscle weakness
legs became numb with little control over them after
    much standing or walking
foot drop from driving car and pushing on gas or brake
pedal
tenderness of specific and general musculature
weakness
cramps
respiratory distress

Pain and Neurosensory Disturbances

neurosensory disturbances were frequently more pro-
    nounced than motor disturbance and were the most
    disabling feature of the illness
mild to severe headaches
frontal headaches
occipital headaches
fronto-occipital headaches
sore extremities
tingling in extremities
numbness or cutaneous anaesthesia
hyperesthesia
paresthesias
pain and aching in feet and toes
neuritis
shooting pains, causalgia
tendon pains, specifically archilles tendon
terrific pain along the spine

Neuropsychiatric

insomnia
extreme irritability
difficulty in concentration
difficulty with memory

Psychiatric

nervousness
apprehension
feeling of depression
emotional instability
depression followed by euphoria
spells of weeping for no apparent cause
emotional upsets varying from slight displays of irritability and impatience to violent manifestations of dislike
to for people and things formerly liked.

communicable disease wards, states that it would be improbable that cases developing over a month after exposure to working on these wards could have escaped opportunities for infection during this time. He also stated that it would appear likely that the incubation period in some individuals might be prolonged, or that repeated exposures to infection were necessary to produce illness in these persons. Gilliam does not comment on the possibility of "well carriers" infecting these patients at a later date.

It is of interest to compare these results to those of the Akureyri epidemic in 1948[19], those of the London Free Hospital epidemic in 1955[20] and that of the wife of Dr. R.K. Davis in the Massachusetts epidemic of 1953[21].

In the Akureyri epidemic, the incubation period was calculated at 5 days[19] and a maximum of 10 days. In the London Free epidemic an incubation period of 5-6 days[20] was given. In the case of Mrs. Davis, she fell ill with typical M.E./CFS 4-5 days after starting to nurse a seriously ill patient with acute paralytic poliomyelitis. Like many of these epidemics, this was a mixed M.E./CFS epidemic. She remained ill with M.E. symptoms for over 20 years. Much later, her husband developed Parkinson's disease.

It would appear that the incubation period is as short as 4 days and that some people who fall ill at approximately 7-10 days may have contracted their illness either from a well carrier or simply through slower development of the illness. It is interesting that these figures are so consistent.

Incubation Period of Epidemic M.E. / CFS	
Epidemic	Incubation Period
Los Angeles	4 -7 days
Akureyri	5 - 10 days
London Free	5-6 days
Pittsfield, Mass	4-5 days

Non-epidemic or sporadic incubation period:

Marinacci, who in 1948 was seeing two non-epidemic cases per month, gives an incubation period of 7-10 days in these cases of what he refers to as Iceland Disease or benign Myalgic Encephalomyelitis[22].

Infectivity

Gilliam notes that, of the 198 cases, 185 were interviewed and, of these 185, 170 (92%) were able to recall a direct contact with a case of poliomyelitis. He writes that this is contrary to the usual experience in careful case investigations during epidemics of poliomyelitis where it is more common to find only about 20% of patients giving a history of direct contact with a case (of poliomyelitis)[23]. The distribution of food stuffs, milk products, water supply and laundry were each independently investigated as a possible source of infection transmission. None was found to be a likely candidate for infection transmission[24]. It was assumed that none of these potential vectors played a role in transmission of the epidemic.

Lumbar Puncture[28]

Nearly all cases in which pressure was recorded showed the spinal fluid to be under increased pressure. Only 3% showed pleocytosis an 16% increased globuline and 28% changes in the colloidal benzoin reaction. It should be remembered that these samples were taken early in the disease process.

Gilliam's Summary[25]

"The observed distribution of the disease is therefore what might have been expected had it been an epidemic of a disease, such as scarlet fever, spread by direct personal contact with cases and carriers. It is quite different from what one would have expected in an epidemic such as typhoid fever, spread by contamination of the hospital water, milk, or food supply. The facts appear to be consistent with an hypothesis of spread by direct personal contact with cases and carriers, with the former playing the most important role. From an epidemiological point of view, the disease was distributed as an infectious disease would be expected to be distributed. Despite the peculiar clinical character of any of these cases, there appear to be good grounds for assuming that the majority of them resulted from infection with the virus of poliomyelitis. Whatever may have been the actual origin and mechanism of spread of this infection, the distribution of the disease was such, both in intensity of risk of attack and in time-sequence, as might be expected had it spread through direct personal contact from the communicable diseases ward and main admitting office."

Family Contacts

Gilliam makes an extremely important observation when he examined the family contacts of employee cases who lived outside of the hospital. He notes that family members of those hospital employees who fell ill during this epidemic, particularly those under the age of 15, developed a secondary attack rate of about twice that of reported cases, and that, when the study was confined to children 15 years of age and younger, the attack rate was three times the expected rate[26]. There is ample evidence of this family spread from both our experience at Nightingale and that of most clinicians who have a large M.E. / CFS practice. However, the only publication that acknowledges such a finding is that of the Mercy San Juan Hospital epidemic that occurred in Sacramento, California in 1975, in which the authors of the epidemic study note that the infection propagated itself through secondary and tertiary contacts[27].

It would appear possible, then, that the patients that developed the M.E. / CFS form of the disease, did so either from contact with infectious poliomyelitis patients, well carriers, or from the pooled adult serum or convalescent serum that was used as prophylactic.

Long Term Chronicity

In his book Applied Electromyography[7] Alberto Marinacci describes the chronic features of the 1934 epidemic. I repeat his comments since so rarely in the medical literature do we find mention of the chronic features of M.E./CFS.

"In 1937, while I was an intern at the Los Angeles County General Hospital I came in contact with many of the epidemic cases, some of whom were (still) hospitalized (three years after the epidemic) and others who were readmitted because of a recurrence of the symptoms. The chief complaints were fatigue, insomnia, impaired memory, emotional instability and hysterical episodes. As these symptoms were often misinterpreted by the attending physicians, many of these cases were labelled as 'malingerer' or 'compensationitis.' This attitude often produced a conflict between the patient and the attending medical staff, and the patients were transferred from clinic to clinic and from department to department."

The first electromyographic evaluation on any of these patients was done during the period 1948-1952, (14 -18 years after the epidemic). Twenty-one patients in all were examined; all were females, the majority being nurses. The main complaints were recurring fatigue, pains and some muscle spasms in the distribution of the cervical and lumbosacral segments. In these cases there was also impaired memory. It was obvious that the chronicity of the 1934 epidemic persisted until at least 1952.

References

1. Private communication between Dr. A. G. Gilliam and Dr. Alexis Shelokov at a Symposium on Epidemic Neuromyasthenia in the mid 1950's, in which Dr. Gilliam related that Dr. James P. Leake, Medical Director, United States Public Health Service and others at NIH attempted to block publication of the report (2).

2. **Public Health Bulletin No. 240,** April 1938, Epidemiological Study of an Epidemic, Diagnosed as Poliomyelitis, Occurring Among the Personnel of the Los Angeles County General Hospital During the Summer of 1934, by A. G. Gilliam, Past Assistant Surgeon, U.S. Public Health Service, Division of Infectious Diseases, National Institute of Health, United States Government Printing Office, Washington: 1938.

3. Private communication between Dr. Marinacci and Dr. Hyde in 1989.

4. Idem, {all idems refer to (2)}, see case histories pages 70-80.

5. Idem, pages 7 & 8.

6. Idem, page 32.

7. Chapter 9, **Applied Electromyography,** Alberto Marinacci M.D., Lea & Febiger, Philadelphia, 1968.

8. Idem page 1.

9. Idem, page 1.

10. Idem, page 2.

11. Idem, pages 4 & 5, also 9-11.

12. Idem, pages 2 & 3, also 48-52.

13. Idem, pages 3 & 4.

14. Bjorn Sigurdsson, Margaret Gudnadottir, Gudmundur Peterson, **Response to Poliomelitis Vaccination**, The Lancet, 15 Febuary, 1958, page 370-371 also

15. Idem, pages 3 & 4.

16. Idem, pages 22 & 23.

17. Holmes, G.P., Kaplan, J.E., Gantz, N.M. et al(1988) **Chronic Fatigue Syndrome; A Working Case Definition**, Annals of Internal Medicine, 108, 387-389.

18. Idem, pages 88-89.

19. Bjorn Sigurdsson, Julius Sigurjonsson, Jon H.J. Sigurdsson, Johann Thorkelsson and Kjartan R. Gudmundsson, **A Disease Epidemic in Iceland Simulating Poliomyelitis**, American Journal of Hygiene, Vol 52, page 222-238.

20. The Medical Staff of the Royal Free Hospital, **An Outbreak of Encephalomyelitis in the Royal Free Hospital Group**, London, in 1955, The British Medical Journal, 19 October, 1957, pages 895- 904.

21. Personal communication between the wife of Dr R.K. Davis and Dr Hyde in 1988 concerning the Pittsfield, Mass. epidemic described by Roy H. Hart, **Correspondence**, New England Journal of Medicine, 1969, vol 281, no 14, page797.

22. Idem, **Applied Electromyography**, page 93.

23. Idem, page 81.

24. Idem, pages 82-84.

25. Idem, pages 68-69.

26. Idem, page 85.

27. In preparation, Ryll E., Chabursky B., Hyde B. **Mercy San Juan Hospital Epidemic**.

28. Idem, page 66.

Chapter 14

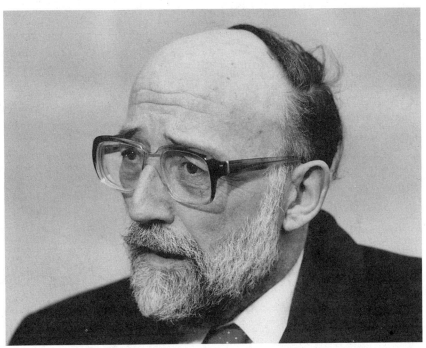

Sir (Ernest) Donald Acheson, KBE

Photograph courtesy of The Times. This classic article is reprinted with the kind permission of The American Journal of Medicine, April 1959, pages 569 to 595. For c.v. please see end of this chapter.

The Clinical Syndrome Variously Called Benign Myalgic Encephalomyelitis, Iceland Disease and Epidemic Neuromyasthenia*

E.D. Acheson, D.M., M.R.C.P.† Washington, D.C.

"Disease is very old and nothing about it has changed. It is we who change as we learn to recognize what was formerly imperceptible."

J.M. Charcot

Recent technical advances have added greatly to the ease with which virological methods may be applied to the study of poliomyelitis and allied infection of the central nervous system. These technics have already borne abundant fruit in the development of a vaccine against poliomyelitis. The accurate appraisal of the preventive value of such a vaccine will depend on our ability to diagnose poliomyelitis accurately. It had long been believed that the clinical features of acute paralytic poliomyelitis were sufficiently characteristic for a confident diagnosis to be made on clinical grounds alone. This confidence has recently been shaken by the finding that the virus of louping-ill (Russian spring-summer encephalomyelitis) may produce a similar clinical picture, even in the United Kingdom[1]. There is also suggestive but incomplete evidence that Coxsackie B, Echo[2] and other viruses[3] may occasionally cause acute flaccid paralysis. The position of "non-paralytic" poliomyelitis is even less secure[4] and the diagnosis can no longer be established on clinical grounds alone.

The purpose of this article is to review a number of obscure outbreaks of paralytic illness, the majority of which were at first confused with poliomyelitis but which were later differentiated on clinical and epidemiologic grounds. Although investigations have been restricted by the fact that no deaths have occurred, the most careful virologic studies have failed to incriminate the polio virus, the Coxsackie or

* From the Department of Medicine, State Univeristy of New York, College of Medicine of New York, and the Department of Medical Services, Maimonides Hospital, Brooklyn, New York. The expenses of the study have been defrayed in part by a grant from the Wallace Laboratories, New Brunswick, New Jersey.
† Radcliffe Traveling Fellow of Oxford University in the United States. Present address: Department of Medicine Central Office, Veterans Administration, Washington, D.C.

Figure 1

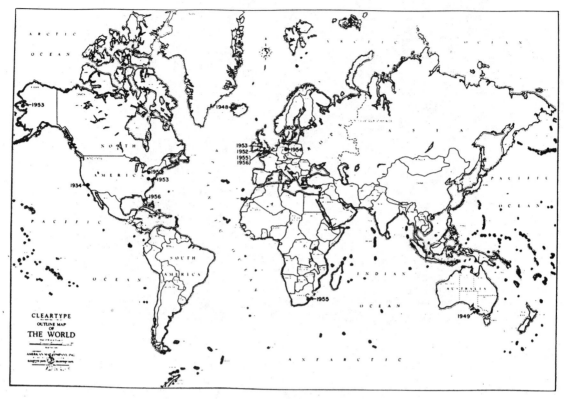

Geographical Distribution of Outbreaks

Echo groups of organisms, or any other known neurotrophic agent. The outbreaks will be compared, and the basis for the view that they constitute a clinical entity will be discussed. Such information as is available about the etiology, prognosis and treatment will be reviewed.

Historical

In the summer of 1934 an epidemic of poliomyelitis struck Los Angeles[5], and many of the sick patients were treated in the Los Angeles County Hospital. Within a few weeks an alarming number of cases of a similar illness had appeared among the hospital staff, particularly in the nurses. As the hospital outbreak developed, certain clinical and epidemiologic features appeared which made the diagnosis of poliomyelitis difficult to sustain. Thus disturbances of sensation and mental symptoms were unduly prominent, and although muscular pain and paresis were the rule, muscular atrophy was a rare sequel. In spite of the fact that no less than 198 cases developed (an attack rate of 4.4 per cent) there were no deaths, and the general trend of the disease was towards complete recovery. A further distinction

from typical poliomyelitis lay in the cerebrospinal fluid, which was normal in fifty-three of fifty-nine cases studied.

After an interval of fourteen years, an epidemic with many features in common was reported in Iceland[6], and later other similar outbreaks occurred in Australia[7], Europe[8-13], the United States[14-16], Alaska[17], and South Africa[18-20]. The names "Iceland disease" (White and Burtch 1954[14]), "Akureyri disease" (Sigurdsson and Gudmundsson 1956[21]), "benign myalgic encephalomyelitis" (Lancet 1956[22]), and "epidemic neuromyasthenia" (Shelokov et al. 1957[15,16]) amongst others have been given to this syndrome. Of the fourteen outbreaks which form the basis of this study, no less than seven have occurred in the staff of hospitals. More than 1,000 persons are known to have been affected up to the present time. The geographical distribution of the outbreaks is shown in Figure 1.

Criteria and Definition

The difficulties in defining a disorder from which no

deaths have occurred, and for which no causative infective or toxic agent has been discovered, are obvious. Recognition has to depend on the clinical and epidemiologic pattern. These features must be sufficiently characteristic to separate the disorder from other conditions. A parallel may be helpful. Von Economo[23] first described encephalitis lethargica on the basis of the clinical triad of fever, stupor and ophthalmoplegia. Although autopsy material was abundant, the pathologic picture was not in itself distinctive and the findings were often insignificant. No etiologic agent or specific diagnostic test was ever found. It was the clinical pattern and the characteristic sequelae which set the seal on the condition as a nosological entity. Epidemic myalgia (epidemic pleurodynia; Bornholm disease) affords a closer analogy. Here the disease became established as a clinical entity[24-26] in spite of the absence of mortality or any specific laboratory test long before the discovery of the Coxsackie group of viruses.

In the instance under discussion, the problem has been attacked by making a clinical and epidemiologic analysis of a number of similar outbreaks in which it has been difficult to sustain a diagnosis of poliomyelitis or any other known infection of the nervous system. All the outbreaks shared the following characteristics: (1) headache; (2) myalgia; (3) paresis; (4) symptoms or signs other than paresis suggestive of damage to the brain, spinal cord or peripheral nerves; (5) mental symptoms; (6) low or absent fever in most cases; (7) no mortality. In addition, (1) a higher frequency in women; (2) a predominantly normal cerebrospinal fluid, and (3)

relapses have occurred in almost all outbreaks. In eleven of the fourteen epidemics symptoms which suggest activity of the disease have persisted for months or years in a few cases, and in eight instances there was an apparent predilection for the nursing or medical professions. Lymphadenopathy was a feature in four outbreaks.

The case for an entity will depend on the distinctiveness of these findings.

Epidemiologic Features

Of the fourteen outbreaks considered in this paper, seven occurred amongst the staff of hospitals; one in an army barracks; two in small towns; two in semi-rural communities, and two in the populations of large cities. The attack rate was measured in eight outbreaks. It varied from 2 per cent* in the Middlesex Hospital Nurses' Home[8] to approximately 20 per cent* in the Nurses Homes at Durban[18] and Coventry[10]. At the Los Angeles County Hospital[5] the attack rate was 19.0 per cent among nurses, and 4.4 per cent for all employees, resident or living out. At the Royal Free Hospital in London[27] the figures were 18.3 per cent for nurses and 8.3 per cent for the whole population at risk. In the small communities at Akureyri in Iceland[6], Seward in Alaska[17] and Punta Gorda in Florida[16], the attack rates were approximately 6 per cent. These attack rates were much higher than usually seen in poliomyelitis.

Ten of the twelve outbreaks in the Northern Hemisphere commenced between April and September.

* The denominator is the total number of nurses employed.

Table 1						
Attack Rates by Sex						
	Males			Females		
Outbreak	Population at Risk	No. of Cases	Attack Rate per 100	Population at Risk	No. of Cases	Attack Rate per 100
Los Angeles 1934	1,779	28	1.6	2,536	168	6.4
Iceland 1948-49	3,339	171	5.1	3,548	294	8.3
Royal Free Hospital 1955	950	27	2.8	2,550	265	10.4
Punta Gorda 1956	497	20	4.0	513	42	8.4

The exceptions were the epidemic in Punta Gorda[16] which commenced in February and the small outbreak in Berlin[11] which began in November. In the Southern Hemisphere the outbreaks began in February (Durban)[19] and August (Adelaide)[7].

On the basis of case to case contact, attempts have been made to fix the incubation period of the disorder. In the Iceland[6], Bethesda[15], Royal Free Hospital[27] and Punta Gorda[16] outbreaks the evidence indicated an incubation period of less than one week, probably five to six days. In Los Angeles[5] the information on this point is incomplete, but a few patients became ill four days after their first exposure, indicating the minimum incubation period. On the other hand, the Middlesex Hospital[8] and Durban[18] reports suggested a longer period of two to three weeks. An incubation period of fourteen days was present in the single case in which isolated contact occurred in the small second outbreak in the Royal Free Hospital in 1956[13].

The general consensus is that the disorder occurs more frequently in women. (Table 1) This is certainly true of the outbreaks in hospital staffs. In the Middlesex[8], Coventry[10] and Durban Hospitals[18] no men were affected, and only one man became ill at Bethesda[15]. In the Los Angeles[5] and Royal Free Hospital[27] outbreaks the attack rates for women were 6.4 per cent and 10.4 per cent respectively, and for men 1.6 per cent and 2.8 per cent. The higher attack rate in women on the staff of a hospital might indicate an occupational hazard rather than a true sex susceptibility. However, outbreaks in the general population confirm the higher incidence in women noted in the hospital cases. White and Burtch[14] regarded the ratio of 15:1 in favor of women in their small series as due to chance. Poskanzer and his colleagues[16] believed that in Punta Gorda, women were affected both more commonly and more severely than men. If the figures for white people and Negroes derived from their house to house survey are combined, the attack rate for women is 8.2 per cent, and for men 4.0 per cent. This female predominance is largely due to a high incidence in Negro women. Sigurdsson[6] found that at Akureyri females were affected more commonly than males in the ratio of 8:5. All patients studied by Fog[9] in Copenhagen were female. In the Alaska[17] outbreak, the syndrome developed in 122 females and 53 males. The attack rates in these two outbreaks cannot be calculated as the population by sexes is not given. Sporadic cases[28-32] are also reported more frequently in women than in men. The single outbreak with a predominance of affected males was that described in a military barracks in Berlin[11]. The patients were all men.

All age groups have been affected from late childhood[6,14,16,17] to the eighth decade[16]. However, many reports stress the high frequency among young adults. In the Los Angeles outbreak[5] the figures show a strikingly selectivity of the disorder for women between the ages of twenty and twenty-nine. In men the relationship to age was irregular. In the Middlesex Hospital[8], Coventry[10], Durban[18], Bethesda[15] and Berlin[11] outbreaks most of the cases occurred in the third decade, but this may be due, in part at least to the composition of the population at risk. Figures from which attack rates may be calculated by age are not given. In the Royal Free Hospital outbreaks[12,13] the incidence was higher in the nineteen to thirty-five age group (11 per cent)* than in older people (4 per cent).* In Iceland[6] the highest incidence was in adolescents aged fifteen to nineteen. Cases in small children have been rare.

A prevalence of poliomyelitis in the area of the outbreak has been noted on several occasions and has made differential diagnosis difficult. The most striking example is the Los Angeles outbreak[5] of 1934. There the cases among the staff occurred after the admission of large numbers of patients with poliomyelitis from the city and the rise and fall of the epidemic in the city corresponded closely with that of the hospital outbreak. Virus studies and autopsy material proved that the city epidemic was poliomyelitis, although there were certain atypical features[5].

However, the clinical characteristics in the cases among the staff differed in important particulars. Coincident outbreaks of poliomyelitis also occurred in Copenhagen[9], New York State[14] and Alaska[17]. In Adelaide[7] and Durban[18], epidemics of poliomyelitis preceded the outbreaks of illness and in Iceland[6] there were a few cases of typical poliomyelitis at the beginning of the outbreak. At Coventry the outbreak occurred amongst the staff of an infectious diseases hospital which was commonly concerned with the treatment of poliomyelitis. In the Middlesex[8], Bethesda[15], Royal Free Hospital[12], Berlin[11] and Punta

* Approximate figures.

Gorda[16] outbreaks there was no known association with poliomyelitis.

Most curious of all the epidemiologic features is the apparent susceptibility of the nursing, medical and ancillary professions. Seven of the fourteen outbreaks have occurred in the staffs of hospitals. In one other[16] a high attack rate among nurses, doctors and their helpers was noted. Thus the attack rate among medical personnel was 40 per cent (sixteen of thirty-eight) as opposed to 6.1 per cent (62 of 1,010) in the community as a whole. In the Los Angeles[5] and Royal Free Hospital[12] outbreaks the attack rates were higher in nurses than in the other hospital staff. In the Middlesex[8], Coventry[10], Bethesda[15] and Durban[18] epidemics the disorder was virtually confined to nurses.

It is recognized that nurses through contact with patients have an increased risk of contracting certain infections. As far as this syndrome is concerned, however, there has been evidence that the nurses might have been infected by patients in only two outbreaks[5,10]. Thus, in Los Angeles[5], cases occurred both earlier and more commonly in those members of the hospital staff who were in close contact with patients with poliomyelitis who had been admitted from the city. On the other hand, the clinical evidence suggests that the illness among the staff was different. In the Coventry Hospital[10], the disorder may have reached the staff by way of the patients. Galpine and Brady[32] were of the opinion that some of the cases admitted immediately prior to the outbreak in the staff in Coventry were not poliomyelitis but an illness identical with that which affected the staff. In the remaining five institutional outbreaks there is no evidence that nurses were infected by patients. Spread in the reverse direction (nurses *to* patients) has either been extremely uncommon[12,15] or absent.

This apparent predilection for medical personnel, particularly nurses, remains one of the most difficult and interesting features of these outbreaks. It should be recalled, however, that a high standard of diagnostic skill is usually available to nurses, and that similar outbreaks in other types of residential institutions may have been unrecorded.

Observations concerning the possible mode of spread are available in nine outbreaks. In eight there is good reason to suppose that the agent responsible was not food- or water-borne. The distribution of cases did not correspond with any source of water or food. In the Iceland outbreak spread occurred along the main traffic route from Akureyri. Instances of spread by personal contact have been recorded[8,13,27] and most authors agree that this is the probable means of dissemination. The best authenticated example is cited by Crowley[27]. A nurse who had attended the first and fourth girls to fall sick in the Royal Free Hospital epidemic became ill six days later. During the incubation period "she had accompanied a surgical case from ward to operating theatre, remained in attendance during the operation, and escorted the case to bed in a different ward. The patient, the ward sister, the theatre sister, a medical officer, a medical student working in the theatre, and the second ward sister all became ill within eight days." In the Bethesda outbreak[15] the discovery of a paracolon organism in the stools of a large proportion of the affected nurses and in a kitchen attendant focussed attention on the possibility of food-borne infection. However, only one doubtful case developed among the patients who were also supplied with food from the same source. The world-wide distribution of the outbreaks (Fig. 1) together with the marked differences in the types of community affected are points against either an insect vector or a toxic agent, both of which have been sought without success.

Clinical Features

An exact numerical comparison of the symptoms and signs reported in the various outbreaks is not possible. Thus in some instances only cases selected on the basis of severity or convenience were examined in detail[6,9,14,16] while in others[5,8,12] in over-all picture of the outbreak was provided. Reports of the Durban epidemic are fragmentary, and it has been necessary to refer to unpublished data[18]. The description of the Adelaide epidemic[7] differs from the rest of the material in that it refers only to cases which were admitted to an isolation hospital from an urban community. Presumably, this would bias the material in favor of severe cases.

Broadly speaking, the epidemic cases have fallen into two groups: patients with definite localized muscular paresis, and those without. Only the former will be described in detail, as it is doubtful whether the latter could be distinguished from many other illnesses in the absence of an epidemic. The frequency of paretic cases in the various outbreaks has varied from about 10 per cent in the Punta Gorda outbreak to 80 per cent in Los Angeles. An approximate over-all figure is 40 per cent.

Mode of Onset. The onset of the illness has usually been abrupt. According to Gilliam's detailed report[5] the onset in the Los Angeles cases was sudden, the most prominent early symptoms being headache and muscular pain, both of which occurred in over two-thirds of all cases during the first three days of the illness. Next in frequency were nausea, which occurred in about half the cases, and sensory disturbances, stiffness of the neck and back in about one-third. Fever, with a temperature in excess of 100°F., was found in only a quarter of all cases and in almost all of these it appeared on the first day of the illness. Muscular tenderness and localized pareses were uncommon initial symptoms, but by the end of the first week they had developed in about half the cases.

In the Akureyri outbreak[6] pains in the neck and back were almost universal in the first few days of the disease. Low fever was also common. Within a few days pains accompanied by paresthesias appeared in the limbs. In the more severe cases fibrillary twitchings of muscles were also noted. In the paralytic cases paresis usually appeared three to seven days after the onset.

According to White and Burtch[14] the onset of illness in the Thousand Islands district of New York State was acute in four and insidious in fifteen of the cases selected for detailed study. The average duration of symptoms prior to the initial examination was twenty-one days. In retrospect, the commonest presenting symptoms were found to have been muscle pain and headache associated with low fever. Coryza, sore throat, cough, nausea and diarrhea were also noted during the first few days. An exact account of the time of onset of paresis was not given, but it seemed likely from the two "representative case reports" that it did not occur before the end of the first week.

In the Adelaide epidemic[7] the onset was abrupt with stiff neck and backache. Headache, pain on moving the eyes, malaise, aching in the limbs and hyperpathia were other common early symptoms. It should be recalled, however, that only patients sufficiently ill

to be admitted to an isolation hospital from a city were dealt with in this report, a striking contrast to the selection of the New York cases.

In the Middlesex Hospital outbreak[8], like the other epidemics involving hospital staffs, the whole population at risk was under close medical supervision throughout. In most cases symptoms appeared abruptly. Headache, malaise and backache were almost invariable, and pain in the limbs occurred early in ten of fourteen cases. Mild pyrexia was present at the onset in nine cases. Vomiting and diarrhea occurred infrequently. In one case there was a definite biphasic illness similar to that which is seen in poliomyelitis.

According to Fog[9] headache associated with low fever was an invariable initial symptom in the Copenhagen patients. In a few it was accompanied by stiffness of the neck or back, nausea, vomiting, dizziness and pain in the limbs.

In the Coventry epidemic[10] the preparetic symptoms were usually insidious and insufficiently severe to make the patients report sick before the onset of paralysis. The premonitory symptoms included sore throat, headache, backache, nausea, chills and lethargy. Paresis developed from two to thirteen days after the onset of these symptoms, usually on the sixth day. In only six of the thirteen patients was fever noted after reporting sick, and in none of these did it exceed 100°F.

In their description of the Bethesda outbreak, which occurred in the staff of a psychiatric hospital, Shelokov and his colleagues[15] confined their detailed description to the twenty-six confirmed paretic cases. Twenty-one of these patients presented with premonitory symptoms before the onset of paralysis. The prodomal illness was characterized by malaise, headache, aches and low grade fever, which lasted from four to six days. Sometimes there was an interval of apparent well-being between the prodomal illness and the paretic manifestations. Occasionally, the prodomal illness was prolonged by the appearance either of acute respiratory or gastrointestinal symptoms, namely, cough, diarrhea, nausea and vomiting.

In the small outbreak in an army barracks in Berlin[11] the patients presented with abrupt onset of headache and low fever. Three days later muscular pains, backache and photophobia appeared.

According to Adnams[18] most of the patients amongst the staff of the Durban Hospital became ill with severe occipital headache, stiffness of the neck, backache and weakness of the muscles of the back and abdomen. Heaviness, weakness and paresthesias in a limb or limbs followed within twenty-four hours. Prodromal symptoms of lassitude, sore throat, vomiting and diarrhea in the preceding ten to fourteen days were sometimes volunteered by the patient, but more frequently were ascertained only by direct questioning. It would appear, therefore, that the prodomal illness in this outbreak was mild in most cases. According to Hill[19] coryza and sore eyes were also occasional prodomal features.

Both in size and in the wealth of clinical detail reported, the Royal Free Hospital epidemic[12] compares with the Los Angeles outbreak of 1934. The following presenting symptoms occurred in at least a third of the 200 patients in whom records were complete. In order of frequency they were headache, sore throat, malaise, lassitude, vertigo, pain in the limbs and nausea. A striking feature was the intensity of the malaise, which was out of proportion to the slight pyrexia. In only nine cases (4.5 per cent) was a temperature over 100°F recorded. On examination the superficial lymph nodes of the neck were enlarged in almost every case, particularly in the posterior triangle. Paralysis and other neurological signs developed toward the end of the first week in many cases. The small second outbreak affecting the Preliminary Training School of the same hospital a year later[13] had a similar pattern of onset.

According to Poskanzer and his colleagues[16] the onset of the Punta Gorda outbreak was insidious, and was marked by fatigue, headache, pains in the back and limbs, depression and instability. The average period between onset and confinement to bed was nineteen days with a range of one to sixty-five days. In half the patients there was a sudden exacerbation of symptoms one to four weeks after the onset.

The Fully Developed Acute Illness. Gilliam's[5] account of the Los Angeles outbreak is of particular interest, not only because of the richness of the clinical detail but because it is the first definitive description of the illness in the literature. The postwar European, Icelandic, Adelaide and Durban epidemics were recorded without knowledge of Gilliam's findings and are unbiased by his interpretation of them. The Los Angeles outbreak therefore affords an ideal basis for comparison with later epidemics.

Severe generalized headache was almost invariable (94 per cent) and was accompanied by some stiffness of the neck or back in two-thirds of the patients. Pain in muscles was also an almost constant feature. The common sites were the neck, shoulders and limbs. It varied in intensity, both from case to case and from day to day, and was usually aggravated by exertion. In severe cases it was agonizing and unresponsive even to opiates. When severe, it was accompanied by exquisite muscular tenderness, tender nerve trunks and by skin sensitivity so that the affected limb required cradles to prevent contact with bed clothes. Muscular twitching, sometimes sufficient to move a whole extremity, was noted and cramps were frequent. Definite paresthesias occurred in 42 per cent of the cases. Low fever, with temperatures which uncommonly rose above 100°F., accompanied these symptoms during the first few days.

Localized muscular weakness developed in 80 per cent of the cases. It was notably variable both in site and in intensity from day to day. Of a total of 152 paretic cases, the weakness was noted within the first fourteen days in 119. In about half it had cleared within four weeks, and in a further 25 per cent within eight weeks. In 12 per cent demonstrable paresis was present three months after the onset.

There is a notable absence of information about the changes in tone, sensation and deep reflexes associated with the paresis. Gilliam admits that full neurological examinations were rarely performed; this was doubtless due partly to the pressure of the epidemic. More important perhaps is the fact that orthopedic surgeons rather than internists had much of the clinical responsibility. As it was, patchy anaesthesia was noted in a few cases, diplopia in thirty-one, facial paresis in three and difficulty in swallowing in six. Other cranial nerve symptoms or signs were found in eleven patients. True vertigo was rare and hyperacusis and deafness were not recorded. Two patients required treatment in a respirator for a short time.

Urinary retention requiring catheterization was a complicating feature in 12 per cent. It was frequently accompanied by constipation. Although these symptoms developed only in the paralytic cases following total immobilization in Bradford frames, Gilliam was satisfied that the time relationships showed that they were a real part of the illness and not an artifact introduced by the mode of treatment.

Gilliam observed the mental symptoms which have been an almost constant feature of more recent outbreaks. Later writers have also shared his perplexity in assessing their significance. In the Los Angeles outbreak they occurred in 30 per cent of the patients. His original description of them deserves direct quotation. "The emotional upsets reported are difficult to interpret. They varied in degree from relatively slight displays of irritability and impatience to violent manifestations of dislike for people and things formerly liked. A common type of upset consisted of crying spells resulting from no known provocation. The emotional upsets of a few individuals were undoubtedly hysterical in nature, but it would be manifestly erroneous to consider as hysteria the emotional instability associated with this illness in all of the cases in which it was present. Other disturbances chiefly consisted of loss of memory and difficulty in concentration. Transient personality changes of varying degrees of severity were relatively common." Coma and reversal of sleep rhythm did not occur. After running a course of four to eight weeks, the illness abated and paresis disappeared in most cases. However, in some cases one or more well defined relapses occurred. The average period of hospitalization was eight weeks.

In the Iceland outbreak[6] paresis was usually confined to a single muscle group, the abductors of the shoulders and the abductors and rotators of the hip being the most commonly affected. Paresis was accompanied by an exacerbation of pain and tenderness in the muscles concerned, together with paresthesias. In severe cases, hyperpathia or anesthesia developed in the affected limb. Coarse muscular twitching was common, but true fasciculation was absent. The paralysed limb was always hypotonic, although reflex changes were reported as variable. Extensor plantar responses were not noted. Cranial nerve palsies were rare and urinary retention was reported in two cases only.

Emotional lability, irritability, depression and lack of concentration appeared in convalescence and were extremely troublesome. The duration of the illness in the milder cases was from two to four weeks and in the more severe cases from two to three months.

In the New York State cases[14], muscular aching often accompanied by head or neck ache was the most consistent symptom. It affected the muscles of the shoulder girdle in seventeen of nineteen cases at some state of the illness, but other muscles were usually involved and pleuritic chest pain was also reported. The aching was invariably accompanied by muscular tenderness and usually by hyperpathia and paresthesias. Muscular weakness, which was common, never coincided with the distribution of the tenderness. The deep tendon reflexes were usually reduced in the weak limb, but atrophy did not develop. Sensory loss was noted in three cases. Marked mental depression occurred in eleven of the nineteen subjects studied.

In the Adelaide outbreak[7] the acute illness was short. Following the development of severe headache and mild generalized muscular aching, widespread paresis occurred. It cleared rapidly after a few days. Cranial nerve palsies, paresthesias and hyperpathia were rare. Retention of urine occurred in a number of cases. A recrudescence of the disease, characterized by hyperacusis, depression and fatigue, often occurred four to eight weeks after the original illness. It was protracted and resistant to treatment.

In the Middlesex Hospital outbreak[8] the characteristic features were "the association of severe muscular pain affecting the back, limbs, abdomen and chest with evidence of mild involvement of the central nervous system in which the weight of the damage appeared to fall on the pyramidal tracts, the posterior columns, and the cranial nerves rather than on the anterior horn cells". Following the prodromal symptoms already described, nine of the fourteen patients experienced sudden onset of pain, tenderness spasm and paresis in the muscles of a limb or limbs associated with paresthesias and hyperpathia. The discomfort was always sufficiently severe to require full doses of analgesics for relief. Any handling of the limb at the bedside was resented and the patient could not bear the weight of the bed clothes upon it. The paresis was usually most marked in the distal muscles and was accompanied by variable reflex changes. The plantar response was frequently extensor on the paralysed side and loss of vibration sense was common in affected limbs. Pleuritic chest pain and urinary retention and incontinence were also prominent features. In the cranial nerves nystagmus was almost invariable, and vertigo, deafness and paresis of the soft palate were also reported. One patient was nursed in a respirator for a short time. In most cases the muscular pain and paresis had disappeared by the end of the third week. Relapses in the second and third weeks occurred in a few cases. Emotional disturbances were common in the acute stage, but did not persist into convalescence[8a].

In Copenhagen[9] the fully developed syndrome was characterized by severe pain and unpleasant paresthesias in the extremities. Definite paresis associated with increased deep reflexes was present in one patient and weakness and clumsiness in several others. Hyperhidrosis and muscular tenderness also occurred in the affected limbs. Nystagmus, diplopia, ptosis and extensor responses were each noted on one occasion. Depression and mental lability were prominent.

In the Coventry cases[10] the onset of paresis was coupled with an exacerbation of headache and pain in the neck and usually first manifested itself by clumsiness and heaviness of a limb. Muscular pain occurred but does not appear to have been severe. Chest and abdominal pain are not described. Tenderness, unsteadiness in response to effort and hyperpathia were often noted. Temporary loss of position sense was found in four patients. The deep reflexes in the affected limb were usually diminished and the plantar responses were flexor. Difficulty in micturition was noted in four cases. Recovery took place in some instances within a month, and in all cases was substantially complete within two months. Lack of concentration and ability to memorize was described as a characteristic symptom in convalescence.

Shelokov's[15] description of the Bethesda outbreak resembles the Coventry epidemic in many ways. The onset of paresis was heralded by an exacerbation of the headache and stiffness of the neck, together with heaviness and numbness in one or more limbs. Myalgia and muscular tenderness were invariable in the paralysed limbs and pleuritic chest pain was also

noted. Paresthesias were common and were sometimes accompanied by changes on formal sensory testing. Nervousness, unprovoked crying spells, difficulty in concentration, undue irritability and anxiety occurred in nineteen of twenty-six patients studied in detail. Nausea, diarrhea, somnolence and insomnia were unusual manifestations of this outbreak. Cranial nerve palsies were not mentioned.

In the Alaska outbreak[17] muscular pain was accompanied by photophobia, hyperacusis, disturbances of taste and extreme anxiety. Paresthesias were common. Use of the affected muscles exacerbated the pain, but marked muscular tenderness did not occur. Tremors in the acute stage were a bad prognostic sign as far as the subsequent development of paralysis was concerned. Muscular weakness was widespread and commonly affected one or the other side of the body exclusively. Incoordination and myoclonic jerks were also seen, and constipation and transient urinary retention were common.

The clinical account of the small Berlin outbreak[11] is incomplete. Severe pains in the limbs with muscular tenderness were invariable. Paresthesias and other sensory changes are not mentioned. Slight muscular weakness unaccompanied by reflex changes developed in three of the seven cases and hyperacusis in two. Depression was a feature in three patients and persisted into convalescence. Conjunctival injection occurred in five patients and an erythematous rash in two.

In the extensive outbreak among the nurses at the Addington Hospital, Durban[18-20] the onset of paresis, backache, shoulder girdle and subcostal pain followed an ill-defined period of prodromal symptoms. Headache, if pre-existing, became very severe at this stage. Weakness of the abdomen and back were so common that the inability to sit up from the supine posture became an important early diagnostic sign. Paresis in a limb was usually accompanied by paresthesias and patchy sensory loss. Posterior column signs were also noted. The deep reflexes were usually altered in a paralysed limb. Although the plantar responses were equivocal on a number of occasions, they were never frankly extensor. Retention of urine occurred in ten cases. Affection of the cranial nerves was rare[19] and was limited to a few instances of facial paresis and perceptive deafness. Mental symptoms were prominent, particularly in the severer cases and included defective concentration and memory, drowsiness, emotional instability and nightmares. In the majority, full recovery occurred within two months. Muscular atrophy was never observed.

In the epidemic at the Royal Free Hospital[12] no clear division of symptoms into those appearing early and late was possible. Neurological manifestations appeared most commonly in the second and subsequent weeks of the disease, but occasionally in the first. The fully developed clinical picture consisted of pain in the neck, back, subcostal region or limbs, out of all proportion to the degree of pyrexia, and general constitutional disturbance, and dizziness. The intensity of the symptoms fluctuated widely from day to day but on occasion the pain required the strongest analgesics for relief. Pyrexia rarely reached 100°F., and there was little tachycardia. Tender enlargement of the cervical lymph nodes was almost invariable. The liver was palpable in 8.5 per cent of cases.

The neurological symptoms and signs which developed in 148 (74 per cent) were believed to form "a characteristic picture that distinguishes this disease from other infections of the nervous system." Hypersomnia, nightmares, panic states, uncontrollable weeping and amnesia were frequent symptoms in the acute state. In six patients severe mental illness developed in which the dominant feature was depression. Two of these had to be committed and subsequently were treated with convulsive therapy; a third took her own life. Cranial nerve lesions occurred in sixty-nine of the 200 fully documented cases, the ocular, facial and acoustic nerves being most commonly affected. Bulbar palsy appeared in eleven cases.

In the limbs, motor weakness occurred in 102 patients and sensory disturbances in eighty-two. The paresis was almost invariably accompanied by pain and marked muscular tenderness and the slightest attempt at active or passive movement was resented. Cutaneous hyperpathia, paresthesias and loss of position and vibration sense were common accompaniments. Spasm, fasciculation and myoclonic jerks occurred less frequently. The paresis was usually most marked in the peripheral muscles and was commonly of hemiplegic distribution. The deep tendon reflexes were sluggish in the early stages and

exaggerated later in the disease. They were never abolished. Frank extensor plantar responses occurred in two cases only, but equivocal or absent responses were common. Muscular wasting occurred in two cases. Bladder dysfunction, including retention of urine, developed in one-fourth of the patients. In the phase of recovery, jerkiness of the paretic limbs in response to voluntary movement was noted and considered to be characteristic. (A similar phenomenon was also noted in the Coventry and Durban outbreaks.)

The clinical picture of the Punta Gorda outbreak[16] was described on the basis of the findings in twenty-one of thirty patients interviewed between May 24 and June 6, 1956, "who presented similar histories of illness, and had no major intercurrent medical problems." It will be recalled that these patients had been ill with vague symptoms for periods ranging from one to sixty-five days. The most prominent general symptom was fatigue coupled with headache, pain in the neck, nausea and vomiting. Depression and impaired memory was present in nineteen, and was associated with terrifying dreams and episodes of crying without provocation. Symptoms suggesting involvement of the central nervous system consisted of paresthesias, unsteadiness, vertigo, blurring of vision and diplopia. The account of paresis is confusing and is recorded as present in eight cases in the text, and in only two cases in the accompanying table. In any case, it appears to have been mild and localized, and other neurological signs were absent. It seems that the illness in Punta Gorda ran a subacute rather than an acute course, and that objective evidence of disease was minimal.

Status of Patients on Discharge from Hospital. In addition to formal follow-up studies, some information is available about the state of health of the patients on discharge from the hospital, and in the case of nurses, about the total time lost from work.

According to Gilliam[5], the average period which elapsed from the onset of illness to return to duty in Los Angeles was 13.6 weeks, but this figure is based on less than half the cases, as 55 per cent of the patients were still on the sick list at the time of his report. When he last observed them, forty-three patients (22 per cent) still had definite localized paresis, and in eighteen this was moderate or severe.

Muscular atrophy was a rare sequel and in the ten cases in which it was noted it was slight. He stated that the irregularities in the course of the disease and the peculiarities of the paresis forbade an accurate estimate of the recovery rate.

Adnams[18] gives an account of the disability rate in the Durban Hospital outbreak six months after the appearance of the last case. Of ninety-eight nurses, fifty had returned to full duty with no apparent sequelae, and a further thirty-two were on duty with "mild or more serious residua." Seven were on sick leave with serious sequelae, seven were on vacation or had resigned, and two had been readmitted to the hospital in relapse. In mild cases full recovery of muscular power occurred within a few days and convalescence, which was punctuated by headache, aching and fatigue, was complete within a month. In moderate cases the return to normal took three to four months. In the severe cases, which fortunately were few, relapses were continuing up to seven months after the onset.

In the Royal Free Hospital outbreak[12], the duration of hospital in-patient treatment was less than one month in 57 per cent; from one to two months in 28.5 per cent; from two to three months in 7.5 per cent and more than three months in the remaining 7 per cent. Convalescence was very prolonged, "and extreme fatigue and general aches and pains made the rehabilitation period extremely tedious and long." A period of six weeks convalescence was found necessary for patients who had been in bed for more than a month. Even when this was completed many patients could work only four hours a day. Four patients still had marked disability at the time of the report, two years after the epidemic. In one patient choreoathetoid movements had developed in her paralysed right hand; two required leg callipers and a fourth crutches.

In the Middlesex Hospital outbreak[8], seven of the fourteen patients showed no physical signs of disease on discharge from the hospital on an average of one month after the onset. Of the remainder, four showed mild pyramidal tract involvement, one had absent position and vibration sense in the right foot, another had mild bilateral deafness of the inner ear, and a third had patchy anesthesia involving the left thigh with marked tenderness of the underlying muscle.

The Aftermath. Relapses: The majority of patients afflicted in these outbreaks have been discharged from the hospital within two months and have returned to work after a period of convalescence prolonged by fatigue, aches and pains, depression and lack of concentration. However, in a proportion which has varied from outbreak to outbreak, relapses or a chronic state of ill health have developed.

Relapses have been a feature of all outbreaks except one (Coventry[10]). They have usually occurred within a week or two of the initial illness, while the patient was still in the hospital, but in some instances they have necessitated a second admission to the hospital. In the New York State cases[14] the timing of the relapses was not described, but they are mentioned indirectly as a feature in common with the Iceland outbreak. In the Punta Gorda outbreak the course was subacute from the onset and exacerbations, rather than relapses, occurred. In five outbreaks[5, 9, 15, 16, 17] relapses or exacerbations of symptoms in women have coincided with menstrual periods. Physical exertion and cold weather have also been incriminated. Most reports indicate that the chance of relapse diminished with the interval after recovery from the initial illness and that recurrences are rare after the end of the third month. However, Deisher[17] described cyclical recurrences in many of his patients up to two and a half years after the first illness, but it is not clear whether these were relapses in apparently healthy people or repeated exacerbations of chronic symptoms. Galpine and Brady[32] have described a second attack three years after a previous similar illness. There had been complete recovery in the interim with perfect health.

The relapses have consisted either of a return of paresis to areas previously affected, or to fresh areas, accompanied in some cases by fresh neurological signs, or simply of fresh muscular pains or mental symptoms. Fever is a frequent but not invariable accompaniment. Little has been added to Gilliam's original description, "Following a recrudescence of constitutional symptoms there was frequently an extension of pain or weakness into muscle groups not previously involved. In many cases the constitutional symptoms during the recurrences were considerably more severe than at onset...The milder "relapses" were sufficiently annoying that all convalescents were constantly "keyed up" in fear they would develop one. There appeared to be no predisposing cause for them, though in many, they were associated with untimely overexertion or with some phase, usually the onset, of menstruation. Cold damp weather frequently increased pain and a sense of ill-being in patients in whom a definite recrudescence was not precipitated. A few of the "relapses" were unquestionably hysterical in nature." It is interesting to compare the description of relapses in the Royal Free Hospital outbreak, which was written without knowledge of Gilliam's account. "There might be periods of two weeks in which the symptoms were mild and fever had disappeared. Such periods were often followed by marked recrudescence of old symptoms and sometimes by the appearance of fresh neurological manifestations. In such relapses further fever and tender enlargement of glands occurred. Relapses occurred in some cases after patients had been fit enough to return to their homes...Functional manifestations in a few cases overlaid the organic picture, particularly in those cases longest in hospital."

The subacute and chronic stages: In seven of the recorded outbreaks, a proportion of the patients has been followed for periods of months or years. Once again the methods of selection have varied and prevent an accurate assessment of the comparative incidence of sequelae and chronic cases. In the Iceland epidemic, fifty-seven (12 per cent) of the 465 patients originally affected at Akureyri were examined seven to ten months after the onset[6]. These patients were not representative of the epidemic as a whole, as 74 per cent of them had been paralyzed whereas the paralysis rate for the whole outbreak was only 28 per cent. Six years after the outbreak Sigurdsson[21] examined thirty-nine of these fifty-seven patients again (thirty-three women and six men) and reported his findings. There is no information as to what had happened to the remaining eighteen. It seems reasonable to suspect that a bias was operating in favor of patients with continued symptoms. The grounds for the selection of eight of nineteen patients for re-examination fifteen months after the New York State outbreak[14] and twelve of fifty patients six months after the Bethesda epidemic[15] are uncertain. The follow-up studies in the Alaska[17] and Punta Gorda[16] outbreaks are important because all patients originally examined were traced and studied after the elapse of two years in the former, and of five months in the latter.

Seven to ten months after the Akureyri outbreak, Sigurdsson and his colleagues[6] found that most of the fifty-seven patients whom they examined had returned to work. However, only six were free of symptoms. Among the remainder, nervousness, fatigue and persistent muscular pains were common, and eleven complained of mild paresis. On examination, nineteen of the patients were found to be free of all objective evidence of disease but in the rest there was a confusing mixture of signs, some of which were thought to represent organic disease and others to indicate hysteria. Localized muscular tenderness was found in nineteen, Paresis in sixteen, muscular atrophy in fourteen and sensory changes in twelve.

Six years later, thirty-nine of these patients were examined again[21]. All had returned to their previous occupations (except one who was suffering from a gastric ulcer), but only five considered themselves completely recovered. Of the remainder, twenty-eight complained of nervousness and tiredness, twenty-four of muscle pains, and eight of loss of memory. Sleeplessness and paresthesias occurred less frequently. Muscular tenderness was found in ten, paresis in nine, and atrophy in six. Unfortunately, both these follow-up studies are lacking in any description of changes in tone, coordination or reflexes.

Two to three years after the acute illness, Pellew[33] interviewed the five Adelaide patients who had originally been chosen for virological studies. In all, there had been emotional instability or lack of concentration for eighteen months to two years, and in four, muscular pains had also been a feature. All five had improved and were well at the time of interview.

Fog[9] describes the enormous fluctuations in symptomatology in his Copenhagen patients during the first two to three months of the illness. Six months after the outbreak, three of the ten patients had returned to their occupations, three were working part time, two were convalescent and two were still in the hospital. None were free of symptoms, but all had improved.

In the Bethesda outbreak[15], none of the twelve patients selected for re-examination three to five months after the onset felt well, although they considered that they were improving slowly. They complained of recrudescences of low grade fever, myalgia, chest pains and localized weakness.

Interrogation of the Punta Gorda patients[16] five months after the original study demonstrated a paucity of signs as compared with symptoms, an over-all tendency towards slow improvement and a fluctuating course. Only one patient was completely well. In the remainder there had been periods of improvement interrupted by exacerbations of symptoms with a definite trend towards recovery. Thus, whereas in the second month of the disease more than half of the patients were confined to bed, only three were thus confined in the sixth month. Symptoms remained common; nervous tensions in eighteen, fatigue in fifteen, and depression in twelve. On the other hand, objective evidence of mental tension (the criteria are not described) was found in only one case. Diminution in sensation was found in ten patients, muscular tenderness in seven and paresis in one.

Deisher[17] appears to have had the unusual opportunity of re-examining all his 175 patients two years after the onset of the illness. Unfortunately, the information derived was incomplete; there are no data available about the number who were free of symptoms or the number who had been unable to resume work, and no description is given of reflex and sensory changes. Of the 175 patients, 110 complained of tiring easily, eighty-one of pain and stiffness, and fifty-seven of muscle weakness (as distinct from "paralysis," which was present in sixteen cases). Emotional instability, tension, poor concentration and memory defects were extremely common. Tremor, incoordination and muscular jerking were also seen.

Summary of the Clinical Features. In all outbreaks prodromal symptoms preceded the development of paresis or other neurological signs, but their severity and duration varied. In eight, the prodromal illness was well defined, and lasted about a week. In the Coventry and Durban cases it was mild and most of the patients presented for treatment in the paretic phase. In the Berlin outbreak the prodrome was sharp but abbreviated, lasting three days. The Punta Gorda outbreak differs in the length and vagueness of the premonitory phase. Most of the patients were not confined to bed until the end of the third week. Information about the length of the prodomal illness in the New York and Alaska cases is incomplete.

Headache has been reported as a presenting feature

in all outbreaks and pain in the neck, back and limbs are also common early symptoms. These complaints and the malaise which accompanies them have been out of proportion to the fever, which is usually slight even at the onset and sometimes absent[8,12,15,16]. Symptoms of an upper respiratory or gastrointestinal disturbance (sore throat, coryza, nausea, vomiting, diarrhea) may also develop at this stage. A definite intermission between the prodromal symptoms and the paretic illness is rare, and has been reported as a constant feature in only one outbreak[15].

Muscular pain, headache or pain in the neck, and paresis have been features of the fully developed syndrome in all outbreaks. In the worst Los Angeles, Middlesex and Royal Free Hospital cases, the myalgia has been agonizing, requiring administration of narcotics for its relief. Its variability both in site and in intensity from day to day has been remarked on a number of occasions. Pain in the limbs has occurred at some stage in most cases, but pain in the shoulders, chest and abdomen is also a prominent feature, and has raised the question of a Coxsackie infection. In the New York State and Coventry cases the discomfort in the limbs scarcely amounted to pain.

With the exception of the New York cases the distribution of the paresis has followed that of the muscle pain and tenderness. Numbness, tingling and in some cases deficiencies of sensation on formal testing have been a feature of all outbreaks except one[11], and usually occurred in limbs affected by paralysis. Hyperpathia, muscular spasm, cramps, tremors and involuntary movements were noted in severely affected patients in about half the outbreaks. The deep reflexes in the paretic limbs may be hyperactive or depressed, but are rarely if ever abolished. Frank extensor plantar responses have been unusual, but equivocal or absent responses are relatively common. Retention of urine requiring catheterization or incontinence has occurred in eight outbreaks, and urinary frequency was a feature of one other.

Symptoms or signs indicating damage to the cranial nerves or their central connections have occurred in nine outbreaks. In six they were uncommon, but in the Royal Free Hospital Middlesex and Los Angeles cases they were relatively frequent. Diplopia, facial paresis, tinnitus, vertigo, inner ear deafness and bulbar involvement have all been reported. Hyperacusis was a feature of no less than five epidemics[7, 8, 11, 12, 17]. Nystagmus was almost invariable in the Middlesex Hospital and Berlin patients, common in the Royal Free Hospital cases, and an unusual finding in four other outbreaks. Mental disturbances, of which depression, emotional lability and lack of concentration are commonest, have occurred in all reported outbreaks. In most instances they appeared during the acute illness[5,8,12,14-18] but in others they first became manifest during convalescence[6,7,10].

Lymphadenopathy was first reported by White and Burtch[14] in four of the New York State cases. It also occurred as a rare feature in the Durban and Middlesex Hospital cases. In the Royal Free Hospital outbreaks it was such a constant feature that the illness was at first diagnosed as infectious mononucleosis. Hepatic enlargement was also noted in a few of these cases.

In most patients recovery has been complete within one to two months. However, in a proportion, which has varied from outbreak to outbreak, the course has been punctuated by relapses. These have involved simply a return of pain and fever in some instances, in others, fresh paresis and other neurological signs, or mental disturbances. In general, even in these patients there has been a trend towards improvement but in some instances a characteristic syndrome of chronic ill health has developed, with cyclical recrudescences of pain, fatigue, weakness and depression, often coincident with menstruation, cold weather and exertion. Objective neurological sequelae, such as muscular atrophy, involuntary movements, sensory loss, deafness and incoordination have occurred in a small minority.

Sporadic Cases

In addition to epidemics, sporadic cases with the familiar clinical features have occurred. The first endemic case in which a diagnosis of "Iceland disease" was made was reported by Hardtke[28]. He described the illness of a forty-one year old female physiotherapist in Indiana in October 1953. She presented with headache, stiff neck, pain in the shoulders and limbs, and incoordination. Within a few days she found that attempted movements or the slightest jolting precipitated agonizing cramp-like muscular spasms against which her only defense

was absolute immobility. She was admitted to the hospital as a poliomyelitis suspect and on examination was found to have questionable weakness of the lower left side of the face and exaggerated unequal reflexes. The cerebrospinal fluid was normal, and in the absence of any flaccid paralysis, a diagnosis of poliomyelitis could not be sustained. A relapse occurred in February 1954, and when examined in July she was found to be depressed, with loss of memory and absent gag reflex on the right, diminished sensation on the left side of the body and persistence of the reflex abnormalities already described. Coxsackie infection was not excluded in this instance, although the combination of neurologic signs with a normal cerebrospinal fluid and a chronic course make this diagnosis unlikely.

In 1956 Ramsay and O'Sullivan[29] reported on eight patients admitted to the Infectious Diseases Department of the Royal Free Hospital from the population of northwest London between April and October 1955, before, during and after the extensive epidemic in the staff of the main hospital. None of these patients, of whom seven were female, had been in contact with the sick nurses.

The onset was generally gradual with headache, pain in the limbs, giddiness and upper respiratory or gastric symptoms. Fever rarely exceeded 100°F. Earache, tinnitus, cramps, muscular twitching, tremors and paresthesias were also noted. On examination, lymphadenopathy occurred in seven; stiffness of the neck, paresis and exaggerated deep reflexes in six; sensory impairment and muscle tenderness in five; and cranial nerve involvement in four. Extensor plantar responses were noted in three cases. Convalescence was protracted. In four cases it was complicated by emotional disturbances. Full virological studies, including the use of tissue culture methods, were carried out in all eight cases and were negative.

Jellinek[30] described two patients on the staff of hospital in Hampshire who suffered from a similar illness in the summer of 1955. Both were females, one a doctor and the other a nurse. Both had headache, stiffness of the neck, fever, myalgia and a variety of neurological signs, including nystagmus (two), facial weakness (one), exaggerated reflexes (two), clonus (one) and sensory changes (one). There were two well defined relapses in each case in which retention of urine, requiring tidal drainage, was a distressing feature. Lymphadenopathy occurred in one case. In both, emotional lability was noted. Repeated examination of the cerebrospinal fluid revealed no abnormality. Virological studies were incomplete.

Galpine and Brady[32] reported seven cases which arose sporadically in the Coventry area in the late summer and fall of 1956, three years after the outbreak in their nursing staff. Four patients were female and three male. The early symptoms (sore throat, lassitude, drowsiness, vomiting, nuchal pain, backache, giddiness and headache) were similar to those reported elsewhere. Paresis was found in all cases and tended to fluctuate and shift. It was usually accompanied by aching, paresthesias and tenderness. Alterations in tone were rare, but twitching, cramps, involuntary movements and tremors occurred. The reflexes were brisk and the plantar responses difficult to obtain. The sensory changes noted included hyperpathia, hypoasthesia, anesthesia and astereognosis. Difficulty in starting micturition occurred in three cases and incontinence in one other. Shotty lymph nodes were found in the posterior triangle of the neck in three. Of six patients who were examined three months after their discharge from the hospital, two had recovered completely. The remainder complained of myalgia, weakness, paresthesias and diminished metal grasp. Examination of the feces in three cases failed to show any evidence of a cytopathogenic agent, and serological tests for poliomyelitis were negative.

In a second paper, Ramsay[31] reviewed his experience with thirty-four patients admitted from northwest London between April 1955 and December 1957. Headache was an almost universal symptom, and pain in the limbs, giddiness and pain in the neck occurred in about half of the patients. Lassitude, subjective sensory phenomena and back pain occurred in about a third, and sore throat, earache and cramps were less frequent. On general examination conjunctivitis and evidence of an upper respiratory infection were noted in one-third, and enlarged lymph nodes in one-fourth of the patients. In the nervous system, definite evidence of paralysis occurred in 50 per cent. Exaggerated deep reflexes, sensory disturbances and muscular tenderness were also prominent. Nystag-

mus and extensor plantar responses were found in about one-fifth. Cranial nerve lesions, tremors and myoclonus occurred in four patients. Low pyrexia was the rule. Results of serological tests for lymphocytic choriomeningitis, mumps, leptospirosis and poliomyelitis were negative in each case. Throat washings and feces were also examined.

Other Unexplained Outbreaks. Other problematic outbreaks have been described which share some of the characteristics already outlined. Bond[34] mentions briefly an outbreak of 463 cases in Tallahassee, Florida, in the fall of 1954. The disease, which was selective for married white women, was characterized by disturbances of mood, transient paresis, parasthesias and relapses. This outbreak, and that reported by Wallis[35-37] from Cumberland, England, are probably similar to those already described but sufficient data have not been published on which to base a definite opinion.

Rose[38] and Wright and Morley[39] have reported epidemics of obscure encephalitis in West Africa, and have referred in their discussions to the outbreaks already described. In the former, which occurred in Sierra Leone, the onset resembled cholera with high pyrexia and prostrating diarrhea and vomiting, and the course was fulminating with terror, severe myalgia and vertigo. Pains around the costal margin similar to those of Bornholm disease were a common feature. A little less than one-third of the patients died. The cerebrospinal fluid was normal.

The outbreak in Nigeria, described by Wright and Morley[39], was characterized by low fever, tremor, aphasia, a normal cerebrospinal fluid and a favorable outcome in all cases. Certain of the epidemiologic features suggested an intoxication.

Other than an unknown etiology, the predilection of the agents for the nervous system, and a normal cerebrospinal fluid, neither of these outbreaks resemble those described in this paper.

McConnell[40] reported sixteen cases of illness among the student nurses of the University Hospital of Pennsylvania in 1945. Severe headache was invariable, hyperesthesia occurred in thirteen, meningism in twelve, and pleurodynia in ten. A diagnosis of epidemic pleurodynia (Borholm disease) was made, although the clinical picture was considered to be atypical. A low grade fever accompanied by "disproportionate severe generalized headache and myalgia" persisted for several weeks in five cases, and in two there were four and five relapses, respectively. Stupor and episodes of loss of consciousness occurred in one patient and sensory loss in another. The sequelae were headache, myalgia and pleuritic pain. Of five patients examined a mild pleocytosis was found in the cerebrospinal fluid in two. The similarities which this outbreak shares with the fourteen already described are obvious. However, in view of the absence of paresis, and the fact that the outbreak preceded the isolation of the Coxsackie viruses which could thus not be excluded in this instance, it has been classified separately.

Hook's[41] report from Hygiea, Sweden, underlines the nosological difficulties in this field in the absence of pathological support. Under the title "Iceland disease" he described four cases in the staff of a hospital in the summer of 1956. The affected persons, of whom two were physicians, worked in a "single room". (It is not clear whether this was a laboratory or a clinic.)

The first patient's illness developed gradually with mild muscular aches, paresthesias and weakness in the hands and feet. The paresis progressed over a period of several weeks and was accompanied by flaccidity and diminished reflexes. Mental depression was a feature in the later stages. Lumbar puncture in the second month of his illness revealed a protein of 60 mg. per cent, with a normal cell count. Electromyography showed the typical picture of denervation and a provisional diagnosis of infective polyneuritis was made. Polio and Coxsackie viruses were searched for without success. Vague illnesses characterized by headache and paresthesias subsequently developed in the patient's family.

The second patient's illness, which developed four weeks later, was acute. Three days after the onset of myalgia and paresthesias she had fever, indefinite stiffness of the neck and weakness of the legs. Within a further four days flaccid paralysis of the lower limbs was virtually complete. It had not regressed eight weeks later, and no fresh signs had developed. Lumbar puncture shortly after the onset showed 44 polymorphonuclear leukocytes, 52 lymphocytes and 90 r of protein. The suspicion that this case was,

in fact, poliomyelitis is not dispelled by the failure to isolate polio virus from the stools in the fifth week. An unconvincing twofold rise in antibody titre against type 2 polio virus was demonstrated between the seventh and twenty-first day. The Coxsackie virus was not found. The third and fourth patients described by Hook suffered indefinite illnesses characterized by fatigue and paresthesias but exhibited no physical signs.

Hook's outbreak is difficult to classify. The localization of four cases to a small segment of a community suggests a common etiology. However, although the second case is clinically consistent with a diagnosis of poliomyelitis, the first with its slowly progressive paraplegia and sensory loss is not. The flaccidity of the paralysis, the failure to improve, and the electromyographic picture of denervation (Case I) are features quite unlike the cases reported from Los Angeles, the Royal Free Hospital and elsewhere. Cases III and IV resemble the milder cases reported from these outbreaks. In our present state of ignorance it may be well to suspend judgment on this outbreak.

Laboratory Investigations

The Peripheral Blood. Examination of the cells of the peripheral blood has been, on the whole, unrewarding. Anemia has not been reported. In eight outbreaks[5,6,8,10,14,16-18] the total and differential white counts have been normal in most cases.

A special study of the leukocytes was made in the first Royal Free Hospital epidemic[12], a total of 750 specimens being examined from more than 400 confirmed or suspected cases. In addition, smears from 138 selected patients were examined by three independent observers. No specific changes were found. In about half the cases, relative lymphocytosis was seen during the early course of the illness. Occasional abnormal lymphocytes (Türk and plasma cell-like forms) were noted in some patients, but the changes characteristic of infectious mononucleosis did not occur. Similar findings have been reported in the endemic cases in the neighborhood of the Royal Free Hospital[29,31]. The authors stress the point that the changes are not specific, and are identical to those seen in virus infections, such as poliomyelitis and the common cold. A relative lymphocytosis was also observed in one-third of the Bethesda cases. The small Berlin outbreak differed in that a polymorphonuclear leukocytosis occurred in all seven patients (range 9,700 to 15,300 cells per cu. mm.).

Information about the erythrocyte sedimentation rate is incomplete. In the Royal Free and Middlesex Hospital outbreaks it was normal. In the Alaska outbreak it was raised in the few patients in whom it was performed.

A positive agglutination reaction to washed sheep erythrocytes (Paul Bunnell test) is extremely uncommon[14] and when present further studies have suggested a remote infection.

The Cerebrospinal Fluid. The cerebrospinal fluid is known to have been examined in 199 cases in eleven outbreaks in which exact figures are available. The number of additional cases examined in the Durban and Alaska outbreaks is not recorded; lumbar punctures were not performed in the second Royal Free Hospital outbreak.

The cells: Normal cell counts (less than 5 cells per cu. mm.) have been the rule in all outbreaks except those in Iceland[6] and Alaska[17]. At Akureyri, two of five patients studied showed mild lymphocytosis, as did three others examined at Reykavik. In Alaska the total number of examinations is not stated but it appears that in two-thirds of those studied counts of 10 to 30 cells were found. In the remaining ten outbreaks in which exact figures are available, lumbar punctures were performed in 194 cases and less than 5 cells were observed in 180 of these (92.8 per cent). In the other fourteen cases (7.2 per cent) the cell counts ranged from 6 to 66 lymphocytes. In sporadic cases the results have been similar. Of twenty-seven cases studied, normal cell counts were found in twenty-five, a mild lymphocytosis in two.

Protein: Protein estimations were made in 194 cases in ten epidemics. In 182 cases (94.6 per cent) concentrations of 40 mg. per cent or less were found, and in the remaining eleven (5.4 per cent) the readings varied from 48 to 85 mg. per cent. In addition, we have the observation that in the Durban outbreak, abnormal concentrations of protein were "very rare." There is no information about the Alaska outbreak. Of twenty-seven sporadic cases examined, protein

concentrations ranged between 50 to 80 mg. per cent in 4 cases; in the remainder the protein concentrations were less than 40 mg. per cent.

Apart from an occasional weakly positive Pandy test, no other abnormalities have been reported in the cerebrospinal fluid.

Creatinuria. White and Burtch[14] studied the excretion of creatine in thirteen patients. In twelve the urinary output was more than 100 mg. daily and in eight of these it exceeded 200 mg. It was considered that the findings could not be explained on the basis of physiological creatinuria as there were no athletes with exceptional muscular development in the group, and only one child. Creatine studies have not been reported by other workers.

Electromyography. Electromyographic studies were performing in two patients in the Copenhagen outbreak in 1952. Unfortunately, no description of the tracings is given. They were interpreted as showing "neurogenic weakness of peripheral or radicular origin." Macrae and Galpine[10] were the authors who first drew attention to a consistent electromyographic pattern in affected muscles on voluntary movement, which has subsequently been confirmed by Richardson[42] and Ramsay[31].

According to Richardson, who studied twenty-eight patients with marked motor involvement from the Royal Free Hospital outbreak, the strength-duration curves of the involved muscles were normal in all cases except one. Nerve conduction measurements were within normal limits. Evidence of lower motor neurone degeneration was therefore exceptional. Similar results were reported by Alexander[43] who performed nerve conduction studies on twenty patients from Durban.

Electromyography early in the disease revealed fasciculation potentials. With the onset of paresis an abnormality of recruitment occurred similar to that which has been described in involvement of the motor units at the level of the cord by Bauwens[44]. On volition, the number of motor unit potentials was severely reduced and in some instances the movement was initiated by prolonged polyphasic potentials. However, the accompanying evidence of nerve fibre degeneration which might be expected in a protracted lesion of the motor neurone was not obtained.

Figure 2A

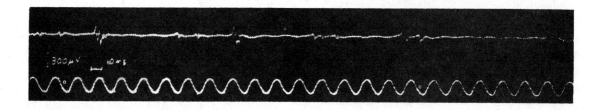

Recording from severely involved tibialis anterior muscle on maximal sustained volition. Recordings with concentric needle electrode and maximal sustained volition.

Figure 2B

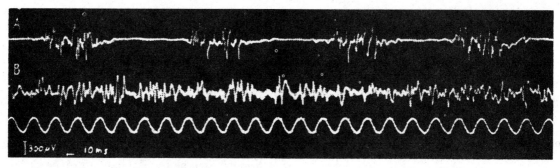

Recordings with concentric needle electrode and maximal sustained volition. A, from weak tibialis anterior muscle. B, from normal contralateral tibialis anterior muscle. Calibration 50 cycles. 300 microvolts. (From Brit. M.J., 2:895, 1957.)

Figure 3

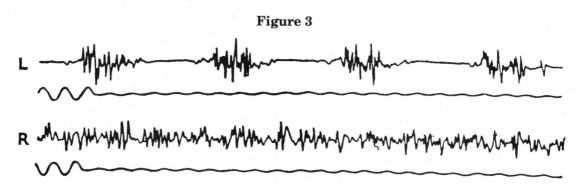

Electromyograms: upper register, from left (affected) tibialis anterior muscle on maximal volition, showing grouping of large polyphasic motor-unit potentials; lower register, from right (unaffected) tibialis anterior muscle on maximal volition, whowing complete interference pattern of normal motor-unit potentials. Calibration 500 and 100 µV at 50 cycles per second. (From Ramsay, A.M. Lancet, 2:1196, 1957.)

During recovery, Richardson found changes similar to those described by Macrae and Galpine[10]. On volition the motor unit potentials were grouped in sequences lasting from 50 to 80 milliseconds, with regular intervals of complete inactivity giving rise to a tremulous contraction at a frequency of 5 to 10 per second. Ramsay and O'Sullivan[29] studied eight sporadic cases and reported similar findings. On electromyographic exploration of affected muscles, voluntary movement produced action potentials in groups of the same duration and frequency as those reported by Richardson. The similarity of the findings in the Royal Free Hospital cases and Ramsay's material is strikingly demonstrated in Figures 2 and 3. In his later review of thirty-four cases, Ramsay[31] reported that twenty-one of twenty-six patients examined electromyographically (including the eight originally described) had shown the changes described. Galpine and Brady[32], reporting seven sporadic cases from Coventry, found a reduction in the number of motor unit potentials and grouping in all five patients examined. Polyphasic and abnormally large potentials were also found.

Electroencephalography. Electroencephalograms have been studied by Fog[9], Ramsey and O'Sullivan[29], Galpine and Brady[32] and Poskanzer et al.[16]. Some non-specific abnormalities were reported in patients with behavior disorders by Ramsay and O'Sullivan. In all other cases the electroencephalogram has been normal.

Etiological Studies

Virology. In view of the dissimilarity of the clinical picture to any known bacterial infection, attention has naturally been focused on isolating a virus as the responsible agent. (Table 2). In nine of the fourteen

Table 2				
Attempts to Isolate Virus				
Location	No. of Cases Examined	Pathological Material Studied	Animal species	Tissue Culture Material
Los Angeles	0	Nil	Nil	Nil
Iceland	12	Blood, C.S.F., feces	Guinea pigs, hamsters, mice, suckling mice, monkeys	
Adelaide	5	Blood, C.S.F., throat washings, feces	Monkeys, suckling mice, weaned mice	Embryonated hen eggs
New York State	17	Feces, throat washings	Monkeys (2), suckling mice (15)	
Middlesex Hospital	3	Feces	Monkeys, suckling mice	Monkey kidney, monkey testicle
Copenhagen	0	Nil	Nil	Nil
Coventry Hospital	5	Feces	Guinea pigs (2), adult mice, suckling mice, monkeys (2), rabbit (1)	Human embryonic muscle and skin; monkey kidney, monkey testis
Bethesda Hospital	?	Blood, C.S.F., throat washings, feces	Suckling hamsters (9), adult mice (26), suckling mice (40)	Human HeLa(28), chorion (20), fibroblasts (10),monkey kidney (28), monkey testicle (31)
Seward, Alaska	0	Nil	Nil	Nil
Berlin	4	Feces	Inoculated into mice and tissue cultures were set up for Coxsackie and polio virus	
Durban Hospital	?		Extensive virologic studies negative	
Royal Free Hospital(1)	?	Blood clots, throat washings feces	Ferrets, guinea pigs, suckling hamsters, adult mice, suckling mice, monkeys	Fertile hen eggs, HeLa cells (9); human embryo brain (2), liver (1), spleen (1), kidney (6), human infant kidney (3), monkey kidney (10)
Punta Gorda	19	Blood clots, throat washings, feces	Suckling mice	HeLa, human liver, monkey kidney
Royal Free Hospital(2)	0	Nil	Nil	Nil

Note: Number of experiments, where given, indicated in parentheses. C.S.F. = cerebral spinal fluid.

Table 3

	Los Angeles	Iceland	Adelaide	New York State	Middlesex Hospital	Copenhagen	Coventry Hospital
A.P.C. virus							
Brucellosis							
Coxsackie				0 (17)			
Encephalitis Eastern Equine	Nil	0 (12)				Nil	
Encephalitis Japanese B	Nil	0 (12)				Nil	
Encephalitis Western Equine		0 (12)					
Encephalitis St. Louis		0 (12)					
Encephalo-myocarditis			0 (5)				0 (10)
Herpes Simplex							
Influenza A		0 (12)					
Influenza B							
Influenza C							
Leptospirosis			0 (5)		0 (8)		0 (10)
Louping Ill							
Lymphocytic Choriomeningitis		0 (12)	0 (5)		0 (8)		0 (10)
Mumps			0 (5)		* (8)		* (10)
Paracolon (Bethesda-Ballerup)							
Polio Virus			0 (5)	0 (17)	3† (10)		0 (10)
Psittacosis							
Q. Fever		0 (12)					
Rabies		0 (12)					
Rickettsia Burneti							
Toxoplasmosis							

	Bethesda Hospital	Seward, Alaska	Berlin	Durban Hospital	Royal Free Hospital (1)	Punta Gorda	Royal Free Hospital (2)
A.P.C. virus	0 (7)				0 (?)		
Brucellosis	† (13)		0 (7)			0 (12)	
Coxsackie	0 (5)						
Encephalitis Eastern Equine				No		0 (12)	
Encephalitis Japanese B				details			Nil
Encephalitis Western Equine				known		0 (12)	
Encephalitis St. Louis						0 (12)	
Encephalo-myocarditis					0 (6)		
Herpes Simplex					0 (?)		
Influenza A			0 (7)		0 (?)		
Influenza B			0 (7)		0 (?)		
Influenza C					0 (?)		
Leptospirosis					0 (?)	0 (12)	
Louping Ill					0 (?)		
Lymphocytic Choriomeningitis						0 (12)	
Mumps					0 (?)	* (12)	
Paracolon	See text						
(Bethesda-Ballerup)						0 (12)	
Polio Virus		† (19)					
Psittacosis					0 (?)		
Q. Fever							
Rabies							
Rickettsia Burneti					0 (?)		
Toxoplasmosis					0 (?)		

*Note: Figures indicate number of positive tests; in parentheses, number of cases studied. * Immune bodies in titres suggesting remote infection found in some cases. † The findings were of doubtful significance and are discussed in the text.*

outbreaks unsuccessful attempts were made to isolate the poliomyelitis and Coxsackie viruses. In the Middlesex Hospital outbreak[8] polio virus Type 3 was isolated from the feces of one case. However, in view of the failure to isolate any detectable antibody from serial specimens of this patient's serum, the extremely unusual clinical picture (bilateral perceptive deafness developed), and a normal cerebrospinal fluid, it was concluded that this virus was probably not responsible for her illness. Table 2 shows that unsuccessful attempts have also been made to isolate other viruses in a number of outbreaks. Particularly extensive investigations were carried out in the Bethesda and Royal Free Hospital epidemics.

In four outbreaks no attempts to isolate a virus were made; one of these was the small second Royal Free Hospital outbreak[13], which was regarded as clinically identical with the large epidemic which had been the subject of extremely extensive virologic studies the previous year. In the Seward outbreak[17] the only investigation performed consisted in random serological studies in nineteen patients who were experiencing subacute symptoms, revealing that the "neutralization titres against the three types of poliomyelitis virus were generally low and showed no consistent pattern." In the Los Angeles[5] and Copenhagen[9] outbreaks no virological studies were made.

Serological studies (Table 3) have also been widely performed. Immune bodies to the mumps virus in titres suggesting remote infection were found in a few cases. In the Bethesda outbreak[15] thirteen serum pairs were examined for antibodies against polio virus. A questionable fourfold rise in the titre occurred in three cases, one against each of the three types of virus. Otherwise, serological tests have been uniformly negative.

Bacterial Studies. In the Bethesda outbreak the prominence of diarrhea as an early symptom directed attention to the possibility of an enteric infection. Organisms of two strains of the Bethesda-Ballerup paracolon group were isolated from feces from twelve of thirty-eight nurses examined and from only one of fifty-four persons who were on the hospital staff at the time of the epidemic and remained well. H and O serum agglutinins against the Bethesda-Ballerup group (at a titre of 1:40 or more) were found in twenty-two of forty-seven affected

nurses and in three of twenty-seven control subjects. In eleven affected nurses a rise and fall in titre was demonstrated during the period of observation. A kitchen girl who had started work one week before the onset of the epidemic was the only person in the entire study who showed both serological strains of organism in her stools. Examination of sixty asymptomatic nurses three to seven months after the end of the epidemic revealed antibody titres in two cases, but no positive cultures.

There is thus strong circumstantial evidence to suggest that the Bethesda-Ballerup paracolon organisms were related to the epidemic of clinical illness among the nursing staff. However, in the absence of other evidence (1) that a disease can be transmitted by these organisms either in man or in animals, (2) or that they produce a neurotoxin, it is premature to conclude that they caused the epidemic. As Shelokov and his colleagues have themselves suggested, the findings may indicate simply that fecal contamination of food was occurring in the hospital kitchen at the time of the epidemic. It is possible that an unknown causative organism was being spread in addition to the Bethesda-Ballerup organism.

It is important to note that attempts to isolate paracolon organisms from patients during the Punta Gorda outbreak were unsuccessful[16].

Poisons. In view of the apparent predilection for hospital staffs, the question has arisen whether or not the disorder may be due to an occupational toxic hazard. This possibility received particular attention in the Royal Free Hospital outbreak[27]. Insecticides, paints and detergents received scrutiny, with negative results. Similar studies were negative in the Durban outbreak[18] and at Bethesda[15].

The Case for a Clinical Entity

It is significant that the first review of the syndrome under discussion was entitled, "Not poliomyelitis"[45]; the second, "A new clinical entity?"[22]. In later articles entitled, "Epidemic myalgic encephalomyelitis"[46], "Benign myalgic encephalomyelitis"[46a] and "Epidemic neuromyasthenia"[15, 16], the authors considered themselves on sufficiently strong ground to describe and name the syndrome. This sequence indicates that the first and minimum requirement in the definition of an entity is the essentially negative one of showing that the syndrome is not an unusual manifestation of a disease already recognized. Later, as evidence accumulates, it may be possible to define the disorder in positive terms.

Poliomyelitis. In nine outbreaks an initial diagnosis of poliomyelitis was made. In favor of this diagnosis were the mode of onset in many cases (headache, pain in the neck and myalgia), the development of paresis and the season of the year. The low or absent fever, so unusual in poliomyelitis at the beginning of the paretic phase, and the rarity of a biphasic illness were at first discounted. However, other atypical features made their appearance in the later stages of the illness in such frequency that the diagnosis of poliomyelitis was withdrawn. In the second and third weeks the distinguishing features were (1) a longer active course with the development of fresh neurological symptoms and signs later than occurs in poliomyelitis, (2) the prominence and persistence of sensory phenomena, (3) the retention or exaggeration of deep reflexes in the paralyzed limbs, and (4) the normal cerebrospinal fluid in most cases.

In some outbreaks the persistence of muscular pain after the development of paresis[47], the occurrence of tremors and involuntary movements, and the high incidence of retention of urine in the absence of severe paralysis[48] were further points against the diagnosis of poliomyelitis at this stage.

The subsequent subacute and chronic course of the disorder, with its mental symptoms and partial or complete remissions and exacerbations, is quite distinct from poliomyelitis which runs its active course within a week of the onset of the major illness. With the exception of the Iceland epidemic, muscular wasting in patients with persistent paralysis has been extremely rare and in such patients no electromyographic evidence of denervation has been found. The over-all mortality in more than 1,000 cases has been nil. From the clinical point of view, the differences from poliomyelitis become progressively clearer as the illness develops.

Epidemiologically, the high attack rates (Table 1) and the predilection of the disorder for small semi-closed communities are also against the diagnosis of poliomyelitis.

The final evidence lies in the laboratory findings. In spite of careful search in ten of fourteen outbreaks, poliomyelitis virus was found in only one case[8] and in this patient no detectable antibodies appeared in the blood.

Other Enteric Viruses. There is now good evidence that enteric viruses of the Coxsackie group[49] cause epidemic pleurodynia[50] and encephalomyocarditis in babies[51]. Viruses of the Coxsackie and Echo groups have also been recovered from cases of aseptic meningitis[52] and lower motor neurone type paralysis.

Scrutiny of reports claiming that they have been concerned in outbreaks of encephalitis in adults shows that objective evidence of damage to the central nervous system has, in fact, been the exception rather than the rule[53, 54].

In the outbreaks reported here certain clinical similarities with epidemic pleurodynia, notably the occurrence of pleuritic chest pain in six outbreaks, of abdominal pain in six, and pain in the shoulders in twelve, stimulated a search for these viruses. In nine outbreaks material was injected into suckling mice with negative results (Table 2); and in five instances[8, 10, 12, 15, 16] tissue cultures of kidney cells from monkeys failed to grow ECHO viruses. In other respects, notably the mental symptoms and the chronicity of some cases, the outbreaks reported here are unlike any that have been found to be associated with Coxsackie or Echo viruses.

Encephalitis Lethargica. The occurrence of tremors, myoclonus or other involuntary movements in a few cases in seven outbreaks raised the question of the reappearance of encephalitis lethargica in epidemic form. Although this disease was notably pleomorphic[55], it has certain distinct clinical and epidemiologic features, which are not shared by any of the outbreaks reported here. According to Von Economo[55] it occurred chiefly in the first three months of the year, was of low infectivity, with no sex predominance and a high mortality. Postencephalitic Parkinsonism occurred in about 30 per cent of all recognized cases. This complication has not been recorded in the illness described here, although one Royal Free Hospital patient had choreoathetoid movements of the right arm with cog-wheel rigidity some months after the acute illness. Involuntary movements have also been reported in the chronic stage in a few of the Alaskan cases[17]. Delinquent behavior, such as occurred after encephalitis lethargica epidemics, has not been described.

The Arthropod-Borne Encephalitides. The various arthropod-borne encephalitides have common epidemiological and clinical features which distinguish them from the syndrome reported here. As might be expected, these diseases occur most frequently in field and forest workers who are exposed to the bites of mosquitoes, ticks, and bird and animal parasites[56], and evidence of spread by personal contact is uncommon. The various types of insect-borne encephalitis share an acute onset with high fever and headache, followed in severe cases by delirium, convulsions, tremors and spastic paralyses. Death occurs within ten days in a variable proportion. A pleocytosis of 100 to 500 cells in the cerebrospinal fluid and a polymorphonuclear leukosytosis in the peripheral blood are characteristic.

The syndrome described in this paper, with its institutional outbreaks, evidence of spread by personal contact[5,6,12], absence of delirium or convulsions, predominantly normal cerebrospinal fluid and absent mortality, is in striking contrast. From the virological point of view, the agents of the insect-borne encephalitides are best recovered from nervous tissue which was not obtained from this material. However, a search for antibodies against some of the known types of encephalitis virus was made in the Iceland[6] and Punta Gorda[16] outbreaks and against louping ill (Russian spring-summer encephalomyelitis) in the Royal Free Hospital cases[12] without success.

Infectious Mononucleosis. A diagnosis of infectious mononucleosis was seriously entertained at the onset of the Royal Free Hospital outbreak[57]. In favor were the known predilection of this disease for hospital staffs, the lymphadenopathy, and the presence of a few atypical lymphoctyes in the peripheral blood in some cases. A wide variety of neurological manifestations have been described in infectious mononucleosis, but these are rare. As the epidemic developed, the overwhelming frequency of neurological symptoms and signs made this diagnosis unlikely, and the failure to demonstrate typical Downey cells or significant titres of heterophile antibodies finally excluded it.

Other Infections. Searches for a wide variety of other agents have been carried out (Tables 2 and 3) without success.

The Question of Hysteria. The question of hysteria has been raised in five outbreaks[5,6,9,12,20] and by Galpine and Brady[32] and Ramsay[31] in the discussion of their endemic cases. Most authors agree that hysterical manifestations have occurred in a few patients[5,9,31], particularly in the later stages,[12] but none has felt that it has contributed significantly to the pattern of the disease.

In an illness in which there has been a selectivity for young women, no mortality, and few positive laboratory findings, it is important to examine the possibility that hysteria may have accounted for part or all of the clinical picture more closely. Epidemic hysteria has been recognized for many centuries as a particular hazard in institutions containing women[58]. It has presented in many bizarre ways from the mass compulsive dancing (St. Vitus Dance) of the middle ages, to the "quaking" of the early Quakers, the fits of Wesley's converts and the effort syndrome of soldiers in the 1914-1918 World War. The form and content of the manifestations depend upon the ideas and fears of the age[59].

No one can seriously contend that every patient in all the outbreaks described in this paper has been hysterical. The presence of definite ocular, facial and palatal pareses, or nystagmus, and of extensor plantar responses in rare instances, and a definite pleocytosis in the cerebrospinal fluid in a few cases indicate organic disease of the nervous system in a minority at least, unless we are to doubt the competence of a number of different observers.

A more reasonable viewpoint would be that the majority of the cases constitute a hysterical reaction to a small number of cases of infection of the nervous system, for example, poliomyelitis. Thus it will be readily admitted that an epidemic of poliomyelitis, such as occurred in Los Angeles in 1934, would produce overwork and emotional strain in the nursing staff of the hospital concerned. Many of the nurses would naturally feel apprehensive about becoming ill with the disease, and might be inclined to misinterpret the minor aches and pains of every day life. With the development of a few genuine cases of poliomyelitis among the staff and the resulting increasing tension, it is possible to envisage an epidemic of hysterical paralysis.

An attractive case could be made for such a hypotheses. The high attack rates in the most suggestible groups of the community, the predilection for hospital staffs, and the association with preceding or concurrent outbreaks of poliomyelitis might thus be explained. Clinically, the absent or insignificant fever, the prominence of sensory phenomena, which are admittedly often of bizarre distribution and content[13,15], the fluctuation of symptoms and signs from day to day, and the high incidence of negative cerebrospinal fluid findings would also fit in with this hypothesis. Further support might be obtained from the peculiar nature of the paresis. Paralysis without the disappearance of tone and deep reflexes and subsequent atrophy on the one hand, or true spasticity and extensor plantor responses on the other, is suspicious of hysteria. As Brain[60] has pointed out, inability of the patient to relax the affected limb in such cases may cause the deep reflexes to appear exaggerated. Tremors on volition and involuntary movements may also be present in such patients. A jerky contraction against resistance is often prominent[60]. If we add muscle pain and tenderness, which are admittedly uncommon in hysterical paralysis, such a description resembles closely the features of the paralysis in the Royal Free Hospital cases[12] which were attributed to a deep subcortical lesion, and is similar to those described in many less detailed reports.

There are also strong arguments against the idea that the syndrome constitutes a mass hysterical reaction to a few cases of poliomyelitis. In the first place, in the minority who had undoubted objective physical signs, the clinical picture was quite unlike poliomyelitis. In this minority, nystagmus[7,8,9,12,18,19], ophthalmoplegia[8,12], facial palsy[5,7,9,12,18,19], palatal paresis[5,8,12] and extensor plantor responses[8,9,12] were recorded, but true flaccid paralysis with absent reflexes did not occur, and subsequent atrophy was recorded with any frequency in only one outbreak[6] and in exceptional instances in two others[5,12]. In addition, these patients shared the other characteristic features, namely myalgia, sensory changes, low pyrexia, mental symptoms, and a chronic or relapsing course, which were experienced by the majority of patients who had no truly objective physical signs.

Thus we would be forced to the conclusion, on this hypothesis, that even the patients with objective findings were also suffering from hysteria. This seems unlikely.

In the second place, the relationship to poliomyelitis is not constant. At the Royal Free Hospital no patient with poliomyelitis had been admitted to the hospital prior to the outbreak, nor was the diagnosis entertained in the initial cases. There was no undue apprehension about poliomyelitis among this hospital staff, but rather about infectious mononucleosis which was the early diagnosis. In spite of this the course of the disease and the type of neurological involvement was similar to that found in Los Angeles. In the Coventry outbreak six of the twelve patients had been nursing poliomyelitis cases for several years, and it is difficult to imagine why such experienced persons should suddenly manifest a hysterical reaction to the fear of this disease. In the Middlesex Hospital, Berlin and Bethesda cases there was no known contact with poliomyelitis and, in the early cases at least, no reason for anxiety about it in the communities concerned.

The mental symptoms which are a constant feature of all the outbreaks are not typical of hysteria. Disorders of consciousness and convulsions such as may be seen in hysteria have been extremely rare. A single grand mal seizure was reported in a small child in Alaska. Shallowness of affect and "belle indifference" have not been seen. On the contrary, depression and undue emotional lability have been the rule. In the acute stage, terrifying dreams, panic states, uncontrollable weeping and hypersomnia occur. In the convalescent stage the prominent features are impairment of memory, difficulty in concentration and depression. These symptoms are more consistent with cerebral damage than with hysteria. Many years ago Von Economo[55] stressed the ease with which the mental symptoms of encephalitis may be confused with those of psychoneurosis. The slight lymphocytosis in the cerebrospinal fluid in two outbreaks[6,17] which shared many other features with the remainder, and the presence of a characteristic electromyogram in cases from three separate localities, are further strong arguments in favor of an organic etiology.

Final points against mass hysteria as a major factor

in the syndrome are the consistency of the course of the illness, and the similarities in the symptoms described, in spite of a wide variation in the types of community affected, from hospital staffs on the one hand to semi-rural and urban populations on the other. The fact remains that in sporadic cases the illness may be extremely difficult to differentiate from hysteria and other types of psychoneurosis[31]. The diagnosis should therefore be reserved, in isolated instances, for patients with evidence of acute damage to the brain or cord, including the characteristic paresis. If not, the syndrome will become a convenient dumping ground for non-specific illnesses characterized by fluctuating aches and pains, fatigue and depression.

The Homogeneity of the Material. The clinical and epidemiologic evidence suggests that the fourteen outbreaks described in this review have not been due to any known neurotropic infection. The virologic evidence supports this contention so far as it goes, but it is incomplete. Thus poliomyelitis and Coxsackie virus were not formally ruled out in four outbreaks, and Echo viruses were not excluded in nine. It might be argued that at least some of the apparent clinical similarities are due to unconscious bias or undue emphasis on the part of observers familiar with the features of previous epidemics. Such bias cannot have contributed towards the striking reported similarities between the Los Angeles and Royal Free Hospital outbreaks[5, 12] because Gilliam's paper was unknown to the British authors. These similarities are even more impressive when it is appreciated that bias was probably operating in opposite directions. In the Los Angeles outbreak the initial diagnosis was poliomyelitis, and the patients were cared for by orthopedists; in the Royal Free Hospital cases the initial diagnosis was infectious mononucleosis, and patients were treated by internists and neurologists. Further independent evidence is supplied by the Copenhagen cases. Fog's paper[9] was not known to the authors of the later Middlesex, Durban, and Royal Free Hospital reports, although once again they share many common features. It seems therefore that the syndrome is not a self-perpetuating medical artefact.

There are also important differences between the outbreaks. The paralysis rate varies from 10 per cent in the Punta Gorda outbreak to 80 per cent in the Los Angeles cases. The Los Angeles, Middlesex, Durban and Royal Free Hospital epidemics differ quantitatively from the remainder in regard to the frequency of neurological signs (other than paresis), notably cranial nerve lesions, hyperpathia, and retention of urine. They share with the Copenhagen cases a high incidence of paresthesias. On the other hand the Royal Free Hospital epidemics stand apart from the remainder because of the very high incidence of lymphadenopathy, which was otherwise limited to a few cases in the New York State, Middlesex[8(c)] and Durban outbreaks. The Iceland and Alaska epidemics differ from the rest in that a slight lymphocytosis in the cerebrospinal fluid was the rule rather than the exception. The length of the illness and the incidence of subacute and chronic cases have also varied.

Two outbreaks in particular stand apart in several important respects from the rest and it is debatable whether or not they should be classified with them. In the small Berlin outbreak[15] the illness was brief, sensory symptoms and signs were absent, and there were no sequelae or chronic cases. A leukocytosis in the peripheral blood was another distinguishing feature. The onset was November, later than in any other outbreak in the Northern Hemisphere. The outbreak at Punta Gorda[16] also began at an unusual time of the year (February). The onset of symptoms was insidious in all cases. Most of the cases were diagnosed on the basis of a house to house survey, presumably by retrospective questioning. Paresis was exceptional, and other objective evidence of disease of the nervous system was extremely uncommon.

In mild cases, when paresis and other signs of neurological involvement are absent, the illness has few differences in its early stages from many short-lived infections characterized by headache and generalized aches. Even in these patients, however, the degree of malaise and the severity of the pains are disproportionate to the disturbance of temperature and pulse. In the convalescent stage in such cases the easy fatiguability, the aches and pains, and the emotional disturbances without definite physical signs lead to difficulty in differentiation from psychoneurosis. Indeed, in the absence of an epidemic such a differentiation may be impossible.

In its epidemic form the illness is distinctive and therefore has a rightful place in medical literature as a clinical entity. Its epidemiological features suggest that it may be an infection. However, in the absence of any pathological evidence it remains uncertain whether it is due to a single agent or to a group of related agents.

As far as sporadic cases are concerned the diagnosis can be made with a degree of certainty only in cases which show all, or nearly all, the characteristics herein described, including paresis and some other objective evidence of neurological involvement which cannot be simulated. Negative virologic studies are also desirable. The diagnosis of less severe sporadic cases must await further knowledge of the pathology and the development of an objective laboratory test. Although further work is required before the electromyographic changes can be regarded as diagnostic, they may provide objective evidence of disease when this is otherwise lacking.

Treatment. No specific treatment is known to affect the course of the disease. Antibiotics were tried in the early stages of the Bethesda outbreak, when the diagnosis was uncertain, and in those patients in the Royal Free Hospital who had complicating intercurrent bacterial infections. No beneficial effect on the basic disease was observed. Steroid therapy has not been tried.

The importance of rest, as early in the disease as possible, and as absolute as practicable, is stressed by many authors[5,12,15,18,19]. Paretic limbs should be immobilized in the correct posture. Local heat may be used to abate pain and spasm. The association of premature rehabilitation with relapse is well described[5,12,18,19] and it is probable that bedrest should be maintained for some time after the disappearance of symptoms.

Symptomatic treatment is important in this painful and protracted disorder. Muscle relaxants such as meprobamate* have been tried[12,15,17] and have relieved muscle pain and tenderness in some cases. The sedative action may also be of value[17].

In a few cases full doses of narcotics may be necessary to control pain[5,8,12].

Complications should be treated as they arise. Retention of urine can usually be controlled by parasympathomimetic drugs such as carbachol[12] but oc-

* Miltown (Wallace Laboratories, New Brunswick, New Jersey).

casionally catheterization or even tidal drainage will become necessary[8,30]. In rare instances of bulbar palsy, tube feeding has been necessary[12]. An artificial respirator has been required for a short time in three cases[5,8]. Shock treatment for severe depression was required in three of the Royal Free Hospital patients[12].

In the subacute and chronic stages constant encouragement and support is essential. The patient may be reassured that the trend is toward improvement and final recovery. Rehabilitation should be conservative, and return to work gradual.

Nomenclature

The wisdom of naming a disorder, the nature of which cannot at present be proved, and which may be due to more than one agent, is debatable. That there are successful precedents is shown by the history of epidemic pleurodynia[24,25,50] and herpangina[4,61], both of which have subsequently proved to be virologic entities. In view of the widespread agreement that the illness described here is clinically recognizable in its own right, at least in severe cases[15,17,22,31,46], various authors have been of the opinion that a name is necessary for reference purposes. Unfortunately there has been no agreement as to what this name should be. White and Burtch[14] suggested "Iceland disease." This has the disadvantage of all eponyms that it gives no inkling to the uninformed of the nature of the disorder. It is also incorrect on historical grounds as the Los Angeles outbreak described by Gilliam is the original account in the literature. The same disadvantages (with the added difficulty of pronunciation) apply to "Akureyri disease" which is preferred by Sigurdsson and Gudmundsson[21].

The first attempt at a descriptive name was made by Fog[9] who suggested "neuritis vegetativa" in the belief that the autonomic nervous system bore the brunt of the damage. A further suggestion was made in an editorial in the Lancet in 1956[22]. It was hoped that the term "benign myalgic encephalomyelitis" would emphasize the absent mortality, the severe muscular pains, the evidence of parenchymal damage to the nervous system, and the presumed inflammatory nature of the disorder. This term has been adopted by Galpine and Brady[32] and Deisher[17] in subsequent articles. It has also been criticized by Sigurdsson[62] and the staff of the Royal Free Hospital[12,27]. Sigurdsson objects that the disease is not always benign, not invariably myalgic, and possibly never encephalomyelitic. Benignity is relative; it seems that "benign" is justified by the fact that there is no other recorded infective disease of the central nervous system without mortality. As various authors have stressed[5, 8,12], the pain in this disease, although not invariably present, may be devastating, and is perhaps the feature which impresses itself most forcefully on the observer. As far as the final term is concerned, the clinical impression that the lesion is central rather than peripheral is supported by the electromyogram. In our present state of ignorance "encephalomyelitis" seems preferable to "encephalopathy" because it conveys the suggestion that the disease is infective in origin, which is almost certainly the case.

In the Royal Free Hospital report it is pointed out that the name fails to describe the involvement of the lymph nodes and liver. As the author has indicated elsewhere[63], a fully descriptive name such as "benign ameningitic myalgic lymphoreticular encephalomyelopathy" is impracticable. Shelokov et al.[15] and Poskanzer et al.[16] have coined the phrase "epidemic neuromyasthenia." The first term is misleading because it suggests that the disorder is confined to epidemics; the second (translated nerve-muscle-weakness) is either meaningless or, if it means anything, suggests a disorder of the muscle end-plate, which is contrary to the electromyographic evidence. The verbal similarity with "neurasthenia" (i.e., psychoneurosis) is particularly unfortunate.

It is unlikely that an adequate term will be found until fresh evidence is available. In the meantime "benign myalgic encephalomyelitis" may act provisionally as a rallying point in the current list of medical literature for patients with the clinical features already described.

Summary and Conclusions

Fourteen outbreaks of a paralytic illness of worldwide distribution are described. Twelve of these have so many epidemiologic and clinical features in common that there is a prima facie case for a single or related group of causative agents.

The epidemiologic features are a high attack rate as compared with poliomyelitis, a predilection for residential communities, a higher attack rate in women than in men, a tendency to occur more commonly in young adults, and the commencement of most outbreaks in the summer months. The evidence is consistent with the hypothesis that the disorder is an infection which is spread by personal contact.

The fact that hospital staffs, particularly nurses, have borne the brunt of seven outbreaks suggests an occupational hazard. An alternative explanation is that the unusual nature of the illness has been noted in such persons because of a higher standard of diagnostic skill at their disposal than is available to the members of other residential communities.

Severely affected patients show a characteristic clinical picture. After an acute or subacute onset with headache, symptoms of a gastro-intestinal or upper respiratory upset, muscular pains and low or absent fever, an unusual type of paresis develops which is rarely associated with the classic signs of lower motor neurone or pyramidal tract involvement. This is often accompanied by paresthesias, sometimes by sensory loss, and occasionally by painful muscular spasms, myoclonus or other types of involuntary movement. As the paresis recovers a curious jerky muscular contraction on volition has been noted in some instances. Involvement of the cranial nerves and the bladder may occur.

Convalescence has been prolonged by fatigue and recurring myalgia but recovery has usually been complete within three months. In a proportion which varies from outbreak to outbreak a well defined state of chronic ill health has developed, characterized by fluctuating myalgia and paresis, partial remissions and exacerbations, and depression, emotional lability and lack of concentration. The major differences within the group of outbreaks lie in the incidence of lymphadenopathy, paresis, and mild lymphocytosis in the cerebrospinal fluid.

Clinical laboratory studies have on the whole proved unhelpful. With the exception of two outbreaks in which a mild lymphocytosis was found, the cerebrospinal fluid has been normal in 95 per cent of cases investigated. An unusual electromyogram has been found in two outbreaks and in some sporadic cases.

No deaths directly attributable to the disease have occurred and the pathology remains unknown. In spite of the widest investigations, no known bacterial or viral pathogen has been incriminated. In particular, there is no evidence that the poliomyelitis, Coxsackie or Echo groups of viruses have been responsible.

Evidence is adduced to show that the outbreaks can be distinguished on clinical grounds from poliomyelitis, encephalitis lethargica, the arthropod-borne encephalitides, epidemic myalgia and infectious mononucleosis. The disorder is not a manifestation of mass hysteria.

It is concluded that the disease is recognizable in its epidemic form on clinical and epidemiologic grounds and therefore may properly be considered a clinical entity. In its sporadic form, which is now well documented, the diagnosis should be reserved at present for severe cases with definite neurological signs including paresis and the characteristic fluctuating course. The disease is probably due to infection by an unknown agent or group of related agents.

The problems of nomenclature and treatment are also discussed.

Acknowledgment: *It is a pleasure to acknowledge the help and encouragement provided by Professor Max Michael, Jr., during the preparation of this paper.*

References

1. Likar, M. and Dane, D.S. An illness resembling acute poliomyelitis caused by the virus of the Russian spring/summer encephalitis louping ill group in Northern Ireland. Lancet, 1: 456, 1958.

2. Hammon, W.M., Yohn, D.S., Ludwig, E.H., Pavia, R.A. and Sather, G.E. A study of certain non-poliomyelitis and poliomyelitis enterovirus infections. J.A.M.A., 167: 727, 1958.

3. Rhodes, A.J. Recent advances in study of virus diseases with particular reference to neurotrophic infections. Report of annual meeting and proceedings of Royal College of Physicians and Surgeons of Canada, p. 40. 1954.

4. Kumm, H.W. Relationship of Echo and Coxsackie viruses to paralytic and non-paralytic poliomyelitis. Journal-Lancet, 77: 469, 1957.

5. Gilliam, A.G. Epidemiological study of an epidemic diagnosed as poliomyelitis occurring among the personnel of the Los Angeles County General Hospital during the summer of 1934. Public Health Bulletin, U.S. Treasury Dept. No. 240, 1938.

6. Sigurdsson, B., Sigurjonsson, J., Sigurdsson, J., Thorbelsson, J. and Gudmundsson, K.R. Disease epidemic in Iceland simulating poliomyelitis. Am. J. Hyg., 52: 222, 1950.

7. Pellew, R.A.A. Clinical description of disease resembling poliomyelitis. M.J. Australia, 1: 944, 1951.

8. (a) Acheson, E.D. Encephalomyelitis associated with poliomyelitis virus: an outbreak in a nurses' home. Lancet, 2: 1044, 1954;

(b) Acheson, E.D. Unpublished data;

(c) Acheson, E.D. Letter. Lancet, 2: 395, 1955.

9. Fog, T. Neuritis vegetativa epidemica. Ugesk. f. laeger, 115: 1244, 1953.

10. Macrae, A.D. and Galpine, J.F. Illness resembling poliomyelitis in nurses. Lancet, 2: 350, 1954.

11. Sumner, D.W. Further outbreak of disease resembling poliomyelitis. Lancet, 1: 764, 1956.

12. The medical staff of the Royal Free Hospital. An outbreak of encephalomyelitis in the Royal Free Hospital group, London, 1955. Brit. M. J., 2: 895, 1957

13. Geffen, D. and Tracy, S.M. Outbreak of acute infective encephalomyelitis in a residential home for nurses in 1956. Brit. M. J., 2: 904, 1957.

14. White, D.N. and Burtch R.B. Iceland disease, a new infection simulating acute anterior poliomyelitis. Neurology, 4: 506, 1954.

15. Shelokov, A., Habel, K., Verder, E. and Welsh, W. Epidemic neuromyasthenia. An outbreak of poliomyelitis-like illness in student nurses. New England J. Med., 257: 345, 1957.

16. Poskanzer, D.C., Henderson, D.A., Kunkle, E.C., Kalter, S.S., Clement, W.B. and Bond J.O. Epidemic neuromyasthenia. An outbreak in Punta Gorda, Florida. New England J. Med., 257: 356, 1957.

17. Deisher, J.B. Benign myalgic encephalomyelitis (Iceland disease) in Alaska. Northwest Med., 56: 1451, 1957.

18. Adnams, J.N. Observations on the epidemic of encephalomyelitis affecting the nursing staff of the Addington Hospital, 1955. Unpublished.

19. Hill, R.C.J. Memorandum on the outbreak amongst the nurses at Addington, Durban. South African M.J., 29: 344, 1955.

20. Clinical meeting of the Natal Coastal Branch. The Durban mystery disease. South African M.J., 29: 997, 1955.

21. Sigurdsson, B. and Gudmundsson, K.R. Clinical findings six years after outbreak of Akureyri disease. Lancet, 1: 766, 1956.

22. Leading Article. A new clinical entity? Lancet, 1: 789, 1956.

23. Von Economo, C. Encephalitis lethargica. Jahrb. f. Psychiat. u. Neurol., 39: 202, 1917.

24. Daae, A. Epidemi i Drangeldal Af Akut Muskelreumatisme Udbredt Uedsmitte. Norsk.mag.f.laegevidensk., 3: 409, 1872.

25. Homann, C. Om En I Kragero Laegedistikt Herskende Snitsam Febersygdom. Norsk.mag.f.laegevidensk., 3: 542, 1872.

26. Sylvest, E. Epidemic Myalgia. London, 1934. Oxford University Press.

27. Crowley, N., Nelson, M. and Stovin, S. Epidemiolgical aspects of an outbreak of encephalomyelitis at the Royal Free Hospital, London, in the summer of 1955. J.Hyg., 55: 102, 1957.

28. Hardtke, J. Iceland disease in Indiana. J. Indiana M.A., 48: 245, 1955.

29. Ramsay, A.M. and O'Sullivan, E. Encephalomyelitis simulating poliomyelitis. Lancet, 1: 761, 1956.

30. Jellinek, J.E. Benign encephalomyelitis. Lancet, 2: 494, 1956.

31. Ramsay, A. M. Encephalomyelitis in Northwest London. An endemic infection simulating poliomyelitis and hysteria. Lancet, 2: 1196, 1957.

32. Galpine, J.F. and Brady, C. Benign myalgic encephalomyelitis. Lancet, 1:757, 1957.

33. Pellew, R.A.A. Further investigations on a disease resembling poliomyelitis seen in Adelaide. M.J.Australia, 2: 480, 1955.

34. Bond, J.O. Letter. Lancet, 2: 257, 1956.

35. Wallis, A. L. An unusual epidemic. Lancet, 2: 291, 1955.

36. Wallis, A.L. Letter. Lancet, 2: 1091, 1955.

37. Wallis, A.L. Letter. Lancet, 2: 146, 1956.

38. Rose, J.R. An outbreak of encephalomyelitis in Sierra Leone. Lancet, 2: 914, 1957.

39. Wright, J. and Morley, D.C. Encephalitis tremens. Lancet, 1: 870, 1958.

40. McConnell, J. An epidemic of pleurodynia with prominent neurologic symptoms and no demonstrable cause. Am.J.M.Sc., 209: 41, 1945.

41. Hook, O. Islandssjuka, Nord.med., 7: 373, 1956.

42. Richardson, A.T. Some aspects of the Royal Free Hospital epidemic. Ann.Phys.Med., 3: 81, 1956.

43. Alexander, J.S. Observations on neuromuscular dysfunction in the Addington outbreak. South African M.J., 30: 88, 1956.

44. Bauwens, P. Variations of the motor unit. Proc. Roy. Soc. Med., 49: 110, 1955.

45. Leading article. Not poliomyelitis. Lancet, 2: 1060, 1954.

46a. Leading article. Epidemic myalgic encephalomyelitis. Brit. M.J., 2: 927, 1957.

46b. Galpine, J.F. Benign myalgic encephalomyelitis. Brit.J.Clin. Practice, 12: 186, 1958.

47. Russell, W.R. Poliomyelitis, London, 1952. Oxford University Press.

48. Weatherley, C.H. and Steigman, A.J. Influence of age and sex on the urinary bladder retention associated with acute poliomyelitis. Am.J.M.Sc., 226: 38, 1953.

49. Dalldorf, G. and Sickles, G.M. An unidentified filtrable agent isolate from the faeces of children with paralysis. Science, 108: 61, 1948.

50. Melnick, J.L. Coxsackie group of viruses. Ann. New York Acad.Sc., 56: 587, 1953.

51. Van Creveld, S. and DeJager, H. Myocarditis in new borns caused by coxsackie virus. Ann.Paediat., 187: 100, 1956.

52. Johnsson, T. Poliomyelitis epidemic in Stockholm in 1953. IV. Acta med. Scandinav., (supp. 316) 154: 33, 1956.

53. Galpine, J.F. and Macrae, A.D. Outbreak of meningoencephalitis; isolation of coxsackie virus. Lancet, 1: 372, 1953.

54. Stanley, N.F. Coxsackie virus infections in Australia with special reference ot their epidemiology. M.J. Australia, 2: 216, 1953.

55. Von Economo, C. Encephalitis Lethargica; Its Sequelae and Treatment. Translated by Newman, K.O. London, 1931. Oxford University Press.

56. Schlesinger, R.W. The Seasonal and Arthropod-Borne Virus Encephalitides, p. 380. Baltimore, 1952. Monographs in Medicine. Williams & Wilkins.

57. Annotation. Outbreak at the Royal Free Hospital. Lancet, 2: 351, 1955.

58. White, A.D. A History of the Warfare of Science with Theology in Christendom, vol. 2, p. 135. New York, 1896. Appleton.

59. Sargent, W. The Battle for the Mind. London, 1957. Heinemann.

60. Brain, R. Diseases of the Nervous System. Oxford, 1955.

61. Zahorsky, J. Herpangina. South. M.J., 13: 87, 1920.

62. Sigurdsson, B. Letter. Lancet, 2: 98, 1956.

63. Acheson, E.D. Letter. Lancet, 1: 834, 1957.

Sir (Ernest) Donald Acheson, KBE 1986

Sir (Ernest) Donald Acheson, KBE 1986, has just retired after holding the post of Chief Medical Officer, Departments of Health and Social Security for Great Britain. It is of notable interest that this principal early M.E. / CFS researcher had risen to become the chief Medical Officer for Great Britain. Dr. Donald Henderson, one of the early American M.E. / CFS pioneers whose work is also in this book, went on to become Dean of Medicine of Johns Hopkins and is presently the White House Chief of Science for the U.S.A. After Sir Donald Acheson graduated from Oxford in 1946 he held numerous senior positions, including Professor of Clinical Epidemiology, University of Southampton, Chairman of Slow Virus Group, Visiting Professor, McMaster University, Canada 1977. He has also held numerous important posts in many universities in the United Kingdom and New Zealand. *The information about Sir Acheson was obtained from the British* **Who's Who** *1992, Collier Macmillian Press, Cambridge, Ontario.*

Chapter 15

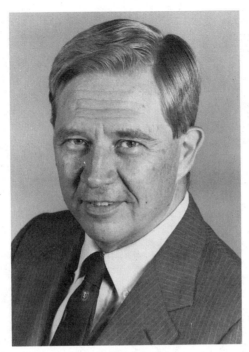

D. Henderson

This article is reprinted with the kind permission of The New England Journal of Medicine, Apr. 9, 1959, Vol. 26, Number 15, pages 757 to 764.

Epidemic Neuromyasthenia - Clinical Syndrome?*

Donald A. Henderson, M.D. † and Alexis Shelokov, MD. ††

Atlanta, Georgia, and Bethesda, Maryland

Dr. Henderson is presently the Associate Director for Life Sciences, Office of Science and Technology Policy in the Executive Office of the President in Washington, D.C. He received his M.D. at the University of Rochester School of Medicine and his M.P.H. at the John Hopkins University School of Hygiene and Public Health. He has also been the recipient of many honorary degrees including Sc.D.s from Yale University, Albany Medical College, University of Maryland and L.H.D. from the State University of New York. In the past, Dr. Henderson has held various positions including Chief, Epidemic Intelligence Service and Assistant to Chief, CDC, and Chief Medical Officer, Smallpox Eradication, World Health Organization, Geneva, Switzerland. He has played an integral part in many societies such as the American Board of Preventive Medicine, American Public Health Association, Royal College of Physicians (Edinburgh), Fellow and the Royal Society of Tropical Medicine and Hygiene, Fellow. Dr. Henderson has been involved in many professional committees which include Institute of Medicine, Board on International Health, Foundation for Development of International Health (Japan), Scientific Consultant and Rotary Foundation of Rotary International, Polio Plus Advisory Committee. Dr. Henderson has been involved in more than one hundred scientific publications dealing primarily with smallpox eradication, epidemiology and immunization.

* From the Communicable Disease Center and the National Institute of Allergy and Infectious Diseases, National Institutes of Health, Public Health Service, United States Department of Health, Education, and Welfare. † Epidemiologist, Epidemiology Branch, Communicable Disease Center, assigned to the Mary Imogene Bassett Hospital, Cooperstown, New York. †† Chief, Laboratory of Tropical Virology, National Institute of Allergy and Infectious Diseases; director, Middle America Research Unit, Canal Zone.

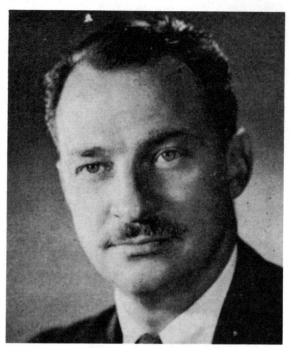

A. Shelokov (No recent photograph was available.)

Dr. Alexis Shelokov was born in Harbin, China and was educated in Gymnasium, China and Stanford University where he obtained his A.B. and M.D. Dr. Shelokov has held many affiliations with institutions, including, Massachusetts Memorial Hospitals, National Institutes of Health, University of Texas, Health Science Center at San Antonio, John Hopkins University School of Hygiene and Public Health and The Salk Institute, where he is presently the Director of Vaccine Research in the Government Services Division. He also holds outside appointments including Adjunct Professor of Epidemiology, School of Hygiene and Public Health, The John Hopkins University and a Member of the Core Group of the Expert Working Group on Biological Toxin Weapons Verification, Federation of American Scientists. Dr. Shelokov's research interests include infectious diseases, tropical medicine, preventive medicine, virology, epidemiology and vaccinology.

Dr. Shelokov's photgraph is courtesy of Industrial Medicine and Science, Vol. 33, Issue #10, pg 716, 1964.

During the past ten years an impressive number of outbreaks of bizarre, clinically similar illnesses have been reported from several areas of the world. The cases have shared the features of a protean symptomatology, including fatigue, headache, alterations in emotional status, aching muscular pain, paresis and paresthesias. Regarding the severity of the illnesses, few significant and consistent physical findings and abnormal laboratory determinations have been noted. The courses of the patients have been unaccountably prolonged and debilitating and marked by frequent exacerbations. Cases have been confined principally to young and middle-aged adults; females have been more frequently and severely afflicted. Although most of the outbreaks have involved the general community, the most notably susceptible have been nurses and physicians. Intensive efforts to characterize these illnesses, etiologically and pathologically, have met with little success.

The illnesses have been termed, variously, "Iceland disease,"[1] "benign myalgic encephalomyelitis,"[2] "Akureyri disease,"[3,4] epidemic vegetative neuritis,"[5] "acute infective encephalomyelitis,"[6] "encephalomyelitis"[7,8] "persistent myalgia following sore throat,"[9] "a disease resembling or simulating poliomyelitis,"[10,11] "atypical poliomyeltis"[12] "encephalomyelitis resembling poliomyelitis,"[13] and, more recently, "epidemic neuromasthenia."[14,15]

Careful appraisal reveals differences among the various epidemics, but most of these concern minor details. The apparent similarity in the courses of illness, the common nature of most symptoms and signs, the remarkable paucity of abnormal laboratory determinations and the similar epidemiologic characteristics suggest a nosologic, if not etiologic, association among the various outbreaks. Reviewed are the epidemics that to us appear to share these basic associations. Included are data from epidemics presently recorded in the literature, reports of several of significance previously overlooked by others and a number of unpublished reports of epidemics obtained from sources as gratefully acknowledged.

History

Attention was focused on this group of illnesses in 1950 by Sigurdsson and his associates,[10] who reported from Iceland an epidemic of over 1000 cases of an illness, superficially simulating poliomyelitis but presenting a number of inconsistent features. Among these were the following: a clinical course marked by easy fatigability, disturbances in sensibility and emotional instability persisting for several years[3]; an inordinately high community attack rate of 6.7 per cent; a morbidity rate twenty times higher among those fifteen to nineteen than those zero to four years of age; and an absence of deaths. Fecal specimens from patients with acute cases injected intracerebrally into rhesus monkeys and by various routes into other laboratory animals, including suckling mice, proved negative. Serums were found negative by complement-fixation tests for the arthropod-borne encephalitides, choriomeningitis, rabies and Q fever, and by hema glutination-inhibition tests for influenza viruses.

Reports of outbreaks of clinically similar but previously unrecognized illnesses followed in succeeding years from England, Australia, South Africa, Denmark, Germany, Greece and in the United States, from Florida, New York, Maryland, Alaska, Connecticut and Massachusetts (Table 1).

Preceding the report of the outbreak in Iceland were 2 epidemics in the United States and 1 in England, all of which, in retrospect, bear it a striking resemblance. Gilliam[12] documents in detail an outbreak in 1934 of 198 cases among personnel at the Los Angeles County General Hospital during which 10 per cent of the 1531 physicians and nurses were afflicted. Occurring concomitantly in Los Angeles and in other areas of California were many cases that were considered typical of paralytic poliomyelitis and a great many others that were not.[24] In addition to a number of hitherto unknown clinical manifestations particularly among adults, epidemiologic appraisal of reported cases revealed an unusually high attack rate,

a low paralytic and case fatality rate and a relative age selection for adults, particularly females.[17] Gilliam believed that the symptomatology among the hospital personnel was not characteristic and that the very high attack rate among the hospital personnel was without parallel in the history of poliomyelitis. He concluded, however, that since classic poliomyelitis prevailed among a large number of the patients with communicable disease in the hospital, the simpler explanation of the facts was that the atypical disease seen among the hospital staff was the same.

Two years later, after studying an outbreak of 32 similar cases among 63 novitiates and candidates at a convent in Fond du Lac, Wisconsin, Armstrong[25] concluded that the disease "is not explainable on the basis of any infection or intoxication with which I am familiar."

Described by Houghton and Jones[9] were 7 cases occurring over a four-week period in the fall of 1939 among young nurses at Harefield Sanatorium in England. The illnesses began with an apparent streptococcal pharyngitis, but after seven to fourteen days, a multiplicity of debilitating symptoms developed, evolving into the clinical picture and course similar to that described elsewhere. The authors were unable to identify the illness and suggested tentatively that an unidentified virus might be the cause.

Epidemics of similar illnesses occurring between 1939 and 1948 are unknown to us. Since almost two thirds of the recorded outbreaks have occurred during or at the end of the usual poliomyelitis season, and since they present a number of clinical features in common with poliomyelitis, misidentification may have occurred. It would be surprising indeed if no outbreaks had occurred in view of the relative frequency of reports since 1948.

Clinical Characteristics

Features in common among cases in these outbreaks are headache and aching pains in the extremities and usually the neck and back, associated with symptoms of paresis in one or more muscle groups. Initial appraisal has suggested to most observers the diagnosis of poliomyelitis. Subsequently the protean

Table 1

APPARENT OUTBREAKS OF EPIDEMIC NEUROMYASTHENIA

Location	Year	No. of Cases Reported	Nature of Outbreak
United States - Los Angeles, California*	1934[12,16-24]	198†	Hospital staff; community.*
United States - Fond du Lac, Wisconsin	1936[25]	35	Convent candidates & novitiates
England - Harefield	1939[9]	7	Hospital staff
Iceland	1948-49[3,4,10]	1090	Community
Australia - Adelaide	1949-51[11,26]	800	Community
United States - Louisville, Kentucky	1950[27]	37	Student nurses
United States - Northern New York	1950[1]	19†	Community
Denmark	1952[5,28]	10†∫	Community
United States - Lakeland, Florida	1959[29]	27†	Community
England - London (Middlesex Hospital)	1952[30]	14	Student nurses
England - Coventry	1953[31]	13†	Hospital staff; community.
United States - Rockville, Maryland	1953[14]	50	Student nurses predominantly; community.§
United States - Tallahassee, Florida	1954[32]	450	Community
United States - Seward, Alaska	1954[33]	175	Community
Germany - Berlin	1955[34]	7	Barracks group
England - London (Royal Free Hospital)	1955[7,8,13,35,36]	300	Hospital staff; community.ƒ
South Africa - Durban	1955[37,38]	140†	Hospital staff, community.
United States - Ridgefield, Connecticut	1955-56[39]	70	Community
United States - Punta Gorda, Florida	1956[15,40]	124	Community
United States - Pittsfield - Williamstown, Massachusetts	1956[41]	7	Community
England - London (Royal Free Hospital)	1956[6]	7	Student nurses
England - Coventry	1956[42]	7	Community
Greece - Athens	1958[43]	27	Hospital staff

* 198 cases at Los Angeles County Hospital documented in detail by Gilliam.[12] From other reports[16-24] large numbers of similar cases seen elsewhere in California.

† Number noted indicates only cases studied. Additional cases known or thought to have occurred.

∫ 10 cases reported in detail by Fog.[5] An additional 70 cases were reported but only sketchily described by Heidemann.[28]

§ Community cases suspected.

ƒ Community cases described by Ramsay and O'Sullivan.[12]

symptomatology, accompanied by emotional instability and depression, a relative paucity of physical findings (and these often of a bizarre nature) and the lack of significant laboratory findings has led to the consideration of psychoneurosis or mass hysteria as the underlying problem. Increasing numbers of remarkably similar cases sharing also the features of protracted debility and recrudescences over months to years have indicated to each investigator an illness foreign to his previous experience.

Although the clinical and epidemiologic descriptions indicate a close relation between epidemics, there are differences in the over-all severity of cases from one outbreak to another and well defined differences in presence or absence of some symptoms and physical findings. For a number of reasons, the differences may be more apparent than real; protean symptomatology makes complete recording of all findings difficult; physical findings are frequently on the borderline of abnormality and may be recorded or disregarded depending on the observer; patients were seen almost at the onset in some outbreaks whereas in others the evaluation was not begun until several weeks of illness had elapsed; and in some cases it is probable that an effort to make the clinical picture conform to some conventional neurologic process unwittingly biased observations. Because of these factors, construction of a comprehensive table that quantitatively compares the symptoms and physical findings among outbreaks is impossible. For purposes of orientation, however, a summary of the more prominent clinical features is presented in Figure 1. These, with other notable aspects of the illnesses, are discussed below in a narrative synthesis that seeks to embody the impressions of other writers and our own about the natural history of these illnesses.

Within each outbreak, there is a spectrum in the severity of illness. Apparently milder cases present some combination of the prodromal symptoms of fatigue, headache, diffuse, aching muscular pain, upper respiratory infection, diarrhea, tension or low-grade fever, most of the symptoms subsiding within a few days or weeks. Because of the uncertainties of diagnosis of such cases, authors, when compiling clinical and epidemiologic statistics, have commonly disregarded these illnesses. The clinical picture discussed relates then principally to the moderate or severe cases.

The onset of illness ranges from a fairly abrupt to a more usual, insidious evolvement of the prodromal symptoms already noted. This phase extends over a period of a few days to several weeks and may be difficult to date precisely. The symptoms may be intermittently or constantly present. A respiratory infection, often reported at the outset, may be accompanied by mild cough or coryza, tender lymphadenopathy most evident in the posterior cervical chain and, rarely, conjunctival injection or pneumonitis. Diarrhea, usually mild and of fairly brief duration, is frequently alluded to, particularly in the early course of the illness.

After a period of days to three or four weeks, there is often an abrupt exacerbation of symptoms accompanied by paresis, paresthesias, changes in emotional status and mentation, and dizziness, nausea or blurring of vision, with, in some patients, even vertigo, projectile vomiting and diplopia. This acute phase persists for one to several weeks and is accompanied by numerous symptoms, many of which are difficult to evaluate in the presence of tension, depression, anxiety and alterations in mentation.

Malaise and fatigability are particularly pronounced and persist long into convalescence. Headache and extremity, neck and back pain are usually present in about that order of frequency. The headache is commonly suboccipital or generalized although other variants are described. It is moderate to very severe in intensity, and usually nonthrobbing in character. The extremity pain is aching, diffuse, poorly localized, and, in general, more frequent in the lower limbs, although in some outbreaks it appears to be more common around the shoulder girdle. Pain is usually present in more than one limb, not uncommonly is asymmetrical and may shift in location. The neck and back pain is of the same general character as that in the extremities. Nuchal pain and a sense of tightness in the nape of the neck or back on extreme forward flexion of the head are usual; nuchal rigidity is not common. Abdominal pain, initially mistaken for peritoneal irritation, has been found, on careful examination, to be related to the abdominal musculature. Pleuritic-type chest pain, occasionally associated with a friction rub, has been related by some observers not to pleural irritation but to lesions in the intercostal or diaphragmatic musculature.

Uniformly present in all outbreaks, although not in all cases, is paresis, which usually begins with the acute illness but may be delayed for a period of days to several weeks. Manifestations of paresis seem to be of two general types. Most common initially is a diffuse weakness of one or more limbs usually accompanied by aching pain and a sense of heaviness in the affected part. Some have commented on this form of paresis as appearing to be more a disinclination than an inability on the part of the patient to contract the muscles. Deep tendon reflexes in the affected extremity range from being moderately hyperactive to depressed but are rarely absent or unilaterally unequal. Weakness of a similar type in the shoulder or hip girdle, back, neck, and abdominal musculature has been observed.

The second form of paresis involves single muscles or muscle groups, more commonly in the hand, arm, lower leg, hip or shoulder girdle, the facial muscles or the external rectus of the eye. Foot drop in a few patients has been mentioned in several epidemics. Although sometimes evident during the early acute phase, weakness in these muscles usually becomes manifest with resolution of the more extensive paresis noted above and appears, in a few cases, to constitute permanent residual damage. Contraction of paretic muscles is often jerky and associated with a coarse tremor. Fibrillary twitching and painful myoclonic spasms of involved large-muscle groups are frequently described. Fasciculations are rarely present. Atrophy of the involved muscles is exceptional despite persistence of measurable paresis.

Involved muscles are commonly tender, either diffusely or in focal, discrete areas. Focal areas of tenderness are stable in location, and relieved sometimes by procaine injection but without evident improvement in strength of contraction of the involved muscle. More diffuse tenderness has been associated with muscles described as edematous, doughy, or rubbery in consistence.

Present from early in the acute phase and often corresponding in distribution to the involved musculature are paresthesias, including numbness and tingling, hypesthesia or hyperesthesia, and, occasionally, anesthesia. Severe hyperesthesia requiring the use of bed cradles has been observed. Characteristically, the paresthesias are shifting in distribution over a period of hours or days and do not usually correspond to a peripheral nerve or root distribution. Cutaneous sensory examination discloses a similar bizarre shifting pattern of areas of marked impairment of touch, pain and temperature or hyperesthesia to touch. Less commonly, cutaneous sensory changes correspond to peripheral nerve or root zones and may be associated with tenderness over nerve trunks, especially the ulnar or sciatic. Anesthesia is rarely observed. Loss of position and vibration sense usually in the lower extremities and corresponding to the distribution of muscular pain and paresis has been seen in a number of outbreaks. The Babinski sign was demonstrated in a very few patients in two of the outbreaks.

Depression, tension and emotional instability have been impressive and among the most incapacitating and persistent symptoms. Repeated episodes of crying without provocation, insomnia, terrifying dreams and difficulty in concentration are probably secondary phenomena. Persons tending to be emotionally labile before illness have appeared to be most severely afflicted.

Mild confusion, impaired memory for recent events, alterations in personality structure, euphoric behavior and tendencies to transpose and "stumble over" words have frequently been observed during the more severe acute phase and during recrudescences, although sometimes persisting into convalescence.

Common also as an initial symptom in the acute phase is "dizziness", which varies in severity from a commonly observed postural giddiness to actual vertigo among fewer cases. Nystagmus on lateral or upward gaze is found accompanying some of the severe illnesses, but , as with numerous other signs, seems to appear and disappear over the course of hours to several days. Persistent vomiting, sometimes projectile in character, commonly accompanies the vertigo. Vertigo rarely persists for more than a few days, but a postural "dizziness" may persist for many weeks or months. Other symptoms much less common but probably related to eighth-cranial-nerve involvement include tinnitus, hyperacusis, and, uncommonly, transient hearing impairment.

Possible involvement of other cranial nerves is suggested by occasional transient facial pareses and the more regularly noted symptoms of blurring of vision or diplopia. These visual symptoms have often been associated with eye pain aggravated by movement, less commonly with photophobia. Most observers have been unable to demonstrate associated ocular-muscle weakness, although paresis of the external rectus with evident strabismus has been seen in some outbreaks. Symptoms of functional impairment of swallowing are not uncommon, but are only occasionally associated with palatal paralysis or regurgitation. Whether this symptom is related to cranial-nerve involvement, some lesion in the deglutitional muscles or emotional factors is not clear. During several outbreaks a few patients were placed in respirators, never for more than a few days. Clear documentation of respiratory embarrassment because of diaphragmatic or bulbar involvement, however, is not reported.

Gastrointestinal disturbances, particularly nausea, are common in the acute phase. These may or may not be related to vertigo. Diarrhea is usual early in the course, and constipation later.

Figure 1

Selected Symptoms and Signs in 23 Outbreaks of Epidemic Neuromyasthenia

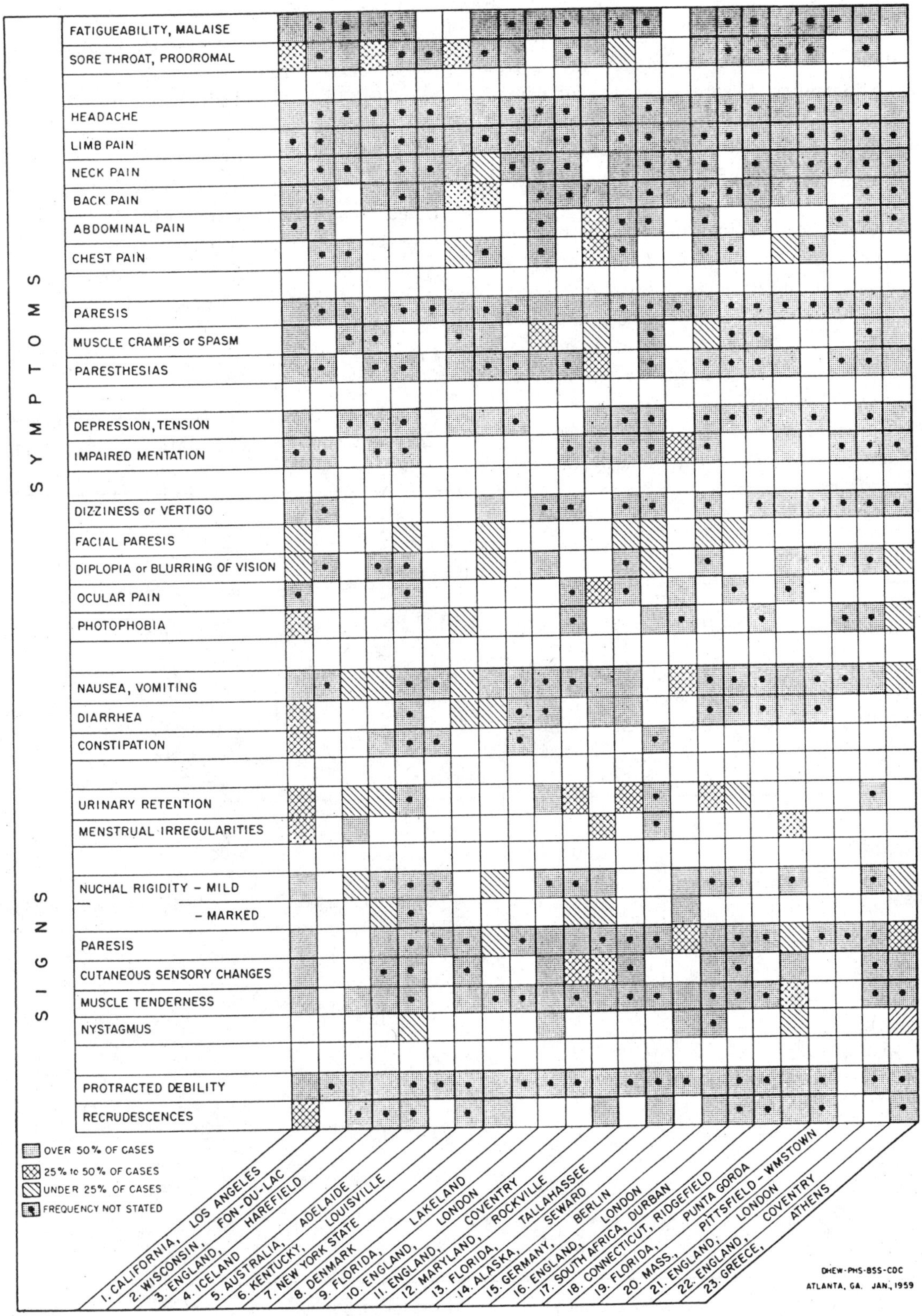

A mild hepatomegaly without splenomegaly in somewhat less than a tenth of the patients was found in the Royal Free Hospital outbreak, but only 1 patient had evidence of jaundice.

Present inconstantly and in small numbers from epidemic to epidemic were symptoms of urinary retention without dysuria but of sufficient severity to require catheterization and occasional tidal drainage. These symptoms subsided within five to six days.

Symptoms suggesting angiospasm have been particularly prominent in several outbreaks and rare or unremarkable in others. Hyperhidrosis, marked pallor and flushing or occasionally cyanosis of the hands or feet, accompanied by numbness and tingling over the affected area and sometimes edema, has been noted in several epidemics. These were so impressive in the Danish outbreak as to suggest primary involvement of the autonomic nervous system.[5]

Menstrual disturbances, including amenorrhea, menorrhagia and disturbances of cycle, have been repeatedly noted.

Throughout most of the illness, the temperature does not exceed 100°F. Early in the course a temperature of 100 to 103°F. occurs in a fourth to a half of the patients, but rarely persists for more than two or three days. Among three groups of carefully studied patients, an instability of body temperature was noted consisting of a variation of two or three degrees over the course of a day but within the normal range. As symptoms subsided, a more normal diurnal temperature fluctuation was assumed.

Course of Illness

After an acute phase lasting a few days to several weeks, there is a slow resolution of symptoms punc-

---

Table 2

Results of Cerebrospinal-Fluid Examination - 17 Outbreaks

Location of Outbreak	No. of Persons Examined	No. of Persons with Pleocytosis*	No. of Cells *per cu. mm.*	Day of Illness	No. of Patients with Elevated Protein	Protein Concentration *mg./100ml.*
California[12]	59	3	12,50,66	0,2,4	18	(12†;6.§)
Wisconsin[25]	2	0				
England[9]	1	0				
Iceland[3,4,10]	8	5	10,18,35 50,80	3,6,4 3,10	4	50,59,75,80
Australia[11]	59	5	44-88	7	2	45,60
Kentucky[27]	3	0				
New York[1]	11	2	27,44	4,12		
Denmark[5]	5	0				
London, England[30]	6	0				
Coventry, England[31]	9	0				
Maryland[14]	25	0			3	48,58,61
Tallahassee, Florida[32]	101	7	"Up to 15"	?		
Germany[34]	7	0			1	85
London, England[8]	18	0				
Punta Gorda, Florida[15]	5	0				
Coventry, England[42]	7	0			3	50,60,80
Greece[43]	4	0			1	66

*>6 cells/cu.mm.   †Trace of globulin   §+test for globulin.

tuated by exacerbations during which all the symptoms initially present may recur in their original, severe form and persist for days to weeks. Exacerbations commonly coincide with increased exertion, with cold or damp weather, in the premenstrual period, with trauma or with upper respiratory infection. The most persistent and incapacitating symptoms are fatigability and malaise, headache, neck, back and extremity pain, paresis, depression, irritability, impairment of concentration and paresthesias.

The protracted debility engendered by the illness is illustrated by studies from several epidemics. Among 198 cases in the Los Angeles County Hospital outbreak, the average time lost from work was fourteen weeks: 24 per cent of the personnel lost more than twenty weeks.[12] Inpatient hospital care among 300 cases from the Royal Free Hospital outbreak extended for periods in excess of a month in 43 per cent.[8]

In the sixth month after onset, studies of 21 patients from the Punta Gorda, Florida epidemic revealed that 5 of the group were confined to bed for one or more days, and definite restriction of activity because of residual symptoms represented 43 per cent of patient days in that month.[15]

A few long-term follow-up studies have been carried out that suggest definite gradual improvement extending over several years' time. Exacerbations or relapses of varying severity, although mimicking the original acute phase of illness, became increasingly milder and of shorter duration.

Re-examination of 8 patients in New York State fifteen months after onset showed none to be completely without symptoms although the symptoms were mild.[1] Muscle pain, easy fatigability and more labile emotional habitus were the principal complaints. An eighteen-month re-examination of patients from the Punta Gorda outbreak revealed all to be much improved or essentially well.[40] Residual symptoms similar to those reported by the New York State patients were noted by some but were so equivocal as to be difficult to ascribe to the original illness.

A six-year follow-up study of 39 cases from the Icelandic epidemic, one of apparently greater initial severity than that in Punta Gorda, revealed that all

patients had returned to work, but only 13 per cent considered themselves free of symptoms.[3]

Laboratory

White-cell counts have been reported as normal in most outbreaks, although ranging in a few patients as high as 14,000. In one series an absolute neutropenia was noted, 4 of 7 patients having total counts below 3000.[42] A relative lymphocytosis (counts of 50 to 60 per cent) during the acute illness was observed in the Maryland outbreak[14]; a low normal neutrophil count and a high normal lymphocyte count were found among half of 138 studied at the Royal Free Hospital.[8] In this outbreak abnormal adult lymphocytes, with cytoplasmic vacuolation, and plasma-cell-like forms, with coarsely reticulated nuclei and deeply basophilic cytoplasm, were frequently noted. The cells were not, however, considered to be those seen in infectious mononucleosis.

Erythrocyte sedimentation rates, when recorded, were rarely elevated. The exceptions were among patients from the Alaska outbreak, two thirds of whom were said to have had higher than normal values[33] and among nurses in the 1939 English outbreak, in which slight elevations were recorded.[9]

With few exceptions, cerebrospinal-fluid examinations have shown slight or no abnormality. In Table 2 are the compiled results from the reports in which the number of lumbar punctures performed is stated. A few cases in each of five outbreaks have shown pleocytosis between the time of onset and the twelfth day. Increased cerebrospinal-fluid protein was found in about the same number although not always in the same patients. Glucose and chloride determinations were normal. Colloidal-benzoin and colloidal-gold determinations in the Los Angeles outbreak showed a mid-zonal elevation in 18 of 59 cases.[12] Since these epidemics have tended to occur during or at the end of the enterovirus season and have sometimes been coincident with epidemics of poliomyelitis, it is conceivable that those with cerebrospinal fluid abnormalities in fact represent cases of poliomyelitis, Coxsackie virus or ECHO meningitis. Conversely, because it is uncommon to see patients early in the course of the illness, transient cerebrospinal fluid changes could be missed in the majority of cases. Interpretation of these data is thus difficult.

Liver-function studies performed in significant numbers in the Maryland[14] and Royal Free Hospital[8] outbreaks revealed but 1 to be notably abnormal in a patient from the latter outbreak who became clinically jaundiced.

Serial twenty-four urinary creatine determinations performed on 10 adult patients from the New York State outbreak revealed initial levels in excess of 100 mg. daily among 9 of the 10, 6 of these returning to normal levels within four to seven weeks. Three patients showed little change during this period; 1 showed an increase from about 230 mg. to 300 mg. per100ml. at four weeks and to 400mg. per 100ml. at seven weeks.[1] Estimations of the serum cholinesterase in 7 patients and cerebrospinal-fluid cholinesterase in 1 patient were normal. Electrophoretic patterns showed no abnormality in these serums.[8]

Heterophil-antibody determinations in several outbreaks revealed no significant elevation except for 1 of 7 patients in the Coventry outbreak[42] and 4 of 121 in the Royal Free Hospital outbreak.[8] Repeat determinations in the latter outbreak revealed, however no change in titers - findings interpreted as indicative only of probable past infection.

Complement-fixation, neutralization and agglutination studies have been wholly unrevealing. Tests for antibodies for the following were reported negative in the various outbreaks: poliomyelitis[1,14,15,26,29,31-33]; lymphocytic choriomeningitis[10,15,26,29-32]; encephalomyocarditis[8,26,31]; Eastern equine encephalitis[10,15,29,32]; Western equine encephalitis[10,15,29,32] St. Louis encephalitis[10,15,29,32]; Japanese B encephalitis[10]; Port Augusta encephalitis[26]; influenza[8,10,29,33]; Q fever[8,10,29];leptospirosis[8,9,15,26,29-31,34]; trichinosis[9,14]; toxoplasmosis[8,15]; adenovirus[8]; herpes simplex[8]; psittacosis lymphogranuloma venerem[8,32]; brucellosis[8,9,25]; tularemia[25]; rabies[10]; typhoid[9,25]; paratyphoid[25]; louping ill[8]; Coxsackie A and B viruses[14]; ECHO virus, Type 6[14]; and *Salmonella typhimurium*.[14] A very few serums with elevated complement-fixation titers for mumps have been observed, but the majority have been negative.[8,15,26,29-32] Tests for cold agglutinins[34] and Wassermann reactions have been negative.[8,9,14] Toxicologic studies carried out in three outbreaks were unrevealing.[14,15,38]

Electroencephalography was performed on 19 patients from five outbreaks.[5,13,15,42,43] Borderline abnormalities of a nonspecific nature were seen in some, but all except 1 were interpreted as being within normal limits. One severely afflicted patient from the epidemic in Greece had a tracing showing paroxysmal or continuous slow-wave activity at high potentials predominating over the frontal leads and sometimes extending simultaneously to all leads.[43] Electrocardiograms obtained on patients in the Maryland[14] and Punta Gorda, Florida,[15] outbreaks were interpreted as normal. Three of 42 in the Royal Free Hospital epidemic showed abnormalities consisting of abnormal T waves in two or more leads and a prolongation of the QT interval in one. Two reverted to normal records. One patient with extensive neurologic abnormalities initially showed isoelectric T waves in Lead 1 and inverted T waves in Lead V_3 that, although improved over an eighteen-month period, were still abnormal at that time.[8]

Electromyographic studies have given conflicting results. Two Danish cases studied four months after onset showed neurogenic paresis of radicular or peripheral origin in isolated, involved muscle groups.[5] Observations in 20 cases from the Durban, South Africa outbreak showed no abnormalities.[38] Among the 1953 Coventry cases, 3 during the fourth to eighth week of illness gave inconclusive evidence of partial denervation of muscle groups.[31] The most consistent evidence of dysfunction was reported among 28 cases studied from the Royal Free Hospital epidemic. Examinations carried out one or two months after onset showed largely unremarkable nerve-muscle excitability and nerve-conduction measurements, but electromyography, in the early stages, indicated some irregularly occurring fasciculation potentials of nor- mal motor-unit potential form. With the onset of paresis, a severe reduction in the number of motor-unit potentials on volitional movement of the affected muscles was apparent, of long duration and polyphasic in some cases. In the less severely involved and, particularly during recovery, the motor- unit potentials were grouped resulting in a tremulous contraction of 5-10 per second that rapidly fatigued. This combination of findings was thought to suggest a myelopathic lesion indicating involvement of the motor unit at the level of the spinal cord. The absence of lower-motor-neuron degeneration in the face of persistence of these lesions could not be explained.[8] Similar myographic findings were reported among 7 patients in the 1956 Coventry outbreak,[42] and 4 of 6 in the 1958 outbreak in Greece.[43]

This article is reprinted with the kind permission of The New England Journal of Medicine, Apr. 16, 1959, Vol. 260, No. 16, pages 814-818.

Epidemic Neuromyasthenia - Clinical Syndrome? (Concluded)*

Donald A. Henderson, M.D.,† and Alexis Shelokov, M.D.††, Atlanta, Georgia

Viral and Bacteriological Studies

The nature of these illnesses has suggested to most a viral etiology, but, despite intensive efforts to implicate such an agent, results have been meagre. Cerebrospinal fluid, feces, throat washings, acute-phase serums and blood clots have been inoculated by a variety of routes into many different laboratory animals and various tissue-culture systems. Despite the frequent use of blind passages, attempts to infect the following animals have thus far proved futile: suckling[1,8,10,14,15,26,29-31,34] and adult mice[8,14,26,29,31]; guinea pigs with[8] and without cortisone[10,26,31]; hamsters[8,10,14,26]; rabbits[26,31]; rats with and without cortisone[15]; ferrets[8]; and cynomologus and rhesus monkeys with[8,27] and without cortisone.[1,8,10,14,27,30,31]

Embryonated hens' eggs of various ages injected into the chorioallantoic membrane, allantoic sack, yolk sack and amnion have yielded negative results.[8,14,26,27,29] Tissue-culture systems employed with similarly negative results include the following: monkey testicle[14,30,31]; monkey kidney[8,14,15,30,31]; HeLa cells[8,14,15]; human-embryo skin[31], brain[8], liver[8,15] and spleen[8]; human-infant kidney[8]; human fibroblast[14]; and human chorioamnion.[8,14]

Positive findings of possible significance are reported by Pellew and Miles[26] from specimens obtained from Australian patients. In their studies throat washings, feces and cerebrospinal fluid from each of 5 patients with acute cases were inoculated in combinations into paired young rhesus monkeys intranasally, and subcutaneously on three successive days. The monkeys inoculated with material from 2 of the 5 gave evidence of illness. One of the 4 had a lowered temperature (95°F.) on the eighth day, and was sluggish. No definite abnormalities were found at post-mortem examination. The remaining monkeys showed sluggishness and abnormal temperatures between the sixteenth and eighteenth days.

One showed wasting, particularly of the hind limbs and tremulousness and was killed on the eighteenth day. Of the remaining 2, 1 died on the twenty-seventh day, and the other recovered by the twenty-sixth day and remained well.

At post-mortem examination, the only gross abnormality was the occurrence of minute red spots along the course of the sciatic nerve in the last 2 monkeys. Microscopical sections showed localized infiltrations of inflammatory cells and exudation of red cells in the sciatic nerves. In the nerve roots close to their point of exit from the spinal canal there was pronounced infiltration with lymphocytes and mononuclear cells. In some of the nerve fibers axon swelling and vacuoles in the myelin sheaths were found. No abnormalities in the brain or spinal cord were detected. The heart muscle of the monkey that died showed severe myocarditis, with widespread infiltration of lymphocytes and mononuclear cells. Passage of a pool of brain, spinal cord, nerve, skeletal and heart muscle from these animals led to no illness in the monkeys inoculated. Repeat inoculation with the original material caused similar symptoms in 2 of 4 monkeys, but passage was again unsuccessful.[26]

* *From the Communicable Disease Center and the National Institute of Allergy and Infectious Diseases, National Institutes of Health, Public Health Service, United States Department of Health, Education, and Welfare.*

†*Epidemiologist, Epidemiology Branch, Communicable Disease Center, assigned to the Mary Imogene Bassett Hospital, Cooperstown, New York.*

††*Chief, Laboratory of Tropical Virology, National Institute of Allergy and Infectious Diseases; director, Middle America Research Unit, Canal Zone.*

Confirmation of these observations has not been forthcoming from other outbreaks.

Because of at least superficial resemblance of these illnesses to poliomyelitis, efforts to isolate a possible etiologic agent have been focused on viral studies. Thorough bacteriologic studies have been reported from the Maryland outbreak only.[14] Results obtained suggest at least a coincidental relation between cases of the disease, isolation from the stool of organisms of the Bethesda-Ballerup paracolon group and rises in serologic titer.

Table 3			
Age-Specific Attack Rates in Two Community-Wide Outbreaks.			
	Rate in Akureyri, Iceland		Rate in Punta Gorda, Florida	
Age	Male Patients	Female Patients	Male Patients (White)	Female Patients (White)
yr.	%	%	%	%
0-9	1.4	2.0	-	-
10-19	11.7	13.2	10.9	10.7
20-49	4.8	11.1	9.1	11.5
50 & over	2.1	2.9	2.0	8.3
Average	5.1	8.3	4.7	8.3

A total of 218 fresh fecal specimens from 113 persons, both ill and well, were painstakingly examined. Specimens were placed in enrichment mediums and then grown aerobically and anaerobically on a variety of selective and nonselective mediums. Obtained were 13 isolates of 2 strains of Bethesda-Ballerup paracolon organisms and 2 isolates of *S. typhimurium*. Serial serum samples from persons from whom the latter organisms were isolated showed no antigen agglutination with these organisms, thus discounting their pathogenic significance.

Isolates of the Bethesda-Ballerup bacilli were obtained only from 12 nurses with the illness and an asymptomatic kitchen helper. One type (antigenic formula, 1a, 1b, 1c: 8, 9) was found in the stools of 7 nurses; the second type (formula, 2a, 1b: [21] 25, 26) was detected in the stools of 5 nurses; both types were isolated from a kitchen helper. Neither of the strains appeared in large numbers in the stools, and neither was isolated from more than two stools of the series obtained from any person.

H and O agglutinins for the freshly isolated strains were found in titers of 1:40 or greater in the serums of 15 of the 26 paretic patients, in 7 of the 24 with "minor illness," in 3 of 27 nurses without illness and in the kitchen helper. Among 11 of the 22 ill nurses showing the presence of agglutinins, there was a rise and fall of antibody titers; in 5, there was a demonstrable rise, and in 3, a fall in the antibody levels (in the remaining 3, single specimens only were available).

Serial serum specimens from 9 patients from the Punta Gorda, Florida, epidemic tested against the two Bethesda-Ballerup strains from the Maryland outbreak showed 1 with falling 0 agglutinins and a 1:160 H agglutination titer that was preceded and succeeded by negative titers in other specimens.[15]

Epidemiology

The epidemiologic features of these illnesses have been uniquely distinctive, and because of the absence of specific pathognomonic findings in the individual case, these features must be regarded as integral to the diagnosis. They include, particularly, the concentration of cases among young and middle-aged adults, the increased frequency and severity of cases among females, the virtual absence of illness among preadolescents and the marked susceptibility of nursing personnel and physicians.

Two epidemics in communities of similar size (Table 3) in which detailed data regarding age-specific attack rates were obtained include the outbreaks in Akureyri, Iceland[10] (population, 6887) and Punta Gorda, Florida[15] (population, 2020). The similarity in attack rates between these two outbreaks is notable. Most heavily afflicted were those between ten and forty-nine years of age. In the Akureyri epidemic, those aged fifteen to nineteen seemed particularly susceptible; in Punta Gorda, it was the group aged thirty to thirty-five. Although the rates indicate a predominance of female to male cases in the ratio of more than 1.5:1, the severity of cases among females in both epidemics was considerably greater. An absence or virtual absence of cases in persons under the age of ten is surprising, and despite intensive search for some minor illness variant among this group in Punta Gorda, none was found. Equally interesting is the decrease in frequency of cases beyond the age of fifty. In the Tallahassee outbreak, a similar age distribution of cases was noted, those age twenty-five to forty-four being most susceptible.[32] All the other outbreaks have involved primarily young and middle-aged adults, principally females.

Suggestive that the disease may be one with which communities have had no previous experience or, at least, to which they have built up no immunity is the remarkable similarity in attack rates in different community epidemics (Table 4). The rates in the Seward, Akureyri and Punta Gorda outbreaks are essentially identical. That in Tallahassee is lower but may be the result of a less homogeneous spread of illness throughout this much larger community. In Table 4, the rates noted for Punta Gorda and Tallahassee are for the white population since Negro rates were somewhat lower in the former and over sixtyfold lower in the latter epidemic despite intensive search in both for cases among Negroes.

The differences noted between the larger and smaller community outbreaks suggest, and other studies support, the necessity of close contact for spread of the disease. With the exception of the outbreaks in Iceland[10] adjacent communities have not become involved, and a spread of illness to surrounding rural areas has been quite uncommon for all outbreaks, including those in Iceland. Outbreaks among groups in intimate contact (Table 5), particularly those living together in dormitories, have produced attack rates considerably in excess of those seen among comparable age groups in community epidemics. A tendency for aggregation of cases by households has been observed in several outbreaks.[10,15,18,32]

Table 4
Attack Rates in Community Epidemics.

Location of Outbreak	Population	Number Ill	Percentage Ill
Akureyri, Iceland[10]	6,887	465	6.7
Seward, Alaska[33]	3,000	175	5.8
Punta Gorda, Florida[15]	1,604*	104*	6.5
Tallahassee, Florida[32]	23,708*	346*	1.5
* White population only.			

Table 5
Attack Rates among Groups in Close Association.

Group	Population	Number Ill	Percentage Ill
Los Angeles student nurses[12]	401	65	16
Wisconsin convent[25]	65	32	49
Akureyri high-school residents[10]	70	34	49
Kentucky student nurses[27]	161	37	22
Maryland student nurses[14]:			
Paretic cases	66	19	29
All cases	66	36	55
Royal Free Nurses Preliminary Training School[7] - 1955	40	8	20
Royal Free Nurses Preliminary Training School[6] - 1956	27	5	19

Disproportionate among the total of outbreaks is the number among hospital groups. Ten[6,7,9,12,14,27,30,31,38,43] of twenty-three epidemics studied dealt principally with cases among hospital personnel, although it is known or believed that cases in the surrounding community were occurring concomitantly in six of these.[7,9,12,14,31,38] Two outbreaks in which studies were principally of community cases, disclosed rates four or five times greater among medical and allied personnel[15,32] than among similar age groups in the general community. Among 275 employees at the Tallahassee Memorial Hospital, 16 cases were reported — an attack rate of 5.8 per cent as contrasted to 1.5 per cent for the white population of Tallahassee fifteen years of age or older. In Punta Gorda, medical and allied personnel had an attack rate of 42 per cent as compared to one of 8.6 per cent for white persons in the community aged ten to sixty-nine. That degree of exposure was probably the principal cause of these differences is further suggested by the virtual absence of cases at the university in Tallahassee, where a large student population of a presumably highly susceptible age resided.

Among those afflicted in major hospital epidemics, the nursing staff and physicians have shown particular susceptibility as contrasted with other hospital personnel. In the Los Angeles County Hospital epidemic[12] three groups within the hospital were delineated: occupations having intimate patient contact; occupations having less regular patient contact; and occupations rarely involving patient contact. Rates for these groups were, respectively, 8.2 per cent (169 cases among 2072 employees), 1.7 per cent (16 cases among 951) and 0.8 per cent (11 cases among 1291). These differences could not be accounted for by age differences between groups. In the Royal Free Hospital[7] outbreak, the rates among nurses, resident domestics, doctors and inpatients and ancillary medical, technical and social workers ranged from 13 to 18.6 per cent whereas among 2060 other employees, the rate was 2.2 per cent.

Analysis of cases among nurses by place of work in the Los Angeles epidemic[12] demonstrated that cases occurred considerably earlier and four times more frequently among those working on the communicable-disease wards and in the main admitting office than among those working elsewhere in the hospital. Further demonstration of the importance of intimate contact is obtained by a comparison of rates between personnel resident at the hospital contrasted to personnel not living on the hospital grounds. Among those resident at the Royal Free Hospital,[7] males experienced an attack rate of 20 per cent, and females one of 19 per cent; among nonresidents, males had a rate of 2.5 per cent, and females one of 6.1 per cent. Among residents at the Los Angeles County Hospital,[12] 9.4 per cent of physicians and 19 per cent of the nurses were afflicted whereas among nonresidents, only 3.1 per cent of physicians and 5.8 per cent of nurses were ill.

Although transmission of the disease to hospital inpatients has been noted,[7,12] the frequency with which this occurs is not known.

The relative restriction of outbreaks by communities or groups in close association has suggested possible common-source exposure to water, foods, or some toxic agent in the environment. Efforts to identify such exposure have been made in several studies, but without success.[10,14,15,32] Additional evidence weighing against a common exposure, at least in community outbreaks, is the very high attack rate accompanied by the uniformly consistent selection of cases by age and sex and the noted predominance of cases among medical and allied personnel. It is difficult to postulate a chemical agent that would produce such an epidemiologic pattern.

The incubation time has been found to be between five and eight days when precise single dates of exposure could be determined.[7,10,12,14,31] Indirect determinations based on patterns of spread of illness and cases with continuing exposure suggest that the incubation period may be longer in some cases, but definite evidence of this is lacking.

Geography and Season

The epidemics are scattered in both latitude and longitude although concentrations are to be noted in the London-Coventry area of England and in Florida. This may reflect better recognition and reporting in these areas or may indicate a tendency for illness to recur in areas in which it is once established. With four exceptions, reported epidemics have been located on or very near salt water. Specific inquiry, however, during two epidemics regarding possibly related factors has been unrevealing.[15,32]

Over half the epidemics have occurred during the summer and particularly during the fall months, often succeeding or overlapping the latter portion of the poliomyelitis season in the particular area. This seasonal predilection accounts in part for the initial confusion in diagnosis between cases of these illnesses and poliomyelitis. The seasonal occurrence is not constant, however. Other epidemics are described that began in the fall and extended through the winter,[17] or appeared in late winter and continued through the spring,[15] in addition to other variants.

The Process, the Name and the Future

Crucial to a definitive classification and understanding of the group of diseases reviewed is a knowledge of the pathophysiology involved. Of this, essentially nothing is known. Deaths that occurred among definite cases during the acute phase or could be directly attributable to the illness have nowhere been reported. Two fatal cases occurring within a year of onset of illness have been noted, both of which occurred months after the initial episode and from unrelated causes. Post-mortem findings were wholly unrevealing.[8] Material for histologic study has almost been nil. The only positive finding reported is a nonspecific reactive hyperplasia found in a biopsied lymph node two weeks after the onset of illness in 1 case.[8]

The symptoms indicate a multiorgan system involvement, but which systems are primarily and which secondarily involved is not clear. There is agreement among investigators that altered functions in either the central or the peripheral nervous system or both must be present to account for many of the symptoms and findings, but confirmation through histologic study is lacking. To define the anatomic sites of lesions on the basis of symptomatology and physical findings is not as yet possible. A multifocal, changing process is postulated. If it involves the central nervous system, it does so in such a way that it rarely, or but briefly, alters the cerebrospinal fluid. Postulates based on these criteria have little precedent from other communicable diseases. A primary myalgic process has been considered likely by most investigators, but no histologic material to confirm this is available and electromyography to date has been confusing.

Etiologically, the Australian studies[26] indicate the possibility of a viral agent, and the Maryland studies[14] implicate a bacterial agent of the Bethesda-Ballerup paracolon group possibly as a toxin-producing pathogen, or perhaps as a fellow traveller with an unknown virus. These represent, as yet, but interesting leads.

In summary, despite intensive study by competent investigators in a number of different areas, the etiology and pathophysiology of these illnesses remains almost a total mystery.

As a group, however, the illnesses share a great number of common features and, both clinically and epidemiologically, present a unique and distinctive appearance. A nosologic relation is strongly suggested. For convenience of reference and identification a single descriptive name would be useful. Originally proposed by White and Burtch,[1] the name "Iceland disease" has been most commonly used in this country. Since this designation, however, has not been used in other countries, and since Sigurdsson, who originally focused attention on these illnesses through his studies in Iceland, objects to it, it seems wise to discard it. Sigurdsson in a counterproposal has suggested "Akureyri disease"[3] named for the medical district in which the studies of his group were concentrated. To date, this has been ignored. In 1956 an editorial in the *Lancet* introduced the term "benign myalgic encephalomyelitis."[2] To those who have observed cases, the illnesses are anything but benign, except in terms of mortality. Encephalomyelitis, additionally, implies knowledge of a central-nervous-system inflammatory process of which there is presently no proof. English studies published since this proposal, with one exception,[42] have ignored this name. In reporting the Danish outbreak, Fog,[5] unaware of similar outbreaks, designated the illness seen in Denmark as "epidemic vegetative neuritis" because of what appeared to him to be major, although not exclusive, involvement of the autonomic nervous system. Objection must be registered to use of this term as well as to that in a recent English report, "acute infective encephalomyelitis,"[6] since both again imply knowledge of an inflammatory process that has not as yet been demonstrated. The latter term, in addition, properly includes essentially all the infectious encephalomyelitides, the etiology of many of which is well established.

To date, there is no agreement on a name, almost every epidemic receiving a different designation. For purposes of referencing and indexing, this presents a chaotic problem. Until an etiologic agent or agents are identified or until the underlying pathophysiologic processes are defined, we recommend use of the name, "epidemic neuromyasthenia."[14,15] This, we believe, meets previous objections and is specifically distinctive within the limits of current knowledge. Use of the word "epidemic" emphasizes the need for epidemiologic as well as clinical appraisal of cases. Diagnosis of a single, sporadic case of illness marked by a protean symptomatology within pathognomonic physical or laboratory findings and presenting many of the features of psychoneurotic illness is fraught with difficulty. Adequately characterizing the most prominent symptoms of the illnesses without reference to the underlying pathologic processes are the terms "neurasthenia" and "myasthenia" or, when linked, "neuromyasthenia."

In the light of the frequency of reports in the past few years, it is probable that further epidemics will occur. In the study of these, particular emphasis must be placed on elucidating the pathophysiologic processes involved, indirectly by electroencephalography, psychometric testing, personality evaluation, electromyography and careful serial physical examination, and more directly through the histologic study of biopsy material, particularly involved muscle, and by autopsy of patients dying early in the disease. Indicated also are intensive bacteriologic, virologic and serologic studies of specimens obtained early in the prodromal phase, especially among those complaining of respiratory illness in whom the full-blown picture of the disease subsequently develops. Previous studies have too often been obliged to deal with specimens obtained many days to weeks after the insidious onset of the prodromal phase. In a community outbreak intensive study of hospital personnel, particularly nurses and student nurses, should be especially fruitful in yielding cases in greater proportionate numbers than among other groups in the population.

Although, from current reports, these illnesses do not appear numerically important on a national scale, the long-term morbidity among those who are ill and the very large percentage involved in a single out break indicate a need for intensive, comprehensive investigation and surveillance of outbreaks as they occur.

We are indebted to Dr. E. Charles Kunkle, professor of neurology, Duke University School of Medicine, for many helpful suggestions in the appraisal and synthesis of material.

References

1. White, D.N., and Burtch, R.B. Iceland disease: new infection simulating acute anterior poliomyelitis. *Neurology* 4:506-516, 1954.

2. Leading article. New clinical entity? *Lancet* 1:789,1956.

3. Sigurdsson, B., and Gudmundsson, K.R. Clinical findings six years after outbreak of Akureyri disease. *Lancet* 1:766,1956.

4. Sigurdsson, B. New clinical entity? *Lancet* 2:98, 1956.

5. Fog, T. Vegetative (epidemic?) neuritis. *Ugesk, f. laeger.* 115:1244-1250,1953.

6. Geffen, D., and Tracy, S.M. Outbreak of acute infective encephalomyelitis in residential home for nurses in 1956. *Brit. M. J.* 2:904-906, 1957.

7. Crowley, N., Nelson, M., and Stovin, S. Epidemiological aspects of outbreak of encephalomyelitis at Royal Free Hospital, London, in summer of 1955. *J. Hyg.* 55:102-122, 1957.

8. Outbreak of encephalomyelitis in Royal Free Hospital Group, London, in 1955. *Brit M.J.* 2:895-904, 1957.

9. Houghton, L.E., and Jones, E.I. Persistent myalgia following sore throat. *Lancet* 1:196-198, 1942.

10. Sigurdsson, B., Sigurjonsson, J., Sigurdsson, J.H., Thorkelsson, J.V., and Gudmundsson, K.R. Disease epidemic in Iceland simulating poliomyelitis. *Am. J. Hyg.* 52:222-238, 1950.

11. Pellew, R.A.A. Clinical description of disease resembling poliomyelitis, seen in Adelaide, 1949-51. *M.J. Australia* 1:944-946, 1951.

12. United States Public Health Service, Division of Infectious Diseases, Institute of Health. Gilliam, A.G. *Epidemiological Study of Epidemic, Diagnosed as Poliomyelitis, Occurring among Personnel of Los Angeles County General Hospital During the Summer of 1934.* 90pp. (*Public Health Bulletin* No. 240.) Washington, D.C.: Government Printing Office, 1938.

13. Ramsay, A.M., and O'Sullivan, E. Encephalomyelitis simulating poliomyelitis. *Lancet* 1:761-764, 1956.

14. Shelokov, A., Habel, K., Verder, E., and Welsh, W. Epidemic neuromyasthenia: outbreak of poliomyelitis-like illness in student nurses. *New Eng. J. Med.* **257**:345-355,1957.

15. Poskanzer, D.C., et al. Epidemic neuromyasthenia, outbreak in Punta Gorda, Florida. *New Eng. J. Med.* **257**:356-364, 1957.

16. Dunshee, J.D., and Stevens, I.M. Previous history of poliomyelitis in California. *Am. J. Pub. Health* **24**:1197-1200, 1934.

17. Leake, J.P., Cedar, E.T., Dearing W.P., Gilliam, A.G., and Chope, H.D. Epidemiology of poliomyelitis in California, 1934. *Am. J. Pub. Health* **24**: 1204-1206, 1934.

18. Van Wart, R., Courville, C., and Hall, E.M. 1934 epidemic of poliomyelitis in Los Angeles: preliminary report on pathological changes in nervous system. *Am.J.Pub.Health* **24**:1207-1209, 1934.

19. Bower, A.G., Meals, R.W., Bigler, M., Ewing, J., and Hauser, V. Clinical features of poliomyelitis in Los Angeles. *Am. J. Pub. Health* **24**:1210-1212, 1934.

20. Stevens, G.M. 1934 epidemic of poliomyelitis in Southern California. *Am. J. Pub. Health* **24**:1213, 1934.

21. Kessel, J.F., Hoyt, A.S., and Fisk, R.T. Use of serum and routine and experimental laboratory findings in 1934 poliomyelitis epidemic. *Am. J. Pub. Health* **24**:1215-1223, 1934.

22. Hart, T.M., and Luck, J.V. Orthopedic aspect of Los Angeles County 1934 poliomyelitis epidemic. *Am. J. Pub. Health* **24**:1224-1228, 1934.

23. Shaw, E.B., and Thelander, H.E. Poliomyelitis in San Francisco. *Am. J. Pub. Health* **24**:1229-1233, 1934.

24. Wilson, J.C., and Walker, P.J. Acute anterior poliomyelitis: orthopedic aspects of California epidemic of 1934. *Arch. Int. Med.* **57**:477-492, 1936

25. Armstrong, C.A. Personal communication.

26. Pellew, R.A.A. and Miles, J.A.R. Further investigations on disease resembling poliomyelitis seen in Adelaide. *M.J. Australia* **2**: 480-482, 1955.

27. Steigman, A.J. Personal communication.

28. Heidemann, H. Increasing occurrence of myositis. *Ugesk. f. laeger.* **114**:1504, 1952.

29. United States Public Health Service, Communicable Disease Center. Unpublished data.

30. Acheson, E.D. Encephalomyelitis associated with poliomyelitis virus: outbreak in nurses' home. *Lancet* **2**:1044-1048, 1954.

31. Macrae, A.D., and Galpine, J.F. Illness resembling poliomyelitis observed in nurses. *Lancet* **2**:350-352, 1954

32. Bond, J.O., Wolff, H.G., and Bistowish, J.M. Personal communication.

33. Deisher, J.B. Iceland disease in Alaska. Paper presented at clinical meeting of American Medical Association, Seattle, Washington, November 27-30, 1956.

34. Sumner, D.W. Further outbreak of disease resembling poliomyelitis. *Lancet* **1**:764-766, 1956.

35. Public health. Outbreak at Royal Free. *Lancet* **2**:351, 1955.

36. Jelinek, J.E. Benign encephalomyelitis. *Lancet* **2**:494, 1956.

37. Hill, R.C.J. Memorandum on outbreak amongst nurses at Addington Hospital, Durban. *South African M.J.* **29**:344, 1955.

38. Alexander, J.S. Observations on neuromuscular dysfunction in Addington outbreak. *South African M.J.* **30**:88-90, 1956.

39. Henderson, D.A., Shelokov, A., Heller, J.H., and Safford, T. Unpublished data.

40. Henderson, D.A., Kunkle, E.C., and Clement, W.B. Unpublished data.

41. Deutaman, W., and Davis, R.K. Personal communications.

42. Galpine, J.F., and Brady, C. Benign myalgic encephalomyelitis. *Lancet* **1**:757, 1957.

43. Daikos, G.K., Garzonis, S., Palaiologos, A., Papadojianakis, N., and Bousraros, G. Personal communication.

Chapter 16

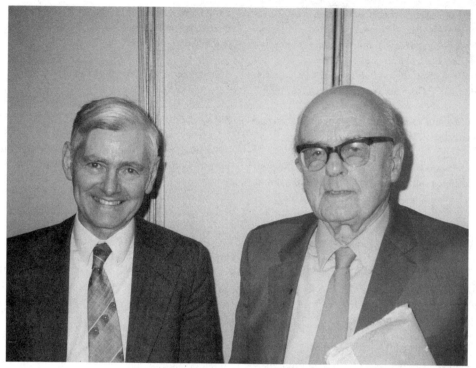

J. Gordon Parish with A. Melvin Ramsay

A Bibliography of M.E./CFS Epidemics

This list was largely based on bibliographies first published by Sir Donald Acheson (see Chapter 14) and also by Drs Henderson and Shelokov (see Chapter 15). They were collected, improved upon and circulated by the British physician, Dr. J. Gordon Parish. I have added some of the more recent epidemics to this list.

The numbering of epidemics up to 1975 is that of Dr. Gordon Parish. Although Dr. Parish may not be in agreement with the additions and deletions to his original compilation, I wish to acknowledge my gratitude for his considerable assistance, the use of his library and the extensive time he shared with me, without which this chapter and much of this book could not have been written. His photograph, shown here, was one of the last photographs taken of Dr. Ramsay.

Byron Hyde, M.D.

1934
Epidemic 1

Los Angeles City and California State, U.S.A.

Gilliam AG, Epidemiological study of an epidemic diagnosed as poliomyelitis occurring among the personnel of the Los Angeles County General Hospital during the Summer of 1934. Public Health Bulletin No. 240 - April 1938. United States Public Health Service, Washington, D.C., Government Printing Office.

Wilson JC, Walker PJ, Acute anterior poliomyelitis: Orthopaedic aspects of California epidemic of 1934.

Archives of Internal Medicine 1936; 54:477-91. (Statistics for California State, description of atypical features including arthopathy.) The following references appeared in the American Journal of Public Health,1934:24, describing the unusual features of the 1934 poliomyelitis epidemic in California, U.S.A.

Dunshee JD, Stephens IM. Previous history of poliomyelitis in California, pp 1197-1200.

Leake JD, Cedar ET, Palmer W, Dearing WP, Gilliam AG, Chope HD. Epidemiology of poliomyelitis in California, 1934 (describes cases in Ruth Protection Home), pp 1204-6.

Van Wart R, Courville C, Hall EM. 1934 epidemic of poliomyelitis in Los Angeles. Preliminary report on the pathological changes in the nervous system, pp 1207-9.

Bower, AG, Meals RW, Bigler M, Ewing J, Hauser V. Clinical features of poliomyelitis in Los Angeles, pp 1210-2.

Stephens GM. 1934 Epidemic of poliomyelitis in Southern California, pp 1213-4.

Kessel JF, Hoyt AS, Fisk RT. Use of serum and routine and experimental laboratory findings in 1934 poliomyelitis epidemic, pp 1215-23.

Hart TM, Luck JV. Orthopaedic aspects of Los Angeles County 1934 poliomyelitis epidemic, pp 1224-8.

Shaw EB, Thelander HE. Poliomyelitis in San Francisco, pp 1229-33.

Pathology: Kessel JF, Van Wart R, Fisk RT, Stimpert FD. Observations on the Virus recovered from 1934-35 poliomyelitis epidemic in Los Angeles. Proc Soc. Exp Biol Med. 1936; 35:326-9.

Electromyography: Marinacci AA, Von Hagen KO. The value of the electromyogram in the diagnosis of Iceland Disease. Electromyogram 1965; 5:241-51.

1936
Epidemic 2

Fond-du-Lac, Wisconsin, U.S.A.

Armstrong G. Report to the Surgeon General, U.S. Public Health Service of the investigation of an outbreak of "Encephalitis" in the St. Agnes Convent, Fond-du-Lac, Wisconsin.

1937
Epidemic 3

Erstfeld, Switzerland

Stahel H. Die Poliomyelitis - Epidemic bei Stab Geb. I.R. 37 and Geb Sch Bat #11, Erstfeld 18-30 Juli 1937. Die Abortiv-Poliomyelitis. Schweiz Med Wochenschr 1938; 68: 86-91.

Gsell O. Abortive Poliomyelitis. Verlag Thieme, Leipzig 1938, 20-1.

Epidemic 4

Frohburg Hospital, St. Gallen, Switzerland

Gsell O. Abortive Poliomyelitis. Leipzig 1938, 13-18. The three Swiss epidemics 3,4 and 6 are summarised in review articles by Gsell O (1958) and Parish JG (1978).

1939
Epidemic 5

Harefield Sanatorium, Middlesex, England

Houghton LE, Jones EI. Persistent myalgia following sore throat. Lancet 1942; 1:196-8.

Epidemic 6

Degersheim, St. Gallen, Switzerland

Gsell O. Abortive Poliomyelitis. Helv Medica Acta 1949; 16:169-83.

1945
Epidemic 7

University Hospital of Pennsylvania, U.S.A.

McConnell J. An epidemic of pleurodynia with prominent neurologic symptoms and no demonstrable cause. Am J Med Sci, 1945; 209: 41-8.

1946-47
Epidemic 8

Iceland

Sigurjonsson J. Poliomyelitis and the Akureyri Disease. Mixed epidemics of poliomyelitis and a disease resembling poliomyelitis with the character of the Akureyri Disease. Nord Med 1959; 61:174-82. (The 1948 epidemic appears to have started in 1947.)

1948-49
Epidemic 9

North Coast Towns, Iceland;
   Akureyri Nov-Dec 1948,
   Saudakrokur Dec 1948- Feb 1949,
   Isafordur Jan-April 1949

Sigurdsson B, Sigurjonsson J, Sigurdsson JHJ, Thorkelsson J, Gudmundsson KR. A disease epidemic in Iceland simulating Poliomyelitis. Am J Hyg 1950; 52:222-38.

Sigurdsson B, Gudmundsson KR. Clinical findings six years after outbreak of Akureyri Disease. Lancet 1956; 1:766-7.

Effect of previous experience of Akureyri Disease on subsequent poliomyelitis epidemic and poliomyelitis vaccination (see Sigurdsson B), Gudnadottir M, Petursson G. Response to poliomyelitis vaccination. Lancet 1958; 1:370-1.

Hyde B, Bergmann S, Chronic Aspects of Akureyri Disease, p 205-215, Post-Viral Fatigue Syndrome. Jenkins & Mowbray, John Wiley and Sons, (1991)

1949-51
Epidemic 10

Adelaide, South Australia

Main Article: Pellew RAA. A clinical description of a disease resembling poliomyelitis seen in Adelaide, 1949-51. Med J Aust 1951; 1:944-6.

Monthly incidence of cases: Jackson JF. 14th Annual General Report South Australia Institute of Medical and Veterinary Science, July 1951 - June 1952;17.

Virus and Animal Studies: Pellew RAA, Miles JAR. Further investigations on a disease resembling poliomyelitis seen in Adelaide. Med J Aust 1955; 42:480-2.

Pappenneimer AM, Bailey OT, Cheever FS, Daniels JB. Experimental polyradiculitis in monkeys. J Neuropath Clin. Neurol 1951; 1:48-62.

1950
Epidemic 11

St. Joseph Infirmary, Louisville Kentucky, U.S.A.

Steigman AJ. An outbreak of an unidentified illness in the Nurses' Training School of St. Joseph Infirmary, Louisville, in Kentucky in October 1950. Report to the National Foundation of Infantile Paralysis, 1951. Data summarised by Henderson DA, Shelokov A, (note review article 2, 1959). Steigman AJ. epidemic neuromyasthenia. N EJM 1969;281:797.

Epidemic 12

Upper New York State

White DN, Burtch RB. Iceland Disease - a new infection simulating Acute Anterior Poliomyelitis. Neurology 1954; 4:506-16.

1952
Epidemic 13

Middlesex Hospital Nurses' Home, London, England

Main Article: Acheson ED. Encephalomyelitis associated with Poliomyelitis Virus. Lancet 1954; 2:1044-8.

Acheson ED. Outbreak at the Royal Free. Lancet 1955; 2:395 (letter giving further details of 1952 Middlesex Hospital epidemic).

Epidemic 14

Copenhagen, Denmark

Main Article/Electromyography: Fog AT. Neuritis Vegitiva Epidemica? Ugeskr Laeger 1953;115:1244-51.

Heidemann H. Ophobet optraeden af myositer (epidemic myositis). Ugeskr Laeger 1952; 114:1504.

Krarup NB. Ophobet optraeden af myositer: poliomyelitis? (Epidemic of myositis: poliomyelitis?). Ugeskr Laeger 1952; 114:1534.

Epidemic 15

Lakeland, Florida, U.S.A.

Henderson DA, Shelokov A. Epidemic Neuromyasthenia-clinical syndrome? NEJM 1959; 260:757-64.

1953
Epidemic 16

Whitley Hospital, Coventry and Coventry District, England

Main Article and Electromyography: Macrae AD, Galpine JF. An illness resembling Poliomyelitis observed in nurses. Lancet 1954; 2:350-2.

Epidemic 17

Chestnut Lodge Hospital, Rockville, Maryland, U.S.A.

Main Article, bacteriological and serological studies: Shelokov A, Habel K, Verder E, Welsh W. Epidemic Neuromyasthenia. An outbreak of poliomyelitis-like illness in Student Nurses. NEJM 1957; 257:345-55. Case Report, Indiana University, Bloomington, Indiana, U.S.A.

Hardtke EF. Iceland Disease in Indiana. J Indiana State Med Assoc 1955; 48:245-50.
Case also described by Acheson ED, see Review article (1), 1959.

Epidemic 18

Jutland, Denmark

Pedersen EP. Epidemic Encephalitis in Jutland. A clinical survey for the years 1952-54. Dan Med Bull 1956; 3:65-75. (Encephalitis with vertigo, Autumn 1953).

1954
Epidemic 19

Tallahassee, Florida, U.S.A.

Bond JO. A new clinical entity? Lancet 1956; 2:256.

Epidemic 20

Seward, Alaska

Deisher JB. Benign Myalgic Encephalomyelitis (Iceland Disease) in Alaska. Northwest Med 1957; 56:1451-6.

Epidemic 21

British Army, Berlin, Germany

Sumner DW. Further outbreak of a disease resembling poliomyelitis. Lancet 1956; 1:764-6.

Review of epidemics

Leading Article
Akureyri 1948 (9) Not Poliomyelitis. Lancet 1954; Adelaide 1949 (10) 2:1060-1. New York State 1950 (12) Middlesex Hospital 1952 (13) Coventry 1953 (16)

Epidemic 22

Liverpool, England

Outbreak involving medical and nursing staff in a Liverpool Hospital.

Comparative Epidemiology: see Official Public Health report for Epidemic 24 (1955).

1955
Epidemic 23

Dalston, Cumbria, England
Wallis AL. An unusual epidemic. Lancet 1955;

2:290. Further details in letters, Lancet 1955; 2:1091 and Lancet 1956; 2:146.

Main account: Wallis AL. An investigation into an unusual disease seen in epidemic and sporadic form in a general practice in Cumberland in 1955 and subsequent years. MD Thesis. University of Edinburgh 1957.
Spread to County Durham: Parish JG. Epidemic malaise. Br Med J 1970; 3:47-8.

Epidemic 24

Royal Free Hospital, London, England

Leading Article: Infectious mononucleosis. Br Med J 1955; 2:309-10. (July 30th, refers to what was first believed to be infectious mononucleosis - glandular fever at the Royal Free Hospital, an error that later was magnified in the USA into the theory that M.E/ CFS was Chronic Epstein Barr disease).

Public Health report. Outbreak at the Royal Free. Lancet 1955; 2:351.

Vital Statistics. Outbreak at the Royal Free Hospital. Obscure nature of infection. Br Med J 1955; 2:442-3.

Compston ND. Epidemic at the Royal Free Hospital. Br Med J 1956; 2:157. (Brief report to the BMA meeting at Brighton).

Official Public Health report and Comparative Epidemiology

Report of the Ministry of Health for the year ended 31/12/55. Part II on the state of the Public Health: Being the Annual Report of the Chief Medical Officer for the year 1955. Her Majesty's Stationery Office; 71-4. Epidemics 13,16,22,24,27.

Main articles: The medical staff of the Royal Free Hospital. An outbreak of encephalomyelitis in the Royal Free Hospital Group, London, in 1955. Br Med J 1957; 2:895-904.

Compston ND. An outbreak of encephalomyelitis in the Royal Free Hospital Group, London, in 1955. Postgrad Med J 1978; 54:722-4. (précis of the previous report).

Geffen D. An outbreak of encephalomyelitis in the Royal Free Hospital Group, 1955. Public Health, 1957; 71;13-24.

Crowley N, Nelson M, Stovin S. Epidemiological aspects of an outbreak of encephalomyelitis at the Royal Free Hospital in the summer of 1955. J Hyg (Camb) 1957; 55;l02-22. (Bacteriological and viral studies, serological tests, heterophile antibody types, lymphocyte changes and biochemical tests).

Electromyography: Richardson AT. Some aspects of the Royal Free Hospital epidemic. Ann Phys Med1956; 3:81-9

Review article: Benign mylagic encephalomyelitis. Lancet 1957; 1:1342.

Epidemic 25

Perth, Western Australia,

Steen AS. Virus epidemic in recurrent waves. BR Med J 1956; 1:235.

Epidemic 26

Gilfach Goch, Wales

Jones TD. Virus epidemic in recurrent waves. BR Med J 1956; 1:348.
Sporadic Cases **Boscombe, Hants, England**

Jelinek JE. Benign encephalomyelitis. Lancet 1956; 2:494-5.

East Ham, London England

Bonomini V, Montuschi E. Benign encephalomyelitis. Lancet 1956; 2:629-30.

Epidemic 27

Addington Hospital, Durban and Durban City, South Africa

Hill RCJ. Memorandum on the outbreak amongst the nurses at Addington Hospital, Durban. S. Afr Med J 1955; 29:344-5.

Association News. Report of the clinical meeting of the Natal Coastal Branch held on 17th May 1955 at the Addington Hospital, Durban. The Durban 'Mystery Disease'. S. Afr Med J 1955; 29:997-8.

Alexander JS. Observations on Neuromuscular dysfunction in the Addington Outbreak. S. Afr Med J 1956; 30:88-90.

Main Article: Hill RCJ, Cheetham RWS, Wallace HL. Epidemic myalgic encephalomyelopathy - the

Durban outbreak Lancet 1959; 1:689-93. (Non-nitrogenous acidity toxic metabolite noted in urine of some patients).

Sporadic cases
Johannesburg, South Africa
July 1954 - March 1955

Jackson AL, Jacobson S, Cooper B. A disease resembling poliomyelitis. Report of an outbreak in Johannesburg. S. Afr Med J 1957; 31:514-7.

1955-6
Epidemic 28

Segbwema, Sierra Leone Oct 1955 - Oct 1956

Preliminary report: Rose JR. A new clinical entity? Lancet 1956; 2:197.

Main Article: Rose JR. An outbreak of encephalomyelitis in Sierra Leone. Lancet 1957; 2:914-6.

Epidemic 29

Patreksfordur and Thorshofn,Iceland Oct 1955 - April 1956

Sigurdsson B, Gudnadottir M, Petursson G. Response to poliomyelitis vaccination. Lancet 1958; 1:370-1 (outline of 1955-6 epidemic and unusual response to subsequent poliomyelitis vaccination.)

Epidemic 30

N.W. London, England April 1955 -September 1957

Main article-electromyography- electroencephalography: Ramsay AM, O'Sullivan E. Encephalomyelitis simulating poliomyelitis. Lancet 1956; 1:761-6.

Royal Free Hospital, Nurses Preliminary Training School May - June 1956

Ramsay AM. Encephalomyelitis simulating poliomyelitis and hysteria. Lancet 1957; 2:1196-1200.

Geffen D, Tracy SM. An outbreak of acute infective encephalomyelitis in a residential home for nurses in 1956. Br Med J 1957; 2:904-6.

1956
Epidemic 31

Ridgefield, Connecticut, U.S.A.

Henderson, DA Shelokov A, Heller JH, Safford T.

Unpublished data, quoted by Henderson DA, Shelokov A. Epidemic neuromyasthenia NEJM 1959; 260:757-64.

Epidemic 32

Punta Gorda, Florida, U.S.A.

Poskanzer DC, Henderson DA, Kunkle EC, Kalter SS, Clement WB, Bond JO. Epidemic neuromyasthenia. An outbreak in Punta Gorda, Florida. NEJM 1957; 257:356-64.

Epidemic 33

Newton-le-Willows, Lancashire, England

Lyle WH. Lymphocytic meningo-encephalitis with myalgia and rash. Lancet 1956; 2:1042-3.

Tyrrell DAJ, Snell B. Recovery of a virus from cases of an epidemic exanthem associated with meningitis. Lancet 1956; 2:1028-9.

Lyle WH. An unfamiliar infectious disease: An account of an outbreak. MD Thesis. University of Manchester.

Main article/virology: Lyle WH. An outbreak of disease believed to have been caused by Echo 9 virus. Ann Int Med 1959; 51:248-69.

Epidemic 34

Pittsfield, Williamstown, Massachusetts, U.S.A

Deutaman W, Davis RK. (Unpublished). Data included in survey by Henderson DA, Shelokov A. Epidemic Neuromyasthenia - clinical syndrome? N Engl J Med 1959; 260:757-64 and 814-8.

Hyde, BM Myalgic Encephalomyelitis (Chronic Fatigue Syndrome): An Historic Perspective, Canada Weekly Report, Health and Welfare Canada, January 1991 Vol. 17S1E, pg 5-8, based upon conversation with Dr Davis, whose wife was a patient in that epidemic.

Sporadic cases, Hygiea, Sweden

Hook O. Data summarised by Acheson ED, see Review article (1) 1959.

Review article - 1 Nomenclature, Leading article. A new clinical entity. Lancet 1956; 1:789-90. (Name "benign mylagic encephalomyelitis" suggested).

Correspondence: Sigurdsson B. Lancet 1956; 2:98.

Review article - 2 Annotation. Encephalitis, meningitis or poliomyelitis. Lancet 1956; 2:1091. (Coxsackie B and Echo Virus infections)

1956-57
Epidemic 35

Coventry, England

Galpine JF, Brady C. Benign myalgic encephalomyelitis. Lancet 1957; 1:757-8. Br Med J 1957; 2:645.

Galpine JF. Benign myalgic encephalomyelitis. Br J Clin Pract 1958; 12:186-90.

Galpine JF. Epidemic malaise. Br Med J 1970; 1:501.

1957
Epidemic 36

Brighton, South Australia

Hicks DA. A new clinical entity. Lancet 1957; 1:686.

Review article - 1 Leading article. Virus meningitis and encephalomyelitis. Br Med J 1957; 1:811-3. (Coxsackie, Echo Virus meningitis and myalgic encephalomyelitis).

Review article - 2 Leading article. Epidemic myalgic encephalomyelitis. Br Med J 1957; 2:927-8.

Review article - 3 Annotation. Benign myalgic encephalomyelitis. Lancet 1957; 2:1208-9.

Nomenclature Acheson ED. Benign myalgic encephalomyelitis. Lancet 1957; 1:834-5.

1958
Epidemic 37

Athens, Greece

Daikos G, Paleologue A, Garzonis S, Bousvaros GA. Papadoyannakis N. Arch Med Sci, Athens 1958; 14:617.

Main Article: Daikos GK, Garzonis S, Paleologue A, Bousvaros GA, Papadoyannakis N. Benign Myalgic Encephalomyelitis. An outbreak in a Nurses' School in Athens. Lancet 1959; 1:693-6. (No reticuloendothelial involvement but periostitis and arthropathy noted; EMG and EEG studies). Review article - 1

Switzerland

Gsell O. Encephalomyelitis myalgic epidemic eine poliomyelitisahnliche Krankheit. Schweiz Med Wochenschr 1958; 88:488-91. (German - summarises epidemics in Switzerland 1937-39).

Review article - 2 Galpine JF. Benign myalgic encephalomyelitis. British Journal of Clinical Practice 1958; 12:186-90.

1958-9

Sporadic cases, S.W. London, England

Price JL. Myalgic encephalomyelitis. Lancet 1961; 1:737-8. (Abnormal ECG, EEG and EGM findings).

1959
Epidemic 38

Newcastle upon Tyne, England

Pool JH, Walton JN, Brewis EG, Uldall PR, Wright AE, Gardner PS. Benign myalgic encephalomyelitis in Newcastle upon Tyne. Lancet 1961; 1:733-7. (EMG studies).

Sporadic cases N.W. London England

Goldwater S. Influenza-like illness. Br Med J 1960; 1:962-3 (arthropathy with effusions prominent).

Review article - 1 Major review of literature: Acheson ED. The clinical syndrome variously called Benign Myalgic Encephalmyelitis, Iceland Disease and Epidemic Neuromyasthenia. Am J Med 1959; 26:569-95. Comparative epidemiology: epidemics 1 California, 7 Pennsylvania, 9 Iceland, 10 Adelaide, 12 New York State, 13 Middlesex Hospital (London), 14 Denmark, 16 Coventry (England), 17 Maryland, 20 Alaska, 21 Berlin, 24 Royal Free Hospital (London), 27 Durban (S. Africa), 28 Sierra Leone, 30 N.W. London, 32 Punta Gorda (Florida), 35 Coventry (England).

Review article - 2 Major review of literature: Henderson DA, Shelokov A. Epidemic Neuromyasthenia - clinical syndrome? N Engl J Med 1959; 260:757-64 and 814-8. Comparative epidemiology: 1 California, 2 Wisconsin (U.S.A.), 5 Harefield (England), 9 Iceland, 10 Adelaide, 11 Louisville (Kentucky), 12 New York State, 13 Middlesex Hospital (London), 14 Copenhagen, 15 Lakeland (Florida), 16 Coventry (England), 17 Maryland, 19 Tallahassee (Florida), 20 Alaska, 21 Berlin, 24 Royal Free Hospital (London), 31 Ridgefield (U.S.A.), 32 Punta Gorda (Florida), 34 Pittsfield (Massachusetts), 35 Coventry (England), 37 Athens.

Henderson and Shelokov introduced the term epidemic neuromyasthenia.

Sporadic cases, England

Kendall RE. The psychiatric sequelae of Benign Myalgic Encephalomyelitis. Br J Psychiat 1967; 113:833-40.

1961

Sporadic case Basel, Switzerland

Gsell O. Encephalomyelitis Basel myalgica benigna, epidemische Pseudoneurasthenie. Schweiz Med Wochenschr 1963; 93:197-200.

1961-2
Epidemic 39

New York State

Albrecht RM, Oliver VL, Poskanzer DC. Epidemic Neuromyasthenia. Outbreak in a convent in New York State. JAMA 1964; 187:904-7.

1964-1966
Epidemic 40

N.W. London

Scott BD. Epidemic malaise. Br Med J 1970; 1:170. Ramsay AM. Hysteria and Royal Free Disease BR Med J 1965; 2:1062.

Ramsay AM. Epidemic neuromyasthenia 1955-1978. Postgrad Med J 1978; 54:718-21.

Epidemic 41

Franklin, Kentucky, U.S.A.

Miller G. Chamberlin R., McCormack WM. An outbreak of neuromyasthenia in a Kentucky Factory - the possible role of a brief exposure to organic mercury. Am J Epidemiol 1967; 86:756-64.

1934-1965

Review of Electromyographic Findings, California

1965-6
Epidemic 42

Galveston County, Texas

Johnson JM, Micks DW. Epidemic Neuromyasthenia Variant? Texas Reports on Biology and Medicine

1967; 25:484.

Leon-Sotomayor L. **Epidemic Diencephalomyelitis**. A possible cause of neuropsychiatric, cardiovascular and endocrine disorders. New York, Pageant Press, 1969.

1967-70

Sporadic cases Edinburgh, Scotland

Innes SGB. Encephalomyelitis resembling benign myalgic encephalomyelitis. Lancet 1970; 1:969-71

1968
Epidemic 43

Fraidek, Lebanon

Mourad S, Chidiac J. Benign Myalgic encephalomyelitis in Lebanon. Leb Med J 1969; 22:735-40.

1969
Epidemic 44

Medical Centre, State University of New York U.S.A.

Damadian R. Unidentified symptom complex. NEJM. 1969; 280:1131. Correspondence: Trimble GX. Epidemic Neuromyasthenia. NEJ M 1969; 281:105; Fisher CM. On Damadian's Ache, 281:106, Epidemic Neuromyasthenia, 281:797-8 Steigman AJ, Hart RH, Adamson JR (criteria for diagnosis).

1970
Epidemic 45

Lackland Air Force Base, Texas, USA.

Graybill JR, Silva J. O'Brien MS, Reinarz JA. Epidemic Neuromyasthenia. A Syndrome or disease? JAMA 1972; 219:1440-3

1970-71
Epidemic 46

Hospital for Sick Children Great Ormond Street, London, England

Dillon, MJ, Marshall WC, Dudgeon JA, Steigman AJ. Epidemic Neuromyasthenia: outbreak among nurses at a children's hospital. BR Med J 1974; 1:301-5.
Correspondence: Epidemic neuromyasthenia. Br Med J 1974; 1:574-5 Wallis GG; Perry FS: 2:276 Parish JG; 2:559 Dillon MJ (Marshall WC, Dudgeon JA: Steigman AJ).

Dillon MJ. 'Epidemic neuromyasthenia' at the Hospital for Sick Children, Great Ormond Street, London. Postgrad Med J 1978; 54: 725-30.

1974

Review article
Parish JG. Epidemic neuromyasthenia: a reappraisal. IRCS J International Research Communications, Medical Science 1974; 2:22-6 (survey of literature to 1974).

1975
Epidemic 47

Mercy San Juan Hospital Sacramento, California

Ryll, E. ; Chabursky, B. (In preparation.) 200 hospital staff in the Sacramento, California hospital fell ill in August September 1975. The epidemic appears to have spread to the children of the hospital staff and from there to the children's teachers. 43 have been seriously disabled with chronic illness from 1975-1992.

1976
Epidemic 48

Southwest Ireland

Preliminary report: Corridan JP, Myalgic Encephalomyelitis. J Irish Med Ass 1976; 69:414. Main article: Corridan JP. Epidemic neuromyasthenia in Southwest Ireland. Postgrad Med J 1978; 54:731-6.

Review article Ramsay AM. Benign Myalgic Encephalomyelitis or Epidemic neuromyasthenia. GP Update 1976; 12:539-42.

1977

Definition Anonymous. Reply to question: "What is Icelandic Disease?" Br Med J 1977; 1:965.

Correspondence: Ramsay AM, Dowsett EG, Dadswell JV, Lyle WH, Parish JG. Icelandic disease (benign myalgic encephalomyelitis or Royal Free Disease) Br Med J 1977; 1:1350.

Epidemic 49

Dallas - Fort Worth, Texas, USA

Shelokov A, Currie DM, Nelson M. 'Epidemic Neuromyasthenia' Texas 1977. Postgrade Med J 1978; 54:741 (Abstract).

Currie DM, Shelokov A. Repetitive stimulation abnormalities in 'epidemic neuromyasthenia': identification and implications. PostgradMed J 1978; 54:746 (Abstract).

1978

First major M.E./CFS Symposium, Royal Society of Medicine London

Lyle WH, Chamberlain RN (eds). 'Epidemic neuromyasthenia 1934-1977; Current Approaches Postgrade Med J 1978; 54:705-74.

Papers: Parish JG. Early outbreaks of 'epidemic neuromyasthenia': 711-7 (comparative epidemiology: 1 California, 3 Erstfeld (Switzerland), 4 Frohburg (Switzerland), 6 Degersheim (Switzerland), 9 Iceland, 10 Adelaide, 12 New York State, 23 Dalston (England).

Ramsay AM. 'Epidemic neuromyasthenia' 1955-78: 718-21 (epidemics 30 and 40 NW London, England).

Compston ND. An outbreak of encephalomyelitis in the Royal Free Hospital Group, London in 1955:722-4. (epidemic 24).

Dillon MJ. 'Epidemic neuromyasthenia' at the Hospital for Sick Children, Great Ormond Street, London: 725-30 (epidemic 46).

Corridon JP. 'Epidemic neuromyasthenia' in Southwest Ireland: 731-6 (epidemic 47).

Ball AP. Disease due to echovirus type 19 in Birmingham, England, 1975: relationship to 'epidemic neuromyasthenia: 737-40.

Shelokov A, Currie DM, Nelson M. 'Epidemic neuromyasthenia', Texas 1977 (abstract): 741.

Richardson, AT. Electromyographic studies of patients with 'epidemic neuromyasthenia' at the Royal Free Hospital (abstract):745.

Currie DM, Shelokov A. Repetitive stimulation abnormalities in 'epidemic neuromyasthenia' (abstract):746.

Sutton RNP. Ill defined neurological diseases of possible viral origin. 747-51.

Pampiglione G, Harris R, Kennedy J. Electroencephalographic investigations in myalgic encephalomyelitis: 752-4.

Behan PO. Post-infectious encephalomyelitis: some aetiological mechanisms: 755-9 (Similarity of features of acute disseminated encephalomyelitis to those of epidemic myalgic encephalomyelitis - epidemic neuromyasthenia).

Cooke WT. The neurological manifestations of malabsorption: 760-2.

Crow TJ. Viral causes of psychiatric disease: 763-7.

Thomas M. Epidemiological approaches to 'epidemic neuromyasthenia': syndromes of unknown aetiology (epidemic myalgic encephalopathies): 768-70.

General discussion: biochemical data. Rundle A (raised lactic dehydrogenase and glutamic oxaloacetic transaminase levels and normal creatinine phosphokinase): Wilkie D (low oxygen uptake of lymphocytes, which are intolerant of chlorimipramine): 771; nomenclature Compson N, Behan PO, Wookey C, Lyle H, Ramsay AM, Richardson AT, Parish JG, Shelokov A: 772-4.

Review article Editorial Epidemic myalgic encephalomyelitis. Br Med J 1978: 1:1436-7. Correspondence 1969 Easton HG; 2:202 Wookey C.

Case Report, Church AJ. Myalgic encephalomyelitis "An obscene cosmic joke" Med J Aust 1980; 1:307-8. Correspondence: 613 Davies GRW: 613-4 Webb J.

1979
Epidemic 50

Southampton, England

May PGR, Donnan SPB, Ashton JR, Ogilvie MM, Rolles CJ. Personality and Medical Perception in Benign Myalgic Encephalomyelitis. Lancet 1980; 2:1122-4. (Outbreak in a girls' school).

Correspondence: Was it "Benign Myalgic Encephalomyelitis"? Lancet 1980; 2:1310 Ramsay AM; 1981; 1:37-8 Goodwin GS, May PGR (Donnan SPB, Ashton JR, Ogilvie MM, Rolles CJ): 221-2 Gosling PJH: 325 Ramsay AM. Myoglobinaemia in Benign Myalgic Encephalomyelitis. Lancet 1981; 1:670 Layzer RB. Myalgic encephalomyelitis: 950-1 Parish JG.

Biochemistry Ramsay AM, Rundle A. Clinical and biochemical findings in ten patients with benign myalgic encephalomyelitis. Postgrad MedJ 1979; 55:856-7. (Raised levels of serum myoglobin and GOT, and reduced level of fasting whole blood pyruvate).

1980

Review articles: Bishop J. Epidemic myalgic encephalomyelitis. Med J Aust1980; 1:585-6 and 609.

Behan PO. Epidemic myalgic encephalomyelitis. Practitioner 1980; 224:805-07.

Kale SA, Jones JV, Poskanzer DC. Icelandic Disease or Epidemic neuromyasthenia. (Questions and Answers). JAMA 1980; 244:2666.

Behan PO, Behan WMH. Epidemic myalgic encephalomy- elitis. In: Rose FC, ed. Clinical neuroepidemiology. Tunbridge Wells: Pitman Medical 1980; 374-83.

1980-81
Epidemic 51

West Kilbridge, Ayrshire, Scotland

Fegan KG, Bell EJ. Myalgic encephalomyelitis in a rural practice in Ayrshire. Communicable Diseases in Scotland 81/2, vii

Fegan KG, Behan PO, Bell EJ. Myalgic Encephalomyelitis - report of an epidemic. J R Coll Gen Pract 1983; 33:335-7.

1980-83
Epidemic 52

Helensburgh, Scotland

Calder BD, Warnock PJ. Coxsackie B infection in a Scottish general practice. J R Coll Gen Pract 1984;34:15-19.

1981-82

Sporadic cases Stirlingshire, Scotland

Keighley Bd, Bell EJ. Sporadic myalgic encephalomyelitis in a rural practice. JR Coll Gen Pract 1983; 33:339-41

1982-84
Epidemic 53

West Otago, New Zealand
This epidemic started in February 1983, at the end of the New Zealand Summer

Poore M, Snow P, Paul C. An unexplained illness in West Otago. N Z Med J 1984; 97:351-4.

Correspondence: West Otago illness. N Z Med J 1984; 97:502.
Snow P. Myalgic encephalomyelitis: 620 Gow PJ:654 Hardman MJ: 698-9
Snow P, Simpson LO (Shard BI, Olds, RJ), Poore M.. (Paul C), Gow PJ: 782Matthew C, Brook-Church AJ (Brook-Church JV): 868 Gow PJ: 1985; 98:20-1
Simpson LO (Shard BI, Olds RJ), Gow PJ, Murdoch JC, Simpson FO: 201-2 Murdoch J.C.

Dunedin and Hamilton New Zealand
Clements CJ. Myalgic encephalomyelitis N Z Med J 1984; 97:458.

1984

From 1984 until 1992 an endemic period ocurred in which an unusually large number of clusters and epidemics of M.E. / CFS have been recognized in North America. After an apparent initial increase in morbidity in 1983 there seemed to have appeared in late summer of 1984 an unprecedented increase of sporadic and epidemic cases across North America. Although certain geographical hot spots seem to have taken up much of the medical interest, this endemic situation probably represents an unusual and unremitting morbidity in all areas of the United States and Canada. Some of the clusters and epidemics are listed.

Epidemic 54

Incline Village, Lake Tahoe Nevada Epidemic August - September

Buchwald D, Cheney P, Peterson D, et al. A chronic illness characterized by fatigue, neurologic and immunologic disorders and active human herpesvirus type 6 infection (1992) 15 Jan, Annals of Internal Medicine, Vol. 116, No. 2, 103-113.

This community epidemic, apparently started in a girls' basketball team, then involved primarily teachers in at least three high schools, and then large numbers of the community. A large number of lay and medical publications have been generated.

Epidemic 55

Chapel Hill, North Carolina

Epidemic amongst members of The North Carolina Symphony Orchestra. Work Prepared by Grufferman, S.; Herberman, R.; Eby, N. Low NKC associated with high yield of lymphoma, astrocytoma, glioma (see this text)

Epidemic 56

Montreal, Quebec-Ontario,Canada

Labour Day epidemic, Montreal, S O'Sullivan, in preparation

Over 500 cases of M.E./CFS documented in Ontario during the August-November 1984 period. Although these cases were recorded from all over Ontario, there seems to be a curious prevalence along the seaway valley from the area of Kingston to Cornwall, Ontario. This endemic was active in all parts of Canada during this period and appears have maintained its activity until the time of writing in 1991.

Review
Gray JA. Some long-term sequelae of Coxsackie B virus infection. J R Coll Gen Pract 1984; 24:3-5.

Nuclear MagneticResonance Study
Arnold DL, Bore PJ, Radda GK,Styles P, Taylor DJ. Excessive intracellular acidosis of skeletal muscle on exercise in a patient with a post-viral exhaustion/ fatigue syndrome. Lancet 1984; 1:1367-9.

Correspondence: Muscle acidosis in post-viral fatigue. Lancet 1984; 2:293 Fulop M, Arnold DL (Bore PJ, Radda GK, Styles P, Taylor DJ), Gow PJ

Review
Murdoch JC. Myalgic encephalomyelitis and the general practitioner. N Z Family Physician 1984; 11:127-8.

1884-1985
Epidemic 57

Truckee, California

Involoving teachers and students, see Paul Levine's chapter, page 201.

1985
Epidemic 58

Lyndonville Epidemic New York

This was an epidemic involving children and adults and was described by Dr David S. Bell in his book **"The Disease With a Thousand Names"**, Pollard Publications, Box 180, Lyndonville NY 14098, 1991.

Sporadic cases
MacWilliam K, Dadswell JV, Tillet H. Antiviral titres, lymphocytic reactions and low IgA levels in patients with recurrent or persistent symptoms. Lancet 1985; 1:764-5.

SMON Epidemic in Japan
Zhi Fang Epidemic in China

See pages 333, 334 for discussion. The status of these two epidemics in relation to M.E. / CFS can only be speculation at this point.

Epidemic 59

Yerington, Nevada Outbreak

See Paul Levine's chapter, pages 201, 202. In the same area an M.E./CFS-like epidemic reputedly occurred in a reservation of American Native People. Information is incomplete on this epidemic.

1986
Epidemic 60

Placerville Outbreak

See Paul Levine's chapter, page 201.

1988
Epidemic 61

Sonora, California

This epidemic started in August 1988. More than 35 children and adults were diagnosed with M.E. in the mountain country 100 miles from Lake Tahoe. Many of these patients were associated in some way with Columbia Community College. This epidemic involved teachers and students and persisted until 1991. (No medical publication to date)

1989
Epidemic 62 ?

Roseville, California

This epidemic was reported by H. Kallis and J. Fever. It started in 1989 at the Rosedale Hospital, Roseville California where 11 or more cases of M.E./CFS were diagnosed among the staff of the 3rd floor of the hospital. Roseville is a town adjacent to Sacramento. Reported in the local newspaper. (No medical report to date).

1990
Epidemic 63

Elkgrove High School, Elkgrove, California

This epidemic occurred among teachers and students at the Elgrove High School, starting in April-May 1990 (in preparation) Chabursky, B. This epidemic was still active in 1991.

The Epidemiology and Methodology of M.E. / CFS

Chapter 17

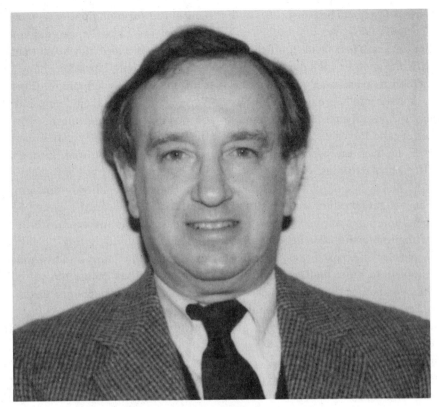

Seymour Grufferman

Epidemiologic and Immunologic Findings in Clusters of Chronic Fatigue Syndrome

Seymour Grufferman, MD, Dr. PH
Chairman,
Department of Clinical Epidemiology and Preventive Medicine, University of Pittsburgh School of Medicine
M-200 Scaife Hall, Pittsburgh, Pennsylvania 15261 USA

Dr. Grufferman is Professor and Chairman of the Department of Clinical Epidemiology and Preventive Medicine at the University of Pittsburgh School of Medicine, as well as a pediatrician and epidemiologist. He has a long-standing research interest in cancer epidemiology, particularly whether viruses play an etiologic role in human cancer. He has done extensive epidemiologic research on the lymphoreticular malignancies and childhood cancer. Recently, he has become interested in the chronic fatigue and immune dysfunction syndrome (CFIDS) and directs the CFIDS Clinic at the University of Pittsburgh.

Abstract

Two discrete outbreaks of chronic fatigue syndrome were studied - one in a symphony orchestra and the other in an elementary school. By studying total defined populations, interesting new information on the epidemiology of the syndrome emerged.

Laboratory investigations of subjects in the two populations revealed significantly lower levels of natural killer cell activity in cases than in non-cases. Additionally, subjects in the two outbreaks were found to have variable patterns of elevation of Epstein-Barr virus antibodies, elevations of antibodies against human herpes virus Type 6 and elevated T4/T8 ratios. Surprisingly, similar abnormalities were found in non-cases who were closely exposed to cases. This would be compatible with a model of inapparent infections in close contacts of cases.

Study of the closeness of contacts between cases and other cases and between non-cases and other non-cases revealed that case-case pairs had significantly closer contacts with one another than did non-case-non-case pairs. This was particularly true for the sharing of eating utensils and bedrooms. Additionally, in the symphony there appeared to be a remarkably increased risk of cancer in cases and their close contacts. However, no such increased occurrence was observed in the school outbreak.

In summary, our investigations show that there are objective laboratory abnormalities consistent with a broad spectrum of immune dysfunction in both cases and in healthy people closely exposed to cases. Furthermore, cases appear to have had significantly closer contact with one another than did non-cases, supporting a model of transmissibility. Additionally, it is possible, but not proven, that there may be an increased risk of cancer in subjects with chronic fatigue syndrome and in their close contacts. Findings in these investigations suggest that the name "chronic fatigue and immune dysfunction syndrome" might be more appropriate for the disease than "chronic fatigue syndrome."

I am going to be talking today about my research group's investigation of two discrete outbreaks or clusters of chronic fatigue syndrome. By studying two very well-defined groups, albeit small groups, including both cases and non-cases, I think we can add another piece of useful information regarding knowledge of the epidemiology of chronic fatigue syndrome. What we have done in essence is to do a total community study in microcosm.

Transmission of Lymphomas

I might begin by telling you how I got involved with chronic fatigue syndrome. I am a cancer epidemiologist by training and by research interest, and in 1985 I reported the story of a family that was very interesting. A woman from South Africa came to visit her family in the U.S. A few days before leaving Africa she became ill with an infectious mononucleosis-like illness. During her stay in the U.S., she visited family members in four different parts of the country and, within six to eleven months, four of the eleven persons exposed to her developed unusual B-cell lymphomas, one of which was a Burkitt's lymphoma in an adult. [1]

One of the surviving patients moved to an area not far from the Lake Tahoe epidemic and sent me a clipping from a local newspaper entitled: "How Mystery Disease Hits Three Teachers". I ignored it. She sent me another clipping. This was about the Yerrington, Nevada, epidemic and was titled: "Mysterious Illness Strikes Another Town". At about that time, Dr. Paul Cheney called me to ask if I would come out and meet with him and with Dr. Dan Peterson regarding the outbreaks and I went out to visit them. Dr. Cheney thought there might be similarities between the events I reported and the outbreak he was involved with in Nevada. Thus, I thought it was intriguing. I didn't think that our epidemic in the family and his epidemic had much in common at that point, but it did make me very receptive to what happened next.

Epidemic in Symphony Orchestra

In the fall of 1986, I was contacted by a member of a symphony orchestra about an outbreak of chronic fatigue syndrome in his group. Fortunately, I had been primed and thought that this would be an interesting outbreak to investigate. This person had read about our investigation of a group of non-Hodgkin's lymphoma patients in the family with a common-source exposure to a relative from Africa who was ill during her visit to the U.S. When one of the symphony members with chronic fatigue syndrome developed a non-Hodgkin's lymphoma, he thought we might be interested in investigating the outbreak. Subsequently, we found eight members of the orchestra who had symptoms of chronic fatigue syndrome.

The first symptoms began in August of 1984; seven affected persons were diagnosed by a local physician as having had acute infectious mononucleosis. Their ages ranged from 31 to 42 years. The eighth case was initially diagnosed as viral meningitis. Her age was 32.

In doing investigations of clusters, one has to be very, very cautious. For example, I make it a point never to talk to any of the patients in a cluster initially because I might lead them with questions to provide answers that I want to get to support my hypothesis. We have a space in the questionnaire which we administered to the orchestra asking "Is there any other information in particular you think we ought to know about?" Through this we obtained the story that one of the members of the orchestra had become ill with a chronic fatigue syndrome-like illness after visiting a relative in South Africa, but before the outbreak in the orchestra. I think that this is probably just a chance finding. Also, he had read the story about our interesting family that was written up in TIME magazine, so probably what we got was just selective recall of events. Nevertheless, it raises the possibility that the outbreak in the symphony could have originated from an exposure in South Africa.

Study Design

Let me describe our study design. When you do an investigation of a cluster it is so easy to lead people to give you the information that you want, that you must collect your data in a structured way. Thus, we used questionnaires rather than interviews of people for initial data collection. This is a very important point; you can structure results any way you want by asking leading questions. Use of a questionnaire also forces you to develop **a priori** hypotheses. In addition to the questionnaire, we did psychological testing using a self-administered scale to rule out depression. We administered a test of fatigability, the "two's and seven's test", which was developed by the U.S. Air Force.

We did immune function assays in Dr. Ronald B. Herberman and Theresa Whiteside's laboratory at the Pittsburgh Cancer Institute. Dr. Herberman is the person who discovered the natural killer cell. (The way this came about is interesting.) I was being recruited from Duke University to the University of Pittsburgh and in a meeting with Dr. Herberman, I told him about this fascinating disease. He pointed out the similarity of chronic fatigue syndrome to a syndrome one of his colleagues, Dr. Aoki in Japan, had reported and called "low natural killer cell syndrome"[2]. The primary symptom of the latter syndrome is severe protracted fatigue. Based on that, we proceeded to do immunologic studies on members of the orchestra.

The human herpes virus Type 6 was reputed to be a possible etiologic agent, so we looked at antibodies to that virus and, of course, we did Epstein-Barr virus (EBV) antibody studies. These were all done in leading research laboratories. HHV-6 studies were done by W. Carl Saxinger, Ph.D. at NIH, and EBV studies were done by Ciro V. Sumaya, M.D. at the University of Texas. All diagnoses were verified by reviewing medical records and past specimens. Dr. Robert Herfkens at Duke University did MRI scans on all eight cases; we found one case with questionable borderline frontal lobe atrophy. I am skeptical about the meaning of this abnormal finding.

Working with me at the time was a very bright third-year medical student, Mary Huang, and a postdoctoral fellow, Dr. Nancy L. Eby, and we came up with what we thought might be a very clever design. I believe we backed into the right approach without realizing what we were doing. We wanted to study the cases, but we thought it would be very nice to have some controls; so Mary Huang said "Why don't we study the non-cases? They would be a perfect match for the cases". That led us to what I believe is our most important set of findings.

The cases were predominantly female and all white (but all of the non-cases are white). One interesting finding that may or may not mean anything is that most of our cases were non-smokers as compared to half of the non-cases. Cigarette smoking is related to natural killer cell activity. Of interest is the observation that most of our patients met the CDC criteria, although I must say it is very difficult to use those criteria when you cannot personally examine the patients and must rely only on medical records; so this was a real problem. However, they do meet the criteria by and large.

We looked at EBV antibody titres in this group and we found, surprisingly, little difference between cases and controls. There are no statistically significant differences between cases and controls with regard to any of the subcategories of EBV antibodies. We also looked at HHV-6 antibodies using Dr. Saxinger's assay, where his ELISA score of 1.0 is the population norm, many of our non-cases were above the population norm but, in general, our cases were somewhat higher.

Abnormal Natural Killer Cell Activity

Of great interest to us were striking abnormalities in natural killer cell activity. Amongst our eight cases we found a mean value of 51 lytic units with a range of 13-114; the mean value concurrently measured in normal controls was 235. But surprisingly, many of our non-cases were low as well. With regard to all of the virological and immunological studies we had done, this was the only marker of disease that was statistically significantly different between cases and non-cases.

We also looked at T4/T8 ratios and found, much to our surprise, high T4/T8 ratios in cases and in controls as well. This was not statistically significantly different between cases and controls, but this was very striking. For example, one of the highest values was a T4/T8 ratio of 11. (The upper bound of normal is usually 2.5 to 3).

Up until now we have heard lots of reports of people presenting data on viral antibodies or measures of immune function. However, few people have put all of the data together to look at the array of laboratory studies on individual subjects. For example, for case number 44, there is very low natural killer cell activity, a very high HHV-6 ELISA score, no antibodies whatsoever against the Epstein Barr virus and a T4/T8 ratio of 11. On the other hand, case 46 has a normal level of NK activity, probably a normal ELISA score for HHV-6, but an elevated EBV IgG VCA and a normal T4/T8 ratio. And as you review our results, what you see is no consistent pattern across these variables.

We can say that NK activity is significantly lower in cases than it is in non-cases, but you can't say the same about abnormal EBV studies, or the T4/T8 ratios, or for the other variables we studied. I think this is the pattern of such findings in the disease and it needs further investigation. I believe Dr. Komaroff has observed this non-pattern in his series as well. The cases of ours that went on to develop cancer were really not much different from our other cases with CFS.

But things became very puzzling to us when we looked at the same array of data for non-cases. I have here some data on selected non-cases (of course, I picked the most interesting ones). As an example of our findings in this group, non-case number 26 has remarkably low natural killer cell activity, a high HHV-6 ELISA score, high IgG VCA, and a borderline-high EBV early antigen titer but a normal T4/T8 ratio. Even though these people have no evidence of

chronic fatigue syndrome, many have the same pattern of abnormalities as do cases in measures of their immune function.

This underscores my statement about the value of studying a total community, because what we are looking at here are the findings in a group of non-affected, but close, contacts of cases. I was skeptical about these very puzzling findings, so we searched for and found another epidemic, this time in a school.

I should point out that we did testing for depression; there were some slight differences between cases and non-cases which were not statistically significant. They were primarily related to the two questions on the SCL 90R: "Do you feel low in energy or slowed down?" and "Do you feel everything is an effort?". Those are symptoms of fatigue which are also symptoms of depression. Similarly, we found no differences in fatiguability between cases and non-cases using the "2s and 7s" test.

Our second investigation was of an elementary school in Ohio. We had identified three clusters. Since we had no grant support, we chose the one closest to home. We didn't know what we might find, but again we found findings similar to those in the orchestra. In several cases, NK activity levels were very low, but we found the same findings in several non-cases. There was no significant difference between NK activity in cases and non-cases. T4/T8 ratios were on average a little bit above normal, but we uncovered some persons with very high values. For example, one person, had a T4/T8 ratio of 66; six months later it came down to 7, still quite high.

When we arrayed the data in the same way as we had done for symphony subjects, we found the same patterns of inconsistent abnormalities in both cases and non-cases that we observed in the symphony. For example, here is a case with low NK activity, a normal T4/T8 ratio, and normal EBV antibody titers. An other person with high EBV antibody titers, had low NK activity, but a normal T4/T8 ratio. Again there was no consistent pattern of abnormalities in cases or in non-cases.

In the school group, we found perhaps even more striking findings in the non-cases than we did in the cases. We attribute this, as a guess, to the fact that these studies were done about a year after diagnosis in the school study whereas the studies were done two to three years after diagnosis in the orchestra outbreak. Again we found close contacts of cases with remarkable laboratory abnormalities, yet no evidence of fatigue. One of the cases in the school was a non-white (half Black, half American Indian) so CFS does occur in non-white people.

To summarize our laboratory findings, we found inconsistent depression of NK cell activity, elevation of T4/T8 cell ratios and what appear to be secondary reactivation antibody responses to the EBV and HHV-6. Similar observations were made in cases and in close work contacts who were asymptomatic. In both cases and contacts, there was no consistent pattern of abnormalities. There is no simple unifying hypothesis which might explain this pattern of laboratory abnormalities. This led me to coin the name "chronic fatigue and immune dysfunction syndrome" in 1987 at a meeting of the (then) National CEBV Syndrome Association in Portland, Oregon. I chose the vague term "dysfunction" because it best fits the diverse and non-specific set of abnormalities observed.

Now, let me address an important question. Is there an increased risk of cancer in persons with the chronic fatigue and immune dysfunction syndrome? One caveat to remember is that my area of research interest is the clustering and possible transmissibility of cancer. I was contacted by the orchestra because they had read in TIME magazine that I reported an unusual cluster of Burkitt's and other B-cell lymphomas in a family exposed to a visitor from Africa. Many of the members of this group had very high EBV antibody titers. So there could be a selection bias built into our study in that I was contacted because there was an occurrence of cancer in the orchestra and there was an outbreak of CFS which was at that time thought to be related to the EBV. When I spoke to the person who contacted me, he was only aware of one B-cell non-Hodgkin's lymphoma; we subsequently uncovered three other cancers. The first case had B-cell lymphoma. She was a 44 year-old woman with the onset of fatigue in 1984. She had an initial diagnosis of acute infectious mononucleosis. The second cancer was a breast cancer in a 38 year-old woman who was a case. This could very well be a chance occurrence. The third tumour was an extremely unusual carcinoma of the

parotid gland, an acinic cell carcinoma. It is one of the least frequent histologic types of parotid tumours and it occurred in a 41 year-old man with no overt symptoms of chronic fatigue syndrome. His wife was also an orchestra member and had chronic fatigue syndrome. Incidentally, the MRI scan of her head was the only one of those done that was read as abnormal with borderline frontal lobe atrophy. The fourth was a glioblastoma multiforme, in a 46 year-old woman with no overt symptoms of chronic fatigue syndrome. She had the highest EBV antibody titers of anybody in our study, but she never had any symptoms which could be construed as chronic fatigue syndrome.

Does this amount to an increased occurrence of cancer? We had complete information available for 58 members of the orchestra. We followed them from the time period 8/1/84 when the first CFS symptoms developed until the end of last year (12/31/89) and within this time window there were four observed cancers. We did an exact computation of the number of cancers we would expect to find in a group of this age/sex/race composition using U.S. national cancer incidence rates and we came up with an expectation of .37 cases. This means that there is almost eleven times more cancer in the group than one would expect. The excess is highly statistically significant. But, would I "hang my hat on it?" My answer is "No." The reason being that we found no such occurrence in the elementary school study. What this suggests is the possibility that there might be an increased frequency of malignancy with chronic fatigue syndrome. It is still an hypothesis - which is a fancy word for a somewhat educated guess. I think that it is urgently necessary to confirm or refute this hypothesis. In the meantime I wouldn't advise anybody to be concerned about an increased risk of cancer based on our findings. There are so many biases that led to my getting involved in this investigation that we have to be extremely cautious in interpreting this preliminary finding.

We can also break down this analysis in terms of the occurrence of cancer in CFIDS cases and in non-cases. There were two cancers in CFIDS cases. We computed the expected value and there are 48 times as many tumours in this group as would have been expected. Again this is statistically significant. For the non-cases the risk was lower; a six-fold increased risk. It was not statistically significant, but we're splitting small numbers here. I'm not sure this means anything except to say that if there is an increased risk of cancer with this syndrome, persons closely exposed to cases probably have an increased risk as well. However, this needs to be confirmed in other studies.

Next my colleagues and I tried to develop a statistical approach to evaluate whether cases had had closer contacts with one another than non-cases had had with other non-cases. This approach is an attempt to assess possible person-to-person transmissibility of CFIDS.

So we created a large grid, listing everyone's name in the orchestra. Next to each name we asked a series of questions such as: Did you know the person? Did you ever perform in a small chamber group together? Did you ever spend time together outside work? Did you travel together in a car or a bus? This is a travelling symphony, which, if CFIDS is an infectious disease, creates an interesting model. It is a low-budget travelling orchestra in which members share rooms, share cars and eat together. They have a smoker's bus and a non-smoker's bus, (remember our earlier finding on cigarette smoking - this could be related to the buses).

We looked at the proportions of subjects answering yes to these questions. Of course everyone knew everyone else, whether they were cases or non-cases. We asked if they played together in a small chamber group and we found that 60% of the case-case pairs had played together in a small group but only 1/3 of the non-case-non-case pairs. This difference was not statistically significant. We asked whether they spent time together outside of work and came up with fairly similar results. We also asked whether they rode together in the same car, and the difference between case-case and non-case-non-case pairs turned out to be statistically significant. When we asked whether people ate together, 90% of case-case pairs did, but so did 76% of non-case pairs.

However, we found that almost 40% of cases had shared an eating utensil with one another case as compared to 16% of the non-case-non-case pairs. This is an intriguing difference which is highly statistically significant. We also looked at sharing of a bedroom and found that 28% of the case-case pairs had shared a bedroom, but only 5% of the non-case-non-case pairs had shared a bedroom, another statistically significant difference. We didn't have enough numbers of subjects to evaluate intimate sexual contact; they're a friendly group, but apparently not all that friendly. Basically what these figures show is that perhaps cases have had closer contact with one another than non-cases have had with one another. There's an alternative explanation of this; that is, if you look to the literature on alcoholism, alcoholics tend to befriend other alcoholics. Perhaps people with chronic fatigue syndrome tend to befriend other people with chronic fatigue syndrome to commiserate or provide moral support. So, these data must be interpreted with caution. The "flip-side" of these findings is that if we had found no such associations, that would be fairly good evidence against the notion of transmissibility of an etiologic agent. Our findings are compatible with an infectious model, but they are also compatible with an assortative friendship model as well. Nevertheless, these are the first data to suggest that there might be person-to-person transmission of an etiologic agent for this disease. This again illustrates the value of doing total community studies where you can look at people with a disease and those around them without disease.

Conclusions

I believe the chronic fatigue and immune dysfunction syndrome is a real disease with objective laboratory abnormalities. One caveat I must state at this point is that these findings are perhaps not generalizable to all chronic fatigue syndrome cases. What I have been talking about here is the form of the disease that occurs in epidemic fashion. In clusters of cases where there is clearly a point epidemic pattern of transmission, I think our conclusions apply.

Depression of natural killer cell activity appears to be the most consistent laboratory abnormality in the syndrome. It was the only one that was statistically significantly different between cases and controls even though the controls (non-cases) had low levels as well.

EBV antibody responses seen in the syndrome probably represent secondary reactivation responses. I think we all know this; I don't have to preach to the true believers. Probably, the same is true of HHV-6.

We have observed subjects over time and have done repeat laboratory tests. The values fluctuate greatly, but these people maintain their laboratory abnormalities over time and they persist for at least two to three years. Dr. Komaroff has longer follow-up data and in his experience these abnormalities persist even longer than they do in our study. We have found that many persons with no fatigue or other symptoms of the syndrome can show the characteristic laboratory abnormalities.

I interpret this to mean that if this is a viral disease, we're talking about a pattern of transmission analogous to that seen with herpes viruses and the EBV, where there are many more inapparent infections than there are apparent infections. If CFIDS does turn out to have a viral etiology, my guess is that you will find that there are many people who have had inapparent infections.

Lastly, there seems to be a markedly increased risk of cancer in persons with the syndrome or in persons closely exposed to others with the syndrome. I don't think that I would say this is definitely a causal association, but I think that there is urgent need to confirm or refute this finding and I won't believe it myself until it is confirmed.

References

1.   Grufferman S, Raab-Traub N, Marvin K, Borowitz MJ, Pagano JS: Burkitt's and other non-Hodgkin's lymphomas in adults exposed to a visitor from Africa. N Engl J Med 313:1525-1529, 1985.

2.   Aoki T, Usuda Y, Miyakoshi H, et al.: Low natural killer syndrome: Clinical and immunologic features. Nat Immun Cell Growth Regul 6:116-128, 1987.

Chapter 18

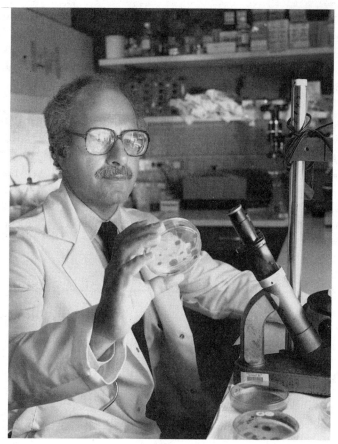

Paul H. Levine

Epidemiologic Aspects of
Chronic Fatigue Syndrome / Myalgic Encephalomyelitis

Paul H. Levine, MD

From the Viral Epidemiology Section, Environmental Epidemiology Branch, National Cancer Institute, National Institutes of Health, Bethesda, MD 20892
Reprint requests to the Environmental Epidemiology Branch, Division of Cancer Etiology, National Cancer Institute, NIH, Executive Plaza North, Room 434, Bethesda, MD 20892

Dr. Levine has been with the National Cancer Institute since 1964, his past positions including Chairmanship of the Immunology-Epidemiology Segment of the Virus Cancer Program, Head of the Clinical Studies Section, Viral Leukemia and Lymphoma Branch, and Chairman of the Viral Oncology Clinical Advisory Group. He has worked for more than 15 years on studies of the Epstein-Barr virus and his current research also includes the epidemiology of human herpesvirus-6 and HTLV-I.

Abstract

There are at least four areas in the study of chronic fatigue syndrome (CFS) where the epidemiologist can make a contribution: (a) disease classification, (b) disease surveillance, (c) identification of risk factors, and (d) evaluation of clinical trials. Disease classification is most critical; the process has been initiated with the working guidelines recently published by Holmes et al, in 1988.[1] One useful aspect of international working groups could be the development of improved guidelines to subclassify CFS using subgroups such as those with or without documented immune dysfunction, etc. Disease surveillance, including the detailed description of individual clusters, is important since this can lead to clues as to specific etiologic agents. A review of published reports suggests that different patterns are associated with various clusters, indicating that different etiologic agents are producing similar but distinguishable syndromes. The identification of risk factors can best be pursued through the development of case-control studies which require a rigid case definition for each study. Our experience indicates that some of the reported risk factors, such as socioeconomic status, may reflect bias in case ascertainment and may be incorrect. Finally, the evaluation of clinical trials is particularly important because of the tendency for the patient population to utilize unproven remedies for the disease based on inadequate data. Several specific projects are suggested whereby clinical as well as laboratory investigators can resolve conflicting data on this disabling enigmatic illness.

Introduction

An attempt to control any disease as complex as the topic of this symposium requires interdisciplinary efforts of clinicians, basic scientists, statisticians, and many others, including the patients who are affected. In this report, I would like to review the role of the epidemiologist, pointing out several areas where either epidemiology has played an important role in our understanding of the chronic fatigue syndrome/myalgic encephalomyelitis (CFS/ME) or where the epidemiologist could be of value in future studies.

First, as documented in this symposium whereby several investigators described their preference for the term *chronic fatigue syndrome* or *myalgic encephalomyelitis* based on their views of pathogenesis, it is quite likely that we are discussing a multiplicity of entities. One extremely important outcome of a meeting such as this could be to clarify and categorize as many of these entities as possible since it is quite clear that the triggering infectious agents vary, as discussed below, and therefore it is quite possible that the pathogenesis and approach to therapy also could vary.

Disease Classification

Disease classification and case definition are extremely critical since little sense can be made of etiologic, diagnostic or therapeutic studies unless we have an agreed upon case definition or, at least with this multifaceted group of illnesses, an agreed upon case categorization. Table 1 lists seven commonly used terms as well as published working definitions and/or descriptions that could serve as a common starting point for investigators in different countries.

Table 1
Currently Used Terms for CFS/ME with Suggested Working Definitions and/or Descriptions
Chronic Epstein-Barr virus (CEBV)—See Refs. 2-7 Chronic fatigue syndrome (CFS)—See Ref. 1 Post-infectious chronic fatigue syndrome (PICFS)—See Ref. 10 Chronic fatigue/immune dysfunction syndrome (CFIDS)—See Ref. 10 Myalgic encephalomyelitis (ME)—See Ramsay, this symposium and Ref. 11 Epidemic neuromyasthenia—See Refs. 12-23 Low natural killer syndrome (LNKS)- See Ref. 23a

The first term, chronic Epstein-Barr virus (EBV) infection (CEBV), sometimes referred to as chronic infectious mononucleosis or chronic active EBV infection, has been considered as being applicable to those patients with chronic fatigue syndrome (CFS), usually post-infectious CFS (see below and Fig 1), with high antibody titers to EBV who also fulfill the criteria for CFS described in the Annals of Internal Medicine.[1] This well-documented disease[2-7] is characterized by elevated IgG antibodies to EBV capsid antigens and early antigen (EA) and may be associated with persistent IgM antibody to EBV VCA. At the National Institutes of Health, Dr. Stephen Straus and his colleagues attempt to document EBV activity by demonstrating increased quantities of EBV in affected tissues by anticomplementary immunofluorosecence or nucleic acid hybridization,[6] but these findings cannot be documented in most clinical settings. An abnormally low antibody titer to an EBV induced nuclear antigen (EBNA-1) has been suggested as being a manifestation of CEBV[8,9] but this

Figure 1

PROPOSED INTER-RELATIONSHIP
OF CHRONIC FATIGUE SYNDROMES

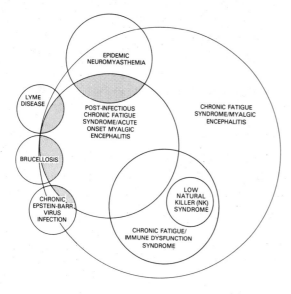

Schematic diagram of inter-relationship among clinical syndromes related to myalgic encephalomyelitis / chronic fatigue syndrome. In this concept, chronic fatigue syndrome and myalgic encephalomyelitis (CFS/ME) are considered to be interchangeable terms for a loosely defined constellation of signs and symptoms. Within the CFS/ME spectrum are two distinct and overlapping groups: a) Chronic fatigue/immune dysfunction syndrome (CFIDS), which is associated with well documented abnormalities of the immune system, and b) Post-infectious CFS/ME which has an acute onset associated with signs and symptoms of an infection. In some cases, the precipitating agent can be identified, as exemplified in this diagram by Lyme disease, brucellosis, and chronic EBV infection. Not all patients with these illnesses have the signs and symptoms of CFS/ME and therefore are not incorporated in the CFS/ME patient population. Similarly, many reports of "epidemic neuromyasthenia" do not fulfill current criteria for CFS/ME and "epidemic neuromyasthenia" also appears to include a heterogeneous group of illnesses. Low natural killer syndrome, which is primarily defined in the laboratory, currently appears to be a subset of CFIDS.

has not been a consistent finding (Pearson, personal communication). Persistent elevated EBV titers alone may not be diagnostic of CEBV, however, since patients with immunological disorders may have elevated antibody titers to a number of viruses.

One of the most important steps toward a case definition for the second widely used term, CFS, was made by Dr. Gary Holmes and his associates in 1988 when they developed a working definition for research purposes.[1] The terms **working definition** and **research purposes** need to be emphasized. The authors fully understood the limitations of their definition and developed it with the understanding that it would require modification with the appearance of new information similar to the evolving Jones criteria for rheumatoid arthritis.

The definition probably continues to be too all encompassing and still allows the inclusion of a multiplicity of diseases; it also does not take into consideration the co-existence of any of the exclusionary diagnoses with CFS. However, since it was specifically developed as a tool for investigators, it provides guidelines for research efforts and it is very encouraging to see so many reports in this symposium referring to these guidelines. Two relevant points to be emphasized are (a) these criteria are *not* adequate for clinical diagnosis in an office setting, and (b) all of the criteria are either symptoms reported by the patient or findings observed by the physician. There are no laboratory tests that are included in these criteria and as you have heard from others in this symposium (see Gupta, Chapter 58, this symposium), there are no laboratory tests at the present time that are diagnostic of CFS.

The third term, post-infectious chronic fatigue syndrome (PICFS), describes a subset of CFS patients whose illness began abruptly after an acute infection. Acute onset is only a minor criterion for CFS[1] and there is some rationale for specifying those patients whose illness began abruptly after an infectious illness. We have offered a definition for PICFS in our recent review of this syndrome,[10] emphasizing our preference for post-infectious rather than post-viral CFS because there are no clear distinctions between the syndrome following a documented viral illness, as with EBV, cytomegalovirus (CMV), or human herpesvirus-6 (HHV-6), as compared with the illness following Brucella or Borrelia burgdorferi (Lyme disease).

Continuing the separation of CFS into subgroups, one major subgroup has been termed chronic fatigue/ immune dysfunction syndrome (CFIDS). It is not appropriate to use CFIDS interchangeably with CFS because there are people with classic CFS who do not have any evidence of immunologic dysfunction. Furthermore, there is considerable uncertainty as to the specific immunologic abnormalities found in this illness. An informative review by Dr. Dedra Buchwald, who summarized the results of 45 papers in a review of PICFS,[10] documented the varying results in laboratory oriented studies and, as also noted by others in the symposium, some of the reasons for these discrepancies are obvious; heterogeneity of case definition and absence of longitudinal studies with clinical/laboratory correlation are two of the most important.

Regarding myalgic encephalomyelitis (ME), since this is a term that is not often used in the United States, it is more appropriate for those evaluating ME patients to provide the current working diagnosis. The definition utilized by Professor Ramsay, presented at the beginning of this conference (see Ramsay, Chapter 7, this symposium), is very appealing since it coincides so closely with the definition of PICFS and, in particular, the case definition we have developed for the Lake Tahoe cluster (see below).[10] As Dr. Peter Snow pointed out in his presentation (see Snow, Chapter 11, this symposium), however, many consider the classic case to be that of Tony Jeffreys, who described her illness in detail in **The Mile High Staircase**.[11] This case report is of great interest because the onset contrasts markedly with that proposed by Dr. Ramsay. Instead of an infectious disease precipitating her illness, Mrs. Jeffreys describes an onset with periodic attacks of abdominal pain not accompanied by evidence of infection. Since Dr. Bell, in his presentation (see Bell, Chapter 19, this symposium), noted a different pattern between his CFS patients with acute and gradual onset, it could be of value if ME investigators maintained separate analyses of patients with acute and gradual onset since they may be distinct entities.

The sixth common term that appears to have merit currently is epidemic neuromyasthenia, which often (but with important exceptions) is a cluster of PICFS cases occurring as an outbreak with a defined onset and a defined conclusion. A careful review of the reports of epidemic neuromyasthenia and related clusters [12-23] reveals that some have the clinical features of CFS as defined by Holmes et al and could therefore be called epidemic CFS but others do not. Dillon et al[21], for example, note that in their outbreak

of epidemic neuromyasthenia in nurses, the total duration of symptoms lasted 6-12 weeks, far less than the six months required for the diagnosis of CFS. Future investigations of apparent outbreaks should carefully document the clinical features in the context of the working definition so that outbreaks of epidemic neuromyasthenia can be documented as either being associated with CFS or representing another illness. In general, the distinction of epidemic CFS from the sporadic cases is very important since the etiologic agents are likely to be different.[10] Herpes viruses such as CMV, HHV-6, and EBV have been documented as causing mononucleosis which can persist as classical CFS. These are ubiquitous herpes viruses to which virtually everyone has been exposed by the age of 10 and therefore it is highly unlikely that the herpes viruses that are associated with the sporadic cases of CFS are in any way related to clusters of disease.

Finally, low natural killer syndrome (LNKS) is an illness described primarily in Japanese patients with prolonged fatigue and low grade fever, often accompanied by upper respiratory signs and symptoms (including pharyngitis and/or tonsillitis) as well as nervous system abnormalities (headaches, dizziness and/or depression)[23a]. The common feature characterizing this illness is low natural killer (NK) cell activity. Thus far, it appears that the laboratory abnormalities appear similar to those described for a large number of patients with CFIDS and therefore LNKS may prove to be a sub-group of CFIDS.

Disease Surveillance

One of the most common questions that epidemiologists are asked regarding CFS is, "How common is this illness?" Because of the variability in defining this syndrome, variations in incidence and prevalence data are likely to occur in different studies. Lloyd et al[24] attempted to determine the prevalence of CFS in an Australian population but used a definition of the syndrome quite different from the CDC definition;[1] only unexplained fatigue lasting greater than six months and neuropsychiatric dysfunction were required for the diagnosis. Of the 28 patients appearing for an interview, 21 (25%) gave no history of an acute onset or evidence of infection, therefore emphasizing the heterogeneity of the study population. The prevalence rate of 37.1 cases / 100,000 estimated in this study, therefore, must be viewed with caution.

A study being conducted by CDC [25] which is still in progress is utilizing the 1988 case definition published by CDC and collaborators[1]. This project, initiated September 1, 1989 in four surveillance sites (Atlanta, GA; Grand Rapids, MI; Reno, NV; and Wichita, KS), has a detailed clinical, psychological and laboratory evaluation which results in four discrete groups of cases based on the features compatible with or inconsistent with the 1988 case definition. Thus far, incidence and prevalence data are not available but of the 250 patients classified by the surveillance system, 42% "suffer from debilitating chronic fatigue without either a likely physical cause or any prior diagnosable psychological condition" and most of these (26% of the total group) meet the 1988 CFS case definition. Since referrals continue from these four areas at a rate of 15-20 per month, useful information from this well defined group is expected.

A somewhat easier surveillance task is the evaluation of clusters, since the symptom complex is likely to be more uniform. Epidemic neuromyasthenia is not a new problem, having been reported as far back as 1934 in Los Angeles[12] and in a number of subsequent publications.[13-23] The careful evaluation of a cluster is most likely to give clues to the etiology of an individual outbreak of CFS because it should allow a better case definition of a relatively defined group of patients. It is quite likely that various outbreaks of CFS have distinct etiologies and, in fact, both the literature and our own experience indicate that multiple agents are likely to trigger epidemic neuromyasthenia. The importance of developing a systematic approach to the evaluation of clusters cannot be overemphasized. There are certain features of the clusters we observed in Nevada and California, described in part elsewhere, [26-29] which illustrate approaches to the evaluation of other clusters, should they be identified. Briefly, as shown in Table 2 and Fig 2, outbreaks of chronic fatigue following an acute

Figure 2

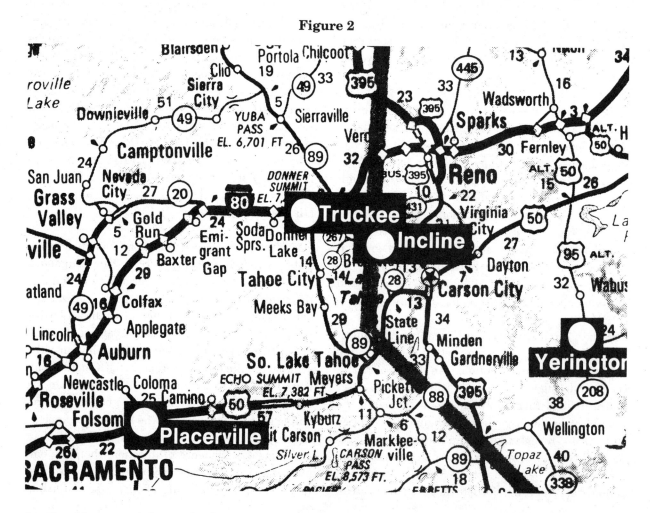

Location of four reported clusters of epidemic CFS investigated in 1986.

Table 2
Chronology of Events in the Nevada/California Cluster

Late 1984 -	Incline Village, NV - first cases of chronic fatigue syndrome reported by Drs. Cheney and Peterson.
Fall 1984 -	Truckee, Calif - Two students noted to have unusually persistent symptoms during an outbreak of infectious mononucleosis.
February 1985 -	Truckee, Calif - First two faculty members affected with chronic fatigue syndrome.
Spring and Summer 1985 -	Incline Village, NV - In March/April, rising case production first noted and Drs. Cheney and Peterson suspect an epidemic of chronic fatigue syndrome. In June, the number of cases peaked.
October/ November 1985 -	Incline Village, NV - Number of new cases notably declined.
Late Fall 1985 -	Yerington, NV - "Outbreak" initially flulike in type, with atypical lymphocytosis and positive mono-spot tests observed in record numbers.
February/ March 1986 -	Placerville, Calif - Outbreak of chronic fatigue syndrome "coincident with a heavy contamination of the local, unfiltered water supply."

infectious episode occurred in four communities within 90 miles of Lake Tahoe between late 1984 and early 1986, the first cluster being identified in the Incline Village, Nevada community by Drs. Daniel Peterson and Paul Cheney.[26,27]

The first epidemiologic investigation of the Lake Tahoe cluster occurred in September 1985 when Dr. Gary Holmes and his colleagues interviewed by telephone 134 patients who had Epstein-Barr virus serology testing between January 1 and September 5, 1985, which was very early in the outbreak. In their report,[28] they concluded that, indeed, there appeared to be an epidemic or an outbreak of CFS and that this outbreak was associated with an elevation of antibodies to Epstein-Barr virus and other viruses as well. In 1986, shortly after the discovery of HHV-6,[30] my colleague Robert Biggar and I went to Incline Village to attempt to develop a case definition for future laboratory studies. The particular goal of this trip was to interview a series of patients from the four sites noted on Fig 2. The original outbreak

identified by Drs. Peterson and Cheney were in the area of their internal medicine practice in Incline Village, NV, an outbreak which appeared almost the same time as another one in Truckee, CA. A separate outbreak was subsequently noted in Yerington, NV, a working class community where farming is the major occupation, and was reported to Dr. Cheney by Dr. Judy Hilbish, a local physician who had noted a high frequency of atypical lymphocytosis in the community hospital laboratory with the concomitant, apparent increase in CFS. The fourth community, Placerville, CA, which is on the other side of the Sierra Nevada Mountains, was brought to Dr. Cheney's attention by one of his patients, and was associated with a giardiasis outbreak documented in local newspapers.[31] The case definition we developed for the Lake Tahoe cluster[10] consisted primarily of an acute onset following signs or symptoms of infection, severe pain (headache and/or myalgia), prolonged fatigue and cognitive dysfunction. This is very similar to the case definition for ME reported by Dr. Ramsay as well as for certain outbreaks of epidemic neuromyasthenia,[18,32] but it is quite different from those reported by other investigators (see below).[13-15, 19, 21] Evidence of concurrent familial infection was one feature of epidemic CFS we observed occasionally in Nevada and California, such as the following:

Family 1 (Truckee, Calif)

This 44-year-old white female school teacher first became ill in June 1985 with fatigue, headache, lymphadenopathy, sore throat, earache and night sweats. Associated symptoms included loss of memory and coordination, sleeplessness, depression, and tingling and numbness in her arms and legs. Evidence of a cognitive disorder included frequent word reversal and loss of ability to type or proofread. Her illness occurred coincidentally with a similar disease in other faculty members. She had previous symptoms diagnosed as mononucleosis in 1963 but had recovered without apparent residual signs or symptoms. Improvement was noted in the spring of 1986 and the patient was able to return to work in September. She has remained fairly well since then, but continues to complain of fatigue and occasional insomnia. Her 12 year-old daughter became ill in May 1985 with fatigue associated with sore throat, lymphadenopathy, headache, myalgia, and an outbreak of oral herpes. However, her illness was severe for only two weeks and recovery was complete within seven months.

Family 2 (Yerington, NV)

This 22-year-old white female, mother of three children and employed in several part-time jobs, suddenly became ill November 25, 1985 noting that "My head felt like it was going to explode." She complained of tightness of her neck, nausea, anorexia and disorientation. There was transient improvement but one month later she relapsed with a sore throat, fatigue and depression. Her symptoms again improved until July 1986 when she had a recurrence of aches, weakness, loss of strength, sore throat and lymphadenopathy. She was treated with Acyclovir with little effect. On July 9 symptoms increased and she became tired, depressed and almost suicidal. In August the headache was still present. When she was interviewed in October 1986 she continued to be depressed and had the feeling of "Not being all here, spacey." In the subsequent ten months she gradually improved and at last follow-up, 2 1/2 years after disease onset, she had recovered almost completely with persistent fatigue her principal remaining symptom.

The patient's brother, a 25-year-old power plant worker, became ill at the same time (November 1985) with fever and aching joints, but his symptoms lasted only two days. Their mother, a 46-year-old bookkeeper, subsequently became ill in December 1985 with a sore throat and a positive mono-spot test. Approximately one week after the onset of symptoms, the mother became anorexic and extremely depressed with crying episodes. She tried to return to work but was unable to concentrate on her accounting. She also noted myalgia and tiredness in her arms, being unable even to lift a laundry basket. Normal activities and concentration on numbers, part of her work as a bookkeeper, were impossible during the course of her illness. Her symptoms gradually diminished over the next year, although at last follow-up she still complained of proximal muscle weakness and loss of concentration.

Although these family studies suggest that a single agent produced CFS in one or two family members and a less severe illness in other family members, it is not possible to determine whether the agent was passed from one family member to another or whether both were infected from a common source. Furthermore, while it is readily apparent that sporadic CFS is not contagious, these family studies also indicate that host factors play a significant role in determining the clinical outcome.

Just as one must have a case definition for the description of a disease, one also needs a case definition for the description of a typical case in a cluster. Table 3 contrasts our case definition with the definition that we find from reading descriptions of some of the other clusters reported in the literature.[12-16,19,21] As noted in Table 3, for example, in one of the classic cases of epidemic neuromyasthenia, designated Iceland disease, a more gradual onset was observed and no cognitive disorder was noted. The groups studied by Shelokov[19] and by Dillon et al[21] reported as epidemic neuromyasthenia also were notable for an absence of changes in cognitive functions, a major feature in Incline Village, Truckee, Yerington, and also in Punta Gorda, FL.[18,32]

Table 3					
Comparative Features of Epidemic Neuromyasthenia Reports					
	Acute Onset	Evidence of Infection		Pain MUSC	Cognitive Disorder
		URI	GI		
Akureyri, Iceland (1948-9) Sigurdsson et al	-	-	-	+	+
Washington, DC (1953) Shelokov et al	+	+	+	+	-
Glasgow, Scotland (1985) Behan et al	+	+	+	+	+
Coventry, GB (1956) Galpine, Brady	+	+	+	+	+
Punta Gorda, FL (1956) Poskanzer et al	+	-	+	-	+
London, GB (1970-1) Dillon et al	+	+	-	+	-
NV/CA (1984-5)	+	+	-	+	+

Identification of Risk Factors

As with disease surveillance, the problems of case definition have caused major difficulties in defining risk factors for CFS/ME. There are, however, some recent data that confirm certain reported risk factors and cast doubts on others.

Age/Race/Sex.—In terms of age, race, and sex, the disease apparently has been diagnosed more often in young white females than any other group. It has a wide age spectrum, being increasingly documented in the pediatric population (Bell, Chapter 19,this Symposium[24,33,34]) and in patients above age 50 (10% of the patients studied thus far by Gunn et al [25]). Racial predisposition is currently uncertain. DuBois reported in 1984[3] that CFS was rarely seen in black patients in his internal medicine practice, which has an almost equal proportion of black and white patients. More recently, in reviewing his case material, Dr. DuBois reported that of approximately 200 patients with CFS that he has seen since 1982, fewer than five were black (DuBois, personal communication). There continues to be the possibility of a referral bias, however, and therefore racial/ethnic predisposition is currently under active investigation.

Socioeconomic Status.— Most articles, particularly in the lay press, will say that CFS/ME is a disease primarily of people in upper/middle socioeconomic groups. Our experience in Yerington, Dr. Snow's in New Zealand (see Snow, Chapter 11,this symposium), and reports from upstate New York ([34]; see Bell, Chapter 19, this symposium) and Australia [24] would suggest that the apparent predominance of patients in upper socioeconomic strata is more a matter of referral patterns than incidence. This illness may be more readily identified in very motivated active individuals, often in a situation where even a moderate change in life style is much more handicapping because of the goals and motivations of the patient. Such a pattern, described in sheepherders by Dr. Snow, may affect the apparent epidemiologic pattern in the United States.

Genetics.—A third risk factor appears to be genetic predisposition, suggested by an association with allergies. Several studies, such as those of Jones and Straus,[7] describe signs and symptoms of allergy in approximately 75% of patients with apparent EBV associated CFS.

Psychologic Predisposition.—The possible importance of psychologic predisposition, which is quite controversial, seems to be well documented in the literature. The series of reports[35-38] on brucellosis and influenza that suggest a psychological role in postinfectious CFS are very informative. Imboden et al, [21,38] stimulated by the finding of a psychological profile suggesting greater depression in patients with more severe brucellosis in the Frederick community [35-37], developed a prospective study evaluating psychologic profiles in a series of 600 subjects prior to the arrival of the Asian influenza outbreak in 1957-58. Their observation that a psychologic profile "characteristic of depression-prone patients" was associated with a more severe course of influenza is frequently cited as evidence for a psychologic predisposition to CFS. As with other aspects of CFS, more standardized psychological and neurological evaluation of patients with this syndrome is needed.

Endocrine Pattern.—Recent data[39] suggest that patients with CFS have impaired activation of the hypothalamic-pituitary-adrenal axis. A study of 30 patients and 72 controls demonstrated mild glucocorticoid deficiency and enhanced adrenocortical sensitivity to exogenous ACTH, among other findings. The authors were unable to define the precise nature of the defect or its etiology, noting that such abnormalities could be compatible with a viral infection.

Evaluation of Clinical Trials

Identification of active therapeutic agents is an important area of research that requires considerable expertise. Thus far, several studies have shown gamma globulin to have temporary benefit in some patients[40,41] and antidepressants may also be efficacious in improving sleep patterns[41] but other agents, such as Acyclovir,[42] have been disappointing. Epidemiologists have played major roles in the development of clinical trials in a number of areas, such as cancer chemotherapy, and their assistance in clinical trials involving CFS could be particularly helpful in view of the importance of case definition, study design, and statistical evaluation of the results. The placebo effect in clinical trials is quite strong[42] and the utilization of the cross-over method whereby the patient serves as his/her own control is one that appears particularly well suited to CFS trials. Anecdotal studies on a few patients or uncontrolled therapeutic trials should be viewed with suspicion in view of the variable course of this illness.

Summary

As our understanding of CFS improves with the multifaceted approach represented by the many studies described in this symposium, it is important that attention be paid to scientific principles. This meeting has shown increased attention to case definition, selection of controls, objective measurements, etc. which have set the stage for improved communication among various disciplines and investigators in various countries. Further standardization of terminology and techniques are now needed to accelerate the collection of useful data. Among the issues to be addressed are: (a) more detailed definition of study populations; (b) standardization of data collection, including neuropsychiatric, as well as immunologic data; (c) development of serum banks with standardized data collection to allow comparison of different populations; (d) development of more detailed protocols for patient identification, perhaps

using the comprehensive center approach that is now being used for cancer patients. Closer communication between investigators in the field and in the laboratory are critical, particularly in the workup of clusters. Laboratory investigators need to alert field workers to the appropriate biologic specimens and field workers need to collect and transmit to the laboratory full clinical and epidemiologic data. Specific check lists should be developed for each cluster, with particular attention to cognitive disorders since these findings are often striking but need to be carefully and systematically evaluated.

Other manuscripts in this symposium have addressed these and other issues important to the control of CFS. The opportunity to facilitate collaborative efforts afforded by symposia such as this one should continue to improve our understanding of this complex problem.

Aknowledgement: *The author thanks Dr. Stephen E. Straus for helpful comments.*

References

1. Holmes GP, Kaplan JE, Nelson MG, et al: Chronic fatigue syndrome: a working case definition. *Ann Int Med* 1988;108:387-389.

2. Tobi M, Morag A, Ravid Z, et al: Prolonged atypical illness associated with serologic evidence of persistent Epstein-Barr virus infection. *Lancet* 1982;1:61-64.

3. DuBois RE, Seeley J, Brus I, et al: Chronic mononucleosis syndrome. *South Med J* 1984;77:1376-1382.

4. Jones JF, Ray CG, Minnich LL, et al: Evidence for active Epstein-Barr virus infection in patients with persistent, unexplained illnesses; elevated anti-early antigen antibodies. *Ann Int Med* 1985;102:1-7.

5. Straus SE, Tosato G, Armstrong G, et al: Persisting illness and fatigue in adults with evidence of Epstein-Barr virus infection. *Ann Int Med* 1985;102:7-16.

6. Straus SE: The chronic mononucleosis syndrome. *J Infect Dis* 1988;157:405-412.

7. Jones JF, Straus SE: Chronic Epstein-Barr virus infection. *Ann Rev Med* 1987;38:195-209.

8. Miller G, Gorgen E, Rowe D, et al: Selective lack of antibody to a component of EB nuclear antigen in patients with chronic active Epstein-Barr virus infection. *J Infect Dis* 1987;156:26-35.

9. Henle W, Henle G, Andersson J, et al: Antibody responses to Epstein-Barr virus-determined nuclear antigen (EBNA)-l and EBNA-2 in acute and chronic Epstein-Barr virus infection. *Proc Natl Acad Sci USA* 1987;84:570-574.

10. Levine PH, Krueger GRF, Kaplan M, et al The post-infectious chronic fatigue syndrome. In: Ablashi DV, Faggioni A, Krueger GRF, et al, eds. *Epstein Barr Virus and Human Disease.* Crescent Manor, NJ:Humana Press; 1989:405-438.

11. Jeffreys T. The Mile High Staircase, Hodder and Stoughton, Auckland, 1982.

12. Gilliam AG: Epidemiologic study of epidemic diagnosed as poliomyelitis, occurring among personnel of Los Angeles County General Hospital during the summer of 1934, bulletin 240. Washington, DC, US Public Health Service, Division of Infectious Diseases, Institute of Health, 1938;1-90.

13. Sigurdsson B, Sigurjonsson J, Sigurdsson JH, et al: A disease epidemic in Iceland simulating poliomyelitis. *Am J Hyg* 1950;52:222-238.

14. White DN, Burtch RB: Iceland disease: a new infection simulating acute anterior poliomyelitis. *Neurology* 1954;4:506-516.

15. Sigurdsson B, Gudmundsson KR: Clinical findings six years after outbreak of Akureyri disease. *Lancet* 1956;1:766-767.

16. The Medical Staff of the Royal Free Hospital: An outbreak of encephalomyelitis in the Royal Free Hospital Group, London, in 1955. *Br Med J* 1957;2:895-904.

17. Galpine JF, Brady C: Benign myalgic encephalomyelitis. *Lancet* 1957;1:757-758.

18. Poskanzer DC, Henderson DA, Kunkle EC, et al: Epidemic neuromyasthenia: an outbreak in Punta Gorda, Florida. *N Engl J Med* 1957;257:356-364.

19. Shelokov A, Habel K, Verder E, et al: Epidemic neuromyasthenia: an outbreak of poliomyelitislike illness in student nurses. *N Engl J Med* 1957;257:345-355.

20. Acheson ED: The clinical syndrome variously called benign myalgic encephalomyelitis, Iceland disease and epidemic neuromyasthenia. *Am J Med* 1959;26:569-595.

21. Dillon MJ, Marshall WC, Dudgeon JA, et al: Epidemic neuromyasthenia: outbreak among nurses at a children's hospital. *Br Med J* 1974;1:301-305.

22. Behan PO, Behan WMH, Bell EJ: The postviral fatigue syndrome—an analysis of the findings in 50 cases. *J Infect* 1985;10:211-222.

23. Henderson DA, Shelekov A: Epidemic neuromyasthenia: clinical syndrome? N *Eng J Med* 1959;260:757-764.

23a. Aoki T., Usuda Y., Miyakoshi H., et al: LNKS: Clinical and immunologic features. *Nat Imun Cell Growth Regul* 1987;6:116-128.

24. Lloyd AR, Hickie I, Boughton CR, et al: Prevalence of chronic fatigue syndrome in an Australian population. *Med J Australia* 1990; 153:524-528.

25. Gunn WJ, Randall B, Connell D: Progress Report: Chronic fatigue syndrome surveillance and long term follow-up system. Centers for Disease Control and Abt Associates, 1991.

26. The Sacramento Bee, *Mystery sickness hits Tahoe,* October 11, 1985, pp Bl.

27. Barnes DM: Mystery disease at Lake Tahoe challenges virologists and clinicians. *Science* 1986;234:541-542.

28. Holmes GP, Kaplan JE, Stewart JA, et al: A cluster of patients with a chronic mononucleosis-like syndrome. *JAMA* 1987;257:2297-2302.

29. Daugherty SA, Henry BE, Peterson DL, et al: Chronic fatigue syndrome in Northern Nevada. *Rev Inf Dis* 1991; 13:S39-S44.

30. Salahuddin SZ, Ablashi DV, Markham PD, et al: Isolation of a new virus, HBLV, in patients with lymphoproliferative disorders. *Science* 1986;234:596-601.

31. Placerville Record, July, 1986.

32. Roueche B, ed. In the Bughouse. In: *The Orange Man.* Boston: Little, Brown and Co.; 1965:95-115.

33. Dale JK, Straus SE: The chronic fatigue syndrome: Considerations relevant to children and adolescents. *Adv in Pediatric Infectious Diseases* 1992;7:63-68.

34. Bell KM, Cookfair D, Bell DS, et al: Risk factors associated with chronic fatigue syndrome in a cluster of pediatric cases. *Rev Inf Dis*; 1991; 13:S32-S38.

35. Trevor RB, Cluff LE, Peeler RN, et al: Brucellosis I. Laboratory-acquired acute infection. *Arch Int Med* 1959;103:381-397.

36. Cluff LE, Trevor RW, Imboden JB, et al: Brucellosis II. Medical aspects of delayed convalescence. *Arch Int Med* 1959;103:398-405.

37. Imboden JB, Canter A, Cluff LE, et al: Brucellosis III. Psychologic aspects of delayed convalescence. *Arch Int Med* 1959;103:406-414.

38. Imboden JB, Canter A, and Cluff LE: Convalescence from influenza. *Arch Int Med* 1959;108:115-121.

39. Demitrack M, Dale J, Straus E, et al: Evidence for Impaired Activation of the Hypothalamic-Pituitary-Adrenal Axis in Patients with Chronic Fatigue Syndrome. *J Clin Endocrinology and Metabolism* 1992; 73:1224-34.

40. DuBois RE: Gamma globulin therapy for chronic mononucleosis syndrome. *AIDS Res* 1986;2:Sl91-S195.

41. Gantz NM, Holmes GP: Treatment of patients with chronic fatigue syndrome. *Drugs* 1989;38:855-862.

42. Straus SE, Dale JK, Tobi M, et al: Acyclovir treatment of the chronic fatigue syndrome: lack of efficacy in a placebo controlled trial. N *Eng J Med* 1988;319:1692-1698.

Children and Students with M.E. / CFS

Chapter 19

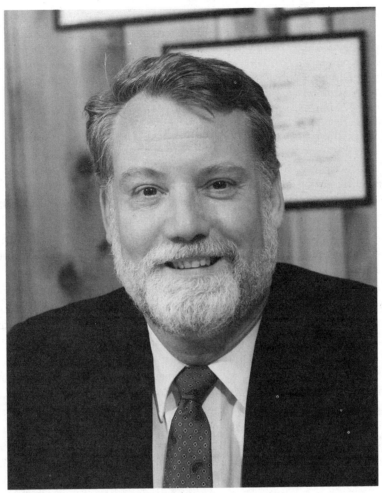

David S. Bell

Children with Myalgic Encephalomyelitis / Chronic Fatigue-Immune Dysfunction Syndrome: Overview and Review of the Literature

David S. Bell MD, FAAP
Department of Pediatrics, Cambridge Hospital and Mount Auburn Hospital, 1493 Cambridge Street, Cambridge, Massachusetts 02139 USA

Dr. Bell has spoken throughout the United States and internationally on M.E. / CFS. His publications on CFS have appeared in numerous journals, including Annals of Internal Medicine, American Journal of Epidemiology, and Journal of Infectious Diseases.

Abstract

Myalgic Encephalomyelitis / Chronic Fatigue Immune Dysfunction Syndrome (ME / CFIDS) is a serious chronic illness that affects children as well as adults, occurring in epidemics or as sporadic cases. In children the illness is rare under the age of five and presents most commonly at puberty. Males and females are equally affected. Long term morbidity is common because of persisting somatic symptoms, prolonged school absence and abnormal cognitive function. The most common misdiagnosis in children with ME / CFIDS is school phobia.

Of the more than fifty epidemics described, many have been community based outbreaks involving large numbers of children. Several of these outbreaks are reviewed, as well as the literature on Juvenile Primary Fibromyalgia Syndrome, which may represent the same condition. The 1985 epidemic in Lyndonville, New York is reviewed, and 104 patients were identified who retrospectively met the current disability and symptom criteria of the Centers for Disease Control. Forty-four patients were children, representing 42% of the total. Of the children, 35% had an acute onset of symptoms while 65% had a gradual onset of symptoms. All children were followed for at least 27 months, and only 8 children (18%) described complete resolution of symptoms and considered themselves well.

I. Overview

Myalgic Encephalomyelitis (ME), also known as Chronic Fatigue-Immune Dysfunction Syndrome (CFIDS) is a discrete clinical entity of numerous signs and symptoms affecting children as well as adults. The majority of published reports concerning ME/CFIDS have concentrated on the adult population, but some studies have reviewed the pediatric presentation[1,2]. The purpose of this paper is to review the clinical presentation of 44 children affected during the Lyndonville, New York outbreak, and to review the literature concerning this illness in children.

In general, the symptoms of ME/CFIDS in children are similar to those of adults. Differences from the adult presentation include a greater incidence of gradual onset of symptoms, and a more equal sex distribution. Children, especially younger children with gradual onset describe less fatigue, perhaps because of a relative lack of a healthy reference activity level. School difficulties are common because of prominent somatic symptoms, prolonged school absence, and cognitive disturbances.

Perhaps the most common misdiagnosis in the school age child is depression or school phobia. While children may manifest emotional symptoms after the onset of their illness, the pattern of these symptoms differs from primary depression. School phobia is frequently diagnosed because of school absence and a relatively normal physical and laboratory examination. However, children with ME/CFIDS fail to show evidence of separation anxiety. In addition, family dynamics are normal, and there is no precipitating emotional event frequently seen in school phobia. The diagnosis of school phobia should not be a "diagnosis of exclusion", and should not be made without evidence of a primary emotional disturbance.

The literature on ME/CFIDS in the paediatric age group has fallen into several categories. The major-

ity of papers are reports of epidemics involving both children and adults. Several reports have emphasized possible etiologic agents and have included data on children as well as adults. Examples of this type of study are the papers implicating Enterovirus and Epstein-Barr virus. There have been several reports on Primary Juvenile Fibromyalgia Syndrome in the rheumatology literature which bear striking similarities to ME/CFIDS. Finally, there have been scattered editorials or case reports concerning ME/CFIDS in children. Papers from this last category will not be discussed in this paper.

The greatest obstacle in evaluating the literature on ME/CFIDS is the varying approach in diagnosis and clinical description. Some authors have concentrated on neurologic symptoms, as in the early clusters associated with acute anterior poliomyelitis. Other descriptions have stressed the rheumatologic symptoms, such as the reports of primary juvenile fibromyalgia syndrome. ME/CFIDS needs to be more precisely defined so that future outbreaks may be quickly recognized and appropriate etiologic and epidemiologic studies may be carried out. The reader is referred to several comprehensive reviews for a more thorough discussion of ME/CFIDS in adults[3-8].

II. Clinical Presentation in Children: Lyndonville, New York

From 1983 through 1987 an outbreak of ME/CFIDS occurred in upstate New York, centered around the rural farming community of Lyndonville on the southern border of Lake Ontario. During this period over two hundred persons developed an illness characterized by a specific symptom complex. Over thirty persons, including at least eight children, have developed the illness since December 1987 and are not included in this survey.

The diagnostic criteria originally used to establish the diagnosis are based upon this specific symptom complex[9]. These criteria were developed in 1986, prior to the current criteria established by the Centers for Disease Control[10]. The 104 patients included in this survey were retrospectively selected so as to conform to the CDC criteria of fatigue severity and symptom pattern. However, the majority have not had the extensive exclusionary laboratory tests as required by the CDC criteria. It is estimated that at least an equal number of persons, not included in this review, developed a similar symptom complex which was mild and/or of short duration.

Table 1
Diagnostic Criteria

1. Symptoms Present for at least 6 months.
 	
2. Six of Eight Major Symptoms
    Fatigue
    Neurologic Symptoms
    Headache
    Joint Pain
    Muscle Pain
    Lymph Node Pain
    Sore Throat
    Abdominal Pain
 	
3. Or 5 of 8 Major plus 2 of 3 Minor Symptoms
    Eye Pain / Photophobia
    Fever / Chills / Night Sweats
    Rash

One hundred four patients were selected, and all met the "Lyndonville Criteria" shown in Table 1. Of the 104 patients, 44 were children, representing 42% of the total. Of these 44 children, 29 (66%) met all eight major symptom criteria, 7 (16%) had seven major symptoms, and 8 (18%) had six major symptoms. 37 children (84%) had at least two of the three minor symptom criteria. In this study, no child required the inclusion of minor symptom criteria to make the diagnosis. Comparison of adults and children in the Lyndonville outbreak showed a similar pattern of symptoms, but children had a greater number of individual symptoms than adults (data not shown).

Seventeen of the children were male (39%) while 27 were female (61%). The majority (66%) had a gradual onset of symptoms over several months, while 34%

had an acute onset of the illness with a "flu-like" illness. There was no sex prevalence observed in the type of onset. Fifteen of the children (34%) were between the ages of 9 and 11 at the time of onset (Table 2). The dates of onset of all cases, adult and children, are presented in Table 3. Twenty nine of the children in this study (66%) have had at least one other family member with a similar symptom complex.

Table 2
Age at Onset, Lyndonville Outbreak
(Children only)

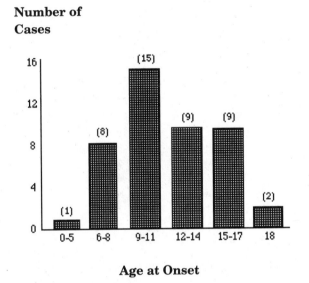

Age at Onset

Table 3
Lyndonville, NY Outbreak: Date of Onset

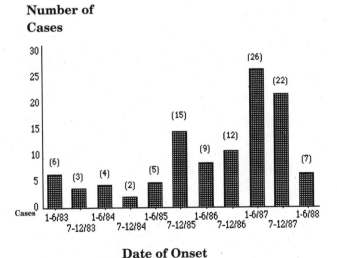

Date of Onset

All children described numerous symptoms which fit a consistent pattern. All complained of marked fatigue and headache, and most had neurologic complaints including loss of short term memory, dyslogia, paresthesias, weakness, dizziness and word finding difficulties. Most had a disturbed sleep pattern characterized by non-restorative sleep and episodes of hypersomnolence, insomnia or both. Other prominent symptoms included joint and muscle pain, abdominal pain, recurrent sore throat, lymphodynia, eye discomfort and sensation of abnormal temperature. The frequency of symptoms in these children is shown in Table 4.

Table 4	
Lyndonville Epidemic Symptoms in 44 Children	
Fatigue	100%
Headache	100%
Neurologic	98%
Memory Loss	70%
Dyslogia	68%
Sore Throat	95%
Abdominal Pain	93%
Muscle Pain	89%
Joint Pain	82%
Lymphodynia	82%
Photophobia	82%
Eye Pain	80%
Rash	80%
"Fever"	68%
Night Sweats	48%
Emotional Change	45%
Chills	43%
Dysuria	27%

In an earlier description of some of the children involved in this epidemic[1], most had marked difficulties in school performance, and many had family and social disruption. School difficulties were most marked in those children with an acute onset of symptoms. Laboratory evaluation in these children revealed that 25% had no antibody to Epstein-Barr virus (EBV).

In a case control study of 21 children and 42 age and sex matched controls[11], three factors significantly separated cases and controls: 1) past history of allergies and/or asthma 2) family members with similar illness and 3) a history of drinking unpasteurized milk prior to onset of illness. Numerous other factors, including socio-economic status, exposure to pesticides, type of drinking water, and location of dwelling (rural or town) were not significant. While cultures of raw milk from cows and goats in the area revealed Camplobacter, Yersinia enterocolitica, Shigella and Salmonella species, there have been no significant outbreaks of illness caused by these pathogens. The link with unpasteurized milk remains unexplained.

III. Epidemics of M.E. / CFIDS

Iceland (Akureyri) Disease

While there have been reports of epidemics of ME/ CFIDS extending back to the 1930's, perhaps the largest and best recognized epidemic to involve children occurred in Akureyri on the Northern coast of Iceland in 1948. The illness, reported by Sigurdsson et al[12], became known as Iceland Disease and affected over 1000 persons, nearly half of them children. The epidemic began in the winter of 1948 with three confirmed cases of acute anterior poliomyelitis and spread rapidly through the town of Akureyri and the surrounding countryside. Overall 6.7% of the town and 0.8% of the rural population became ill. Children were prominently involved and children in the 15 to 19 year old age group had the highest attack rate. Women were more commonly affected than men except in children where the incidence was nearly equal. Multiple cases were seen within households, and more than 30% of the cases occurred in the upper grade schools. The illness was felt to be infectious with an incubation period of 5 to 7 days.

Clinical descriptions emphasized neurologic symptoms stemming from the original assumption that poliovirus was the cause. The acute course was characterized by low grade fever, malaise, paresthesias, exhaustion, and sweating. Flaccid and asymmetric paresis would occur, occasionally followed by atrophy. Little or no respiratory or gastro-intestinal symptoms were noted. The course was prolonged and marked by relapses with many cases being bedridden for months. Eye discomfort, memory loss, sleep disturbance, emotional lability and arthralgias occurred. Follow-up of fifty seven cases seven to ten months later showed that only 11% had become totally well. Most patients resumed work, but 19% had residual weakness. Fatigue occurred in 37% while 42% had "nervousness." Attempts to isolate an infectious agent were not successful.

Adelaide, Australia Epidemic

At almost the same time, an epidemic of classical poliomyelitis occurred in Adelaide, South Australia[13] affecting 1350 persons. During the epidemic, however it became clear that another illness was present which did not fit the diagnostic expectations of polio. This variant affected children, with 45% of all cases being under 15 years of age. The onset of this illness would be either abrupt or gradual. It was characterized by "lassitude", muscle aching and weakness, headache, sore throat, abdominal symptoms, paresthesias, fever, blurring of vision and urinary retention. A chronic course was common among these patients with muscle pain, psychologic symptoms, and poor concentration predominating. There were no deaths. This illness varied from acute anterior poliomyelitis in several respects: 1) the CSF was normal 2) rapid improvement of weakness but prolonged recovery 3) prominent psychologic symptoms, dyslogia, and myalgia. A variant of poliovirus was proposed to be the cause.

Kingston / Upper New York State Epidemic

Another epidemic of "Iceland Disease" involving children was described by White and Burtch in 1953 in northern New York State[14]. The first cases presented in the summer of 1950 and were assumed to be acute anterior poliomyelitis or abortive poliomyelitis. However, because of prominent dysesthesias and muscle aching and the absence of marked weakness and wasting, the illness was subsequently assumed to be Iceland disease.

Forty seven patients were described, eleven of whom were considered to have true poliomyelitis. Of the remaining, nineteen were chosen for intensive study, fifteen women and 4 men ranging in age from nine to forty five years of age. The onset was more commonly gradual than acute. Prominent symptoms included muscle aching, transient weakness without wasting, transiently decreased tendon reflexes, paresthesias, headache, photophobia, depression and lymphadenopathy. Personal contact seemed to be involved in the spread of this illness, and family clustering was noted. In one family five of seven children were ill. Two of eleven patients had abnormal CSF with elevations in cell count and protein. Elevated urinary creatinine excretion was present in most of thirteen tested. At follow up fifteen months later, no patient was entirely well, although most had improved.

The Cumberland, England Epidemic

In 1955 a physician, Dr. A. L. Wallis, in Cumberland noted a large epidemic of Iceland Disease, or Royal Free Disease as it was then called, and described his findings in a paper which was submitted as a doctoral thesis[15]. The epidemic involved 233 persons over a six month period, half of them children. Males were affected more frequently than females among children while in adults this ratio was reversed. It appeared to be an infectious illness with a 5 to 7 day incubation period. Most cases were mild, resolving within one month, but some patients had extended illness marked by relapses and remissions.

The most prominent symptoms included fatigue, headaches, myalgia, dizziness, "dry throat", tender and enlarged lymph nodes, sore eyes and blurred vision. Other symptoms included abdominal discomfort, diarrhea, nausea, dysesthesias, night sweats, sleep disturbance, and difficulty with concentration. There were no obvious differences in the pediatric presentation from that of adults.

The Punta Gorda, Florida Epidemic

In 1957 an epidemic of ME/CFIDS occurred in Punta Gorda, Florida[16] involving 21 persons, several of them children. The onset was insidious with fatigue, headache, neck pain and mental confusion with exacerbations from one to four weeks after onset. Nineteen patients were hospitalized or bed ridden. Follow-up after five months demonstrated a prolonged, irregular course. In a community survey, there were no cases identified under the age of 9, while eleven cases from ages 10-19 were identified, an attack rate of 7.7%.

The Great Ormond Street Epidemic

In 1978, Dillon[17] describes an outbreak of ME/CFIDS involving 145 adults which occurred in 1970 at the Hospital for Sick Children, Great Ormond Street,

London. In a supplementary note, seven children were described with what appeared to be the same illness. The report detailed the symptoms of five boys and two girls, with the average age of onset 11.7 years. The children had a protracted course, and two were still ill two years after onset. There appeared to be contact with other family members with the same constellation of symptoms. Prominent symptoms were headache, fatigability, lethargy, back and muscle pains, sore throat, nausea, abdominal pains. On physical examination, pharyngitis, lymphadenopathy and mild pyrexia were noted. It is of interest that in the primary epidemic, which affected 15% of the nursing staff and 3% of the medical staff, no inpatient children were noted to have become ill.

In 1980 May et al[18] described an epidemic in Southampton and attempted specifically to address the lingering questions of psychogenic origin which had persisted in the twenty years since the Royal Free epidemic. The outbreak occurred in spring of 1979 in the Southampton Girls' School and was studied using a personality questionnaire. Forty five children became ill, with an average age of 13.2 years. They had 8.1 separate symptoms and were bed-ridden 14.2 days, many with a prolonged convalescence. With the exception of one child with mononucleosis, virologic studies were negative.

The conclusions of this study were that 1) there was no evidence of stress as a predisposing factor 2) "Altered medical perception" was a factor in diagnosis while "neuroticism" was not. Also of interest was that of the children considered "well" at the time of the epidemic, many had fatigue, myalgia, sore throat, and headache.

Ayrshire Epidemic

In January 1980 an outbreak of ME/CFIDS occurred in Ayrshire[19] involving 22 cases, two of whom were children aged 8 and 10. The specific symptoms for the children were not recorded but symptoms of the patients in general were similar to other descriptions. It was noted that 82% had elevated neutralizing antibody titers to Coxsackie B virus.

West Otago Epidemic

The West Otago, New Zealand outbreak of 1982[20], subsequently called the "Tapanui flu", involved 28 cases. Thirty six percent were children under the age of 15, 3 between the ages of 5 and 10, and 7 between 10-15 years of age. All had fatigue and mood changes, and most had abdominal pains, joint and muscle pain, headache and change in sleep pattern.

IV. Sporadic ME/CFIDS - Enterovirus, Epstein-Barr virus

There have been numerous reports describing ME/CFIDS in studies which have concentrated on possible specific etiologic agents. In the United States, these papers have tended to concentrate on Epstein-Barr virus, while experience in Great Britain, Australia, and New Zealand have concentrated on the enteroviruses. In one paper, DuBois and his colleagues[21] described 2 children among 14 patients who were selected because of prominent fatigue, fever, myalgia, depression, pharyngitis and lymphadenopathy. Epstein-Barr virus anti-Early Antigen was noted to be higher in patients than in controls.

Sporadic Cases

The following year, Jones et al[22] published a paper involving forty four patients, eighteen of whom were children under 15 years of age. The cases appeared to be sporadic rather than epidemic. The report demonstrated elevated Epstein-Barr virus anti-Early Antigen antibodies, with 39 of 44 elevated compared to healthy controls. Both of these papers described ME/CFIDS to a medical audience who had been largely unaware of reports of ME in other countries.

In 1985 Salit[23] described fifty patients with sporadic postinfectious neuromyasthenia, 5 of whom were adolescents. The study is of interest as a systematic attempt was made to identify the organism responsible for the initial infectious episode. The results suggested an association with the following agents: EBV in 16; Coxsackie B virus in 4; Giardia lamblia in 2; Mycoplasma pneumoniae in 2; Toxoplasma gondii in 2; Hepatitis A virus in 1; Herpes zoster virus in 1; Cytomegalovirus in 1 and unknown in 22. One patient had evidence of simultaneous infection with both EBV and Coxsackie B virus.

Two recent papers have attempted to look at the epidemiology of ME/CFIDS from the perspective of laboratory testing requests. In a study by Ho-Yen[24] 381 cases were diagnosed retrospectively based upon information contained in virology requests. Based upon this data, they concluded ME/CFIDS is very common in children, perhaps more common than infectious mononucleosis, and that boys are as likely to be affected as girls. In a separate paper, Wilson and co-workers[25] presented 39 children with a clinical diagnosis of ME evaluated for antibodies to Coxsackie B virus. The clinical symptoms of the children involved were fatigue, myalgia, headache, limb pain, anorexia, weakness and extended school absence. Males and females were equally affected.

V. Primary Juvenile Fibromyalgia Syndrome

Note has been made of similarities between ME/CFIDS and Primary Fibromyalgia Syndrome (PFS)[26], with similarities in symptomatology, sleep physiology and immunology. In a few papers involving PFS in children[27-31], symptoms other than muscle tender points have been described. It is possible that Primary Fibromyalgia Syndrome represents a group of patients with ME/CFIDS where muscle tenderness is the most prominent symptom.

In February 1985, Yunus and Masi[27] described a group of 33 children who presented for rheumatological evaluation as having Juvenile Primary Fibromyalgia Syndrome (JPFS). These evaluations were conducted along the same lines as adult PFS with detailed descriptions of "tender points" and joint symptoms, but also included a description of accompanying symptoms. The average age was 12.3 years at onset with a predominance of females (31 female, 2 male). Of these children the following was observed: generalized aches and pains 97%; stiffness 79%; subjective soft tissue swelling 61%; waking up tired 100%; poor sleep 67%; general fatigue 91%; anxiety 70%; depression 55%; chronic headaches 54%; paresthesias 36% and irritable bowel symptoms 27%. No mention was made of cognitive difficulties, type of

presentation (acute or insidious), muscle weakness; sore throat or lymphatic pain.

Physical examination demonstrated "tender points" on muscle palpation. Routine laboratory studies were "normal", but immunological studies were not performed. At follow-up of an average of 18.8 months, complete recovery was seen in 5%, improvement in 55%, while 40% retained moderate symptoms. The authors emphasized that while the symptoms of anxiety and depression were present, they did not appear to be etiologic, and none of the children had school phobia. They emphasized the need for accurate diagnosis.

VI. Conclusions

This illness, called Myalgic Encephalomyelitis (ME), Chronic Fatigue Syndrome (CFS), or Chronic Fatigue-Immune Dysfunction Syndrome (CFIDS), appears to affect children as frequently as it does adults. However, attention has been directed primarily toward adults with this disorder, perhaps because of several factors: 1) The illness in children may be milder 2) children may be more "adaptable" to chronic symptoms 3) a gradual onset of symptoms is more common in children thus making diagnosis more difficult, and 4) an adult who has lost the ability to support a family commands more attention than a child with prolonged school absence. While considerable discussion has revolved around hysteria, depression and school phobia, there has been no evidence in any of the published studies in children to suggest these factors as etiologic.

Several common factors are observed in the studies of ME/CFIDS in children: 1) The presence of a specific pattern of symptoms, 2) Nearly equal sex distribution, 3) High attack rate at puberty, 4) High family incidence, 5) School, family and social disruption, and 6) Prolonged morbidity. Clearly, more studies on the pediatric population are indicated.

VII. References

1. Bell DS, Bell KM. The post-infectious chronic fatigue syndrome: diagnosis in childhood. In Ablashi DV, Faggioni A, Kreuger GRF, et al (eds). **Epstein-Barr Virus and Human Disease.** Clifton, NJ: Humana Press 1989; 412-7.

2. Gordon N. Myalgic Encephalomyelitis. *Dev Med & Child Neurol* 1988;30:673-82.

3. Acheson ED. The clinical syndrome variously called benign myalgic encephalomyelitis, Iceland disease, and epidemic neuromyasthenia. *Am J Med* 1959; 26:569-95.

4. Behan PO, Behan WMH: Epidemic Myalgic Encephalitis. In **Clinical Neuroepidemology** Clifford F, Ed., Pitmans 1980; 374-383.

5. Henderson DA, Shelokov A. Epidemic neuromyasthenia-Clinical Syndrome. *N Eng J Med,* 1959, 260 : 757-64.

6. Komaroff AL. Chronic fatigue syndromes: relationship to chronic viral infections. *J Virol Methods* 1988; 21: 3.

7. Behan PO, Behan WMH. Postviral Fatigue Syndrome. CRC (Critical Reviews in Neurobiology) 1988 4:2; 157-178.

8. Ramsay AM. **Myalgic Encephalomyelitis and Postviral Fatigue States**. 1988 2nd Edition; London: Gower Medical

9. Bell DS, Bell KM. Chronic fatigue syndrome: diagnostic criteria.[letter] *Ann Intern Med.* 1988. 109 (2):167.

10. Holmes GP, Kaplan JE, Gantz NM, Komaroff AL, Schonberger LB, Straus SE, et al. Chronic fatigue syndrome: A working case definition. Ann Intern Med 1988;108:387-89.

11. Bell KM, Cookfair D, Reese P, Bell D, Cooper L. Risk Factors with chronic fatigue syndrome in children. [Abstract]. *Am J Epidemiol.* 1988; 128:899.

12. Sigurdsson B, Sigurjonsson J, Sigurdsson JH, Thorkelsson J, Gudmundsson KR. A Disease Epidemic in Iceland simulating Poliomyelitis. *Am J Hyg.* 1950; 52: 222-238.

13. Pellew RAA. A Clinical description of a disease resembling poliomyelitis, seen in Adelaide, 1949-1951. *Med J Aust* June 1951; 944-6.

14. White DN, Burtch RB. Iceland Disease A New Infection Simulating Acute Anterior Poliomyelitis. *Neurology* 1954; 4:506-516.

15. Wallis AL. An Investigation into an unusual disease in Epidemic and sporadic form in a general practice in Cumberland in 1955 and subsequent years. University of Edinburgh doctoral Thesis 1957..

16. Poskanzer DC, Henderson DA, Kunkle EC, Kalter SS, Clement WB, Bond JO. Epidemic neuromyasthenia: An outbreak in Punta Gorda, Florida. *N Eng J Med* 1957; 257:356-64.

17. Dillon MJ. Epidemic neuromyasthenia at the Hospital for Sick Children, Great Ormond Street. London. *Postgrad Med J* 1978; 54: 757-64, 814-8.

18. May PBR, Donnan SPB, Ashton JR, Ogilvie MM, Rolles CJ. Personality and medical perception in benign myalgic encephalomyelitis. *Lancet* 1980, ii; 1122-4.

19. Fegan KG, Behan PO, Bell EJ. Myalgic Encephalomyelitis-report of an epidemic. *J Roy Col. Gen. Pract.* 1983: 33; 335-337.

20. Poore M ,Snow P, Paul C. An Unexplained Illness in West Otago. *N Z Med J* 1984; 97:351-4.

21. DuBois RE, Seeley JK, Brus I, Sakamoto K Ballow M, Harada S Bechtold TA. Chronic Mononucleosis syndrome. *South Med J.* 1984, 77: 1376.

22. Jones J J, Ray C G, Minnich L L, Hicks MJ, Kibler R, Lucas DO. Evidence for active Epstein-Barr virus infection in patients with persistent, unexplained illnesses: elevated anti-early antigen antibodies. *Ann Intern Med.* 1985; 102:1-6.

23. Salit IE. Sporadic postinfectious neuromyasthenia *Can Med Assoc J* 1985; 133: 659-63.

24. Ho-Yen Darrel.The epidemiology of post viral fatigue syndrome. *Scott Med J* 1988; 33(6):368-9.

25. Wilson PM, Kusumaker V, McCartney RA, Bell EJ. Features of Coxsackie B virus (CBV) infection in children with prolonged physical and psychological morbidity *Psychosom Res* 1989; 33(1): 29-36.

26. Buchwald D, Goldenberg DL, Sullivan JL, Komaroff AL. The "chronic active Epstein-Barr virus infection" syndrome and primary fibromyalgia. *Arthritis Rhum,* 1987; 30:1132-6.

27. Yunus MB, Masi AT. Juvenile primary fibromyalgia syndrome. *Arthritis Rheum* 1985; 28 138-145.

28. Calabro JJ. Fibromyalgia (Fibrositis) in Children. *Am J Med* 1986; 81 (Suppl 3A): 57-9.

29. Yunus MB, Aches and pains: is it juvenile fibromyalgia syndrome? *Diagnosis* August 1984; 93-102.

30. Pellegrino MJ, Waylonis GW, Sommer A. Familial occurrence of primary fibromyalgia. *Arch Phys Med Rehabil* 1989; 70: 61-3.

31. Cicuttini F, Littlejohn GO. Female adolescent rheumatological presentations: the importance of chronic pain syndromes. *Aust Paediatr J* 1989; 25: 21-4.

General Review

Chapter 20

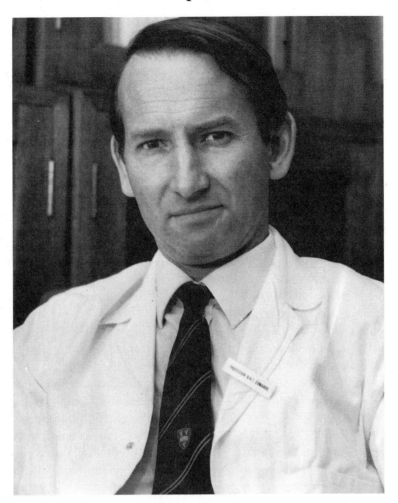

Richard H.T. Edwards

A Multidisciplinary Approach to Investigating and Treating Patients with Chronic Fatigue

Richard H.T. Edwards, PhD, FRCP, University of Liverpool Muscle Research Centre, Department of Medicine, University of Liverpool, P.O. Box 147, Liverpool L69 3BX United Kingdom

Acknowledgements: The research programme into the physiology of muscle fatigue directed by the author has at various times been supported by the Wellcome Trust, Muscular Dystrophy Group of Great Britain and Northern Ireland, ICI Pharmaceuticals and Mersey Region Health Authority. The outstanding work of the research collaborators cited is specially acknowledged.

Previous to Professor Edwards' present position as Head of the Department of Medicine at the University of Liverpool, he was the Co-Director of the Jerry Lewis Muscle Research Centre at the Royal Post-graduate Medical School, Honorary Consultant Respiratory Physician to the Hammersmith Hospital, Professor of Human Metabolism at the University College Hospital Medical School in London, and past President of the European Society for Clinical Investigation. Professor Edwards was awarded the Robert Bing Prize of the Swiss Academy of Medical Sciences for development of new techniques for analyzing muscle weakness and fatigue.

Introduction

The constellation of symptoms comprising the 'Chronic Fatigue Syndrome' (CFS) are well known and were the subject of a recent Oxford Consensus Meeting [1]. There, CFS was defined as a syndrome characterised by disabling mental and physical fatigue, of definite onset (i.e. not life long) and associated with other symptoms e.g. myalgia, mood and sleep disturbance. As a matter of practical definition the diagnosis can be made if fatigue has been present for more than six months and for more than fifty percent of the time. The condition may overlap with the (acute onset) postviral fatigue syndrome[2] in which there is evidence (corroborated by laboratory studies) of past or continuing viral infection[3]. The condition (Table 1) currently known as 'Myalgic Encephalomyelitis' (M.E.) bears some similarity to the 'Effort Syndrome' (as it was known to Sir Thomas Lewis earlier this century)[4] as one of a group of disorders manifesting the symptoms of weakness, fatigue and exercise intolerance[5].

Table 1
Summary of Myalgic Encephalomyelitis from the ME Association
Onset - Viral infection (Epidemic or scattered cases) Headache Sore throat General aches and pains Dizziness Chronically - Profound fatigue Muscle weakness Muscle tenderness Coldness of extremities Impaired memory and concentration Intense malaise and extreme debility Relapses usually triggered by periods of excessive physical or mental activity. Advice: Rest

---

Other symptoms are loss of ability to concentrate, disturbed sleep, dizzy spells and disturbances of the autonomic system causing such effects as feeling feverish or cold. Patients with postviral fatigue syndromes (including M.E.) fall into this category. Our work over several years[6,7,8,9] provides a systematic physiological analysis of muscle fatigue. Clinical investigations and exercise testing show evidence of a physiological basis for symptoms such as breathlessness or palpitations as a feature of "unfitness" due to lack of exercise[5, 10, 11]. A detailed study was carried out to investigate the possibility of a persistent viral infection and a further study was done to explore, within the context of a General Medical Clinic, the possible psychological factors underlying, perpetuating or amplifying the impairments in mental or physical performance. The results of these comprehensive studies suggest a means of explaining the mechanisms of symptom production (irrespective of the actual cause: viral or psychogenic) to provide a basis for positive diagnosis, reassurance and sympathetic, confident management.

Objective Studies of Muscle Structure and Function

The physiological basis of human muscle fatigue was the subject of a Ciba Foundation Symposium[12] in which the relative importance of 'central'[13,14] and 'peripheral'[15,16] mechanisms in the genesis of fatigue and, in the case of the latter, the importance of "metabolic" or "electrical" factors in various types of exercise was debated. A clinically relevant classification is whether the fatigue (defined as failure to sustain force or power output) is of central origin i.e. due to a failure to maintain the recruitment of high threshold motor units or peripheral, due to failure of neuromuscular transmission, sarcolemmal excitation, or excitation-contraction coupling (Table 2).

Our earlier studies included a review of 109 patients presenting with the symptom of unexplained myalgia[17]. A large proportion of these patients could now be classified as having M.E. Exclusion of the cases of inflammatory or metabolic myopathy on the basis of percutaneous muscle biopsy with studies of histomorphology and histochemistry[18, 19] showed then, as now, that M.E. patients have few significant pathological abnormalities in muscle or, if they do occur, the changes are such as may be seen on percutaneous biopsy in the large population of normal subjects (especially athletes) studied by ourselves and others[20] in the UK, North America and Scandinavia. Among the reported abnormalities including minor atrophic changes are sometimes those reported ("moth-eaten" Type I fibres) as occurring in the related syndrome of 'Primary Fibromyalgia'[21, 22].

Table 2
Physiological Definitions and Classification of Human Skeletal Muscle Weakness and Fatigue[8,9]

Weakness - Failure to generate force
(N.B. In maximally activated contractions, force is directly proportional to the cross-sectional area of the contractile elements of the muscle).

Fatigue - Failure to sustain force or power output

Causes of Fatigue

Type of Fatigue	Definition	Possible Mechanism
Central	Less force with 'maximal' voluntary contractions than with maximal electrically stimulated contractions or as evidenced by the 'Twitch Interpolation Technique'	Failure to sustain maximal recruitment of of motor units or firing frequency.
Peripheral	Same force loss with voluntary as with electrically stimulated contractions	
	a) High Frequency Fatigue	Impaired neuromuscular transmission or conduction of muscle action potential
	b) Low Frequency Fatigue	Impaired excitation-contraction coupling

The EMG evidence of abnormal jitter[23, 24] and the occasionally observed evidence of a resolving viral polymyositis[25] are not diagnostic and neither can adequately explain the symptom of fatigue which, when analysed systematically (Table 2), is found to be 'central' rather than a consequence of any 'peripheral' impairment of muscle[26]. There is no appreciable muscle wasting other than that which might be attributed to inactivity in the most severe cases and there is usually no evidence of weakness as tested with brief (5 sec) maximal voluntary contractions though some patients may fail to achieve maximal

activation of their muscle as indicated by the 'Twitch Interpolation Technique'[15, 27]. The possible objection of using the Adductor Pollicis as a model for the function of larger muscle groups and the limitation of the electrical stimulation technique for the assessment of fatigue induced by isometric contractions[26] have been overcome in subsequent studies[28] in which objective measurements were carried out in the quadriceps after fatiguing cycle ergometer exercise.

The recovery from exercise was followed with repeated assessments of muscle function over the next 48 hours to check whether the symptom of prolonged fatigue after exercise could be attributed to some delayed or slowly recovering physiological process but there was no evidence of undue fatigue (when compared with age and sex matched normal controls) at the end of exercise nor a slower rate of recovery. Muscle function was normal when patients were complaining of the protracted fatigue after exercise. The reported abnormal tendency to develop intracellular acidosis with moderate aerobic exercise in muscle as demonstrated by magnetic resonance spectroscopy in a patient with postviral fatigue syndrome[29] is scarcely surprising given the observed (nonspecific) reduction in mitochondrial enzyme activity[30] seen in chronic fatigue patients (Figure 1, courtesy of Dr P MacLennan). In this connection, it has proved interesting to make a comparison with the metabolic and physiological responses to exercise seen in patients with a biochemically defined defect of mitochondrial oxidative metabolism. Such a 'paradigm' case was studied in detail[31,32]. Other useful indicators of muscle inflammation or damage (ESR and plasma creatine kinase activity respectively) are invariably normal or not raised to the levels indicative of actual muscle pathology in CFS patients.

The symptom of fatigue before exercise could not be logically attributable to any metabolic defect of muscle, even if a specific one had been described, because it is characteristic of metabolic myopathies[18] that pain and fatigue occur during and after but not before exercise. From these considerations, it can be concluded that there is insufficient evidence to attribute the fatigue of CFS to any form of primary myopathy. Even if 'secondary' changes in muscle occur, they cannot logically be held responsible for the symptom of fatigue since objective testing shows muscle function to be normal[26, 28].

Formal Exercise Testing may reveal abnormal responses in acute viral or bacterial infections[34, 35] but, in CFS patients, testing usually reveals a reassuring response to submaximal power outputs, but a reduction in the maximal work rate, achieved usually with a submaximal heart rate indicating cessation of exercise before reaching the physiological limit[11, 36]. Rating of Perceived Exertion (RPE) with the Borg scale reveals that CFS patients rate submaximal power outputs higher than normal suggesting an increased 'gain' for the perception of physiological signals associated with exercise. It is worth determining that there is a postural element i.e., that patients may feel more fatigued by sitting or standing for a long period and better if lying horizontal.

Evidence of postural hypotension or of a dependent shift of blood volume is easy to seek at the bedside by measuring pulse rate followed by blood pressure first in the lying then standing posture[5]. The former is obvious while the latter is indicated by an excessive rise (more than 20 beats per minute) in pulse rate. This will be helpful in planning treatment, for the patient taking sufficient exercise to reap the therapeutic benefit. In such cases the following may be tried: a) support stockings (or tights) to reduce pooling of blood in dependent capacitance vessels; b) Dihydroergotamine as a venoconstrictor to achieve the same purpose; c) Fludrocortisone to increase sodium retention and thus achieve blood volume expansion and a small rise in resting mean blood pressure.

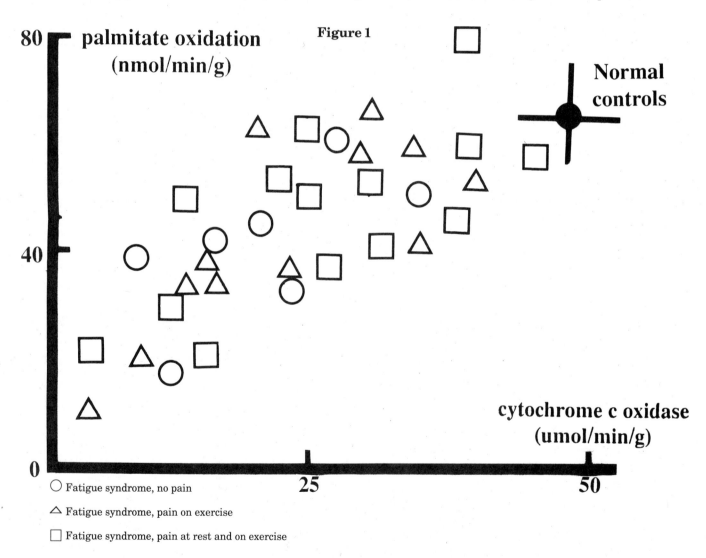

Figure 1

○ Fatigue syndrome, no pain

△ Fatigue syndrome, pain on exercise

□ Fatigue syndrome, pain at rest and on exercise

Mitochondrial enzyme activities in patients with myalgia and chronic fatigue showing non-specific general reduction in activity. (Results from patients attending Muscle Clinic at the Royal Liverpool Hospital - analyses by techniques published previously (30). Normal control values are means +/- S.D.; n=13)

Viral Aetiology

A seriously considered possible aetiology of the disease is that there is a persistent viral infection in the muscles and elsewhere. Present evidence points to the enteroviruses[3, 37, 38] and the assumption is that there is an inadequate immune response to the infecting virus. The suggested impaired response may quite possibly involve the T-cell response as cell-mediated immunity is important in control to prevent persistence of virus infection, but eventually this fault is rectified and the patient recovers. Definite evidence of viral infection has been found in a variable proportion of patients in that there may be high IgM antibody titres to Coxsackie viruses, indicating recent infection[24]. Viral protein has been found in the serum of patients and Coxsackie virus has also been isolated from the stools of patients. Circulating immune complexes containing IgM have also been found in a fair proportion of patients[37]. Viral RNA has been found in muscle biopsies of patients with postviral fatigue syndrome[39, 40].

There is no doubt that a viral infection can be a precipitating factor or a complication of a reduced immunity as when active Epstein Barr virus was reported to occur in PVFS[41]. We considered it would be interesting to compare[41] CFS patients with patients with muscle diseases who were also involved in the psychological assessment. Circulating immune complexes containing IgG and IgM and the lymphocyte proliferation in response to Concanavilin A and to Coxsackie B virus were determined but there were no changes which could lend support to the belief that there could be a specific viral aetiology for CFS. It is evident that there is a substantial proportion of patients who do not have any history or other evidence of viral infection.

A very similar constellation of symptoms to those complained of by CFS patients may be seen in the 'Post Polio Syndrome'[43] (interestingly a consequence of another enterovirus infection) and after head injury[44]. If a viral aetiology is found to be important at least in some patients, it is possible that the feature common to several aetiologies is diffuse (microscopic) brain damage which has significant psychological if not psychiatric consequences.

Psychological and Psychiatric Assessment in CFS

The psychological/psychiatric aspects of CFS are a matter of current debate especially as to whether M.E. is a new entity or 'neurasthenia' in a new guise[45, 46]. What is needed now is a systematic unbiased assessment of the present psychological health of CFS patients and then to seek to identify 'risk factors' in terms of underlying personality traits as suggested in the case of the 'Post Polio Syndrome'[47] and susceptibilities, with attention to initiating stressful life events and the developing factors which subsequently determine illness behaviour.

Structured interviews were carried out in consecutive CFS patients and in ambulant patients with myopathy (Becker and Facioscapulohumeral muscular dystrophy and inactive polymyositis) of similar age distribution. Scores on a questionnaire to measure mental fatigue, Spielberger's State Trait Anxiety Inventory, Hospital Anxiety and Depression Scale and Present State Examination/Catego were used as the main outcome measures[48]. Psychiatric symptoms were significantly more common in CFS patients than those with myopathy. A variety of psychiatric diagnoses were made (Table 3) supporting the belief that fatigue is a common nonspecific psychiatric symptom. Whether any or all of these can be attributed to being the cause or the consequence of the CFS is not known.

Table 3
Psychiatric Diagnoses in Chronic Fatigue Syndrome
Summary Results[47] **The breakdown is as follows:**

Depression	24%
Phobic Anxiety State	12%
Somatoform Disorders	6%
Anxiety State	6%
Subcases of Anxiety and Depression	27%
'Pure' Chronic Fatigue Syndrome without associated psychiatric diagnosis	25%
Chronic Fatigue with associated psychiatric diagnosis	75%

An Integrated Physiological Interpretation

There may be grounds for suggesting[49] that the psychosomatic disorder manifested in the CFS is an example of 'Somatisation'[50] where the thresholds for distinction between physical and psychiatric illness have become blurred. That patients with CFS have heightened perception of physiological signals during exercise is evident as may be observed of the heightened cutaneous and muscle sensibility on clinical examination. Evident too is the tendency for patients to suffer from the consequences of consciousness of hitherto unconscious (automatic) central motor control functions[51]. Thus walking very slowly may deprive the patient of the learned automaticity of the motor skills, including balance and coordination necessary for normal gait. Failure to relax antagonists compromises the function of agonists and may cause muscle pain due to inappropriate use. Similarly the 'nonrestorative sleep' which may also affect immune responsiveness[52] can be associated with myalgia on waking, or before exercise may result in continued activity of a small percentage of muscle fibres with physiological and metabolic overuse to a degree which is seen in the related condition of 'Primary Fibromyalgia'[21, 22]. CFS may thus be more a true functional disorder i.e. a disorder of physiological regulations rather than a disease resulting from a discrete pathology. It is clear however that lesions of the brain can result in a striking increase in the conscious effort necessary to perform simple, familiar everyday tasks[53]. Such an explanation is useful for operational purposes in designing and explaining a positive programme of support and rehabilitation.

A Positive Approach to Management

The first step is to convince the patient that there is no mystery concerning the origin of their symptoms; they are 'real' and not 'imaginary' in that they have a recognizable physiological basis. Next it is necessary to adopt a firm "the buck stops here" approach to management so that the commitment of the patient may be engaged. The multidisciplinary approach currently used in my medical clinic covers assessments of the relevant medical conditions, viral and immunological screens as well as percutaneous muscle biopsy and measurement of muscle function. Coupled with this is the formal assessment of the psychological/psychiatric state. The rehabilitation programme encompasses detailed explanations of the pathophysiology in layman's terms and instruction on relaxation and control of breathing[54].

Finally, there is guidance on the proper conduct of a graduated exercise programme designed to overcome the effects of inactivity[55] and to re-educate motor performance skills. Exercise is also valuable in returning autonomic controls which are often disturbed in CFS, e.g. postural control of heart rate and blood pressure, thermal regulation involving skin blood flow and control of sweating. Sometimes it may be helpful to recommend that the patient keeps an activity diary in which the day's physical and mental exertions are recorded together with a note as to the extent of physical and mental fatigue such as in the diary currently available from the M.E. Association. It may also be useful to give encouragement to seek to regularise sleep patterns, if possible without the use of drugs such as hypnotics or antidepressants[2, 56] (though in our experience this has helped only a small proportion of CFS patients) by going to sleep and waking (if necessary by setting an alarm clock) at a set time so that diurnal physiological rhythms may be kept as normal as possible.

If a patient finds an exercise session too much, either on a given day or is unable to continue with the programme on subsequent days, the intensity of the exercise chosen initially was too great and should be reduced. It is not accepted however that exercise is harmful to the extent that patients have to stay in bed for days or weeks afterwards; no known physiological disturbance or medical condition does this. In such an event a search must be made into the psychological reaction to the exercise and why such a low physical stress appears to impede progress in rehabilitation. Certainly it is well known that muscles have a great capacity to adapt to increased use[57] with benefit to peak performance but especially endurance and this can provide a valuable positive feedback on the road to recovery.

CFS can be of very variable duration ranging from months to many years, but eventually most people do recover[24]. In this, a close working relationship with physiotherapists is important[5, 54].

Finally, it is important to educate doctors and health

professionals that CFS is a condition which can be diagnosed on positive grounds and not just by excluding others. It is not necessary to refer patients for complex, expensive investigations of muscle. It is not a primary muscle disease and it would be to the patients' advantage for them to be given sympathetic but firm reassurance and confident advice on their first contact with the medical profession.

References

1. **Editorial. Consensus on research into fatigue syndrome.** Brit Med J (1990) 300: 832.

2. Smith DG. **Understanding ME.** (1989) London: Robinson Publications.

3. Yousef GE, Bell EJ, Mann GF, Murugesan V, Smith DG, McCarthy RA and Mowbray JF. **Chronic enterovirus infection in patients with postviral fatigue syndrome.** Lancet (1988) i: 146-150.

4. Lewis T. **The soldier's heart and the effort syndrome.** London: Shaw & Sons 1918.

5. Newham D and Edwards RHT. **Effort syndromes.** Physiotherapy (1979) 65: 52-56.

6. Edwards RHT, Young A, Hosking GP, and Jones DA. **Human skeletal muscle function: description of tests and normal values.** Clin Sci Mol Med (1977) 52: 283-290.

7. Edwards RHT and Jones DA. **Diseases of skeletal muscle.** In: Handbook of Physiology: Skeletal Muscle. Eds Peachey D, Adrian RH & Geiger SR. American Physiological Society. Baltimore: Williams & Wilkins (1983) pp 633-672.

8. Edwards RHT. **New techniques for studying human muscle function, metabolism, and fatigue.** Muscle & Nerve (1984) 7: 599-609.

9. Jones DA and Edwards RHT. **Muscle strength and metabolism.** In: Recent Achievements in Restorative Neurology 2: Progressive Neuromuscular Diseases. Ed M Dimitrijevic, B Kakulas and G Vrbova. (1986) Basel: Karger. 123-138.

10. Riley MS, O'Brien CJ, McCluskey DR, Bell NP and Nicholls DP. **Aerobic work capacity in patients with chronic fatigue syndrome.** (1990) In press

11. McCluskey DR. **Aerobic work capacity in patients with Chronic Fatigue Syndrome.** The Nightingale (1990) 1 (3): 21 (Abstract).

12. Edwards RHT. **Human muscle function and fatigue.** In: Human Muscle Fatigue: Physiological Mechanisms. (Ciba Foundation Symposium 82) London: Pitman Medical, (1981) pp 1-18.

13. Waller AD. **The sense of effort: an objective study.** Brain (1981) 14: 179-247.

14. Bigland-Ritchie B, Jones DA, Hosking GP, Edwards RHT. **Central and peripheral fatigue in sustained maximum voluntary contractions of human quadriceps muscle.** Clin Sci (1978) 54: 609-614.

15. Merton PA. **Voluntary strength and fatigue.** J Physiol (1954) 123: 553-564.

16. Cooper RG, Edwards RHT, Gibson H and Stokes M. **Human muscle fatigue: frequency dependence of excitation and force generation.** J Physiol. (1988) 397: 585-599.

17. Mills KR and Edwards RHT, Gibson H and Stokes M. **Human muscle fatigue: frequency dependence of excitation and force generation.** J Physiol. (1988) 397: 585-599.

18. Mills KR, Newham DJ and Edwards RHT. **Muscle Pain.** In : Textbook of Pain Ed Wall PD and Melzack R. (Second Edition) Edinburgh: Churchill Livingstone (1989): pp420-432.

19. Dietrichson P, Coakley J, Smith PEM, Griffiths RD, Helliwell TR and Edwards RHT. **Conchotome and needle precutaneous biopsy of skeletal muscle.** J Neurol, Neurosurg. Psychiat. (1987) 50: 1461-1467.

20. Doyle D. **Muscle biopsies in Postviral Fatigue Syndrome.** The Nightingale (1990) 1 (3): 9 (Abstract).

21. Henriksson KG, Bengtsson A, Larsson J, et al. **Muscle biopsy findings of possible diagnostic importance in Primary Fibromyalgia (Fibrositis, Myofascial Syndrome).** Lancet (1982) ii: 1395.

22. Henriksson KG. **Muscle pain in neuromuscular disorders and primary fibromyalgia.** Eur J Appl Phsyiol (1988) 57: 348-352.

23. Jamal Ga, Hansen S. **Electrophysiological studies in the post-viral syndrome.** J Neurol, Neurosurg, Psychiat. (1985) 48: 691-694.

24. Behan PO, Behan WMH and Bell EJ. **The postviral fatigue syndrome an analysis of the findings in 50 cases.** J. Infection (1985) 10: 211-222.

25. Schwartz MS, Swash M, and Gross M. **Benign postinfection polymyositis.** Brit med J (1978) 2: 1256-1257.

26. Stokes MJ, Cooper RG and Edwards RHT. **Normal strength and fatiguability in patients with effort syndrome.** Brit med J (1988) 297: 1014-1017.

27. Chapman SJ, Edwards RHT, Greig C, Rutherford O. **Practical application of the Twitch Interpolation Technique for the study of voluntary contraction of the quadriceps muscle in man.** J Physiol (1984) 353: 3P.

28. Gibson H, Carroll N, Coakley J and Edwards RHT. **Recovery from maximal exercise in Chronic Fatigue States.** Eur. J. Clin. Invest. (1990) 20: A29.

29. Arnold DL, Bore PJ, Radda GK, et al. **Excessive intracellular acidosis of skeletal muscle on exercise in a patient with a post-viral exhaustion/fatigue syndrome.** Lancet (1984) i: 1367-1369.

30. Wagenmakers AJM, Kaur N, Coakley JH, Griffiths RD and Edwards RHT. **Mitochrondrial metabolism in myopathy and myalgia.** In "Advances in Myochemistry" ed G. Benzi. London: John Libby Eurotext pp. 219-230.

31. Edwards, RHT, Wiles CM, Gohil K et al. **Energy Metabolism in Human Myopathy.** In: Disorders of the Motor Unit. Ed D Schotland. New York: John Wiley. (1982) 55: 715-728.

32. Griffiths RG and Edwards RHT. **Energy metabolism in human muscle studied by 31P MRS**. In: Biochemical aspects of physical exercise. Ed. G. Benzi, L Packer and N Siliprandi. Amsterdam: Elsevier (1986) pp 261-272.

33. Wiles CM, Jones DA, and Edwards RHT. **Fatigue in human metabolic myopathy.** In: Human Muscle Fatigue: Physiological Mechanisms. (Ciba Foundation Symposium 82) London: Pitman Medical (1981) 264-282.

34. Friman G. **Effect of acute infectious disease on isometric muscle strength.** Scand J Clin Lab Invest (1977) 37: 303-308.

35. Friman G. **Effects of acute infectious disease on circulatory function.** Acta Med Scand (1977) Supp 19: 40-41.

36. Carroll N, Gibson H, Coakley J and Edwards RHT. **Cycle ergometry in patients with chronic fatigue syndromes.** Eur. J. Clin. Invest. Suppl. (1990) 20: A29.

37. Mowbray JF. **Evidence for chronic enterovirus infection in ME.** (1990) The Nightingale 1 (3): 22 (Abstract).

38. Calder BD, Warnock PJ, McCartney RA & Bell EJ. **Coxsackie B viruses and the post-viral sydrome: a prospective study in general practice.** J. Roy. Col. Gen. Prac. (1987) 37: 11.

39. Archard LC. **Molecular virology of muscle disease: Persistent virus infection of muscle in patients with postviral fatigue.** The Nightingale (1990) 1 (3): 5 (Abstract).

40. Archard LC, Bowles NC, Behan PO, Bell EJ and Doyle D. **Postviral Fatigue Syndrome: Persistence of enterovirus RNA in muscle and elevated creatine kinase.** J Roy Soc Med (1988) 81: 326-329.

41. Hotchin NA, Read R, Smith DG and Crawford DH. **Active Epstein-Barr virus infection in post-viral fatigue syndrome.** J Infection (1989) 18: 143-150.

42. Milton JD, Edwards RHT and Clements GB. **Immune responsiveness in Chronic Fatigue Syndrome.** Postgrad. Med. J. (1991) 67: 532-537.

43. Halstead LS, Wiechers DO, Rossi DC. **Late effects of poliomyelitis: Case reports.** In: Late Effects of Poliomyelitis. Eds Halstead LS & Wiechers DO Miami: Symposia Foundation, (1985).

44. Lishman WA. **Physiogenesis and psychogenesis in the 'Post Concussional Syndrome'.** Brit J Psychiatry (1988) 153: 460-469.

45. David AS, Wessely S and Pelosi AJ. **Postviral fatigue syndrome: time for a new approach.** Brit Med J (1988) 296: 696-699.

46. Wessely S. **Old wine in new bottles: Neurasthenia and 'ME'.** Psychological Medicine (1990) 20: 35-53.

47. Bruno RL and Frick NM. **Stress and "Type A" behaviour as precipitances of Post-polio sequelae: the Felican/Columbia Survey.** In: Research and Clinical Aspects of the Late Effects of Poliomyelitis. Eds. Halstead LS & Wiechers DO Birth Defects: Original Article Series. (1987) 23, (4), pp 145-155.

48. Wood GC, Bentall RP, Gopfert M and Edwards RHT. **A comparative psychiatric assessment of patients with Chronic Fatigue Syndrome and Muscle Disease.** Psychol. Med (1991) 21,619-628.

49. Edwards RHT. **Muscle Fatigue and Pain.** Acta Med. Scand. (1986) Suppl. 711: 179-88.

50. Lipowski ZJ. **Somatization: A Borderland between Medicine and Psychiatry.** CMAJ. (1986) 135. 609-614.

51. Granit R. **Constant Errors in the Execution and Appreciation of Movement**: Brain (1971) 95: 649-660.

52. Moldofsky H. **The significance of sleep- wave physiology and immune functions to chronic fatigue syndrome (CFS) and Fibromyalgia.** The Nightingale 1 (3): 22 (Abstract).

53. Brodal A. **Self-observation and Neuro-anatomical considerations after a stroke.** Brain (1973) 96: 675-694.

54. Harvey J. **Breath of Fresh Air on Chronic Fatigue.** Therapy Weekly. (1990) 16: 6.

55. Greenleaf JE, and Kozlowski S. **Physiological consequences of reduced physical activity during bed rest.** Exercise and Sport Sciences Reviews. (1982) 10: 84-119.

56. Vallings R. **Myalgic Encephalomyelitis - A Consideration of Treatment.** The New Zealand Family Physician. (1989) Summer 9-13.

57. Saltin B and Gollnick PD. **Skeletal muscle adaptability: significance for metabolism and performance.** In: Handbook of Physiology: Skeletal Muscle. Eds Peachey D, Adrian RH & Geiger SR. American Physiological Society. Baltimore: Williams & Wilkins (1983) pp 555-631.

Chapter 21

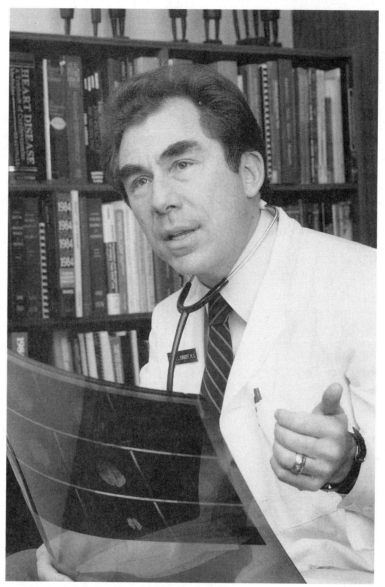

Anthony L. Komaroff

A Review of Myalgic Encephalomyelitis / Chronic Fatigue Immune Dysfunction Syndrome / Post-Viral Fatigue Syndrome (M.E. / CFIDS / PVFS) in America

Anthony L. Komaroff, MD Department of Medicine, Brigham and Women's Hospital,   Harvard Medical School, Boston MA

This work was supported by grants 1R01AI26788 and 1R01AI27314 from the National Institute of Allergy and Infectious Diseases, and grants from the Minann and Rowland Foundations.

Dr. Anthony Komaroff is an academic general internist who has been studying ME / CFIDS / PVFS for the past six years. He follows a large group of patients with this illness, and has an active program of research. He has been primarily interested in studying possible etiologic agents, and neuroimmunologic dysfunction in this syndrome.

Abstract

Myalgic encephalomyelitis (M.E.), chronic fatigue immune dysfunction syndrome (CFIDS), and post-viral fatigue syndrome (PVFS) are characterized by chronic, debilitating fatigue lasting greater than six months, with associated chronic and recurrent fever, pharyngitis, myalgias, adenopathy, arthralgias, difficulties in cognition and disorders of mood. In the majority of patients, the illness starts suddenly with an acute, apparently infectious illness. In such cases, the term "post-viral" fatigue syndrome (PVFS) is often used. Preliminary work suggests that various laboratory abnormalities may be seen more often in patients with CFS than in healthy individuals, including atypical lymphocytosis, monocytosis, elevation of heptocellular enzymes, low levels of antinuclear antibodies, elevated levels of IgG, elevated numbers of B cells, elevated CD4/CD8 T cell ratio, and low levels of immune complexes. Preliminary clinical and serologic studies suggest an association of CFS with enteroviral infection, Epstein-Barr virus (EBV) and the recently-discovered human herpesvirus-6 (HHV 6). No viral agent has yet been shown to play a causal role in the illness.

It is likely that this illness can be triggered by a heterogeneous group of forces and circumstances. An attractive model is: immune dysfunction is produced as a consequence of exogenous lymphotropic viruses, environmental toxins, stress or depression; the immune dysfunction leads to the reactivation of dormant, latent infectious agents; the reactivated infectious agents produce morbidity through cytodestructive action; the immunologic response to exogenous and endogenous agents, such as the elaboration of various cytokines, may also produce some of the morbidity of the illness; both a past atopic history, and a past history of major affective disorder, may make an individual vulnerable to this illness.

M.E./CFIDS/PFS: A Description

Practising physicians frequently see patients seeking care for the complaint of chronic fatigue. Most of the time, formal or informal evaluation leads to the conclusion that the patient is depressed, or anxious, or both. On unusual occasions, the patient may be suffering from a well-recognized "physical" disease such as an occult malignancy or thyroid disease.

Yet another subgroup of patients with chronic fatigue, presumably a small fraction, do not fit the pattern of any recognized physical disease, but do have features that suggest an "organic" disorder. Over the past 100 years, the medical literature has included descriptions of several ill-defined clinical syndromes that produce chronic fatigue: neurasthenia[1], post-viral fatigue syndrome[2], chronic mononucleosis[3-5], severe chronic active EBV infection[6,7], myalgic encephalomyelitis[8,9], fibrositis or fibromyalgia[10,11], and more recently chronic fatigue syndrome[12]. Dr. Hyde discusses this history in more detail. In recent years, there has been much speculation that these syndromes may be secondary to chronic viral infection. The syndromes go by different names, but share so many clinical and laboratory features that some believe they may be the same illness: that is, they may share a final common pathogenetic pathway. In this manuscript, I will assume that they are all the same illness, and refer to them all by the shorter name, chronic fatigue syndrome (CFS).

In my judgment, the similarities in the clinical descriptions of patients in all these groups are more impressive than the differences. The average patient is in his or her thirties, but the age at onset ranges from childhood to the elderly. Approximately 70% of the patients are women. The patients generally are middle-class, but all socioeconomic groups are represented. The main symptom is fatigue. Some patients are regularly bedridden or shut-in, unable to work. Many can work only part-time. Before they became ill, the patients perceived that they typically were more energetic than most of their friends.

In contrast to most patients seen in a general practice with chronic fatigue, the great majority of patients with CFS experience the **sudden onset** of an illness that then becomes chronic. Typically, the patients with chronic fatigue syndrome state that their chronic illness began on a particular day, with an acute "infectious" illness characterized by fever, pharyngitis, adenopathy, myalgias and related symptoms. Often, the onset is a respiratory tract infection characterized by sore throat, cough, myalgias and fever. Sometimes the onset is a gastrointestinal infection, with the predominant symptoms being nausea, diarrhea, and vomiting. Sometimes both respiratory and gastrointestinal symptoms are present. On occasion, the initial illness is acute infectious mononucleosis, with the classic clinical, hematologic and serologic findings. On occasion, the initial illness is dominated by neurologic findings: headache, photophobia, marked cognitive disturbance, profound vertigo and ataxia, visual impairment, paresis, or seizures.

This acute illness never seems to fully resolve. While its character may change over time, and its severity may vary, a state of chronic ill health ensues. The principal symptoms, and their frequency, are summarized in Table 1.

Table 1	
Frequency of Chronic Symptoms and Signs*	
Symptom / Sign	Frequency
Fatigue	75-100%
Low-grade fever	60-95%
Myalgias	30-95%
Depression	70-85%
Headaches	35-85%
Pharyngitis	50-70%
Impaired cognition	50-70%
Sleep disorder	15-70%
Anxiety	50-70%
Adenopathy	40-60%
Nausea	50-60%
Arthralgias	40-60%
Diarrhea	30-40%
Cough	30-40%
Odd skin sensations	30-40%
Rash	30-40%
Weight loss	20-30%
Weight gain	50-70%
Low basal body temperature (95.0 - 97.6F)	10-20%

*Adapted from the experience of the author, plus others[16-18].

In our experience, two particularly remarkable findings are chronic post-exertional malaise and recurrent, often drenching night sweats. The post-exertional malaise is characterized not only by symptoms that could represent deconditioning, pain and weakness of the involved muscles, but also by exacerbation of "systemic" symptoms, e.g., fever and adenopathy.

The patients state that these symptoms and others were typically not a chronic problem in the years before the onset of their illness, but became common after the illness began. We ask patients to make this distinction explicitly. Here are the frequency of several common chronic symptoms after the illness began vs. before the illness began: arthralgias (76% vs. 6%); morning stiffness (62% vs. 3%); distractibility (82% vs. 4%); forgetfulness (71% vs. 2%); dizziness (61% vs. 4%); paresthesias (52% vs. 2%); sleep disorder (90% vs. 7%); irritability (68% vs. 4%); depression (66% vs. 7%).

In our experience, patients with acute neurologic events (primary seizures, ataxia, focal weakness, transient blindness) have clinical and laboratory findings very similar to those of the larger group of patients with chronic fatigue, except for the neurologic events themselves.

On past medical history, the only clearly striking finding is a high frequency of atopic or allergic illness (in approximately 50%), as was first highlighted by Jones and his colleagues[13,14], and confirmed by Straus[15].

On physical examination, unusual and abnormal findings are observed in 15-50% of our patients: fevers; unusually low basal body temperature (below 97 F); posterior cervical adenopathy; and abnormal tests of balance (Romberg and tandem gait).

On standard hematologic testing, preliminary evidence indicates that results outside the normal range are seen in 15-50% of patients: relative lymphocytosis and relative lymphopenia; atypical lymphocytosis; monocytosis; and elevated sedimentation rate. These results have not yet been formally compared to results in a control group of healthy patients.

Standard serum chemistry testing is remarkable only for modestly elevated transaminases on one or more occasions in a quarter of the patients we have seen. None of these patients has had serologic evidence of active infection with hepatitis A, B or C virus.

On immunologic testing, we and others[14,16-21] have found evidence of subtle and diffuse dysfunction: partial hypogammaglobulinemia (25-80%); partial hypergammaglobulinemia (10-20%); low levels of autoantibodies, particularly antinuclear antibodies (15-35%); low levels of circulating immune complexes

(30-50%); elevated ratios of helper/suppressor T-cells (20-35%); reduced EBV-specific cytotoxic T-cell activity; reduced in vitro synthesis of interleukin-2 and interferon by cultured lymphocytes; increased IgE-positive T and B cells; deficient functional activity of natural killer cells; anergy or hypoergy by skin testing; and elevated levels of various cytokines. Some investigators have found increased levels of circulating interferon, whereas others have not. Straus demonstrated a significant increase in levels of leucocyte 2', 5'-oligoadenylate synthetase activity, an enzyme induced during acute viral infections[18].

Viruses and Chronic Fatigue Syndrome

As each of the chronic fatigue syndromes we have discussed has found its way into the medical literature, it has brought with it the speculation that the illness was initiated by an infectious agent. The speculation has centered most often on viruses, although Salit has suggested that non-viral infectious agents also can trigger a similar post-infectious malaise[22].

Myalgic encephalomyelitis was thought for some time to be produced by a less virulent strain of poliovirus. Recently Mowbray has kept alive the possibility that enteroviral infection may indeed be associated with some cases of CFS, by demonstrating circulating enteroviral antigen more often in patients than in control subjects[23]. Archard has found enteroviral RNA in muscle from patients, as well[24].

Antibody to Epstein-Barr virus has been measured in many patients, and higher levels of VCA-IgG and EA-Ab generally have been found in patients than in healthy control subjects; also, antibody to EBNA is absent in 10-30% of patients, whereas this is thought to be quite unusual in seropositive healthy individuals[16-18,25]. Moreover, it has been shown that antibody to EBNA-1 is absent in 10-30% of patients; it is absent more often in the more severely ill patients. Absence of antibody to EBNA-1 is very rarely seen in patients convalescing from acute infectious mononucleosis, or in patients with cancer. It is, however, seen frequently in children with AIDS[26].

In the few cases of CFS that start with acute infectious mononucleosis, it is reasonable to assume that EBV may be playing a central role in the CFS. In other cases, there is no strong evidence that EBV plays a **primary** role in the pathogenesis of CFS: most patients have normal antibody levels to EBV. Furthermore, there is clinical and laboratory evidence that other herpesviruses also can be reactivated in this illness; antibody to measles virus also may be higher[27]. Therefore, it seems most likely that the EBV serologic results in most patients with chronic fatigue syndrome represent **secondary** evidence of some immunologic perturbation, rather than a primary pathogenetic role for EBV. Nevertheless, secondary reactivation of EBV may not be just an epiphenomenon, as will be discussed shortly.

The recently-discovered human herpesvirus-6 is an interesting candidate for a pathogenetic role in some cases of chronic fatigue syndrome, primarily because it is lymphotropic and gliotropic[28-30]. There appears to be a serologic association of this virus with both chronic fatigue syndrome and fibromyalgia[31-33], although some studies have not found such an association. Studies to assess active replication of HHV 6 are now underway. At this time, the evidence seems most consistent with the hypothesis that this virus may be secondarily reactivated in this syndrome, as are other viruses; however, a primary role for HHV-6 in the pathogenesis of this illness remains possible.

In this decade of the human retroviruses, it was inevitable that there should be some speculation linking retroviruses to chronic fatigue syndrome. We and others have found no evidence that any of the known human retroviruses are involved with this syndrome. Furthermore, we have found no evidence of reverse transcriptase activity in the supernatants of primary lymphocyte cultures from a number of our sickest patients. Nevertheless, our diagnostic assays could have failed to recognize a retrovirus that was not T-lymphotropic, and/or was primarily lytic.

CFS and Psychological Illness

Most patients seeking medical care for chronic fatigue probably are suffering from a primary affective disorder (depression and/or anxiety), and probably do not have CFS[34,35].

What is the role, if any, of affective disorders in CFS? This is a difficult issue to study, since the affective disorders are defined in part by symptoms that could also reflect a "physical" illness. Our experience suggests that most patients with CFS perceive themselves as becoming **secondarily** depressed and/or anxious following the (usually sudden) onset of their illness: 80-90% initially deny suffering from depression or anxiety in the years prior to their illness. Yet more intensive interviewing by a trained interviewer, using the Diagnostic Interview Schedule, suggests that affective illness predated the onset of CFS in a somewhat greater number of patients (unpublished data).

Even if it were true that patients with CFS more frequently have an affective disorder that predates the onset of chronic fatigue, what might that mean? The classic Descartian notion of mind-body duality has led some to conclude that the symptoms in patients with CFS reflect no physical abnormality, just a heightened awareness of and concern about physical sensations, possibly coupled with a desire to attribute their dysfunctional state to a physical illness.

I am more inclined to view affective disorders as biologically-determined disorders of neurochemistry. "Mind" and "body" are not separate and discrete, but linked. Neurochemical disorders can affect immune function and, in turn, neurochemistry can be perturbed by the immune system. Biological forces that increase the likelihood of affective disorder also may increase vulnerability to disorders of immunity. In patients with CFS, who have a current and/or past affective disorder, and who also have evidence of

immune dysfunction and active viral infection, it may never be possible to determine whether the affective disorder, the immune dysfunction or the viral infection came first. Rather, the practical question is what form of therapy will be most effective: psychotherapy, pharmacotherapy of the affective disorder, "immune modulating" pharmacotherapy, anti-microbial therapy, or some combination of these.

A Model For The Pathogenesis of CFS

Knowledge about CFS is limited. The available data permit many models, but provide strong support for none of them. My own current view of this illness is reflected in Figure 1. At the core of CFS, I suspect, is an immunologic disturbance that allows reactivation of latent and ineradicable infectious agents, particularly viruses. The reactivation of these viruses may only be an epiphenomenon. However, I feel it is more likely that, once secondarily reactivated, these viruses contribute to the morbidity of CFS — directly, by damaging certain tissues (e.g., the pharyngeal mucosa), and indirectly, by eliciting an on-going immunologic response. In particular, the elaboration of various cytokines (e.g., interferon-alpha and interleukin-2) as part of this on-going immunologic war may produce many of the symptoms of CFS — the fatigue, myalgias, fevers, adenopathy, and even the disorders of mood and cognition. This is suggested by the finding of increased levels of various

Figure 1

Current Favorite Model

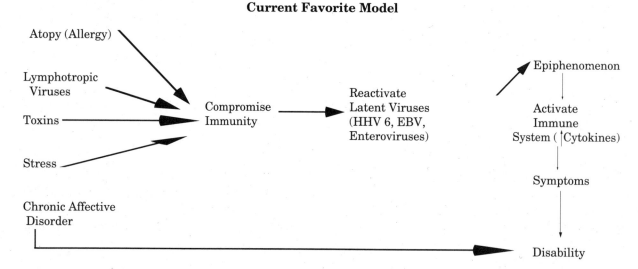

cytokines in CFS and related conditions[36-38], and the experience with infusing cytokines made by recombinant DNA techniques for various therapeutic purposes[39-45].

Whatever the course, the symptoms of CFS lead to some degree of debility in every patient. As with any illness, the degree of debility must be due, in part, to psychological factors.

What triggers the immune dysfunction in the first place? It is likely that many factors could do so: an atopic diathesis, exogenous lymphotropic infectious agents, environmental toxins, stress and, as argued earlier, the biology of an underlying affective disorder. It seems unlikely that a single explanation, such as a single infectious agent, explains this complex illness.

References

1. Paul O. DaCosta's syndrome or neurocirculatory asthenia. Br Heart J 1987;58:306-15.

2. Behan PO, Behan WMH, Bell EJ. The postviral fatigue syndrome — an analysis of the findings in 50 cases. J Infect 1985;10:211-22.

3. Isaacs R. Chronic infectious mononucleosis. Blood 1948;3:858-61.

4. Komaroff AL. The "chronic mononucleosis" syndromes. Hosp Pract 1987;22:71-5.

5. Straus SE. The chronic mononucleosis syndrome. J Infect Dis 1988;157:405-12.

6. Edson CM, Cohen LK, Henle W, Strominger JL. An unusually high-titer human anti-Epstein Barr virus (EBV) serum and its use in the study of EBV-specific proteins synthesized in vitro and in vivo. J Immunol 1983;130:919-24.

7. Schooley RT, Carey RW, Miller G, et al. Chronic Epstein-Barr virus infection associated with fever and interstitial pneumonitis. Clinical and serologic features and response to antiviral chemotherapy. Ann Intern Med 1986;104:636-43.

8. Acheson ED. The clinical syndrome variously called benign myalgic encephalomyelitis, Iceland disease and epidemic neuromyasthenia. Am J Med 1959;4:569-95.

9. Henderson DA, Shelokov A. Epidemic neuromyasthenia — clinical syndrome. New Engl J Med 1959;260:757-64.

10. Yunus M, Masi AT, Calabro JJ, Miller KA, Feigenbaum SL. Primary fibromyalgia (fibrositis): Clinical study of 50 patients with matched normal controls. Sem Arth Rheum 1981;11:151-71.

11. Goldenberg DL. Fibromyalgia syndrome: An emerging but controversial condition. JAMA 1987;257:2782-7.

12. Holmes GP, Kaplan JE, Gantz NM, et al. Chronic fatigue syndrome: A working case definition. Ann Intern Med 1988;108:387-9.

13. Olson GB, Kanaan MN, Gersuk GM, Kelley LM, Jones JF. Correlation between allergy and persistent Epstein-Barr virus infections in chronic-active Epstein-Barr virus-infected patients. J Allergy Clin Immunol 1986;78:308-14.

14. Olson GB, Kanaan MN, Kelley LM, Jones JF. Specific allergen-induced Epstein-Barr nuclear antigen-positive B cells from patients with chronic-active Epstein-Barr virus infections. J Allergy Clin Immunol 1986;78:315-20.

15. Straus SE, Dale JK, Wright R, Metcalfe DD. Allergy and the chronic fatigue syndrome. J Allergy Clin Immunol 1988;81:791-5.

16. DuBois RE, Seeley JK, Brus I, et al. Chronic mononucleosis syndrome. South Med J 1984;77:1376-82.

17. Jones JF, Ray CG, Minnich LL, Hicks MJ, Kibler R, Lucas DO. Evidence for active Epstein-Barr virus infection in patients with persistent unexplained illnesses: Elevated anti-early antigen antibodies. Ann Intern Med 1985;102:1-7.

18. Straus SE, Tosato G, Armstrong G, et al. Persisting illness and fatigue in adults with evidence of Epstein-Barr virus infection. Ann Intern Med 1985;102:7-16.

19. Tosato G, Straus S, Henle W, Pike SE, Blaese RM. Characteristic T cell dysfunction in patients with chronic active Epstein-Barr virus infection (chronic infectious mononucleosis). J Immunol 1985;134:3082-8.

20. Caligiuri M, Murray C, Buchwald D, et al. Phenotypic and functional deficiency of natural killer cells in patients with chronic fatigue syndrome. J Immunol 1987;139:3306-13.

21. Murdoch JC. Cell-mediated immunity in patients with myalgic encephalomyelitis syndrome. NZ Med J 1988;101:511-2.

22. Salit IE. Sporadic postinfectious neuromyasthenia. Can Med Assoc J 1985;133:659-63.

23. Yousef GE, Bell EJ, Mann GF, et al. Chronic enterovirus infection in patients with postviral fatigue syndrome. Lancet 1988;1:146-50.

24. Archard LC, Bowles NE, Behan PO, Bell EJ, Doyle D. Postviral fatigue syndrome: persistence of enterovirus RNA in muscle and elevated creatine kinase. J Royal Soc Med 1988;81:326-9.

25. Tobi M, Morag A, Ravid Z, et al. Prolonged atypical illness associated with serologic evidence of persistent Epstein-Barr virus infection. Lancet 1982;1:61-64.

26. Miller G, Grogan E, Rowe D. Selective lack of antibody to a component of EB nuclear antigen in patients with chronic Epstein-Barr virus infection. J Infect Dis 1987;156:26-35.

27. Holmes GP, Kaplan JE, Stewart JA, Hunt B, Pinsky PF, Schonberger LB. A cluster of patients with a chronic mononucleosis-like syndrome: Is Epstein-Barr virus the cause?. JAMA 1987;257:2297-2302.

28. Salahuddin SZ, Ablashi DV, Markham PD, et al. Isolation of a new virus, HBLV, in patients with lymphoproliferative disorders. Science 1986;234:596-601.

29. Josephs SF, Salahuddin SZ, Ablashi DV, Schacter F, Wong-Staal F, Gallo RC. Genomic analysis of the human B-lymphotropic virus (HBLV). Science 1986;234:601-3.

30. Ablashi DV, Salahuddin SZ, Josephs SF, et al. HBLV (or HHV-6) in human cell lines. Nature 1987;329:207.

31. Buchwald D, Saxinger C, Goldenberg DL, Gallo RC, Komaroff AL. Primary fibromyalgia (fibrositis) and human herpesvirus-6: a serologic association. Clin Res 1988;36:332A.

32. Komaroff AL, Saxinger C, Buchwald D, Geiger A, Gallo RC. A chronic "post-viral"fatigue syndrome with neurologic features: serologic association with human herpesvirus-6. Clin Res 1988;36:743A.

33. Ablashi DV, Josephs SF, Buchbinder A, et al. Human B-lymphotropic virus (human herpesvirus-6). J Virol Meth 1988;21:29-48.

34. Kroenke K, Wood DR, Mangelsdorff AD, Meier NJ, Powell JB. Chronic fatigue in primary care. Prevalence, patient characteristics, and outcome. JAMA 1988;260:929-34.

35. Manu P, Lane TJ, Matthews DA. The frequency of the chronic fatigue syndrome in patients with symptoms of persistent fatigue. Ann Intern Med 1988;109:554-6.

36. Wallace DJ, Margolin K. Acute-onset fibromyalgia as a complication of interleukin-2 therapy. Arth Rheum 1988;31:S24.

37. Peter JB, Wallace DJ. Abnormalities of immune regulation in the primary fibromyalgia syndrome. Arth Rheum 1988;31:24.

38. Cheney PR, Dorman SE, Bell D. Interleukin-2 and the chronic fatigue syndrome. Ann Intern Med 1989;110:321.

39. Muss HB, Costanzi JJ, Leavitt R, et al. Recombinant alpha interferon in renal cell carcinoma: a randomized trial of two routes of administration. J Clin Oncol 1987;5:286-91.

40. Quesada JR, Talpaz M, Rios A, Kurzrock P, Gutterman JU. Clinical toxicity of interferons in cancer patients. J Clin Oncol 1986;4:234-43.

41. Erstoff MS, Kirkwood JM. Changes in the bone marrow of cancer patients treated with recombinant interferon alpha 2. Am J Med 1984;76:593-6.

42. Rosenberg SA, Lotze MT, Muul LM, et al. A progress report on the treatment of 157 patients with advanced cancer using lymphokine activated killer cells and interleukin 2 or high dose interleukin 2 alone. N Engl J Med 1987;316:889-905.

43. Belldegrun A, Webb DE, Austin HAI, et al. Effects of interleukin 2 on renal function in patients receiving immunotherapy for advanced cancer. Ann Intern Med 1987;106:817-22.

44. Denicoff KD, Rubinow DR, Papa MX, et al. The neuropsychiatric effects of treatment with interleukin 2 and lymphokine activated killer cells. Ann Intern Med 1987;107:293-300.

45. Ettinghausen SE, Puri RK, Rosenberg SA. Increased vascular permeability in organs mediated by the systemic administration of lymphokine activated killer cells and recombinant interleukin 2 in mice. J Nat Cancer Inst 1988;80:178-188.

Chapter 22

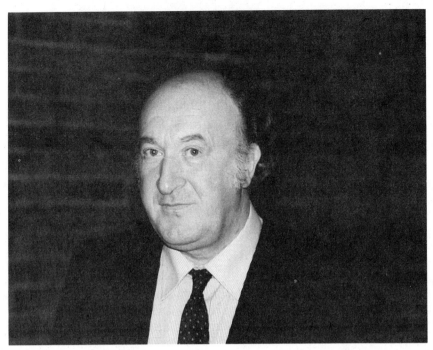

Peter O. Behan

Post-Viral Fatigue Syndrome Research in Glasgow
A Review of Lectures given by Professor Peter O. Behan

Review by The Nightingale Research Foundation Staff

The following is a review of some of the work of Peter O. Behan M.D. and his associates in Glasgow, Scotland. Dr. Behan is Professor of Clinical Neurology at the University of Glasgow at the Institute of Neurological Sciences, Southern General Hospital, Glasgow. His ideas represent years of experience and the joint work of his team , perhaps the best funded and the most dedicated clinical and scientific group studying M.E. / CFS in Europe. Dr. Behan is preparing his own chapter for this book but it has not arrived at the time of printing. The following chapter is taken from Dr. Behan's speeches over the past three years and does not represent his most recent research and publications (see following page). Although we have made every effort to reproduce Professor Behan's ideas in a manner to be consistent with his various speeches, we do not pretend that this chapter represents Professor Behan's present views on Post Viral Fatigue Syndrome (PVFS). The world of PVFS, M.E. / CFS is undergoing continual flux, with new discoveries announced almost monthly. We refer the reader to the Index Medicus for the most recent papers from Dr. Behan's group.

Nowhere in his writings or speeches can we find a precise definition of PVFS. However, the elements in the encapsulated definition that we publish here have been discussed by Professor Behan and we have salvaged them from several of his speeches and papers. It may not be his exact and present formulation.

Dr. Peter Behan was born in County Kildare, Ireland, studied at Leeds University in the Midlands in England and did his doctorate at Harvard. He and his wife Dr. Wilhelmina Behan, reside in Glasgow. Dr. Behan refers to M.E. / CFS as Post-Viral Fatigue Syndrome (PVFS). He feels that the U.S. term, CFS, is too broad and inclusive.

Dr. Behan's research interest has included the immunological aspects of muscle and nervous diseases. He is a co-author of the text, Clinical Neuroimmunology, and is editor of the Journal of Neuroimmunology. He serves on the editorial board of Autoimmunity and is a member of the Medical Advisory Board, Epidemic ME Association of London, the Association of British Neurologists and the British Society of Immunology.

Post-Viral Fatigue Syndrome (PVFS) Definitions
Preconditions

Post-Viral Fatigue Syndrome (PVFS): Unless you start with some reference point, such as a definite or probable **initial precipitating viral infection**, it is difficult to know what you are studying.

(1) The disease should have as its onset a viral infection, preferably with laboratory evidence of this infection.

(2) PVFS is an endemic disorder occurring sporadically and occasionally occurring in epidemics.

(3) The patient should have a prior well-adjusted, premorbid personality with a good past work record.

(4) PVFS results in a 50% or more reduction in the individual's ability to carry out previous levels of work, school or social abilities.

PVFS Defining Characteristics:

Essential Features

(1) There is central fatigue (arising in the brain) with poor exercise tolerance.

(2) There is hypothalamic dysfunction.

(3) There is sleep disturbance that, in a child, frequently resembles sleeping sickness.

Frequently Occurring Features

(4) There may be myalgia in a specific topographical distribution. The usual areas are the neck, trapezius and intercostal muscles. This pain in some cases simulates heart disease because the pain is so severe and so acute.

(5) There are sometimes psychiatric symptoms that mimic endogenous depression with a diurnal variation

(6) Gastrointestinal symptoms are common and may be synonymous with irritable bowel syndrome

(7) Cardiac symptoms may occur, usually with a very rapid pulse and with missing beats. On objective testing, some patients are found to have infection or disturbance of the myocardium or pericardium.

(8) Idiopathic cyclic oedema is common in women with monthly periodic weight gains of up to 12 lb.

(9) Vestibular symptoms may occur. They do not have true vertigo but have difficulty or imbalance in walking

Exclusions: to define the research population clearly, patients should be excluded if they have:

(1) a previous or pre-existing history of psychiatric disease
(2) any other organic illness not associated with PVFS
(3) any pre-existing chronic infectious illness

The following review of Dr. Behan's research group's work is based upon lectures given in:

Los Angeles, California in 1990,[1]
London England, 1990,[2] and in
Hamilton Ontario in late 1991.[3]

Some of the original tapes are available on request from Dr. Jay Goldstein[4] in California, and Miriam Gallacher, of the Hamilton Wentworth M.E. Association in Hamilton Ontario.[5] Transcripts are available from The Nightingale Research Foundation.[6] We have made every effort to record as faithfully as possible, either the exact words or intent of Dr. Behan's statements. For more extensive review articles on the Glasgow group's work, see references 7 and 8.

Abnormal EMG Studies

In the London epidemic of 1955 abnormal EMG studies[9,10] were noted, but there was criticism from some sources that these abnormal findings could possibly be self-induced artifacts simulating disease.

Dr. Jamal[11], senior neurophysiologist in Professor Behan's research centre, perfected a technique invented by Professor Stalberg of Sweden[12] and demonstrated that patients with PVFS who had a lesion either in the nerve, the terminal dendrites or in the neuromuscular junction, developed "jitter". Jitter represents a lack of congruity in the action potentials of two proximate muscle fibres. Professor Behan notes that these findings are extraordinarily abnormal and highly significant in 75% of 40 patients studied. The importance of this finding is that jitter is entirely objective and cannot be simulated.[13] This test merely points out that there is something wrong with the muscle, but it doesn't tell you what's wrong.

Immunological Abnormalities

Professor Behan recently stated that immunological abnormalities are not specific, that there are not any basic primary immune abnormalities; they are secondary to other events.

(Immune abnormalities are discussed in detail in his excellent paper, The postviral fatigue syndrome[7]. Dr. Behan notes under immunological results that in vitro lymphocyte function was highly abnormal. bmh)

Also in the paper by L. Morrison[14], Dr. Behan's group writes:

"These phenotypic changes provide laboratory evidence of immunological abnormalities in this syndrome, and, we suggest, may be consistent with persistent viral infection."

HLA Study (human leukocyte antigen)

Professor Behan's group has studied the genetic make-up of patients who develop PVFS since there may be an increased susceptibility among patients who possess certain DR antigens. This would explain why the illness may have some familial origin or clustering.

PVFS may be expressing a specific epitope (antigenic determinant) in the FHC region. This change can be induced in normal individuals with the introduction of interferon.

Dr. Behan's group conducted a study of 100 patients in a tissue typing laboratory in Glasgow to see if there was any association with Class 1 or Class 2 HLA antigens. They were not able to find any association.

They also looked at hypo-reactivity because it is known that there is a hypo-reactivity to certain viral vaccines in PVFS. Again they found no homozygosity in the DR antigen cluster and there was no lymphocyte hyporeactivity.

Professor Behan notes that individuals in Holland have claimed that there is a specific monoclonal antibody that reacts with the DR region. It doesn't react with DP, DQ or DR, but is said to be a marker for activated lymphocytes and to act on cells from patients with Post-Viral Fatigue Syndrome. Professor Behan's group received the monoclonal antibody from the originators and tested it and found no association whatsoever. In fact, it was totally inactive in the cases they have looked at.

Normal Interleukins

Professor Behan noted that Dr. Smith of the Medical Council Research Unit measured reaction time of interferons, and the various effects of interferon on the brain. Professor Behan's group wanted to know if there was any relationship of circulating interferon, circulating interleukins or cytokines either in the CSF or in the serum. Were there inhibitors of these substances present that would allow them, for example, avoid detection? The measurement of all of these interleukins both in the cervical spinal fluid and in the serum was entirely negative in Behan's group's study.

(This appears to be a reversal of Dr Behan's position, where certain enormous interleukin increases were observed and noted at the CIBA conference in London in 1989. bmh) [15]

Abnormal Muscle Biopsy

Professor Behan observes that the muscle looks normal even to an experienced muscle pathologist, However when one looks at it very carefully, there is a difference in the distribution of muscle fibre types that can be measured. In addition there is an abnormality of the mitochondria, that become very large and deformed.

Seventy percent of muscle tissue from biopsies of both children and adult PVFS patients were shown to have type 2 predominance with type 2 atrophy. They have not found that type 2 fibre atrophy occurs with disuse even with patients with their leg in a plastic cast. He notes that an Australian researcher has published that disuse does not cause type 2 predominance nor does it cause type 2 fibre atrophy. Professor Behan states that if you look carefully at the muscle, you will find the occasional muscle fibre necrosis, but it occurs without any cellular reaction.

They observe occasional paracrystaline inclusions in muscle biopsies.

(This material is published in The post-viral fatigue syndrome ,1984[8]in which the authors note there were widely scattered necrotic muscle fibres without any sign of inflammatory reaction and increased size and numbers of type 2 fibres. Mitochondria were increased with occasional tubular inclusions . bmh)

Abnormal Mitochondria and Myalgia

Professor Behan notes that mitochondria are related to cellular energy and that they can be adversely affected by acute viral infections, by alcohol, by toxic processes such as strychnine and they are adversely affected in PVFS patients suggesting that there is some derangement of the energy-producing mechanisms of the cell.

He also notes that electron microscopy at the muscle membrane level in the sub-sarcolemal portion reveals grossly abnormal swollen mitochondria and extraordinary inclusions of fat. Small compartments occur in these mitochondria. This mitochondrial compartmentalization syndrome occurs with small hyalin matrix bodies in the compartments. Some mitochondria look entirely necrotic. The number of abnormal mitochondria with abnormal para-crystaline inclusion bodies bear a direct statistical relationship to the patients with myalgia.

Professor Behan finds that there is an aberration of the interdigitalization of the cristi. This type of pathological mitochondrial anatomy is sometimes seen in patients with severe febrile viral infections. The role of the mitochondria in the contribution to the disease process is not known.

Abnormal Muscle and Liver Mitochondria

In the literature, particularly with chicken pox,

there are cases of fat lipid storage myopathy, which means the mitochondria have packed in following a viral infection. In Ray's syndrome, following varicella, influenza B, as well as in coxsackie and other enteroviruses, patients also develop mitochondrial abnormalities in muscle liver and in the brain. Now we have looked at the mitochondria both of muscle and the mitochondria of liver and both of them are abnormal in our typical PVFS cases.

In summary: In mitochondrial myopathies, which are inherited, recent reports show that in several syndromes that there are lesions in the mitochondria of the hypothalamus and that there are quite distinct neuro-endocrine abnormalities. Professor Behan believes that this might explain the mitochondria lesions they have found in muscle. Similar lesions of course can be seen in the brain and specifically can occur in the hypothalamus.

Dr. Behan's , as yet unpublished, grossly abnormal mitochondria are very similar to the abnormal mitochondria shown by Dr. Elaine DeFreitas in her Sarasota, Florida speech of March 1992. These were greatly enlarged with abnormal cristi and possible viral inclusion. This is similar if not identical to Professor Behan's findings.

Magnetic Resonance Spectrography (MRS)

PVFS muscle demonstrates massive early lactic acidosis that is persistent in over 40 cases examined by Professor Behan's group[3]. The Ph falls considerably and the ADP remains normal after exercise indicating that there is something wrong with the chemistry of breaking down glycogen into sugar to give energy. The cause is not known but this could suggest that there is an enzyme derangement in the actual cell within the mitochondria. However, although they can measure this muscle abnormality it is not of great enough severity to account for the degree of fatigue in PVFS. He believes that the fatigue is caused primarily by a neurotransmitter abnormality in the brain and to a lessor degree by a peripheral muscle derangement.

Dr. Behan notes that NMR was carried out on a number of PVFS patients at Oxford University. They exhibited early excessive and persistent lactic acidosis after exercise. There was low intercellular PH and normal ATP after exercise, indicating excessive glycolytic activity. There was obviously a muscle cell metabolic lesion to cause this.

Verifiable information comes from a paper published by D. Arnold[16] *[This paper referred to a single patient who fell ill with chicken pox. To my knowledge, there has been no publication of the 40 positive cases mentioned by Dr. Behan . bmh.(Also see chapter, this text concerning MRS that is essentially in agreement with Dr. Behan's observations.)]*

Water Loading Test

Professor Behan states that there are similarities between PVFS and Addison's disease. Addison's disease is a disease in which there is failure of the adrenal glands to produce steroids. These cases, if they were very severe, would have died before the advent of steroids, but if they were sub-clinical, then they would have complained of depression, asthenia, weakness and fatigue. They would be identical to the symptomatology he finds in Post-Viral Fatigue Syndrome. There is a test for this defect called the water loading test.

According to Professor Behan, like Addison's disease patients, PVFS patients compared to normals tend to be unable to excrete a given water load in a specific time. If cortisone is given, PVFS patients still show this defect whereas Addison's patients will return to a normal excretion pattern. This is a reasonable screening test, in that it tends to be persistently abnormal.

Professor Behan states that it is a simple test that requires no expertise. This group studied a series of 18 consecutive PVFS cases who came to their clinic.

These patients were hospitalized and made to fast overnight. Smoking was not permitted. They were asked to empty their bladder immediately before the test and to lie flat throughout the test unless they were to void. At 8:00 AM, 8:15 AM and 8:30 AM, they took 500 mls. of body temperature water. The urine was then collected every hour for three hours. A normal result occurs if the output is greater than 80% of normal capacity at the end of three hours.

Their results were found to be very abnormal.

When they looked at patients with organic disease, such as diabetes mellitis, multiple sclerosis with brain stem lesions or in sarcoidosis, the test was positive.

In eighteen patients examined:

9 were very abnormal,
3 were borderline,
4 were unable to take the test, and,
2 were normal.

Professor Behan states that if you give these patients an injection of steroid, fluid output will return to normal if they have Addison's disease and stay abnormal for PVFS.

Hypothalamic Hormone Abnormality

According to Professor Behan, that the problem appears to be that the hypothalamus in PVFS patients must have receptors that turn off a hormone called the antidiuretic hormone (ADH). When this hormone is turned off the kidneys excrete urine. The levels of ADH in PVFS patients follows a very irregular pattern. This hormone comes from the area of the supraoptic and paraventricular nucleus in the hypothalamus. There is a derangement in this area in PVFS patients. It appears to be the same derangement found in irritable bowel syndrome and also idiopathic cyclic oedema.

He notes that Professor of Neurology Dr. Raymond Adams at the Mass. General Hospital, at Harvard, in his textbook on neurology advocates it as a simple test for differentiating organic from functional fatigue.

Abnormal Hypothalamic-Pituitary-Adrenal Axis

Professor Behan observed that when they looked at hypothalamic pituitary adrenal axis tests, these patients are also extraordinary. Six of the eighteen cases had very high basal cortisone levels, one of four of them had high basal prolactin levels. They have subsequently collected a number of cases investigated for prolactinoma. There have been high basal gonadotrophin levels in one, and a flat gonadotrophin response in another one and no hypoglycemia response when you have used double the amount of insulin that you would normally use in six. So this test indicates that there is something the matter with the hypothalamus in a subtle way. These results are striking. There is something wrong in the hypothalamus pituitary adrenal axis.

Rat models indicated hypothalamic changes in the region of the paraventricular nucleus. When the brains of PVFS patients who had committed suicide or the brains of patients who had suffered from poliomyelitis years before were examined, they had similar brain injury in the area of the paraventricular nuclei.

(This material discussing the abnormal hypothalamic hormones was reviewed by Dr Peter Behan in a symposium in Los Angeles, exactly 23 months prior to the paper published by Demitrack and Steven Straus in December 1991.[18] The authors in that paper gave no mention of Dr Behan's paper. bmh.)

Enterovirus Sequences in PVFS Muscle

Professor Behan's group asks the question: are there enterovirus sequences in PVFS muscle? They investigated muscle for sequences of the coxsackie virus B genome using oligo-peptide sequences. Forty out of a hundred cases were positive.

Their probe and primers were taken from the region of the oligo nucleotide sequences The non-transferable region was the sight chosen for the polymerase chain reaction. The reason for choosing this site was that this site has 80% homology with other enteroviral types.

First they checked if their probe was working by infecting normal tissue culture cells with various enteroviruses. Others were infected with measles virus and others with nothing. Then in a blinded fashion they were able to check if their probe could separate enterovirus RNA in cell cultures from that containing abnormal measles cultures. Their probe proved successful.

He states that RNA was extracted from a PVFS muscle biopsy. They then did agarose gel visualization of 28 and 18 S RNA bands to see that one had pure RNA. The next step was a complementary DNA PCR amplification of an endogenous gene. This is a housekeeping gene, a tyrosine kinase gene. If this was present, then they did PCR amplification of this gene. They then did complementary DNA PCR amplification of the enterovirus sequences using the primers mentioned.

The products were looked at by agarose gel, athenium bromide stain and slot block assays and by hybridizations to both the internal probe of P 32, and dysontogenic.

If one looks at the various coxsackie, polio and echo viruses, for the sequences observed, one can see those that are positive. Professor Behan notes that the controls were entirely negative.

An agarose analysis of the various enteroviral PCR products to the various coxsackie and entero viruses were positive.

A slot blot analysis of enterovirus PCR products probed with digoxygenin labelled internal probe, the P2 was also positive.

In another series of polio, echo and various other entero-viruses showing the PCR product, a very distinct band occurs right acrossin a certain blot analysis of the previous gel probed with digoxygenin labelled P2 probe. The slot blot assay of human muscle PCR products was probed with the radioactive P32 labelled P2 probe.

Strict precautions against contamination were followed including using different laboratories, different pipettes, control tubes with unaffected RNA and no RNA in sequences, so there was no question of contamination, nor of carrying products across.

They continue to examine to find which cells are affected. Are they muscle cells, macrophages or other cells? Professor Behan states that muscle cells and also certain white blood cells were involved.[7]

Some of this material was published in the Gow paper[17] that noted that:

"Overall, significantly more patients than controls had enteroviral RNA sequences in muscle, 53% v. 15%. ...Conclusions- Persistent enteroviral infection of muscle may occur in some patients with postviral fatigue syndrome and may have an aetiological role."

(Dr .Behan noted that the 53% recovery resulted from a single needle muscle biopsy per patient and when more than one needle biopsy was made per patient the yield of virus recovery was actually higher. This is not noted in the paper. bmh)

Lymphocyte Protein Synthesis Abnormalities

When one cultures lymphocytes, with vita hema-glutanin, and measure the incorporation of radio-labelled iso-lucine over the first 24 hours, there is virtually a flat curve when compared to controls. Simply, patients with PVFS lymphocytes do not incorporate as much leucine as healthy controls. Professor Behan notes that Professor Peters in London has shown a similar feature in muscle cells with a failure to incorporate protein at normal anticipated levels. This suggests that something is wrong with intracellular protein synthesis but it does not tell you what is wrong.

Parkinson's Disease

Occasionally, Professor Behan's group observe young patients who, after a viral infection, develop all of the symptoms of PVFS, but in addition get Parkinson's disease. He mentioned a clear cut case in a 19 year old girl from Belfast and a 21 year old woman from Dundee. They have collected a series of them. He states that the Parkinson's disease lasts for about a year or so and they look exactly the same as old people in a geriatric home with Parkinson's disease.

In Akureyri, in northern Iceland it has been found that there is a statistical increase in Parkinson's disease in the patients who fell ill with PVFS in 1948.

This disease is related to dopa and also to 5-hydroxytryptamine receptors.

(Associated Parkinson's disease is not always as innocuous as mentioned here. Dr Behan does not mention the children who fell ill with classical Parkinson's disease in the Akureyri area epidemic in 1948, and then went on after a few years, to die of Parkinson's disease before reaching adulthood.[19] We have also noted what appears to be an increased incidence of Parkinson's disease in spouses of M.E./ CFS patients but we have not done a good statistical investigation.bmh)

5-Hydroxytryptomine

Professor Behan's group came up with the idea that there was an intense perturbation or abnormality of some of these hormones, in particular, the neurotransmitter 5 hydroxytryptomine. They then tried a relatively harmless substance, a 5 HT agonist, that

affects these receptors to PVFS patients *(We believe this may have been buspirone. bmh)* He states that within 10 minutes of receiving this chemical, these PVFS patients became intensely ill during the next hour or two with diarrhoea, vomiting, sweating, collapse and mood changes. When they gave this drug to 20 normal patients, who did not have PVFS, absolutely nothing happened to them.

They then gave this drug that acted on the hypothalamus of PVFS patients and measured their prolactin levels. Within 10 minutes their prolactin levels started to rise in a grossly abnormal manner. Again, when they gave this drug to normal non-PVFS patients there was no abnormality in their prolactin response.

It is Dr. Behan's opinion that, in PVFS patients, there are gross abnormalities of 5-hydroxytryptamine and possibly L-dopa. This could explain their blood abnormalities, their sleep dysfunction, their depression. These same substance may be abnormal in M.S. patients.

Serotonin, 5-Hydroxytryptamine Agonist

Professor Behan states that there is a problem in treatment for this defect. Since the body has been deprived of a normal level of 5-hydroxy-tryptomine for many years and will have altered its normal homeostasis, introduction of these agents will then create abnormal clinical responses until you get back to your previously healthy levels. He believes that drug trials will be very difficult in that initially they will cause these patients to be worse. However they would expect that after 2-4 weeks the patient should begin to feel better.

If a 5 HT agonist is given to a normal person, the symptoms of PVFS can be reproduced. 5HT1 blockers appear to have some benefit in the treatment of PVFS patients. Hopefully, the results of Professor Behan's trial will tell quite clearly that it works. In his hands, at the moment, these medications seem to be highly advantageous in a very large number of people.

Other treatments to date that they have tried have been to no avail.

*[**It is my understanding** that Dr Behan has mentioned to individuals in Ontario that the two pharma-*

ceuticals that he is presently investigating and which he believes hold promise for PVFS patients are the following:

(1) Sertraline Hydrochloride, (Pfizer) known as Zoloft in North America and Lustral in Great Britain. This is a serotonin (5 hydroxytryptomine) reuptake inhibitor. It down regulates brain norepinephrine and serotonin receptors in animals. It is marketed as an antidepressive.

(2) Buspirone Hydrochloride (Bristol-Myers-Squibb) known as Buspar in Canada. This is marketed as an anxiolytic. It has an affinity for brain D2 Dopamine receptors and acts both as an agonist and antagonist and on the 5HT1A receptors where it acts as an agonist.

If a trial of these medications is to be considered, please take note of the initial effects of this drug noted above. Medical supervision is essential. Also a forthcoming publication anticipated from Dr. Behan should further clarify this information. bmh]

Essential Fatty Acids

Professor Behan's group has found abnormalities in essential fatty acids in PVFS patients It is known that essential fatty acids can be useful in diabetic neuropathy in humans and greatly improve cardiac dysregularities in mice. In PVFS patients essential fatty acids can be helpful but are not a cure.

In the paper by Behan et al[20], the authors stated that:

"At one month, 74% of patients on active treatment and 23% of those on placebo assessed themselves as improved over the baseline....At three months the corresponding figures were 85% and 17%, since the placebo group had reverted towards the baseline state, while those in the active group showed continued improvement. There were no adverse events. We conclude that essential fatty acids provide a rational, safe and effective treatment for patients with post-viral fatigue syndrome."

Magnesium

Dr. Behan stated in Hamilton, Ontario that the whole question of magnesium treatment is bogus and it would be a waste of time even to consider it.

This statement is made on the basis of a lot of debate, a lot of experimentation and a lot of talking to people who really know and have experience of treating with magnesium. Professor Behan reiterates that "it is total utter bogus and of no value whatsoever. It is beyond me, why the editor of *The Lancet* allowed the paper to be published."[3]

Immunizations

Professor Behan was asked, does immunization have any effect on someone who has postviral fatigue syndrome? He stated that there have been no studies done on this, so there's no one to his certain knowledge who can authoritatively say yes or no, but "we have seen some patients, particularly those who have received hepatitis (B) immunizations, who get much worse. We've also seen them get much worse following yellow fever." He stated that if you wanted to be immunized and it's of no importance whether you're immunized or not, then he would stay away from it. But if it's essential, if you're going to an area where diseases were endemic, in the jungle in Africa or in South America, then clearly you should require immunization, but other than that it would be very prudent to leave it alone until further information is available.[3]

Pregnancy

Professor Behan stated that he knew of no effect on unborn children (*of mothers who have been ill prior to pregnancy with PVFS*). Several of his patients have asked whether they should they become pregnant or not. A few of them have been made much worse, in that their symptoms have obviously caused great distress during the pregnancy, but by far the greatest response has been that the illness has disappeared, usually by about the 3rd month of pregnancy. There are innumerable cases on record where the illness has cleared up totally and completely in some, unfortunately in others it has come back. He also stated that some of them have developed quite severe post-natal depression, but generally speaking, pregnancy has an excellent effect on them.

Professor Behan notes that pregnancy has an excellent effect on several disorders including certain cases of multiple sclerosis, some cases of myasthenia gravis, and some more autoimmune diseases. But when you go back and analyse it, people have not been able to predict who are the ones who are going to get better and who are the ones who may in fact even get worse.[3] Generally speaking, they tend to get better.

Children

Professor Behan noted that in children below the age of 7 or 8, PVFS is extremely rare. They don't seem to be affected. If they are affected, they behave in a different way. But after the age of 7, they certainly are affected and the symptoms in children are identical to the symptoms in adults.

He noted that there was an outbreak of this illness in a small community in Scotland and it was the children who brought it to the attention of the physicians insofar as the school teachers at school noticed that a number of their pupils had difficulty with their schooling. He relates how their schooling fell off dramatically. He recounted that in those cases that he had seen, the mothers mentioned that their children had aches and pains. If they were good at athletics, that fell off extraordinarily, and they refused to play games. He observed that in Scotland these children were handed over to psychologists and to psychiatrists who said it was a matter of behaviour, and the net result is that these children did in fact, in his opinion, suffer enormously and were never treated properly.

Further Diagnostic Criteria

To complement the diagnostic statements made by Dr. Behan and reconstructed into the two tables at the beginning of this chapter, please also refer to the Diagnostic Criteria in Dr. Jamal's paper in this text (Chapter 47).

References

1. National Conference on Chronic Fatigue Syndrome and Fibromyalgia, Feb 16 - 18, 1990 Los Angeles, California 1990.

2. London England, 27 October 1990, Lecture given to the members of the M.E. Association of Great Britain.

3. St Joseph's Hospital , Hamilton Ontario, 21 September 1991, Lecture to several of the M.E. Associations of Southern Ontario, organized by Miriam Gallacher of the Hamilton Wentworth M.E. Association, 90 Malton Drive, Hamilton, ON L9B 1E9 Canada.

4. Jay Goldstein M.D., Director of Chronic Fatigue Syndrome Institutes of Anaheim Hills and Beverly Hills, 500 South Anaheim Hills Rd., Suite 206, Anaheim Hills, CA 92807 USA.

5. Miriam Gallacher, R.N., Hamilton-Wentworth M.E. Association

6. The Nightingale Research Foundation, 383 Danforth Ave., Ottawa, Canada, K2A 0E1.

7. Behan P, Behan W and Bell E, The postviral fatigue syndrome, an analysis of the findings in 50 cases, Journal of Infection, (1985) 10, 211-222.

8. Behan P, Behan W, Post-viral fatigue syndrome, CRC Critical Reviews in Neurobiology, (1988) Vol 4, Issue 2, pages 157-178.

9. Medical Staff of the Royal Free Hospital, An outbreak of encephalomyelitis in the Royal Free Hospital Group, London, in 1955, The British Medical Journal, (1957) October 19, pages 895-904.

10. Richardson AT, Some aspects of the Royal Free Hospital epidemic, Annals of Physical Medicine,(1956) July, pages 81-9.

11. Jamal G, Hansen S, Electrophysiological studies in the post-viral fatigue syndrome, Journal of Neurology, Neurosurgery and Psychiatry 91985) 48; 691-694.

12 Stalberg E, Ekstedt J, Broman A, The electromyographic jitter in normal human muscles, Electroenceph. Clin. Neruophysiol., (1971) 31: 429-438.

13. Dr Jamal's paper, see this book, Chapter 40.

14. Morrison LJA, Behan W, Behan P, Changes in natural killer cell phenotype in patients with post-viral fatigue syndrome, (1991) Vol 83, pages 441-6.

15. CIBA London Conference, CIBA Foundation, 41 Portland Place, London, England, October 11, 1988.

16. Arnold D, Radda G, Bore P, Styles P, Taylor D, Excessive intracellular aidosis of skeletal muscle in a patient with a post-viral exhaustion/fatigue syndrome, The Lancet (1984) 23 June, 1367-9.

17. Gow J, Behan W, Clements G, Woodall C, Riding M, Behan P, Enteroviral RNA sequences detected by polymerase chain reaction in muscle of patients with postviral fatigue syndrome, BMJ, (1991), 23 March, Vol 302, 692-6.

18. Demitrack M, Dale J, Straus E, et al: Evidence for Impaired Activation of the Hypothalamic-Pituitary-Adrenal Axis in Patients with Chronic Fatigue Syndrome. *J Clin Endocrinology and Metabolism* 1992; 73:1224-34.

19. Bergmann private communication with B. Hyde, Reykjavik, Iceland, 1988.

20. Behan P, Behan W, and Horrobin D, Effect of high doses of essential fatty acids on the postviral fatigue syndrome. Acta Neurol Scand (1990) 209-216.

Evaluating the M.E. / CFS Patient

Chapter 23

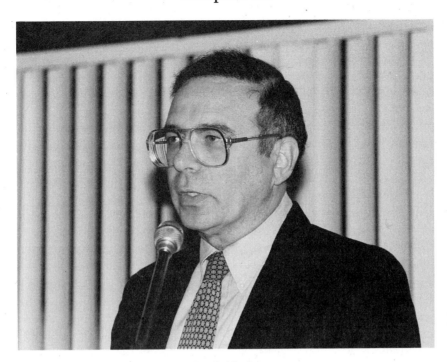

Jay Goldstein

How Do I Diagnose a Patient with Chronic Fatigue Syndrome?

Jay Goldstein, MD
Director, Chronic Fatigue Syndrome Institutes of Anaheim Hills and Beverly Hills
Anaheim Hills, California, 92807 USA

Dr. Jay Goldstein has been involved in research on Chronic Fatigue Syndrome and treatment of patients with this disorder for several years. He has coordinated a team of researchers who study the disease from the level of viral DNA to functional examinations of the brain. Viewing the symptoms of Chronic Fatigue Syndrome as a cascade of dysregulation of immunotransmission, he has tried to develop rational scientific therapies based on this hypothesis. Struck with the similarity in presentation of Chronic Fatigue Syndrome and Fibromyalgia, he has recently been attempting to unify approaches to both of these difficult problems. Dr. Goldstein was the recent organizer of the highly successful LA symposium on CFIDS / Fibromyalgia.

When I first began to see such patients, I believed their symptoms were so distinctive that no other illness could produce them. I now realize that a small percentage of patients will have other disorders, and that I cannot depend on the patient's previous physician to necessarily have ruled them out. Autoimmune diseases, primary sleep disorders and pelvic pathology are probably the main illnesses to have been overlooked. The physician must do a thorough history and physical examination unless the patient is warned in advance that it is the responsibility of his referring or primary care physician to do so, and that I will be functioning only as a consultant.

There are several symptoms which may serve to distinguish Chronic Fatigue Syndrome from other illnesses. Virtually all of the symptoms can be understood if the disease is viewed as a limbic encephalopathy in a dysregulated neuroimmune network:

1) **The fatigue is made worse by exercise.** Very few patients report feeling better after strenuous exercise. There are probably fatigue receptors in the limbic system which are dysfunctional. They may be stimulated by cytokines which are produced in increased amounts by exercise. In Chronic Fatigue Syndrome, the quantities or types of cytokines pro-

duced may be abnormal or the receptors for them may be dysregulated. In many individuals, the cytokines may begin a cascade of immunochemical events, since severe fatigue or exacerbation of all the CFS symptoms do not begin for several hours after exercise, or perhaps not until the next day.

2) **Cognitive dysfunction is extremely common.** Impairment of short-term memory, a hippocampal function, is most frequently seen. Sometimes the symptoms are obvious, other times it may manifest by the patient's admission that he goes into another room and frequently forgets why he did. Getting lost while driving, impaired concentration and difficulty in word finding are often discussed.

3) **Mood disorders are also quite common.** A recent onset of panic disorder, which is probably a limbic derangement, is rather diagnostic. Premorbid mood disorders may indicate a poor prognosis, as may length and severity of illness, and also the absence of an acute precipitating event, especially an infectious one with documented physical and laboratory abnormalities.

4) **A disorder of initiating and maintaining sleep is characteristic.** A patient will state, "I can't shut my mind off no matter how tired I am." Sleep fragmentation and non-restorative sleep are typical. Hypersomnia is more frequently encountered in the initial stages of the illness. Frequent vivid nightmares are common.

5) **Intermittent blurring of vision** with normal ophthalmalogic examination is the most frequently cited visual complaint, along with photophobia.

6) **Few CFS patients are able to tolerate alcohol.** A small amount, even a few sips will make patients intoxicated, sleepy, produce severe hangovers, and even relapses. If the mode of action of alcohol on the brain were better understood, the pathophysiology of CFS would be also. In mouse embryo hippocampal neurons, ethanol specifically inhibits NMDA receptor activation. Such inhibition may contribute to the neural and cognitive impairment associated with intoxication and the NMDA receptor involved in CFS.

7) **Malaise and myalgia** are characteristic of nu-merous diseases, but very few diseases produce recurrent sore throats, even though examination of the oropharynx is usually normal.

8) **Nasal allergy is a common premorbid disorder which is usually exacerbated by the onset of CFS.** Are nasal mucosal mediators such as substance P, somatostatin, histamine, and calcitonin gene-related peptide subject to retrograde axonal transport into the limbic system via the piriform cortex?

9) The presence of the **18 tender points of fibromyalgia** is the only reliable physical finding in Chronic Fatigue Syndrome. They should be examined in each patient suspected of having the disorder. If they are present, the diagnosis of Chronic Fatigue Syndrome can be made with much more confidence.

10) **Night sweats**, although seen in other diseases, are also quite common in Chronic Fatigue Syndrome and are probably caused by impaired hypothalamic temperature regulation.

11) **Premenstrual Syndrome (PMS)**, usually severe, is almost uniformly encountered in women with Chronic Fatigue Syndrome. Many of the symptoms are similar to Chronic Fatigue Syndrome, and PMS is probably a hormonally entrained cyclic disorder of limbic gonadal steroid receptors.

12) **Other disease associations** such as irritable bowel syndrome, polycystic ovarian disease, thyroiditis, and endometriosis are probably part of the Chronic Fatigue Syndrome. Loss of libido and erectile dysfunction are also quite typical. It is a rare woman with Chronic Fatigue Syndrome who has not had hair loss, usually diffuse and non-scarring.

13) **Dyspnea on minimal exertion**, air hunger and hyperventilation are frequently seen. I believe these symptoms are a result of abnormal input from the central nucleus of the amygdala to the pneumotaxic centre in the pons. Single pulse stimulation of this nucleus results to an immediate switch to inspiration.

14) **Complaints of sensitivities** (not allergies) to medications, food and environmental agents are quite common. It is possible that some antigens may be directly transported from the oropharynx to the brain, that abnormal antigen presentation may occur in the

TREATMENT APPROACHES

1) Anti-infective

Antiviral agent against reactivated herpes viruses if detected by culture or PCR.
Other antiviral agents for "Agent X"
Antibiotics to treat sinusitis, borrelia, mycoplasma
Antifungal drugs for possible candida GI invasion
Antiparasitic for Giardia and other possible agents

2) Immunomodulatory

H-2 blockers
Ampligen
Kutapressin
Gamma globulin, IM or IV
Lentinan & LEM
Thymic hormones
Transfer factor
Isoprinosine
DTC
Peptide T
Alpha interferon
Herbal Products, e.g. echinacea, astragalus
Graduated exercise
Gamma linoleic acid
Zinc
Antihistamines   )—
Steroids and cromlyn sprays....)— For allergic
Hyposensitization....................)— rhinitis
Allergen avoidance
Sinus Surgery
Leuprolide acetate (Lupron)

3) Neuromodulatory

Improving DIMS and alpha-delta sleep with TCA's, fluoxetine, trazodone, ritanserin.

H-2 Blockers
Cognitive-behavioural therapy
Antidepressants and strategies for treatment-resistant depression: Lithium, buspirone, thyroid hormone, MAOI's
Anticonvulsants: carbamazepine, valproate, clonazepam
Calcium channel blockers
Biofeedback
Altering trigeminal nerve afferents to thalamic nuclei
Cognitive restructuring techniques
Acupuncture
$MgSO_4$ to block the NMDA receptor and as a vasodilator
Naltrexone
Precursor therapy
Pain management
Nutritional counselling
Hydergine and other nootropics
S-adenosyl methionine
Vitamin B-12
Diamox
Amantadine and ACE inhibitors to raise encephalin levels
Cyclobenzaprine (Flexeril) for Fibromyalgia
Leuprolide acetate (Lupron)

4) Other

Multivitamins
Antioxidants
Coenzyme Q10
Resting
Avoid sunshine, immunizations, alcohol, stress, over-exertion
DHEA

---

limbic system of the CFS patients, and that there is a dysregulated limbic response to substances such as insulin, alpha fibroblast growth factor, interleukin-1 beta, and tumour necrosis factor alpha which are secreted post prandially. Some patients report feeling better after they eat, often only with certain types of foods. Others are unable to eat almost anything without a worsening of symptoms. Exogenous psychotropic substances in foods, such as opioids or benzodiazepines, may play a role.

Laboratory investigations can be done in levels:

Level I: **Rule out other diseases.** This caution can be taken to great extremes, with $5,000 lab bills and imaging of virtually every body part. My Level I includes a CBC, urinalysis, SMA-20, thyroid profile with TSH, sedimentation rate, antinuclear antibody, ferritin, HIV serology, and a multitest CMI

skin test for delayed hypersensitivity. CFS patients usually have very low sed rates. I do not do routine chest x-rays, although occult neoplastic disorders or sarcoidosis, as well as fungal diseases could be missed. If the patient has the proper geographic exposure, I will do Lyme titers, and stools for ova and parasites. In a patient without significant lymphadenopathy, I do not order viral titers for anything.

Level II: **Autoimmune investigation.** I order a lupus panel to investigate the possibility of autoimmune diseases. Antithyroid antibodies, when present in high titers, may indicate subclinical hypothyroidism, particularly important when contemplating thyroid hormone augmentation of antidepressant therapy. The presence of circulating immune complexes is another indication of immune dysfunction. Serum copper is often elevated, although ceruloplasmin and 24-hour urine copper are normal. None of my patients has yet had a low red blood cell magnesium. IgA levels and IgG subclasses are ordered if I am contemplating gamma globulin therapy.

Level III: **Immune system investigation.** I like to know if my patient has an activated immune system and how he might respond to immunomodulatory therapy. I order IL-2 receptor levels because patients with elevated levels may respond better to intravenous immunoglobulin, soluble T-8 receptor levels, a T cell "Levy" panel, and a natural killer cell function assay. I order a single lymphocyte immune function assay if Kutapressin treatment is to be considered. I find T and B cell subsets and mitogen stimulation tests in general to not be helpful. Viral cultures and PCR for putative CFS-associated agents are available to me now and, hopefully, will be generally disseminated in the future. Sensitivity testing of anti-viral drugs may also be important.

Level IV: **Brain Imaging.** Brain functional imaging is an important part of my workup if the patient's insurance will pay for it or if the patient can afford it. Topographic brain mapping is useful if I am considering anticonvulsant or stimulant therapy.

All of these brain mapping techniques are functional or physiological. In this regard, scanning before and after exercise provides more information consistent with the patient's disease process. BEAM (QEEG) scanning is an excellent preliminary step and not overly expensive. SPECT scanning is helpful diagnostically and detects mid-brain as well as the cortical features of the disease process, and also may justify vasodilator therapy with calcium channel blockers, Diamox, or magnesium sulphate, which also produces a voltage-dependent block of the NMDA receptor. PET scanning can also suggest other areas of the brain amenable to neuropharmalogic intervention. All of these modalities are helpful in documenting an organic mental disorder.

Level V: **Neuropsychological testing**, if it reveals the characteristic encoding deficit seen in CFS, will be helpful diagnostically and will also suggest appropriate cognitive restructuring intervention.

Testing with the MMPI can reveal a typical CFS profile. Functional capacity evaluation by an occupational therapist is helpful if the patient will be applying for disability as well as suggesting approaches for retraining and conditioning.

Dr. Goldstein's CFS Symptom checklist

This symptom checklist is not sufficient to diagnose Chronic Fatigue Syndrome unless other disorders have been ruled out by appropriate assessment.

A.   Did your illness begin:
          _____abruptly
          _____gradually
          _____about how long ago?

B.   Did your illness begin with a flu-like episode?
          _____yes
          _____no
                  If yes: were lab tests done?_____
                          what tests?_____
                          were abnormalities found?_____

Were you treated for psychological problems prior to the onset of this illness?

          _____yes
          _____no
                  If yes: psychotherapy? _____yes _____no
                  medication:_____

Rate the severity of your symptoms from 0 to 10.

1._____Fatigue (100%) - usually made worse by physical exercise.

2._____Cognitive function problems (80%)
          _____a) attention deficit disorder
          _____b) calculation difficulties
          _____c) memory disturbance
          _____d) spatial disorientation
          _____e) frequently saying the wrong word

3._____Psychological problems (80%)
          _____a) depression
          _____b) anxiety - which may include panic attacks
          _____c) personality changes- usually a worsening of a previous mild tendency
          _____d) emotional lability (mood swings)
          _____e) psychosis (1%)

4._____Other nervous system problems (100%)
          _____a) sleep disturbance
          _____b) headaches
          _____c) changes in visual acuity
          _____d) seizures
          _____e) numb or tingling feelings
          _____f) dysequilibrium
          _____g) lightheadedness - feeling "spaced out"
          _____h) frequent unusual nightmares
          _____i) difficulty moving your tongue to speak
          _____j) ringing in ears
          _____k) paralysis
          _____l) severe muscular weakness
          _____m) blackouts

        _____n) intolerance of bright lights
        _____o) intolerance of alcohol
        _____p) alteration of taste, smell, hearing
        _____q) non-restorative sleep
        _____r) decreased libido
        _____s) twitching muscles ("benign fasciculations")

5._____Recurrent flu-like illnesses (75%) - often with chronic sore throat.

6._____Painful lymph nodes - especially on sides of neck and under the arms (60%).

7._____Severe nasal and other allergies - often worsening of previous mild problem (40%).

8._____Weight change - usually gain (70%).

9._____Muscle and joint aches with tender "trigger points" or fibromyalgia (65%).

10._____Abdominal pain, diarrhea, nausea, intestinal gas- "irritable bowel syndrome" (50%).

11._____Low grade fevers or feeling hot often (70%).

12._____Night sweats (40%).

13._____Heart palpitations (40%).

14._____Severe premenstrual syndrome - PMS (70% women).

15._____Rash of Herpes Simplex or Shingles (20%).

16._____Uncomfortable or recurrent urination - pain in prostate (20%).

17._____Other symptoms
        _____a) rashes
        _____b) hair loss
        _____c) impotence
        _____d) chest pain
        _____e) dry eyes and mouth
        _____f) cough
        _____g) TMJ syndrome
        _____h) mitral valve prolapse
        _____i) frequent canker sores
        _____j) cold hands and feet
        _____k) serious rhythm disturbances of the heart
        _____l) carpal tunnel syndrome
        _____m) pyriform muscle syndrome causing sciatica
        _____n) thyroid inflammation
        _____o) various cancers (a rare occurrence)
        _____p) periodontal (gum) disease
        _____q) endometirosis
        _____r) easily getting out of breath ("dyspnea on exertion")
        _____s) symptoms worsened by extremes of temperature
        _____t) multiple sensitivities to medicines, food and other substances

* Some of the above statistics were compiled with the assistance of data provided by Daniel Peterson, M.D. and Paul R. Cheney, M.D., Ph.D.

Chapter 24

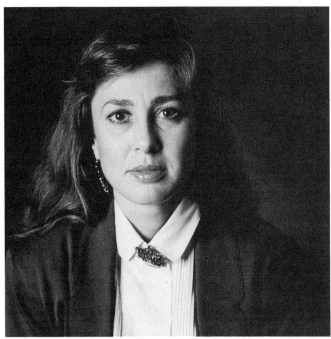

Dedra Buchwald

The Evaluation of Adults with Chronic Fatigue:
A Review of Laboratory and Psychological Findings

Dedra Buchwald, MD Department of Medicine, University of Washington Seattle, Washington

Dr. Buchwald received her medical degree from the University of California, San Diego and completed a Kaiser Fellowship at Brigham and Women's Hospital, Harvard Medical School. After completion of her post-graduate training, she assumed her current academic position at the University of Washington in the Department of Medicine, Division of General Internal Medicine. She presently directs the Chronic Fatigue Clinic and the Refugee Clinic at Harborview Medical Center, a major university-affiliated teaching institution. Dr. Buchwald has received external support for her work on Chronic Fatigue Syndrome and has authored and co-authored articles on various aspects of this illness.

This work was supported by grant RO1A126788 from the National Institute of Allergy and Infectious Diseases and by a Young Investigator Award from the National Alliance for Research on Schizophrenia and Depression.

During the past several years, much attention has been focused on an illness called chronic fatigue syndrome (CFS). CFS is a disabling systemic illness characterized by severe persistent fatigue often associated with fevers, pharyngitis, myalgias, headache, neurocognitive difficulties, sleep disturbances and depression. Although the cause of CFS remains obscure, findings from a growing body of literature suggest that immunological abnormalities, infectious agents, particularly viruses, and psychological factors may play important roles. The following is a review of these findings and recommendations for the evaluation of adults with chronic fatigue.

Laboratory Findings

1. Standard Laboratory Tests

Although a diversity of laboratory abnormalities have been reported (mostly in uncontrolled studies), there have been no consistent findings associated with CFS. On standard hematologic testing, leukocytosis and leukopenia are each seen in approximately 20% of patients[1-3] (AL Komaroff, unpublished data; AL Komaroff, D Buchwald, unpublished data). A relative lymphocytosis has been described in up to 71% of patients[2,4-8] (AL Komaroff, unpublished data). Atypical lymphocytes have been reported in 0-30%[2,4,5,7,9-12] (AL Komaroff, unpublished data; AL Komaroff, D Buchwald, unpublished data) and in serial studies, in about 50% of patients (AL Komaroff, unpublished data). Similarly, in one series, 48% of patients demonstrated monocytosis (AL Komaroff, unpublished data). Some investigators have reported elevated erythrocyte sedimentation rates in CFS patients[2,4,6,7,12,13] and approximately 15% have positive heterophile or monospot tests[5,6,8,10,12,13]. Other standard testing has revealed that 20% of patients have modestly elevated transaminases[6,8,12,14] (AL Komaroff, unpublished data; AL Komaroff, D Buchwald, unpublished data).

Table 1

Frequency of Selected Laboratory Abnormalities in Adults

Hematologic

Leukocytosis	0 - 21%
Leukopenia	0 - 26%
Lymphocytosis	0 - 71%
Atypical lymphocytes	0 - 30%
Positive heterophile	0 - 50%

Immunologic

Positive antinuclear antibodies	0 - 32%
Decreased immunoglobulin classes	4 - 100%
Increased immunoglobulin classes	11 - 40%
Circulating immune complexes	0 - 73%
Increased T4/T8 ratio	30 - 40%
Decreased T4/T8 ratio	2 - 100%
Anergy	0 - 54%
Decreased number of natural killer cells	0 - 73%
Decreased natural killer cell function	0 - 100%

2. Immunologic Abnormalities

Unusual and often conflicting findings have been noted in many immunologic studies (Table 1). Of the various circulating autoantibodies reported, the most common are antinuclear antibodies, detected in up to a third of patients[7,8,10-12,16] (AL Komaroff, unpublished data; AL Komaroff, D Buchwald, unpublished data). They are typically found in low concentrations without other evidence for lupus. Studies of immunoglobulin levels have yielded inconsistent findings as both decreased, and less commonly increased, immunoglobulins of the IgA, IgD, IgG or IgM class have been reported[3,6,7,12,14,18,19] (AL Komaroff, unpublished data; AL Komaroff, D Buchwald, unpublished data). An average of 53% of patients have low levels of circulating immune complexes[4,5,12] (AL Komaroff, unpublished data), but only a minority of patients show depressed complement[4-7] and none have clinical manifestations of immune-complex mediated disease. A mitogen-induced diminution in immunoglobulin synthesis in vitro has also been reported in 10% of CFS patients.

Several groups have noted abnormalities in the lymphokine and interleukin responses of CFS patients. Leukocyte activity of the interferon-induced enzyme, 2'5'-oligoadenylate synthetase was elevated in a small number of CFS patients[12,20] and circulating interferon has been infrequently detected[1,5,10,12,21,22]. Although one study found reduced synthesis of gamma interferon and interleukin-2 by mitogen-stimulated lymphocytes[23], others have found elevated interleukin-2 levels in CFS[24].

Abnormalities of lymphocyte number and function have also been noted. Both elevated and diminished numbers of T4 and T8 cells[4,25] (AL Komaroff, unpublished data) and increased and decreased T4/T8 ratios have been found[1,6,9,10,25] (AL Komaroff, unpublished data; AL Komaroff, D Buchwald, unpublished data). As with T-cells, both increased and decreased numbers of B-cells have been reported[5,21] (AL Komaroff, unpublished data; AL Komaroff, D Buchwald, unpublished data). In studies of lymphocyte function, up to 54% of patients are anergic[3,5,6,12,26], and significantly delayed hypersensitivity to multiple antigens has been demonstrated[26]. Decreased responsiveness in vitro to standard mitogen stimulation assays has also been reported[1,4,5,8,10]. A recent controlled study found a significant reduction in the display of CD3, a common membrane structure found on T cells[27]. Since CD3 interacts with antigen and is considered important in the transduction of T cell activation signal, this finding suggests a mechanism for the T cell dysfunction observed in CFS.

Natural killer cell deficiencies in CFS have been confirmed in a number of independent laboratories. Decreased numbers of natural killer cells and reductions in the normally dominant (NKH1 positive-T3 negative) subset have been reported in up to 73% of patients[1,4,28]. Natural killer cell function has been found to be increased[11], decreased[1,23,28] and normal[5] as measured by cytolytic activity against a number of different target cell lines. Diminished cytolytic activity resistant to interleukin-2 stimulation, particularly against Epstein-Barr virus infected cells, has been documented in many patients with CFS[28]. These abnormalities of natural killer cell phenotype and function are interesting given the central role played by these cells in viral infection, particularly infections with the herpes virus family.

3. Infectious Agents

CFS has been reported following infections with several different agents[7]. Although early studies linked Epstein-Barr virus and CFS, further investigations and evidence from two seroepidemiologic surveys have indicated that Epstein-Barr virus is unlikely to be an etiologic agent in most cases of CFS[29,30,31]. Many studies have found elevated IgG to viral capsid antigen and early antigen, generally in the absence of IgM to viral capsid antigen[2,3,5,8,10,12-14,16,19,32-35]; however, there is extensive overlap between patients and healthy control subjects. A low or absent antibody to the nuclear antigen, thought to be an unusual finding in healthy seropositive individuals, has been found in some CFS patients[5,8,10,12-14,19].

The enteroviruses have also been implicated as possible etiologic agents in CFS. Two intriguing studies report finding circulating enteroviral antigen[36,37] and IgM complexes in the majority of patients, and isolation of the virus in 22%[37]. Moreover, enteroviral nucleic acid has been found in muscle cells more often in patients with CFS than in control subjects[38].

It has been suggested that several latent viruses — herpes simplex, cytomegalovirus, measles virus[33] and human herpesvirus-6[39,40] — may be reactivated in patients with CFS. If true, it is unclear whether this reactivation of latent viruses contributes to the morbidity of CFS, or whether it is an epiphenomenon. In addition, several investigators have found no evidence of infection with human T-cell lymphotropic virus or human immunodeficiency virus[1,3,16] (AL Komaroff, unpublished data; AL Komaroff, D Buchwald, unpublished data).

4. Allergy Testing

Allergies are a common feature of CFS[10,12,41,42]. Several investigators have explored this association in adults and found increased cutaneous reactivity to allergens, increased levels of circulating IgE and IgE-bearing T and B cells, greater lymphocyte responsiveness to allergens and increased numbers of Epstein-Barr nuclear antigen bearing B cells in response to stimulation with specific antigens[43,44]. The mechanisms linking allergy and CFS remain unknown.

5. Muscle Studies

Muscle studies of chronic fatigue following a viral infection have demonstrated normal muscle enzymes[4] and the absence of antibodies to the acetylcholine receptor[45]. Most patients studied had muscle biopsies showing type II fiber atrophy or necrosis, tubular and mitochondrial structural abnormalities[4,46] and 75% had abnormal single fiber electromyography[45]. Excessive intracellular acidosis by nuclear magnetic resonance spectroscopy has also been reported[4,47]. In contrast, studies of metabolic and enzymatic markers of muscle activity in CFS demonstrated no evidence of a defect in the intermediary energy pathway[48]. Likewise, normal muscle strength, endurance and recovery[49,50] and normal cardiac function at rest[51] have been documented by a variety of techniques . However, on graded exercise testing (which is effort dependent), CFS patients have a markedly limited exercise capacity characterized by an inability to achieve their target heart rate, a lower exercise heart rate and an abbreviated exercise duration.

In summary, the laboratory abnormalities observed in adults with CFS are diverse, sometimes conflicting and frequently modest in degree. While some findings have been consistently reported by multiple investigators, others have been noted by only one group and await confirmation. The most interesting laboratory findings in CFS are those involving the immune system. While there is evidence of diffuse immunologic dysfunction, with some parameters reflecting deficient function, and others indicating hyperactivity, it has not been shown that these findings explain symptomatology of CFS, nor correlate with changes in symptoms over time. It also remains to be seen whether these findings distinguish CFS patients from those with other illnesses which can present with a similar clinical picture. Most likely, when more systematic "blinded" studies using healthy control subjects are performed, some of the "abnormalities" currently thought to be characteristic of CFS will disappear.

Psychological Findings

Some early reports describe neuropsychologic symptoms in young adults with prolonged illness following infectious mononucleosis or other acute infections[52-55]. The reports which heralded the current interest in CFS describe depression and "psychosocial problems" as prominent components of the syndrome[10,12]. Although psychological distress was presumed to result from the stress of chronic illness or from neurotoxic effects of viral infection, subsequent investigations have suggested a role for psychologic factors. At present, controversy remains regarding a primary or secondary role for psychiatric disorder in CFS.

Recent investigations have consistently found a high prevalence of psychiatric disorder, primarily depression, in adult CFS patients (Table 2)[11,56-61]. Those studies, which included control groups, demonstrate a higher prevalence of psychiatric disorder in patients than in control subjects. Among those with both chronic fatigue and psychiatric disorders, approximately half experienced an episode of the psychiatric disorder prior to the onset of chronic fatigue[58,60,61]. Furthermore, in a specialty fatigue clinic, it was found that 95% of patients did not meet the Centers for Disease Control criteria for CFS[56,57]. Over 70% of the excluded patients had fatigue symptoms severe enough to meet criteria, but each was excluded because the psychiatric disorder was thought to be responsible for the fatigue syndrome.

Recommended Evaluation

A detailed history, careful physical examination, and selected laboratory tests are indicated in all patients with chronic fatigue that is significantly affecting daily activity. Although no laboratory tests are diagnostic in CFS, a reasonable laboratory test battery to evaluate patients with possible CFS would include: a complete blood count, with manually performed differential white blood cell count; erythrocyte sedimentation rate; chemistry panel; thyroid function tests; antinuclear antibodies; in some cases, circulating immune complexes and immunoglobulin levels (IgG, IgA and IgM) may be warranted. Extensive serological testing for viruses is not usually helpful in identifying a causal link between fatigue and persistent or reactivated viruses. Consideration must be given to a psychological evaluation, searching, in particular, for anxiety and depression. Whenever possible, the use of a comprehensive standardized, interviewer-administered instrument such as the Diagnostic Interview Schedule is recommended. This evaluation should be useful in supporting a diagnosis of CFS, or in ruling out other diseases that produce chronic fatigue.

Table 2					
Frequency of Psychiatric Dysfunction in Adults					
Author	Assessment Used	Psychiatric Disorder in CFS		Psychiatric Disorder in Controls	
		Current	Lifetime	Current	Lifetime
Manu (56,57)	DIS	59%	77%	N/A	N/A
Kruesi (58)	DIS	N/A	75%	N/A	N/A
Wessely (59)	SADS	72%	N/A	36%	N/A
Taerk (60)	DIS	67%	N/A	N/A	29%
Katon (61)	DIS	45%	86%	6%	48%

DIS - National Institute of Mental Health (NIMH) Diagnostic Interview Schedule
SADS - Schedule for Affective Disorders and Schizophrenia

Note added in proof

Klimas[62] has recently reported multiple abnormalities of cellular immunity in 30 CFS patients, including a diminution in natural killer cell cytotoxicity, gamma interferon production and lymphoprolifera-tion after mitogen stimulation. Other findings were an increase in the percentages of suppressor-cyto-toxic T cells, activated T8 cells and number of B cells and a decrease in the suppressor- inducer subset of T4 cells.

References

1. Aoki T, Usuda Y, Miyakoshi H, Tamura K, Herberman RB. Low natural killer syndrome: Clinical and immunologic features. Nat Immun Cell Growth Regul 1987;6:116-28.

2. Kaslow JE, Rucker L, Onishi R. Liver extract-folic acid-cyanocobalamin vs. placebo for chronic fatigue syndrome. Arch Intern Med 1989;149:2501-3.

3. Lloyd AR, Wakefield D, Boughton CR, Dwyer JM. Immunological abnormalities in the chronic fatigue syndrome. Med J Aust 1989;151:122-4.

4. Behan PO, Behan WMH, Bell EJ. The postviral fatigue syndrome - an analysis of the findings in 50 cases. J Infect 1985;10:211- 22.

5. Borysiewicz LK, Haworth SJ, Cohen J, Mundin J, Rickinson A, Sissons JGP. Epstein- Barr virus-specific immune defects in patients with persistent symptoms following infectious mononucleosis. Quarterly J Med 1986;58:111-21.

6. DuBois RE, Seeley JK, Brus I, Sakamoto K, Ballow M, Harada S, Bechtold TA, Pearson G, Purtilo DT. Chronic mononucleosis syndrome. South Med J 1984;77:1376-82.

7. Salit IE. Sporadic postinfectious neuromyasthenia. Can Med Assoc J 4385;133:659-63.

8. Tobi M, Morag A, Ravid Z, Chowers I, Weiss VF, Michaeli Y, Ben- Chetrit E, Shalit M, Knobler H. Prolonged atypical illness associated with serological evidence of persistent Epstein-Barr virus infection. Lancet 1982;1:61-4.

9. Hamblin TJ, Hussain J, Akbar AN, Tang YC, Smith JL, Jones DB. Immunological reason for chronic ill health after infectious mononucleosis. Br Med J 1983;287:85-8

10. Jones JF, Ray G, Minnich LL, Hicks MJ, Kibler R, Locas DO. Evidence for active Epstein- Barr virus infection in patients with persistent, unexplained illnesses: elevated anti-early antigen antibodies. Ann Int Med 1985;102:1-7.

11. Gold D, Bowden R, Sixbey J, Riggs R, Katon WJ, Ashley R, Obrigewitch R, Corey L. Chronic fatigue: A prospective clinical and virologic study. JAMA 1990;264:48-53.

12. Straus SE, Tosato G, Armstrong G, Lawley T, Preble OT, Henle W, Davey R, Pearson G, Epstein J, Brus I, Blaese RM. Persisting illness and fatigue in adults with evidence of Epstein-Barr virus infection. Ann Int Med 1985;102:7-16.

13. Kroenke K, Wood Dr, Mangelsdorff AD, Neier NJ, Powell JB. Chronic fatigue in primary care: prevalence, patient characteristics, and outcome. JAMA 1988;260:929-34.

14. Roubalova K, Roubal J, Skopovy P, Fucikova T, Domorazova E, Vonka V. Antibody response to Epstein-Barr virus antigens in patients with chronic viral infection. J Med Virol 1988; 25:115- 22.

15. Lane TJ, Manu P, Matthews DA. Prospective diagnostic evaluation of adults with chronic fatigue. Clin Res 1988;36:714A.

16. Prieto J, Subira ML, Castilla A, Serrano M. Naloxone-reversible monocyte dysfunction n patients with chronic fatigue syndrome. Scand J Immunol 1989;30:13-20

17. Weinstein L. Thyroiditis and "chronic infectious mononucleosis." N Eng J Med 1987;317:1225-6.

18. Read R, Spickett G, Harvey J, Edwards AJ, Larson HE. IgG1 subclass deficiency in patients with chronic fatigue syndrome. Lancet 1988;1:241-2.

19. Tosato G, Straus S, Henle W, Pike SE, Blaese RM. Characteristic T cell dysfunction in patients with chronic active Epstein-Barr virus infection (chronic infectious mono-nucleosis). J Immuno 1985;134:3082-8.

20. Morag A, Tobi M, Ravid Z, Revel M, Schattner A. Increased (2'- 5')-oligo-a synthetase activity in patients with prolonged illness associated with serological evidence of persistent Epstein-Barr virus infection. Lancet 1982;1:744.

21. Ho-Yen DO, Carrington D, Armstrong AA. Myalgic encephalitis and alpha-interferon. Lancet 1988;1:125.

22. Lloyd A, Abi Hanna D, Wakefield D. Interferon and myalgic encephalomyelitis. Lancet 1988;1:471.

23. Kibler R, Lucas DO, Hicks MJ, Poulos BT, Jones JF. Immune function in chronic active Epstein-Barr virus infection. J Clin Immunol 1985;5:46-54.

24. Cheney PR, Dorman SE, Bell DS. Interleukin-2 and the chronic fatigue syndrome. Ann Intern Med 1989;110:321.

25. Linde A, Hammarstrom L, Smith CIE. IgG subclass deficiency and chronic fatigue syndrome. Lancet 1988;1:885-6.

26. Murdoch JC. Cell-mediated immunity in patients with myalgic encephalomyelitis syndrome. NZ Med J 1988;101:511-2.

27. Subira M, Castilla A, Cireira M, Prieto J. Deficient display of DC3 on lymphocytes of patients with chronic fatigue syndrome. J Infect Dis 1989; 160:165-6.

28. Caligiuri M, Murray C, Buchwald D, Levine H, Cheney P, Peterson D, Komaroff AL, Ritz J. Phenotypic and functional deficiency of natural killer cells in patients with chronic fatigue syndrome, J Immunol 1987;139:3306-13.

29. Hellinger WC, Smith TF, Van Scoy RE, Spitzer PG, Forgacs P, Edson RS. Chronic fatigue syndrome and the diagnostic utility of antibody to Epstein-Barr virus early antigen. JAMA 1988;260:971-3.

30. Horwitz CA, Henle W, Henle G, Rudnick H, Latts E. Long-term serological follow-up of patients for Epstein-Barr virus after recovery from infectious mononucleosis. J Infect Dis 1985;151:1150-3.

31. Lamy ME, Favart AM, Cornu C, Mendez M, Segas M, Burtonboy G. Study of Epstein Barr virus (EBV) antibodies: IgG and IgM anti-VCA, IgG anti-EA and IgG anti-EBNA obtained with an original microtiter technique: -Serological criterions of primary and recurrent EBV infections and follow-up of infectious mononucleosis; - Seroepidemiology of EBV in Belgium based on 5178 sera from patients. Acta Clin Belgica 1982;37:281-98.

32. Buchwald D, Sullivan JL, Komaroff AL. Frequency of 'chronic active Epstein-Barr virus infection' in a general medical practice. JAMA 1987;257:2303-7.

33. Holmes GP, Kaplan JE, Stewart JA, Hunt B, Pinsky PF, Schonberger LB. A cluster of patients with a chronic mononucleosis-like syndrome: Is Epstein-Barr virus the cause? JAMA 1987;257:2297-2302.

34. Hotchin NA, Read R, Smith DG, Crawford DH. Active Epstein-Barr virus infection in post-viral fatigue syndrome. J Infect 1989;18:143-50.

35. Waters-Peacock N, Wray BB, Ades EW. A prospective study: Evaluation of the antibody-dependent cell mediated cytotoxicity assay in chronic active Epstein-Barr syndrome. J Clin Lab Immunol 1988;27:11-2.

36. Halpin D, Wessely S. VP-1 antigen in chronic postviral fatigue syndrome. Lancet 1989;1:1028-9.

37. Yousef GE, Bell EJ, Mann GF, Murugesan V, Smith DG, McCartney RA, Mowbray JF. Chronic enterovirus infection in patients with postviral fatigue syndrome. Lancet 1988;1:146-7.

38. Archard LC, Bowles NE, Behan PO, Bell EJ, Doyle D. Postviral fatigue syndrome: persistence of enterovirus RNA in muscle and elevated creatine kinase. J Royal Soc Med 1988;81:326-9.

39. Komaroff AL, Saxinger C, Buchwald D, Geiger A, Gallo RC. A chronic "post-viral" fatigue syndrome with neurologic features serologic association with human herpes virus-6. Clin Res 1988;36:743A.

40. Wakefield D, Lloyd A, Dwyer J. Human herpes virus 6 and myalgic encephalomyelitis. Lancet 1988;1:1059.

41. Jones JF, Straus SE. Chronic Epstein-Barr virus infection. Ann Rev Med 1987;38:195-209.

42. Straus SE, Dale JK, Wright R, Metcalfe DD, Allergy and the chronic fatigue syndrome. J Allergy Clin Immunol 1988;81:791-5.

43. Olson GB, Kanaan MN, Gersuk GM, Kelley LM, Jones JF. Correlation between allergy and persistent Epstein-Barr virus infections in chronic-active Epstein-Barr virus infected patients. J Allergy Clin Immunol 1986;78:308-14.

44. Olson GB, Kanaan MN, Kelley LM, Jones JF. Specific allergen-induced Epstein-Barr nuclear antigen-positive B cells from patients with chronic-active Epstein-Barr virus infections. J Allergy Clin Immunol 1986;78:315-20.

45. Jamal GA, Hansen S. Electrophysiological studies in the post-viral fatigue syndrome. J Neurol Neurosurg and Psychiatry 1985;48:691-4.

46. Warner CL, Cookfair D, Meffuer R, Bell D, Ley D, Jacobs L. Neurologic abnormalities in the chronic fatigue syndrome. Neurol 1989;39 (suppl):420.

47. Arnold DL, Bore PJ, Radda GK, Styles P, Taylor DJ. Excessive intracellular acidosis of skeletal muscle on exercise in a patient with a post-viral exhaustion/fatigue syndrome. Lancet 1984;1:1367-9.

48. Byrne E, Trounce I. Chronic fatigue and myalgia syndrome: mitochrondrial and glycolytic studies in skeletal muscle. J Neurol Neurosurg Psychiatry 1987;50:743-6.

49. Lloyd AR, Hales JP, Gandevia SC. Muscle strength, endurance and recovery in the post-infection fatigue syndrome. J Neurol Neurosurg Psychiatry 1988;51:1316-22.

50. Stokes MJ, Cooper RG, Edwards RHT. Normal muscle strength and fatigability in patients with effort syndromes. Br Med J 1988;297:1014-7.

51. Montague TJ, Marrie TJ, Klassen GA, Berwick DJ, Horacek BM. Cardiac function at rest and with exercise in the chronic fatigue syndrome. Chest 1989;95:779-84.

52. Greenfield NS, Roessler R, Crosley AP. Ego strength and length of recovery from infectious mononucleosis. J Nerv Ment Dis 1959;129:125-28.

53. Bender CE. Recurrent mononucleosis. JAMA 1962;182:954-6.

54. Issacs R. Chronic infectious mononucleosis. Blood 1948;3:858- 61.

55. Kasl SV, Evans AS, Niederman JC. Psychosocial risk factors in the development of infectious mononucleosis. Psychosom Med 1979;41:445-6.

56. Manu P, Lane TJ, Matthews DA. The frequency of the chronic fatigue syndrome in patients with symptoms of persistent fatigue. Ann Intern Med 1988;109:554-6.

57. Manu P, Matthews DA, Lane TJ. The mental health of patients with a chief complaint of chronic fatigue: a prospective evaluation and follow-up. Arch Intern Med 1988;148:2213-17.

58. Kruesi MJP, Dale J. Straus SE. Psychiatric diagnoses in patients who have chronic fatigue syndrome. J Clin Psychiatry 1989;50:53-6.

59. Wessely S, Powell R. Fatigue syndromes: a comparison of chronic "postviral" fatigue with neuromuscular and affective disorders. J Neurol Neurosurg Psychiatry 1989;52:940- 8.

60. Taerk GS, Toner BB, Salit IE, Garfinkel PE, Ozersky SO. Depression in patients with neuromyasthenia (benign myalgic encephalitis). Int J Psychiat Med 1987;17:49-56.

61. Katon WJ, Buchwald DS, Simon GE, Russo JE, Mease PJ. Psychiatric illness in patients with chronic fatigue and rheumatoid arthritis. J Gen Intern Med 1991; 6:277-85.

62. Klimas NG, Salvato FR, Morgan R, Fletcher MA. Immunologic abnormalities in chronic fatigue syndrome. J Clin Microbiol. 1990; 28:1403-10.

Chapter 25

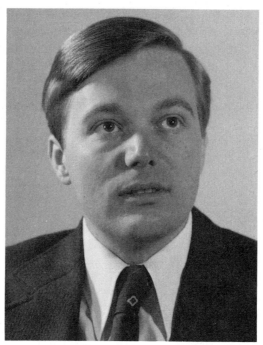

Alexander C. Chester

Chronic Fatigue of Nasal Origin: Possible Confusion with Chronic Fatigue Syndrome

Alexander C. Chester III, MD, FACP
Clinical Professor of Medicine, Georgetown University Medical Center
Foxhall Internists, PC
Suite 348, 3301 New Mexico Avenue, NW, Washington, DC 20016 USA

Dr. Chester has studied at Georgetown University, Washington, University of Salzburg, Austria as well as Columbia University, New York. Dr. Chester has been involved in many societies, including The Osler Society, National Kidney Foundation, Council on Clinical Nephrology, Dialysis and Transplantation and The Clinico-Patholgical Society. Dr. Chester has held many prestigious positions including the President of The Osler Society and he presently holds the position of the Secretary and Treasurer of the Hippocrates-Galen Society.

William Osler described three types of fatigue. The first is a weakness experienced in the muscles and limbs caused by neurologic or muscle illness. The second, a "lassitude felt on slight exercise" is associated with systemic disease. Finally, a "painful weariness" or the feeling of being "knocked out" after minimal exertion is the type generally noted in unexplained chronic fatigue.[1]

The last type of fatigue is characteristic of both chronic fatigue syndrome (CFS) and fatigue of nasal origin.[2,3] Upper respiratory complaints are noted in both. Unlike CFS, nasal disease with its related sinusitis, is eminently treatable and should be thoroughly considered in the differential diagnosis of unexplained fatigue. Additionally, failure to treat could result in the severe complications occasionally associated with sinusitis.

Conversely, sinusitis has been noted as the initial symptom of CFS and may serve as a possible trigger. The possibility that nasal problems can precipitate a more complex disease, possibly of viral origin, is suggested by an outbreak of multiple sclerosis following sinusitis.[4]

In the practice of general internal medicine, chronic fatigue is responsible for approximately 25% of visits.[5] Less than half of these are clarified with a diagnosis leaving the syndrome of unexplained chronic fatigue as one of the largest problems in the outpatient population.[6] Psychologic explanations are often suspected but proof or consensus is lacking. Unlike the fatigue of a typical organic illness, however, the patient does not in general feel best in the morning, "wearing down" as the day goes on. Moreover, unlike most physical illnesses, there are no known laboratory markers. The physical examination is likewise unremarkable.

All agree that psychologic problems are often present in the fatigued but they are considered by many the result, rather than the cause of the physical problems. Clearly, depression can cause fatigue but generally this fatigue is characterized by a lack of desire and motivation rather than a pronounced "painful weariness". Little is written on this pervasive problem of unexplained fatigue and research is minimal. Without objective means, such as laboratory findings, all studies and treatment results are suspect.

In the United States, publications in 1985 linking the Epstein Barr Virus to a severe form of unexplained fatigue reintroduced the subject as one in need of serious scientific investigation. The abnormal viral titer, despite later controversy, supported a nonpsychologic origin of the problem and stimulated study. Symptoms were analyzed with much greater scrutiny and a syndrome characterized by severe fatigue was defined by consensus. Not designed to be inclusive, nor proposed as a definite and unique entity, the CFS definition is useful in clinical research. This syndrome is relatively uncommon and its relation to the much more frequent problem of unexplained fatigue is unknown.

CFS is associated with a very high incidence of allergic disorders. Up to 90% of this population documents complaints consistent with IgE mediated allergic disease.[7] Indeed, many of the symptom criteria needed to establish the diagnosis of CFS are consistent with a nasal or sinus origin: sore throat, tender cervical lymph glands, headache, dizziness, etc.

The following abstract offers preliminary results of a study examining unexplained fatigue and explaining its relationship to allergic, nasal, and sinus complaints.

Abstract

An outpatient population of 307 consecutive patients under the age of 40 was interviewed, examined and tested. Significant unexplained fatigue for greater than one month, unrelieved by rest, was noted in 68 patients (study group). Findings were compared to the remaining 239 (control).

Women contributed 60% of the study group and 41% of the control (p<.01). The overall population was overwhelmingly white and generally upper middle class, 45% women and 55% men. The mean duration of fatigue was 35.0+/- 7.8 months (+/- SE) and mean age 30.3 years in the study group and 30.6 years in the control.

Fatigue intensity was divided into 3 groups: incapacitating, those able to work less than half time; severe, those who must restrict activity and never feel well; moderate, those who occasionally feel well and/or do not restrict activity. Mild fatigue was not included in the study. Characteristics are summarized in Table 1.

Table 1				
Fatigue Severity and Characteristics				
	No. of Pts.	Women (%)	Sudden Onset (%)	Following a URI (%)
Total Study Group	68	60	37	19
Incapacitating	3	33	100	100
Severe	23	70	35	13
Moderate	42	57	33	17
Control	239	41	N.A.	N.A.

Depression is more common in the study group, 35% vs. 10% (p<.001), increasingly common with increasing severity. Questioned about their own opinion regarding the cause, patients more mildly affected were more likely to consider a psychologic origin. Type A behavior pattern by self-assessment, was not significantly more common in the study group (49%) than the control (48%). Major life changes in the last 2 years were noted in 6l% of the study group and 47% of the control.

Findings on physical examination, complete blood as count, sedimentation rate, urinalysis, and chemical profile were similar. No significant differences were noted in blood pressure, orthostatic blood pressure change, pulse, or weight. Eosinophil, lymphocyte, and monocyte counts were similar.

The rhinologic symptoms of chronic fatigue are described in Table 2. Those with unexplained fatigue often had nasal and head complaints. A sense of dysequilibrium and feeling of generalized "heavy headedness" was common. Facial pressure over the frontal and maxillary sinuses was also more frequent was nasal stuffiness. The sore throat and tender cervical adenopathy may be related to postnasal

Table 2		
Rhinologic Symptoms of Chronic Fatigue		
	Study Group (%)	Control (%)
Pharyngitis	19	8 $p < .05$
Facial Pressure	54	13 $p < .001$
Nasal Stuffiness	74	40 $p < .001$
Cervical Adenopathy	34	5 $p < .005$
Heavy Headedness	65	8 $p < .001$
Allergic History	68	46 $p < .005$
Dysequilibrium	65	3 $p < .001$

Table 3		
Additional Symptoms of Chronic Fatigue		
	Study Group	Control
Myalgias/arthralgias	37%	3% $p < .005$
Perception of fever	29%	2% $p < .001$
Irritability	34%	17% $p < .05$
Forgetfulness	39%	10% $p < .001$
Difficulty thinking	30%	8% $p < .005$
Sleep disturbance	29%	7% $p < .005$

Table 4
Treatment
Cephalexin 500 mg four times daily for 1 week (if the patient fails to improve: Doxycycline 100 mg twice daily for 1 week following Cephalexin)
Xylometazoline 0.1% nasal spray three times daily for 3 days
Pseudoephedrine 60 to 120 mg twice daily
Nasal steam inhalations for 20 minutes, three times daily
Resume former sleeping habits
Elimination of beer, wine and milk products

Table 5

Charactertistics of Responders

	Control	Study Group % of	
		Responders	Non- Responders
No. of pts.	239	31	37
Age (yrs.)	30.6	32.5	29.2
Women (%)	41	74	49
Durational fatigue (mo.)	N.A.	23.3	43.3 (N.S)
Sudden onset of fatigue (%)	N.A.	42	32

Table 6

Fatigue Severity and Response

	Total No. of Pts.	No. (%) of Responders	No. (%) of Non-responders
Incapacitating	3	1 (33%)	2 (67%)
Severe	23	11 (48%)	12 (52%)
Moderate	42	19 (45%)	23 (55%)
Total	68	31 (46%)	37 (54%)

drip, a common complaint. The incidence of additional CFS symptom criteria are noted in Table 3. Table 4 lists the treatment directed at the nasal symptoms. The response to treatment was noted in Table 5. Of the 68 examined 31 (46%) responded as feeling completely well or generally well and much improved. This result was sustained over the 5 month observation period and not associated with a relapse that failed to respond to the original regimen in less than one week. Women were somewhat overly represented in the responders but not significantly so. Forty-two percent of the responders and 32% of those who failed to do so had a sudden onset of their fatigue. Eight of the 13 (62%), whose problems started with an upper respiratory infection, were cured.

As shown in Table 6, each of the 3 levels of fatigue contributed somewhat similarly to the responders. Responders did not differ from non-responders in the presence of nasal or sinus symptoms. Many were, however, unaware of symptoms prior to the initiation of therapy when the extent of nasal blockage became obvious in retrospect. Nasal and sinus symptoms responded along with complaints of achiness and depression in those whose fatigue resolved.

Twenty-six percent of those who became well had depression which in all cases lifted, vs. 41% of those who remained fatigued. The initial perception of the problem as physical was noted in 74% of the responders and 59% of the non-responders.

Duration of Fatigue

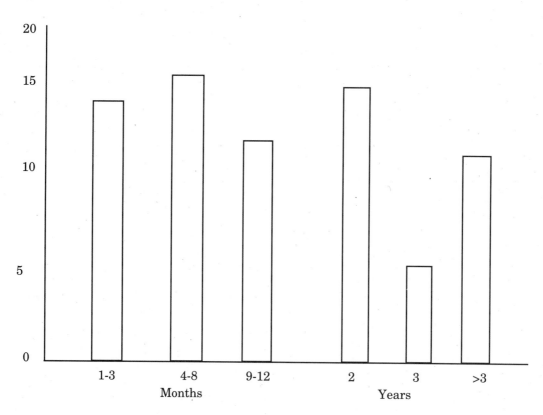

264

Discussion

The symptoms of unexplained chronic fatigue, as well as the much less common chronic fatigue syndrome are similar. Both often occur suddenly. Many of the symptom criteria for CFS are noted more commonly than control in those with unexplained chronic fatigue. They share a preponderance of nose and throat symptoms as well as an allergic history.

Chronic fatigue of nasal origin may easily be confused with CFS. Both induce a fatigue that is often characterized by upper respiratory complaints. A nasal origin may not be obvious with the etiology apparent only after a gratifying response to sinusitis treatment.

CFS does not respond to such treatment but curiously may be initiated by a sinusitis. The mechanism by which this relatively common infection occasionally precipitates CFS may be the same as that involved in an apparent outbreak of multiple sclerosis following sinusitis.[7] Perhaps a viral disease is activated by a nasal mechanism.

A nasal origin of systemic problems received significant attention for the first time in the latter 19th century. Extensive literature described fatigue due to nasal disorders and documented headaches, depression and multiple additional symptoms as the consequence of nasal obstruction. Removal of a small growth or straightening of the septum often caused a cure. This perplexing phenomenon was explained on the basis of a nasal reflex. Voltolini had recently demonstrated that asthma could occasionally be cured by the removal of even a tiny nasal polyp. A similar reflex was postulated to explain "nasal fatigue".

In 1898, Walter A. Wells reported 10 cases representing neurological and mental manifestations of nasal disease.[8] They were characterized by extraordinary fatigue with neurologic and musculoskeletal symptoms. At the time the linkage of nasal symptoms and fatigue associated with the lack of motivation was well-accepted enough to be termed "aprosexia nasalis".[9] Sigmond Freud's close friend and personal physician, Wilhelm Fliess, wrote extensively on nasal reflexes.[10] Although many were apparently fanciful, the proved systemic effects of the nose were more scientifically investigated by Dr. Maurice Cottle years later.[11]

Approximately 50 years ago observers noted fatigue, nasal stuffiness, headaches, achiness, inattention, depression, etc. in children were cured by the elimination of milk or certain foods in the diet. All symptoms reappeared with the re-introduction of the offending food. Rowes' list of "allergic toxemia" symptoms includes most CFS symptom criteria.[10] Unfortunately, the tension-fatigue syndrome, as it was called, has suffered the problems of all purported food allergies. Organized medicine was skeptical of testimonials unaccompanied by adequately controlled studies.

Expanding on the theme, Randolph analyzed the problems of allergies and fatigue more broadly in 1945.[11] Upon questioning University of Michigan nursing students, he noted fatigue unrelieved by rest in 52% of those with an allergic history and only 5% of those without. The chronic sore throat and tender glands were also a common finding in the allergic and fatigued. Many responded well to dietary modifications. A keen observer, Randolph managed to predict the future in his title, "The Coincidence of Allergic Disease, Unexplained Fatigue, and Lymphadenopathy; Possible Diagnostic Confusion with Infectious Mononucleosis".

Although the association of nasal disorders and fatigue has been either discounted or overlooked for most of the 20th century, it is now re-emerging, albeit, with a different emphasis. Dr. Peretz Lavie documents sleep disorders in many with even mild nasal obstruction.[12] Micro-arousals and brief periods of awakening occur throughout the night resulting in non-restorative sleep. Surgical correction or medical therapy of the allergic swelling generally reverses the associated fatigue.

Conversely, Moldofsky reports abnormal sleep studies in those with post-viral fatigue syndrome.[13] He postulates that an underlying psychologic arousal state during sleep may cause the fatigue.

Whatever the mechanism a nasal and related sinus disorder of acute or subacute onset would explain many of the confusing features of unexplained fatigue: (1) the lack of routine laboratory abnormalities, physical findings, mortality; (2) the fluctuation of symptoms with weather changes, emotional states, dietary manipulations; (3) the puzzling and often acute variability of symptoms; (4) the onset after an upper respiratory infection including the apparent epidemic nature; (5) the high incidence of allergic and nasal symptoms.

Nasal, allergic, and sleep disorder should be thoroughly searched for and treated in all the fatigued individuals. The proportional contribution of these problems to chronic fatigue remains to be clarified, but will be done so, only when considered.

References

1. Osler W. **A System of Medicine**. Vol. VIII. Diseases of the Nervous System. London: Oxford University Press, 1910.

2. Holmes GP, Kaplan JE, Genty NM, et al: Chronic fatigue syndrome: a working case definition. Annals Int Med 1988: 108: 387-389.

3. Goldman JL, Blaugrund SM, Shugar JM, eds. The Principles and Practice of Rhinology: A Text on the Diseases and Surgery of the Nose and Paranasal Sinuses. New York, NY: John Wiley and Sons; 1987.

4. Gay D, Dick G, Upton G. Multiple sclerosis associated with sinusitis: case controlled study in general practice. Lancet 1986; 1: 815-819.

5. Kroenke K, Wood DR, Mangelsdorff DA, et al. Chronic fatigue in primary care. JAMA 1988; 260: 929-934.

6. Jerrett WA. Lethargy in general practice. Practitioner 1981; 225: 731-737.

7. Behan PO, Behan WMH and Ben EJ. The post-viral fatigue syndrome—an analysis of findings in 50 cases. J Infec 1985; 10: 211-222.

8. Wells WA. Some Nervous and Mental Manifestations Occurring in Connection with Nasal Disease. Am J Med Sci 1898; 116: 677-692.

9. Guye D. On aprosexia, being the inability to fix the attention and other allied troubles in the cerebral functions caused by nasal disorders. Br Med J. 1889; 2: 709-711.

10. Fliess W. **Die Nasale Reflexneurose: Vehandlungen des Kongresses fur Innere Medizine**. Wiesbaden: JF Bergman, 1893.

11. Barelli PA, Loch WE, Kern EB, et al, eds. Rhinology. **The Collected Writings of Maurice H. Cottle, M.D.** Amer Rhin Soc, 1987.

12. Speer F. The allergic tension-fatigue syndrome in children. Int Arch Allergy. 1958; 12: 207- 214.

13. Rowe AH. Allergic toxemia and fatigue. Ann Allergy 1950; 8: 72-84.

14. Randolph TG. The coincidence of allergic disease, unexplained fatigue and lymphadenopathy; possible diagnostic confusion with infectious mononucleosis. Am J Med Sci. 1945; 209: 306- 314.

15. Lavie P. Nasal obstructions, sleep and mental function. Sleep, 1983; 6: 244-246.

16. Whelton C, Saskin P, Salit I and Moldofsky H. Post-viral fatigue syndrome and sleep (abstract). Sleep Res. 1988; 17: 307. 1988.

The Infectious Origins of M.E. / CFS

Chapter 26

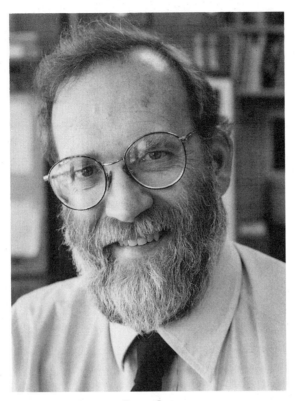

James Jones

Possible Role for Epstein-Barr Virus (EBV) in the Chronic Fatigue Syndrome (CFS)

James Jones, MD
Associate Professor of Pediatrics, National Jewish Center for Immunology and Respiratory Department of Medicine, 1400 Jackson Street, Denver, Colorado 80206 USA

Dr. Jones was educated at Duke University and the University of Texas Medical Branch, with extensive research training and clinical experience. Dr. Jones actively participates in numerous organizations such as the American Association for the Advancement of Science, American Society for Microbiology, American Academy of Pediatrics, American Academy of Allergy to name a few, and has won the James W. McLaughlin and the NIH New Investigator Awards. Since 1983, he has held the position of Senior Staff Physician in the Department of Pediatrics at the National Jewish Center for Immunology and Respiratory Medicine. Dr. Jones' interests lay, in particular, in immunology, immunodeficiency diseases, host response to virus infections and definition and pathogenesis of Chronic Fatigue Syndrome (Epstein-Barr virus).

The signs, symptoms and consequences of the chronic fatigue syndrome may be considered those of an acute infection that does not resolve. This concept is strengthened by the frequent occurrence of the syndrome following an illness of sudden onset. Of course, there are some obvious differences, such as the absence of fever and the lack of specific organ involvement. What are some possible reasons that these generalized symptoms that are the products of the host's response to the infection or immune injury persist or recur for such long periods of time?

One group of reasons would include persistence of the infection or reactivation of a latent infection with continued attempts by the host to control infection. Another set of reasons would include persistent production, or lack of inhibition of production, of mediators responsible for symptoms even though the infection *per se* had resolved. A third explanation would include alteration of mediator target organ function even though the infection is controlled and mediator production has ceased.

This discussion will focus on the infectious agent EBV, and address its persistence or reactivation as a trigger for inducing CFS.

EBV is a prime candidate for triggering CFS. First, CFS may follow acute infectious mononucleosis (IM)[1]. Secondly, there is a considerable literature that suggests IM may have a prolonged course with exacerbations[2]. Thirdly, as a member of the herpes virus family, EBV achieves a latent infection state in all infected people, and may be reactivated in some. Reactivation may be followed by disease in some persons, but may occur in the absence of illness as detected by maintenance of antibodies to certain viral proteins[3].

An appreciation of the life cycle of this virus is necessary to continue the discussion. The reader is referred to a review of this topic by Werner and Gertrude Henle and Evelyn Lennette for details[4]. Initial infection of pharyngeal epithelial cells and/or B lymphocytes leads to production of virus particles. These newly produced virons continue to infect naive cells until host responses intervene. Instead of all cells allowing complete replication of virus and subsequent cell death, some lymphoid cells are transformed so that they replicate indefinitely with the virus remaining in a circular or episomal stage throughout the life of the cell. The dual process of cell lysis with new virus production and prolonged life of EBV transformed cells continues until intervention by host responses. These responses control replication of virus by neutralization of free virus, killing infected cells and preventing outgrowth of transformed cells. Some cells containing latent virus escape the surveillance and go on to allow replication of new virons that subsequently infect naive cells, thus continuing the cycle.

One series of events that reflect the host's response to infection are antibody responses. Table 1 depicts the order in which viral antigens are produced versus the order in which antibodies are produced. It is this progression of combined events that has allowed modelling of acute, convalescent or reactivated EBV disease. The full cycle of virus replication yields proteins known as Epstein-Barr nuclear antigens (EBNA), early antigens (EA), and viral capsid antigens (VCA). Even though EBNAs are produced first during virus replication, antibodies directed against

these proteins are the last to be observed. Since viral antigens need to be processed before specific immune responses can be made, EBNAs must be hidden from the host until responses to cytoplasmic or membranous proteins are made. It is thought that these events correspond to specific killing of infected cells by immune T cells[5].

Table 1
Appearances of EBV Antigen and Respective Antibodies

Antigen	Antibody
Epstein-Barr Nuclear Antigen	anti-VCA
Early Antigen	anti-EA
Viral Capsid Antigen	anti-EBNA

These defense mechanisms are not absolute, however, because cells containing virus in its latent state (or circular episomal form of viral DNA are not totally removed. Cells with this form of the virus persist indefinitely with virus replication occurring with cell division. For unknown reasons, circular episomal forms of the virus may change to the linear form, accompanied by new virus production[6]. Failure to control this reactivation, as occurs in immunosuppressed persons, allows unbridled growth of infected B cells and leads to a variety of lymphoproliferative diseases[7].

Table 2
Koch-Evans Postulates

1. **Postulate A**. The syndrome is part of a spectrum of host responses following exposure to a putative agent.

2. **Postulate B**. Measurable host immune responses occur in affected individuals that are known to be important in the resolution induced specific illness.

3. **Postulate C**. There is a genetic predisposition for the syndrome.

4. **Postulate D**. The illness and its apparent causes make "biological and epidemiologic sense".

Table 3			
AI	Alcohol intolerance	HS	Hand swelling
ANX	Anxiety	IN	Incoordination
ARTH	Arthralgia	LOA	Loss of appetite
BD	Bladder dysfunction	MOOD	Mood swings
CH	Chills	MP	Myalgia
DBP or SP	Dreams of being paralyzed or sleep paralysis	NS	Night sweats
DEP	Depression	NV	Nausea / vomiting
DC	Difficulty concentrating	OSS	Odd skin sensations
DEAR	Diarrhea	PAR	Paresthesias
IZ	Dizzy	POB	Pain on breathing
DS	Difficulty sleeping	PHO	Palpitations
EAR	Earache	RASH	Rash
ES	Eyelid Swelling	SLN	Swollen lymph nodes
FAT	Fatigue	SP	Stomach pain
FVR	Fever	STL	Sensitivity to light
HCI	Heat / cold intolerance	ST	Sore throat
HEAD	Headache	TS	Trouble sleeping
HL	Hair loss	WL	Weight loss

The above events were detected for the most part in persons with acute mononucleosis and in their progression to resolution. Thus, IM is the current model for EBV infection, even though only 1/3 of seropositive persons have had this syndrome.

We are testing the hypothesis that clinical, viral and immune phenomena seen in IM occur in CFS. Four of Koch-Evans postulates are being tested (Table 2). First is that the syndrome is part of a spectrum of host responses following exposure to a putative agent. When one becomes ill, local and systemic host processes and local consequences of the infection *per se* alter baseline physiology and lead to what patients call illness and to what physicians call signs and symptoms. Systemic responses such as malaise, headache, fatigue, sleep disorder, anorexia and trouble concentrating are produced by a large number of mediators, e.g., interferon, and are not unique to specific organisms[8]. Some viruses are more likely to produce systemic symptoms that others, just as some patients become more ill than others. The pharyngitis and cervical lymph node swelling that are the hallmarks of primary IM are obviously not specific for that syndrome. But patterns and frequencies of symptoms are more frequently recognized in some illness versus others. Table 3 lists 36 common symptoms described by patients as recorded in 1985 by Jones, et al[1]. The presence or absence of these symptoms, their consistency and whether their presence caused major problems are being addressed in the present study. In addition, the subjects were asked to quantitate daily primary symptoms on a scale of 0-4, ranging from absence of the symptoms to incapacitation due to the symptom. These primary symptoms include: sore throat, lymphadenopathy, headache, fatigue, joint aches, muscle aches, nerve tingling, depression, loss of abstract thinking, sleep disturbances.

The second postulate is that measurable host responses occur during this infection with the corollary that one can identify unique responses by looking at certain aspects of immune function. Specific antibody generation against VCA, EA and EBNA antigens as described above is one such measure. Another phenomenon that occurs during acute EBV infection is the outgrowth of infected B cells due to transformation by the virus. Subsequent control of this process by a variety of nonspecific and specific immune responses follows during convalescence and recovery[5]. The sum of these processes is tested by culturing PBL mononuclear cells with the result that cells from patients with acute illness transform and cells from persons with resolved IM or well persons with antibodies to EBV, but with no history of IM, do not routinely transform[9]. The host responses that control outgrowth can be abrogated by removal of T cells or the addition of the immunosuppressant agent, cyclosporin A.

Table 4						
Population Groups Under Study and their number per year						
Group Number*	**I**	**II**	**III**	**IV**	**V**	**VI**
EBV Seropositive	+	+	+	+	+	+
2 yr History CFS Symptoms	+	-	-	+	+	-
Hx Infectious Mononucleosis	50%	-	100%	50%	50%	33%
% with history of IgE allergy (year 1)	82	30	77	77	55	67
EA antibody titer	≥80	NR†	NR	<80	<10	NR
n year 1	22	18	18	18	11	6

* I= cases; II-VI=controls; II, III=well; IV, V chosen on basis of anti-EA titer; VI blood relative of I=genetic control
† no requirement for entry

Two additional Koch-Evans postulates are that there is a genetic influence on disease expression and that the whole process makes biological sense. Genetic questions may be asked on different levels. For example, is there a genetic propensity for production of high anti-EBV antibodies that bears no relationship to the level of illness? Or, is there an underlying disease process that might influence symptom production?

One caveat must be stated at this time. Since only one third of persons who are seropositive to EBV had IM, the immune responses associated with IM may be peculiar to that group and not representative of the at large response to the virus.

Results

Table 4 recapitulates the 6 groups that encompass the study. Each patient was followed for one year. They have 4 different collections of samples of virus samples as well as immunologic tests as well as clinical findings. One interesting thing in this table is that in the first year of study, 50% of persons in group 1 had a history of IM. By definition all in group 3 did and 50% had had IM in patient control groups 4 and 5, whereas only 1/3 of the relatives had IM and, of course, in group 2 by definition no one had had IM. We had some trouble in collecting certain family controls (group 6), and the number of persons that we could find who did not have antibodies to the early antigen (group 5) was also quite low. This approach should allow us at the end of this 3 year study to do a variety of statistical analyses to determine if any of these factors are meaningful or not.

Figure 1 depicts the symptoms addressed in the enrolment questionnaire. One of the key things that has been criticized about this syndrome, at least in the United States, is that everybody has these symptoms. The figure suggests that the patients (groups I, IV, V), because of selection, obviously had the

Table 5		
Log2 Anti-EBV Titers		
Group n	**VCA**	**EBNA**
	mean ± SD (SEM)	
I 22	10.83 ± 0.49 (0.10)	6.17 ± 1.09 (0.23)
II 18	9.91 ± 0.82 (0.19)	6.41 ± 0.87 (0.21)
III 18	10.19 ± 0.90 (0.21)	6.74 ± 1.02 (0.24)
IV 18	10.59 ± 0.55 (0.13)	6.34 ± 0.91 (0.21)
V 11	8.59 ± 3.10 (0.93)	5.64 ± 2.22 (0.67)
VI 16	11.20 ± 0.99 (0.40)	6.67 ± 1.22 (0.50)
	EA-D	**EA-R**
I 22	3.36 ± 3.10 (0.66)	5.44 ± 2.60 (0.55)
II 18	2.64 ± 2.46 (0.58)	4.61 ± 2.25 (0.53)
III 18	1.78 ± 1.79 (0.42)	6.06 ± 1.91 (0.45)
IV 18	2.62 ± 3.23 (0.76)	4.15 ± 2.66 (0.63)
V 11	0.47 ± 0.66 (0.20)	4.60 ± 2.88 (0.90)
VI 16	3.38 ± 3.10 (1.27)	4.75 ± 2.90 (1.18)

Figure 1A

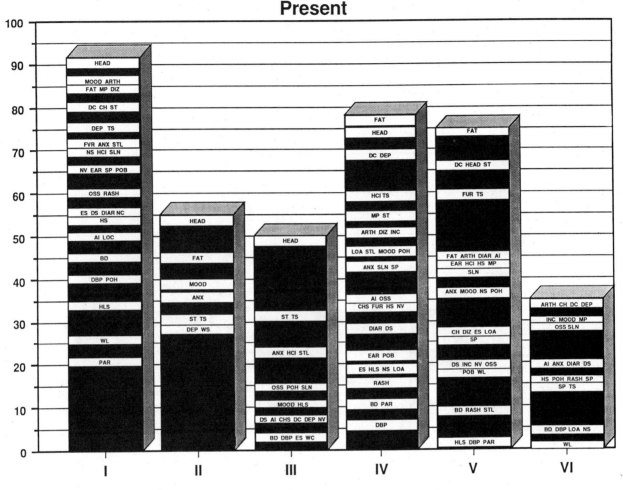

presence of more symptoms. But it also suggests that healthy controls at various times have headaches, fatigue, mood changes and so forth at some point in time during their history. If you ask, however, whether this problem was constant or not, obviously the patients are different than the controls. And if you ask if this is a major problem in daily life, then there is obviously a difference in patients from in controls. Even though controls may have these symptoms they certainly don't cause them a lot of trouble. This prospective analysis of these issues, obviously suggests patients are different from well people.

If one examines antibody levels, key issues are whether antibodies to EBV are elevated or are in any way peculiar in patients vs controls. Table 5 displays the analysis of the first year of the study. Antibodies to the early antigen (components that are produced

during replication) are detected by immunofluorescence in 2 patterns, a diffuse pattern in which you see these antigens expressed throughout the infected cell and a restricted pattern that is primarily nuclear. There are some interesting differences among the groups. First, that patients in group 1 had high early antigen antibody titers whereas group 4 had low anti-early antigen antibody titers reinforces the concept of patients selection for this study. The important things are the differences between the healthy controls and the family controls. Family controls, even though the number is somewhat small, had titers that were equivalent to the cases, suggesting that at least in those families there may be a genetic component in the magnitude of antibody response. Patients with IM had lower levels of the early antigen diffuse pattern, the components seen during active or reactivated infections, than did the

Figure 1B

Constant

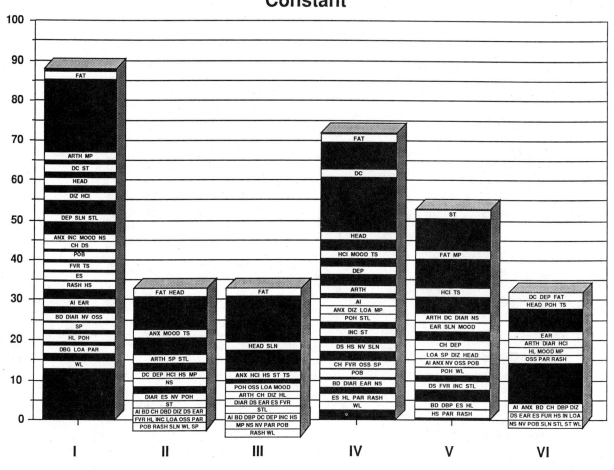

Table 6
Correlation Between Symptom Scores and Laboratory Values

Symptom	Group	anti-VCA		anti-EA-D		anti-EBNA
Depression	IV			0.0001*	0.80**	
Fatigue	IV			0.002	0.57	
Headache	IV			0.001	0.62	
Loss of thinking	IV			0.001	0.62	
Arthralgia	IV			0.002	0.56	
	I			0.03	0.043	
Myalgia	IV			0.003	0.54	
	V					0.01 0.65
Pain	V	0.03	0.53			

* p value   ** Pearson correlation coefficient

other controls. If one looks at the restricted components one sees that patients with an IM history have the highest titers, supporting previous observations[10]. These data suggest that with resolution of acute illness, patients make antibodies to the early antigen restricted, whereas with active disease you make antibodies to the diffuse components. The anti-viral capsid antigen and the anti-EBNA titers are not terribly informative. The magnitude of these responses are similar among the groups. Absence of anti-EBNA antibodies may be meaningful because approximately 15% of individuals with CFS do not make anti-EBNA[1]. If one looks at EBV antibody titers over time, the groups do not separate out in terms of anti-VCA or anti-EBNA but the anti-early antigen data may be important. However, we need to analyze more persons to see if that is the case.

Figure 1C

Major

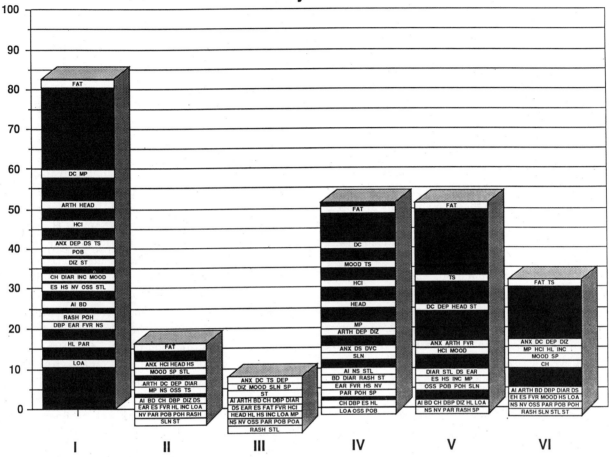

One thing that has been questioned throughout the recent resurrection of interest in these patients is the nature of relationships between antibody titer and disease activity. Table 6 compares an analysis of changes in anti-early antigen antibodies, anti-viral capsid antigen and anti-EBNA in a positive manner with positive increases in symptom scores. The patients recorded daily in a log the magnitude of symptoms on a 0-4 scale. In subjects in group 4, the group that did not have markedly elevated anti-EBV titers upon entry into the study, there is a high correlation between increase in depression, fatigue, headache, loss of thinking, arthralgia and myalgia, with an increase in symptoms to the anti-early antigen antibodies. These observations would support reactivation of an active infection in these persons.

One previous study that may have addressed CFS suggested that antibody titers to other viruses in this syndrome are also elevated[11]. If that hypothesis is true, there would have been increased titers in group 1 patients and group 4 patients vs groups 2 and 3, which contain the well controls (Table 7). If you look for antibodies against herpes simplex for example, you do not see that is the case. If you follow this all the way across there is no difference in the magnitude of antibody titers in these patients vs controls, except perhaps in the infectious mononucleosis control group, where anti-CMV titers are much lower.

Another component testing both the first and second postulates is spontaneous transformation. The test for spontaneous transformation is a variation on the theme of a screeing skin test. Although specific populations of effector cells or other mechanisms of inhibiting outgrowth phenomena are identified, it

Table 7							
Mean Antibody Titers (log$_2$) to Other Infectious Agents							
Group	(n)	HSV	VSV	CMV	Infl A	Adeno	*M. Pneu*
I	13	0.7	5.6	2.8	1.3	0.9	1.4
II	13	0.5	5.0	3.4	2.7	1.6	2.5
III	11	1.0	5.2	0.4	2.0	0	0.8
IV	8	0.6	5.7	2.6	1.4	0.2	0.6

tests immunity to EBV. In an open study in which we enrolled 250 patients vs 60 controls, there was a 30% transformation rate in these 250 patients and 3% in the controls. In the prospective study, (Table 7) peripheral blood cells underwent spontaneous transformation in 32% in group 1, and 27% in group 4, similar to the open population, whereas in persons who had no history of infectious mononucleosis we found 1 out of 18, or 5%, and 2 out of 18, or 11%, in those that had infectious mononucleosis, suggesting again a 30% transformation in patients versus 5-8% in controls[9]. There appears to be an abnormality in control or prevention of outgrowth in patients with symptoms.

Salivary excretion rate is measured by diluting saliva and adding it to cord blood lymphocytes. This method, which is the time honored approach for looking for excretion of this virus, showed slightly higher values in group 1 but very much the same throughout the entire study population. Twenty percent is the average excretion rate in the literature unless you undergo great care in identifying the target cells[12]. Using the polymerase chain reaction technique, we found about 40% presence of virus in saliva across all of the groups. Contrary to spontaneous transformation, these tests did not support differences among groups in testing populations.

We also compared natural killer cell activity across these groups, again with 2-4 specimens per person, and found no real differences in natural killer cell activity. If one compares spontaneous transformation to natural killer cell activity, there is no correlation between decreased or increased natural killer cell activity and the presence or absence of transformation either in patients or controls. Thus, this test of postulate 2 showed no differences among groups.

We also asked in these patients that do transform, whether or not viral genome patterns are different[9]. The overall pattern is that the viral genome patterns from patients are similar. In the Bam HI H portion of the gene some heterogeneity in the size of the fragments is present. Whether or not that is meaningful is not clear, but overall there is certainly no specific viral strain pattern associated in these patients. Another approach to determining whether there is active disease in the patients whose cells transform is identification of the form of the viral gene in the spontaneous cell lines. If the viral DNA is circular, the virus is in its latent state. If viral DNA is present in linear and circular form, the virus is capable of lytic replication and infection of new cells. We found that 19 persons in the open study and another 3 persons in the control study had virus in the lytic replication form. A number of patients have had multiple cultures in which the viral gene has been in linear form.

The presence of viral DNA in linear form in cell lines obtained from patients does not necessarily mean that these subjects were undergoing active infection. An additional approach is analysis of antibody production by an antibody test that identifies patterns of response directed against a number of viral proteins. When this test was applied to the patients that transformed, a number had antibody patterns that reflected active infection[9].

In terms of the third postulate, the paucity of group VI subjects precluded strict analysis of a genetic tendency toward higher antibody responses, but a trend was present. An additional finding, however, may be of more interest. Table 4 also displays the incidence of IgE-mediated allergy in these subjects.

It is apparent that symptomatic subjects (either CFS or infectious mononucleosis patients) were allergic more frequently than healthy, EBV seropositive persons who did not have a history of IM. The underlying immunological factor(s) that allow expression of allergy might, therefore, influence expression of CFS or symptomatic IM.

Summary

The preliminary data described here support the concept that differences in host response to EBV occur in patients with CFS versus control subjects.

These differences occur at the antibody level and at the cell-mediated immunity level, as well as at the clinical level. Whether these differences are associated with disease production, however, remains unclear. The data only partially support the hypothesis that clinical and laboratory findings in CFS are similar to those described during infectious mononucleosis. Equally important, the data open the question of a role of allergy in the production of CFS.

These issues must be addressed before testing of the fourth Koch-Evans postulate, that the whole thing makes sense, is possible.

References

1. Jones, J.F., Ray, C.G., Minnich, L.L., Hicks, M.J., Kibler, R., and Lucas, D.O. (1985). Evidence for active Epstein-Barr virus infection in patients with persistent, unexplained illnesses: Elevated anti-early antigen antibodies. Ann Int Med. 102:1-7.

2. Straus, S.E., Relapsing, recurrent and chronic infectious mononucleosis in the normal host., in Epstein-Barr Virus and Associated Diseases, P.H. Levine, et al., Editor. 1985, Martinus Nijhoff: Boston. p. 19-33.

3. Rickninson, A.B., On the biology of Epstein-Barr virus persistence: A reappraisal., in Immunobiology and Prophylaxis of Human Herpesvirus Infections, C. Lopez, et al., Editor. 1990, Plenum Press: New York. p. 137-146.

4. Henle, W., Henle, G., and Lennette, E.T. (1979). The Epstein-Barr virus. Sci. Am. 241:48-59.

5. Wallace, L.E., and Murray, R.J., Immunological aspects of the Epstein-Barr virus system., in Advances in Viral Oncology, G. Klein, Editor. 1989, Raven Press:New York. p. 219-236.

6. Miller, G., Epstein-Barr virus: Biology, pathogenesis and medical aspects., in Virology, B.N. Fields and D.M. Knipe, Editor. 1990, Raven Press: New York. p. 1921-1958.

7. Giller, R.H., and Grose, C. (1989). Epstein-Barr virus: The hematologic and oncologic consequences of virus-host interaction. Crit Rev Oncol Hematol. 9:149-195.

8. Adams, F., Quesada, J.R., and Gutterman, J.U. (1984). Neuropsychiatric manifestations of human leukocyte interferon therapy in patients with cancer. JAMA. 252:938-941.

9. Jones, J.F., Streib, J., Baker, S., and Herberger, M. (1991). Chronic fatigue syndrome: I. Epstein-Barr virus immune response and molecular epidemiology. J Med Virol. 33:151-158.

10. Horowitz, C.A., Henle, W., Henle, G., Rudnick, H., and Latts, E. (1985). Long-term serological follow up of patients for Epstein-Barr virus after recovery from infectious mononucleosis. J. Inf. Dis. 151:1150-1153.

11. Holmes, G.P., Kaplan, J.E., Stewart, J.A., Hunt, B., Pinsky, P.F., and Schonberger, L.B. (1987). A cluster of patients with a chronic mononucleosis-like syndrome. Is Epstein-Barr virus the cause? JAMA. 257:2297-2302.

12. Miller, G., Niederman, J.L., and Andrew, G. (1973). Prolonged oropharyngeal excretion of EB virus following infectious mononucleosis. N. Engl. J. Med. 288:229-232.

Chapter 27

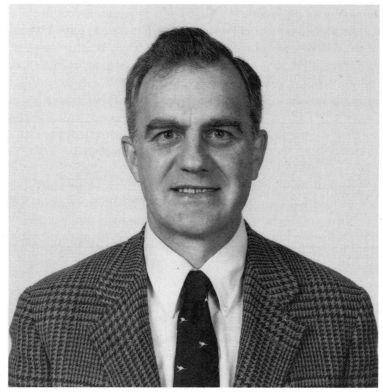

W. John Martin

Detection of Viral Related Sequences in CFS Patients Using the Polymerase Chain Reaction

W. John Martin M.D., Ph.D., Professor of Pathology, USC School of Medicine, Los Angeles California 90033

Dr. Martin received his medical training at the University of Sydney, Australia and his PhD at the Walter and Eliza Hall Institute, Melbourne, Australia. Dr. Martin is a pathologist with interest in the application of molecular technology to diagnostic medicine. He has helped pioneer the clinical use of the polymerase chain reaction for the detection of latent viral infection. Dr. Martin is the Chief of the Immunology / Molecular Pathology Unit of the LAC / USC Medical Centre. He is also Professor of Pathology at the USC School of Medicine.

Introduction

The chronic fatigue syndrome (CFS) refers to an illness characterized by unexplained fatigue lasting beyond 6 months which results in greater than 50% reduction in an individual's normal level of activity[1]. The pathophysiology of this illness is poorly understood with many conflicting theories and few substantiated facts. An exciting new technology, termed the polymerase chain reaction. (PCR), has recently become available to investigate whether some forms of this disease are associated with a persistent viral infection. This paper will provide a brief overview of the PCR technique and will describe some of the preliminary findings using PCR assays in CFS patients.

Polymerase Chain Reaction (PCR)

PCR refers to enzymatic amplification of a defined DNA sequence[2,3]. It requires the following reactants: target DNA containing the sequence to be amplified; oligonucleotide primers complementary to the flanking regions, on opposing DNA strands, of the particular segment of double stranded DNA to be replicated, DNA polymerase enzyme, deoxynucleotide triphosphates (dNTP) and buffer. The PCR is performed in a thermal cycling machine. PCR proceeds by denaturing the double stranded DNA molecule by heat; and cooling in the presence of the oligonucleotide primers. Because of their high concentration and greater mobility in solution, the primers bind more rapidly to the target DNA than the slower reannealing process exhibited by the larger complimentary DNA strands. The primer DNA complex provides a substrate for DNA polymerase. In the presence of dNTP, the polymerase will extend the primers in a DNA synthesis reaction. Each newly synthesized strand will be complimentary to the template DNA and will acquire at its 3' end, the sequence complimentary to the other primer used in the PCR. On reheating, the newly formed hybrids will denature, thereby providing two additional template molecules during the next primer annealing step. With each successive cycle of heating, primer annealing and primer extension, there will be an exponential increase in the targeted segment of DNA. Eventually, the reaction will become rate limiting due mainly to competition between primer binding and reannealing of the greatly amplified single DNA molecules synthesized during the PCR. In a typical reaction, however, amplification in the order of 106 fold can be achieved in form 25-30 cycles. The specifically amplified PCR product will be of uniform size corresponding to the distance separating the 5' ends of the two primer binding sites on the opposing strands of the target segment of DNA. It can be identified by electrophoresis in agarose gels and further characterized by a hybridization reaction using a labeled probe reactive with the amplified sequence.

PCR has been applied to the detection of an ever increasing number of human pathogens. Examples include; human papillomavirus[4], human immunodeficiency virus-1[5] and -2[6], human T lymphotrophic virus type I and type II[7], cytomegalovirus (CMV)[8], herpes simplex virus (HSV)[9], Epstein-Barr virus[10], human herpesvirus-6 (HHV-6)[11], hepatitis B virus[12], B16 parvovirus[13], JC and BK viruses[14], rubella virus[15], mycobacteria[16], Toxoplasmosis gondii[17], Trypanosoma cruzi[18], and malaria[19]. PCR can be applied to the detection of virtually any pathogen for which even limited DNA (or RNA) sequence information is known and in which a specimen of infected tissue can be readily obtained.

PCR assays can be positive in the absence of detectable antibody responses[20,21] PCR assays can also be more discriminative than conventional serology. Thus, most clinical serological reactions are directed against a mixture of antigenic epitopes which can be variously shared by closely related pathogens. Thus, for example, it is difficult to distinguish HIV-1 from HIV-2 or HTLV-I from HTLV-II by serology, yet such distinctions can be readily made on the basis of PCR amplifications of type specific genetic sequences[6,7]. Recently, PCR analysis has led to the detection of different strains of EBV[22], HBV[23] and of Plasmodium vivax malaria[19].

Conventional culture techniques have been established to more or less provide a broad screen for a range of microorganisms. In principle, PCR can also be used as an initial screen for major categories of pathogens. The primer sets required would need to be reactive with conserved regions of bacterial, viral or fungal genomes. Moreover, the PCR and subsequent hybridization reactions may need to be run at a lower than normal stringency. This approach is especially suited for the detection of new types of pathogens[24].

Application of PCR to CFS Patients

We were interested in applying the PCR to study patients diagnosed as having CFS. We initially chose primer sets reactive with a sequence contained in a recently described herpesvirus termed human herpesvirus-6. Two sets of primers were synthesized based on data kindly provided to us by Dr. S. Josephs working in Dr. Gallo's laboratory. Blood samples obtained from patients seen by Dr. Jay Goldstein were processed by simple lysis and proteinase K digestion. Following the PCR, the products were dot blotted onto a nylon membrane and probed with an oligonucleotide representing a region of the HHV-6 genome that would have been amplified. Blood from healthy donors rarely, (<1%), gave a discernable positive hybridization reaction following PCR amplification. With a known isolate of HHV-6, strong 3+ to 4+ responses were obtained. Furthermore, the HHV-6 amplified products were easily detectable on agarose electrophoresis and had the expected sizes as predicted from the regions of homology with the primer sets. We next examined over 100 blood samples from CFS patients. Detectable 1+ to 2+ responses were seen in only 3-5% of the patients tested in different assays. The PCR products from CFS patients were not easily visualized on agarose electrophoresis. The variability between assays reflected on the critical importance of the temperatures at which the PCR and subsequent hybridization steps were performed. By lowering the temperatures of primer annealing and primer extension and by performing hybridization at lower than normal stringency, we were able to obtain weak but detectable responses in up to 20% of CFS patients tested. Unfortunately, the reactivity of the positive samples appeared to deteriorate with storage, even at -20°C. The data were suggestive, but certainly not conclusive, that CFS patients may harbor a virus related to, but distinguishable from, HHV-6.

We next tested a set of PCR primers reactive with the late antigen of CMV[8] for potential cross-reactivity with all known human herpesviruses. Again under conditions of reduced stringency, CMV, EBV, HHV-6 and HSV gave a clearly discernible hybridization signal. Using similar PCR conditions, clinical testing was performed on normal individuals, CMV infected individuals, and CFS patients. While no responses were seen with the normal individuals, positive, but weak, responses were seen with a significant number of CFS patients (approximately 20-30% in different groups tested). The responses seen in CFS patients were far less impressive than those obtained in CMV infected individuals. Furthermore, none of the CFS patients gave positive PCR when tested with a second set of primers reactive with sequences within the immediate-early (I-E) gene of CMV[8]. There was also a lack of reactivity with a set of EBV specific primers or with HHV-6 primers run under highly stringent conditions.

Although, the PCR findings distinguished CFS patients, as a group, from normal individuals, and possibly distinguished some CFS patients from others, the data were difficult to interpret. If the detectable sequences are of CMV, EBV or HHV-6 origin, the data would suggest that the virus is incomplete and only partially represented. More likely, the data reflect a new virus with partial DNA sequence homology with herpesviruses. The low stringency conditions used would allow cross-priming to distantly related viral and even normal cellular DNA sequences. Analyses of agarose gels confirmed that cross-priming was occurring since multiple diffuse bands were seen with DNA from both normal individuals and CFS patients. Even though there was no hybridization to amplified products from normal DNA, the results in the CFS patients could not be confidently ascribed to a specific type of virus.

An ongoing study has provided support for the view that some CFS patients may have a persistent neurological infection with an atypical virus. A patient with dysphasia, dyspraxia and an MRI scan showing periventricular lesions, recently underwent a stereotactic brain biopsy to exclude lymphoma. Instead, the biopsy showed mild gliosis associated with demyelination. On electron microscopy, enveloped viral particles were seen. The findings with PCR have closely approximated those seen with the CFS patients. Thus, a positive but weak response occurred with the HHV-6 and the cross-reactive CMV reactive primer sets when tested on the brain biopsy sample and on the CSF from this patient. Interestingly, all of the routine chemistries on the CSF, including testing for myelin basic protein, were normal. Attempts to further characterize this neurotropic, virus are in progress.

Discussion

The PCR technology represents a major breakthrough in efforts to detect persistent viral infections. Highly specific assays can be performed providing the exact DNA or RNA sequence is known. The stringency, and, therefore, the specificity of the assay has to be compromised when one is searching for an unknown virus using primer sets matched for a known virus. The logical progression is to amplify a product using the cross-reactive primer set; sequence the amplified product; and synthesize perfectly matched primer sets based upon the sequence data.

The preliminary results suggest that the first goal has been achieved. The PCR assay has also provided evidence for neurological disease associated with a persistent atypical viral infection. Clinically, one can distinguish two major sub-groups of CFS patients on the basis of whether the patient has neurological evidence for a thought-processing (cognitive) disorder. Patients with this form of CFS often complain of dysphasia and dyspraxia and have an impediment of short term memory. They appear to have a defect in processing and in expressing higher intellectual functions. Fatigue in these patients may be less prominent and, certainly is less distressing, than the neurological defect. This type of illness may often have an acute onset and follow a fluctuating clinical course. The other broad category of disease manifestation is primarily one of a "rapid draining of energy". It may have features in common with fibromyalgia. Although there may be an acute origin, some of these patients have a life-long pattern of illness. As the PCR technology becomes increasingly applied to CFS patients, it should be possible to test the validity of this distinction and determine if it is based on the type and location of a persistent viral infection.

Acknowledgement:

I wish to thank Dr. Jay Goldstein for allowing me to test some of his patients. I also wish to thank Dr. Rick George, Peymon Javaherbin, Jeanette Santiago, Victor Ramirez, Keith Callahan and Anton Mayr for helping to process blood samples and in establishing the PCR assay for HHV-6. The work was supported by a grant from DiaTech (Cooperative Agreement DPE-5935-A00-5065-00 between the Program for Appropriate Technology in Health and the U.S. Agency for International Development).

References

1. Holmes GP, Kaplan JE, Grantz NM, et.al. Chronic fatigue syndrome: A working case definition. Ann Intern Med 1988; 108:387-389.

2. Mullis KB, Faloona FA Specific synthesis of DNA in vitro via a polymerase catalysed chain reaction. Meth Enzymol 1987; 255:335-350.

3. Saiki RK, Gelfand DH, Stoffel S, et al. Primer directed enzymatic amplification of DNA with a thermostable DNA polymerase. Science 1987; 239:487-491.

4. Shibata D, Arnheim N, Martin WJ. Detection of human papillomavirus in paraffin embedded tissue using the polymerase chain reaction. J Exp Med 1988; 158:225-230.

5. Hufert FT, Laer Dv, Schramm C, et al. Detection of HIV-1 DNA in different subsets of human peripheral blood mononuclear cells using the polymerase chain reaction. Arch Virol 1989; 106:341-345.

6. Rayfield M, Cock KD, Heyward W, et al. Mixed human immunodeficiency virus (HIV) infection in an individual: Demonstration of both HIV type 1 and type 2 proviral sequences by using polymerase chain reaction. J Infect Dis 1988;158:1170-1176.

7. Ehrlich GD, Glaser JB, LaVigne K, et al. Prevalence of human T-cell leukemia/lymphoma virus (HTLV) Type II infection among high-risk individuals: Type specific identification of HTLVs by polymerase chain reaction. Blood 1989;74:1658-1664.

8. Shibata D, Martin WJ, Appleman MD, et al. Detection of cytomegaloviral DNA in peripheral blood of patients infected with human immunodeficiency virus. J Infect Dis 1988;158:1185-1192.

9. Boerman RH, Arnoldus FR, Raap AK, et al. Polymerase chain reaction and viral culture techniques to detect HSV in small volumes of cerebrospinal fluid, an experimental mouse encephalitis study. J Virol Meth 1989;25:189-197.

10. Saito I, Servenius B, Compton T, et al. Detection of Epstein Barr virus by polymerase chain reaction in blood and tissue biopsies from patients with Sjogern's syndrome. J Exp Med 1989;169:2191-2197.

11. Bushbinder A, Josephs SF, Ablashi D, et al. Polymerase chain reaction amplification and in situ hybridization for the detection of human B-lymphotropic virus. J Virol Meth 1988;21:191-197.

12. Kaneko S, Feinstone SM, Miller RH. Rapid and sensitive method for the detection of serum hepatitis B virus DNA using the polymerase chain technique. J Clin Microbiol 1989;27:1930-1933.

13. Salimans MM, van de Ryke FM, Raap AK, et al. Detection of parvovirus B19 DNA in fetal tissue by in situ hybridization and polymerase chain reaction. J Clin Path 1989;42:525-529.

14. Arthur RR, Dogostin S, Shah KV. Detection of BK virus and JC virus in urine and brain tissue by the polymerase chain reaction. J Clin Microbiol 1989;27:1174-1179.

15. Carman WF, Williamson C, Cunliffe BA, et al. Reverse transcription and subsequent DNA amplification of rubella virus RNA. J Virol Meth 1989;25:21-29.

16. Hance AJ, Grandchamp B, Levy-Frebault V, et al. Detection and identification of mycobacteria by amplification of mycobacterial DNA. Mol Microbiol 1989;3:843-849.

17. Burg JL, Grover CM, Pouletty P, et al. Direct and sensitive detection of a pathogenic protozan, Toxoplasma gondii, by polymerase chain reaction. J Clin Microbiol 1989;27:1787-1792.

18. Moser Dr, Kirchhoff LV, Donelson JE. Detection of Trypanosoma cruzi by DNA amplification using the polymerase reaction. J Clin Microbiol 1989;27:1477-1482.

19. Rosenberg R, Wirtz RA, Lanar DE, et al. Circumsporozoite protein heterogeneity in the human malaria parasite **Plasmodium vivax**. Science 1989;245:973-976.

20. Farzadegan H, Polis M, Wolinsky SM, et al. Loss of human immunodeficiency type I (HIV-1) antibodies with evidence of viral infection in asymptomatic homosexual men. Ann Int Med 1988;108:785- 790.

21. Thiers V, Nakajima E, Kremsdorf D et al. Transmission of hepatitis B from hepatitis-B-seronegative subjects. Lancet 1988;ii:1273-1276.

22. Sixbey JW, Shirley P, Chesney PJ, et al. Detection of a second widespread strain of Epstein-Barr virus. Lancet 1989;ii:761-765.

23. Carman WF, Jacyna MR, Hadziyannis S, et al. Mutation preventing formation of hepatitis B e antigen in patients with chronic hepatitis B infection. Lancet 1989;ii:588-590.

24. Mach DH, Sninsky JJ. A sensitive method for the identification of uncharacterized viruses related to known virus groups: Hepadnavirus model system. Proc Nat Acad Sci USA 1988;85:6977-6981.

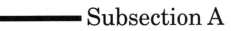

The Enteroviral Theories

Chapter 28

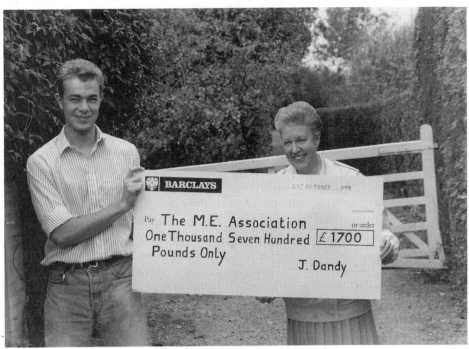

Betty Dowsett

This paper is reprinted with the kind permission of The Macmillan Press, Dowsett et al., Postgraduate Medical Journal, 1990, 66, 526-530.

Myalgic Encephalomyelitis (M.E.) - A Persistent Enteroviral Infection?

E.G. Dowsett[1], A.M. Ramsay[2], R.A. McCartney[3] and E.J. Bell[3]

1 Basildon and Thurrock Health Authority, Basildon Hospital Essex, 2 Royal Free Hospital, London and
3 Enterovirus Reference Laboratory, Regional Virus Laboratory, Ruchill Hospital, Glasgow, UK

Dr. Dowsett graduated in Medicine at Edinburgh University and, after several years in General Practice, went on to study Microbiology, Immunology and Virology at the London School of Hygiene and Tropical Medicine, Chelsea Polytechnic and Ewoll Technical College, Surrey. She was appointed Consultant Microbiologist to the Harrisgey group of hospitals, London in 1967 and to the Basildon/Murrock Area Health Authority, Essex in 1973. For 25 years she has combined her interests in hospital infections and epidemiology with providing an open access clinic in infectious diseases for General Practitioners and Hospital colleagues, during the course of which she has investigated several local epidemics of Myalgic Encephalomyelitis. Her collaborations with Dr. Ramsay began in 1976 and, at the time of his death, they were engaged in a joint study of 436 patients who had suffered from this illness for more than 10 years. Dr. Dowsett was elected President of the M.E. Association in succession to Dr. Ramsay and, in addition to her clinical work, chairs a working party on young people (25 years and under) with M.E., and coordinates a support group for M.E. patients. This is a collaborative study with the "Neuro carc" project pioneered by Dr. L. J. Findley, consultant Neurologist at the Regional Neurology Centre, Harold Wood and Oldchurch Hospitals, Essex.

(Please see Chapter 7 for Dr. Ramsay's photograph and curriculum vitae.)

Summary:

Myalgic encephalomyelitis is a common disability but frequently misinterpreted. Amongst 6,000 patients referred for general microbiological diagnosis between 1975 and 1987, 420 cases were recognized. Coxsackie B neutralization tests, in 205 of these, demonstrated significant titres in 103/205 (50%), while of 124 additionally investigated for enteroviral IgM, 38/124 (31%) were positive. This illness is distinguished from a variety of other post-viral states by an unique clinical and epidemiological pattern characteristic of enteroviral infection. Prompt recognition and advice to avoid over-exertion is mandatory. Routine diagnosis, specific therapy and prevention, await further technical advances.

Introduction

Since 1934, myalgic encephalomyelitis (M.E.) has been increasingly reported from socially developed countries and temperate regions of the world. Endemic prevalence alternates with periodic epidemics, showing a curious predilection for female staff of health care and teaching institutions.[1] Maximum incidence in both sexes occurs in the third decade. M.E. is a multisystem syndrome including nervous, cardiovascular, endocrine and other involvement, distinguished by severe muscle fatigue following trivial exertion. Other characteristics include high morbidity, low mortality, a prolonged relapsing course and variation in intensity of symptoms within and between episodes, tending to chronicity.[2,3] Conventional technology is limited in demonstrating abnormalities and this has hitherto permitted misinterpretation of the symptoms as psychogenic.[4,5] Historically, a marked similarity to non-paralytic poliomyelitis in respect of prodrome, seasonal and geographical incidence[1-3] caused diagnostic confusion. The return of a local family from holiday with a poliomyelitis-like illness (of whom 3 subsequently developed M.E.), prompted collaboration between the authors.

Patient selection

We adopted the following clinical criteria for investigation of M.E.: a syndrome commonly initiated by respiratory and/or gastro-intestinal infection but an insidious or more dramatic onset following neurological, cardiac or endocrine disability occurs. The pathognomonic features are: a complaint of general or local muscular fatigue following minimal exertion with prolonged recovery time; neurological disturbance, especially of cognitive, autonomic and sensory functions; variable involvement of cardiac and other systems; a prolonged relapsing course. Four hundred and twenty patients, fulfilling these criteria, were selected for further investigation amongst 6,000 patients with heterogeneous infections referred to one of us (EGD) between 1975 and 1987. Patients with M.E. comprised approximately 7% per annum of all who attended; 324/420 (77%) were referred from general practice and 96/420 (23%) from other hospital specialities in Essex and South London, including cardiology, endocrinology, neurology and psychiatry.

Clinical investigation

To elicit the essential features of this multisystem syndrome and ensure a comparable history, examination, and investigation for selected patients, a detailed questionnaire was devised with a scoring system weighted for the above diagnostic criteria. When tested on normal adults and clinic patients with other chronic diseases, none achieved scores in the M.E. range. Cognitive disturbances in patients with M.E. were readily elicited by failure to complete the questionnaire without assistance. Muscular fatigue was demonstrated by repeated activity such as weight raising on a block or climbing several flights of stairs, and myalgic foci by careful palpation of affected muscles with the finger tip. Standard methods were used to elicit other clinical signs.

Laboratory investigation

Tests included: routine haematological and biochemical screening; Paul Bunnell, Monospot or Epstein-Barr virus (EBV) IgM; rheumatoid factor, liver and cardiac enzymes, thyroid function, blood glucose; bacterial and viral culture; serological tests for streptococcal infection, brucellosis, toxoplasmosis, legionella, hepatitis A and B, cytomegalovirus, rubella, respiratory syncytial virus and parvovirus. Specialist technology was introduced as it became available but did not include EBV reactivation.

Coxsackie B virus (CBV) serology

Neutralizing tests (NT) to CBV1-5 were estimated using the Microlitre method described elsewhere.[6] Titres of 512 and above were regarded as indicative and of 256 as suggestive, of recent CBV infection. After 1985, only sera positive by the μ antibody capture ELISA technique were tested by NT.

Immunology

Tests for immune complexes were performed as described elsewhere[8] and autoimmune screening by standard immunofluorescence methods.

Results

Epidemiological characteristics

Age, sex, occupation : Of 420 patients with M.E., 307 (73%) were female and 113 (27%) male. The average age at onset was 32.3 years (range 7-64 years):

Patients with M.E. seen	Profession	Non M.E. patients seen
172 (41%)	health care or teaching	4%
109 (26%)	clerical, administrative or other professional posts	21%
88 (21%)	skilled or unskilled manual occupations	12%
51 (12%)	not gainfully employed, including children, pensioners, housewives	63%

See Table 1.

Season and type of prodromal illness :   A distinct prodrome occurred in 340/420 (81%) patients:
-characterized by a respiratory/gastrointestinal or 'flu-like illness in 277/340 (81%)
- lymphadenopathy and summer/autumn onset in 218/340 (64%).

Alternative prodromal presentations in 63/340 (19%) included:
- acute neurological
- visual or psychotic episodes
- myo/pericarditis
- pleurodynia
- exanthems
- enanthems
- thyroiditis
- orchitis
- mesenteric adenitis.

The remaining patients, 80/420 (19%) described an insidious onset, 105/340 (31%) reported a similar illness in family or occupational contacts not invariably followed by M.E.

In eleven families, an incubation period of 2 - 5 days for the prodrome was noted, but subsequent recognition of M.E. varied from a few days to 6 months.

Table 1			
Age at onset of M.E.			
Age group	Males	Females	Total
< 10 years	3	12	15 (3.5%)
11 - 15	5	14	19 (4.5%)
16-20	15	40	55 (13%)
21-25	12	26	38 (9%)
26-30	8	30	38 (9%)
31-35	22	58	80 (19%)
36-40	20	56	76 (18%)
41-45	13	33	46 (11%)
46-50	6	15	21 (5%)
51-55	3	9	12 (3%)
56-60	4	10	14 (3.5%)
> 60 years	2	4	6 (1.5%)
Total	113	307	420

Clinical characteristics

Duration of illness at first attendance of 420 patients:

Less than 12 months in 38 patients (9%)
1-2 years in 139 (32%)
3-10 years in 198 (47%)
11-20 years in 33 (8%)
21-60 years in 17 (4%)

Severity of illness:
improving in 130 (31%)
fluctuating in 84 (20%)
a steady level of disability in 105 (25%)
no remission or worse in 101 (24%).

Symptoms and signs   (Table 2) Symptomatology in M.E. is characteristically varied between age groups and episodes. Our study includes a number of families followed up from the prodromal illness, when the nature and frequency of symptoms may differ greatly from those recorded in individuals who subsequently develop M.E.

Relapse of M.E. :   Known precipitants included

physical and mental stress in all 420 patients (100%),
intercurrent infection in 176 (42%),
climatic change or hot baths in 50 (12%),
surgery, immunization, hormonal disturbance in
38 (9%),
psychoactive, antiarthritic or steroid drugs in 21 (5%).

Laboratory results

Haematology and biochemistry

Screening tests were normal with the following exceptions: 55/420 (13%) had leucocyte counts below normal range (3,500 x 10^9/1) with occasional atypical lymphocytes and 22/420 (5%), abnormal liver function tests, of whom two had hepatitis A. Two further patients had undiagnosed persistant hyperbilirubinaemia.

CBV serology

The sera of 205 patients with diagnostic features of M.E. seen before 1985, were tested by NT: 68/205 (33%) had titres indicative and 35/205 (17%) suggestive of recent CBV infection. Subsequently, 124 patients were additionally tested by the enteroviral IgM ELISA system. Applying the diagnostic criteria established by McCartney et al.,[7] 38/124 (31%) had evidence of recent/active enteroviral infection. Sixteen patients in our study, who were retested annually for three years, showed persistently raised CBV NTs and intermittently positive enteroviral IgM .

Other viral investigations

Inter current viral infections occurred in 12 patients with positive enteroviral serology (not serological cross reactions). EBV IgM was positive in three patients; hepatitis A, respiratory syncytial virus and parvovirus in two cases each; influenza B, varicella, rubella, one case each.

Immunology

128/276 (46%) of patients tested had evidence of circulating immune complexes, but only 15/420 (4%), antinuclear, thyroid or muscle antibodies.

Discussion

Differentiation of the M.E. syndrome from other forms of post-viral debility

Table 2		
Symptoms and signs in 420 patients with M.E.		
Commonly found (> 50%)	*No.*	*%*
Muscle fatigue	420	100
Emotional lability†	411	98
Myalgia††	336	80
Cognitive disturbance†††	323	77
Headache	310	74
Giddiness, disequelibrium	302	72
Autonomic dysfunction††††	289	69
Auditory disturbances*	289	69
Reversal of sleep rhythm	268	64
Visual disturbances**	260	62
Parasthaesia, hypo &hyperasthaesia	256	61
Intercostal myalgia/weakness	247	59
Fasciculation, spasm, myoclonus	239	57
Clumsiness***	235	56
Less commonly found(<50%)	*No.*	*%*
Gastrointestinal symptom****	205	49
Disturbance of micturition§	160	38
Recurrent lymphadenopathy§§	152	36
Arthralgia	118	28
Orthostatic tachycardia	88	21
Recurrent abacterial conjunctivitis	68	16
Orchitis/prostatism in young males	15/113	13
Seronegative polyarthritis	42	10
Vasculitic skin lesions	42	10
Myo/pericarditis	34	8
Positive Romberg sign	25	6
Thyroiditis in female patients	15/307	5
mesenteric adenitis§§§	5	1
Paresis and muscle wasting	3	1

†Includes frustration, elation, depression; ††characteristically affects limbs, shoulder girdle, spinal muscles; †††memory, concentration, anomia, dyslexia; ††††especially circulation and thermoregulation; *hyperacusis, deafness, tinnitus; **mainly loss of accomodation, photophobia, nystagmus; ***usually due to impaired spatial discrimination; ****nausea/disturbance of intestinal motility; §frequency incontinence, retention; §§enlargement, recurrent after prodrome.; §§§surgical intervention for abdominal pain.

In our opinion, two major errors are responsible for the present confusion surrounding the case definition, aetiology and diagnosis of M.E.[9] First, there has been a failure to distinguish the syndrome from postviral debility following Epstein-Barr mononucleosis, influenza and other common fevers. Compared with M.E., these lack the dramatic effect of exercise upon muscle function, the multi-system involvement, diurnal variability of symptoms and prolonged relapsing course. Laboratory tests can distinguish chronic mononucleosis[10] and other infections which, as our results show, may occasionally co-exist with M.E. and, by their immunosuppressive effect, precipitate relapse. Second, there has been a failure to recognize the unique epidemiological pattern of M.E., which, from earliest accounts, has lead to confusion with non-paralytic poliomyelitis.

The epidemiological features of M.E. require explanation

Polio viruses (Types 1 - 3) are the best known examples of a group of 69 enteroviruses which, by faecal/oral spread, commonly lead to asymptomatic childhood infection. The epidemiology of poliomyelitis remained enigmatic until virus isolation from carriers demonstrated the link between paralytic cases. In 1948, the non-polio enteroviruses (NPEV) were shown to be causative agents of illness previously designated as 'non-paralytic poliomyelitis'. Reports of NPEV isolation from individual cases[1,2,11] or serological evidence of NPEV infection[5,12,13] occur in many published accounts of M.E. Our study also supports association of the M.E. syndrome with NPEV. Thirty three per cent of 205 patients tested had CBV NTs indicative of infection - a figure comparable with that for enterovirus - associated myocarditis.[14] Seasonal distortion was excluded by the observation that 37/75 (49%) of those attending in Winter and Spring had significant CBV NT compared with 66/130 (51%) of those attending in Summer and Autumn. Moreover, 31 % of our patients tested had positive enteroviral IgM tests compared with 12% of normal blood donors tested simultaneously in South London by the same technique.[15]

The geographical epidemiology of enteroviral infection depends entirely upon the interaction of climate and hygiene. Virtually all children born in hyperendemic tropical areas lacking sanitation, acquire immunity in early life.   Conversely, many adults in temperate zones with seasonal and hygienic limitation of enterovirus circulation, lack immunity. Post-pubertal infections tend to be severe and lead (as in poliomyelitis) to the paradox of overt adult infection and epidemics in affluent societies with cool climates. It is only in these geographical areas that

epidemic M.E. has been described. Sixty four per cent of our patients with a prodrome reported Summer/Autumn onset, while in 34/420 (8%), travel to an endemic area at any season was an antecedent factor. The peak incidence of M.E. is in the third decade and Table 1 indicates that a minority of our patients developed M.E. before puberty or after 45 years (when a less hygienic childhood may have afforded natural immunity). In this country, asymptomatic children, especially when diapered, are the main dispersers of infection. Male infants are more susceptible than female and possibly acquire earlier immunity. These factors do much to explain the sex ratio of M.E., the earlier onset and higher incidence in women (Table 1), the secondary cases in family and school contacts and the curious predisposition of health care and teaching staff.

Multi-system clinical involvement in patients with M.E.

Most enteroviral infections are biphasic. A non-specific prodromal illness precedes, by an interval, infection of target organs. Host factors, such as age, physical and mental stress, climatic change, hormones, immunosuppression, anti-inflammatory drugs, surgery and immunization, contribute to this outcome.[16] The onset of illness and relapse in our patients was significantly associated with similar events. Enteroviruses exhibit an extensive cell tropism. Symptoms are protean within the family and community, depending upon the age and susceptibility of the host as well as the strain and virulence of the virus. Enteroviral syndromes which range from trivial to severe, include: respiratory, gastrointestinal, muscular and neurological infections, exanthems, enanthems, conjunctivitis, arthritis, diseases of endocrine and lymphatic glands. All of these are encountered in the prodrome of M.E. In Autumn 1976, at the beginning of our survey, 488/814 (60%) of all viruses associated with neurological manifestations notified to the Public Health Laboratory Service, were identified as NPEVs.[17] This could well explain the common neurological and encephalitic features of M.E. The psychological disturbances in our patients differed from classical depression in that all but three patients had a normal premorbid personality, volition was preserved, weight and appetite disturbance minimal and treatment with antidepressant drugs ineffectual in 123/420 (29%) of patients in whom it had been tried. Moreover, neurophysiological research using cognitive event-related potentials has shown prolonged latencies in M.E. - an abnormality *not* present in patients with depression.[18]

Exercise related morbidity in M.E.

Coxsackie viruses are characteristically myotropic and enteroviral genomic sequences have been detected in muscle biopsies from patients with M.E.[19] Exercise related abnormalities of function have been demonstrated by nuclear magnetic resonance[20] and single fibre electro-myography[21] including a failure to coordinate oxidative metabolism with anaerobic glycolysis causing abnormally early intracellular acidosis, consistent with the early fatiguability and the slow recovery from exercise in M.E.

Coxsackie viruses can initiate non-cytolytic persistent infection in human cells.[22] Animal models demonstrate similar enteroviral persistence in neurological disease,[23] myopericarditis[24] and the deleterious effect of forced exercise on persistently infected muscles.[25] These studies elucidate the exercise-related morbidity and the chronic relapsing nature of M.E.

Diagnostic pitfalls in enterovirology

A symptomatic enteroviral carriage is common (it is the rationale for oral polio vaccine) and caution is required in the interpretation of conventional laboratory tests or case/control studies. Virus isolation (unless from a sequestered site) may lack significance and the difficulty is compounded by an early and abundant neutralizing response. Acid dissociation of the virus from neutralizing antibody has been

used to permit direct culture and the production of a monoclonal antibody (5 D 8/1), directed against a viral protein component (VPI) exclusive to enteroviruses, has demonstrated persistent bowel infection leading to systemic disease with VPI antigen, free or bound to antibody, in the circulation of patients with M.E.[8] Of 40 patients in our study referred for VPI testing, 20 had positive results.

Conclusions

Clinical, laboratory, and epidemiological data support the suggestion that M.E. is a complication in non-immune individuals of widespread subclinical NPEV infection.

M.E. predominantly affects the most socially and economically active section of society. Misinterpretation of this common illness as psychogenic delays the early recognition mandatory for modification of life style which may avoid progression to chronic disability. Other forms of therapy are disappointing.[26] Despite the use of prophylactic anti-enteroviral drugs in animal research[27] the control of enteroviral infection in humans still depends upon immunization and measures to improve public hygiene.[28]

Acknowledgements

We should like to thank Dr. Morgan Capner, Kings College Hospital, Professor J. E. Banatvala, St. Thomas's Hospital, and Dr. D.A. Gamble, Epsom Public Health Laboratory for assistance with some CBV tests. We are indebted to Dr. D. Bainbridge, The London Hospital and Professor J.F. Mowbray, St. Mary's Hospital for all the immunological studies.

References

1. Acheson, E.D. The clinical syndrome variously called benign myalgic encephalomyelitis, Iceland Disease and epidemic myasthenia. Am J Med 1959, 26: 569- 595.

2. Behan, P.O. & Behan, W.M.H. Postviral fatigue syndrome. CRC Crit Rev Neurobiol 1988, 4: 157- 178.

3. Ramsay, A.M. Post viral fatigue syndrome. - The Saga of the Royal Free Disease, London. Gower Medical Publishing, 1986 (M.E. Association, P.O. Box 8, Stanford le Hope, Essex SS 17 8EX).

4. McEvedy, C.P. & Beard, A.W. Royal Free Disease Epidemic of 1955 - a reconsideration. Br Med J 1970 1: 7 - 11.

5. Winbow, A. Myalgic encephalomyelitis presenting as a psychiatric illness. Br J Clin Soc Psych vol 1986, 4: 30- 31.

6. Bell, E.J. & McCartney, R.A. Study of Coxsackie B virus infections 1972-1983. J Hyg Camb 1984, 93: 197-203.

7. McCartney, R.A., Banatvala, J.E. & Bell, E.J. Routine use of (L antibody-capture ELISA for the serological diagnosis of Coxsackie B virus infections. J Med Virol 1986,19:205-212.

8. Yousef, G.E., Bell, E.J., Mann, G.F. et al. Chronic enterovirus infection in patients with post viral fatigue syndrome. Lancet 1988, i: 146- 149

9. David, A., Wessley, S. & Pelosi, A.J. Post viral fatigue syndrome - time for a new approach. Br Med J 1988, 1: 696-698.

10. Hotchin, N.A., Read, R., Smith, D.G. & Crawford, D.H. Active Epstein-Barr virus infection in post viral fatigue syndrome. J Infect 1989, 18: 143 - 150.

11. Lyle, W.H. An outbreak of disease believed to have been caused by an Echo 9 virus. Ann Intern Med 1959, 51: 248 - 269.

12. Keighley, B.D. & Bell, E.J. Sporadic myalgic encephalomyelitis in a rural practice. J R Co U Gen Pract 1983, 33: 339-341.

13. Calder, B.D., Warnock, P.J., McCartney, R.A. & Bell, E.J. Coxsackie B viruses and the post viral syndrome - a prospective study in general practice. J R Cog Gen Pract 198 7, 37: 11 - 14.

14. Bell, E.J., Irvine, K.G., Gardiner, A.J.S. & Rodger, J.C. Coxsackie B infection in a general medical unit. Scott Med J 1983, 28: 157-159

15. Muir, P., Tilzey, A.J., English, T.A.H., Nicholson, F., Signy, M. & Banatvala, J.E. Chronic relapsing pericarditis and dilated cardiomyopathy: serological evidence of persistent enterovirus infection. Lancet 1989, i: 804-807.

16. Loria, R.M. Host conditions affecting the course of Coxsackievirus infections. In: Bendinelli, M. and Friedman, H. (eds). Coxsackieviruses. A General Update. Plenum Press, New York and London, 1988, pp. 135-157.

17. Epidemiological Research Laboratory PHLS - Viruses associated with neurological manifestations. Communicable Disease Report, 1976: No. 48, page 1.

18. Prasher, D., Smith, A. & Findley, L. Sensory and cognitive event - related potentials in myalgic encephalomyelitis. J Neurol Neurosurg Psychiatry, 1990, 53: 247 - 253.

19. Archard, L.C., Bowies, N.E., Behan, P.O., Bell, E.J. & Doyle, D. Post viral fatigue syndrome; persistence of enterovirus RNA in muscle and elevated creatine kinase. J R Soc Med 1988, 6: 326-329.

20. Arnold, D.L., Radda, G.K., Bore, P.J. & Styles, P. Excessive intracellular acidosis of skeletal muscle on exercise in a patient with post viral exhaustion/fatigue syndrome. Lancet 1984, i: 1367 - 1369.

21. Jamal, G.A. & Hansen, S. Electrophysiological studies in the post viral fatigue syndrome. J Neurol Neurosurg Psychiatry 1985, 48: 691 -694.

22. Matteucci, D., Paglianti, F., Giangregorio, A.M., Capobianchi, M.R., Dianzani, F. & Bendinelli, M. Group B Coxsackie viruses readily establish persistent infections in human lymphoid cell lines. J Virol 1985, 56: 651 - 654.

23. Miller, J.R. Prolonged intra cerebral infection with polio virus in asymptomatic mice. Ann Neurol 1981, 9: 590- 596.

24. Banatvala, J.E. Coxsackie B viral infections in cardiac disease. In: Waterson, A. P. (ed.) Clinical Virology, Churchill-Livingstone, Edinburgh, London 1983.

25. Reyes, M.P. & Lerner, A.M. Myocarditis. Clinical and experimental correlates. In: Bendinelli, M. and Friedman, H. (eds) Coxsackiesviruses. A General Update. Plenum Press, New York, London, 1988, pp. 253 - 270.

26. Vallings, R. Myalgic encephalomyelitis - a consideration of treatment. The New Zealand Family Physician 1989, 16: 9-13.

27. McKinlay, M.A., Frank, J.A. Jr., Benziger, D.P.&Steinberg, B.A. Use of WIN 51711 to prevent Echo virus type 9 induced paralysis in suckling mice. J Infect Dis 1986, 154: 678 - 681.

28. Dowsett, E.G. Human enteroviral infections. J Hosp Infect 1988, 11: 103-115.

Chapter 29

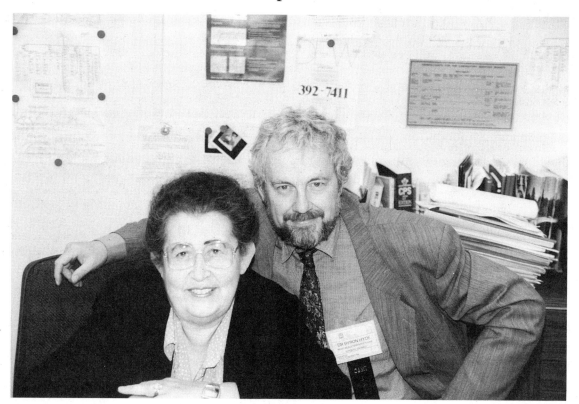

Bernadette McLaughlin with Byron Hyde

This article is reprinted with the kind permission of Health and Welfare Canada, Proceedings of a Workshop, January 1991, Vol 17S1E, pages 51-55.

Virology Laboratory Diagnosis of Chronic Fatigue Syndrome

B. McLaughlin, MD
Laboratory Services Branch, Ontario Ministry of Health,
Box 9000, Terminal A, Toronto, Ontario M5W 1R5 Canada

The Virology Laboratory of the Laboratory Services Branch, Ontario Ministry of Health, is in a somewhat unique position. The facility is a large laboratory providing services to a province of 9,500,000 inhabitants. It is the only virology laboratory except for six teaching hospitals, which test mostly their own patients, and one of only two laboratories testing for Epstein-Barr virus (EBV).

As previous speakers have discussed virology laboratory findings of different viruses in chronic fatigue syndrome (CFS), to avoid repetition, I will look at our global numbers and at the trends we have observed in our population over the last 9 years. Data on 2 types of viruses, EBV and enteroviruses, will be reviewed.

Epstein-Barr Virus (EBV)

Tests done in the last 9 years show a steady increase in demand for EBV testing (Table 1), with a cumulative total of 138,646 specimens. These vary with the age of the population tested and significant titres vary with the laboratory doing the test. We use a standard immunofluorescence technique, with a commercial kit for viral capsid antigen (VCA)-IgG, and prepare our own slides for the other markers. Viral capsid antigen-IgG is assayed at dilutions 1/80 to 1/640 (in children, the starting dilution is 1/20). Early antigen (EA) (R&D) are screened at dilution 1/40, as this is the dilution at which we found clinical and statistical differences.

Figure 1

EBV Serology: Nine-Year Period
(138,646 specimens)

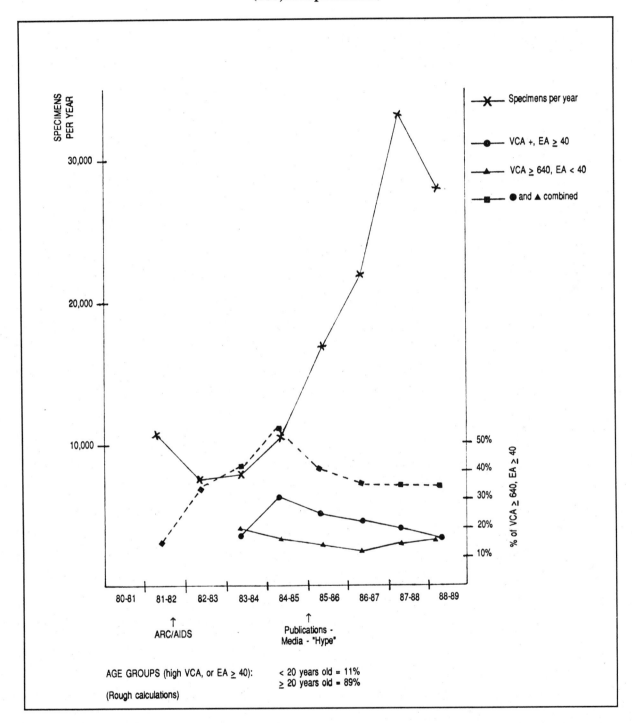

Roughly 80% of the tests we receive are from adults, and more than 99% of adults over 39 years of age are VCA-IgG positive. For this reason the tests chosen for adults are VCA-IgG and EA (EBNA) and VCA Immunoglobulin M (IgM) are done mostly in children and teenagers, where primary infections are suspected.

Figure 2

**Enteroviruses Isolation and Serologic Diagnostic Results
(3,225 viruses) Over Nine Years from Ontario Patients**

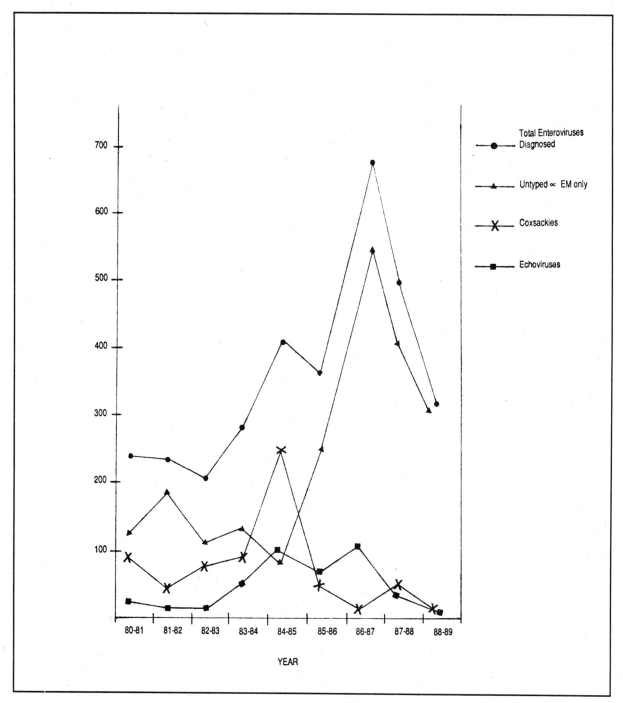

We consider an EA ≥ 40 to indicate a recent, or relatively recent active infection (primary or reactivation); a VCA ≥ 640 with EA < 40, a relatively recent active infection but less recent; positive VCA-IgMs have been positive only rarely in our adults; EBNAs have been almost constantly positive in adults, indicating those high VCAs or present EAs were due to reactivations. It is very difficult to interpret EBV serology significance in cases with "fatigue" of more than six months' duration, or of several years' duration.

Table 1					
EBV Serology of Ontario Patients: A Nine-Year Review					
	Total Tested	VCA+ EA ≥ 40	VCA ≥ 640 EA < 40	Sero- Conversions	IgM VCA+
1981-82	11,492	1,676			
1982-83	7,419	2,688			
1983-84	7,878	1,540	1,652		
1984-85	10,600	3,499	1,953		
1985-86	16,835	4,335	2,706		
1986-87	22,409	5,193	2,633	39	31
1987-88	33,734	6,984	5,292	42	16
1988-89	28,669	5,193	4,891	56	59
138,646					

Figure 1 shows the large, steady increase in demand for the test. The media's influence on demand has been very noticeable following programs on TV and radio, and publications in popular magazines and newspapers on chronic fatigue, chronic EBV infections, the "Yuppie Plague", "Lake Tahoe Disease," etc.

If we look at the *percentage* of significant results (Figure 1), we see that specimens with VCA ≥ 640 with EA < 40, and specimens with EA ≥ 40 represent about equal numbers in 1983-84. The percentage of EA ≥ 40 increases while the EA < 40 decreases in 1984, 1985, 1986, and 1987. In 1988-89 (Table 2), they are restored to the proportions of 1983-84. It seems that between 1983 and 1988 the number of recent reactivations was higher. Although it is impossible to draw accurate conclusions from such data, it seems that some event occurred between 1983 and 1988 to cause EBV reactivations.

Table 2							
EBV Serology of Ontario Patients: March, April, May 1989							
Age	VCA < 40 EA < 40	40-320 128<40	≥640 < 40	40-320 ≥ 40	≥ 640 ≥ 40	Sero- Conversions	IgM	Total
≤ 14	232	180	47	10	29	2	3	503
15-20	150	341	109	33	49	3	4	689
21-25	50	274	75	22	38	0	0	459
26-30	39	325	130	40	78	0	0	612
31-35	36	273	132	40	73	0	1	555
36-40	19	218	123	41	90	1	0	492
> 40	64	583	284	83	177	1	0	1,192
Total	**687**	**2,605**	**1,095**	**309**	**622**	**7**	**8**	**5,373**
%	12.7%	48.4%	20.3%	5.7%	12.3%	0.1%		

Table 3

Nine Years of Enterovirus Isolation Results from Ontario Patients

	80/81	81/82	82/83	83/84	84/85	85/86	86/87	87/88	88/89	Total
Combined (C.V.I. & S.)										
Coxs A, nt	5			6						11
Coxs A 9	14	6	14	8	13	18	7	21		101
Coxs B 1				3				1		4
B 2	9	14	4	10	17	11	1	4	3	73
B 3	31	2	13	6	28	10	3	17	4	114
B 4	30	15	36	13	27	3	1	8		133
B 5	6	8	2	22	160	1	1	3	4	207
B 6			1							1
	95	**45**	**70**	**68**	**245**	**43**	**13**	**54**	**11**	**644**
Combined (C.V.I. & S.)										
Echo 2				1					1	2
3		3	2	1		2	5			13
5		3			43			2	5	53
6	2	3	3	1	7	1		5	1	23
7	1					6	71		1	79
9	5	1	2	11	13	22	6	10	2	72
11	8	5	4	25	15	23	18	6	1	105
13		1								1
14			1	1	1		2	5		10
17	2	1		5						8
18								6		6
21	3									3
22						10				10
24				1		2				3
25				1						1
29	1								1	2
30			5	7	8					20
	22	**17**	**17**	**54**	**87**	**66**	**102**	**34**	**12**	**411**
V.I. only										
Polio 1			1,v						1,w	2
2	1,v		1,v		2,v					4
3		4,v	6,v	2,v						12
	1	**4**	**8**	**2**	**2**	**0**	**0**	**1**	**1,v**	**19 (1w, 18v)**
V.I. only										
EMOnly						99	266	90	111	566
	124	172	109	138	78					621
Ent, nt						149	290	321	192	952
	124	**172**	**109**	**135**	**78**	**248**	**556**	**411**	**303**	**2,139**
TOTAL	**242**	**238**	**204**	**262**	**412**	**361**	**671**	**500**	**327**	**3,225**

Legend

nt = not typed   v = vaccinal   w = wild   V.I. & S. = Virus Isonation & Serology
EM = Electron Microscopy

Enteroviruses

Dr. Byron Hyde has earlier discussed the etiologic significance of polio, coxsackie and echoviruses as causes of CFS. We reviewed the enteroviruses diagnosed in our laboratory during the last 9 years. A total of 3,225 (Table 3) diagnoses were made. These are virus diagnoses made by isolating viruses in cell cultures while some were detected only by electron microscopy. They represent mostly cases of viral meningitis, "summer flu," sore throat, fever, myalgia, pleurodymia, febrile rashes, and diarrhea, and they were essentially detected in late summer and early winter. Typing of these enteroviruses is time-consuming and was not always done, but we see a peak of Coxsackie B5 in 1984-85 and Echovirus 7 in 1986-87.

Figure 2 shows the increase in enterovirus detection between 1984 and 1987, with a decline in 1987-88. Enteroviruses are always present in Ontario, with type variations and epidemic peaks varying from year to year, which again makes interpretation of these data difficult. Serology for polio and coxsackie in patients said to be suffering with CFS was analyzed for the first 6 months of 1989 and showed frequently high titres for polio, especially Polio 3 (Table 4). The

results are difficult to interpret in the absence of precise clinical or immunization history, which we were unable to collect.

Discussion

The laboratory data reviewed here are of 2 different types. For EBV, the number of specimens received were certainly influenced by the media, and the percentage of significant results were provided by the laboratory. For enteroviruses, the number of actual viral isolates from clinical specimens should not have been influenced by media "hype" but should reflect the epidemiologic patterns of these viruses.

Still, both EBV reactivations and enteroviruses infections increased between 1983 and 1987, a phenomenon that seems to confirm the impressions of Dr. Mildon and Dr. Hyde in their review of their Ontario patients. It is impossible to draw further conclusions from these very general data, but they do merit further investigation.

Editor's note*: The marked clinical increase of M.E. / CFS noted in Canada between 1984-1987 cannot be explained by the Ontario Ministry of Health's relative lack of increase of EBV findings, but could be explained by the observed increased Coxsackie B viruses in 1984 and marked increase in Echo viruses in 1984-87. Dr. McLaughlin and Dr. Yousef, neither aware of the other's work, both noted Coxsackie B5 and Echo 11 as the major enteroviral infectious agents during the period under their particular and unrelated studies.*

Dr. McLaughlin notes significant indications of Echovirus 7, 9 and 11. She apparently did not test for Echo 1. Dr. Yousef also notes specific increased recovery of Echo 1, 9 and 11. Echo 11 appears to be specifically correlated with the same type period of 1985-1987 by both researchers. The sum total of positive enteroviral tests are more consistent with the 1984-1987 M.E. / CFS epidemic than any individual enterovirus. This correlation does not confirm that enteroviruses were the cause of the 1984-1987 M.E. / CFS epidemic but does place the enteroviral group of viruses as potential causes of this epidemic period.

Table 4
Chronic Fatigue / Myalgic Encephalomyelitis Enterovirus Serology January - June 1989

High Titres to 1 or 2 Viruses (≥1:512)

Polio 1	1
Polio 2	3
Polio 3	18
Coxsackie B2	1
Coxsackie B3	3
Coxsackie B4	3
Echovirus 9	1
	30
Total tested	1269
% with High Titres	11%

Chapter 30

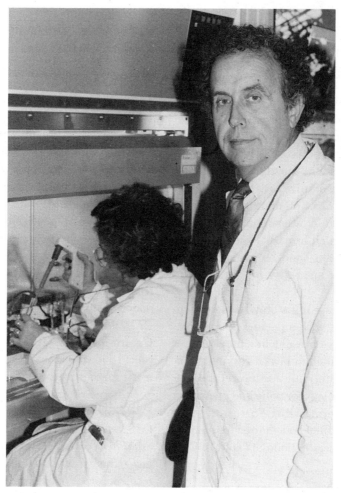

Mauro Bendinelli

The Immunosuppressive Effects of Group B Coxsackievirus Infections

Mauro Bendinelli, MD, PhD and Donatella Matteucci, BS
Virology Section, Department of Biomedicine, University of Pisa. Address: Dr. M. Bendinelli, Dipartimento di Biomedicina, Via S. Zeno 35, 56127 Pisa, Italy.

In addition to his academic position, Dr. Bendinelli is Director of the Department of Biomedicine and head of the Clinical Virology Unit of the University of Pisa as well as being Professor of Microbiology. His main research interests are: pathogenesis and immunopathogenesis of viral infections; immunobiology of Coxsackieviruses and retroviruses; viral-induced immunodeficiencies. Dr. Bendinelli is also the Co-editor of the series "Infectious Agents of Pathogenesis" for Plenum Press, New York, as well as several scientific journals.

D. Matteucci has been a research assistant at the Virology section of the Department of Biomedicine of the University of Pisa since 1976. Her research interests include: interactions of murine retroviruses and coxsackieviruses with the host's immune system, mechanisms of coxsackievirus persistence in infected cells, biology and pathogenesis of feline immunodeficiency virus and other feline retroviruses.

1. Introduction

Group B coxsackieviruses (CBV) encompass six different serotypes that belong to the genus **Enterovirus** of the family **Picornaviridae**. These impor-tant human pathogens are small, naked icosahedral, positive single-stranded RNA viruses that usually cause common enteric infections throughout the world but may also produce a wide range of well characterized acute clinical illnesses, including aseptic meningitis and other diseases of the central nervous system, acute myocarditis and pericarditis, and epidemic pleurodinia (also known as epidemic myalgia or Bornholme disease). In addition, CBV have been implicated in the etiology of a number of other infections such as congenital malformations, acute pancreatitis and orchitis, exanthemata, chronic cardiopathies, and type 1 diabetes (Bendinelli and Friedman, 1988). Recently, they have been considered as possible etiological agents of myalgic encephalomyelitis (M.E.) (Bell et al., 1988).

CBV-induced Immune Deficiency

One aspect of CBV pathogenecity that, until recently, had been entirely overlooked is their detrimental action on the functions and integrity of the immune system. Recent studies, however, have clearly shown that experimentally infected mice may present a markedly reduced immune response to unrelated antigens and a severe degree of lymphoid involution, and that human lymphocytes exposed to CBV in vitro also exhibit a reduced responsiveness. In addition, in vitro studies have shown that, with the exception of serotype 6 (CBV-6), CBV can readily establish carrier-type persistent infections in cultures of immortalized human lymphocytes. These data may be relevant to the etiopathogenesis of M.E., as from the very beginning it has been suspected that the disease is associated with disordered regulation of the immune system (Behan et al., 1985).

This paper summarizes the studies performed in mice in the attempt to understand the mechanisms underlying CBV-induced immune deficiency and then reviews published evidence suggesting that CBV can be immunosuppressive in humans.

2. Animal Studies

In early experiments, adult random bred Swiss mice were infected with the six CBV, as well as with three group A coxsackievirus (CAV) serotypes, and then challenged with unrelated immunogens. Animals infected with CBV-1, 3, 6 and CAV-15 exhibited a reduced antibody responsiveness. CBV-3 also suppressed the ability of mice to mount a normal cell-mediated contact sensitivity response to the skin sensitizer oxazolone (Bendinelli et al., 1975).

Subsequent studies were carried out using adult inbred BALB/c mice infected with CBV-3. Using monodispersed spleen cells stimulated in vitro with selected antigens, it was observed that, within a few days from infection, primary antibody responses to thymus-dependent antigens were depressed by 50 to 80%. In contrast, secondary responses to the same antigens were essentially spared (Bendinelli et al., 1982).

Attempts to understand the mechanisms for the reduced immunoresponsiveness of infected spleen cell cultures yielded the following results:

i. spleen cells responded well to thymus-independent antigens and, when supplemented with non-B cells from uninfected mice, also to thymus-dependent antigens;

ii. activated nonspecific T suppressor cells were present in the infected spleens, although the level of suppressive activity detected in individual mice did not correlate with the degree of immunodepression exhibited by the same animals;

iii. supplementing with splenic or peritoneal macrophages from normal mice restored the responsiveness of infected spleen cell cultures;

iv. adding splenic macrophages from infected spleens did not reintegrate the responsiveness of macrophage-depleted spleen cell cultures from normal or infected animals;

v. addition of cell-free CBV-3 to normal spleen cultures did not reproduce the immunosuppressive changes exhibited by spleen cells obtained from infected mice.

Taken together, these findings indicate that CBV-3-induced immunosuppression is sustained by defects in the ability of accessory cells to cooperate normally with lymphocytes and, possibly, also to the activation of nonspecific T suppressor cells. In contrast B lymphocytes do not seem to represent a major target of immunosuppression (Bendinelli et al., 1982).

In addition to such functional alterations, the immune system of CBV-infected mice undergoes a marked anatomical involution. Thymus, spleen and lymph nodes gradually lose weight and cellularity. Histologically, the thymus showed an early depletion of cortical thymocytes and loss of distinction at the corticomedullary junction, followed by cellular depletion of the medulla. In the peripheral lymphoid organs, cellular depletion was characterized by a parallel decline of the various cell classes and subclasses studied, except for an early temporary rise of T cells with suppressor phenotype. Fibrosis was the eventual outcome in all organs (Matteucci et al., 1985).

How the functional and anatomical alterations of the immune system observed in CBV infected mice are generated remains an enigma. A direct adverse effect of locally replicating virus, due to viral cytopathology or less obvious changes, is generally believed to contribute to the genesis of many virus-induced immune deficiencies (Specter et al., 1989). However, attempts to grow CBV in freshly harvested murine lymphoid cells were unsuccessful. Moreover, infectious center assay detected few, if any, productively infected cells in central and peripheral lymphoid organs. Only the bone marrow contained substantial numbers of virus-producing cells (Matteucci et al., 1985).

Direct immunofluorescence with monoclonal antibody to CBV-3 evidenced production of viral molecules in scattered cells (usually less than 1%) whose nature remained elusive (Garzelli et al., 1988). It seems possible that virus-infected cells are a small subpopulation of lymphoid cells or blood vessel cells or other cell types (Easton and Eglin, 1988). In this context, it is worth mentioning that in vitro the murine lymphoid cell line YAC-1 could be persistently infected with CBV-3 (Cao and Schnurr, 1988) in a manner similar to the human lymphoid cell lines discussed below. In these cultures, infection was perpetuated by a minority of susceptible cells whereas most of the cells were resistant to the carried virus. It is therefore possible that murine lymphoid cells are inherently resistant to CBV but become susceptible under particular physiological conditions. Even if one assumes that local viral replication in a few cells is responsible for immunosuppression and lymphoid involution, it remains to be established how the damage is amplified. Two possibilities come to mind: one is that the infected and presumably lysed cells have important trophic functions (Garzelli et al., 1989). The other is that local infection triggers

a chain of progressive autoaggressive events. Interestingly, attempts to alleviate the lymphoid involution by administering a number of immunopotentiating compounds led to a paradoxical exacerbation of manifestations (Matteucci et al., 1985). Similar results were obtained by treating mice with bacterial lypopolisaccharide (LPS), a well known polyclonal B cell activator (unpublished data).

Recently, we have investigated the role played by selected cytokins in the generation of the immune derangements produced by CBV-3 infection in mice. The amounts of interleukin (IL) 2 and gamma-interferon (IFN) produced by concanavalin A stimulated spleen cells were reduced in the early stages of infection but highly enhanced after the onset of lymphoid involution. At this time IL 1 production by LPS-treated adherent spleen cells was also enhanced. Basal titres of circulating tumor necrosis factor (TNF)-alpha were transiently increased early after infection, while LPS-induced levels remained considerably increased for several days. Serum from infected mice inhibited the proliferation of lymphoid cells in vitro at higher dilutions than that of normal mice, but this activity could not be attributed to TNF-alpha. On the other hand, the administration of anti-murine TNF antibody failed to protect mice against CBV-3-induced lymphoid involution and lethality. Thus, although it could not be excluded that altered cytokine physiology might play a major role in CBV-3-induced immunological damage, no single alteration appeared responsible for lymphoid involution (Bendinelli et al. 1990).

3. Human Studies

To the authors' knowledge, there are no published reports on the behaviour of standard clinical immunology parameters in CBV-infected patients. Neither is there evidence that CBV can replicate extensively in the lymphoid organs of humans. In fact, the histopathology of human lymphoid tissues during CBV infections is generally poorly understood. There are, however, scattered clinical reports indicating that these viruses can worsen concomitant infections and facilitate disease production by opportunistic agents. An example is the case of fulminant pulmonary coccidioidomycosis described in a child co-infected with CBV-4 (Gururaj et al., 1984).

Recently, studies have been performed on the ability of human peripheral blood mononuclear cells (PBMNC) exposed to CBV in vitro to support viral replication and to effect their normal functions. In one study, it was found that CBV-3 replication in human PBMNC was essentially restricted and could not be enhanced by mitogen stimulation. Polyclonal blastogenic and antibody responses of lymphocytes were not significantly affected (Hyypia et al., 1988). In similar studies by us, a considerable degree of variability was observed in the permissiveness of PBMNC from individual donors to the six CBV serotypes. Such variations appeared unrelated to donor age and gender and showed no relation to the presence and titre of anti-CBV neutralizing antibody in the donor sera. PBMNC presented a reduction of mitogen-driven proliferation whose extent varied from 20 to 50%, again depending not only on viral serotype and dose but also on the PBMNC donor. The depressive effect of CBV-6 was particularly pronounced and consistent. Suppression was not mediated by the antiproliferative properties of IFN produced by the PBMNC in response to CBV challenge, as it could not be prevented by the addition of high titre anti-alpha and/or beta-IFN antibodies. The suppression was only partially reversed by the addition of large amounts of recombinant human IL 2 (Conaldi et al., 1988).

The cell type(s) among human PBMNC which support a low degree of CBV replication is still unclear. By immunofluorescence, it was found that viral antigens were mostly located in adherent cells (Hyypia et al., 1988). It should be noted, however, that human lymphoid cells may be permissive for CBV replication. We examined the response of a number of lymphoid cell lines of the B and T lymphocyte lineage to infection by the six CBV immunotypes (Matteucci et al., 1985). The outcome of infection varied but complete restriction of CBV replication was infrequent. Among the virus-cell combinations studied, variation in permissiveness was reflected in the peak titre of virus produced as well as in the time of first detection of progeny virus and in the time of peak yield (that ranged between day 1 and 4). Variation was also observed in the effects on cell viability. CBV-6 was the only immunotype which regularly led to complete destruction of the cultures. The other CBV caused partial or minimal damage. In many instances, no visible adverse effects on cell culture viability or

proliferation were evident over the entire period of incubation, despite the high viral titres produced. This was of interest because CBV are generally considered highly cytocidal, as virions are liberated in a burst when the host cell lyses at the end of the replication cycle.

On the whole, lines of B-lymphocytic origin appeared somewhat more susceptible to CBV infection than T-cell lines and their permissiveness appeared to be independent on the presence of the Epstein-Barr virus genome that reportedly influences B cell susceptibility to other viruses (Creager et al., 1981). A further level of variation was observed when the lymphoid cells were exposed to different clones of a same CBV immunotype. At 37°C all clones grew well, even though the effects on culture viability varied considerably, but certain small plaque clones proved unable to replicate significantly at 39.5°C.

Several days after CBV infection, many lymphoid cell cultures were still producing virus but showed no morphologic changes or loss of proliferative capacity. By passaging these cultures serially, long-term persistent infections were readily established. The infected cells continued to grow and shed high titres of virus for months and years. For example, the MOLT-4 cell line persistently infected with CBV-3 is still propagated in our laboratory after over 5 years from its establishment.

In earlier studies performed with nonlymphoid cells, CBV had shown no tendency to persist unless virus inhibitors were added exogenously (reviewed in Bendinelli and Friedman, 1988). Lymphoid cell lines may liberate IFN and other lymphokines spontaneously or following induction. However, exhaustive attempts to demonstrate virus inhibitors during the acute and persistent phases of CBV infection in MOLT-4 cells were unsuccessful. Persistence in these cells was shown to be maintained by a carrier culture mechanism involving virus spread through the medium and replication among a minority of susceptible cells that appeared to emerge continuously from a population of resistant cells. The genetic or phenotypic basis of the MOLT-4 cell heterogeneity that permits a permanent virus-cell equilibrium have however remained unclear. As permissiveness to CBV and other picornaviruses is known to be controlled mainly at the absorption-penetration step (reviewed in

Crowell et al., 1988), differences at this level might be implicated.

Akin viruses which have been shown to give persistent infections in vitro include the three polioviruses and echovirus type 6. In lymphoid lines, polioviruses were shown to establish a carrier culture mechanism (Carp, 1981) but, in neuroblastoma cells, the mechanism seemed different since viral antigens could be detected in all the cells of the persistently infected cultures (Colbère-Garapin et al., 1989). Echovirus 6 persistence was described in the human amnion WISH cell line and appeared to be maintained by a steady state mechanism in which all the cells contained defective genome-size viral RNA which was synthesized continuously and incorporated into defective virions unable to infect cells because they were devoid of two structural proteins (Righthand and Blackburn, 1989).

Generally, viral persistence is a dynamic process. In all the above systems, as well as in CBV infected human lymphoid cells, viral persistence was associated with evolution of the persisting virus and of the persistently infected cells. For example, the human MOLT-4 lymphoid cell line persistently infected with CBV-3 remained normally susceptible to unrelated viruses but became progressively more resistant to the parental virus and, to a lesser extent, to other CBV serotypes. On the other hand, during persistence, the virus evolved an increased cytopathogenicity for the original MOLT-4 cells and a reduced ability to replicate in other cell lines. The virus recovered from the media of persistent cultures also differed from the parental virus in the size of plaques produced on indicator cells, in the ability to replicate at supraoptimal temperatures and in animal pathogenicity. Although these changes did not seem to contribute significantly to the establishment of persistence as they evolved gradually while the conditions leading to persistence were already established within a few days after virus infection, they may be instrumental in the stabilization and maintenance of the carrier state.

In vitro models of viral persistence have provided important clues to the understanding of how viruses are implicated in the generation of chronic and progressive diseases. Persistence of infectious CBV in vivo has never been unequivocally demonstrated even though prolonged virus shedding is not rare. This may reflect the fact that the presence of persistent or latent virus infections in intact tissues may be extremely difficult to demonstrate. However, CBV persistence has been implicated in the genesis of chronic CBV-induced cardiomyopathies both in animal models and in humans and CBV specific RNA sequences have been detected in chronically diseased hearts by dot blot or in situ hybridization (Archard et al., 1988; Kandolf et al., 1988). Furthermore, related viruses such as echoviruses have been shown to produce long-term infections of the CNS (Griffith et al., 1977). The cell type(s) where CBV might persist in vivo is still undetermined but lymphoid cells are likely candidates as many viruses have been shown to persist preferentially in lymphoid tissues of chronically infected hosts (Specter et al., 1989). It may be of clinical interest that CBV persistence in lymphoid cells could be terminated by treatment with virus-specific antibody and, even more effectively, with IFN (Bendinelli et al., 1987).

4. Closing Remarks

For many years, CBV were believed to produce only acute infections and to induce tissue damage and disease exclusively by direct cytopathology. As recently discussed in several reviews (Bendinelli and Friedman, 1988; Wolfram and Rose, 1989), it is now increasingly recognized that CBV infections do instead share many complexities traditionally associated with infections by enveloped viruses which are generally considered more sophisticated pathogens. They can persist for prolonged periods and possibly indefinitely in patients, produce subtle changes of infected cells, cause chronic pathology, trigger immunopathological damage to infected tissues, and initiate autoimmune phenomena. Thus, while many aspects of pathogenesis remain little understood, there is no doubt that, in CBV infections, the immune system plays a much more complex role than it was originally thought. A detailed understanding of the interactions CBV establish with the host's immune system might provide clues to the etiology and pathogenesis of several cryptogenesic diseases, including M.E.

References

1. Behan P.O., Behan W.M.H., and Bell E.J., 1985, The post viral fatigue syndrome - An analysis of the findings in 50 cases, J. Infect. Dis.10, 211-222.

2. Bell J.E., Assaad F., and Esteves K., 1988, Neurologic disorders, In Coxsackievirus. A General Update (Bendinelli M., and Friedman H., eds.), Plenum Press Corporation, New York, pp. 318-337.

3. Bendinelli M., and Friedman H.(eds.), 1988, **Coxsackieviruses: A General Update**, Plenum Press Corporation, New York, p. 430.

4. Bendinelli M., Matteucci D., Conaldi P.G., and Soldaini E., 1990, Bacterial endotoxin as a probe to investigate virus-induced immunodeficiencies. **Adv. Exp. Med. Biol.** 256: 511-523.

5. Bendinelli M., Matteucci D., Toniolo A., Patanè A.M., and Pistillo M.P., 1982, Impairment of immunocompetent mouse spleen cell functions by infection with coxsackievirus B3, J. Inf. Dis. 146: 797-805.

6. Bendinelli M., Ruschi A., Campa M., and Toniolo A., 1975, Depression of humoral and cell-mediated immune responses by coxsackieviruses in mice. Experientia 31: 1227-1229.

7. Cao Y., and Schnurr D. S., 1988, Persistent infection of YAC-1 cells by coxsackievirus B3, J. Gen. Virol. 69: 59-65.

8. Carp R.I., 1981, Persistent infection of human lymphoid cells with poliovirus and development of temperature-sensitive mutants, Intervirology 15: 49-56.

9. Colbère-Garapin F., Christodoulou C., Crainic R., and Pelletier I., 1989, Persistent poliovirus infection of human neuroblastoma cells, Proc. Natl. Acad. Sci. 86: 7590-7594.

10. Conaldi P.G., Matteucci D., Soldaini E., Guidi M., and Bendinelli M., 1988, Interactions of group B coxsackieviruses with immunocytes, In **New Concepts in Viral Heart Disease; Virology, Immunology and Clinical Management** (Schulteiss H.-P., ed.), Springer-Verlag, Berlin, pp. 195-204

11. Eglin R.P., 1988, The detection of coxsackievirus RNA in cardiac tissue by in situ hybridization, J. Gen. Virol. 69: 285-291.

12. Garzelli C., Basolo F., Matteucci D., Prabhakar B.S., and Toniolo A., 1989, Picornavirus-induced immunosuppression, In **Virus induced Immunosuppression** (Specter S., Bendinelli M., Friedman H., eds.), Plenum Press Corporation, New York, pp. 217-234.

13. Griffith J.S., Katz S.L., and Moore M., 1977, Persistent enterovirus infections in agammaglobulinemia. in **Microbiology 1977** (Schlesinger D., ed.) American Society for Microbiology, Washington, D.C.

14. Easton A. J., Gururaj V.J., Marsh W.W., and Aiyar S.R., 1984, Fulminant pulmonary coccidioidomycosis in association with coxsackie B4 infection, Clin. Pediatr.24: 406-408.

15. Hyypia T., Vainionpaa R., and Akerman K., 1988, Interaction of measles and coxsackie B3 viruses with human peripheral blood mononuclear cells, **Proc. 9th European Immunology Meeting**, Rome, 14-17 September.

16. Matteucci D., Paglianti D., Giangregorio A.M., Capobianchi M.R., Dianzani F., and Bendinelli M., 1985, Group B coxsackieviruses readily establish persistent infections in human lymphoid cell lines, J. Virol. 56: 651-654.

17. Matteucci D., Toniolo A., Conaldi P.G., Basolo F, Gori Z., and Bendinelli M., 1985, Systemic lymphoid atrophy in coxsackievirus B3-infected mice: Effects of virus and immunopotentiating agents, J. Inf. Dis. 51: 1100-1108.

18. Righthand V.F., and Blackburn R.V., 1989, Steady-state infection by echovirus 6 associated with nonlytic viral RNA and an unprocessed capsid polypeptide, J. Virol. 63: 5268-5275.

19. Specter S., Bendinelli M., and Friedman S., 1989, **Virus-induced immunosuppression**, Plenum Press Corporation, New York, p. 477.

20. Wolfram L.J., and Rose N.R., 1989, Coxsackievirus infection as a trigger of cardiac autoimmunity, Immunol. Res. 8: 61-71.

Chapter 31

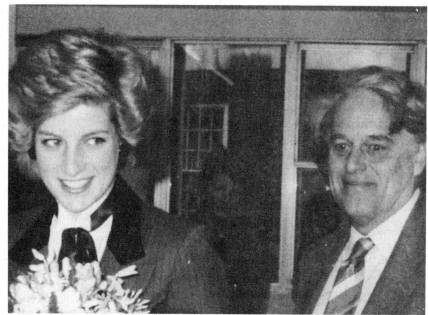

H.R.H. The Princess of Wales and James Mowbray
Photograph courtesy of Zhang Hong Yi

Evidence of Chronic Enterovirus Infections in M.E.

James F. Mowbray, FRCP
Professor of Immunopathology, Department of Immunopathology, St. Mary's Hospital Medical School
Norfolk Place, London W2 1PG, England

Dr. James Mowbray is an Immunologist with special interests in transplantation and reproductive Immunology as well as problems of chronic virus infections. He showed 10 years ago that the enteroviral antigens in the blood of patients with ME and viral myocarditis were the same. His research group have shown that a material fraction of ME patients have chronic infection with enteroviruses which could be recovered from the GI tract using special techniques. Dr. Mowbray has very wide experience of viral / immunological studies of ME patients and their management.

Editor's note: Since neither Dr. Mowbray nor Dr. Yousef have sent their manuscripts, the following is a transcript taken from a tape recording of Dr. Mowbray's lecture at Cambridge, and then corrected by Dr. Mowbray. We have reproduced Dr. Yousef's published paper that corresponds roughly to his Cambridge paper. For a better review of Dr. Mowbray's group's important work, please refer to Chapter 32 of this text and also **Post-Viral Fatigue Syndrome***, 1991, John Wiley & Sons, Jenkins and Mowbray.*

What I want to do first is to try to explain what I'm talking about and then discuss the evidence that has accumulated in my laboratory over the last few years, largely about enteroviruses in M.E.

If we were to consider all fatigue syndromes, there would be a lot of potential candidates. Within all fatigue syndromes, we would find some non-infectious ones and infectious ones. We would find things like cancer, which produces a fatigue syndrome.

We're all aware of some chemical causes of fatigue syndromes. Interestingly, one of them is germanium, a heavy metal which is actually being used by some people as a treatment for M.E. Germanium toxicity produces serious renal involvement. Renal damage produces myalgia, diminished muscular effort capabilities and certain cognitive difficulties. It looks a little bit like M.E., but is clearly of a chemical nature. Cancer, particularly cancer chemotherapy produces severe muscle fatigue symptoms. But we're really concerned with the infectious fatigue syndrome. The oldest and best established of those is tuberculosis and those of you who lived in the era when tuberculosis was a common disease know that it produced severe prostrating fatigue with extremely poor muscle capability throughout the disease. But one of the things I wanted to point out is that as the infection got better, these symptoms decreased.

Giardiasis is a condition with which a number of patients return from other parts of the world. It is an infection which produces a severe fatigue syndrome. This may be very protracted because it is a chronic illness. Now, in order to produce a chronic fatigue syndrome caused by an infection, the infection must be chronic. There are not many chronic virus infections. So, if you were to look at the virus caused chronic fatigue syndrome which we call ME or post infectious, protracted viral infectious syndrome, there would not be very many candidate viruses, and the viruses which appeared out of the woodwork are those which have the capability of producing long term chronic infection. I don't mean latent or dormant but active infection. Something like the flu is not going to produce a disease for more than a few days. Yet, if we were to look at the acute illness of flu, it has much of the characteristic symptomatology found in the more protracted chronic fatigue syndrome.

Now the definition that I am concerned with of ME has those things: There is muscle fatigue on exercise, with slow recovery going to the point of exhaustion. It sometimes takes days or weeks to recover after severe exhaustion. There are also cognitive difficulties, difficulties in concentration, short term memory and particularly nominal dysphasia which I think is a thing always worth looking for as the patients frequently don't notice it. Their families and their medical attendants may notice it more frequently.

One of the very few physical signs in this condition is that they frequently show very slow accommodation, particularly from near gaze to the distance. This may be associated with hippus during the time of re-accommodation, in which the pupil is seen to expand and contract over a period of fifteen - thirty - sixty seconds before it finally settles down.

So that's the group of patients we've been concerned with. We have not minded whether they've had an acute onset with a flu-like illness or an insidious onset. In terms of rates of recovery and virology and all the other things we've looked at, there does not seem to be any striking difference between the two groups. Now it has already been suggested today that possibly there might be mediators of some of the symptoms as a result of an infection, or as somebody earlier said, as a result of an immune response. Well, both virus infections and immune responses generate cytokines. Lymphokines, those things specifically associated with immune response, can occur with agents other than viruses. However, the alpha and beta interferons are produced by virus infected cells, not by the immune response to them. It appears that alpha interferon as well as gamma interferon which is produced by lymphocytes, both produce on administration the well-known interferon toxicity syndrome which is produced by giving pure interferon. It had been described very accurately by one of the patients who was receiving the treatment as being just like a flu but without the bunged-up nose. They got all the other things; the difficulties in thinking, the myalgia, the anhedonia, (the lack of pleasure in life while they've got it) and really all the symptoms, with the exception of the severe muscle pain limiting exercise. They've got all of those as a result of the administration of either gamma or non-gamma interferon. So it may be that a virus infection by infecting cells may result in the interferon production. The immune response to it will result in the production of other things such as interleukin 1 and interleukin 2, which has been referred to this morning, although interleukin 2 doesn't really produce as much in the way of symptoms as does recombinant interferon.

Part of this syndrome is pain in muscle and in joints as well as simply in muscle, and that was one of our very early starting points in looking at patients who had ME and also happened to have myocarditis. We found that most of them had circulating complexes with IgM antibodies bound to an antigen. Those, of course, are the sort of complexes which are most frequently associated with polyarthralgia. The joints may be mediated by complexes. A lot of the central nervous system effects may be mediated by cytokines of various kinds. But there is always the possibility that virus infection of the central nervous system or virus infection of the muscle may produce the effect locally as well. And in the enteroviruses we have a group of viruses which have, although they are found in the enteron (they're found in the gastrointestinal tract), are myotropic and neurotropic and some of the strains are also cardiotropic. So they're quite good candidates and the only problem would appear to be that it was assumed that chronic virus infection with enteroviruses was a rarity. You see enteroviruses, unlike most other sorts of viruses, have no mechanism for integration into the nuclear material in the cell and they have no mechanism for dormancy. So the only way to keep the infection going is by having active infection of cells, cell death, release of infectious particles, infection of new cells, and a cycle continuing that way. You cannot have latency. So if you find evidence that there is virus protein around, for instance, it means that there must be virus replication around. It's quite different from a situation of the herpesviruses, which in fact integrate and may lie dormant for eighty years before appearing as reactivation of a herpes zoster virus.

Now, what was the evidence, apart from the outbreaks, that there were enteroviruses involved in ME? There was evidence from neutralizing antibody titres with people saying "Oh yes, look, some of them have very high titres against whatever few neutralizing antibodies were looked at" (usually against five or occasionally six coxsackie B viruses out of a possible 72 enteroviruses). Circulating immune complexes we found were present in about 2/3 of the patients whether they had myocarditis or not. And then Professor Banatvala's development of IgM anti-entero viral antibodies really made a lot of difference because it was now possible to get some idea whether the infection was continuing or recent. The presence of neutralising antibody shows only the past history of the patient. It then became obvious that there were IgM anticoxsackie antibodies in a significant fraction of the ME patients whenever you looked at them. They were there month by month, or year by year, suggesting that the infection was continuing.

If we actually look at the neutralising antibody, there's a paper that Professor Banatvala and I actually never got around to finishing as the evidence was pretty poor. The best evidence is from a study of one hundred extremely carefully worked out patients with ME in which the neutralizing titres to one of the Coxsackie B viruses that the highest neutralizing titre is recorded here, and there is the matched group

of control patients who were matched for living on the same road, the same sex, and same decade of age. You see it's pretty unimpressive. Fairly impressive maybe for the few patients here and there, but for the most part it was pretty poor evidence. If you are not concerned with an outbreak where you isolate the particular strain, it was not very good evidence that they've got better immune responses (higher antibody levels) to Coxsackie B than the rest of the population. You could say that, as there are over 70 serotypes of enteroviruses, that they don't have the other one, but there is no evidence to prove that supposition.

So we set out to try and see if we could show that the patients were infected with a virus. To do that, we looked at the normal cyclic of virus which is in the gut. And, as Betty Dowsett said earlier on, you cannot isolate viruses normally in enteroviral infection for more than a few weeks, because of the development of IgA antibodies secreted into the gut, which are neutralizing antibodies. This neutralizes the virus so that you can't calculate it.

So we had to develop a technique for finding the virus in the presence of antibody. What we did was to take enteroviruses and deliberately neutralize them with IgA antibodies (human IgA antibodies from human breast milk of people who had a lot of anti entero antibodies), then taking the neutralized virus to an acidic wash, so that the antibody would come off the virus again. Since the viruses are gastro-intestinal viruses, they can infect through the stomach. They don't mind the acid condition. So separate the antibody from the virus. Then, in the alpha-centrifuge, centrifuge the virus to the bottom, leaving the antibody at the top and culture the bottom. Doing this, we were able to get enterovirus isolates from people.

Only in a very few people did we get isolates just by culturing the feces directly, the reason being that the studies were done in the beginning of May 1986 to the beginning of May 1987 and the summer enterovirus season in Britain doesn't really start until the end of May continuing to the end of October. The weather then becomes too cold for the survival of enteroviruses in the population and they disappear to warmer climates for the winter (like much of the population at home). If you go to Central Africa, you'll meet maybe three or four or five enteroviruses a year. In

Britain, you generally only meet one, unique to the summer cold, and you meet it between the end of May and the end of October.

So we chose a time when they weren't around very much and we took patients with ME and matched controls and what happened was that, in two of the patients and two of the controls, direct viral cultures were possible. They were probably people who had transient intestinal carriage even though they were a bit early in the season. They did not have evidence that virus proteins were present in the blood and the virus was not recoverable subsequently. So these are those with transient carriage. However, we did find in 22% of the patients that it was possible to culture a virus (only after removing *neutralizing antibody*). So they had an infectious virus and they had symptoms for a minimum of two years and a maximum of twenty-six years in this group. Most of them demonstrated enteroviral infection lasting between two and eight years.

That shows that they had a virus but it doesn't show that they were persistently infected with a virus, which is part of Koch's postulate; the disease has to be associated with a virus and it has to be associated both in time and geographically, and the removal of the virus would be associated with disappearance of symptoms. But there's always the chance that someone could get the infection but you can't, for some reason, culture it. So we went back a year later and did the same thing again. In each patient in which we cultured a virus for two years, it was the same serotype of virus. I think that's a vital recording element that you would expect to have, that it is, a persistent infection with that virus. It is not a reinfection occurring at intervals.

Monoclonal Antibody

The other thing we did was to develop a monoclonal antibody which detected one of the virus proteins. That protein is not very variable between all of the enteroviruses and there is on it one epitope, which is the same in all enteroviruses. We have developed a monoclonal antibody against that epitope. So then if you look at the small RNA virus, it makes one messenger strand, one protein. The protein is then keyed by protealytic in the enzymes within the cell and also coded for by the virus. It splits into frag-

ments and of these fragments, one of them, the VP1, one of the captured proteins, is then used for the architecture of the virus and one spot of this doesn't do anything. So now we can have an antibody which will react with the VP1 of any enterovirus; echoes, coxsackie A, coxsackie B, polio, it reacts with all of them. This just shows you on a dot-blot that it doesn't react with a lot of controls, but reacts to a whole slew of enteroviruses.

Now using that antibody, label the antibody with Peroxidase and add it to a blood sample that contains antibodies to VP1, and may contain VP1 itself if there is an infection there. If there is an infection there and the antigen is there, if we look at the labelled enterovirus and wait long enough, the complexes will dissociate and reassociate and the labelled antibody will become incorporated into the complex. Then, using polyethylene glycol under carefully controlled conditions, you can precipitate the complex and leave the free antibody behind. You've made half your label. From that you can calculate how much VP1 there was present in the sample. This technique proved useful because it was possible to do a lot of assays and detect any enterovirus. Whereas, if you were to look for even things like IgM antibodies to enteroviruses, you would need to do thirty or forty tests to cover the whole range of overlapping antigenicity to the enteroviruses.

Looking back at what we published after we had done the culture work, looking at the amount of VP1 label that was precipitated, in any patient, a lot of patients were above three standard deviations above the normal and there were quite a few below, this being the normal control range and these being other inflammatory and infectious disease samples that were coming in to the department at the time. One of those is a patient with the condition called epidemic mastoiditis or viral labrynthitis. Some other of those patients would also prove to be positive and it looks quite likely that some of those epidemic labrynthitis outbreaks might happen to be going through viruses.

Now I said we frequently found people with circulating/renewing complexes in ME. This was our starting point some eight or nine years beforehand. You will see that, if you take the ones who are complex positive, a lot of them have VP1 detectable. If you take the ones that are complex negative, there are only a couple. Normal controls have hardly any.

Now let's look at the ones who are "culture positive" or "culture negative", having acidified the virus preparation in the stool. You will see a capture of positive ones with two exceptions of VP1 positive and a capture of negative. There are some positives that are a bit low level. There may have been too little virus there for us to capture them into. Those two negatives are the two who had virus cultures which were positive without acidification. Another thing was that in people who had the virus for a few days it was passing through, it was not a chronic infection. They just had intestinal carriage at the time.

So, getting back to where I was, we had a technique for measuring the virus present in the blood and it could only be there if there was an infection there. There was no dormancy or latency not an antibody. It's like measuring hepatitis B surface antigen and hepatitis. It may find the virus.

We have samples that came from Tony Komaroff, a physician in New York, some from Byron Hyde, and a rather poor selection of US normals, but we found in this, as we had in the UK samples, that there's quite a big fraction of people who were positive on all of the series except the chap in New York. It's hidden behind the controls, but he managed to do something which is very difficult to do, which is take a number of people with the syndrome and not find any of them with high VP1. I never did ask him what the secret of his success is but I would quite like to know.

I'm going to mention cross-postulates. Well, here is the last of the cross-postulates that I really wanted to talk about. I'm showing two patients on whom we have done serial VP1's as they recover. You can ask the patients if they're better and they'll tell you. If you do so and if you have some markers for improvement, you will find that the correlation of the VP1 with improvement is quite considerable. In other words, as their symptoms increase, the amount of virus protein detected in their blood also increases. Some patients (they are the subjects of a still incomplete trial) respond extremely well to IgG (normal or pooled human IgG). The chap in green in the back didn't have anything. You can see that over the months his VP1 level is falling as he responds.

Treatment with IgG

This man had an injection of IgG given at that time

and he was virtually symptom free existence for about six weeks. He then went on to regular IgG treatment. But you will see at the time after the IgG is given, the VP1 disappears, and will recur, if not in four weeks, then it will be back in eight weeks to essentially the same level it was before.

So, there is agreement between the level of VP1 and the degree of symptoms. If you take people who have been better, or pretty nearly better, whose VP1's have fallen down to levels we can't detect who then go out and overdo it and exhaust themselves, it's one of those relapses. Now, time after time, we find we can get their VP1 better although it had disappeared previously. So, Koch's postulate is to a large extent verified.

The other one that Koch stated is that, in the organism, the infection is where the disease is. Well, of course that's clearly not true if you think of tetanus or diphtheria. But one would like to know whether the virus is present, in the tissues involved, in the brain, and in the muscle. It is easy to get muscle biopsies, difficult to get brain samples. Here we have a muscle of a patient with adult polymyositis. Yousef and David Eisenberg show, in a paper, how adult polymyositis had enteroviruses. And here you will see muscle cells in a very inflamed muscle area frequently stained with Peroxidase,-Peroxidase which is on the monoclonal antibody and is looking for VP1 and finds VP1 over there as an infection, a very acute infection. There's virus replication, there's damage going on, muscle enzymes are high, cellular infiltration is present and you will find virus present there easy to see.

If, however, we look in the ME patient's muscle, we will not find any VP1 infected muscle or muscle cell with VP1. If, however, we use a probe for the virus RNA which has biotin on it, you can stain the tissue for the viral RNA and get peroxidase stain if the viral genes are there in the muscles. You can then see infected cells (those infected by virus) and they are rare. They represent 1/100 to 1/200 fibres only, that have virus detectable in them. So that any change in muscle performance due to virus infection would not be expected to involve a decrease in the total muscle function. That is one of the reasons why, for those of you who heard Richard Edwards last night, it's so important to realize that the actual performance of the muscle is normal. It is the neuromuscular work which is the problem. But the changes in muscles are present and we found them (Len Archard is going to be talking much more extensively about that this afternoon) but there is virus only in a very few muscle cells. So in at least one of the sites it's there in a large fraction of the patients with ME, and as the ME goes away, the virus goes away and indeed we've never been able to get positive virus cultures from people after recovery either.

I think the evidence for enteroviruses as a main cause of ME is very good. I think Koch's postulates are pretty well answered. Were there an appropriate anti-viral gene therapy, you could complete the proposition by saying I will treat the patients, make them lose their virus, and see if the disease gets better. And that is the sort of approach we're going to have to use, no matter which virus is considered.

I've skipped over a slide which is the result of work by Dorothy Crawford and David Smith and they've studied reactivation of Epstein Barr virus in the same group of patients (a very well worked out group of M.E. patients) who had also been studied by us for the enteroviruses. The result is really quite striking - 65% of them have high levels of detectable VP1 and in the remaining 35%, 20% of them have early Epstein-Barr IgG and some high VCA antibodies as evidence of reactivation. But none of them has both which makes causality from a virus infection much more likely than that some strange alteration in the immune response that made them liable to pick up a couple of viruses. That still leaves 15% in which no evidence of Epstein-Barr virus or an enterovirus was obtained, and that may be due to sensitivities in the technique, or it may be due to other viruses which might cause M.E.

Possible Viral Cause of M.E.

But I would stress that if you're going to show causality and more than one virus is involved, you should only find one virus in each patient and if you find two or three viruses together in each patient, then you would suggest that maybe some sort of immunodepression was going on. But, at the moment, that is not the situation, so: enteroviruses first, Epstein-Barr virus next, and we don't know about the remaining 15%. Thank you very much.

Chapter 32

This article is reprinted courtesy of The Lancet, Ltd., GE Yousef, GF Mann, DG Smith, EJ Bell, V Murugesan, RA McCartney, JF Mowbray, "Chronic Enterovirus Infection in Patients with Postviral Fatigue Syndrome", © The Lancet Ltd., January 23, 1988, i:146-50.

Chronic Enterovirus Infection in Patients with Postviral Fatigue Syndrome

G.E. Yousef, G.F. Mann, D.G. Smith, E.J. Bell, V. Murugesan, R.A. McCartney, J.F. Mowbray

Department of Pathology, St. Mary's Hospital Medical School, London; Enterovirus Reference Laboratory and Regional Virus Laboratory, Ruchill Hospital, Glasgow; London School of Hygiene and Tropical Medicine; and General Practice, Horndon-on-the-Hill, Essex

Summary

76 patients with the postviral fatigue syndrome (PVFS) and 30 matched controls were investigated. Virus isolation was attempted from concentrated faecal samples by direct culture and after acid dissociation of virus from antibody. Positive cultures of enteroviruses were obtained from 17 (22%) patients and 2 (7%) controls. An enterovirus-group-specific monoclonal antibody, 5-D8/1, directed against the VP1 polypeptide, was used to detect enteroviral antigen in the circulation, either free or complexed with antibody. VP1 antigen was detected in the serum of 44 (51%) of a further group of 87 PVFS patients. The number of patients positive for VP1 antigen was greater (42/44) when IgM complexes were detectable than when they were not (2/23). 1 year later, the 17 patients of the first group of 76 with positive cultures were again studied. The same virus was again isolated from 5 (29%), 13 (76%) had detectable IgM responses to enteroviruses, and 9 (53%) were positive for VP1 antigen in the serum. These results show that chronic infection with enteroviruses occurs in many PVFS patients and that detection of enterovirus antigen in the serum is a sensitive and satisfactory method for investigating infection in these patients.

Introduction

An association between previous infection with Coxsackie B viruses and the chronic postviral fatigue syndrome (PVFS), also called myalgic encephalomyelitis, has been suspected.[1] Similar associations have been reported between these viruses and recurrent perimyocarditis and chronic peripheral muscle disease,[2-4] mainly on the basis of retrospective findings of significantly increased titres of neutralising antibodies to Coxsackie B viruses.[5]

These viruses are myotropic and involved in acute muscle disease.[6] Persistent enterovirus infection has now been demonstrated by the detection of genomic sequences of Coxsackie B virus in muscle biopsy samples from patients with dermatomyositis, polymyositis, and chronic myocarditis.[7,8] Chronic enterovirus infection has also been reported in cases of chronic myopathy and myositis.[4,9] Significant levels of IgM antibodies specific for Coxsackie B virus have been found in patients with chronic PVFS,[10] which strengthens the serological evidence for a role of enteroviruses in this syndrome. We report here chronic enterovirus infection in a group of patients with PVFS.

Subjects and Methods

Subjects

The patients had a history of at least 6 months and up to 12 years of excessive muscle fatigue on exercise accompanied by myalgia, with or without an acute viral infection at onset. All patients had dysphasia, difficulty with concentration, and short-term memory, and most had difficulty in accommodation. No patient had evidence of neurological disease, and physical examination was normal. When possible the patients enlisted a neighbour of similar age and sex to act as a control.

Isolation of Viruses from Faeces

Stool specimens were obtained from 76 PVFS patients (group A) and 30 controls during the third week of May, 1986. Specimens reached the laboratory within 24 h of collection and were stored at -70°C.

100 ml of a 20% faecal suspension was prepared from every specimen and the supernatant clarified.[11] Supernatants were centrifuged at 150 000 g for 2 h and the pellets resuspended in 4 ml of 'Medium 199' (Gibco). Virus was cultured by two techniques, direct culture and with acid centrifugation.

Flasks of Vero cells and Hep2 cells were drained of growth medium, inoculated with 0.5 ml of the concentrated faecal sample, and the inoculum adsorbed for 2 h at room temperature. The inoculum was decanted, and 30 ml of maintenance medium (Melnick B)[11] added to the flasks which were then incubated at 37°C. The cultures were examined daily for a viral-induced cytopathic effect (CPE) for 3 weeks, during which time two blind passages were done. Positive flasks were harvested when 75% CPE was seen. For acid centrifugation, 1.5 ml 0.1 mol/1 glycine/HC1 buffer, pH 2.4, was added to 2.5 ml of the concentrated sample and the pH readjusted to 2.4 with 0.5 mol/1HC1 before incubation at room temperature for 3 h. The acidified mixture was centrifuged over a 30% sucrose cushion at pH 2.4 for 2h at 150 000 *g*. The optimum concentration of sucrose required for separation of virus and antibody had been determined previously. The supernatant and sucrose were removed and the pellet was resuspended in 1 ml medium 199. The suspension was adjusted to pH 7 by addition of 0.5 mol/1NaOH, and then inoculated into two flasks.[1]

The sensitivity of the system for dissociating IgG and IgA neutralising antibodies from virus had been determined before use. Suspensions of Coxsackie B2 virus containing 100 plaque-forming units per ml were neutralised by overnight incubation at 4°C with dilutions of previously titrated serum or breast-milk from a lactating woman who was hyperimmune to Coxsackie B2 virus. The neutralised suspensions of the virus were treated[2] and "plaqued" by the technique of Dulbecco.[12] The overall efficiency of virus recovery after acid centrifugation was 50%, estimated by plaque counts.

All positive cultures were presumptively identified by the characteristic morphology of enterovirus-induced CPE and by electron microscopy,[6] and confirmed by indirect immunofluorescence with a monoclonal antibody, 5-D8/1, directed against the enteroviral group-specific protein of VP1.[13] Intersecting antiserum pools were used to identify the serotypes of the isolates by a standard neutralisation test.[14]

Stool samples were obtained 12 months later from all the patients from whom enteroviruses were isolated, and the entire process of virus isolation and identification repeated. 36 normal healthy individuals matched by age, sex, and geographical location were included at this time as a new set of controls.

Detection of Immune Complexes

Circulating IgM immune complexes in serum samples obtained from a different series of 87 PVFS patients (group B) were estimated by precipitation with 2% polyethylene glycol (PEG). Precipitated IgM was measured by single radial immunodiffusion against monospecific antibody to human IgM.[15] Positive samples were those with precipitated IgM more than 2 SD above the mean of 612 normal healthy controls.

Detection of Enterovirus-specific IgM Antibodies

Enterovirus-specific IgM responses in patients with positive stool cultures were measured by the μ-antibody-capture ELISA for Coxsackie B IgM.[10] These assays were done 12 months after the initial virus isolation.

Figure 1

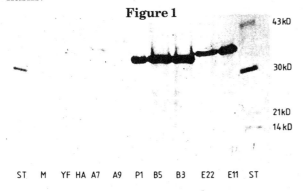

ST   M   YF HA A7   A9   P1 B5   B3   E22 E11 ST

Figure 1 - Western blots of proteins from a range of enteroviruses and other unrelated viruses probed with 5-D8/1 molecular antibody.

Enterovirus peptide reacting with 5-D8/1 has molecular wight of 34-37 kD and has been shown by radioimmunoprecipitation to be VP1.
ST= molecular weight standards, M=measles, YF=yellow fever, HA=hepatitis A, A7=Coxsackie A7, A9=Coxsackie A9, P1=poliovirus I, B5=Coxsackie B5, B3=Coxsackie B3, E22=Echo-22, and E11=Echo-11.

Characterisation of Monoclonal Antibody 5-D8/1

The monoclonal antibody 5-D8/1, produced against heat-inactivated Coxsackie B5 virus, reacted with the VP1 polypeptide of all tested enteroviruses except hepatitis A virus. This antibody specifically detects a single enteroviral protein, and the antibody does not react with any virus that is not an enterovirus (fig 1).[13] In a separate study, 5-D8/1 was used to screen 130 field isolates of a wide range of enteroviruses in a dot-blot enzyme immunoassay. 95% of the isolates were conveniently and correctly identified as enteroviruses.[16]

Table 1
Virus Isolation from Faeces of PVFS Patients

(Group A) and Contols		
Culture technique	PVFS patients (n=76)	Controls (n=30)
No. of patients:		
After direct culture	2 (3%)	2 (7%)
Only after acid centrifugation	15 (20%)	0*
Total	17 (22%)	2(6.7%)

*PVFS vs controls: x^2= 5.9, p<0.01

Detection of Enterovirus Antigen in Serum

The technique[17] for the detection of antigens that are free or in circulating immune complexes was modified by use of peroxidase-labelled 5-D8/1 as detector instead of rabbit polyclonal antibody. Briefly, 100 µl samples of serum were incubated with 10 µl of peroxidase-labelled monoclonal antibody for 5 days at 4°C. PEG in EDTA buffer, pH 7.6, was added to a final concentration of 2%. After a further 2 days at 4°C the samples were centrifuged, the precipitate washed with 2% PEG, and its enzyme content measured. Results were expressed as the percentage of the labelled antibody that was precipitated. 87 group B sera were studied with sera from matched normal controls.

VP1 antigen detection tests were also done on the sera of all group A patients with positive cultures after acid centrifugation and compared with the results from 16 group A patients who were culture negative.

Results
Virus Isolation

Results of attempts to isolate virus from the 76 patients in group A with PVFS and 30 controls are shown in Table 1. 12 of the 17 enteroviruses isolated after acid centrifugation produced visible CPE only after a second passage in cell culture. In May, the month when the first stool samples were collected, some acute enterovirus infections (both overt and subclinical) would be expected in the population. This is shown by the positive findings after direct culture without acid centrifugation in 2 PVFS patients and 2 controls. While acid dissociation and centrifugation resulted in the isolation of viruses from a further 15 PVFS patients, neither of the 2 controls became positive.

3 of the 4 isolates recovered by direct culture were identified as Coxsackie B5 (table 2), which suggests a predominance of this particular serotype at the time the samples were obtained. The remaining direct isolate was an echovirus type 11. Table 2 shows that subgroups of enteroviruses other than Coxsackie B are also associated with PVFS. Despite their characteristic CPE, enteroviral morphology under electron microscopy, and positive reaction with 5-D8/1, 2 isolates could not be serotyped by National Institutes of Health, World Health Organisation, and Colindale antiserum pools, which cover all enteroviruses other than types 68-71.

The 17 patients with positive stool cultures were studied again after 12 months. 5 (29%) were still yielding the same virus (assuming that the untyped enterovirus isolated from patient 14 in 1987 was the same as that isolated in 1986). Neither of the 2 patients from whom virus was isolated previously by direct culture, before acid centrifugation, was positive in 1987. The 2 controls who had been negative for VP1 antigen were still negative when tested 12 months later.

IgM Responses to Enteroviruses

13 of the 17 culture-positive group A patients (76%)

still had detectable enterovirus IgM antibodies 12 months after the isolation of virus from their faeces (table 2). Most patients (9/13) showed heterotypic responses, a well-known finding in enterovirus infections.[18,19] Both patients from whom virus was isolated by direct culture in 1986 had no detectable enterovirus-specific IgM response in 1987.

IgM Complexes and Enterovirus Antigens in Serum

IgM circulating immune complexes were detected in 64 of 87 group B sera (74%) from the second group of patients and 42 of the 64 had detectable enterovirus antigen in the serum (fig 2). 2 of 23 patients (9%) without IgM complexes also had detectable antigen in their circulation, possibly complexed with IgG. Thus a total of 44 (51%) patients were positive for enterovirus antigen. All positive patients were retested after 4 months and 39 (89%) were still positive. No controls were positive for enterovirus antigen. The difference in frequency of detection of VP1 antigen between the PVFS patients and controls was significant (p<0.001).

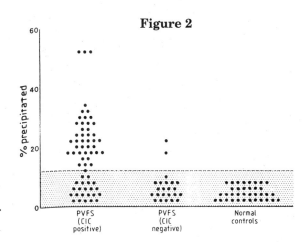

Figure 2

Figure 2 - Detection of VP1 antigen in serum by enzyme immunoassay.

64 PVFS patients from group A were positive for IgM circulating immune complexes (CIC) and 23 were negative. Cut-off level for positive samples was three SD above mean of 36 normal controls.

Table 2						
Correlation of Results in 76 PVFS Patients (Group A) and 30 Controls in May, 1986, and 12 Months Later						
	May, 1986			May, 1987		
	Isolate					
Group	Direct	Acid centrifugation	VP1 antigen	Acid centrifugation isolate	VP1 antigen	Enterovirus-specific IgM antibody
PVFS:						
1	None	CB5	+	None	+	Heterotypic
2	None	Echo-1	+	None	-	-
3	None	CB2	+	CB2	+	Monotypic
4	CB5	CB5	-	None	-	-
5	None	CB3	+	None	+	Heterotypic
6	None	Echo-11	+	None	+	Heterotypic
7	None	CB1	+	CB1	+	Heterotypic
8	None	CB2	+	CB2	+	Monotypic
9	None	CB2	+	None	-	Monotypic
10	None	CB5	+	None	-	Heterotypic
11	None	CB4	+	None	+	Heterotypic
12	None	Echo-9	+	None	-	-
13	None	CB1	+	None	-	Heterotypic
14	None	Untyped	+	Untyped	+	Heterotypic
15	None	Untyped	+	None	-	Monotypic
16	Echo-11	Echo-11	-	None	-	-
17	None	CB4	+	CB4	+	Heterotypic
Contols:						
1	CB5	CB5	-	NT	-	NT
2	CB5	CB5	-	NT	-	NT

NT= not tested

VP1 antigen was detected in the sera of the 15 group A patients who were culture positive only after acid centrifugation but not in the 2 patients in whom virus was detected by direct culture (fig 3). 7 of 16 culture-negative patients had detectable VP1 in the serum, but the level of antigen was low.

Figure 3

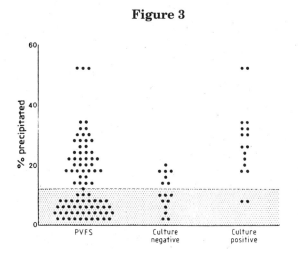

Figure 3 - VP1 antigen in serum of PVFS patients.

Figure shows 87 PVFS patients from group B, and from group A, 17 PVFS patients with positive faecal culture (see table 1) and 16 of 59 with negative faecal culture.

Discussion

Several studies have suggested that infection with enteroviruses is causally related to PVFS.[1,21] The association of PVFS with known outbreaks of enterovirus infection, usually Coxsackie B viruses, has reinforced this view.[22] Nevertheless many investigators felt that the persistence of symptoms was not due to continued infection, but was a functional sequelae of the initial viral infection. In vitro evidence has shown the persistence of enteroviruses in different cell lines,[23,24] which makes it possible to postulate that even the highly lytic enteroviruses are potentially capable of inducing chronic infection in vivo. This was confirmed by reports demonstrating persistent enterovirus infection in association with chronic human muscle and cardiac disease.[7,8]

The association of detectable IgM complexes and VP1 antigen in the serum of the PVFS patients in our study was high. Our assay can detect the viral protein both free or complexed with antibody. Why is there such a strong association between antigen and IgM complexes? In the presence of IgM antibody VP1 probably generates detectable amounts of IgM complexes, as long as the antigen persists in the circulation.

When we substituted an enterovirus-group-specific monoclonal antibody for the rabbit polyclonal antiserum previously used for antigen detection in serum, the amount of precipitated enzyme-labelled antibody was increased from a maximum of 1.5% to over 50%, which makes the test more sensitive and more reproducible. All but 2 patients with positive stool cultures had significantly increased levels of VP1 antigen in the circulation, and although 7 of 16 of those with negative cultures had detectable antigen, it was present at low concentration. The fact that 89% of the patients with detectable levels of VP1 were still positive 4 months later indicates a prolonged infection.

The methods we used to culture the virus effectively removed bound neutralising antibodies from the virus. Overall the technique yielded positive cultures in 17/76 PVFS patients, and 2/30 normal controls. This suggests that enterovirus infection plays an important role in the aetiology of PVFS. This is supported by our finding that acid centrifugation of the faecal samples enhanced the recovery of viruses from the PVFS patients but had no effect on samples from the controls.

Attempts to isolate virus from faecal samples of PVFS patients by direct culture, the conventional method used in clinical virology, were consistently negative, probably because antibodies (predominantly IgA) in the gut neutralise the virus. Acidification, however, dissociates the antibody from the virus, which is acid resistant.[11] The now viable viruses are then pelleted by centrifugation through 30% sucrose leaving the antibody above. Where viruses were cultured before acidification, no VP1 antigen was detected in serum. This suggests transient viral carriage rather than systemic infection.

When investigations were repeated 1 year later, 5 of 17 patients still had positive cultures, of the same serotype as before. 13 of the 17 still had enterovirus-specific IgM antibodies and 9 had detectable VP1 antigen in their serum. This is strong evidence for the persistence of virus infection for at least 1 year.

Viral antigen detection in the serum is a more sensitive test for demonstrating enteroviral infection in PVFS than virus isolation. In fact clinical monitoring of these patients showed that the correlation between clinical improvement and disappearance of both VP1 antigen and IgM complexes from the circulation was high (data not shown).

We thank the ME Association for financial support for some of this work.

Correspondence should be addressed to J.F.M., Department of Pathology, St. Mary's Hospital Medical School, London W2 1PG.

References

1. Calder BD, Warnock PJ. Coxsackie B infections in a Scottish general practice. J R Coll Gen Pract 1984; 34: 15-19.

2. Koontz CH, Ray CG. The role of Coxsackie group B virus infections in sporadic myopericarditis. Am Heart J 1971; 82: 750-58.

3. Rose HD. Recurrent illness following acute Coxsackie B4 myocarditis. Am J Med 1973; 54: 544-48.

4. Tang JT, Sedmack GV, Siegesmund KA, McCreadie SR. Chronic myopathy associated with Coxsackie type A9. N Engl J Med 1975; 292: 608-11.

5. Keighley BD, Bell EJ. Sporadic myalgic encephalomyelitis in a rural practice. J R Coll Gen Pract 1983; 33: 338-41.

6. Melnick JL. Enteroviruses. In: Evans AS, ed. Viral infections of humans. New York: Plenum, 1982: 187-251.

7. Bowles NE, Richardson PJ, Olsen EGJ, Archard LC. Detection of Coxsackie-B-virus-specific RNA sequences in myocardial biopsy samples from patients with myocarditis and dilated cardiomyopathy. Lancet 1986; i: 1120-23.

8. Bowles NE, Dubowitz V, Sewry CA, Archard LC. Dermatomyositis, polymyositis, and Coxsackie-B-virus infections. Lancet 1987; i: 1104-07.

9. Jehn UW, Fink MK. Myositis, myoglobinaemia, and myoglobinuria associated with enterovirus echo type 9 infection. Arch Neurol 1980; 37: 457-58.

10. McCartney, RA, Banatvala JE, Bell EJ. Routine use of µ-antibody capture ELISA for the serological diagnosis of Coxsackie B virus infections. J Med Virol 1986; 19: 205-12.

11. Melnick JL, Wenner HA, Phillips CA. The enteroviruses. In: Lennette EH, Schmidt NJ, eds. Diagnostic procedures for viral, rickettsial, and chlamydial infections. 4th ed. Washington: American Public Health Association, 1979: 471-534.

12. Dulbecco R. Production of plaques in monolayer tissue culture by single particles of an animal virus. Proc Nat Acad Sci USA 1952; 38: 747-69.

13. Yousef GE, Brown IN, Mowbray JF. Derivation and biochemical characterisation of an enterovirus group-specific monoclonal antibody. Intervirology (in press).

14. Grist NR, Bell EJ, Follett EC, Urquhart GED. Neutralisation tests. In: Diagnostic methods in clinical virology. Oxford: Blackwell, 1979: 81-94.

15. Burton-Kee J, Morgan-Capner P, Mowbray JF. Nature of circulating immune complexes in infective endocarditis. J Clin Pathol 1980; 33: 653-59.

16. Yousef GE, Mann GF, Brown IN, Mowbray JF. Clinical and research application of an enterovirus group-specific monoclonal antibody. Intervirology (in press).

17. Dambuyant C, Burton-Kee J, Mowbray JF. Demonstration of two disease specific antigens in circulating immune complexes. Clin Exp Immunol 1979; 37: 424-32.

18. King ML, Shaikh A, Bidwell D, Voller A, Banatvala JE. Coxsackie-B-virus-specific IgM responses in children with insulin-dependent (juvenile-onset; type I) diabetes mellitus. Lancet 1983; i: 1397-99.

19. Pugh SF. Heterotypic reactions in a radioimmunoassay for Coxsackie B virus-specific IgM. J Clin Pathol 1984; 37: 433-39.

20. Bell EJ, McCartney RA, Basquill D, Chaudhuri AKR. µ-Antibody capture ELISA for the rapid diagnosis of enterovirus infections in patients with aseptic meningitis. J Med Virol 1986; 19: 213-17.

21. Calder BD, Warnock PJ, McCartney RA, Bell EJ. Coxsackie B viruses and the post-viral fatigue syndrome: a prospective study in general practice. J R Coll Gen Pract 1987; 37: 11-14.

22. Fegan KG, Behan PO, Bell EJ. Myalgic encephalomyelitis: Report of an epidemic. J R Coll Gen Pract 1983; 33: 335-37.

23. Matteucci D, Paglianti M, Giangregorio A, Capobianchi M, Dianzini F, Bendinelli M. Group B Coxsackieviruses readily establish persistent infections in lymphoid cell lines. J Virol 1985; 56: 651-54.

24. Frank A, Schmidt EV, Smith RE. Persistent infection of rat insulinoma cells with Coxsackie B4 virus. Arch Virol 1986; 87: 143-50.

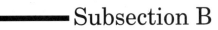

The Retroviral Theories

Chapter 33

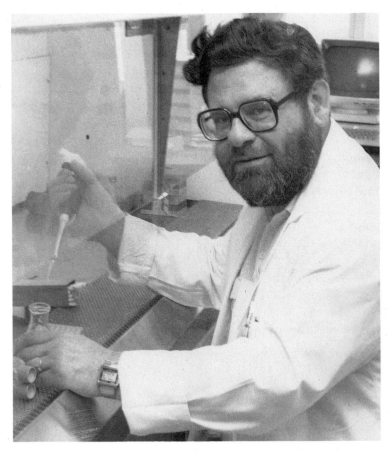

Michael J. Holmes

A Retrovirus Aetiology for CFS?

Michael J Holmes, MD

Senior Lecturer, Department of Microbiology, University of Otago, P.O. Box 56, Dunedin, New Zealand

Dr. Holmes is a clinical immuno-virologist who qualified in Medicine at Liverpool, then spent seven years with the British Antarctic survey. After spells at the UK Common Cold Unit and the Clinical Research Centre, Harrow, he submitted his MD thesis and went to work for NASA on the Viking project. He is now Senior Lecturer at Otago Medical School, New Zealand and has been working on the peripheral blood cytology of CFS for the past four years. In 1986-87, work by Dr Holmes was the first to suggest the possibility of reverse transcriptase activity in CFS T cell cultures. (Several local graduate study papers were written describing this discovery.)

This discussion paper is offered more as a vehicle for airing limited findings and inferential material rather than for making any hard claims that we have established a retrovirus aetiology for CFS. The data are provocative and, in the light of other contemporary observations, would seem to hold up very well. I am, however, still 'flying a kite'. The findings we have rest on the results of a limited pilot study run in July and August 1986. It was shelved when funds ran out and, though we have been trying to obtain more ever since, they have not yet been forthcoming.

Briefly, we took 6 of the CFS patients referred to my laboratory by professor Murdoch of the Department of General Practice, Otago Medical School, in Dunedin, New Zealand, age and sex-matched them with 6 controls, and set up a series of matched patient and control lymphocyte cultures from specimens of peripheral blood taken by venepuncture from the antecubital vein.

Lymphocytes were separated on a Ficoll-Conray interface and cultured for extended periods in an attempt to demonstrate evidence of chronic infection by a lymphotropic virus. Cultures were examined fro cytopathic effects in the lymphocytes, evidence of the presence of structures resembling virus particles and by assay of the culture supernatants for the presence of reverse transcriptase using an assay modified in this laboratory to enhance its sensitivity.

Before setting up the cultures, cytospin preparations were made and phenotyped by immuno-peroxidase labelling, according to the method of Moir and colleagues[1].

The cultures were sampled with each media change, aliquots of the supernatants tested for reverse transcriptase (RT) activity by conversion of the mixed oligonucleotide to its deoxy form in the presence either of magnesium or manganese ions. Duplicate experiments using the deoxy form of the oligonucleotide were carried out to assess the possi-

ble non-specific effects of cellular nucleases. All specimens were tested in triplicate, blind and randomised with the controls. A positive control of caprine arthritis-encephalitis virus RT derived from infected goat synovial membrane primary cell cultures was included with each experiment.

From each specimen, aliquots of cells were removed from the MLC for thin-section low power electron microscopy (EM) of the cellular morphologies. The EM preparations were not examined at high power for virus particles since at this time the machine was faulty and losing definition at higher magnifications.

A Powerful RT Inhibitor

Our findings were puzzling. At 6 days, that is, just before we added mitogen, RT activity was detected in culture supernatants from 4 out of the 6 patients at

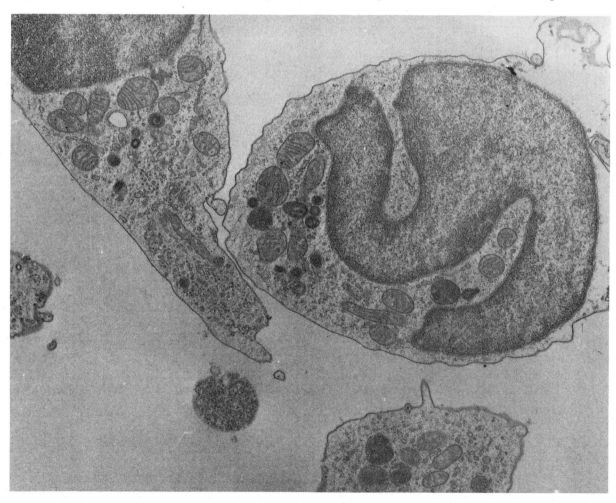

Abnormal Convoluted Nucleus of a Mononuclear Cell from a M.E./CFS patient. This would be similar to what would be expected from an HIV/ARC syndrome patient.

levels from 1.5 to 4 times those of controls. Since each retrovirion has only two molecules of RT, this inferred that a significant quantity of virus was being produced, especially when the replication rate of this group is normally so slow. The DNA oligonucleotide controls were very low, so we were confident of our technique. However, at subsequent samplings the RT levels of the whole group were lower than those of the negative controls. It was not until some time later that we identified a powerful inhibitor in the mitogen preparation.

Abnormal Mononuclear Cells

The EM morphology studies also proved suggestive. In the earliest samples we found a proportion of mononuclear cells with convoluted nuclei comparable to those described in the ARC syndrome. These were not present in controls.

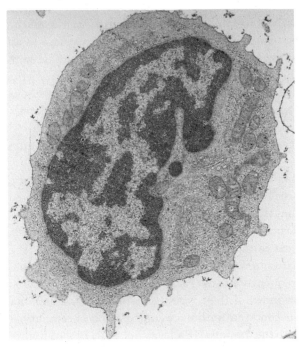

Mononuclear Cell, Normal Control (1986)

At 6 days some of the mononuclear cells had begun to develop vacuoles which had a reticular appearance and which also we were unable to observe in the controls. Later specimens began to show degenerative changes which we did not observe in controls, although cell losses began to increase by day 14 in both patient and control groups.

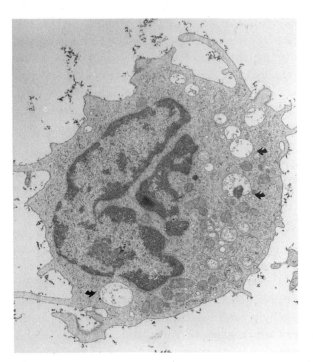

Vaculated Mononuclear Cell, CFS patient (1986)

The only other finding from this pilot study was a T helper cell cytopenia in the CFS patients which we later confirmed in more extensive investigations.

I would like to draw your attention to these observations in a broader context. The RT activity we recorded is not decisive but certainly merits further consideration and the apparent abnormalities we found in the white cells themselves would also benefit from a closer scrutiny. Within the limits of the trial we could scarcely have found anything more suggestive of retrovirus activity that was still consistent with the symptomatology of CFS. However, we would like to propose a retrovirus aetiology for CFS based not only on this pilot but on the train of deductive observation which led us to consider it in the first place.

**Coxsackie Virus and Candida Albicans
as Opportunists**

First, I would ask you to consider the various pathogens from *Candida albicans* to coxsackie-viruses which have been proposed as causative agents. Practically all of them are highly persistent or latent organisms which tend to be found in immunologically embarrassed patients. They are not classical opportunists but they are not far off. Many human retroviruses appear to favour lymphoid cells as targets. If we have one here, it would be thoroughly in keeping with those others which we know to infect humans. The dilemma of the various other candidates for the agent of CFS would then be resolved. Instead of rivals, they become epiphenomena in a condition now recognised as including immune dysfunction.

Interferon Poisoning

We were impressed by our patients' own descriptions of their condition as 'Poor man's AIDS' and, when we compared symptomatology, were even more impressed by the similarities to the ARC syndrome. This has been given a new impetus here by my colleague, Dr. Cheney's, report of the very high levels of activity recorded in the 2'-5' oligosynthetase pathway, which suggests that a lot of interferon (IFN) is being made. Further, Dr. Andrew Lloyd and his colleagues have pointed out the striking similarities of CFS symptoms to IFN poisoning. Let us consider, therefore, the possibility that our patients are making a lot of interferon.

A Chronic Persistent RNA Virus

If the CFS symptoms are due to IFN poisoning, they must have a prolonged stimulus to sustain IFN induction. They must, in fact, have a chronic infection. It must also be an intracellular infection, because IFN is induced only by the presence of foreign nucleic acids *inside* a cell. Furthermore, the most powerful IFN inducers are RNAs. In this scenario we therefore have a chronic, persistent, lymphotropic, RNA virus. We also have a plethora of low-grade, persistent, opportunist, epiphenomena which suggests a degree of immune dysfunction and we now have independent serological evidence of the latter.

A Possible Retrovirus

Now, a virus which induces IFN production normally kills the host cell after a varying period of virus production. Before this happens, however, IFN can diffuse to neighbouring cells rendering them less amenable to infection. Also, during virus production, the cell becomes immunologically 'visible' and thus subject to immune surveillance. Unless a cell is latently infected with a non-productive virus infec-

tion it is destroyed, and this is the basis of the cell-mediated immune response. The production of IFN can therefore be seen, in one aspect, as an interim measure to contain an infection until host defenses can be mobilised to control it. This does not happen in CFS for years, although it seems to eventually. And there is one group of viruses which can make an immunologically invisible DNA provirus copy of themselves which is inserted into a host cell chromosome, namely the Retrovirus.

This provirus copy can lie latent for a long time and is activated only when the host cell reads the frame under the impression it is making a bit of RNA to do some housekeeping job like making a protein. What it actually does is make a new infectious virus which can then induce IFN production. A significant percentage of CFS sufferers relate the onset of their condition to a "dose of 'flu" and indeed, one of the names for CFS is Post-viral Fatigue Syndrome. If an activated lymphocyte is reading provirus frames and accidentally making retroviruses in response to an antigenic challenge, this would be compatible with the CFS picture. Furthermore, many of our patients describe relapses as triggered by an acute infectious episode, which would also be explicable in the same way.

Absence of Common Colds in CFS patients

As a coda to the suggestion that CFS patients are producing sustained levels of IFN, we have noted that the majority of our patients maintain that they do not suffer from common colds during their illness. This is such a feature of the condition that the patients, without any reference to clinical opinion, frequently cite the reappearance of common colds as an index of their recovery. Admittedly this is an anecdotal datum but it would certainly be compatible with the waning of IFN levels, as would be the absence of common colds while IFN levels were sustained.

Finally, there is the strange biphasic nature of the condition: limited outbreaks with a persistent intercurrent trickle of cases. This would also be consistent with a retrovirus aetiology. The RT is an enzyme which forces a reaction the 'wrong way'. It is much easier to make RNA from DNA than vice versa and the DNA copies are not good. They are *low-fidelity* copies (which accounts for the rapid antigenic evolution of HIV). Every so often, therefore, a nastier strain is going to appear, but, because of the essential genetic instability of the virus, it is unlikely to persist for long. This would cause the limited outbreaks. Apart from HIV, the majority of retrovirus infections seem to be occult and this would also be compatible with the sporadic cases which are seen.

The sporadic cases would therefore represent the tip of the iceberg in a largely silent endemic or epidemic situation. The majority of infections would be occult and the unlucky patients would be those who triggered a whole series of latently infected cells with an ill-timed acute infection or an unhappy mutation with a bad provirus copy.

We therefore propose a retrovirus aetiology for CFS. Moreover, we propose a retrovirus which would bear the same sort of relationship to the more severe ones (such as those associated with AIDS and leukemia), that a common cold virus bears to its first cousin, paralytic poliomyelitis. We also suggest that it is likely to cause a high proportion of occult infections and that it is likely to be lymphotropic.

References

Moir, D.J., Ghosh, A.K., Abdulaziz, A., Knight, P.M. and Mason, D.Y. (1983). "Immunoenzymatic staining of haematological samples with monoclonal antibodies." **Brit. J. Haem. 55**: 395-410

Retrovirus Particles (Presumed), Isolated and Grown by Dr. M. Holmes, from CFS patients

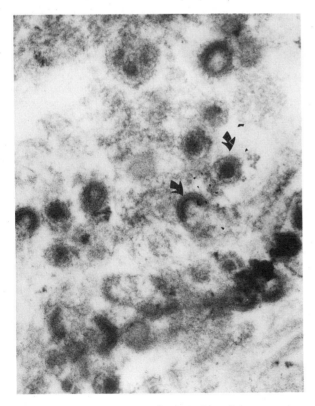

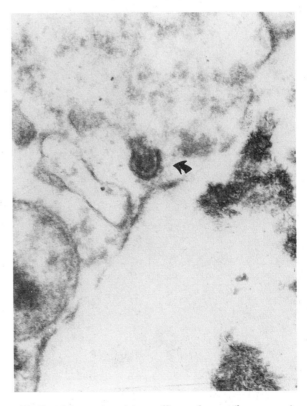

(1) Immature and maturing virions   (2) Particle approaching cell membrane (low power)

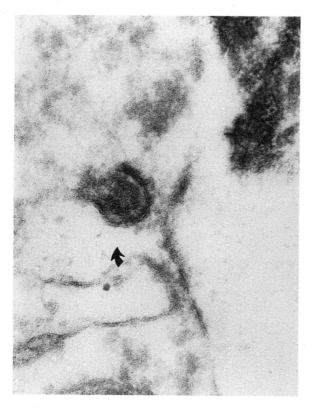

(3) Particle approaching cell membrane (high power)

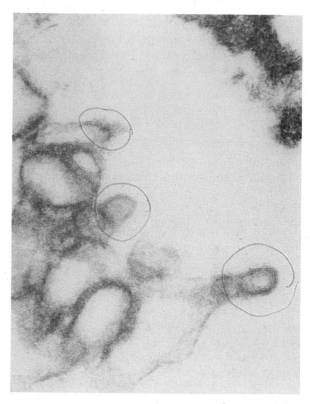

(4) Particle budding across cell membrane. Note similarity of to budding retroviral particles of Dr. DeFreitas.

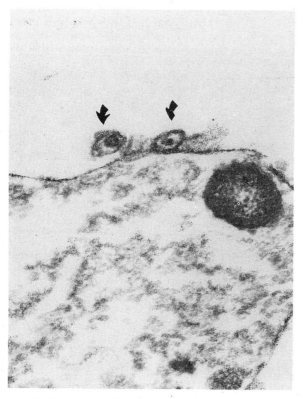

(5) Viral particles outside of cell membrane

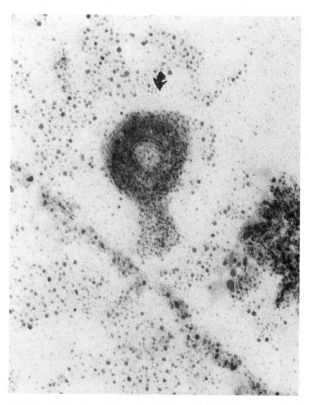

(6) Particles just detached from the cell membrane (high power)

Chapter 34

Viral Infection in CFS Patients

W. John Martin, MD, PhD, Department of Pathology, USC School of Medicine, Los Angeles, California, 90033

(Please see Chapter 27 for Dr. Martin's photograph and curriculum vitae.)

Introduction

As outlined in the preceding manuscript (see Chapter 27)[1], the use of a low stringency polymerase chain reaction (PCR) had provided evidence for persistent viral infection in several patients diagnosed as having the chronic fatigue syndrome (CFS). The viral sequences were detected in patients' blood using a set of PCR primers reactive with regions of the gene coding the gp 64 late antigen (LA) of human cytomegalovirus (CMV)[2]. Actual infection with CMV was considered unlikely, however, since PCR probing for other CMV related genes gave negative results. Moreover, the CMV LA reactive primers were not specific for CMV but could amplify various regions within other human herpesviruses, including human herpesvirus-6, Herpes simplex virus, Epstein-Barr virus and varicella zoster virus.

Support for a viral origin of CFS, and for a spectrum of CFS related disorders ranging from mild illness to profound neurological disturbance, was provided by studies on a stereotactic brain biopsy on a woman with an unexplained progressive dysphasia. The brain biopsy tested positive for the CMV cross-reactive sequences by PCR. Enveloped viral particles were seen within the cytoplasm of neural cells. The nature of the virus could not be determined although the appearance was considered consistent with an atypical herpesvirus or a retrovirus.

These studies have been extended since the time of the Cambridge Symposium. Progress has been made in both the use of low stringency PCR for viral detection and in the cultivation of a novel cytopathic virus from a large number of patients with CFS and with related neurological and neuromuscular diseases.

Polymerase Chain Reaction

The finding of viral particles in a PCR positive brain biopsy specimen led to efforts to identify other patients with unexplained neurological illnesses. In addition to the generic herpesviral PCR probes, the laboratory also used primers designed to amplify the tax gene of human T lymphotropic virus (HTLV) types I and II. Again, the PCR assays using the HTLV primers were run under conditions of reduced stringency so as to detect the possible presence of HTLV related sequences. The actual primers and detecting probe used differed only slightly from those described by Ehrlich and colleagues[3].

The PCR assays were established such that extracts of blood from normal healthy donors would consistently yield negative results by dot blot hybridization on PCR products. Multiple PCR products of varying sizes were, however, visualized on ethidium stained agarose gels when DNA from normal individuals was used as template. A strong positive hybridization by dot blot and a well defined band of the expected size were readily identified when HTLV I infected cells were used as the source of template DNA in the PCR. Blood samples from several CFS patients gave weak, but positive, dot blot hybridization signals. On Southern blot analysis, the reactive PCR products were shown to be of varying sizes and not to correspond to those seen with the positive HTLV control. The diagnostic utility of this assay was critically dependent of standardizing the exact assay conditions each time new primers and detecting probe were synthesized. Only in this way could there be the assurance of conditions that would not yield positive hybridization results with blood from normal individuals. Both positive and negative controls were run in each assay.

The results using the HTLV primers generally paralleled those using the CMV LA primers. Thus, while there were no positive responses seen when testing normal individuals, several patients gave clearly positive results. Of particular interest was the striking findings of CMV-LA and HTLV positive PCR results in a patient with severe residual neurological impairment three years following an atypical encephalitis-like illness. A clinical diagnosis of Herpes simplex encephalitis had been made but only after several days in hospital. The clinical diagnosis had been delayed because of essentially normal findings on examination of the cerebrospinal fluid (CSF). The individual responded poorly to Acylovir therapy. Similar PCR findings were encountered in a 6 months old child in whom an encephalopathic illness slowly developed. By PCR, a 4+ response was seen with the HTLV primer set and a 2+ response with the CMV-LA primer set. Yet the CSF chemistry was unremarkable. Detailed clinical descriptions of these and other cases will be presented elsewhere. The findings did, however, prompt an intense effort to attempt to culture virus from PCR positive CFS patients.

Viral Culture

A CFS patient repeatedly tested positive using both sets of PCR primers. The patient's illness was initially characterized by intense headaches, generalized myalgia and fever. She was hospitalized with an admitting diagnosis of encephalitis / meningitis. Her CSF examination, however, was unremarkable. The patient was treated with antibiotics which were discontinued after she developed watery diarrhea which subsequently subsided. The patient was discharged after 7 days with a clinical diagnosis of unexplained viral infection. Since that time she has experienced severe fatigue necessitating elimination of weekend social activities and a marked reduction in her capacity for normal work. Her cognitive functions have become impaired especially her capacity to name items (dysnomia). Her short term memory is also defective. Moreover, she has near complete amnesia for the period of hospitalization and for events immediately preceding her initial illness. Her blood was cultured on a variety of cell lines including human fibroblasts. A cytopathic effect (CPE), characterized by the formation of rounded cell syncytia with prominent lipid inclusions was noted. The CPE is not typical of any of the commonly isolated viruses in clinical laboratories. Nor do the affected cells stain using commercially available typing antisera. The viral infected cells were examined by electron microscopy. Numerous enveloped viral particles were seen within intracytoplasmic vacuoles. Non-enveloped, developing viral particles, were seen within the nucleus. The CPE and electron micrographic appearances were suggestive of foamy or spumaviruses[4].

We have repeatedly cultured the same virus from this individual as well as from her CSF. Virus producing a similar type of CPE in culture has been cultured from a number of additional patients referred for testing because of CFS-like illness. The rate of viral positivity has varied somewhat depending on the referring clinician. It has ranged from 40% to over 70%. Although, the culture results have yet to be correlated with clinical features, we know of no viral culture positive patients in whom the symptoms were considered to be vague and questionable. Nor have we seen positive cultures from normal, asymptomatic individuals.

Discussion

The culture findings add considerable support to the evidence from PCR that many CFS patients are persistently infected with a virus that shares some features with both herpesviruses and retroviruses. This could be explained by a recombinant virus containing both retroviral and herpesviral sequences. Possibly, the herpesviral related sequences could impart spumaviral and neurovirulence characteristics to an otherwise non-neurovirulent retrovirus. This suggestion would also be consistent with the findings reported by DeFreitas and her colleagues of HTLV-II gag region sequences in blood of CFS patients[5]. The exact classification of the foamy-cell inducing viruses that have been cultured from CFS patients will best be decided on the basis of sequencing data and efforts towards this goal are underway.

The virus has been grown from CSF and this result, along with positive PCR findings on CSF, strongly suggest actual viral infection of the brain in CFS patients. This would readily explain the cognitive impairment experienced by a large number of CFS patients. It also underlies the concept that CFS may represent a spectrum of viral associated neurological diseases. Continued studies on the viruses which we have cultured should help identify stategic approaches to therapy and help unravel many of the questions concerning the pathogenesis of CFS.

Acknowledgement

I wish to thank Khalid Ahmed, Li Cheng Zeng, Manju Roy, Anton Mayr and Peymon Javaherbin for helping to establish the viral culture and PCR assays. The work was supported by funds from CFIDS Association, Inc., North Carolina.

References

1. Martin WJ. Detection of viral related sequences in CFS patients using polymerase chain reaction. Proceedings of the Cambridge Symposium (this issue).

2. Shibata D, Martin WJ, Appleman MD, et al. Detection of cytomegaloviral DNA in peripheral blood of patients infected with human immunodeficiency virus. J Infect Dis 1988; 158:1185-1192.

3. Ehrlich GD, Greenberg S, Abbott MA. Detection of human T-cell lymphoma / leukemia viruses in "PCR Protocols: A Guide to Methods and Applications". Ed Innis MI, Gelfand DH, Sninsky JJ, and White TJ. Academic Press 325-336; 1990.

4. Hooks JJ, Gibbs CJ. The foamy virus. Bacteriol Rev 1975; 39:169-185

5. DeFreitas E, Hilliard B, Cheney PR, et al. Retroviral sequences related to human T lymphocytotropic virus type II in patients with chronic fatigue immune dysfunction syndrome. Proc Natl Acad Sci USA. 1991; 88:2922-2926.

Chapter 35

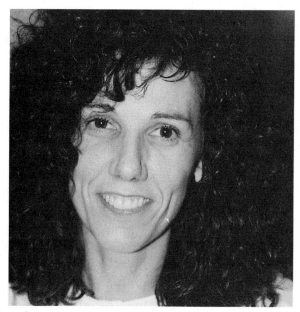

Elaine DeFreitas

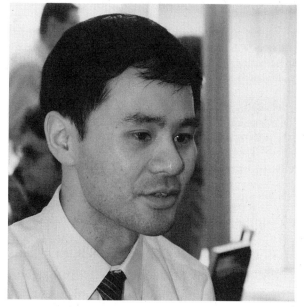

Hiroshi Terunuma

The Search for a Retrovirus in CFS/CFIDS

Elaine DeFreitas, PhD, Hiroshi Terunuma, MD, PhD
The Wistar Institute, 3601 Spruce Street, Philadelphia, PA 19104 USA

The following chapter was first published by the Gulfcoast CFIDS Association, March 1992, Sarasota, Florida in the form of audio and video cassettes, which was then distributed by that society. We have attempted to reproduce the text and visual materials to the best of our abilities. All of this material is based upon a public speech given by Elaine DeFreitas to the press and public in Sarasota, Florida in March of 1992 at a conference entitled, CFIDS, Advances in Research and Treatment. Over 500 antendees were present.

A scientifically more correct version of this chapter has been submitted and we believe will be published at the same time as this book by the Proceedings of the National Academy of Sciences, U.S.A. We suggest that researchers refer to the NAS publication as well as **The CFIDS Chronicle**, *published by the CFIDS Association of North Carolina, who funded this research and who will also be publishing a perhaps more complete version of the material for their members. We highly recommend that the readers of this text refer to these two associations as our material is not an authorized version.*

In her speech, Dr. DeFreitas noted Dr. Paul Cheney, Dr. Hiroshi Terunuma, Dr. David Bell and Dr. Gerd Maul were instrumental in the success of this project. Financial support from the CFIDS Association in Charlotte, NC and the ongoing efforts of Marc Iverson were responsible for the project's financing. She also noted the important collaboration of Edward Kiggundu, Dian Sankey, Subrata Ghosh, Brian Shank and Brendan Hillard.

Dr. DeFreitas received her Master's degree from the University of Florida and her doctoral degree from the Pennsylvania State University. She received post-doctoral training at the National Jewish Research Center for Immunology in Denver, Colorado. Dr. DeFreitas is an Associate Professor at the Wistar Institute in Philadelphia and Associate Professor of pathology at the University of Pennsylvania. As principal investigator of a research team, she has presented evidence of an HTLV-II like virus associated with CFS, which was subsequently published in Proceedings of the National Academy of Sciences in April 1991.

Dr. Terunuma received his M.D. and Ph.D. from the Tohoku University School of Medicine in Japan. After his residency in Neurology at the Nakamura Memorial Hospital in Sapporo, Japan, Dr. Terunuma became Assistant Professor at the Tohoku University School of Medicine. Following this, Dr. Terunuma undertook his current position as Associate Scientist at the Wistar Institute. Dr. Terunuma has authored and co-authored many articles with his main research interests lying in the mechanisms of neuronal tissue damage in vitro and in vivo in HTLV-I infection and the isolation and cDNA cloning of a retrovirus-like agent from patients with chronic fatigue immune dysfunction syndrome (CFIDS).

The Cheney-Bell-DeFreitas-Terunuma Retrovirus

Unfortunately we have been requested by Dr. DeFreitas not to publish this excellent verbatim chapter. Accordingly, we have replaced the space in the book with a review chapter, that discusses some of the fundamentals of the retroviral theory of M.E. / CFS and some of the problems associated with this concept. If the Cheney-Bell-DeFreitas-Terunuma group is correct, they have made an astounding breakthrough. If permission is given prior to printing, we will print this remarkable chapter in the addendum of this text.

Chapter 36

The Search for A Retrovirus in M.E. / CFS, A Review

Byron Hyde, M.D.
(Please see Chapter 5 for Dr. Hyde's photograph and curriculum vitae.)

Many distinguished and eminent researchers have voiced considerable and voluble criticism of the role, if any, of a retrovirus association with M.E./CFS. Some of the adherents of the retrovirus theory pose another question: are there one or two different retroviruses? This retroviral controversy will either rapidly evaporate as did the American based EBV, Cytomegalic Virus and HHV6 theories of M.E. / CFS or it will continue to be an explosive issue over the next few years. If the retroviral theory proves to be correct, in even a small group of individuals, it will not only change the way we think about M.E. / CFS, but it may also alter our present concept of the pathogenesis of many diseases.

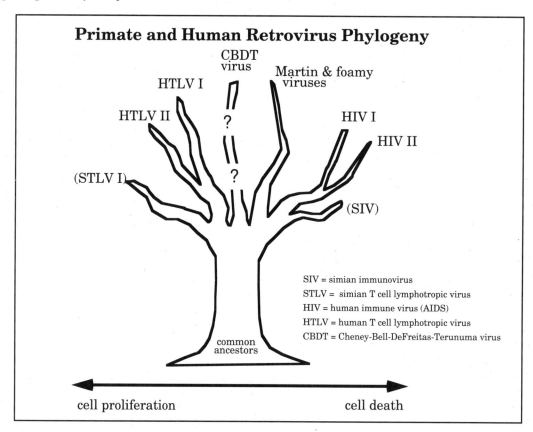

Primate and Human Retrovirus Phylogeny

SIV = simian immunovirus
STLV = simian T cell lymphotropic virus
HIV = human immune virus (AIDS)
HTLV = human T cell lymphotropic virus
CBDT = Cheney-Bell-DeFreitas-Terunuma virus

Human and Simian Retrovirus

The above is a schematic representation of the relationship of the various human and monkey retroviruses.[1]

The M.E./CFS retrovirus discovered by the Cheney-Bell-DeFreitas-Terunuma (CBDT) group and the foamy retrovirus (spume) discovered by Dr. John Martin would be placed genealogically in a homeostatic position between the HTLV and HIV retroviruses. The HTLV virus family causes cell proliferation and various leukemic and lymphomatous malignancies and the HIV family causes cell death.

In effect, we believe this would make the possible Cheney-Bell-DeFreitas-Terunuma virus (CBDT virus), a "perfect virus", that is, this virus neither kills the cell nor the individual but occupies certain cells or organelles in the host. They would exist in a homeostatic position that would interfere with the secondary functions of the cell, i.e. activity, production of hormones and chemicals, conducting information, but would not interfere with the primary functions of the cell, i.e. survival, maintenance and reproduction. Since these CBDT viruses are potentially ready to survive as long as the host, they would have a longer period in which to propagate into other hosts. In theory, this type of virus represents a near perfect parasite.

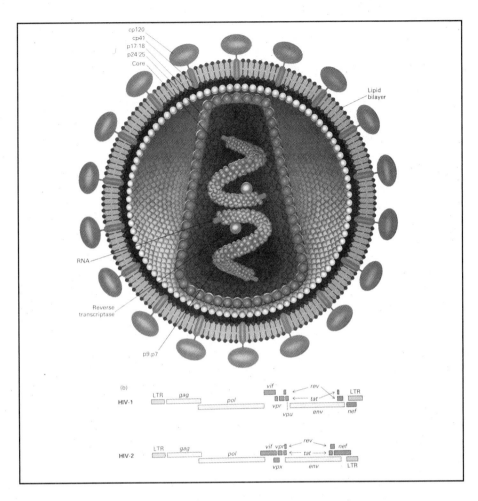

The First Human Retrovirus

From Molecular Cell Biology, Second Edition, by Darnell, Lodish and Baltimore. Copyright (c) 1990 by Scientific American Books, Inc. Reprinted by permission.

The above could be a schematic diagram of any retrovirus.

Disbelief in the Retrovirus Link

When I first raised the question of a retrovirus link to M.E. / CFS with a prominent retrovirologist in the Canadian Government, there was an expression of incredulity. When Dr. Behan spoke in Hamilton in September 1991, he was even more to the point. The following is a direct quotation:

Behan's Criticisms of a Retrovirus Link

"What happens in America, due perhaps to the extraordinary structure of government and the extraordinary structure of getting grants, is that when people make any form of a discovery, instead of them sending the paper to the most reputable journal and then letting their university, in the appropriate time, make the press announcement, they jump in, have their photograph taken and the announcement goes over Newsweek, Time, television and the poor fool of a patient looking at the television says "Hurrah, a major discovery has been made."

"This occurred last year in Japan, when people from the Wistar Institute in Philadelphia claimed that in fact there was a virus in this condition, that was related to a retrovirus. Retroviruses are those viruses, for example, that give rise to AIDS. "

"These are the data as they were reproduced in a very prestigious paper, The Proceedings of the National Academy of Sciences." Dr. Behan then showed a copy of the PNAS report. He then went on to say:

"Now, in a word, we repeated this work. We first of all contacted the doctor who made the discovery and asked if we could have the primers, the substances that she used. We had our own primers for a retrovirus, but if we had her primers, there could be no argument that we would repeat the experiment identically to what she had; we would use the same enzymes and everything. We repeated this experiment and the (reputed retroviral) band was in both normal controls and in patients, there was no difference."

"In other words, what the woman is claiming at the Wistar Institute was bogus."

These are pretty strong words and, as you can see they were said with conviction. I strongly recommend that those interested obtain a copy of this informative recording. It can be obtained from Mariam Gallacher, Hamilton-Wentworth.[2]

It is in the nature of some physicians to be always certain, even when they are most wrong.

When I was a medical student 25 years ago, and continuing until the early 1980's, there was an overly confident belief that retroviruses could not infect humans. In the brief period of 1983 to 1985, with the discovery of the HTLV and HIV series of human retroviruses, it became obvious that retroviruses were not only capable of creating disease in humans, but that these retroviral diseases gave every indication of creating an absolute personal and public health disaster. Thus in the blink of an eye, an idea of human retroviruses went from one of open contempt to one of absolute belief and major public anxiety. A similar pattern may emerge with the possible CBDT retrovirus. It is an unanswered puzzle that I leave to time and to the reader's intuition to resolve.

The Players

There were initially four players in this retrovirus theory: Michael Holmes in 1986, Paul Cheney in 1989, Elaine DeFreitas in 1990 and John Martin also

in 1989-90. Michael Holmes and John Martin both have retroviral papers in this text and I refer you to these chapters. I discussed the Holmes material with Paul Cheney in 1989 and at that time he appears to have already been convinced of the possibility of a retrovirus. To my knowledge, Paul Cheney first spoke with Michael Holmes in person in 1990 at the Cambridge Symposium.

Although I assume that Dr. Cheney has put a considerable amount of his own funds into this research, he, Dr. DeFreitas and Dr. Martin are all financed in part and have been intimately dependent upon funding from the CFIDS patients group in North Carolina.

Michael Holmes, New Zealand

It is not surprising that in 1986, when Michael Holmes in New Zealand first found an indication of reverse transcriptase activity in the blood of M.E./CFS patients, no one believed him. The University of Otago was certainly not willing to fund research into uncovering a possible new retrovirus in M.E./CFS, a disease that for many simply "did not exist." Nevertheless, in New Zealand, Dr. Holmes continued to have his students study the possible M.E./CFS retrovirus that he had discovered.

It should be recalled that one of the first retroviruses discovered was in sheep. When Dr. Holmes first started to investigate the blood of M.E./CFS patients, the disease was then called Tapanui Flu in New Zealand. Tapanui Flu is discussed in this book by Dr. Snow.

The illness started in February and March, 1983 in the New Zealand highlands among sheep farmers who first noted a new illness in their sheep. The sheep were aborting their lambs. This was a major economic concern for these sheep farmers. This illness in the aborting sheep was investigated but, to my knowledge, resulted in no obvious cause of illness being discovered. This epidemic in New Zealand appears to be the first mention of what perhaps developed into the 1984-1987 pandemic of M.E./CFS.

At the same time, the sheep farmers started falling ill with Tapanui Flu or M.E./CFS. There was no reason to believe at that time that the association of aborting sheep and ill farmers was any more than coincidental. The aborting sheep, who were not obviously ill, were apparently slaughtered, and sent to market around the world. This association of sheep farmers with M.E./CFS and ill sheep, provoked Dr. Holmes to investigate the possibility of a retrovirus.

Unfortunately, in 1986-7, a major conservative reaction against health funding and research negatively affected medical funding, both in New Zealand and around the world. There were no funds made available for research into a disease that, to many governments and physicians, was merely a joke, and at the very best, simply represented a nuisance factor.

Paul Cheney, Lake Tahoe, Nevada

Dr. Cheney was one of those medical pioneers who with Dr. Dan Peterson first noted and investigated the Lake Tahoe epidemic in 1984. Initially, the Lake Tahoe outbreak was considered to be an Epstein-Barr virus epidemic and in The United States it was believed that M.E./CFS was caused by EBV. However, by the time of the First International Symposium on Immunobiology and Pathogenesis of Persistent Virus Infections, held in Atlanta in April 1987, this belief was finally put to rest. In America, there was a brief fling with the possibility that cytomegalic virus (CMV), and then human herpes virus 6 might represent a potential cause of M.E./CFS. All of these theories have faded away.

SMON and the Inoue-Melnick Virus

This left few players in line to fill the role of a possible viral cause. The enterovirus family theory was then, as now, still strongly ensconced in Great Britain along with the little known and mysterious Inoue-Melnick virus theory. Although the legal consensus is that SMON disease was due to a toxic medication reaction, Inoue believes that the Inoue-Melnick virus (IMV) was the probable cause. In Japan IMV was thought to have some homology to the ILT virus that produced laryngo tracheitis in chickens.

The SMON epidemic appears to have been preceded by a viral infection that caused an acute gastroenteritis or colitis with marked conjunctivitis. This gastroenteritis was then treated by a common, across-the-counter drug called Mexiform in Canada, but with a pharmaceutical name of Di-iodo-hydroxy-quin. It appears that only those Japanese patients who had an infectious gastroenteritis and who also took this medication developed SMON. Yet millions of individuals with similar GIT infections around the world took this medication without any apparent ill effect. Was it due perhaps to some terrible synergy, possibly supported by some genetic or dietetic feature unique to the Japanese, that resulted in this SMON infection in Japan? In this specific Japanese population there occurred an M.E./CFS-like illness that caused not only the classical features of severe M.E./CFS but also paralysis, blindness and death in the many severely affected individuals.

Only Inoue was successful in culturing this virus in Japan where its very existence was met with much disbelief. It was described as a very unstable herpes or herpes-like virus. Then, in Texas, the famous Nobel Prize winning Professor Joseph Melnick also succeeded in isolating the virus and formulating subtypes. General lack of interest or persistence of an associated pathological entity and perhaps the fact that Di-iodo-hydroxy-quin was removed from the market by the pharmaceutical company has caused a disappearance of this virus from scientific scrutiny.

The Inoue-Melnick virus was a mysterious beast that was recovered only by these two eminent virologists. There can be no doubt that they had a virus, but the true identity and pathophysiology of this virus family is far from clear.

Although it was classified by Inoue and Melnick as a probable member of the herpes family, today, over 20 years later, it appears in no obvious published list of herpes viruses. Some physicians in England, notably Dr. Gordon Parish, still adhere to this virus as a potential cause of M.E./CFS. I am not aware if the Inoue-Melnick virus has ever been studied for possible reverse transcriptase activity.

It is curious that when Dr. John Martin first identified the virus that he has now classified as a retrovirus, he also believed it was a herpes virus. In fact, when he laid down his speech in Cambridge he believed he was dealing with a new and unusual herpes virus. This is no criticism of the work of John Martin. These scientists work with starvation budgets and their material evolves from speculation, to increasingly educated guesses, to provable science. Good science requires speculation and the evolving of knowledge; it also requires funds to proceed upon those speculations.

The Zhi Fang Epidemic

In our list of M.E. / CFS epidemics we have listed neither the SMON epidemic in Japan nor the Zhi Fang epidemic in China. Though no suggestion is made that the Zhi Fang epidemic has a retroviral aetiology, there is an association with SMON virus in case fatality rate. However, in time period, symptom picture and in family disease spread, it resembles the California-Nevada clusters described by Cheney/Peterson. The Zhi Fang epidemic occurred from April to October in Zhi Fang village, in Yanhe county of Guizhou province, China in 1985. The morbidity was considerable, with one fifth of the people in the village becoming ill. The case fatality was 12%.

The presentation was identical to that of epidemic M.E./CFS, with dizziness, malaise, myalgia and only low fevers. Rarely was the temperature elevated. Some patients had wandering myoclonus and tenderness with severe sweats. The severely ill patients usually died in 2-5 days.

A second epidemic occurred in another village in 1986. The benign cases appear identical to the M.E./CFS clusters observed in California-Nevada in the same years. Those that died more closely resembled those afficted by the SMON epidemic, although there was no report of conjunctivitis in China. Again the authors associated this epidemic with a curious, non-typical enterovirus.

The Cheney-Bell-DeFreitas-Terunuma Virus

Dr. Cheney, who had moved to North Carolina after the Lake Tahoe epidemic, became increasingly interested in the possibility that a retrovirus might be the cause of M.E./CFS and went to see Dr. Elaine DeFreitas to see if she would investigate the possibility of retroviral activity in these patients. It appears that initially she refused to accept a retrovirus cause of M.E./CFS as a realistic possibility, but she then became interested and eventually acquiesced. This resulted in her group's joint discovery of a novel retrovirus and the presentation on September 4, 1990 at the 11th International Congress of Neuropathology, Kyoto, Japan. The announcement was as follows and was first reported in the CFIDS Chronicle of September 1990.

This abstract is reprinted with the kind permission of the CFIDS Chronical, September, 1990.

Evidence of Retrovirus in Patients with Chronic Fatigue Immune Dysfunction Syndrome

E. DeFreitas, B. Hilliard, P. Cheney, D. Bell, E. Kiggundu, D. Sankey, Z. Wroblewska, and H. Koprowski. (The Wistar Institute, Philadelphia, PA, 10620 Park Road, Charlotte, NC, 15 Lake Avenue, Lyndonville, NY, USA.)

The chronic fatigue immune dysfunction syndrome (CFIDS) is a recently recognized organic illness with hematological and neurological symptoms. Once thought to be caused by Epstein-Barr virus (chronic EBV syndrome), it is now well accepted to have a different but unknown etiology. Recently, numerous immunologic T cell and NK cell abnormalities have been described in CFIDS patients. These data, coupled with the findings of abnormal brain MRI scans in some CFIDS patients, have prompted us to evaluate the role of a human retrovirus in this disease. Two populations of CFIDS patients, adults and children from two geographic areas of the US, were examined for serum antibodies to HTLV by Western blot, for the presence of HTLV proviral DNA in peripheral blood (PB) cells by PCR, and for viral RNA by *in situ* hybridization. All samples were coded and the investigator blinded. Using criteria for positivity of antibody to both "gag" and "env" gene products, 41% of CFIDS patients were positive compared to 6% of healthy controls from the same geographic area. The majority of patients were positive for certain HTLV sequences by PCR while none of the 20 healthy controls were. A small percentage of preactivated PB cells from several CFIDS adult and pediatric patients were also positive for a segment of human retroviral RNA by high stringency *in situ* hybridization.

Presented at the 11th International Congress of Neuropathy, Kyoto, Japan, September 4, 1990.

This was followed up by a similar paper published in the Proceedings of the National Academy of Sciences.

The title and abstract were as follows:

(extracted from Proc. Natl. Acad. Sci. USA, 88:2922-2926, April 1991, Medical Sciences.)

Retroviral Sequences related to human T-Lymphotropic virus type-II in patients with chronic fatigue immune dysfunction syndrome

(Epstein-Barr virus syndrome/infectious mononucleosis/myalgic encephalomyelitis/polymerase chain reaction/*in situ* hybridization)

Elaine DeFreitas, Brendan Hilliard, Paul R. Cheney, David S. Bell, Edward Kiggundu, Diane Sankey, Zofia Wroblewska, Maria Palladino, John P. Woodward, and Hilary Koprowski

The Wistar Institute, 3601 Spruce Street, Philadelphia, PA 19104

Contributed by Hilary Koprowski, November 13, 1990

Abstract

Chronic fatigue immune dysfunction syndrome (CFIDS) is a recently recognized illness characterized by debilitating fatigue as well as immunological and neurological abnormalities [Straus, S.E. (1988) J. Inf. Dis. 157, 405-412]. Once thought to be caused by Epstein-Barr virus, it is now thought to have a different but unknown etiology. We evaluated 30 adult and pediatric CFIDS patients from six eastern states for the presence of human T-lymphotropic virus (HTLV) types I and II by Western immunoblotting, polymerase chain reaction, and *in situ* hybridization of blood samples. The majority of patients were positive for HTLV antibodies by Western blotting and for HTLV-II *gag* sequences by polymerase chain reaction and *in situ* hybridization. Twenty nonexposure healthy controls were negative in all assays. These data support an association between an HTLV-II-like virus and CFIDS.

Why was such early data published?

The problem as I see it becomes evident. There has been no real money for research in M.E./CFS. The CFIDS group and their patient supporters are dedicated to finding a cause and eventually a cure for M.E./CFS. However, they do not have the millions of dollars or necessary funds to mount a proper and successful research programme. I believe that the scientists who have become involved are as honest as any other scientists, if not more so. These announcements were probably made so that the CFIDS Association members would continue to contribute funds and also stimulate government funding for this research. It is of interest that, in the recent $6,000,000 NIH funding of M.E/CFS research, not one penny was allotted to an investigation of the retroviral theory.

Curiously, one of the three grants went to a specialist in stress. By the definition of Dr. Peter Behan, stress would have been ruled out as a cause of M.E/CFS. All of us would agree that stress can cause illness, but that is not Postviral Fatigue Syndrome and it is not M.E./CFS.

More criticisms of the Retrovirus Theory

In his Hamilton speech[4], Dr. Behan also stated that when his Glasgow group used the same probe they found that it would stick to any form of normal DNA in either controls or patients. In other words, the DeFreitas probe adhered to normal human protein. Dr. Behan's group then took primers from many leading retroviral laboratories in the world, modified and unmodified, and were still not able to repeat Dr. DeFreitas' work.

Dr. Behan summed up his remarks on the retroviral theory and its protagonists as follows:

"People who have no expertise, or nothing to offer and who are charlatans rip off patients left, right and centre by bogus claims. This is one of the things that in fact affects me enormously when I see how patients have been ripped off right, left and centre by bogus charlatans. This (the retroviral theory) falls into that particular category of very poor research, very poor results, and keeps hitting the media and causing nothing but distress." [4]

Are Dr. Behan's comments correctly founded ? Only time and adequate research funding will answer that question. In part it may have been answered in the two papers that we have produced in this text.

Conjecture on the Economic Consequences of a New Viral Discovery

The following speculations are those of the staff of The Nightingale Research Foundation and are not necessarily the views of any other publishers or distributors other than the Nightingale Research Foundation.

However, there is another side to this story that should be discussed. There are so many people ill with M.E./CFS that they would give any amount of money to recover their health. Discovery of the viral cause of M.E./CFS will possibly result in a commercial test and possibly a cure. Such an initial discovery will potentially make a very few researchers incredibly wealthy. If any of these researchers believe that their discovery is valid, they will behave accordingly to protect their patents on this virus.

Thus, it would not be financially rational for the CBDT group or Dr. Martin to have given the keys of the kingdom to Dr. Behan or anyone else unless they had first unravelled the virus and patented it. Have they done that?

From the speech of Dr. DeFreitas in Sarasota[5], it is my understanding that some of the viruses are situated within the mitochondria and that this viral material is routinely thrown away with the supernatant. Is this the cause of Dr. Behan's failure to recover the virus? Is the problem of an inhibitor that apparently dogged the work of the CBDT group also a problem in his research?

Proprietary Rights

Just prior to the departure of Drs Cheney, DeFreitas and Bell for Kyoto, Japan for the September 1990 Congress, it became apparent that the proprietary rights of the CBDT discovery might now belong to the Wistar Institute. As I understand it, this meant that neither Dr. DeFreitas nor Dr. Cheney would receive any personal financial gain from any discovery. Reputedly, when the patent for this virus was applied for by Wistar, they omitted naming Dr. Cheney as co-discoverer, although he had developed the concept and brought the idea and much of the source material to Wistar. In effect, if this sequence of events is correct, Wistar's actions, probably unintentionally, might well disenfranchise Dr. Cheney's major proprietary role in this discovery and thus would block him from any financial gain.

Financial gain is essential if these scientists are to continue their research. If this information is essentially true, as we believe it is, this would explain why Dr. Behan was not given all of the information.

Apparently, research funds going to Dr. DeFreitas and Wistar from the CFIDS Association were abruptly halted or reduced. It seems that, perhaps for various reasons, Dr. Kaprowski, (Dr. DeFreitas' superior and one of the research team), was relieved of his job as were two of the project workers. With decreased funds and workers, and with a potential legal fight concerning ownership of the CBDT virus, all research came to an abrupt slowdown.

A Retrovirus Inhibitor

As mentioned by Dr. Holmes in his paper (see chapter 34), he had discovered that a powerful RT inhibitor existed that blocked laboratory reproduction of this virus. As if the legal matters were not enough, CBDT group had also apparently run into the same or similar problem and was having trouble generating sufficient virus for rapid analysis and study. Meanwhile, Dr. Martin had found a way around the inhibitor and was producing large quantities of this retrovirus material.

It seems that the legal, financial and technical problems have eased up a bit, and some funding has apparently been resumed by CFIDS. It could scarcely be enough. Decoding of major parts and sequencing of the viral structure have continued. Whatever they have found at the time of my writing has caused considerable excitement.

Dr. John Martin

To go back a little, in 1988 - 1989, Dr. John Martin discovered what appeared to be an unusual herpes virus in some M.E./CFS patients. Again, there were very few funds with which to fully investigate this virus. Dr. Martin persisted in his research and what he first believed was an unusual herpes virus proved to be something else entirely. (See two chapters of Dr. Martin) With further funds slowly becoming available, more research led to the belief that one was dealing with a foamy or spume retrovirus.

Spume retroviruses were first isolated as contaminates of tissue culture, particularly monkey kidney cell culture and were believed to be a possible contaminate from the original monkey. This family of virus was reputedly found as a contaminate in early polioimmunization preparations.[6] I am told it routinely shows up and causes problems in the cultures of the viral laboratory of Sick Children's Hospital in Toronto.[7] This is a chilling thought if these preparations are being used to develop immunizations. Although this theory is still being discussed, others believe the Martin virus may be a hybrid virus, partially a retrovirus but sharing some non-retroviral characteristics. This makes one think of the work of Dr. Archard who believes that there is something very unusual about the enterovirus that he has recovered from M.E./CFS patients. Although he makes no suggestions that there is reverse transcriptase activity, he is notably curious about the altered status of the enterovirus sequences he has discovered.[8]

In a way, a retrovirus is already a hybrid, in so much as the capsule of the retrovirus is actually an adsorption product that comes from the host animal's cellular "skin", that attaches to the retrovirus core when it "buds" out from the human cell.

The anxieties and the professional and financial restraints are enormous. It is hard to imagine that these three research groups have not found a retrovirus, and which they believe appears to play a role in M.E./CFS patient pathology. They are recovering this virus from M.E./CFS patients but not from healthy, non-contact controls. To date, neither the enterovirus, nor any herpes viruses associated with M.E./CFS can claim such a clear indication of a direct association with M.E./CFS patients but none with healthy, non-contact controls.

The Cheney-Bell-DeFreitas-Terunuma Virus (CBDT) Discoveries

The following notes were abstracted from public statements by Dr. Elaine DeFreitas at the Sarasota Symposium. The wording is that of Nightingale staff.

1. The foamy (spume) virus of Dr. Martin and the HTLV-II-like virus recovered by the Drs Cheney-Bell-DeFreitas-Terunuma group (CBDT) appear to be different viruses. The gag protein of spuma viruses is 30,000 and that of the CBDT virus is 27-28,000.

2. The C.V. Herst Oncore Analytics (Houston, Texas) test is for the HTLV-like CBDT virus and not the reputed spuma virus identified by Dr. Martin.

3. Some of the proteins made by a herpes virus are similar to the Tax and Rex and so can amplify the replication of known retroviruses. This is of interest since the 1948 Akureyri epidemic was associated with a herpes like viral eruption. This fact has not been hitherto discussed in the literature.[9]

4. The CBDT group was not able to recover HTLV-I from M.E./CFS patients nor their family contacts. Thus HTLV-I was not a causal agent.

5. When the same search was made for an HTLV-II agent in M.E./CFS patients some weak association was discovered. In other words what they were recovering did not appear to be HTLV-II but there was some homology or similarities between the two different viruses.

6. Using umbilical cord blood from healthy

newborns, CBDT has never been able to recover this HTLV-II-like virus or any indication of it.

7. In healthy adult controls, CBDT was never able to recover any indication of the presence of this HTLV-II-like virus.

8. CBDT, employing specific prolene binding site primers for HTLV-I and II on CBDT virus positive patients, supplied by Dr. Bell and Dr. Cheney, were unable to demonstrate the presence of this prolene region suggesting that neither HTLV I nor II were present. Thus the CBDT virus was neither HTLV I or HTLV II.

9. Positive M.E./CFS patients do not have a precipitated protein band at 24,000 as in HTLV I and II but at 27-28,000, as well as a faint band at 13-14 and 11-12.

10. The size of the gag protein most resembles that of one of the 11 Simian D retroviruses.

11. Only one apparently healthy control had a similar configuration but that patient had no band at either 13-14 or 11-12. This patient was perfectly well with no history of M.E./CFS.

12. Nine months later and after she had fallen ill with M.E./CFS, CBDT found that this same patient had developed both the 13-14 and the 11-12 band. In other words, if Dr. DeFreitas is correct, M.E./CFS may occur initially as a dormant phase with no ongoing clinical evidence of disease.

13. CBDT was able to recover and grow the CBDT virus that was located in a search of each of T-cell lines, B-cell lines and macrophages.

14. CBDT was able to isolate closed circular virus forms (frequently found in simian D retroviruses).

15. They also observed exceedingly large deformed mitochondria, with a damaged organization of the cristi and in the centre of these mitochondria there appear to be virus particles. CBDT state that if this injury to mitochondria proves to be consistent, then this could explain the rapid fatigue of the muscle and brain of these patients.

It should be noted that Dr. Peter Behan has also demonstrated these unusual and large mitochondria as has Dr. Michael Holmes. Dr. Behan has discussed and shown projections of this unusual mitochondria expression at each of his meetings that I have attended over the past three years.

16. CBDT also discussed a search for possible retroviral contamination of the laboratory. No contamination was found.

17. I was of the impression that the viral material was recovered from the supernatant rather than the usual precipitated material.

18. Close examination of electron micrographs of the tissue/blood cells of M.E./CFS patients by the CBDT group has resulted in the revelation of three particles rather than a single distinct particle. It is my understanding that these three different particles may appear in the same patient sample. They were:

Source Material	Particle Recovered	Size in Nanometers
Extracellular T-cell, B-cell, & macrophage lines	CBDT virus	90 nm
Intracellular T-cell, B-cell, & macrophage lines	particle of enterovirus size	25 nm
Intramitochondrial tissue	Crystaline-like formation	37 nm

Retrovirus are characterized by a sperical virion of 80-100 nm diameter that could be consistent with the extracellular viral findings.

Enterovirus (polio, coxsackie, echo and numbered virus) are characterized by a isosahedral virion of 27 nanometers that could be consistent with the intracellular viral findings. EM measurements of virus size are always approximates.

Human herpes virus are characterized by a donut shaped virion of 150-200 nm. The CBDT reported no such herpes particle size finding.

19. If the initial and largely unpublished information presented by DeFreitas in Florida (March 1992) and Terunuma in California (April 1992) is found to be a consistent pattern in M.E./CFS infection, then we are dealing with a complex infectious process involving a virion of 90 nm that is within the range of a retroviral particle and slightly smaller than an HTLV II-like virion (100 nm). The second virion is stated to be 25 nm in size or slightly smaller than the range of a typical enteroviral virion (27 nm). Are we observing a combined retroviral immune injury that facilitates a chronic enterovirus infection? Dr. Michael Holmes envisaged exactly such a discovery. See his paper, Chapter 33 this text. The 37 nm, apparently crystalline, intramitochondrial body remains a mystery at the time of writing.

I remind the reader that some of the material in this chapter has not yet been published and has been taken from material presented at symposia. Until this material appears in a peer review journal, it should be considered speculative.

This material that was abstracted from a speech by Elaine DeFreitas presented at the Sarasota Symposium in March of 1992 and by Hiroshi Terunuma at the Third Annual Conference on CFS and the Brain, Bel-Air, California, April 1992, appears, at the moment, to be very difficult to refute. The one question that is troubling me is that it appears that both the CBDT group and John Martin's group are each finding high positive results in large numbers of M.E./CFS patients that they are surveying. It would appear that either one, or both, must be in error, or that two retroviruses are present in M.E./CFS. This is highly unlikely.

Two other labs that I have talked to reputedly also have evidence of this virus. Only time, further scientific evidence and peer scrutiny will tell who is correct: Dr. Behan, those who believe in a retroviral theory, or both groups. As Dr. Walter Gunn recently states in Science: "There is every likelihood that it *(a retrovirus)* will be confirmed eventually."[10]

References

1. Based upon a schematic drawing presented by Dr. Elaine DeFreitas at the Sarasota, Gulf Coast CFIDS Symposium, March 1992.

2. Miriam Gallacher, Hamilton-Wentworth Support Group, 90 Malton Drive, Hamilton, Ontario.

3. Zhang, L.B., Jiang, Y.Z., Mo, H.M., et al. A new disease associated with enterovirus; studies on the aetiology of "Zhi Fang" Disease. Chinese Acad Prev Med, Chinese Journal of Virology 1987;3(1):95-98.

4. Hamilton Symposium at St. Joseph's Hospital, organized by Miriam Gallacher and the Hamilton-Wentworth M.E. Association, Hamilton, Ontario.

5. idem (1).

6. Hooks, J., Gibbs, C. The Foamy Viruses, Bacteriological Reviews, American Society for Microbiology, Sept. 1979;39, no. 3:169-185 (see page 182).

7. Sick Children's Hospital, spume virus, personal communication with virologist from SCH.

8. Dr. Archard, personal communication with Dr. Hyde and also noted at the Cambridge Symposium, 1990.

9. Personal communication between Asgeir Johanesson, Mayor of Reykjavik, Iceland and Dr. Hyde in May, 1988.

10. Editorial, Science 1991;254:1727.

The Skeletal Muscle as Target

Chapter 37

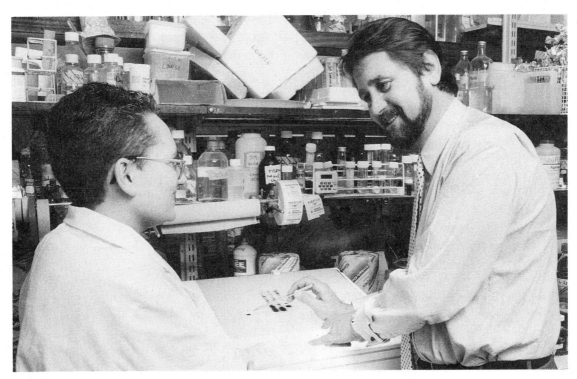

Louise Cunningham and Leonard C. Archard

Molecular Virology of Muscle Disease: Persistent Virus Infection of Muscle in Patients With Postviral Fatigue Syndrome

Leonard C. Archard, PhD and Louise Cunningham, PhD
Dept. of Biochemistry, Charing Cross & Westminster Medical School, St. Dunstans Road, London England W6 8RF

Dr. Archard is a Microbiology graduate with a doctorate in Virology. He held a World Health Organization Research Fellowship associated with the smallpox eradication campaign and a subsequent appointment as Lecturer in Virology at St. Mary's Hospital Medical School, London. He is now a Senior Lecturer in Biochemistry at Charing Cross and Westminster Medical School, London.

Dr. Cunningham is a Microbiology graduate with a PhD in Molecular Virology. She has been working in Dr. Archard's laboratory on the molecular basis of virus persistence in PFS for four years.

Our interest in virus-induced muscle disease includes the syndrome of Post-Viral Fatigue Syndrome (PFS). **PFS patients are a sub-set of patients who present with one of the spectrum of illness which collectively are called Chronic Fatigue Syndrome (CFS).**

PFS is characterized by chronic, excessive muscle fatiguability after moderate exercise, with a prolonged recovery period and follows a demonstrated or presumed viral infection. PFS patients were included in our studies only if other causes of fatigue were excluded and symptoms were present for more than 6 months. These patients generally show little histopathology and few clinical signs. Unlike acute inflammatory muscle disease, neither infectious virus nor virus-specific antigens have been demonstrated, although persistence of virus genetic material can be demonstrated (see below).

We have used molecular hybridization techniques to search for enterovirus-specific nucleic acid sequences in muscle biopsy samples from PFS patients compared to control samples. The probe we used was a 0.85 kb cDNA derived from near the 3' end of the genome of Coxsackievirus B2 (CBV2), corresponding approximately to nucleotides 6550 to 7400. This region includes the sequences from the 3' untranslated region, and part of the viral RNA-dependent RNA polymerase gene which are conserved among the enteroviruses (Stalhandske et al 1984) and so the probe is group-specific and detects the RNA of enteroviruses other than that of Coxsackie B viruses (Bowles et al 1989).

Experiments were controlled using a cell specific probe, 7B6 (Kaczmarek et al 1985), which detects a cell-cycle independent of mRNA. Quantitative slot blot hybridizations were carried out as described previously (Bowles et al 1986). Briefly, muscle samples were solubilized by digestion with 1 mg/ml proteinase K and 0.5% SDS, in the presence of 500 units/ml of RNasin (human placental ribonuclease inhibitor) to prevent RNA degradation. The nucleic acids were deproteinized and ethanol precipitated. After redissolving in water, the RNA was selectively denatured using 7.5% formaldehyde in 6 x SSC at 65°C for 15 minutes, blotted onto duplicate nitrocellulose filters and immobilized by baking. Blots were prehybridized for 5 hours in 6 x SSC, 0.5% SDS, 5 x Denhardt's solution and 100 µg/ml denatured salmon sperm DNA at 65°C, and hybridized overnight in the same solution as above with the addition 1 x 10^6 CPM/ml of ^{32}P labelled probe, at a specific activity of between 1 and 3 x 10^9 DPM/µg, complementary to either virus RNA or 7B6 mRNA. The blots were washed to high stringency, (0.1 x SSC, 0.1% SDS) to remove most of the non-specific signal with the virus probe, and autoradiography performed using Hyperfilm MP at -70°C. Hybridization signals were quantitated by scanning densitometry. The signal is proportional to the amount of RNA loaded onto the filter (Bowles et al 1989) and clinical samples were compared to controls by dividing the signal obtained with the enterovirus probe by the signal obtained with the 7B6 probe. This hybridization index (HI) gives a measure of the relative amount of enterovirus RNA compared to the amount of cellular RNA in any sample. The mean and standard deviation of the negative control samples was then calculated and compared with the results for the clinical samples. Samples with a value of HI exceeding the mean of negative controls by three standard deviations are considered positive for persistence of enterovirus RNA (p=< 0.0015).

Using this method, we have detected enterovirus RNA in 34 of 140 (24%) of PFS muscle biopsy samples compared to none of 152 normal or pathologically irrelevant controls (108 normal biopsy samples, taken to exclude various conditions; 28 pathological biopsy samples including 24 Inclusion Body Myositis; 2 samples obtained from orthopaedic surgery and samples from 14 post mortem procedures) p=<0.001. Representative data is shown in Figure 1.

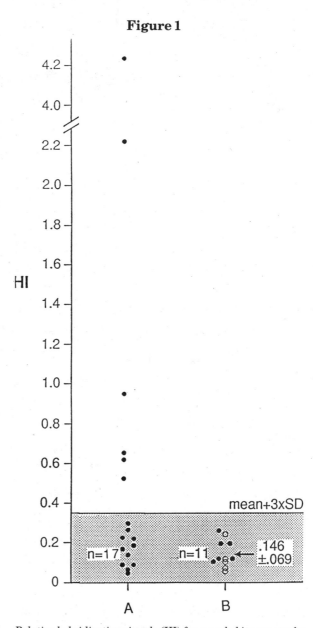

Figure 1

Relative hybridization signals (HI) for muscle biopsy samples with the enterovirus group-specific probe. Group A are samples from PFS patients. Group B are normal or pathologically irrelevant controls. Samples from group A in the shaded area are negative, those above positive for enteroviral RNA (HI more than 3 x SD in excess of the mean of the controls).

We have used the same hybridization probes to investigate muscle biopsy samples from 60 cases of histologically proven inflammatory muscle disease. Enterovirus RNA was detected in biopsies from 4 of 24 (17%) cases of adult polymyositis and 14 of 36 (39%) cases of juvenile dermatomyositis, compared to the same control samples described above. As our PFS patients date their muscle fatiguability to a prior "viral" illness, this suggests that chronic muscle fatiguability associated with persistent enterovirus infection may be a sequela of a previous enteroviral myositis.

Epstein-Barr viruses (EBV) have also been implicated in PFS by retrospective serology (Straus et al 1985). For this reason, an EBV specific probe was used to examine muscle biopsy samples from PFS patients for EBV DNA. The EBV gene probe used was a 3.4 kb RsaI fragment, subcloned, using BamHI linkers, into a pUC9 vector from the 5.1 kb EBV BamHI K restriction fragment. This non-repetitive sequence encodes part of the EBV nuclear antigen 1 (EBNA-1). Some EBV gene probes show cross hybridization with human DNA: this is not the case with the EBNA 1 probe described here (Archard et al 1989). Using this probe, we detected persisting EBV DNA in a 8 of 76 (10.5%) PFS samples compared to none of 48 normal or pathological controls (Figure 2) (P=<0.001). These PFS patients were a subset of those already examined for the presence of enteroviral RNA sequences. No sample was positive for both enterovirus and Epstein-Barr virus sequences.

EBV is a B-lymphotrophic virus of primates, but fusion of lymphocytes to other cell types is known, for example, to epithelial cells in nasopharyngeal carcinoma. This may be a mechanism by which EBV can enter many cell types lacking specific receptors, including myocytes. All the biopsies from the PFS patients in this study were reported negative for the presence of an inflammatory infiltrate. However, it is possible that small numbers of EBV transformed B-lymphocytes are present in the samples and if EBV DNA was present in sufficiently high copy number, these could produce a detectable EBV-specific hybridization signal. Whether the EBV DNA sequences detected are present in myocytes or in B-lymphocytes is not known as the **in situ** hybridization data are not yet available.

In the case of persisting enterovirus infection, single stranded riboprobes of either polarity were used to determine the relative abundance of the positive genomic strand and negative template strand of enteroviral RNA. A cDNA corresponding to nucleotides 5900-6900 (the first 2/3 of the polymerase gene) of Coxsackie B2 virus was cloned into a riboprobe vector in both orientations and probes were produced by transcription of the linearized template using SP6 RNA polymerase. By cloning the cDNA fragment in both orientations, cRNA probes complementary to either the positive or negative strands of enteroviral RNA can be produced by transcription. Using the same polymerase ensures equivalent transcription and radiolabelling of the resulting RNA probes. As before, the RNA probes are enterovirus

Figure 2

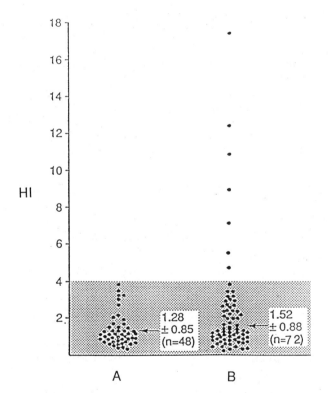

Relative hybridization signals (HI) for muscle samples with EBV probe. Group A are normal or pathologically irrelevant controls. Group B are samples from PFS patients. Those in shaded area are negative, those above positive for EBV DNA (HI greater than 3 x SD in excess of the mean of the controls).

group-specific. Cultured cells (LLCMK2) were infected with CBV2 and total RNA extracted after NP-40 lysis to follow patterns of enteroviral RNA synthesis in productive cytolytic infection. The RNA was denatured and blotted in triplicate. The blots were

Figure 3

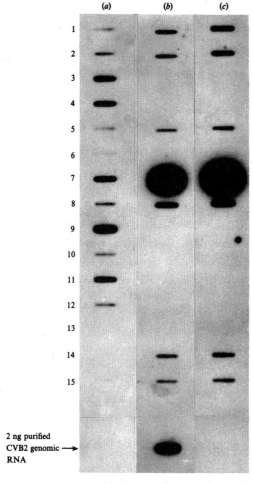

RNA extracted from muscle biopsy samples from patients with PFS was blotted in triplicate and hybridized with single stranded riboprobes specific for (a) 7B6 control, (b) positive genomic strand or (c) negative template strand of enteroviral RNA. Only the probe complementary to the positve strand detected purified CVB2 genomic RNA. Samples 1,2,5,8,14 and 15 are positive for enteroviral RNA and in all cases hybridization signals with riboprobes complementary to either positive or negative strands of enteroviral RNA are approximately equal.

Figure 3 is reprinted courtesy of the Journal of General Virology, 71, 1399-1402, June 7, 1990.

pre-hybridized in 50% formamide, 2 x SSC 0.1 % SDS, 2.5 x Denhardt's solution and 100 μg/ml salmon sperm DNA at 55°C for 5 hours. Riboprobes were added at 0.5-1 x 10^7 CPM/ml, hybridization continued over night and the blots washed stringently at 70°C. By hybridization with probes complementary to either the positive or negative strands of enteroviral RNA, we have shown that synthesis of positive strand RNA predominates over that of negative strand by a factor of at least 100-fold (Cunningham et al 1990). This agrees with other published data (Rotbart et al 1988). In contrast, when RNA was extracted as described previously from muscle biopsies from PFS patients, the two strands of enteroviral RNA were present in similar amounts (Cunningham et al 1990). Representative data is shown in Figure 3 and suggests that virus persistence in these cases results from a defect in the control of RNA synthesis.

Persistence of virus in muscle is clearly a pathological situation: these data suggest that enteroviruses are major aetiological agents of PFS but that other viruses can be involved. Thus, persistent infection of the affected tissue may be the pathogenetic mechanism of muscle fatiguability. Our recent data on non-inflammatory heart muscle disease have shown similar abnormal ratios of positive to negative strands of enteroviral RNA. This suggests that the mechanism of enteroviral persistence is the same in both forms of non-inflammatory muscle disease (Archard et al 1990; Archard et al 1991).

This is the first demonstration of an abnormality in enteroviruses in a pathological situation. In normal replication, enteroviruses replicate cytolytically and so attract an inflammatory response. In PFS there is no such histopathology but persisting viral RNA can be detected by hybridization. We suggest that, during initial infection, mutations occur which impair both the normal replication of viral RNA and the subsequent production of infectious virus and that this results in virus persistence. How such persisting, defective viruses cause muscle fatiguability and the other symptoms of PFS is not yet known.

References

Archard LC, Peters JL, Behan PO, Doyle D, Mackett M, Bowles NE. (1989) Post viral chronic fatigue syndrome: Persistence of Epstein-Barr virus DNA in muscle. In: Ablashi DV et al., (Eds) Epstein-Barr Virus and Human Disease II. Humana Press, Clifton, N.J: pp439-444.

Archard LC, Bowles NE, Cunningham L, Freeke CA, Morgan-Capner P, Olsen EGJ, Banner NR, Rose ML, Yacoub MH, Meany BT & Richardson PJ (1990) Enterovirus RNA sequences in hearts with dilated cardiomyopathy: a pathogenetic link between virus infection and dilated cardiomyopathy. In: Baroldi et al. (Eds) Advances in cardiomyopathies. Springer Verlag, Berlin: pp194-198.

Archard LC, Bowles NE, Cunningham L, Freeke CA, Olsen EGJ, Rose ML, Meany B, Why HJF & Richardson PJ (1991) Molecular probes for detection of persisting enterovirus infection in human heart and their prognostic value Eur. Heart J (in press)

Bowles N.E., Richardson P.J., Olsen E,G. & Archard L.C. (1986) Detection of Coxsackie-B-virus-specific RNA sequences in myocardial biopsy samples from patients with myocarditis and dilated cardiomyopathy. Lancet i 1120-1123

Bowles N.E., Rose M.L., Taylor P., Banner N.R., Morgan-Capner P., Cunningham L, Archard L.C. & Yacoub M.H. (1989). End-stage dilated cardiomyopathy: persistence of enterovirus RNA in myocardium at cardiac transplantation and lack of immune response. Circulation 80 1128-1136.

Cunningham L, Bowles NE, Lane RJM, Dubowitz V & Archard LC. (1990) Persistence of enterovirus RNA in chronic fatigue syndrome is associated with the abnormal production of equal amounts of positive and negative strands of enteroviral RNA. J Gen Virol 71 1399-1402.

Kaczmarek L., CalabrettA B. & Baserga R. (1985) Expression of cell-cycle-dependent genes in phytohemaglutinin stimulated human lymphocytes. Proc. of Natl. Acad. Sci. USA 82 5372-9.

Rotbart H.A., Abzug M.J., Murray R.S., Murphy N.L. & Levin M.J. (1988) Intracellular detection of sense and antisense enteroviral RNA by in situ hybridization. J Virol. Methods 22 295-301.

Stalhandske P.O.K., Lindberg M. & Pettersson U. (1984). Replicase Gene of Coxsackievirus B3. J Virol. 51 742-746.

Straus SE, Tosato G, Armstrong G, et al. (1985) Persisting illness and fatigue in adults with evidence of Epstein-Barr virus infection. Ann Intern Med 102: 7-16.

Chapter 38

Neuromuscular Abnormalities In Patients With Chronic Fatigue Syndrome

Carolyn L. Warner, MD, Dent Neurologic Institute and Department of Neurology, SUNY at Buffalo School of Medicine

Reid R. Heffner, Jr., MD, Departments of Neurology and Pathology SUNY at Buffalo School of Medicine

Diane Cookfair, PhD, Department of Social and Preventive Medicine, SUNY At Buffalo School of Medicine

Dr. Carolyn Warner is a specialist in the diagnosis and treatment of neuromuscular disease, and serves as Acting Chief of the Laboratory of Clincial Electrophysiology at the Dent Neurologic Institute in Buffalo, New York. In 1984, Dr. Warner was selected as a Muscular Dystrophy Association Fellow in Neuromuscular Disease, a fellowship which was completed at the Columbia University Neurologic Institute. In addition to her work concerning ME, she is currently conducting research concerning cerebrospinal fluid and serum androgens in amyotrophic lateral sclerosis and spinal muscular atrophy.

Abstract

Muscle biopsy and/or EMG abnormalities have been reported for M.E. patients from Scotland and Australia, but similar data have not been published for M.E. patients from the United States. We performed muscle biopsies on 25 M.E. patients with myalgias. The majority also underwent quantitative EMG and nerve conduction studies. All were from one geographic region in the Northeastern United States. The majority of patients had normal neurologic examinations; only one had proximal muscle weakness, which was mild.

Several patients had abnormal muscle biopsy findings, including one or more of the following: muscle inflammatory infiltrates without fiber necrosis or regeneration; type II fiber atrophy; type II fiber atrophy without fiber necrosis or regeneration; type II fiber atrophy and predominance; and nonselective fiber atrophy. Other neuromuscular abnormalities included over 20% polyphasic motor units on quantitative EMG (47%), and mild elevations in serum creatinase kinase (3 patients). These findings will be compared with neuromuscular abnormalities which have been reported for patients with other chronic disease as well as other published data from M.E. patients.

Introduction

Myalgias are one of the most common symptoms described by individuals with chronic fatigue syndrome (CFS). Patients also report generalized weakness and extreme fatigue following exercise that is out of proportion with the activity undertaken. These symptoms suggest the possibility of neuromuscular involvement in this syndrome. Muscle biopsy and EMG abnormalities have been reported for patients from Great Britain and Australia, but similar data have not been published for CFS patients from the United States[1-4]. We studied a series of CFS patients with myalgias in order to determine if they had a neuromuscular abnormality.

Methods:

Patients

A total of 25 females and 6 males, (age range 18-48; mean age 36) underwent detailed neuromuscular evaluation. The 31 patients included in the study were accrued over a 3 year period from among 57 CFS patients who had been referred for neurologic evaluation due to their prominent neurologic symptoms. Duration of illness ranged from 8 months to 19 years with a mean of 4.7 years.

All patients included in the study met the Center for Disease Control (CDC) criteria for chronic fatigue syndrome[5]. None had serologic evidence for syphilis, Lyme disease or myasthenia gravis. The majority underwent HIV testing, which was negative; none had risk factors for AIDS. Patients who underwent detailed neuromuscular testing included all those patients with prominent complaints of muscle pain, extensive fatigue, and weakness who agreed to undergo muscle biopsies. Histories and neurologic examinations were obtained on the 57 adult referred patients. Of the 57, 3 did not have prominent myalgias, 15 did not wish to undergo muscle biopsy, and 8 were excluded because they did not meet the CDC criteria for CFS. Examinations and histories for those CFS patients who did not wish to undergo muscle biopsy were not substantially different from those of patients who agreed to comprehensive neuromuscular evaluation.

All patients experienced chronic debilitating fatigue, severe enough to result in a marked reduction in activity levels. Neuromuscular, other neurologic symptoms, and non-neurologic symptoms are listed in Table 1. Myalgias, which were an entry criteria for the study, were prominent and severe enough to cause cessation of normal activity and a sensation of weakness. Intermittent paresthesiae were usually burning and migratory. Headaches were chronic and diffuse. Visual complaints included blurring, diplopia, photophobia, and transient photisms or scotomatas. Dysequilibrium included brief episodes of true vertigo as well as a chronic sensation of being "off-balance".

Table 1
Symptom Prevalance

Neuromuscular and Neurologic Symptoms	
Symptom	Percent*
Myalgia	100
Paresthesias	100
Weakness	100
Headache	100
Visual symptoms	100
Dysequilibrium	90
Tinnitus	74

Non-Neurologic Symptoms	
Symptom	Percent
Sore throats	100
Fever, chills, sweats	94
Swollen or painful nodes	94
Migratory arthralgias	94
Abdominal Pain	87

* N = 31

Laboratory

Laboratory tests included thyroid profile, routine chemistries and blood counts, ANA, ESR, and creatine kinase. All but 2 patients had nerve conduction studies of at least 2 motor and 2 sensory nerves performed at 37°C on a Nicolet Viking. Proximal and distal muscles were studied by concentric needle EMG. Twenty-three patients agreed to additional quantitative motor unit analysis of 20 motor units in the extensor digitorum communis (EDC); 8 underwent single fiber studies of the same muscle including 20 fiber pairs. All patients had muscle biopsies of a proximal muscle.

Muscle biopsy specimens were processed for paraffin section and electron microscopy. Frozen unfixed muscle was used for enzyme histochemistry and immunofluorescence studies. Paraffin sections were stained with H & E, Masson trichrome, and PAS. Cryostat sections were stained with ATPase at pH 9.4, NADH-TR, Modified Gomori Trichrome and myoadenylate deaminase; sections also were analyzed by direct immunofluorescence for IgG, IgA, IgM, C3, C4, and properdin. Ultra thin sections were stained with saturated uranylacetate and 1% lead citrate.

Results:

Clinically, none of the patients had a history of myoglobinuria, relationship of fatigue to diet, or the "second wind" phenomenon that can be seen in some of the metabolic myopathies. The majority of patients had normal neurologic examinations; none had pathologic reflexes, Babinski's sign, or absent reflexes. Of the 31 patients included in the study, two had mild biceps weakness, 2 had mild distal weakness, 1 had intermittent facial myokymia, and 1 had sparse fasciculations in normal strength muscles. Four patients exhibited a markedly positive Romberg, 2 had intermittent vocal cord paralysis, and one had mild left sided weakness and sensory loss.

Routine laboratory tests were entirely normal with these exceptions: four patients had mildly elevated serum creatine kinase (CK) (2 times the upper limit of normal), 5 patients had elevated sedimentation rates (ESR) ranging from 32 to 72 and 1 had borderline hyperthyroidism. The abnormal ESR and thyroid profiles reverted to normal on repeat testing.

Several patients had abnormal muscle biopsy findings (Table 2). Muscle inflammatory infiltrates were seen in 23% or 7/31 patients. These infiltrates were in a perivascular as well as endomysial distribution, and composed mainly of mature lymphocytes (Fig. 1). No necrosis or regeneration of muscle fibers was seen. The structure of the vessel walls was well maintained. Type II fiber atrophy was seen in 15/31 patients. In 2 patients, this finding was associated with Type II fiber predominance. These fibers were not only small but were also more angulated than normal. In another 3 patients, nonselective, or Type I and II fiber atrophy was seen. None of the muscle biopsy specimens showed evidence for myoadenylate deaminase deficiency. Deposits of immunoglobulin and complement were not detected by immunofluorescence and no viral particles, abnormal lipid deposits, or abnormal mitochondria were seen on microscopy.

All sensory and motor nerve conduction studies including F-waves were normal and no spontaneous activity was seen on needle EMG. Quantitative motor unit analysis showed over 20% polyphasic motor units in 13 of the 28 patients, only one of whom had an increased mean motor unit potential duration. Another one had a decreased MUP duration. Six out of 8 had normal single fiber studies of the extensor digitorim communis muscle. In 2, the mean MCD's were normal, but 2/20 fiber pairs had jitter over 55u sec. No blocking was seen.

Discussion

We found type II fiber atrophy in 48%, and inflammatory infiltrates in 23% of the 31 muscle biopsies.

The muscle inflammatory infiltrates we found were scattered and non-specific but suggest a possible infectious or immune-mediated disorder. Inflammatory infiltrates are seen in the idiopathic inflammatory myopathies, a group of disorders including polymyositis, dermatomyositis, and connective tissue associated myositis. These inflammatory myopathies are usually associated with elevated CK levels, proximal muscle weakness, and spontaneous activity as well as short duration motor units on EMG, findings which were rare in our patients.

Type II fiber atrophy is a non-specific abnormality. It can be seen in a number of conditions including disuse, acute denervation, myasthenia gravis, polymyalgia rheumatica, remote effects of systemic malignancy, collagen vascular disease, steroid use, and rapid weight loss[6]. Of the patients included in this study, none had clinical or EMG evidence for acute denervation, myasthenia gravis, or any history of malignancy. None had lost weight, were on steroids, or were bedridden, although all were relatively sedentary compared to their pre-illness functioning. The Type II atrophy seen was probably due to disuse. Type II atrophy has been reported in several Australian CFS cases with persistent myalgias[2]; Behan et al have also found occasional Type II atrophy in CFS patients[1], however, in their study, scattered non-selective atrophy was seen in about 30% of patients, and Type II hypertrophy and predominance were seen in another 30%. They did not find inflammatory infiltrates.

Are there tests to predict which subset of patients will have abnormal muscle biopsies?

Two of four patients with elevated serum CK had inflammatory infiltrates on muscle biopsy, and five of the patients with inflammatory infiltrates had normal serum CK. Muscle enzyme elevations were thus only marginally useful in predicting the presence of inflammatory infiltrates. Neither clinical exam for proximal weakness nor symptom prevalence were helpful. The percentage of polyphasic motor units on EMG also did not correlate with muscle biopsy findings. Of the 17 patients with Type I or II atrophy, 8 had increased numbers of polyphasic motor units and 7 had normal motor units. Only one patient had a mildly elevated CK, shortened mean motor unit potential duration suggesting a myopathy, and inflammatory infiltrates.

Because of the difficulty in sorting out the pathogenesis of many of the neurologic symptoms in these patients, 26 of the 31 patients also underwent spinal fluid analysis. Ten of these patients had mildly elevated IgG synthesis rates, and one of these had oligoclonal bands in the spinal fluid. Another patient had oligoclonal bands in the serum and spinal fluid. This last patient was the only one of the 7 with muscle inflammatory infiltrates who also had abnormal spinal fluid. The patients with spinal fluid abnormalities were clinically indistinguishable from those patients with inflammatory infiltrates.

Table 2	
Laboratory Evaluations	
Blood Tests	**Number**
Elevated Creatine Kinase	4/31
Elevated ESR	5/31
Muscle Biopsy Results	
Inflammatory infiltrates	7/31
Type II atrophy	15/31
Non-selective Atrophy	3/31
Quantitative EMG Results	
Increased polyphasic motor units	13/28
Increased MUP duration	1/28
Decreased MUP duration	1/28

Conclusion

Inflammatory infiltrates were seen in 23% of patients studied. Unlike the inflammatory myopathies, the infiltrates did not cause muscle fiber necrosis or loss of muscle fibers, did not cause large CK elevations, EMG changes suggesting myopathy, or significant weakness. The infiltrates were scattered, mild, and did not correlate with the severity of the fatigue or myalgias experienced by 100% of the patients studied.

A number of authors have now reported immunologic abnormalities in patients with CFS[7,8]. Klimas et al have found a pattern of immunologic abnormalities compatible with chronic viral reactivation. The presence of inflammatory infiltrates in the patients we studied also suggests an infectious or immune-mediated disorder.

References

1. Behan PO, Behan WMH: Post-viral fatigue syndrome CRC Critical Reviews in Neurology Vol 4, 165, 1988.

2. Byrne E, Trounce I, Dennett X: Chronic relapsing myalgia (? post viral): clinical, histological, and biochemical studies. Aust NZ Med Vol 15:305-308, 1985.

3. Jamal GA, Hansen S: Electrophysiological studies in the postviral fatigue syndrome. J Neurol, Neurosurg and Psych: 48:691-694, 1985.

4. Archard LS, Bowles NE, Behan PO, Bell EJ, Doyle D, Postviral fatigue syndrome: persistence of enterovirus RNA in muscle and elevated creatine kinase. J Royal Soc Med 81:326-329, 1988.

5. Holmes GP, Kaplan JE, Gantz NM et al. Chronic Fatigue Syndrome: A working case definition. Ann Intern Med 108:387-389, 1988.

6. Mastaglia FL and Walton J: **Skeletal Muscle Pathology.** Churchill Livingston, New York, New York 1982.

7. Caligiuri M, Murray C, Buchwald D et al. Phenotypic and functional deficiency of natural killer cells in patients with chronic fatigue syndrome. J Immunol 139:3306-3313, 1987.

8. Klimas NG, Salvato FR, Morgan R, and Fletcher MA. Immunologic Abnormalities in Chronic Fatigue Syndrome. J of Clin Microbiol 28:1403-1410, 1990.

Chapter 39

An Account of 100 Muscle Biopsies in Epidemic Myalgic Encephalomyelitis (EME)

By D. Doyle MD, Dept of Neuropathology, Institute of Neurological Sciences, Southern General Hospital, Glasgow

Dr. Doyle was born in Edinburgh and educated at the University of Edinburgh. He has held appointments in obstetrics, medicine, clinical surgery, anatomy and surgical neurology. In 1963, Dr. Doyle was the recipient of the Richard Brown Research Scholarship. He invented microvascular surgical methods, introduced peritoneoscopy and made innovative clinical and pathological studies in neurological trauma. From 1963 to 1971, he held appointments in neuropathology and general pathology in Edinburgh and London and has held his present position as Neuropathologist at Southern General Hospital for 20 years. His interests include experimental medicine and chemistry, aviation and the Royal Scottish Piping Society.

Introduction

Prominent symptoms in patients with EME are muscle weakness and feelings of tiredness on effort which would previously have been well within their ability. There are often complaints that severe lassitude follows periods of physical work which may persist for several days. It was thought reasonable to take muscle biopsies from such patients in investigating the nature of their disorder and also to exclude the possibility of some other recognisable clinical entity which would have been masked by the clinical presentation.

The study of these patients proceeded at the same time as the evaluation of muscle biopsies from patients with all types of neuro-muscular disorders in the West of Scotland and were evaluated against an experience of about 1,500 biopsies examined personally over almost 20 years.

Materials and Methods

Patients diagnosed as having EME were subjected to muscle biopsies. The first ten patients had open biopsies of vastus medialis but subsequently needle biopsies of vastus lateralis were done. It was not thought justified to do open biopsies for the studies envisaged and there was also a need to economise on theatre time because of the potentially large numbers of patients.

All of the biopsies, open and needle[3], were done with local anaesthesia only. No premedication or sedation was used. Most of the patients were outpatients and were able to leave hospital soon after the biopsy was done. Sutures were used to close the open biopsy wounds while adhesive "Neat-seal" closures were used for the 4mm wounds made for the needle biopsies. No complications of the techniques were reported i.e. there was no wound infection and no haematomas were generated.

The patients biopsied were between 24 and 63 years. The sexes were equally represented.

The biopsy samples were handled immediately after removal by a Medical Laboratory Scientific Officer in the theatre. The MLSO prepared blocks for freezing and subsequent transverse sectioning. The samples were rapidly frozen in isopentane cooled with liquid nitrogen then transferred to a cryostat chamber at -40°C for cutting sections. Some samples, and the cryostat block, after sectioning, were stored at -80°C and could be retrieved as required for other purposes or for repeat sectioning.

Frozen selections were examined by light microscopy after standard laboratory techniques[6] had been applied for staining (Haematoxyolin and eosin, HE; Van Gieson, VG; and Gomori's Trichrome) and histochemical methods (Oil-red-O, ORO; Sudan Black B, SBB; Periodic acid Schiff, PAS, with and without diastase; ATPase, preincubated at pH's 4.3, 4.6 and 9.4; succinic dehydrogenase; muscle phosphorylase; phosphofructokinase, PFK; adenylate monophosphate deaminase,[9] AMPDA; and cyto-chrome oxidase by several methods). This routine allowed an assessment of stained cytological details, collagen amounts, muscle fibre typing and distribution, the quantities of lipid and glycogen in muscle fibres and the activities of key enzymes in glycogen and energy metabolism.

For electron microscopy, small pieces of muscle were immersed in glutaraldehyde (2%) in pH7.4 phosphate buffer - freshly prepared. The samples were processed to araldite, cut on a LKB III ultratome and examined after staining with lead and uranyl acetate in a Philips 201 electron microscope. Photographs were taken on strip film - 35 mm - at several magnifications paying particular attention to mitochondria, the quantities of glycogen and lipids and the presence of any inclusion material.

Motor end plates were examined in five of the open biopsies by cholinesterase histochemistry and in all of the open biopsies by the methylene blue supravital staining method.[4,5] The terminal innervation ratio was calculated by counting motor end plates and the number of terminal axons supplying them. Motor end plates were found in five of the biopsies in electron microscopy.

Results:

Light Microscopy

Muscle Fibre Types

It was not possible to quantitate the fibre types by number or size at the time when these biopsies were processed. It may be possible to do this quantitation using image analysis but the results quoted are the results of direct examination. It was possible to check the relative fibre sizes using a micrometer eyepiece and this was necessary because, with highly contrasting images, illusory effects are readily achieved.

The proportions of type 1 and 2 muscle fibres varied considerably from patient to patient but were generally consistent in several small samples taken from one patient. The proportions of type 1 and 2 fibres were judged against an experience of many hundreds of needle and open biopsies from vastus lateralis and vastus medialis.

Forty two of the patients had a **numerical preponderance of type 2 fibres** whereas our experience of this muscle is for equal representation of both types. Abnormal fibre type grouping was noted in 10 patients where clustering of type 2 fibres was noted often in association with numerical preponderance. There was insufficient evidence in all of the cases to suggest an abnormality of innervation. Generalised type 2 fibre atrophy was found in only one patient.

Six patients had a numerical preponderance of type 1 muscle fibres but this was less obvious than the situation with type 2 predominance.

Relative Enlargement of type 2 fibres in comparison with type 1 fibres was observed in 18 cases and relative enlargement of type 1 fibres in comparison with type 2 fibres was seen in 4 biopsies. In these situations of relative enlargement, the largest fibres of either type were thought to be conspicuously larger than the largest of the fibres of the other type and, if the largest fibres were subtracted, the sizes of the other muscle fibres were of usual distribution or of roughly equal size spectrum.

Hypertrophy of type 1 and type 2 fibres was noted in two patients, both of whom had bulky muscles and powerful-looking physiques although they were symptomatically incapacitated.

Abnormalities of Single Fibres were the surprising features in this series of biopsies. Single fibre necrosis[2], affecting one or two fibres in a section was found in only three cases. There was no associated inflammatory cell infiltration or vascular abnormality.

Twenty cases had examples of solitary fibres which were usually less than half of the diameter of the smaller fibres in the biopsy. These stained strongly with eosin but were not distinguished apart from by size in other stained or histochemical preparations. Some of these fibres had a broad margin of peripheral cytoplasm with the contractile protein in the centre.

There was a possibility that one such fibre was undergoing necrosis. When examined for RNA content, no increase was observed with methyl green pyronin staining. The nature of these fibres was not clear. They had a distinctive appearance, unlike any situation except for some resembling muscle fibres at tendinous insertions. This did not seem to be the explanation for their morphology because the narrowness and the unusual internal morphology extended through many serial sections (tendinous insertional parts of muscle fibres change their architecture over very short lengths). In the several serial sections through which these fibres could be followed, there was no evidence, in light microscopy, of any feature related to virus incorporation.

Electron Microscopy

Of the 100 biopsies, 70 showed no abnormalities of any type. The finding of abnormalities of diverse types in 30 patients was a much greater incidence than expected. In the diagnostic series of biopsies (over 1,500), in my experienc , after removing all of the biopsies with diagnostic features, an incidence of non-specific abnormalities ess than 10% has been found. That is to say, if a biopsy is taken for speculative, diagnostic purposes and no diagnosis can be made on the biopsy by light or electron microscopy, the incidence of non-specific abnormalities is about one third of that in this series of patients with EME.

In the open muscle biopsies, where motor point samples were taken, intramuscular innervation details were readily found. In the needle biopsies, however, comparable information was only haphazard. A striking feature in both types of biopsy was that some, generally solitary, myelinated axons were surrounded by **multiple Schwan cell lamellae.** No evidence of myelin abnormality was found in any of the samples which, because of their small size and optimal fixation, gave excellent morphological details.

Atrophic muscle fibres with diminution and disarray of contractile protein were found in 10 biopsies. This was half of the incidence of atrophic fibres in the light microscopy but probably represents a sampling situation (see discussion).

Cytoplasmic "inclusions" of the fibrillary, peripheral, medium-electron dense type were found in 6 cases. One further case had small, rounded, lamellar bodies and one had a very small portion of an inclusion which resembled part of a "finger print" inclusion.

Z-Streaming was seen in 6 cases, usually peripherally in the fibres.

Unstructured Central Cores were found in 4 biopsies although the light microscopy had not suggested their presence.

A single **mitochondrial crystalline** inclusion was found in one biopsy.

Mitochondrial Morphology and Function There were no cases in which there was evidence of mitochondrial hyperactivity, not even in the biopsy in which there was the single mitochondrial crystalline inclusion. The range of activities of succinic dehydrogenase was similar to that in the general run of muscle biopsies, there being no suggestion of consistently deviant mitochondrial activity. Electron microscopy showed variations of mitochondrial morphology which could not be related to abnormalities of function. The distribution and number of mitochondria showed some variation but, critically, these could be explained usually by fortuitous section planes.

Other Enzyme Activities There was no evidence of abnormal muscle phosphorylase or phosphofructokinase activity or of any related abnormalities of glycogen content. Although histochemistry for lipid handling enzymes was not done, there was no suggestion of any relevant abnormality in the amounts of lipid in its several storage forms.

Motor End Plates were assessed by light and electron microscopy. The terminal innervation ratio was almost 1:1 giving no evidence of collateral axonal sprouting in the cases in which adequate numbers of end plates could be seen. There was no light microscopic evidence of ultraterminal sprouting or of abnormally large or small end plates. Electron microscopy, however, showed, in three cases, end plates comprising widely spaced primary synaptic folds with highly complex secondary folds. One biopsy had normal-looking end plates on all of the muscle fibres examined.

Correlation with Enterovirus Studies No correlation was found between the light or electron microscopic findings and the evidence for persistence of enterovirus components obtained by Dr. L. Archard[1] who was sent samples of all these biopsies. A few of his positive results coincided with the biopsies with atrophic fibres but there was no demonstrable association as equal numbers had positive results for enteroviruses and no atrophic fibres in the biopsy sample. Also, several biopsies gave negative results but had atrophic fibres.

Discussion

The great majority - about 70% of these biopsies, taken from a series of patients categorised but not otherwise classified as having EME, were normal. The most striking finding in the study was the **incompletely atrophic muscle fibre** with central contractile protein and peripheral cytoplasm. This, occurring as a solitary muscle fibre, is a novel finding. No relationship to metabolic, innervation or viral phenomena could be established. It was possible that one such fibre could have been undergoing necrosis. The presence of this type of fibre seems to have slight diagnostic value but, as there may be only one such fibre among several hundred normal-looking fibres, it is understandable that the incidence of even a single example in a biopsy depends on the size of the sample. The larger, open biopsies showed this type of fibre almost constantly while many of the needle biopsies did not. It is possible that larger samples in all cases would lead to a higher yield of this feature. None of the other features described above has any specific connotation. The Schwann cell lamination or onion-skinning of solitary axons is interesting in relation to the possibility of a motor end plate disorder. The end plates also had a lamination of Schwann cell cytoplasm and basement membrane overlying them but the changes in the end plates - wide separation of primary synaptic folds and increased complexity of secondary folds- is not a known diagnostic combination. The latter is similar to published prints of the motor end plate in the Eaton-Lambert syndrome[10,7,8].

The absence of any evidence of mitochondrial or other metabolic abnormality is disappointing because it does not open any doors to rational therapy. Other functional biochemical studies may, however, yield more information. The original description of the type 2 muscle fibre changes led to the interesting work of Rada and colleagues using analytical nuclear magnetic resonance to follow the intra-muscular pH and energy utilisation. Further studies of this type are awaited with interest.

Summary

1. Muscle biopsies have been done in patients with Epidemic Myalgic Encephalomyelitis.

2. Abnormalities have been found in light and electron microscopy in 30% of cases only.

3. Solitary muscle fibres with incomplete atrophy, central contractile proteins and peripheral cytoplasm are thought to have diagnostic relevance. This type of pathology was found almost constantly in larger, open biopsies while many of the needle biopsies did not reveal such pathology. Less frequently, Schwann cell lamination or onion-skinning of solitary axons were observed. In these cases, end plates also had Schwann cell lamination with wide separation of primary synaptic folds and increased complexity of secondary folds.

4. No evidence of mitochondrial or metabolic dysfunction has been found.

5. No evidence of morphologically abnormal mitochondria has been found.

6. There is no correlation between microscopic findings and the results of enterovirus probe studies.

Conclusions

Needle biopsies may yield abnormalities such as incompletely atrophic muscle fibres of the type described above but as the samples are small and the abnormalities dispersed there may be no abnormality in a biopsy. Open biopsies give the possibility of studying larger areas of muscle and of studying the motor end plates and terminal innervation where abnormalities are suggested.

No evidence of mitochondrial or other enzyme dysfunction has been found. The variability of muscle fibre type, numerical and size proportions should, if representative of muscle organisation throughout the body, give corresponding metabolic patterns in analytical NMR or other methods of studying whole body or muscle compartment metabolism.

The incidence and variety or non-specific abnormalities in electron microscopy, being much higher than expected, may be evidence of a previous, transient muscle disorder or of a subtle, continuing process.

Acknowledgements

Thanks are due to: Mr. R. Houston, M.L.S.O. who did most of the frozen section work; Miss J. Morrison who typed the manuscript; Mrs. Janice Stewart who prepared the electron micrographs; and Mrs. C. Eadie and Mrs. J. Cunningham who prepared the illustrations. The biopsies were from patients of Dr. P.O. Behan whose enthusiasm is acknowledged.

References

Pearce A. G. E. (1980) "Histochemistry, Theoretical and Applied" 4th Edn. Churchill Livingstone

1. Archard, L., Behan P. O., Doyle, D. J. Roy. Soc. Med. 1988

2. Aström, K.E., Adams, R. D., (1981) in "Disorders of Voluntary Muscle" 165-174 Ed. Walton, J., Churchill Livingstone.

3. Bergström, J. (1962) Scand. J. Clin. Lab. Invest. 14 (Suppt 68) 1-110.

4. Coërs, C. (1952) J. Neurol, Neurosurg, Psychiat. 15:211.

5. Dogiel, A. S. (1902) Archiv f. Mikr. Anat. 59:1.

6. Dubowitz, V. (1985) Muscle Biopsy, 2nd Edn. Ballière Tindall.

7. Engel A. G., Santa, T, (1971) Ann. NY Acad Sci 183:46 Harriman, D. G. F., Currie, S., 1974 In "Troisiemes Journees Internationales de Pathologie Neuromusculaire". Eds Serratrice, H. et al. p 138.

8. Engel, A. G., Angelini, C., Gomez, M.R. (1972) Mayo Clinic Proc. 47-377.

9. Fischbein, W. N., Armbrustmacher, V. W., Griffin, J. L. (1978) Science 200: 545-548.

10. Lambert, E. H. (1966) Ann. NY Acad. Sci. 135:367.

Chapter 40

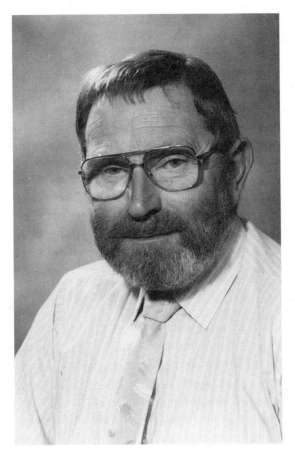

David Halliday

Whole Body and Muscle Protein Synthesis in Myalgic Encephalomyelitis

D. Halliday, MD, Nutrition Research Group, Clinical Research Centre, Watford Road, Harrow HA1 3UJ UK and P.J. Pacy, MD, London School of Hygiene and Tropical Medicine, Keppel Street, London

Dr. David Halliday is head of the Nutrition Research Group at the Clinical Research Centre (MRC) in Harrow UK. He also holds a visiting professorship in human metabolism at the University of Limburg, Maastricht, Holland. Following his doctorate degree in body composition and malnutrition (Kingston, Jamaica), Dr. Halliday lectured in Biochemistry at the Middlesex Hospital Medical School for four years before joining the Medical Research Council. His major interest has been to employ stable isotopes as metabolic probes to quantitate aspects of amino acid and protein kinetics in the whole body, tissues and individual proteins in health and disease. His special interest has been the quantitation of muscle protein fractional synthetic rates in muscular dystrophies.

Dr. P.J. Pacy is a Senior Lecturer in Clinical Nutrition at the London School of Hygiene and Tropical Medicine.

Abstract

A predominant clinical feature of patients with Myalgic Encephalomyelitis (M.E.) is severe muscle weakness although rarely muscle wasting. Previous observations in these patients have revealed a significant reduction in muscle RNA content although not total protein. This is indicative of impaired muscle protein synthesis. The aim of the present study was to quantitate whole body leucine kinetics and quadriceps muscle protein fractional synthesis rate (MPSR) in nine (8F, 1M) M.E. patients. Whole body leucine kinetics were determined from an 8h primed continuous infusion of L-[1-13C]leucine. MPSR was calculated from the increase in 13C-leucine enrichment in mixed muscle protein, obtained from percutaneous muscle biopsies taken 6h apart during the infusion (first biopsy at 2h). Plasma 13C-ketoisocaproic acid was taken to represent precursor pool labelling. Whole body leucine kinetics were similar to those of age, weight and sex matched controls. In contrast, mean MPSR in M.E. patients was lower (p<0.05) than published control values. However more critical examination of the data revealed that only three of the seven available values could be considered below the normal range.

Introduction

Myalgic Encephalomyelitis (M.E.) as a disease entity was recognised by the Department of Health and Social Security in the United Kingdom in 1987[1]. It is associated with a wide range of symptomatology and encompasses many medical disciplines as exemplified by the scope of these Proceedings. However the diverse and non-specific nature of symptoms which frequently incapacitate sufferers has led some physicians to cast doubt on the nature of the illness[2].

Complaints relating to the musculo-skeletal system have tended to focus attention towards the effect of M.E. on various aspects of muscle function and structure. To date, research into various aspects of muscle physiology are far from clear cut. Clinically, while severe muscle weakness is a frequent feature, muscle wasting is rarely observed. This implies that significant immobility is unlikely to be a factor in the disease process as this has been reported to result in rapid loss of muscle mass[3,4]. Several groups have examined muscle histology in M.E. In one of the first such reports Behan reported abnormal histology in all 20 individuals studied[5]. The most common abnormality was the presence of necrotic fibres with no inflammatory response. It is possible that such findings reflect impaired immunity. In a much smaller study of two patients Type II fibre atrophy was noted[6].

More recently, in marked contrast to these findings, Teahon and colleagues[7] failed to document any consistent abnormalities. The most consistent finding was of combined Types I and II fibre hypertrophy which occurred in 4 out of 30 individuals. The significance of this observation remains to be established. Staining of the muscle for several enzymes involved in glycolysis indicated that myophosphorylase, phosphofructokinase and lactate dehydrogenase were all normal. Further evidence that muscle glycolysis is not impaired is provided by the finding of normal lactate production during anaerobic exercise of the forearm in these subjects[8]. Interestingly, Peters and colleagues[9] reported reduced total RNA/mg DNA in M.E. patients (n=22, 0.54 ± 0.14 mg) than matched healthy controls (n=26, 0.64 ± 0.14 mg, p<0.05; all figures are mean±SD). In contrast, total protein/mg DNA were comparable in both groups. As ribosomal RNA comprises at least 80% of total muscle RNA10 these findings are suggestive of impaired protein synthesis. The aim of the present study was to further examine this possibility by directly measuring fractional muscle protein synthesis as well as that of whole body protein by means of stable isotope methodology.

Materials and Methods

Subjects

Nine subjects (8 female; 1 male) were recruited from the M.E. society. They had all been diagnosed as suffering from M.E. for at least six months. At the time of study they claimed to be weight maintaining, the disease had been stable for several months and they had taken no regular medication for at least the preceding month. The clinical details of the subjects were as follows: age 45.6 ± 10.2 years; weight 62.6 ± 11.2 kg; body mass index 22.0 ± 2.9 kg/m^2. There was no evidence of abnormal renal or liver function on routine biochemical variables. The patients were admitted to hospital for the study. An age, sex and weight matched control group was recruited. The clinical details of the six females and two males were, age 46.9 ± 13.6 years; weight 64.5 ± 9.9 kg; body mass index 24.3 ± 3.7 kg/m^2. These individuals were not admitted to hospital. All individuals gave informed consent after the nature of the protocol had been explained to them. The protocols were similar, although it was not considered ethical to perform muscle biopsies on the controls. No financial incentive was offered to them for their participation in the study. Ethical approval was obtained from Northwick Park Hospital Ethical Committee.

Materials

L-[1-¹³C] leucine (99 atom percent) and NaH¹³CO₃ (99 atom percent) were purchased from Cambridge Isotopes (Woburn, Massachusetts, USA). Isotope solutions of both materials were prepared in 150mmol/l sodium chloride and rendered sterile and pyrogen free by Nothwick Park Hospital Pharmacy.

Study Design

All subjects were studied in the post-absorptive state following a 12-14 hour overnight fast. An intravenous catheter was inserted in each arm. One in a superficial forearm vein for the infusion of the L-[1-¹³C] leucine tracer, the other into a vein in the dorsum of the contralateral hand for sampling arterialised blood (plasma ketoisocaproate). Zero samples were taken before the tracer infusion to determine the baseline ¹³C-enrichment. Priming doses of NaH¹³CO₃ (0.16 mg kg⁻¹h⁻¹) and L-[1-¹³C] leucine (0.9 mg kg⁻¹h⁻¹) were injected and followed immediately by the continuous infusion of L-[1-¹³C] leucine (1.0 mg kg⁻¹h⁻¹) for 8h.

Two hours into the leucine infusion, a muscle biopsy was performed under local anaesthesia (2% lignocaine) using a Bergstrom biopsy needle[12]. Some 150-200 mg wet weight muscle tissue was obtained from the lateral aspect of the thigh, approximately 15 cm above the knee joint. All visible fat was removed from the tissue which was immediately frozen in liquid nitrogen to await analysis. A second biopsy was obtained 6h later from the same leg some 10cms from the original site. Arterialised blood and expired air samples were collected every 30 min from 2 to 8h during the infusion. Subjects' expired air was initially collected in a 2L latex bag and duplicate 20ml aliquots rapidly transferred to 20 ml Vacutainers (Beckton Dickinson, Rutherford, New Jersey). The subjects lay quietly throughout the study, and indirect calorimetry was performed during alternate hours using a ventilated hood system[13]. From this measurement the subjects total CO₂ production rate was obtained.

Analytical Procedure

Plasma [¹³C]-alpha ketoisocaproate (KIC) enrichment was used to represent intracellular leucine labelling of the precursor pool for protein synthesis[14,15]. KIC enrichment was measured by selected ion monitoring gas chromatography-mass spectrometry in the chemical ionisation mode. Plasma KIC concentration was determined simultaneously employing ketovaleric acid as internal standard[16]. Enrichment of ¹³CO₂ in expired air was measured by isotope ratio mass spectromety (IRMS)[17]. Separation of the protein-bound amino acids prior to the measurement of L-[1-¹³C] leucine incorporation into the quadriceps muscle has been described previously[18]. Volatile amino acid isobutyl esters were separated on a packed column, with argon as carrier gas, and collected distal to a stream splitter (99:1) by condensation in a liquid nitrogen-cooled 'U' tube. The isolated pure dry leucyl ester was hydrolysed to the free acid; the leucine decarboxylated by the Van Slyke ninhydrin reaction, and the ¹³CO₂ enrichment measured by IRMS.

Calculation

Whole-body leucine kinetics were calculated using a steady-state two pool model in which the leucine flux (Q_L) is calculated from the rate of dilution of the infused tracer by the unlabelled tracee, thus

$$Q_L = i \left[\frac{Ei}{Ep} \right] - 1$$

where i is the rate of infusion of 13C-leucine (µmol kg⁻¹h⁻¹), Ei is the enrichment of the infused tracer, and Ep is the enrichment of the plasma KIC at plateau. The reciprocal pool model exhibits several advantages when compared with calculations based on the use of plasma [¹³C]-leucine enrichment. KIC enrichment reflects more precisely total leucine flux[14,15], is metabolically the more immediate precursor of leucine oxidation[19], minimises sample-site error[15,20], and closely resembles intracellular muscle [¹³C]-leucyl tRNA enrichment[21]. Leucine oxidation was calculated from the excretion rate of ¹³CO₂ and the plasma plateau enrichment of KIC in the following manner;

$$F^{13}CO_2 = \frac{FCO_2 \times E^{13}CO_2 \times 44.6 \times 60}{body\ wt\ (kg) \times 0.81 \times 100}$$

where FCO_2 is the CO_2 production rate (ml min-1), $E^{13}CO_2$ is the plateau $^{13}CO_2$ enrichment, 44.6 x 60 converts CO_2 ml min^{-1} to µmol h^{-1}, 0.81 relates to the CO_2 retention is the bicarbonate pool of the body[22] and the 100 converts the whole to a fraction. Whole body leucine oxidation (µmol kg^{-1}h^{-1}) was then derived from;

$$F^{13}CO_2 \left[\frac{1}{Ep} - \frac{1}{Ei} \right] \times 100$$

In the postabsorptive steady state, Q_L = breakdown = oxidation + the non-oxidative component of leucine flux (synthesis).

Fractional muscle protein synthetic rate (ks) was calculated from;

$$ks\ (\%h^{-1}) = \frac{En\ muscle}{En\ KIC \times time\ between\ biopsies} \times 100$$

where En muscle is the observed increase in [^{13}C] leucine enrichment in muscle protein between the two biopsies. The calculation relies on the assumption that the incorporation of the tracer into muscle protein is linear during the period of plasma KIC plateau enrichment. This has been established for several proteins such as albumin[23] and VLDL apolipoprotein B100[24,25].

Table 1

Whole body leucine kinetics (µmol kg^{-1} h^{-1}) and results of indirect calorimetry (ml min^{-1}) in Myalgic Encephalomyelitis (n=9) and matched controls (n=8).

	ME patients	Controls
Breakdown	87 ± 13	89 ± 10
Synthesis	71 ± 10	72 ± 8
Oxidation	16 ± 4	17 ± 3
KIC concentration (µM)	25 ± 6	18 ± 7
O2 uptake	211 ± 40	212 ± 22
CO2 production	161 ± 34	161 ± 19
RQ	0.76 ± 0.04	0.77 ± 0.03

Figures are mean ± SD. No statistical differences were observed.

Results

Whole body leucine kinetics were determined by steady state kinetics. The mean coefficient of varia-tion (mean/SD) for plateau plasma ^{13}C KIC enrichment in the ME patients was 3.5 ± 0.9% (range 2.2 to 5.0%) while for expired breath $^{13}CO_2$ was 4.4 ± 1.6% (range 3.2 to 7.5%). The respective values in the control individuals were 4.7 ± 2.0 (range 2.8 to 8.2%) and 4.9 ± 1.5% (range 2 to 6.8%) respectively. These data provide evidence of the validity for use of a steady state approach. The whole body leucine data for both groups is shown in Table 1. This clearly demonstrates that there were no abnormalities of whole body leucine metabolism in the ME patients. Likewise indirect calorimetry was similar in both groups. This implies not only a comparable post absorptive state at the time of study but that ME does not apparently effect resting energy expenditure.

Table 2

Individual post absorptive quadriceps fractional muscle protein synthesis

(%/h) in Myalgic Encephalomyelitis patients (n=7)

F	0.0308
F	0.0286
F	0.0396
M	0.0527
F	0.0263
F	0.0471
F	0.0402
mean	0.0379
SD	0.0099

95% Confidence Intervals 0.0287 - 0.0471

Control values (mean ± SD) from published data. 95% Confidence Intervals in brackets.

0.046 ± 0.012	(0.033 -0.059)	Ref 4
0.046 ± 0.012	(0.040 - 0.052)	Ref 31
0.046 ± 0.011	(0.039 - 0.053)	Ref 32

Although all nine individuals had muscle biopsies performed, data are available in seven only. Table 2 documents the individual and mean fractional quadriceps muscle protein synthesis rates in the seven subjects. For comparative purposes we have quoted data published in the literature generated by a similar approach. Overall mean fractional quadriceps muscle protein synthesis was lower than control values (p<0.05). However, when the individual results are examined it is apparent that only three patients had values considered lower than that of previously published controls.

Discussion

This study revealed that patients with stable Myalgic Encephalomyelitis had significantly lower fractional muscle protein synthesis rates than values from healthy controls reported in the literature. However a more critical examination of the data suggests that depressed muscle protein synthesis occurred in only three of the seven patients. Interestingly, there appeared no correlation with the patients self-assessment of the severity of the disease and muscle protein synthesis. In addition, the patient deemed most affected by the disease process on clinical grounds had a normal value.

These results are dependent upon the validity of both the technique used to calculate fractional muscle protein synthesis rate as well as the use of historical control data. With regard to the first of these, the continuous infusion method, which was developed originally in animals[26] has been widely employed in human studies. A potential problem with such an approach is the necessity for enrichment measurement of the precursor pool for protein synthesis i.e. amino acyl tRNA. Very recent evidence suggests that there is a good deal of agreement between enrichment of muscle leucyl tRNA and plasma KIC[21]. This implies that, as in the case of the current study, the theoretical mismatch between enrichment of the inaccessible tRNA pool and accessible plasma compartment does not present a major source of error when plasma plateau ^{13}C-KIC is used during continuous infusion of L-[1-^{13}C] leucine. However, other evidence appears to cast doubt on such a conclusion. Flooding doses of the amino acid tracer have been used to minimise differences between extra and intracellular enrichment with that of aminoacyl tRNA[27]. This frequently used method in animal studies has been extended to human in vivo studies[28,29].

Fractional quadriceps MPSR generated by this technique is approximately twice that obtained from the continuous infusion method. To date there appears to be no satisfactory explanation for such a discrepancy. Evidence suggests that the flooding dose method

does not promote muscle protein synthesis[30]. Thus there remains some concern about the validity of the quantitative nature of fractional quadriceps MPSR in the ME patients and controls. The second issue relates to the use of historical controls which we accept is a less than ideal means of generating comparative data. However, we deemed that it was not ethical to subject controls to the invasive procedure of two muscle biopsies. Of the paper quoted to represent control values the mean age was significantly lower at 29[31] and 27[32] years than the M.E. patients. In the other the mean age of 36[4] was not only more comparable but suggested that over the age range of 20 to 55 years MPSR remains relatively constant. A further consideration is that all these data have been generated in men. However there appears no sex difference in fractional MPSR in the fed state[31] or post absorptive whole body leucine kinetics[33]. Fractional MPSR is a major determinant (approximately 30%) of whole body protein synthesis[32,34,35,36] so this latter observation provides further, albeit indirect, evidence against significant differences of quadriceps MPSR between the sexes. Thus we believe it is acceptable to utilise such historical data in a qualitative fashion.

The present study fails to confirm the RNA data which implies impaired protein synthetic process in the majority of M.E. patients. This is perhaps not surprising given the diverse aetiology of the pathological process. Whole body leucine kinetics were very similar in the matched M.E. and control subjects as was resting energy expenditure. Both these observations are suggestive that M.E. is not associated with any general derangement of protein synthesis.

In summary, the results of this study suggest that M.E. is not associated with general impairment of protein metabolism. In contrast, in some patients, quadriceps MPSR appears decreased although its prediction was not possible on clinical grounds.

We believe this observation is not a secondary phenomenon resultant upon immobilisation as this results in rapid and pronounced wasting of muscle mass which was not a feature in the M.E. patients. These preliminary results suggest that further work is required to document the frequency of this finding and to evaluate whether a graded exercise regimen might improve this variable and aid recovery.

References

1. DHSS. Handbook for Delegated Medical Practitioners. HMSO 1988.

2. Coakley JH. Myalgic Encephalomyelitis and muscle fatigue. Brit Med J 1989; 298:1711-1712.

3. Jaffe DM, Terry RD & Spiro AJ. Disuse atrophy of skeletal muscle. J Neurol Sci 1978; 35:189-200.

4. Gibson JNA, Halliday D, Morrison WL, Stoward PJ, Hornsby GA, Watt PW, Murdoch G & Rennie MJ. Decrease in human quadriceps muscle protein turnover consequent upon leg immobilisation. Clin Sci 1987; 72:503-509.

5. Behan PO, Behan WMH & Bell EJ. The post-viral fatigue syndrome - an analysis of the findings in 50 cases. J Infect 1985.

6. Byrne E, Trounce I & Dennett X. Chronic relapsing myalgia (? post-viral):Clinical, histological and biochemical studies. Aust New Zeal J Med 1985; 305-308.

7. Teahon K, Preedy VR, Smith DG & Peters TJ. Clinical studies of post-viral fatigue syndrome (PVFS) with special reference to skeletal muscle function. Clin Sci 1988; 75:45P (Abstract).

8. Wagnemakers AJM, Coakley JH & Edwards RHT. The metabolic consequences of reduced habitual activities in patients with muscle pain and disease. Ergonomics 1988; 31:1519-1527.

9. Peters TJ & Preedy VR. Pathological changes in skeletal muscle in ME:implications for management. In Post-Viral Fatigue Syndrome. (Eds. Jenkins R & Mowbray J) John Wiley & Son Ltd. Chichester. 1991 p 137-146.

10. Young VR. The role of skeletal and cardiac muscle in the regulation of protein metabolism. In:Mammalian Protein Metabolism. Ed Munro HN. Academic Press, New York 1970; 4:586-674.

11. Abumrad NN, Rabin D, Diamond MP & Lacy WW. Use of a heated superficial hand vein as an alternative site for the measurement of amino acid concentrations and for the study of glucose and alanine kinetics in man. Metabolism 1981; 30:936-940.

12. Bergstrom J. Muscle electrolytes in man determined by neutron activation analysis on needle biopsy specimens:a study in normal subjects, kidney patients and patients with chronic diarrhoea. Scand J Clin Lab Invest 1962; 14 (Suppl 68) 1-110.

13. Garrow JS & Webster JD. A computer-controlled indirect calorimeter for the measurement of energy expenditure in one or two subjects simultaneously. Hum Nutrit:Clin Nutrit 1986; 40:315-321.

14. Schwenk, WF, Beaufrere B & Haymond MW. Use of reciprocal pool specific activities to model leucine metabolism in humans. Am J Physiol 1985; 249:E646-E650.

15. Layman DK & Wolfe RR. Sample site selection for tracer studies applying a unidirectional circulatory approach. Am J Physiol 1987; 253:E173-E178.

16. Ford GC, Cheng KN & Halliday D. The analysis of (1-13C) leucine and (13C)KIC in plasma by capillary gas chromatography / mass spectromety in protein turnover studies. Biomed Mass Spectrom 1985; 12:432-436.

17. Halliday D & Read WWC. Mass spectrometric assay of stable isotopic enrichment for the enrichment for the estimation of protein turnover in man. Proc Nut Soc 1981; 40:321-334.

18. Read WW, Read MA, Rennie MJ, Griggs RC & Halliday D. Preparation of CO2 from blood and protein-bound amino acid carboxyl groups for quantification and 13C-isotope measurements. Biomed Mass Spectrom 1984; 11:400-403.

19. Wolfe RR, Goodenough RD, Wolfe MH et al. Isotopic analysis of leucine and urea metabolism in exercising humans. J Appl Physiol 1982; 52:458-466.

20. Thompson GN, Pacy PJ, Ford GC et al. Relationships between plasma isotopic enrichments of leucine and ketoisocaproic acid during continuous infusion of labelled leucine. Europ J Clin Invest 1988; 18:639-643.

21. Watt PW, Lindsay Y, Scrimgeour CM et al. Isolation of amino acyl-tRNA and its labelling with stable-isotropic tracers: use in studies of human tissue protein synthesis. Proc Natl Acad Sci 1991 (in press).

22. Allsop JR, Wolfe RR & Burke JF. Tracer priming the bicarbonate pool. Am J Physiol 1978; 45:137-139.

23. Pacy PJ, Read M & Halliday D. Influence of insulin on albumin and non-albumin protein fractional synthetic rates in post-absorptive Type 1 diabetic patients. Eur J Clin Nut 1990; 44:343-349.

24. Cohn JS, Wagner DA, Cohn SD, Millar JS & Schaefer EJ. Measurement of very low density and low density lipoprotein apoliopoprotein B-100 and high density lipoprotein apo A-1 production in human subjects using deuterated leucine. J Clin Invest 1990; 85:804-11.

25. Venkatesan S, Pacy PJ, Wenham D & Halliday D. Very-low-density-lipoprotein-apolipoprotein B turnover studies in

normal subjects: a stable isotope study. Trans Biochem Soc 1990; 18:1192-1194.

26. Waterlow JC & Stephen JML. The effect of low protein diets on turnover rates of serum, liver and muscle proteins in the rat, measured by continuous infusion of L-(14C) lysine. Clin Sci 1968; 35:287-305.

27. Henshaw EC, Hirsch CA, Morton BE & Hiatt HH. Control of protein synthesis in mammalian tissues through changes in ribosomal activity. J Biol Chem 1971; 246:436-446.

28. Garlick PJ, Wernerman J, McNurlan MA et al. Measurement of the rate of protein synthesis in muscle of postabsorptive men by injection of a 'flooding dose' of (1-¹³C) leucine. Clin Sci 1989; 77:329-336.

29. Garlick PJ, Wernerman J, McNurlan MA & Heys SD. Organ-specific measurements of protein turnover in man. Proceedings of Nutrition Society 1991; 50:217-225.

30. McNurlan MA, Essen P, Heys SD et al. Measurement of protein synthesis in human skeletal muscle: further investigation of the flooding technique. Clin Sci 1991; 81:557-564.

31. Halliday D, Pacy PJ, Cheng KN, Dworzak F, Gibson JNA & Rennie MJ. Rate of protein synthesis in skeletal muscle of normal man and patients with muscular dystrophy: a reassessment. Clin Sci 1988; 74:237-240.

32. Nair KS, Halliday D & Griggs RC. Leucine incorporation into mixed skeletal muscle proteins in humans. Am J Phsysiol 1988; 254:E208-E213.

33. Inculet RI, Stein TP, Peacock JL et al. Altered leucine metabolism in noncachectic sarcoma patients. Cancer Res 1987; 47:4746-4749.

34. Lobley GE, Milne V, Louie JM et al. Whole body and tissue protein synthesis in cattle. Brit J Nutrit 1980; 43:491-502.

35. Tomas FM, Ballard FJ & Pope LM. Age-dependent changes in rate of myofibrillar protein degradation in humans as assessed by 3 methylhistidine and creatine excretion. Clin Sci 1979; 56:341-346.

36. Pacy PJ, Nair KS, Ford C & Halliday D. Failure of insulin infusion to stimulate fractional muscle protein synthesis in Type 1 diabetic patients. Diabetes 1989; 38:618-624.

Chapter 41

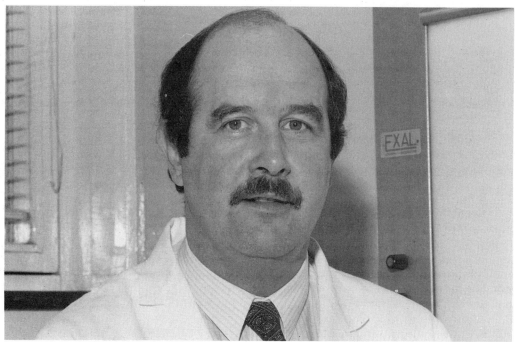

D. R. McCluskey

Exercise Testing in Patients with Chronic Fatigue Syndrome

D.R. McCluskey, MD and M. Riley, MD
Dept of Medicine, Queen's University and Royal Victoria Hospital, Belfast.

In addition to his academic position, Dr. McCluskey is Consultant Physician and Consultant Clinical Immunologist to the Royal Victoria Hospital and Royal Belfast Hospital for Sick Children.

Dr. M. Riley is a Research Fellow in the Royal Victoria Hospital, Belfast.

Summary

Using an exercise treadmill, we have compared the aerobic work capacity of patients with Chronic Fatigue Syndrome to that of a group of normal subjects and a patient control population. Our findings indicate a definite and demonstrable impairment of work capacity together with an abnormality of perceived exertion in patients with this disorder. However, no abnormality in muscle function or metabolism could be detected.

Introduction

Chronic fatigue syndrome (syn: myalgic encephalomyelitis, Royal Free disease, post viral fatigue syndrome), is characterised by complaints of unexplained weakness, lethargy, and post exercise fatigue together with a multiplicity of other symptoms which often include neuropsychiatric features[1].

The onset of symptoms usually follows an acute viral illness in the form of either an upper respiratory infection or gastroenteritis. Patients complain of persisting flu-like symptoms for many months or years for which no definite cause can be found. Enteroviruses, particularly the Coxsackie groups, have been regarded as the putative agents[2]. The Herpes group have also been suggested as putative agents. The most prominent and consistent symptom is that of muscle fatigue which results in limited exercise capacity and profound post exercise weakness and tiredness. Using an exercise treadmill we have studied a group of patients with presumed chronic fatigue syndrome in an effort to develop an objective measurement of their aerobic work capacity. We also attempted to determine whether there was any demonstrable abnormality in response to exercise in comparison to healthy individuals or a patient control group (irritable bowel syndrome patients).

Materials and Methods

Subjects

Three groups of subjects matched for age, sex, and ideal body weight were studied (Table 1). Subjects were excluded from the study if they were suffering from any other medical condition or taking drugs known to affect work performance.

Group 1 (Chronic Fatigue Syndrome Patients)

Since there is no definitive laboratory test, the diagnosis of chronic fatigue syndrome is made by a process of exclusion of other organic disorders together with a clinical history. Thirteen patients (3 men and 10 women) attending an immunology clinic, who met the Centre for Disease Control criteria[3] for CFS were randomly selected for study. All patients had symptoms for >6 months (mean 31 mths range 6-78) with onset following an acute pyrexial illness.

Group 2 (Healthy Control Subjects)

A group of 13 sedentary normal healthy individuals (10 females & 3 males) were selected from the general population for study.

Group 3 (patient control group)

Five women and two men attending the gastroenterology clinic of the Royal Victoria Hospital, and who fulfilled the diagnostic criteria[4] for irritable bowel syndrome(IBS) were selected for study.

Exercise Testing

After an initial familiarisation exercise test approximately one week prior to the study, all subjects reported to the laboratory 2-3 hours after a light meal. A teflon cannula was inserted into an antecubital vein and following 15 minutes supine rest, samples were withdrawn for resting lactate, creatine kinase (CK), phosphate, and glucose levels. Subjects then underwent a symptom-limited treadmill exercise test to a Bruce protocol, modified by adding an initial stage at 5% gradient, with on-line measurement of respiratory gas exchange. They were encouraged to exercise until they were unable to continue. At peak exercise, blood was again withdrawn for the measurement of lactate, CK, phosphate and glucose. In addition, during the final minute of each exercise stage, and after 3 minutes recovery post exercise, a sample was withdrawn for measurement of lactate. After the exercise test subjects were asked to indicate the degree of subjective difficulty, at peak exertion, on a Borg score[5].

All CFS patients returned approximately 18 hours after the exercise test for repeat determination of creatine kinase and phosphate levels.

All exercise testing was performed by the same investigator (MR) who was blind to the experimental group of the subject under investigation.

Activity Score

Subjects were asked to complete a visual analogue scale relating to their overall general capability for physical activity corresponding to periods just prior to their illness, and prior to the exercise testing. They were also asked to indicate on a similar scale the level of activity they reasonably aspired to (Fig 1).

Table 1		
Demographic details of subjects tested		
	Total Number (males)	Age Years (SD)	Weight Kg (SD)
CFS	13 (3)	34 (6.1)	64 (11.2)
NORMALS	13 (3)	34 (4.8)	65 (13.8)
IBS	7 (2)	28 (6.7)	60.9 (9.9)

All Tables show results as Mean Standard Deviation

| | | **Figure 1** | | |

Activity Score

Measurement of Gas Exchange

Minute ventilation was measured using a vane turbine placed on the inspiratory side of a non-rebreathing respiratory valve circuit (dead-space 88ml) in conjunction with a ventilometer (PK Morgan UK). Expired O_2 and CO_2 concentrations were determined by paramagnetic and infrared analysis respectively and minute O_2 consumption (VO_2) and CO_2 production (VCO_2) calculated on-line by an Ericsson microcomputer. Details of this method have been previously reported[6]. Respiratory exchange ratio (RER) was calculated as VCO_2/VO_2. It rises with increasing lactic acidosis as buffering occurs through increased CO_2 elimination, and thus serves as a non-invasive indication of the extent of anaerobic metabolism[7,8]. End-tidal CO_2 was measured by an end-tidal analyser (Engstrom, Sweden), expired air being sampled by a fine-bore tube inserted into the mouthpiece just in front of the mouth.

Statistical Analysis

Variation among groups was tested using analysis of variance. Where this showed a p value of <0.05 further between group comparisons were performed using the Scheffe test.

Blood Sampling and Assays

The venous cannula was flushed with 0.9% saline.

Lactate samples were precipitated immediately in 8% perchloric acid and the supernatant assayed by an enzymatic colorimetric method (Sigma St.Louis, Mo.) Blood glucose, creatine kinase and phosphate were measured using a Cobas Bio nephelometer (Roche Diagnostica, Welwyn Garden City).

Results

All subjects completed the exercise tests uneventfully. In the CFS group, 12 stopped because of fatigue and 1 because of dyspnoea. Ten normal subjects stopped due to fatigue, with 3 due to dyspnoea. In the IBS group, 5 stopped because of fatigue, 1 developed chest tightness without ECG changes and one stopped due to light-headedness (Blood pressure remained normal).

Group 1 subjects attained lower treadmill times and peak achieved VO_2 (pVO_2) compared with subjects in either group 2 or 3. Despite this, their perceived exertion scale was higher than the other two groups (Table 2) and no differences were seen in the peak RER achieved among the groups. No significant differences in these parameters could be demonstrated between group 2 and group 3 subjects. Peak heart rate and lactate levels were also similar. End-tidal CO_2 values both at rest and during exercise were similar in all groups, indicating no tendency to hyperventilation.

Table 2			
	CFS	NORMAL	IBS
Treadmill Time (s)	672 (109)**	849 (52)	902 (91)**
PVO2	31.8 (5.3)*	37.9 (5.1)	42.6 (7.0)**
RER	1.14 (0.1)	1.19 (0.1)	1.13 (0.05)
Peak Heart Rate	177 (18)	182 (7)	189 (5)
BORG	8.2 (1.9)**	6.6 (0.8)	5.3 (1.3)
Peak Lactate	4.25 (1.5)	5.37 (1.2)	5.73 (0.9)
End Tidal CO2 at rest	34.8 (4.4)	35.8 (5.2)	32.1 (5.0)
End Tidal CO2 at peak	34.9 (5.3)	36.3 (5.4)	33.6 (4.5)

$* \ p < 0.06$ $** \ p < 0.001$
relative to controls

Responses at peak exertion in the groups of subjects tested.

Figure 2

Heart Rates at Different Stages of Exercise

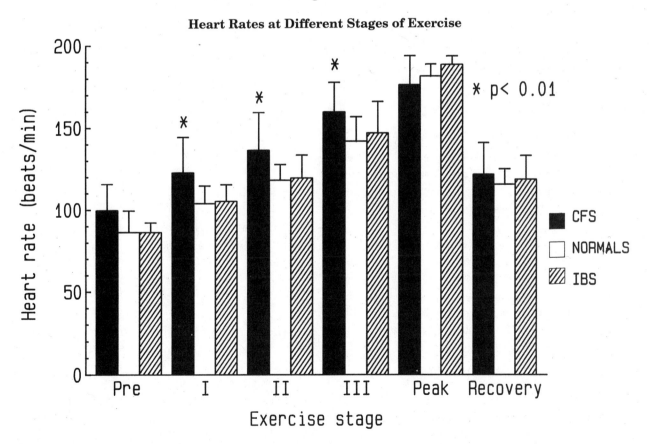

*Heart rates at different stages of exercise testing. *p<0.01 compared to control. Bars show mean standard deviation.*

Figure 3

Serum Lactate Levels at Stages of Exercise Testing

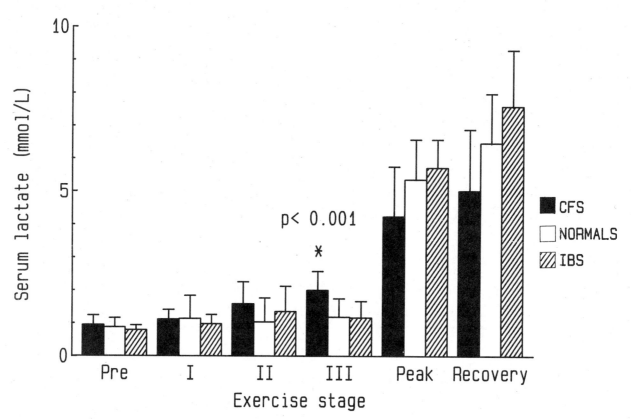

*Blood lactates at different stages of exercise testing. *p<0.001 compared to control. Bars show mean standard deviation.*

Submaximal Heart Rate and Lactate

Heart rate (Fig 2) and lactate (Fig 3) values are shown corresponding to rest and the end of the first three exercise stages. These were the stages completed by all subjects and therefore were used to compare responses at equal absolute workloads.

Overall, heart rate was greater in group 1 subjects at submaximal exertion p<0.05. Similarly, blood lactate was greater in this group (p<0.05), although this difference only became apparent at stage 3. During recovery from exercise, lactate levels were found to be higher in group 3, reflecting the greater workload achieved.

Glucose

No significant differences were apparent among the groups either before or at peak exercise. No group showed any significant change in blood glucose with exercise.

Creatine Kinase

No significant differences in CK were seen among the groups and there was no significant change following exercise.

Phosphate

Phosphate levels were significantly higher at peak exercise in all groups compared to resting values. While there were no inter-group differences among the resting levels, the rise with exercise was significantly less in the CFS patients when compared with the IBS patients, but not with the normal controls. The 18 hour level showed a return to baseline in the CFS group.

Table 3

	CFS	Normal	IBS
Glucose mMols			
Rest	5.1 (1.0)	4.9 (1.2)	4.9 (1.0)
Peak	5.2 (0.9)	5.3 (1.1)	5.5 (1.0)
Creatine Kinase			
Rest	65.2 (23.1)	92.1 (40.3)	88.9 (68.4)
Peak	71.6 (23.4)~~	103.9 (52.4)~	71.3 (20.8)
18 hour Post	65.8 (22.7)		
Phosphate			
Rest	1.0 (0.2)	1.1 (0.2)	1.2 (0.1)
Peak	1.2 (0.2)~~*	1.42 (0.2)	1.6 (0.2)
18 hour Post	1.0 (0.1)		

* $p < 0.05$ compared to control value
~$p < 0.01$ compared to resting value
~~$p < 0.001$ compared to resting value

Blood sugar, muscle enzymes and metabolites at different stages of exercise testing

Activity Scale

Patients with CFS indicated in a VAS score a greater capability for activity prior to the onset of their illness than in the control population (Table 4), but the level was not significantly different from the patients with IBS.

Both of the patient groups indicated reduced activity levels at the time of testing. Normal controls and patients with IBS aspired to a greater level of activity than they had so far achieved, but patients with CFS indicated a level similar to their former status.

Discussion

This study demonstrates that patients with chronic fatigue syndrome do indeed have a lower exercise tolerance than either normal sedentary subjects or patients with irritable bowel syndrome. The reduction in peak achieved VO2 indicates that this is due to a decreased aerobic work capacity and not simply to decreased walking efficiency on the treadmill.

The main reason for the impaired exercise performance would not seem to lie in diminished motivation, as no significant differences were observed in peak heart rate or respiratory exchange ratio amongst the groups.

Significant differences in submaximal heart rate and lactate levels were seen. Comparisons made at the same absolute treadmill workloads (stages I-III) showed a significant trend to higher lactates and heart rates in the CFS group, following the pattern observed in deconditioned subjects[9,10]. In contrast to Montague et al[11], we found no tendency for impaired heart rate responses. Previous studies have demonstrated biochemical and structural abnormalities of muscle in patients with CFS[12,13,14]. Many of these studies were uncontrolled and their findings may, at least in part, be the consequence of deconditioning.

Many muscle disorders exhibit abnormalities of muscle enzymes in the serum[15], which are frequently exacerbated by exercise. We could find no such abnormalities in creatine kinase levels.

Serum phosphate at rest was similar in all groups and though the CFS patients showed a smaller rise with exercise compared to the IBS patients, this may be on the basis of the lower absolute workload achieved.

The stable blood glucose levels pre- and at peak exertion indicate that this is not a limiting factor to exercise.

Table 4			
	CFS	Normal	IBS
Before Illness	7.8 (2.0)*	------------	6.5 (2.0)
Current Level	2.3 (1.6)*	5.7 (1.5)	3.4 (1.1)*
Aspired Level	7.9 (1.5)	7.3 (1.1)~	7.9 (1.8)~

$* \; p < 0.05$ compared to normal controls
$\sim \; p < 0.05$ compared to original status

Exercise Capability (visual analogue score)

Our finding of normal end-tidal CO_2 concentration both at rest and at peak exercise is contrary to the possibility that patients with CFS hyperventilate, as has previously been suggested as a contributory factor to their symptoms[16].

The CFS patients perceived their peak exercise workload to be significantly greater than the other groups (Table 2). Objectively, their relative exertion was not greater as evidenced by the equal peak heart rate response, respiratory exchange ratios and lower peak serum lactates. Possible explanations could be that there is over activity of gamma afferents from muscle endplates resulting in greater perception of stretch[17,18], or alternatively a difference in exercise perception at a higher cerebral level. The results of the activity scores cast an interesting light on the patients' perception of their capability. In general, the scores did not relate to objective measures of exercise capacity such as treadmill time or PVO2.

Patients with CFS invariably indicated a high previous level of activity and a reduced current level, with an aspiration to be restored to their former level. It is of interest that the patients with IBS also claimed reduced exercise capacity, but their objective indices on testing were similar to the normals. Both normals and patients with IBS aspired to exercise levels greater than they had before. Our data would suggest that either patients with CFS were extremely fit prior to their illness, or that they have an altered perception of their premorbid activity level.

In summary, CFS patients exhibit impaired exercise capacity despite increased perceived exertion. We have found no evidence for deficient cardiovascular response or peripheral muscle function other than that which would be expected as a result of deconditioning. However other mechanisms such as muscle fibre atrophy or depletion of muscle enzymes may give similar findings and would merit further investigation.

References

1. Behan PO, Behan WHM, Bell EJ. The post-viral fatigue syndrome - an analysis of findings in 50 cases. J Infect 1985; 10, 211-222.

2. Bell EJ, McCartney RA, Riding MH. Coxsackie B viruses and myalgic encephalomyelitis. J Roy. Soc. Med. 1988; 81, 329-331.

3. Holmes GP, Kaplan JE, Gantz NM, Komaroff AL, Schonberg LB, et al. Chronic fatigue syndrome; A working case definition. Ann. Int. Med. 1988; 108, 387-389.

4. Manning AP, Thompson WG, Heaton KW, and Morris AF. Towards positive diagnosis of the Irritable Bowel. Br. Med J. 1978; 653-654.

5. Borg GAV. Psychophysical bases of perceived exertion. Med. Sci. Sports Exerc. 1982; 14: 377-381.

6. Elborn JS, Stanford CF, Nicholls DP. Reproducibility of cardiopulmonary parameters during exercise in patients with chronic cardiac failure. The need for a preliminary test. Eur J Cardiol 1990 (In Press).

7. Clode M, Campbell EJM. The relationship between gas exchange and changes in blood lactate concentrations during exercise. Clin Sci 1969;37:263-272.

8. Jones NL. Clinical Exercise Testing, 3rd edn, Philadelphia, WB Saunders, 1988: Chap. 10.

9. Saltin B, Blomqvist B, Mitchell JH, Johnston RL, Wildenthal K, Chapman CB. Response to submaximal and maximal exercise after bedrest and training. Circulation 1968; 38(suppl 7): 1-78.

10. Holloszy JO, Booth FW. Biochemical adaptations to endurance exercise in muscle. Ann. Rev. Physiol. 1976; 38: 263-291.

11. Montague TJ, Marrie TJ, Klassen GA, Bewick DJ, Horacek BM. Cardiac function at rest and with exercise in the chronic fatigue syndrome. Chest 1989; 95: 779-784.

12. Arnold DL, Radda GK, Bore PJ, Styles P, Taylor DJ. Excessive intracellular acidosis of skeletal muscle on exercise in a patient with a post-viral exhaustion/fatigue syndrome. Lancet 1984; i : 1367-1369.

13. Archard LC, Bowles NE, Behan PO, Bell EJ, Doyle D. Post viral fatigue syndrome: Persistence of enteroviral RNA in skeletal muscle and elevated creatine kinase. J Roy Soc Med 1988; 81: 326-329.

14. Byrne E, Trounce I. Chronic fatigue and myalgic syndrome: mitochondrial and glycolytic studies in skeletal muscle. J Neurol. Neurosurg. Psychiatry 1987; 50: 743-746.

15. Beaudet AL. The Glycogen Storage Diseases: in Harrison's Principles of Internal Medicine, 11th. edn, Braunwald E et al.eds, New York, McGraw-Hill 1987: p1648.

16. McEvedy CP, Beard AW. Royal Free epidemic of 1955: a reconsideration. Br Med J 1970; 1:7-11.

17. Woods JJ, Furbush F, Bigland-Ritchie B. Evidence for a fatigue-induced reflex inhibition of motorneuron firing rates. J Neurophysiol 1987; 58:125-137.

18. Stokes MJ, Cooper RG, Edwards RHT. Normal muscle strength and fatiguability in patients with effort syndromes. Br. Med J 1988; 297:1014-1017.

The Heart as Target

Chapter 42

Cardiac and Cardiovascular Aspects of M.E./CFS that may be secondary to Neurological or Psychological Involvement, A Review

Byron Hyde, M.D., Anil Jain, M.D.

Patients with M.E / CFS often complain of cardiac symptoms. Several of the recorded M.E. / CFS epidemics also document cardiac irregularities. Other than in the unpublished work of Dr. Richardson of Newcastle-upon-Tyne[1] and Dr. Peter Behan,[2] there is little mention of either severe or long-term cardiovascular pathology in M.E. / CFS. A good many of the cardiac findings noted here, e.g. postural hypotension, are clearly neurological or normal variants.

If the enteroviruses are a major cause of M.E./CFS, as is believed in Great Britain[3], one would expect that the multitude of enterovirus cardiopathies already reported in the literature[4] would form a part of the pathology of M.E./CFS. The paucity of cardiac papers on M.E./CFS may simply be due to the fact that there are no such serious short or long-term cardiac problems. Contrarily, this may simply indicate that, when any serious cardiac or cardiovascular M.E./CFS symptom becomes more prominent, these patients are simply rediagnosed by that major symptom.

For instance, patients who fall ill with M.E./CFS routinely develop minor seizure disorders while a very few develop grand mal or Jacksonian seizure activity. These latter individuals are often diagnosed as epileptic and are treated for their seizure activity and the cognitive changes, muscle pain and fatigue are simply misinterpreted as either being part of an epileptic clinical personality or a medication reaction. If neurological or muscular abnormalities exceed a certain limit, a diagnosis other than M.E./CFS is given. We undoubtedly see the same pattern with cardiac dysfunction. Until much better and specific testing for M.E./CFS is available to the general physician, the question of where the spectrum of M.E./CFS disease stops cannot be seriously answered.

Visibility

It is difficult to observe pathology or variation of any sort unless one looks first with the mind. M.E./CFS is a blind spot in the mind of most cardiologists. The following case illustrates some of the problems of visibility.

A male nurse who fell ill with M.E./CFS during the Lake Tahoe epidemic went on to develop a myocardial infarct. Although this is now a well documented legal case[5], it is not in the medical literature and probably never will be. Was this man's myocardial infarct related to his M.E./CFS? The court ruled it was, but there is insufficient evidence in the medical literature to make significant and conclusive comparisons. There is little chance that the immediate future will better clarify this situation. Why?

First, so few cardiologists even are acquainted with the existence of M.E./CFS as a physical illness that it would be most unusual for a cardiologist or cardiac centre to make the association between cardiac disease and M.E./CFS and then develop a series of such relations that would be publishable.

Second, a myocardial infarct can easily be sufficient grounds for a disability pension whereas an M.E./CFS case might have to go to court to achieve payment of a justifiable disability claim. Yet this is simply a case of perception. A post-myocardial infarct patient is often disabled for only a short period whereas an M.E./CFS patient may be not only chronically disabled but as disabled as a patient with terminal malignancy. Any M.E./CFS physician would know this, but any physician would also know that it will be the cardiac patient who obtains the disability pension.

Is there a relation to this man's myocardial infarction and his M.E./CFS? Let us return to that question after the following.

In this review paper we will look briefly at:

(1) unpublished cardiovascular information,
(2) the acute changes noted in the literature,
(3) recent published findings.

The Unpublished Record

John Richardson has studied many thousands of Myalgic Encephalomyelitis patients since 1953. Based upon his clinical observations and knowledge of families, sometimes running through three and even four generations, he has come to certain beliefs listed below.[1]

In the first weeks of M.E./CFS illness there may occur a sudden change in the cardiac status of the previously well patient, manifested by:

(1) frequent precordial and myocardial chest pain

(2) frequent supraventricular and other arrhythmias

(3) frequent mild to severe problems of postural hypotension

(4) frequent change of B.P. to hypotensive state

(5) rare abrupt onset of normal range B.P. to malignant hypertension

(6) frequent vasomotor abnormalities

(7) rare sudden death due to irregular cardiac rhythm

(8) injury to chordae tendinae resulting in mitral valve prolapse

(9) pericarditis

(10) myocarditis

In the chronic stages of M.E./CFS, Dr. Richardson notes an increase in cardiomyopathies and valvular disease well above what one would expect in a normal non-M.E./CFS population. He notes an increase in cardiac deaths due to these illnesses and a tendency for these deaths to be more common amongst men with M.E./CFS than with women. In the few cases of children born of mothers who fall ill with M.E./CFS while pregnant, he notes an unusual number of major cardiac newborn birth abnormalities. He finds no increase in cardiac birth abnormalities in newborn children of women who have become pregnant, and who were already ill with M.E./CFS.

Dr. Richardson also notes that there is an unexpected temporal increase in many of these cardiac manifestations in other family members who do not have M.E./CFS.

Dr. Richardson stipulates a rider to these observations. Newcastle-Upon-Tyne has in the past been an industrial area, with most of the male jobs involving heavy labour, with few social benefits and a tendency towards relatively large families. Men who fall ill with M.E./CFS have tended to return to work after a few days of illness, otherwise their families would not

have been fed, clothed and housed. This may have resulted in an abnormal increase in damage to a heart muscle already vulnerable and under attack from an acute viral infection. Perhaps, if the patient had been put to bed, he would have eventually recovered without significant sequelae. This is not just clinical supposition. There is a strong basis for this belief of work potentiated heart damage in the literature.

The majority of British M.E./CFS physicians who believe in the infectious origin of this disease, believe that the enteroviruses are the major provoking cause of this illness. Dr. Eleanor Bell provides an excellent review of this subject.[6]

It is well known that enteroviruses may cause chronic cardiac disease as well as major neurological injury. Kandolf states that *"...enteroviruses are capable of causing dilated cardiomyopathy of sudden onset or lead to a variety of cardiac arrhythmias"*[7]. Utilizing mouse models, Wilson and again Reyes demonstrated that Coxsackie infected mice, forced to swim to the point of exhaustion during the acute phase of infection, developed chronic heart disease whereas Coxsackie virus infected mice, of suitable genetic stock, who were allowed to rest during the acute phase, did not develop chronic heart disease.[8,9] Woodruff indicates that severity of disease decreases with age.[10]

The Literature

The 1934 Epidemic

There is a notable and total lack of any cardiovascular information in Gilliam's 90 page study.[11] The questionnaire utilized by Gilliam requested neither blood pressure nor any cardiovascular observation but was directed single mindedly to epidemiological and neurological aspects of illness. This avoidance of general medicine is for all purposes true for all of the publications surrounding the 1934 epidemic. The papers are almost entirely written by epidemiologists, orthopedists and neurologists. In Bower's 1934 paper, there is mention of arrhythmias and a sudden lowering of blood pressure.[12] Bower was one of the rare internists who looked at these patients. Also Wilson and Walker in their 1936 paper[13], reviewing 100 hospitalized patients from that epidemic, write that: *"Vasomotor and trophic disturbances were almost constant findings...with coldness and cyanosis. It was the impression of most observers that a generalized disturbance of vasomotor control occurred in these patients."* They also note that approximately 4% of the adults had associated thrombophlebitis.

The 1948 Epidemic

The 1948 Akureyri epidemic described by the epidemiologist Bjorn Sigurdsson[14], and all subsequent Iceland papers are similarly without mention of any cardiovascular effects. In both the 1934 and 1948 epidemics this lack of cardiovascular information is probably due to professional restriction to their own areas of expertise. Both epidemics were believed to be polio-like or polio-related illnesses and classical anterior poliomyelitis was well known for its associated cardiac pathology.

The 1955 Epidemics

London Free Hospital

It was not until the general medical staff of the London Free Hospital reported on the 1955 epidemic that we start to see observations of cardiovascular abnormalities. They reported that changes occur early and tend to improve over a period of time. Cardiac complaints were noted by 7 of 42 patients, but only 4 had abnormal physical findings on examination.[15] It is impossible to know whether these were variations that could have been recorded in a normal population. Findings included:

(1) sinus tachycardia of 115
(2) abnormal T waves in 2 or more leads
(3) prolongation of Q-T interval
(4) only 1 patient had an abnormal ECG 18 months after onset

The 1955 Cumberland Epidemic

The 1955 Cumberland epidemic actually preceded the 1955 Royal Free epidemic by several months. Dr. Wallis, the author of the thesis on the Cumberland epidemic[16] was the first physician to truly discuss and publish the cardiological findings and his findings were as follows:[17]

Myocarditis in the Acute Phase:

The heart rate was accelerated during the course of the illness and the rate was raised out of proportion to any pyrexia that might be present. Tachycardia was considered to be a diagnostic feature.[17]

In three cases a persistent tachycardia developed; the rate varied from 120-150 per minute and dyspnoea occurred on slight effort, cyanosis of the lips and oedema of the ankles appeared. The heart sounds were soft, the blood pressure was lowered. The heart was not enlarged. These effects persisted for over 12 months. A fourth case resolved in 4 months.[17]

Blood Pressure:

In four cases there was a persistent rise in blood pressure to 180-220/110-130. These slowly lowered over a period of many months.[17]

Venous Thrombosis

Two women experienced deep femoral vein thrombosis 8-10 days after the time of onset.[17] This is of interest since, in the Mercy San Juan, California epidemic, venous thrombosis or superficial venous congestion was a frequent finding.[18]

The 1965 Galveston Epidemic

This epidemic in Texas in the Summer of 1965 was documented by cardiologist Dr. Luis Leon-Sotomayor[19]. Dr. Leon-Sotomayor now distinguishes this form as a possible subtype of epidemic neuromyasthenia, then one of the names for M.E./CFS. This epidemic is important for several reasons. It is the only M.E./CFS-like epidemic in the literature reviewed specifically by a cardiologist. His book **Epidemic Diencephalomyelitis**[18] is a gold mine of information and should be read by every serious student of M.E./CFS. This review discusses 50 patients, 18 males and 32 females, 9 of whom were black, shattering the myth that American blacks do not fall ill with M.E./CFS. The age distribution was between 10 and 72 years, dissipating two other beliefs that children and the aged do not fall ill with M.E./CFS. Several of these patients were students. Some of the cardiovascular symptoms that he mentions are as follows:[20]

Cardiovascular Symptoms in 50 Patients	
Symptom	Numbers involved
(1) Angina-like pain	50/50
(2) Vascular headaches	50/50
(3) Orthostatic hypertension	50/50
(4) Orthostatic tachycardia	50/50
(5) Edema	45/50
(6) Nasal stuffiness	39/50
(7) Acrocyanosis	38/50
(8) Dyspnoea	35/50
(9) Transient hypertension	32/50
(10) Syncope	10/50
(11) Hypertensive crisis	5/50
(12) Hypotensive crisis	5/50

He notes the following long-term cardiovascular residuals[21] that last for more than 6 months.

Long Term Residuals	
Vascular headaches	18/50
Hypertension	5/50
Orthostatic hypotension	4/50

Dr. Leon-Sotomayor notes the following electrocardiographic abnormalities that were found initially in these patients.[22]

Electrocardiographic Abnormalities	
ECG Alterations	Number of Patients
(1) Orthostatic sinus tachycardia	50
(2) Sinus arrhythmia	30
(3) Unstable T-wave syndrome	25
(4) Positive valsalva test	25
(5) Prominent U-wave	20
(6) Premature atrial contractions	18
(7) Premature ventricular contractions	16
(8) Early repolarization phenomena	14
(9) False positive masters	10
(10) False positive Masters Test	5
(11) Depressed T-U Segment	1
(12) Cardiac arrhythmias	
(a) wandering pacemaker	5
(b) paroxysmal auricular fibrillation	3
(c) paroxysmal atrial tachycardia	2
(d) paroxysmal ventricular tachycardia	1
(13) Conduction disturbance	
(a) intraventricular conduction defect	2
(b) transient complete right BBB	2

Blood pressure[23]. Only a sample of the cardiovascular findings are given here and it is important for the physician to refer to the text of Dr. Leon-Sotomayor who writes:

The recording of blood pressure in the recumbent, sitting and standing positions showed reversal of the normal findings. Instead of the usual rise in the systolic component of the blood pressure which one normally gets upon assuming the erect position, there was an elevation of the blood pressure in the recumbent position and hypotension in the standing position. Transient hypotension was occasionally followed by an exaggerated overshoot of blood pressure to higher levels. These observations are similar to those described in patients with pheochromocytoma."[23]

Dr. Peter Behan also notes the following cardiac observations.

In his pamphlet published in 1990 by the British M.E. Association, Diagnostic and Clinical Guidelines for Doctors, he states:

Those patients who present with chest pains often develop a rapid pulse with ectopic beats and indeed several of these have been sent to us by cardiologists with a proven diagnosis of myocarditis."[24]

In his CRC article published in 1988 he notes:[25]

"Evidence of cardiac involvement may be seen, usually in the cases with vertiginous symptoms. Palpitations, severe tachycardia with multiple ectopic beats and occasional dyspnoea may occur suddenly."

In his lecture at CIBA House in London in 1988[2], Dr. Behan drew the audience's attention to the fact that using SPECT scan techniques, his team was able to regularly demonstrate micro-capillary perfusion defects in the cardiac muscle of M.E./CFS patients as well as in mouse models that Dr. Behan's group had succeeded in developing. Unfortunately, to my knowledge, these findings have not been published.

Recent Publications

Cardiac Function at Rest and with Exercise in the Chronic Fatigue Syndrome, Terrence J. Montague et al[26]

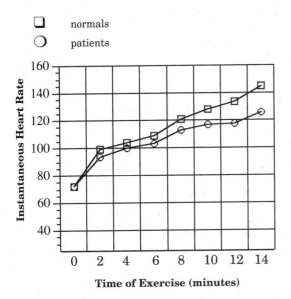

□ normals
○ patients

Figure: Group mean (±1SD) instantaneous heart rate (in beats per minute) in two groups at rest (time 0) and at each two minutes of exercise protocol.

(Approximation of graph from Montague[26], reproduced with the kind permission of Chest 1989; 95:782.)

In the last few years, there has been little published associating M.E./CFS with cardiovascular abnormalities. Montague et al in two recent papers[26,27] published in Chest[26], gives some interesting and appropriate insight into part of the pathophysiology of M.E./CFS cardiac dysfunction. Quoting his 1988 paper in Chest, dealing with post viral cardiac dysfunction, but not M.E./CFS, Montague states:

(1) *"In a previous comprehensive study of patients with community-acquired viral illnesses of several etiologies, we found evidence of cardiac abnormalities during the acute phase, which largely disappeared by six weeks of follow-up. Our findings included segmental wall motion abnormalities in a few patients and small pericardial effusions and altered primary ventricular repolarization properties in the majority of patients. We concluded that acute viral illnesses produce widely prevalent but clinically inconsequential cardiac effects."[28]*

(2) The abstract of this second paper on M.E./CFS concludes with the statement: *"Thus, patients with chronic fatigue syndrome have normal resting cardiac function but a markedly abbreviated exercise capacity characterized by slow acceleration of heart rate and fatigue of exercising muscles long before peak heart rate is achieved. Although not conclusive,*

the data are compatible with latent viral effects on the cardiac electrical and skeletal muscle tissues; the peripheral effects appear greater than the cardiac effects."[26]

Dr. McCluskey (see Chapter 40, this text) studied 13 M.E./CFS patients and could not confirm this finding.

(3) Montague's second paper studied 41 consecutive adult patients who presented with post viral fatigue syndrome either in Cardiology or the Infectious Disease Unit of Victoria General Hospital in Halifax. The population consisted of 28 women and 13 men between the ages of 20 and 59, i.e. 68% women and 32% men. The group had been ill for an average period of 14 months when first seen at the hospital. No indication is given of how long it took for the assembled patients to be passed through the system.

Abnormal Ventricular Cavity Size

The paper[27] notes that approximately 10% of the patients, i.e. 4, had an abnormal ventricular cavity size. In reality, table 1 indicates that there were only three. **They were all males.**

Ventricular Ectopic Beats[27]

VEBs (ventricular ectopic beats) were demonstrated in 22 of the 41 subjects. However the report suggests that only those individuals with over 100 VEBs per 24 hours should be considered clearly pathological. There were only 4 such patients, and they had an astonishing average of 2145 VEBs per minute. Again if we realize that these 4 represented a mixed group of acute and chronic cases of M.E./CFS and that most cardiac abnormalities tend to disappear or significantly decrease once the patients have recuperated from 3-12 months, then only 3 of the 4 cases of grossly abnormal VEBs were chronic. **All of these three chronic cases were males.**

Pericardial Effusion[27]

Montague mentions that 5, (over 12%) of the M.E./CFS group had a previously unrecognized pericardial effusion. Unfortunately, it is not noted if these were chronic cases nor was there any indication of their sex. Curiously, 2 reputedly normal controls also had a pericardial effusion. One wonders if these abnormal controls were family members of an M.E./CFS patient.

Unfortunately, the number of patients is not large but it is highly suggestive from Montague's findings that, although only 32% of his M.E./CFS sample were males, they made up 100% of the major cardiac pathology encountered, (and whose sex is recorded in his study). It is unfortunate that Montague did not point this out in his paper. It is also unfortunate that he did not publish the individual blood pressures of his subjects so that we could compare these with controls. Nor did he segregate the hypertensive M.E./CFS from normotensive patients and controls. This excellent clinical study is totally consistent with John Richardson's unpublished work.

Animal Model

Pellew[29] and Behan[2] are the sole researchers to describe cardiac disease in an animal model. Pellew's paper involved monkeys injected with human M.E./CFS sera. Pellew notes that examination of the heart muscle of the monkey showed severe myocarditis with widespread infiltration, mainly with lymphocytes and mononuclear cells. One of the monkeys appears to have died due to the acquired infection and others were sacrificed.

Nightingale Clinic
Cardiovascular Observations

Over the past 5 years we have seen over 6000 patients at our clinic who had M.E./CFS. We have not had the means to do intensive systemic cardiac workup as have Leon-Sotomayor and Montague. We can however make the following observations concerning cardiac status.

Many of the patients who complain of arrhythmias have normal heart rhythm when we examine them. It is possible that these reputed arrhythmias may in reality be chest wall muscle fasciculations.

Cardiac-like symptoms are frequent in the first month of illness and decrease markedly during the recuperation period. By 3-12 months these cardiovascular and cardiac complaints tend to become less frequent. They include:

Early Symptom Complaints:
(1) angina-like pain
(2) orthostatic and activity related tachycardia
(3) postural hypotension
(4) severe shortness of breath with exertion
(5) syncope
(6) various arrhythmias
(7) pheochromocytoma-like symptom picture
(8) vascular headaches
(9) autonomic system dysfunction with vasomotor instability

Physical findings frequently observed in this group include:

Physical Findings:
(1) below expected nocturnal bradycardia
(2) below normal systemic blood pressure
(3) acute onset of malignant hypertension in a few
(4) muffling of heart sounds in a few
(5) sinus arrhythmia
(6) ventricular premature beats
(7) various ECG transient abnormalities
(8) superficial venous congestion
(9) peripheral oedema
(10) in children, what appears to be an apparent abnormally high occurrence of mitral valve prolapse. In one cluster, the majority of seven M.E./CFS girls aged from 8-16 had ausculatory signs suggestive of mitral valve prolapse.

Chronic M.E./CFS patients.

Cardiac features do not appear to be a significant health risk in the vast majority of our chronic M.E./CFS patients. Pain and discomfort resembling cardiac angina is not uncommon but, in our estimation, is not obviously cardiac related.

We have noted a "brick wall effect" in some patients, particularly when they forget their limitations and run up stairs rather than walk. These patients complain of severe chest pain and shortness of breath as if suddenly stopped by an invisible barrier. They frequently have to sit on the stairs for a while. The Montague effect may be active here, in which a heart with normal gross vascularization, fails to speed up to meet required cardiovascular demands.

It is also possible that some of these patients who on physical examination complained of diaphragmatic pain, had virally related diaphragmatic muscle injury. It is possible that some of them also have intercostal muscle dysfunction.

Fewer than 5% of the chronic M.E./CFS patients attending our clinic have significant cardiac findings. We have not compared these to controls in the normal non-M.E./CFS population. We can assume that those M.E./CFS patients with grossly abnormal hearts, if they occur, are already in the hands of cardiologists and that it is clearly not to their advantage to be diagnosed as M.E./CFS patients.

Slightly more than 5% appear to have developed malignant hypertension at the onset of their M.E./CFS disease. Those most likely to show this change frequently had mild unstable hypertensive disease prior to falling ill with M.E./CFS. We have not noticed a decrease in blood pressures with time in these hypertensive patients as has Leon-Sotomayor. They tend to be recalcitrant to treatment.

Most of the chronic cardiovascular complaints appear to be systemic and to be related to vasomotor instability, fibromyalgia and other striated muscle dysfunction, vascular headaches, blood pressure changes, hypothalamic and thyroid epiphenomena. It is possible that there is pituitary-adrenal axis dysfunction in some of these patients.

Arrhythmias are frequently noted in the first few weeks of illness, then decrease in frequency, only to return in a chronic form 20 years later in some patients.

Summary

Although the various researchers mentioned in this review differ both in their level of investigation and sophistication, their findings tend to support each other. Only in the area of mitral valve prolapse and neonatal cardiac pathology is there insufficient published evidence to make a serious judgement.

We believe that cardiological symptoms, probably due to intrinsic and/or CNS changes, are common in the first weeks of illness and that, in the vast majority of patients, these symptoms and findings rapidly disappear. They are rarely if ever investigated.

This pattern is suggestive of an acute infectious process that tends to progress through a recovery stage.

We are in agreement with Montague et al who suggest that these cardiac findings tend to resemble what one would expect in an illness provoked by an acute viral infection.

We believe that pericarditis and myocarditis occur more commonly than one would expect in early M.E./CFS, particularly in males, and should be carefully looked for. We also believe as Behan that the possibility of microcapillary cardiac dysfunction exists and should be examined for during the first year of illness, particularly during the first months.

We believe that M.E./CFS is a cause of cardiac incapacity in very few chronic patients. Cardiovascular discomfort may be of concern, may be considerably disabling to many patients, but the fact that this disease does not represent a sizeable death risk is not a recommendation for early exercising of these patients.

We believe that much of the chronic cardiac symptomology apparent to patients is not cardiac related but is muscular, neurosensory or hypothalamic in origin.

We have observed no deaths attributable to cardiac causes in some 6000 chronic M.E./CFS patients over a period of up to 5 years. This may be due to the fact that they never occurred or that they were diagnosed as cardiac deaths and that the history of M.E./CFS was simply dismissed as a neurosis.

We believe that M.E./CFS represents a possibility of serious cardiac injury primarily in patients who exercise or maintain exhaustive work efforts during the first weeks of onset of their illness. It is possible that some of these patients who die and others that develop major cardiac changes are never recognized as M.E./CFS.

While we believe that serious heart disease is infrequent in M.E./CFS patients, when it occurs, it tends to manifest itself largely in males. Since they have a cardiac diagnosis that accounts for fatigue, they are selectively separated from those individuals searching for a diagnosis and so we do not see them. If they are pensionable due to a diagnosed cardiac problem, a diagnosis of M.E./CFS might be dangerous for their financial health.

Professionals in the nursing, teaching and medical fields and women with active families may tend to return to work during this first six week period and many may never cease work at all at home, thus potentially creating a physical injury to the myocardium, cardiac pacemaker cells or their autonomic control. No long term study of possible cardiac dysfunction in this group exists in the literature.

Certain epidemics may demonstrate more cardiac pathology than others.

Many British researchers believe that enterovirus infection is the major cause of M.E./CFS. Laboratory work has already confirmed that enteroviruses are capable of causing M.E./CFS like disease.

Enterovirus infections are able to cause

(a) chronic host infection
(b) major or no cardiac disease depending on the virulence of the viral subtype,
(c) cardiac injury dependent upon the sex and level of physical activity of the subject during the acute infectious stage,
(d) cardiac disease depending upon the immunological variability of the host, and
(e) depending upon the age of the host, variations in disease severity.

In the enterovirus family, i.e. polio, coxsackie or echovirus or numbered serotypes, we have a perfect viral model to explain the

(a) age variation
(b) sex variation
(c) obvious resistance of some family members, and
(d) the effect of physical activity and occupation in creating chronic M.E./CFS illness in the host.

Although this chapter reviews only the cardiac aspects of M.E./CFS illness, enteroviruses are primarily considered to be neurotropic viruses. There is no reason to believe that males and females are not infected in equal numbers. If this is the case, then it is possible that the same enterovirus that caused M.E./CFS in a greater proportion of woman can cause cardiac disease in a greater proportion of men.

We suggest that with both CNS and CVS disease, chronicity may be provoked by maintaining strenuous exercise and work levels during the acute and recovery stage of the viral illness. Early patient activation may represent serious cardiovascular danger to some patients. The strange concept of waiting six months to diagnose a classical case of M.E./CFS is unnecessary and fraught with potential danger to the patient. Such a diagnostic delay may create legal consequences for the physician. Physicians who take an early aggressive approach in physically activating these acute stage patients may do so at both their and their patient's peril.

Critique of this Review

Neither author is a cardiologist. Accordingly, we asked Ottawa cardiologist, Dr. Evan Patrick to do a critical review of this chapter. His comments are as follows:

When you come to page 378 and the No. 4 finding (positive valsalva test) that you felt are related to heart disease all the of the findings are in fact quite non-specific. ST T changes in particular (including QT duration) can be due to a wide variety of causes: chemical, neurological, psychoneurotic, and even affective disorders. In all of these cases the findings would be transient, consequently such findings cannot be used to attribute a myocardial factor. When you come to "angina-like pain" (page 378) the commonest mimic of angina of effort is in fact a myalgia rather than myocardial inflammatory process. Most of the other symptoms listed in the table that I am referring to are not cardiac at all. They are nevertheless vascular in many cases though this may be related again to neurological causes. The ECG abnormalities in the next table list a large number of "alterations" which are in fact normal variants. APBs and VPBs for instance up to about 100 or more a day are perfectly normal in healthy individuals. Early repolarization, false positive Master's test, sinus arrhythmia, etc. are all normal variants. Consequently they are not infrequently present. When we get to paroxysmal atrial fibrillation or atrial tachycardia we are perhaps getting to something a little more substantial. Transient complete RBBB is a very common finding if one looks for it and may in fact be another normal variant though this has not been described as such. Looking down the other half of that page, Dr. Peter Behan omits to mention that anybody who has chest pains and gets anxious about it gets a rapid pulse and may indeed get ectopic beats. This can occur whether or not there is a myocarditis. When you come to the "microcapillary perfusion defects" near the bottom of the page, these can occur in normal people also and are not evidence of disease as such. They can be a problem for me clinically because they may give rise to a false positive thallium exercise study on occasion.

References

1. Richardson J., Lecture in Newcastle-upon-Tyne, October 1988.

2. Behan P., CIBA London Conference, CIBA Foundation, 41 Portland Place, London, England, October 11, 1988.

3. Dowsett, B., Chapter 7, this text.

4. Bendinelli & Friedman, **Coxsackie Viruses, A General Update**, Plenum Press, 1988.

5. Legal action in Incline Village, Nevada in 1990 concerning disability and relationship of M.E./CFS to myocardial infarct.

6. idem (4) Bendinelli & Friedman, chapter, Bell E. Assaad F, Esteves K. Neurological Disorders, pages 319-337.

7. idem Bendinelli, page 293, Kandolf R., The Impact of Recombinant DNA Technology on the Study of Enterovirus Heart Disease.

8. Wilson F.M. et al, Residual pathologic changes following murine coxsackie A and B myocarditis, Am J. Pathology, 1969 55: 253-265.

9. Reyes M.P., A mouse model of dilated-type cardiomyopathy due to coxsackievirus B3, 1981, J. Infectious Diseases 144: 232-236.

10. Woodruff J.F., Viral myocarditis, 1970, Am. J. Pathology, 101: 1427-479.

11. Gilliam A.G., (1938) **Epidemiological study of an epidemic, diagnosed as poliomyelitis, occurring among the personnel of the Los Angeles County General Hospital during the summer of 1934**, United States Public Heath Bulletin No. 240, pages 1-90.

12. Bower A.G., Meals R.W., Bigler M., Ewing J.,Hauser V., Clinical Features of Poliomyelitis in Los Angeles. p 1211 , American Journal of Public Health, Vol 24, No 12, Dec. 1934.

13. Wilson J., Walker P., Acute Anterior Poliomyelitis. Archives of Internal Medicine, Vol. 57, No. 3, March 1936, pp.477-492.

14. Sigurdsson B.,Sigurjonsson J., Sigurdsson J.H.J., Thorkelsson J & Gudmundsson K.R. (1950) A disease epidemic in Iceland simulating poliomyelitis, American Journal of Hygiene, 52, 222, page 227.

15. The medical staff of the Royal Free Hospital, An Outbreak of Encephalomyelitis in the Royal Free Hospital Group, London, in 1955, Br. Med. J., 1957; 2:896.

16. Wallis A.L., **An investigation into an unusual disease seen in epidemic and sporadic form in a general practice in Cumberland in 1955 and subsequent years**, Doctoral Thesis submitted to University of Edinburgh (1957).

17. idem (16) Wallis, page 87.

18. Ryll E., Chabursky B., Mercy San Juan epidemic (paper in preparation).

19. Leon-Sotomayor L., **Epidemic Diencephalomyelitis**, Pageant Press, 1969.

20. idem (19) Leon-Sotomayor L, page 66.

21. idem (19) Leon-Sotomayor, page 70.

22. idem (19) Leon-Sotomayor, page 75.

23. idem (19) Leon-Sotomayor, page 71.

24. Behan P., Diagnostic and Clinical Guidelines for Doctors. This is also available from Miriam Gallacher, Hamilton Wentworth M.E. Association, Hamilton, Ontario.

25. Behan P., Behan W., Post viral fatigue syndrome, a review. CRC Reviews. Cleveland, Ohio: CRC Press, 1988.

26. Montague T., Marrie T., Klassen G., Bewick D., Horacek B.M. Cardiac Function at Rest and with Exercise in the Chronic Fatigue Syndrome,Chest, Vol 95, p 779-784, April 1989.

27. Montague, T.J, Bewick D.J., Marrie T.J., McNutt E.J., Spencer C.A., Tremayne H.K. et al, Cardiac Effects of community-acquired viral illness. Chest 1988; 94:919-25.

28. idem (27) Montague T. page 779.

29. Pellew, R.A., Miles J.A.R. Further Investigations on a Disease Resembling Poliomyelitis seen in Adelaide. The Medical Journal of Australia, Sept. 24, 1955, 480-482.

Neurology

Chapter 43

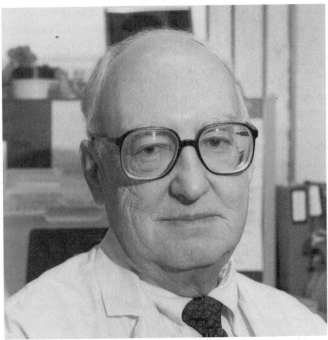

Charles M. Poser

The Differential Diagnosis Between Multiple Sclerosis and Chronic Fatigue Postviral Syndrome

Charles M. Poser, MD

Department of Neurology, Harvard Medical School, and Neurological Unit, Beth Israel Hospital, Boston, Massachusetts

Dr. Charles Poser has been interested in diseases of the white matter for many years and has published extensively in the areas of multiple sclerosis and the neurological complications of viral diseases and immunizations (encephalomyelitis). He headed the team which proposed the new diagnostic criteria for MS which have now been almost universally adopted. Dr. Poser was Chairman of the Department of Neurology at the University of Vermont college of Medicine from 1968 to 1981, and Professor of Neurology at Boston University from 1981 to 1984 before assuming his current positions.

Introduction

It is not unusual for individuals suffering from the chronic fatigue post-viral syndrome (CFPVS) to be given the diagnosis of multiple sclerosis (MS). This is often due to the fact that paresthesiae, a common complaint in MS, are frequent presenting symptoms of CFPVS. In addition, abnormalities of the cerebral white matter may be seen by magnetic resonance imaging (MRI), and in rare instances, oligoclonal bands (OB) have been found in the cerebrospinal fluid (CSF).

In recent years, it has unfortunately become custom-ary for some physicians, including neurologists, to base their diagnoses of MS exclusively upon the results of laboratory procedures such as the MRI, evoked potentials and CSF examination. Despite the introduction of, and increase in the availability of such ancillary diagnostic procedures, the diagnosis of MS is a clinical one based upon its clinical and pathological characteristics which demand that both dissemination in space (multiple lesions) and in time (relapses and remissions) be present. Therefore, the history of the disease remains of paramount importance.

The Clinical History of MS

Many problems arise in the interpretation of historical data provided by the patient and/or his/her family[16]. Some symptoms may be interpreted as being part of the basic illness while others are overlooked: one of the most common examples is the woman patient who has been diagnosed as having a bladder infection while in reality urinary frequency, urgency and incontinence are important symptoms of a neurogenic bladder, a manifestation of MS. The converse is also frequent. It is extremely common for MS patients to have symptoms which may sound bizarre to an inexperienced physician because they fail to conform to anatomical boundaries or physiological concepts, they may be extremely transient, lasting for no more than minutes or seconds, and most importantly cannot be confirmed by objective findings. This is particularly true with the frequent complaints of numbness and tingling (paresthesiae) which often are not associated with demonstrable alterations of sensation. Exaggeration of symptoms, a subconscious phenomenon which has been called hysterical hyperbole, may also mislead the examiner: the physically impossible complaint of triple, or even quadruple, vision may actually be based upon a true diplopia. The patient's way of expressing his complaints must be carefully interpreted. Many patients use the term numbness to describe what is actually weakness and vice versa. Those who complain of blurred vision must be asked if clarity of the image occurs when either eye is closed suggesting, if it does, a mild degree of true diplopia rather than an alteration of visual acuity.

Some symptoms are rarely called to the physician's attention because their importance and significance are not appreciated. Bladder problems, and in particular sexual dysfunction, are rarely mentioned by patients but must be pursued by physicians since they may be of importance not only in establishing the diagnosis but in providing treatment. Cognitive, psychological, and psychiatric disturbances are considerably more frequent in MS than realized and may actually precede more physical problems.

In approximately two-thirds of MS patients the disease pursues an intermittent course characterized by relapses and remissions. Care must be taken to attempt to determine the exact nature of the relapses, if they are true exacerbations rather than pseudo-exacerbations, the latter being the appearance of new symptoms, or the recurrence of previously experienced ones, resulting from a known, recognizable alteration of the external environment or the internal milieu, such as heat, fever, and intercurrent infections (most frequently of the bladder), unusual emotional stress, fatigue, dehydration or electrolyte disturbances. While pseudo-exacerbations are important in that they will bring out signs and symptoms which may help meet the criterion of dissemination in space, they have no significance in fulfilling the basis for the other criterion of dissemination in time. For that, a true exacerbation is required, one that cannot be ascribed to some trigger, and which must last for at least 24 hours. However, a viral infection, or trauma to the head, neck or back, may result in the reappearance of symptoms, but may also lead to the formation of new plaques and the emergence of new signs and symptoms, thus constituting a true exacerbation[17].

Table 1A

Diagnostic Criteria for Multiple Sclerosis*

CATEGORY	ATT	CLN	PCL	CSF
Clinically definite				
1.	2	2		
2.	2	1	& 1	
Laboratory supported definite				
1.	2	1	or 1	+
2.	1	2		+
3.	1	1	& 1	+
Clinically probable				
1.	2	1		
2.	1	2		
3.	1	1	& 1	
Laboratory supported probable				
1.	2			+

ATT= attack   CLN= clinical evidence
PCL= paraclinical evidence   CSF= OB or raised IgG

* Poser et al[24]

+---+

Table 1B

**Diagnostic Criteria for
Multiple Sclerosis***

General considerations and definitions:

Age of onset: 10-59 years

Manifestations characteristic of multiple sclerosis and not attributable to another condition.

The diagnosis must be made by a physician experienced in clinical neurology.

Attack: A symptom of neurological dysfunction with or without objective confirmation lasting more than 24 hours. May be subjective and anamnestic. Two attacks must involve different parts of the CNS and be separated by at least 1 month.

Clinical evidence: Abnormalities of the neurological examination performed by a competent examiner. Two lesions must be anatomically separate.

Paraclinical evidence: Demonstration by means of various tests of the existence of a CNS lesion which has not produced signs of neurological dysfunction but may or may not have caused symptoms. Such tests include evoked response studies, neuro-imaging, hot bath test, urological and neuropsychological investigations.

Laboratory supported: Requires the presence of at least 2 IgG oligoclonal bands, or evidence of increased production of IgG in the CSF, with a normal IgG fraction and no oligoclonal bands in serum.

* From Poser et al[24]

+---+

Diagnostic criteria for multiple sclerosis

A number of diagnostic schemes have been proposed during the past 25 years, the most recent criteria being those proposed by Poser et al[24] in 1983 which have come into general use. They are based upon the two major characteristics of dissemination in space and in time. It is important to emphasize that **both** criteria are of equal importance. It is unfortunately quite common for physicians to apply **only** the criterion of dissemination in space, more often than not based upon the presence of multiple abnormalities of the MRI but overlooking the need for dissemination in time. Table 1 describes the diagnostic criteria.

These diagnostic criteria were designed primarily for use in epidemiologic surveys and other research projects. Therefore, they are more stringent than usually required in clinical practice. Nevertheless, they provide reasonable but not absolute assurance about the accuracy of the diagnosis of MS.

The signs and symptoms of MS

MS characteristically involves particular areas of the central nervous system, thus giving rise to signs and symptoms which reflect such involvement. MS affects the central nervous system, i.e. the brain and spinal cord, and only with extraordinary rarity, the peripheral nervous system; thus, the appearance of clinical and/or electrodiagnosis evidence of peripheral nerve damage is an almost totally reliable means of excluding the diagnosis.

While it is possible for a patient to have multiple sclerosis and yet to have a completely normal neurologic examination, a situation which seems to be

Table 2

Signs and Symptoms of Multiple Sclerosis in 1271 Patients*

Site and type of involvement	Initially %	Total course %
Pareses	42.9	87.6
Sensory changes	40.7	87.0
Visual alterations	35.9	66.1
Cerebral symptoms	31.0	39.2
Brainstem &/or cerebellar signs	22.5	81.6
Spasticity &/or Babinski sign	19.4	85.1
Diplopia	12.7	33.9
Sphincter &/or sexual dysfunction	9.6	63.2
Fifth &/or seventh cranial nerve	6.9	23.1

*: Adapted from Bauer[3]

Table 3	
Signs and Symptoms in 157 Cases of Autopsy-Proven Multiple Sclerosis*	
SIGNS	%
Spasticity and/or hyperreflexia	98
Babinski sign	92
Absent abdominal reflexes	82
Dysmetria or intention tremor	79
Nystagmus	71
Impairment of vibratory sensation	61
Impairment of position sensation	52
SYMPTOMS	%
Muscle weakness	96
Ocular problems (altered vision or diplopia)	85
Urinary disturbance	82
Gait ataxia	60
Paresthesiae	60
Dysarthria or scanning speech	54
* Modified from Poser et al[22]	

an episode represents acute disseminated encephalomyelitis (ADEM) rather than MS.

As indicated in Table 1, there must be, at one time or another during the period of observation, well documented, or reliably recorded evidence of clinical involvement of the central nervous system as manifested by abnormal neurologic signs. The most frequent signs and symptoms seen initially in a large series of German MS patients[3], as well as the frequency with which these abnormalities are encountered during the entire period of observation are listed in Table 2. Except for the sensory changes and some of the cerebral symptoms (which include cognitive and psychological alterations), the presence of these signs and symptoms are of great value in differentiating CFPVS from MS. For comparison, Table 3 summarizes the symptoms and signs noted during their lifetime by at least half of 157 MS patients from the United States, Great Britain and Norway in whom the diagnosis was confirmed by postmortem examination.[22]

Laboratory Procedures

The traditional lumbar puncture for examination of the CSF has become rarely necessary because of the introduction of noninvasive procedures. A few white cells, predominantly lymphocytes, are frequently present but should not be misinterpreted as necessarily signifying activity of the disease process. The total protein is rarely elevated and a content above 100 mg.% should cause some degree of doubt regarding the accuracy of the diagnosis. The elevation of the CSF immunoglobulin G (IgG) is found in approximately 60 to 70% of patients. The most reliable formula for interpreting its meaning remains the percent of total protein with an upper limit of 13-15%. Oligoclonal bands which, in some specialized laboratories, reach the 95% positive response, rarely rise above the 60-70% range in the usual clinical or commercial laboratories. At least **2 bands** must be seen in the CSF and **no bands** may be present in the serum in order to have this test be relevant and confirm the diagnosis of MS. Oligoclonal bands may be found in the CSF of many other conditions, including some which may be quite difficult to differentiate from MS[8]. The measurement of myelin basic protein is of no value whatsoever since it may be found increased in the CSF in any condition of the nervous

quite disturbing to many physicians who are unaware of this fact, such a situation is relatively rare. It is considerably more common to find the more typical signs of the disease such as nystagmus, cerebellar incoordination, ataxia, spasticity, hyperreflexia, abnormal plantar responses and sensory disturbances, principally of vibration and position senses.

Because of the natural history of the illness, i.e., the fact that different parts of the nervous system may be involved and become symptomatic at different times, the diagnosis most often must be based upon a period of clinical observation which may last for months or even years. In fact, it is extremely imprudent to give the patient the diagnosis of multiple sclerosis after a single attack since the chances are 3 out of 4 that such system which causes destruction of myelin. It can be used only as an indicator of myelinoclastic activity when it is elevated because its absence does not rule out such activity.

Evoked potentials are completely nonspecific and may be abnormal in many other conditions beside MS[7]. Brainstem auditory evoked responses have a very poor yield even in the presence of definite brainstem abnormalities; somatosensory evoked responses are of little value in general while visual evoked responses are by far the most important in that they will document involvement of the optic nerve and/or chiasm in as many as 75% of MS patients who have never had any signs or symptoms of lesions of the visual system.

The MRI seems to have become the touchstone for the diagnosis of MS for many clinicians despite the now well recognized fact that areas of increased signal intensity in the cerebral white matter may be present in ADEM, central nervous system AIDS, Lyme disease, neurobrucellosis, sarcoidosis, HTLV-I associated paraparesis, collagenopathies, trauma, migraine, and small strokes[15,19]. In general, but certainly by no means definitively, the lesions of MS are periventricular in location, while in other conditions they have a tendency to occur more at the periphery, i.e. near the cortex. It has been proposed that at least 4 unidentified bright objects, (UBO's) be present, 2 of which must be periventricular, not counting those of the anterior angles of the lateral ventricles which show increased signal intensity in almost every adult[18]. With increasing use of this procedure, it is becoming apparent that as many as 10% of patients with definite MS have normal brain MRI's, and an even greater proportion of spinal cord exams.

Table 4 summarizes the value of various laboratory procedures in the differential diagnosis of multiple sclerosis. Obviously, MRIs, EPs and CSF OBs are of no value in such differentiation.

The complaints of extreme and quite characteristic fatigue, paresthesiae and dizziness are the manifestations of CFPVS which are most likely to suggest the diagnosis of multiple sclerosis. The excessive tiredness exacerbated by even minor exertion, lack of energy and easy fatiguability of the MS patients are

identical to those seen in CFPVS. The paresthesiae are often of a different type: in the CFPVS they have a tendency to have a burning, painful component and to have a migratory characteristic, i.e. involving one part of the body one day and another part the next. Such sensory complaints are most unusual in MS. It is also extremely rare for patients with CFPVS to have specific complaints indicating underlying neurologic dysfunction such as diplopia, incoordination and true gait ataxia (as opposed to the very common complaint of "difficulty with balance"), or exhibit abnormalities of the neurologic examination such as nystagmus, internuclear opthalmoplegia, sustained clonus, or Babinski signs.

Table 4				
Laboratory Differential Diagnosis of Multiple Sclerosis				
	MRI (1)	VEP (2)	OCB (3)	PNM (4)
Multiple sclerosis	+	+	+	-
Disseminated vasculomyelinopathy	+	+	+	+
Devic syndrome	+	+	+	+
HTLV-1 associated paraparesis	+	+	+	+
Nervous system AIDS	+	+	+	+
Neurobrucellosis	+	+	+	+
Neuroborreliosis (Lyme)	+	+	+	+
Neurosarcoidosis	+	+	+	+
Chronic fatigue postviral syndrome	+	+	+	+
Nervous system lupus	+	+	+	+

Not all these tests will be positive in all cases.

(1): Magnetic resonance imaging

(2): Visual evoked potentials

(3): CSF oligoclonal bands

(4): Peripheral nerve and/or muscle involvement

The diagnosis of the chronic fatigue post-viral syndrome

Various recommendations have been made in an attempt to delineate signs and symptoms which would define the CFPVS, in addition to the now classical generalized fatigue; these include mild pyrexia, sore throat, painful lymph nodes in the neck or the axillae, generalized headaches and sleep disturbances[10].

Additional features have subsequently been proposed by other authors consisting of abdominal symptoms, flu-like complaints, itchy bottom, skin rash, vaginal symptoms, ear complaints, tinnitus, gum trouble, painful hernia, breast swelling and nettle rash[6,26]. Goodwin[9] further expanded the syndrome by adding orthostatic tachycardia, abnormal coldness of the extremities, episodes of sweating and pallor, constipation and bladder disturbances, as well as biochemical abnormalities consisting of raised urinary creatine, low serum pyruvate, raised serum myoglobin or an abnormal electropheretic pattern with raised IgM.

Considering these various criteria, it is abundantly clear that none of them can legitimately be considered part of the array of signs and symptoms which usually characterize MS; in fact, their very presence would be sufficient by themselves to exclude the latter diagnosis from serious consideration.

> The recommendation[10] that a long list of conditions and diseases be excluded before diagnosing CFPVS reflects an inappropriate and inordinate dependence upon laboratory procedures which, more importantly, would require a truly gigantic, time consuming and extremely expensive (and probably fruitless) investigation. A detailed history obtained by an astute and experienced clinician, will, in almost all instances establish the correct diagnosis.

What is most characteristic about CFPVS in differentiating it from multiple sclerosis, is the presence of myalgias and arthralgias not mentioning the systemic symptoms which may of course be absent, or escape the attention of the neurologist. The problem of the differential diagnosis between CFPVS and MS is best illustrated by the report by Warner et al[28]

which serves the double purpose of describing the deceptively positive results of various laboratory tests, but at the same time emphasizing the importance of investigating the very characteristic and diagnostic electrophysiological and pathological abnormalities of muscle in CFPVS (Table 5).

Table 5
Neurologic Abnormalities in the Chronic Fatigue Syndrome*

14 patients

SYMPTOMS

Headache	13	Myalgia	13
Weakness	14	Dysequilibrium	11
Visual complaints	12	Paresthesiae	12
Tinnitus	10		

SIGNS
Neurologic exam normal except for mild weakness in 1 pt.

TESTING

CSF protein >	5/13	CSF IgG synthesis >	3/6
CSF cells >	2/13	VEP latency >	2/11
Abnormal EEG	1/13	Abnormal MRI	1/13

NEUROMUSCULAR ABNORMALITIES

Over 20% polyphasic motor units (quant. EMG)	7/10
Inflammatory infiltrates	3/11
Type II fiber atrophy	6/11
Type II fiber predominance	2/11
Nonselective fiber atrophy	2/11

NCT and BAERs all normal

* From Warner et al[28]

The relationship between CFPVS and MS

The vexing question which remains unresolved is the nature of CFPVS. Could it be a mild, mostly systemic form of MS, or an abortive form of chronic disseminated encephalomyelitis (CDEM)?

> It is well recognized that in all three conditions, a viral infection or an immunization may precede a bout of illness[1,5,17]. The latter is of particular significance in CFPVS which has been reported after immunizations against tetanus, cholera, influenza and typhoid[14] and more recently after vaccination against hepatitis B[27].

This would indicate that rather than being a persistent viral infection, CFPVS represents an immune-mediated response to a variety of agents[5]. It has been demonstrated that elevated antibody titers against different viruses are found in CFPVS patients[11] and that the ubiquitous Epstein-Barr virus is not the only possible culprit, if indeed it plays any role at all in this disease. This is a situation which is most reminiscent of what is believed to exist in MS[17, 29]. Traces of viral DNA or RNA, as reported by some authors in CFPVS[2], as well as other evidence of viral infection have also been found in blood, bone marrow, CSF and brain tissue of MS patients[17, 20]. A viral etiology for MS has been claimed at various times, the most recent candidate being the retrovirus HTLV-I although the evidence is, as in all the other instances, quite tenuous[20, 25]. On the other hand, the possibility in CFPVS of a persistent, specific, viral infection with a continuous, contemporaneous immune response, which exists in conditions such as subacute sclerosing panencephalitis, chronic rubella encephalitis, AIDS and HTLV-I associated parapesis[21] cannot yet be dismissed.

Neurological abnormalities have been recorded in some cases of CFPVS[1]. It is not inconceivable that these cases were in reality instances of MS or CDEM[12], that the preceding infection or vaccination caused the clinical appearance of a hitherto asymptomatic case of MS, or the initiation of CDEM, or even that CFPVS and MS may co-exist. Naturally, it is also possible that CFPVS does in fact, cause alterations of the central nervous system resulting in abnormalities of the neurologic examination as well as changes in MRI and in visual evoked potential studies[28].

No post-mortem examinations of cases of CFPVS have been reported to date and the final answer to this dilemma will to have to await the description of whatever abnormalities, if any, are discovered.

Despite the clinical and laboratory[28] similarities between the two, the following features of CFPVS would tend to suggest that it is not the same as MS: the tendency of CFPVS to occur in epidemics[1,4], no such event having been convincingly described in MS[23]; the striking involvement of muscle[13, 28], the characteristic myalgias and arthralgias, and the plethora of systemic manifestations.

Bibliography

1. Acheson E: The clinical syndrome variously called benign myalgic encephalomyelitis, Iceland disease and epidemic neurasthenia. Am J Med 1959; 26: 569-595.

2. Archard L, Bowles N, Behan P et al: Postviral fatigue syndrome: persistence of enterovirus RNA in muscle and elevated creatine kinase. J Roy Soc Med 1988; 81: 326-329.

3. Bauer H: Problems of symptomatic therapy in MS. Neurology 1978; 28 (2): 8-20.

4. Behan P: Epidemic myalgic encephalomyelitis. Practitioner 1980; 224: 805-807.

5. Behan P, Behan W, Bell E: The postviral fatigue syndrome - an analysis of the findings in 50 cases. J Infect 1985; 10: 211-222.

6. Bowman S, Brostoff J, Newman S et al: Postviral syndrome - how can a diagnosis be made? A study of patients undergoing a Monospot test. J Roy Soc Med 1989; 82: 712-716.

7. Courjon J, Mauguiere F, Revol M (eds): **Clinical applications of evoked potentials in neurology**, New York, Raven, 1982

8. Ebers G: Cerebrospinal fluid electrophoresis in multiple sclerosis. In: Poser C et al (eds): **The Diagnosis of Multiple Sclerosis**, New York, Thieme-Stratton, 1984: 179-184.

9. Goodwin C: Was it benign myalgic encephalomyelitis? Lancet 1981; 1:37.

10. Holmes G, Kaplan J, Gantz N et al: Chronic fatigue syndrome: a working case definition. Ann Int Med 1988; 108: 387-389.

11. Holmes G, Kaplan J, Stewart J et al: A cluster of patients with a chronic mononucleosis-like syndrome. JAMA 1987; 257: 2297-2302.

12. Innes S: Encephalomyelitis resembling benign myalgic encephalomyelitis. Lancet 1970; 1: 969-971.

13. Jamal G, Hansen S: Electrophysiological studies in the postviral fatigue syndrome. J Neurol Neurosurg Psychiat 1986; 48: 691-694.

14. Lloyd A, Wakefield D, Boughton C et al: What is myalgic encephalomyelitis? Lancet 1988; 1: 1286-1287.

15. Ormerod I, Miller D, McDonald W et al: The role of NMR imaging in the assessment of multiple sclerosis and isolated neurological lesions. Brain 1987; 110: 1579-1616.

16. Poser C: The diagnostic process in multiple sclerosis. In: Poser C et al (eds): **The diagnosis of multiple sclerosis**. New York, Thieme-Stratton, 1984: 3-13.

17. Poser C: The pathogenesis of multiple sclerosis: a critical reappraisal. Acta Neuropathol 1986; 71: 1-10.

18. Poser C: Diagnostic criteria for multiple sclerosis: an addendum. Ann Neurol 1987; 22: 773.

19. Poser C: MR in the diagnosis of multiple sclerosis. AJNR 1987; 8: 733.

20. Poser C: Viruses, multiple sclerosis and HTLV-I. In: Roman G et al (eds): **HTLV-I and the nervous system**, New York, Liss, 1989; 373-384.

21. Poser C: Notes on the pathogenesis of subacute sclerosing panencephalitis. J Neurol Sci 1990; 95: 219-224.

22. Poser C, Alter M, Sibley W et al: Demyelinating diseases. In: Rowland L (ed) **Merritt's Textbook of Neurology**, 7th edition, Philadelphia, Lea & Febiger, 1984: 593-611.

23. Poser C, Hibberd P, Benedikz J et al: Analysis of the "epidemic" of multiple sclerosis in the Faroe Islands. Neuroepidemiol 1988; 7: 168-180.

24. Poser C, Paty D, Scheinberg L et al: New diagnostic criteria for multiple sclerosis. Ann Neurol 1983; 13: 227-231.

25. Poser C, Roman G, Vernant J: Multiple sclerosis or HTLV-I myelitis? Neurology,1990; 40: 1020-1022.

26. Spracklen F: The chronic fatigue syndrome (myalgic encephalomyelitis) - myth or mystery? S Afr Med J 1988; 74: 448-452.

27. Waisbren B: Personal communication, 1990.

28. Warner C, Cookfair D, Heffner R et al: Neurologic abnormalities in the chronic fatigue syndrome. Neurology 1989; 39(Suppl 1): 420.

29. Woyciechowska J, Dambrozia J, Leinniki P et al: Viral antibodies in twins with multiple sclerosis. Neurology 1985; 35: 1176-1180.

Chapter 44

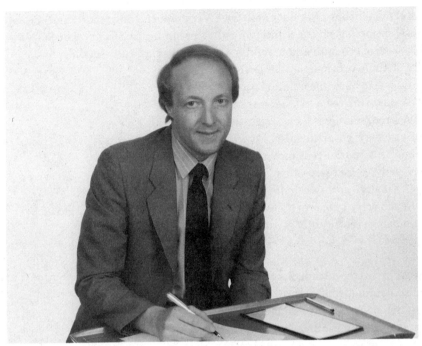

Russell J. M. Lane

Neurological Features of Myalgic Encephalomyelitis

Russell J.M. Lane BSc MD MRCP, Consultant Neurologist, Regional Neurosciences Centre, Charing Cross
Hospital, London W6 8RF, England
Presented at the First World Symposium on Myalgic Encephalomyelitis Cambridge, England April 10-12,
1990

Dr. Lane is a Consultant Neurologist at the Regional Neurosciences Centre, Charing Cross Hospital in London. He trained in Neurology with Lord Walton at the University of Newcastle Upon Tyne and with Professor Allen Roses at Duke University. Prior to his present appointment, he was a Wellcome Senior Research Fellow in Clinical Sciences in Newcastle and at the University of Liverpool. His specialist interest is in neuromuscular diseases and he has published a number of papers on muscular dystrophies, myositis, myasthenia and muscle energy metabolism.

'M.E.', myalgic encephalomyelitis, now more usually and perhaps correctly referred to as Chronic Fatigue Syndrome (CFS)[1], is an identifiable condition comprising a triad of cardinal features: **fatigue, neuropsychological symptoms and multiple somatic complaints.** Of these, fatigue and neuropsychological symptoms are usually predominant; the frequency and severity of other symptoms varies considerably. There is no generally agreed definition of the phenomenon, but a reasonable working description might be

A syndrome of chronic fatigue and malaise usually accompanied by subjective weakness, myalgia, reduced exercise tolerance and excessive post-exertional fatigue, and other symptoms, such as alterations in mood and problems with memory and concentration, without explanation after routine investigation.

The purpose of this paper is to examine the extent to which **neurological symptoms** experienced by CFS sufferers may have a definable basis in terms of clinical evidence of alteration in structure and function of the nervous system.

Fatigue

The nature of the fatigue experienced by CFS patients is extensively discussed elsewhere in this volume. Suffice to say here that it seems to have both physical and mental dimensions. Patients may try to distinguish these, reporting physical fatigue as lassitude, tiredness, lack of strength and inability to perform physically at their previous level, or what they anticipate that level to be, while mental fatigue may be described as vague drowsiness, anergia, and disinterest. However, recent studies have suggested that such distinctions may be artificial[2]. *Fatiguability* is also prominent; patients complain that mental or physical activity increases their fatigue disproportionately. Finally, *post-exertional fatigue* is common, in that such activity exerts a 'cost', with fatigue and myalgia being significantly greater over the following day or so.

Opinion regarding the extent to which such symptoms may be attributed to neuromuscular dysfunction is divided. Some studies have failed to demonstrate abnormalities in static or dynamic muscle strength, physiological evidence of muscle fatigue on repetitive stimulation or biochemical evidence of metabolic abnormalities in muscle tissue samples from such patients[3-5], while others have shown abnormalities of neuromuscular transmission[6] and energy metabolism[7]. These discrepancies may reflect population heterogeneity, or the fact that abnormalities of muscle metabolism in CFS may be more readily identifiable after extended exercise, in keeping with the patients' complaints.

For example, we have studied changes in venous blood lactate levels in CFS patients in a sub-anaerobic threshold exercise test[8]. Briefly, patients were asked to pedal an exercise bicycle for 15 minutes at a work rate of 90% of their predicted anaerobic threshold, based on their age, sex and weight, and venous lactate samples were measured at rest, at the end of the test and 30 minutes later. The test has established limits of sensitivity, and was abnormal in all cases of mitochondrial myopathy studied[8]. In a cohort of 44 consecutive CFS cases, we found 22 (50%) to have abnormal SATET results (Fig 1). This indicates that the regulation of metabolic function in muscle in response to relatively mild exercise is abnormal in some CFS patients, although it does not provide insight as to the *cause* of this defect. However, our group has also demonstrated the presence of persistent enteroviral RNA sequences in muscle biopsy samples from a number of these patients

(reference 9 and see Archard Chapter 37), raising the intriguing possibility that these two observations are pathogenetically linked.

Figure 1

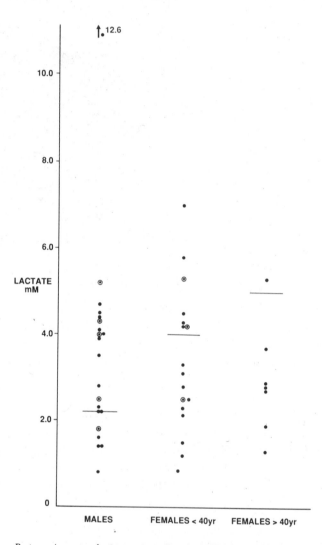

Post-exercise venous lactate concentrations in 44 CFS patients in the sub-anaerobic threshold exercise test (SATET). Horizontal bars indicate normal upper limits (set beyond the established upper 99% confidence limits). The rings indicate cases positive for defective enterovirus sequences on muscle biopsy extracts by slot-blot hybridisatic...

Neuropsychological disorders

These comprise changes in **mood and emotion**, such as depression, anxiety, introspection and hypochondriasis, emotional lability, irritability and anhedonia; subjective changes in **'intellectual capacity'** such as memory disorder, problems with concentration, language disturbances (eg difficulty in finding the right word); and other problems such as **sleep disturbance** (usually initial insomnia and hypersomnia). We routinely perform a simple psychometric screen on our patients (Table 1), looking for evidence of significant depression, overall decline in intellectual capacity, vocabulary skills, memory and concentration. To date, among 22 patients so tested, none has shown significant decline from general estimated pre-morbid capacities.

Table 1
Neuropsychological Screening Tests Performed on CFS Patients

National Adult Reading Test Predicted WAIS-R IQ from NART error score	NART Pred WAIS-R
Logical Memory sub-test of Wechsler Memory Scale	Log Mem
Delayed (30') Logical Memory Scale	Delayed LM
Vocabulary Scaled score from Object Naming Score	Obnm Vocab
Word Fluency for F, A, S	Word Flu
Forced Choice Words from Recognition Memory Test	FCW
Forced Choice Faces from Recognition Memory Test	FCF
Trail Making Tests A and B	Tr Mak
Present State Examination	PSE
Beck Depression Inventory	Beck

A considerable proportion (50%) showed a curious discrepancy between visual and verbal memory function (Forced Choice Words v Forced Choice Faces), verbal memory being much worse than visual, which seems to mirror the patients' complaints; a further 20% performed badly on both verbal and visual memory tasks. However, the exact significance of this observation remains unclear at this point. Surprisingly few patients showed evidence of 'depression' on the Beck Depression Inventory (Table 2).

Table 2
Results of 'Forced Choice Words' and 'Forced Choice Faces' Tests in CFS

PATIENT	FCW%	FCF%	SATET	HYBRIDISATION
CB	75	69	-	+
FB	<5	50*∫	-	-
JC	37	95*	-	-
HC	93	97	-	-
DG	25	10	+	+
GH	5	58*	+	
PK	5	5∫	+	-
JL	21	10	+	-
SM	21	90*	+	-
JM	6	67*	+	-
NP	17	50*	-	-
SR	56	17	-	+
S-C	5	50*	-	-
VS	37	95	-	-
NS	<5	75*	-	-
PS	<5	25*	-	-
AT	25	58*	+	+
LT	37	25	-	-
LW	25	75*	-	-
RC	95	95	+	+
JW	90	50	+	-
SB	95	90∫	-	-

* SIGNIFICANT DISCREPANCY

∫ BECK DEPRESSION SCORE > 15

Multiple Somatic Complaints

A large number of other symptoms may be reported, involving every system in the body. The most prominent are:

Neuromuscular - Myalgia, weakness, cramps, muscle twitching.

Neurological - Headache, visual disturbances, paraesthesiae, hypersensitivity to tactile stimuli.

Gastrointestinal - Sore throat, abdominal discomfort, features suggestive of irritable bowel syndrome.

Other problems - such as arthralgia and tender, swollen lymph nodes.

Neurological symptoms

The **neurological** manifestations of sporadic cases of CFS differ markedly from those observed in some of the previously described 'epidemics' of M.E. Such cases presented acutely with constitutional features suggestive of infection, followed by a neurological syndrome with motor and sensory components, such as numbness, paralysis and ataxia. In the Royal Free epidemic[10] for example, 'hard' neurological signs were observed in a high proportion of cases. However, there was little laboratory evidence to support the view that these signs resulted from damage to the nervous system. More that 30 years later, Thomas[11] examined some of the patients from that epidemic who had persistent neurological symptoms and found either evidence of other identifiable conditions, such as multiple sclerosis, or features to suggest that persistent weakness was 'functional'. A recent review of survivors of 'Akureyri disease', 40 years after the outbreak[12], found persistence of CFS symptoms in 8 of 10 patients studied, two having recovered completely; only one case showed neurological signs, of abnormal visual saccades and Rombergism.

In our own series of cases, which were highly selected for the possibility of an 'organic' basis for their fatigue syndrome, the incidence of even minor neurological signs was low (Table 3). In this series, all patients had a chief complaint of fatigue, fatiguability and exercise intolerance as discussed above, and all were extensively investigated to exclude other medical or primary psychiatric causes. Of the neurological symptoms mentioned, subjective **disturbances of memory and concentration** were frequent, supporting the observation of memory deficits encountered in the Forced Choice Words and Faces test (Table 2).

Headache

Headache was a common complaint but was rarely a prominent symptom. It seemed to have migrainous qualities in some cases, but was more often described as dull and generalised, without characteristic qualities.

Visual disturbances

One patient had dysthyroid eye disease but was euthyroid at the time of investigation; we were un-

able to define a common cause for the quite frequent complaint of 'visual disturbance' mentioned by sufferers. Eyelid myokymia is not uncommon on initial examination of CFS patients, who are often under considerable emotional strain.

Table 3
Comparison of Frequency of Neurological Symptoms in Chronic Fatigue* and Hyperventilation Syndromes*

Symptom	CFS (n=47) %	HVS (n=78) %
Giddiness	na	59
Paraesthesiae	32	36
Loss of consciousness	(1 case)	31
Visual disturbances	28	28
Headache	47	22
Ataxia	0	18
Tremor	na	10
Tinnitus	na	3
Memory loss	55	na
Reduced concentration	66	na
Cramp	19	na
Twitching	25	na

na- not assessed

Based on *present series and +Perkin 1986[14]

Sensory disturbances

While acroparaesthesiae were fairly common on direct enquiry, sensory disturbance was rarely a spontaneous complaint in our patients. Only one patient was found to have sensory deficit on examination.

A 46 yr. old naval Lieutenant-Commander presented in November 1985 with a flu-like illness from which he recovered. Three weeks later he developed pain and paraesthesiae in his legs, followed by numbness, and was found to have decreased sensation to spinothalamic modalities in a glove and stocking distribution, with preserved reflexes and motor function. CSF protein was normal. These symptoms persisted and were increasingly accompanied by fa-

tigue and other features typical of CFS. On investigation in our Unit, he was found to have a small fibre axonal neuropathy on neurophysiological studies, IgM antibodies to Coxsackie B3 in blood, and enteroviral RNA sequences were identified in his muscle biopsy extracts. SATET was normal, however.

Reflex changes

Occasional patients were encountered who exhibited hyperreflexia and even ankle clonus, but no patient exhibited hard evidence of pyramidal tract damage such as hypertonicity or Babinski signs.

Fasciculation

Muscle twitching and cramps were noted by a number of patients, and fasciculation was observed in one case at presentation. However, this patient had no electromyographic denervation or other features of anterior horn cell disease and was considered to have benign fasciculations.

Other signs

A small number of our cases were felt to have rather prominent lymph nodes and one patient was originally referred to our hospital with a mild persistent 'pyrexia of unknown origin', which ultimately could not be explained except as part of her CFS.

Conclusions

The incidence of neurological symptoms in CFS is high, but neurological signs, even of non-specific type, are rarely encountered. It is possible that symptoms and signs such as paraesthesiae, fasciculation, cramp, light-headedness and non-specific headaches in CFS patients are manifestations of hyperventilation syndrome (HVS) which is a common accompaniment of this condition[13]. Indeed, the incidence and nature of the neurological symptoms encountered in CFS were very similar to those observed independently in a large series of patients with HVS[14] (Table 3). The demonstration of a reproducible neurological abnormality in a patient complaining of symptoms compatible with CFS should prompt an exhaustive search for an alternative diagnosis.

References

1. Holmes G, Kaplan J, Gantz N et al. Chronic fatigue syndrome: a working case definition. Ann Int Med 1988; 108: 387-389.

2. Wessely S, Powell R. fatigue syndromes: a comparison of chronic 'post- viral' fatigue with neuromuscular and affective disorders. J Neurol Neurosurg Psychiat 1989; 52: 940-948.

3. Stokes M, Cooper R, Edwards RHT. Normal strength and fatiguability in patients with the effort syndrome. British Medical Journal 1988; 297: 1014-1018.

4. Byrne E, Trounce I. Chronic fatigue and myalgia syndrome: mitochondrial and glycolytic studies in skeletal muscle. J Neurol Neurosurg Psychiat 1987; 50: 743-746.

5. Lloyd AR, Hales JP, Gandevia SC. Muscle strength, endurance and recovery in the post-infection fatigue syndrome. J Neurol Neurosurg Psychiat 1988; 51: 1316-1322.

6. Jamal GA, Hansen S. Electrophysiological studies in patients with the post-viral fatigue syndrome. J Neurol Neurosurg Psychiat 1985; 48: 691- 694.

7. Arnold D, Bore P, Radda G, Styles P, Taylor D. Excessive intracellular acidosis of skeletal muscle on exercise in a patient with post-viral exhaustion/fatigue syndrome. Lancet 1984; i: 1367-1369.

8. Nashef L, Lane RJM. Screening for mitochondrial cytopathies: the sub-anaerobic threshold exercise test (SATET). J Neurol Neurosurg Psychiat 1989; 52: 1090-1094.

9. Archard LC, Bowles NE, Behan PO, Bell EJ, Doyle D. Post-viral fatigue syndrome: persistence of enterovirus RNA in muscle and elevated creatine kinase. J Roy Soc Med 1988; 81: 326-329.

10. Medical Staff of the Royal Free Hospital. An outbreak of encephalomyelitis in the Royal Free Hospital Group, London, in 1955. British Medical Journal 1957; ii: 893-906.

11. Thomas PK. Postviral fatigue syndrome. Lancet 1987; ii: 218-219.

12. Hyde B, Bergmann S. Akureyri disease (myalgic encephalomyelitis) forty years later. Lancet 1988; ii: 1191-1192.

13. King JC. Hyperventilation - a therapist's point of view: discussion paper. J Roy Soc Med 1988; 81: 532-536.

14. Perkin GDP, Joseph R. Neurological manifestations of the hyperventilation syndrome. J Roy Soc Med 1986; 79: 448-450.

Chapter 45

Chronic Fatigue Syndrome: Limbic Encephalopathy in a Dysfunctional Neuroimmune Network

Jay A. Goldstein, MD, Director, Chronic Fatigue Syndrome Institute, 500 South Anaheim Hills Rd., #128, Anaheim Hills, California 92807 USA

(Please see Chapter 23 for Dr. Goldstein's photograph and curriculum vitae.)

Abstract

Chronic Fatigue Syndrome can be viewed as a multi-causal disorder of the neuroimmune network which occurs in genetically predisposed individuals. Infectious agents, probably viral, may activate the immune system and dysregulate the central nervous system, particularly the temporolimbic area. Many symptoms are neurologic and the fatigue appears to be central, not peripheral. Since the symptoms fluctuate and can be altered by neuropharmacological intervention, they may be mediated by neuroimmune transmitter substances. A latent infection or predisposition may be triggered by a number of possible stimuli: infectious, traumatic, post-surgical, toxic, childbirth, or severe emotional stress such as would be seen in child abuse or post-traumatic stress disorder.[1] If the neuroimmune system is viewed as a network, then it could possibly be disrupted by agents influencing the network in various locations. Thus, it would be possible to treat Chronic Fatigue Syndrome with neuropharmacologic, immunomodulatory and anti-infective modalities, particularly since it increasingly appears that lymphocytes and neural cells share many receptor systems. Most of the symptoms of Chronic Fatigue Syndrome can be explained on the basis of a limbic encephalopathy.

The "limbic system" includes the septum, substantia innominata, amygdala, piriform cortex, and hippocampus. These structures are the only cortical areas to receive major projections from the hypothalamus. Through neural and hormonal mechanisms, the hypothalamus can coordinate electrolyte balance, basal temperature, metabolic rate, autonomic tone, sexual phase, circadian oscillations, and immunoregulation. The hypothalamus is essentially the head ganglion of the internal milieu and is also a major generator of drives and instincts that promote the survival of the self and the species. The limbic structures help to regulate memory and learning, drive modulation, the integration of affect and experience, and the higher control of hormonal balance and autonomic tone. The limbic system, therefore, helps to maintain internal homeostasis as well as the associated operations necessary for preservation of the self and the species.

Heteromodal, or generalized association areas, along with paralimbic structures, mediate the relationship between internal needs and the realities of the external world. Thinking, memory and experience alter instinctual responses and basic drive states to make the organism more effective in dealing with a complex environment. Limbic structures receive their most extensive connections from the hypothalamus and paralimbic areas. The paralimbic areas include the temporal pole, the caudal orbitofrontal cortex, the anterior insula, the cingulate gyrus, and the parahippocampal gyrus. Lesions in the paralimbic structures do not generally produce as profound an impairment as lesions in the limbic system in memory and learning, channelling of drive and affect, and of the higher control of autonomic tone.[2] Other areas involved in limbic circuitry include the limbic and paralimbic thalamic nuclei, the mesolimbic area, nucleus accumbens, habenula, and midbrain tegmentum.

Cognitive tasks as well as emotional states are associated with specific patterns of autonomic activity. A disturbance in the relationship between mental events and autonomic activity is thought to be a crucial factor in the pathogenesis of psychosomatic disease. The integration of mental states with patterns of autonomic activation is strongly influenced by the paralimbic areas of the brain, probably through multisynaptic pathways, especially from the paralimbic area to the amygdala through the stria terminalis to the hypothalamus and brainstem, and also from the amygdala to the nucleus of the solitary tract and to the dorsal motor nucleus of the vagus. There are also pathways from the insular cortex directly to the nucleus of the solitary tract and from the hippocampus to the pons.

In temporolimbic epilepsy, a model for limbic disorders, paralimbic structures and the amygdala integrate mental states with autonomic response patterns. If there is an epileptic focus in these structures, this would explain the frequency of autonomic discharges and visceral sensations, particularly pain in the abdomen, in patients with temporolimbic epilepsy. It may, therefore, be possible to treat Chronic Fatigue Syndrome, in which overt temporolimbic epilepsy is fairly uncommon, but **temporolimbic dysfunction** is prominent, by altering cognitive states with cognitive behavioral therapy, modifying limbic function with biofeedback approaches and possibly influencing limbic neural activity by extracranial electrical stimulation. Limbic neural input through the midbrain could also be modulated with devices that could modify neural input to the mesencephalon, for example, through trigeminal nerve transmission.

The amygdaloid complex can be divided into basolateral and corticomedical nuclear groups, the corticomedial subdivison being more primitive. Corticomedial efferents are partly crossed. If bilateral inputs from each amygdala can reach the hypothalamus, peripheral manifestations of limbic dysfunction would not necessarily be lateralized. This principle is also applicable to involvement of other limbic structures.

The various symptoms of Chronic Fatigue Syndrome appear to be very confusing to the casual observer. They seem to have no physiologic commonality and are, therefore, often put into the "black box" of depression as a way of explaining the inexplicable. "Hysteria" may also be another term that is used to explain the generation of this apparently bizarre symptom complex.[3] The mechanisms of the disease can be explained almost entirely if patients are viewed as having a limbic encephalopathy.

If we explore some of the functions of the limbic system it becomes apparent that dysfunction of this region can provide a plausible explanation of symptom generation. The limbic system has distinct receptors and this fact can probably explain the occurrence of limbic encephalitis, one of the paraneoplastic encephalomyelitides, in which the limbic system structures develop an inflammatory infiltrate and a patient presents with disorders of a limbic nature in association with a neoplasm.[4] It is known, as well, that there are specific viral receptors for herpes simplex virus-I in the medial temporal lobe. HSV-I can apparently cause a subclinical infection there and this sort of infection has been speculated to be a cause of temporolimbic epilepsy from which much of our information about limbic function in the human being is derived. Although different pathophysiologies are involved, reduced temporal lobe volume has been described in MRI scans of patients with temporolimbic epilepsy, schizophrenia and affective disorder.[5] Temporal lobe volume has not been reported in patients with Chronic Fatigue Syndrome.

There is considerable information about limbic encephalitis produced by Borna virus in animals[6] and perhaps humans.[7] Antibodies to the virus have been detected in a percentage of patients with affective disorders but not in controls. The spread of a murine neurotropic coronavirus through the olfactory pathway into the limbic system has been demonstrated[8] and a monoclonal antibody to limbic system neurons has been developed.[9] There is current interest in the association of neurotropic spumavirus with Chronic Fatigue Syndrome.[10] About 50% of patients are culture positive in blood and/or CSF, and none of the controls. Virus is seen intraneuronally on brain biopsy, and there is no inflammatory response, even though there is minimal gliosis. Of interest is a report of transgenic mice which express human foamy virus genes. Nerve cell degeneration with tissue atrophy and reactive gliosis were described most prominently in the telencephalon and the CA3 layer of the hippocampus.[11] A viral gene product was thought to be responsible for the neurotoxicity.

There apparently is a fatigue receptor in the medial temporal lobe. When stimulation of the medial temporal cortex through an electrode has been performed in awake patients with temporolimbic epilepsy at the Montreal Neurologic Institute, it has been observed that some of them report a profound feeling of fatigue.[12] It is not known, of course, whether the receptor can be localized in the medial temporal lobe, whether it is elsewhere in the limbic system, or whether it is a multisynaptic type of response.

It is known that levels of various cytokines are increased with exercise.[13] Since many believe that Chronic Fatigue Syndrome, particularly the post-viral kind, is associated with abnormal levels of cytokines,[14] it is a compelling hypothesis that abnormal limbic response to cytokine levels may be involved in post-exertion symptom generation. Reports of cytokine receptors in the central nervous system have primarily concerned interleukin-1 (IL-1). The areas of high density of the IL-1 receptor mRNA are in the granule cells of the dentate gyrus of the hippocampus,[15] although their function is speculative at present. The other hippocompal regions displayed little or no signal above background. The localization of IL-1R mRNA in the granule cells of the hippocampal dentate gyrus corresponds to that of high affinity binding sites for 125 I-recombinant human IL-1 alpha in mouse brain with characteristics similar to those of IL-1 receptors in immune cells.[16] IL-1 receptor antagonist mRNA has been localized in rat brain. It is present in the hypothalamic paraventricular nucleus, the hippocampus, cerebellum and blood vessels where IL-1 receptors have been previously described.[17] High levels of IL-1 antagonist in CFS may block high levels of IL-1 and may modulate its stimulation of CRH, as well as the effect of IL-1 to stimulate production of GH, TSH and somatostatin. IL-1 also inhibits the secretion of prolactin and LH, and the presence of a receptor antagonist could elevate levels of these substances. If CFS is characterized by low levels of CRH, which stimulates sympathetic nervous system function as well as ACTH secretion, IL-1 antagonist in the brain could be a mediator of a neuroendocrine-immune connection.

A decrease in regional cerebral blood flow is characteristically seen in the temporal and inferior frontal lobes in SPECT scans of patients with Chronic Fatigue Syndrome. This regional cerebral hypoperfusion is paradoxically increased after exercise in these patients.[18] PET scans have been performed in patients with Chronic Fatigue Syndrome and compared to those with major depressive disorder. The Chronic Fatigue Syndrome patients have lower metabolic rates in the hippocampus and amygdala, as well as in the caudate nucleus, the pre-motor cortex and the anterior cerebellum.[19] Amygdalar dysfunction could result in the autonomic abnormalities seen in these patients. Cognitive dysfunction is a well known symptom of Chronic Fatigue Syndrome and it probably, at least in part, is due to a hippocampal dysfunction. A deficit in encoding, or the making of new memories, has been postulated on the basis of neuropsychologic testing and evoked response data.[20] The cerebellum has been implicated in learned motor and autonomic responses.[21] The pre-motor cortex supplies one-third of the descending motor fibers and is involved in the planning and programming of movement performance. The ventromedial caudate is part of the limbic striatum. The location of the suprachiasmatic nucleus in the hypothalamus might be responsible for the cyclic nature of many symptoms as a result of limbic and paralimbic dysregulation. Affective disorders, irritability and panic attacks are thought to be a result of limbic dysfunction and antidepressants, one of the primary current neuropharmacologic treatment modalities for Chronic Fatigue Syndrome,[22] alter receptor regulation in the hippocampus and amygdala more than anywhere else in the brain.[23]

Sleep disturbances are very common in Chronic Fatigue Syndrome, and REM and non-REM sleep are regulated, in part, by limbic structures, especially non-REM sleep which is regulated in part by the anterior hypothalamus and the diagonal band of Broca, a septal nucleus.[24] The alpha EEG form of sleep architecture is frequently found in fibromyalgia[25] and Chronic Fatigue Syndrome, impelling some physicians to treat their patients as if they had a primary sleep disorder. In alpha EEG sleep there is a superimposition of alpha waves on the architecture normally seen in non-REM slow wave sleep.

Vertigo is another common symptom of Chronic Fatigue Syndrome. The superior and the posterior parts of the temporal lobe contain an area that responds to vestibular stimulation. Epileptic activation of this area may occur inducing vertigo or a sense of disequilibrium.[26] There are direct connections from the temporal lobe to the cochlea which may account for the tinnitus that many patients experience.[27]

Intolerance of alcohol is an extremely common, almost pathognomonic symptom of Chronic Fatigue Syndrome. The N-methyl-D-aspartate (NMDA) receptor is inhibited by ethanol. In mouse embryo hippocampal neurons, ethanol specifically inhibits NMDA receptor activation. Such inhibition may contribute to the neural and cognitive impairment seen in Chronic Fatigue Syndrome.[28]

Nasal allergies are often noted and direct innervation of mast cells has been demonstrated.[29] Their function could be influenced by the limbic system and the autonomic nervous system and some of the limbic concomitants of nasal allergies could be explained by retrograde axonal transport of mediators secreted by the nasal mucosa into the piriform cortex. These mediators would include substance P, somatostatin, calcitonin gene-related peptide, leukotrienes, vasoactive intestinal peptide and histamine.[30]

Weight gain, which is also very frequent in chronic stages, could be explained by alteration of the limbic modulation of the autonomic nervous system of brown fat thermogenesis, a way of dissipating caloric intake by heat radiation. Mice infected with Borna virus become very obese, a condition presumed to be a result of neuropathologic changes in the hypothalamus.[31]

Premenstrual syndrome (PMS) is almost always seen in women with Chronic Fatigue Syndrome and, if PMS had been present prior to the onset of the illness, it becomes much worse. Many of the symptoms of PMS are quite similar to those of Chronic Fatigue Syndrome. It is known that estrogen and progesterone and their metabolites are highly concentrated in various limbic system structures.

Patients with temporolimbic epilepsy have numerous hormonal problems similar to those seen in Chronic Fatigue Syndrome. Patients with this form of epilepsy also have an exacerbation during the premenstrual period. Some authorities believe that premenstrual syndrome is a rapid cycling disorder which is entrained to hormonal fluctuation.[32] The depression which is seen in patients with PMS may have an abnormality in cortisol function,[33] however, unlike the depression seen in Chronic Fatigue Syndrome.[34] CRH testing suggests a **central hypocortisolemia**, a state which may be common to most neurasthenic conditions.

Environmental illness is often seen in patients with Chronic Fatigue Syndrome. The sensitivity to odors which often can cause an exacerbation of all symptoms may be explained by a dysregulation of the piriform cortex. Unusual sensitivity to other substances may be explained by abnormal limbic antigen presentation which is now known to occur in stressed rats and also by direct transport of substances from the oropharynx to the brain. Many patients report feeling good or bad after they eat certain types of food. This may be due to the reaction of the limbic system to insulin and certain peptides and amino acids that are transported into the brain as well as alpha fibroblast growth factor, interleukin-1 beta, tumor necrosis factor alpha, and other cytokines which may increase post-prandially. It has been demonstrated that there is direct autonomic nervous system innervation of lymphoid organs. This peptidergic and nonadrenergic innervation is mainly associated with T lymphocyte-dependent areas.[35] It is possible that limbic alteration of this directed autonomic nervous system innervation may be involved in the observation that recurrent flu-like illnesses can be caused by stressful situations. It also may be possible that the lymphocytes in the lymphoid organs may secrete neurotransmitters which can be transported back to the central nervous system.

Considering the generation of pain, particularly that of fibromyalgia, a condition frequently associated with Chronic Fatigue Syndrome, it has been demonstrated that the insular and the paralimbic areas have higher levels of endogenous opioid receptors than other areas. The periaqueductal gray area in the midbrain tegmentum is also thought to be part of the limbic system. It controls pain sensation to a large extent and receives projections from other limbic structures, including the limbic striatum.[36] Descending pathways from these areas may be involved in the pathogenesis of fibromyalgia, particularly since it has been demonstrated that patients with fibromyalgia have increased levels of substance P in their cerebrospinal fluid.[37] We have also noted anterior cerebellar abnormalities in the PET scans of many patients. One does not usually think of cerebellar function as being influenced by the limbic system. However, the paleocerebellum, in which the anterior lobe is located, is involved in maintenance of tonus in the muscles. Some of these fibers project to the reticular nuclei in the ventral midbrain tegmentum,[38] part of the limbic system. One of the hypotheses of the pathophysiology of fibromyalgia is alteration of gamma neuron excitability. Gamma neurons are regulated by the firing of cerebellar fibers which can be modulated by the reticular nuclei. The amygdala, caudate, and pre-motor cortex are also involved in modulation of gamma neuron activity.[39]

The limbic system is involved in immunoregulation. Lesions of the amygdala, hippocampus, septum and hypothalamus can cause an alteration in lymphoid cell number and activation.[40] Learning through classical conditioning can also serve an immunoregulatory function.[41] This finding was one of the first to exemplify the relationship between the brain and the immune system.

A number of disorders which have found to be associated with temporolimbic epilepsy are also, perhaps, seen with increased frequency in patients with Chronic Fatigue Syndrome. Polycystic ovarian disease, endometriosis, dysfunctional uterine bleeding, infertility, impotence and decreased libido are known to occur in temporolimbic epilepsy. Some of these hormonal abnormalities have not responded to hormone therapy but have responded to anticonvulsants.[42] Consideration is also being given to using hormonal therapy for temporolimbic epilepsy.

The autonomic preganglionic neurons in the spinal cord and lower brain stem receive direct and indirect limbic connections. The limbic system mediates both affective and cognitive processes is involved in the response to stressors in affective disorders and integrating sensory input from the outside world as well as the inside world.

Limbic regions respond to immunizations or to cytokines by altered neuronal activity or altered monoamine metabolism.[43] Alpha interferon, for example, has been shown to alter neuronal activity in the anterior hypothalamus and the dorsal hippocampus. Respiratory disorders are fairly common in Chronic Fatigue Syndrome, namely, dyspnea on exertion, air hunger, and hyperventilation. Some[44] have stated that the symptoms of Chronic Fatigue Syndrome are **caused** by hyperventilation, and perhaps some of the patients with Chronic Fatigue Syndrome do hyperventilate. The reason why they might hyperventilate, however, has not been examined. The respiratory disorders of Chronic Fatigue Syndrome might also be explained by limbic encephalopathy. The most massive projection to the parabrachial pontine area, also known as the "pneumotaxic" area, arises from the central nucleus of the amygdala. Single pulse stimulation of the central nucleus of the amygdala results in an immediate switch to inspiration.[45] Since the amygdala may not be functioning properly in patients with Chronic Fatigue Syndrome this dysfunction may cause the respiratory abnormalities that we see in Chronic Fatigue Syndrome.

Numerous other symptoms such as irritable bowel syndrome, cardiac arrhythmias, abnormalities in temperature control and the occurrence of hypesthesias and dysesthesias could also be explained on the basis of a limbic encephalopathy.

A good hypothesis explains observations in the simplest manner possible and also lends itself to verification by testing. The concept that Chronic Fatigue Syndrome is a limbic encephalopathy in a dysregulated neuroimmune network postulates that no matter what the cause of the syndrome, the symptoms are transduced through the limbic system. With this hypothesis in mind, it should be possible in the future to have more directed diagnostic investigation and more coherent approaches to treatment that would be, perhaps, antiviral if the notion of a viral encephalopathy resulting in limbic dysfunction proves to be true for certain patients. Agents could be developed to block the effects of viral neurotoxic gene products. The use of immunodulatory, neuropharmacologic and other approaches to alter limbic input and output would also be appropriate.

References

1. deLoos WS. Psychosomatic manifestations of chronic post-traumatic stress disorder. In: Wolf ME, Mosnaim AD. Posttraumatic stress disorder: Etiology, phenomenology and treatment. Washington: American Psychiatric Press, 1990.

2. Mesulam MM. Principles of behavioral neurology, Philadelphia: FA Davis, 1985.

3. Doane BK. Clinical psychiatry and the physiodynamics of the limbic system. In: Doane BK and Livingstone KF, eds. The limbic system: Functional organization and clinical disorders. New York: Raven Press, 1986.

4. Newman, NJ, Bell IR, McKee AC. Paraneoplastic limbic encephalitis. Biol Psychiatry 1990; 27:529-542.

5. Altschuler LL, Conrad A, Hauser P, et al. Reduction of temporal lobe volume in bipolar disorder: a preliminary report of magnetic resonance imaging (letter). Arch Gen Psychiatry 48:482-483, 1991.

6. Ludwig H, Bode L, Gosztony G. Borna disease: a persistent virus infection of the central nervous system. Prog Med Virol 1988; 35:107-151.

7. Amsterdam JD, Winokur A, Dyson W. Borna disease virus: a possible etiologic factor in human affective disorders? Arch Gen Psychiatry 1985; 42:1093-1096.

8. Lavi E, Fisman PS, Highkin MK. Limbic encephalitis after inhalation of a murine coronavirus. Laboratory Investigation 1988; 58(1):31-36.

9. Levitt P. A monoclonal antibody to limbic system neurons. Science 1984; 223:229-231.

10. Martin, WL. Submitted for publication.

11. Bothe K, Aguzzi A, Lassman H, Rethwilm A, Horak I. Progressive encephalopathy and myopathy in transgenic mice expressing human foamy virus genes. Science 1991; 253:555-557.

12. (Karpati G. Presented at: Workshop on Research Directions for Myalgic Encephalomyelitis / Chronic Fatigue Syndrome, Vancouver, Canada, May 11, 1991.)

13. Simon HB. Exercise and human immune function. In: Ader R, Felten DF, and Cohen N, eds. Psychoneuroimmunology, second edition. San Diego: Academic Press, 1991.

14. Cheney PR, Dorman SE, Bell DS. Interleukin-2 and the Chronic Fatigue Syndrome. Ann Intern Med 1989; 110:321.

15. Cunningham ET, Wada E, Carter DB, Tracey DE, Battey JF, DeSouza DB. Localization of interleukin-1 receptor messenger RNA in murine hippocampus. Endocrinology 1991; 128(5):2666-2668.

16. Takao T, Tracey DE, Mitchell WM, DeSouza EB. Interleukin-1 receptors in mouse brain: characterization and neuronal localization. Endocrinology 1990; 127:3020-3078.

17. Licino J, Wong M-L, Gold PW. Localization of receptor antagonist mRNA in rat brain. Endocrinology 129(1):562-564, 1991.

18. (Mena I. Study of cerebral perfusion by neuri-SPECT in patients with Chronic Fatigue Syndrome. Presented at: Chronic Fatigue Syndrome: Current Theory and Treatment, Bel-Air, California, May 18, 1991.)

19. (Lottenberg S, Solano M, Abel A, Goldstein JA, Paddie D, Buchsbaum M. Presented at: Annual Meeting, American Psychiatric Association, New Orleans, May 16, 1991.)

20. (Sandman C. How Chronic Fatigue Syndrome affects memory. Presented at: Chronic Fatigue Syndrome: Current Theory and Treatment, Bel-Air, California, May 18, 1991.)

21. Thompson RF. The neurobiology of learning and memory. Science; 1986; 233:941-947.

22. Goldstein JA. Chronic Fatigue Syndrome. The Female Patient 1991; 16(1):39-50.

23. Hoyenga KB, Hoyenga KT. Psychobiology: The neuron and behavior. Pacific Grove, California: Brooks/Cole, 1988.

24. Jones BE. Basic mechanisms of sleep-wake states. In: Kryger MH, Roth T, Dement WC. Principles and practice of sleep medicine. Philadelphia: WB Saunders, 1989.

25. Adams RD, Victor M. Principles of Neurology, fourth edition. New York: McGraw-Hill, 1989.

26. Valzelli L. Approach to neuroanatomical and neurochemical psychophysiology. Littleton, Massachusetts: John Wright, 1980.

27. Moldofsky H. Non-restorative sleep and symptoms after afebrile illness in patients with Fibrosistis and Chronic Fatigue Syndromes. J Rheumatol (suppl) 1989; 19:150-153.

28. Lovinger DM, White G, White FF. Ethanol inhibits NMDA-activated ion current in hippocampal neurons. Science 1989; 243:1721-1724.

29. Stead RH, Dixon MF, Bramwell NH, et al. Mast cells are closely apposed to nerves in the human gastrointestinal mucosa. Gastroenterology 1989; 97:575-585.

30. Goetzl EJ, Turck CW, Sreedharan SP. Production and recognition of neuropeptide by cells of the immune system. In: Ader R, Felten DF, Cohen N, eds. Psychoneuroimmunology, second edition. San Diego: Academic Press, 1991.

31. Ludwig H, Bode L, Gosztonyi G. Borna disease: a persistent virus infection of the central nervous system. Prog Med Virol 1988; 35:107-151.

32. Reid RL. Premenstrual syndrome. New Eng J Med 1991; 324(17):1208-1210.

33. Parry BL, Gerner RH, Wilkins JN, et al. CSF and endocrine studies of premenstrual syndrome. Neuropsychopharmacology 1991; 5(1): In press.

34. (Demitrack MA, Dale JK, Gold PW, Chrousos GP, Straus SE. Neuroendocrine abnormalities in patients with chronic fatigue syndrome. Presented at: The National Meeting, American Society of Clinical Investigators, 1990.)

35. Felten SY, Felten DL. Innervation of lymphoid tissue. In: Ader R, Felten DF, Cohen N, eds. Psychoneuroimmunology, second edition. San Diego: Academic Press, 1991.

36. Nauta HJW. A simplified perspective on the basal ganglia and their relation to the limbic system. In: Doane BK and Livingston KF, eds. The limbic system: Functional organization and clinical disorders. New York: Raven Press, 1986.

37. Vaeroy H, Helle R, Forre O, et al. Elevated CSF levels of substance P and high incidence of Raynaud's phenomenon in patients with fibromyalgia: new features for diagnosis. Pain 1988; 32:21-26.

38. Adams RD, Victor M. Principles of Neurology, fourth edition. New York: McGraw Hill, 1989.

39. Hulliger M. The mammalian muscle spindle and its central control. Rev Physiol Biochem Pharmacol 101:1-110, 1984.

40. Roszman TL, Cross RJ, Brooks WH, Markesbery WR. Neuroimmunomodulation: Effects of neural lesions on cellular immunity. In: Guillemin R, Cohn M and Melnechok T, eds. Neural modulation of immunity. New York: Raven Press, 1985.

41. Ader R, Cohen N. The influence of conditioning on immune responses. In: Ader R, Felten DF, Cohen N, eds. Psychoneuroimmunology, second edition, San Diego: Academic Press, 1991.

42. Mesulam, MM. Principles of Behavioral Neurology. New York: Raven Press, 1985.

43. Besedovsky HO, DelRey A. Physiological implications of the immune-neuro-endocrine network. In: Ader R, Felten DF, Cohen N, eds. Psychoneuroimmunology, second edition, San Diego: Academic Press, 1991.

44. Rosen SD, King JC, Wilkinson JB, Niton PG. Is chronic fatigue syndrome synonymous with effort syndrome: J Royal Soc Med 1990; 83 (12):761-764.

45. Harper RM. Neurophsyiology of sleep. In: Hypoxia, exercise, and altitude: proceedings of the third Banff international hypoxia symposium, New York: Alan R Liss, 1983:65-73.

M.E. / CFS and the Peripheral Nervous System

Chapter 46

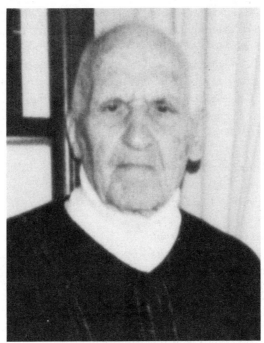

Alberto Marinacci

An Historical Review of
the Electromyographic Features of Post-Infectious M.E. / CFS

Byron Hyde MD, with kind assistance of Alberto Marinacci, M.D. and Karl Von Hagen, M.D.

(Please see Chapter 5 for Dr. Hyde's photograph and curriculum vitae.)

Abstract: *This short paper reviews the Electromyographic findings of Alberto Marinacci, A. Melvin Ramsay and A.T. Richardson. This paper also includes an interview with Dr. Marinacci and Dr. Karl Von Hagen in 1988 concerning sporadic M.E./CFS. Abnormal findings can be demonstrated in post-infectious M.E./CFS and possibly in insidious onset M.E./CFS. These findings are more likely to be discovered in the period immediately following the onset of illness. In many cases, demonstrable electromyographic changes are self-limiting. The findings may relate to transient or minor injury but not destruction of the anterior horn cells. Notes are also included from an interview Dr.Marinacci granted me in January 1988. Dr. Marinacci uses the term "atypical poliomyelitis" in describing M.E./CFS.*

Alberto Marinacci MD, Past Associate Professor of Neurology, School of Medicine, University of Southern California, Los Angeles.

Alberto Marinacci was an intern and later a resident in Neurology at the Los Angeles County General Hospital. He became one of the most renowned electromyography experts in the United States and published several texts on the subject. He employed a Universal Electromyographic Survey Machine, that is no longer utilized, to take his measurements. In many ways it may have been a more precise machine than those used today. However, its application consumed up to half a day or more per patient. Although it apparently gave a more thorough understanding of underlying pathology, it was not cost efficient.

In his book *Applied Electromyography*[1] Alberto Marinacci describes the chronic features of the 1934 Los Angeles epidemic. I repeat his comments since so rarely in the medical literature do we find mention of the chronic features of M.E./CFS.

"In 1937, while I was an intern at the Los Angeles County General Hospital I came in contact with many of the epidemic cases, some of whom were (still) hospitalized (three years after the epidemic) and others who were readmitted because of a recurrence of the symptoms. The chief complaints were fatigue,

insomnia, impaired memory, emotional instability and hysterical episodes. As these symptoms were often misinterpreted by the attending physicians, many of these cases were labelled as 'malingerer' or 'compensationitis'. This attitude often produced a conflict between the patient and the attending medical staff, and the patients were transferred from clinic to clinic and from department to department.

The first electromyographic evaluation of any of these patients was done during the period 1948-1952, (14-18 years after the epidemic). Twenty-one patients in all were examined; all were females, the majority being nurses. The main complaints were recurring fatigue, pains and some muscle spasms in the distribution of the cervical and lumbosacral segments. In these cases there was...impaired memory.[2]"

All 21 cases examined electromyographically showed evidence of mild long-standing, lower motor neurone affection. This was quite different from many patients who had residual poliomyelitis contracted in the 1934 epidemic. These cases all showed a different electromyographic picture, consisting of highly complex motor units. These findings were in patients that would today be considered as marked or severe M.E./CFS.

When Marinacci examined sporadic cases he found further interesting features of M.E./CFS. These results wouldhave spread across the spectrum from self-limiting to major or severe forms of M.E./CFS. His comments indicate the following findings could be anticipated using similar technology.

Spinal Cord Pathology

Patients who fall ill with acute post-infectious M.E./CFS symptoms will demonstrate abnormal electromyographic changes in the first few weeks, that is, early in the acute phase of the disease. These electromyographic changes will be consistent with widespread radiculopathy with about 10% complex motor units, few fibrillations and positive sharp waves in the paraspinal muscles, the girdles and all limbs.

After a few weeks, these electromyographic changes will decrease and after 6 months the electromyographic studies will be essentially normal if the patient has recovered and will show changes as noted above in chronic persisting disease.

It is important to note that Marinacci was using excellent, but labour intensive technology that is no longer available, the Universal Electromyography machine. As computerized machines develop, we will undoubtedly be able to obtain better readings on M.E./CFS consistent with or even better than the labour intensive EMG of Marinacci.

Electromyographic Findings in:

Anterior Poliomyelitis

EMG changes in poliomyelitis differ from those found in M.E./CFS. In anterior poliomyelitis, the anterior horn cells undergo two specific changes developing as, (a) the altered or sick cells, and/or (b) the destroyed cells.

(a) The sick cells : produce highly polyphasic activity which is irreversible for they have been recorded for as long as 65 years after the onset of the disease.

(b) The destroyed cells: result in true paralysis of the affected muscle with profuse denervation activity recorded. The EMG findings are profound and irreversible.

M.E./CFS

In M.E./CFS the EMG changes are mild and in the majority of cases (non chronic cases) are microscopically reversible. There may well be persistance of physiological damage.

In acute cases of M.E./CFS, during the first 2 weeks of illness one may find only polyphasic motor units which have almost normal amplitude.

After a period of three weeks, one finds scattered fibrillation and positive sharp waves which usually follow a plurisegmental distribution. These same findings are usually found in the recurrent cases.

In chronic cases, the few fibrillation potentials are no longer detectable and positive sharp waves may be found. High polyphasic and some giant motor units are present. These changes also follow a segmental distribution.

In the group of cases examined where the electromyogram recorded 5-10% abnormalities, 80% recovered over a period of 18 months. In about 5% of the cases, complaints and abnormal electromyographic findings persisted for about 3 years before a complete recovery could be confirmed. Three percent of the cases had a recurrence of the symptoms.

It is apparent that there is injury of the anterior horn cells in acute M.E. /CFS and that, depending upon the degree of injury, these changes tend to improve over a variable period of time, most showing complete EMG restoration. M.E./CFS produces minor reversible changes in the lower motor neurones which can be detected only by EMG.

Interview with Dr. Alberto Marinacci and Dr. Karl Von Hagen

Q. I first asked Dr. Marinacci if he still knew any of the original physicians who had fallen ill in the 1934 epidemic. **A.** Dr. Marinacci discussed a physician friend of his who prior to the illness, had been a football player for Notre Dame, but after contracting M.E./CFS his muscular fatigue was at times so great that he was unable even to turn a light-switch on. He was at times unstable and unable to face reality. He was able to work only with extreme difficulties.

Q. Were there any total recoveries in any of the 1934 patiets that Dr. Marinacci had treated? **A.** He stated that those patients whom he followed continued to suffer, yet their life expectancy did not appear to diminish. He also noted that those who may have recovered would have been less likely to seek his services.

Q. What were the most recurrent problems in the 1934 patients? **A.** "Their loss of recent memory. At times, they were quite incapable of piecing things together. Frequently these patients were sent to me as neurotics or as people with psychotic breakdowns but, in reality, they were atypical poliomyelitis. One nurse whom I last saw in 1980 had not improved since 1934 and still suffered from pain and fatigue."

Dr. Marinacci's associate, Dr. Von Hagen, replied **A.** "Emotional instability was a frequent finding, but in all of them there would be weakness, sometimes pain and in one nurse that I had followed for a long time, there were contractures. They were disabled.

Very few made a complete recovery. If you saw any of them without a history you would call them psychoneurotic."

Q. What did they believe was the cause of the illness? **A.** Both Dr. Marinacci and Dr. Von Hagen believed that there had been changes in CNS function as a result of the infection but that part of their illness was related to an alteration of the myelin sheath in which the axon was perhaps changed but not destroyed. This would be consistent with the pathological report in this book concerning the sural nerve biopsy of a 1984 epidemic patient.

Sporadic Cases: In addition to the 1934 cases, both Dr. Marinacci and Dr. Von Hagen saw approximately two new, non-1934 cases per month. The incubation period was no longer than 7-10 days. Most of these patients gave a history of exposure to some infection. Approximately half of them gave a history of becoming ill while outside of California, in such places as Mexico, South America, the Orient or after major crowd exposure. Presumably, many of these patients had received immunization just prior to their trip. By 1965 they had seen approximately 330 sporadic cases, some of whom were followed for up to 16 years. The findings of these sporadic patients that were chronic and persistent, were similar to those of the 1934 cases and consisted of all or any of the following:

Description of Sporadic Cases:

1. altered psychic function with impaired memory, emotional instability and hysterical outbursts;
2. extreme muscular fatigue and often pain;
3. sensory changes that included both skin sensitivity changes and altered hearing;
4. affection of the autonomic nervous system, fast pulse, gastric and urinary complaints.

They have a feeling of low fever, followed by headaches and pain, especially in the neck and back and later radiating to one or more extremities. Frequently the pain is accompanied by sensory changes, paresthesias and hypothesia. The pains tend to subside but the neuromuscular symptoms are reactivated on the slightest exertion. The patients complain of fatigue and tiredness out of all proportion to their apparent illness, which is noted even when the patient is confined to bed.

On many occasions the patients complain of tiredness of the eyes on reading, and the vision becomes blurred. Gastric symptoms are frequent and there is an increase in anticipated pulse rate. Transient paresthesias in one or more limbs is common. These symptoms are usually labeled by their referring doctor as neuromyasthenia or neurasthenia or hysterical, neurotic or psychotic personality.

Neurological examination may show varying degrees of hypoalgesia and hypothesia, usually in a segmental or nerve trunk distribution. Minimal decrease of vibration sensation and also a slight decrease of deep sensibility may be noted. Pathological reflexes are rare. The mental symptoms are the most characteristic.

The majority of the acute cases tend to recover within 3-6 months. Some go on to a chronic phase. The patient has symptoms similar to those of the acute phase but they may continue for months or even years with periods of improvement of short duration as in the 1934 epidemic.

Recurrent Phase: Some patients who recover after 3-6 months may have recurrences, even after many years.

A. Melvin Ramsay, M.D.
Past Consultant Physician in Infectious Diseases, Royal Free Hospital, London, England

A.T. Richardson, M.D.
Department of Physical Medicine and Rheumatology, Royal Free Hospital, London

Dr. Ramsay was involved, in a major way, in the investigation of the staff who fell ill with M.E. at the Royal Free Hospital in London, England in 1955[4] and their subsequent care. Until his death in 1990, Dr Ramsay produced numerous papers and a book on Myalgic Encephalomyelitis[5]. He was perhaps the best loved Myalgic Encephalomyelitis treating physician in Britain. He was both learned and wise. He was kind and generous with his time to both patient and physician. No one who knew this man does not regret his passing.

The second author, Dr. Richardson, published extensively on the subject of M.E. in the late 1950's and was obviously working in close contact with Dr. Ramsay. Although their joint publications are based upon the same Royal Free Hospital patient group, their papers suggest that different individuals within the same epidemic were tested. The consistency of their resulting papers is therefore not surprising. What is interesting is that their joint work closely resembles the findings of Marinacci who, although in greater detail, published very similar results. Marinacci's EMG observations come from a different population and were originally described in 1948[6]. It should be remembered that the findings of Gilliam in the L. A. Epidemic[7], were buried in Public Health Bulletin No 240 and, until rediscovered by Dr. Alexis

Shelokov in the late 50's, were unknown to the general medical public[8], including those at the London Free Hospitals. This congruity of findings suggests a similar disease process.

In the 1970's, there was a suggestion by Drs McEvedy and Beard[9], that these EMG findings were contrived either by the patients or their physicians. Careful examination of McEvedy's actual contrived tracings will show that they are not congruent with the pathological tracings. Neither have other professionals been able to duplicate the actual findings of normal patients by purposeful manipulation. I went to see Dr McEvedy at his London home in 1988. He confirmed earlier conversations that I had had with Dr Ramsay, indicating that he had never actually examined any of the London Free patients. Furthermore, he could not recall if he had actually examined any of the patients he discussed in reports of reputed epidemics he had published concerning girls' schools in England.

Ramsay describes the EMG changes as follows[9]: *"Weak muscles showed abnormality of motor unit activity only on volition. The number of motor-unit potentials was reduced (reduced interference pattern) with a tendency to occur in groups of up to 6 potentials."* This grouping of large polyphasic motor-unit potentials was also noted by Marinacci who, however, described normal amplitude. Ramsay describes them as follows:

"Many were of long duration (up to 15 m.sec.). In some instances where muscle weakness was severe, all the residual motor units were abnormal and grouped, the volitional pattern being distinctive".

"These observations are commonly described in so-called myelopathic lesions when there is involvement of the motor unit at the level of the cord, a finding common in vascular lesions of the cord, anterior poliomyelitis and other conditions[4]." However in these conditions, there is also lower motor neurone degeneration and this has rarely been described in M.E.

Dr. Richardson notes that: *"Electrodiagnostic investigation of 28 cases failed to show any signs of lower motor neurone degeneration except in one case. Electromyelograms were normal in four, but in the remainder showed a profound disturbance of volition characterized in severe cases by a reduction in the number of motor-unit potentials even to discrete motor-unit activity, the individual potentials often being polyphasic, and in the less severely involved muscles , and particularly during recovery, by group ing of these motor-unit potentials"[11].*

At Nightingale, although abnormalities are sometimes found, we have not found EMG studies a useful conjunct in the diagnosis of either epidemic or sporadic M.E./CFS. Possibly, with a dedicated in-house EMG facility, this might prove otherwise.

References

1. Marinacci M.D., Alberto, Chapter 9, **Applied Electromyography**, Lea & Febiger, Philadelphia, 1968

2. Idem, page 91, **all idems refer to 1. Marinacci above**

3. Idem page 95-96

4. Medical Staff of the Royal Free Hospital, An Outbreak of Encephalomyelitis in the Royal Free Hospital Group, London, in 1955, (1957) 19 October, British Medical Journal, 896-905

5. **Myalgic Encephalomyelitis/ Postviral Fatigue Syndrome**, The Saga of the Royal Free Disease, Gower Medical Publishing, London, 1986, A. Melvin Ramsay MA MD

6. Idem, page 91

7. **Public Health Bulletin No. 240**, April 1938, Epidemiological Study of an Epidemic, Diagnosed as Poliomyelitis, Occurring Among the Personnel of the Los Angeles County General Hospital During the Summer of 1934, by A. G. Gilliam, Past Assistant Surgeon, U.S. Public Health Service, Division of Infectious Diseases, National Institute of Health, United States Government Printing Office, Washington: 1938.

8. Private communication between Dr. A. G. Gilliam and Dr. Alexis Shelokov in the mid 1950's, in which Dr. Gilliam first discussed the 1934 L.A. epidemic with Dr. Shelokov.

9. McEvedy, C.P., Beard, A.W. The Royal Free Epidemic of 1955: A Reconsideration, British Medical Journal, (1970) January 3, pages 7-11.

10. Ramsay, A. Melvin, O'Sullivan, E. Encephalomyelitis Simulating Poliomyelitis, (1956) 26 May, The Lancet, pages 761-764

11. Richardson, A. T., Some Aspects of the Royal Free Hospital Epidemic, (1956) July, Annals of Physical Medicine, pages 81-89

Chapter 47

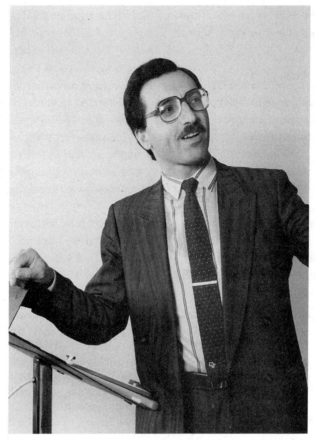

Goran A Jamal

Evidence for Organic Disturbance in the Post Viral Fatigue Syndrome: Neurophysiological Studies

Dr. Goran A Jamal, MD PhD MRCP MB ChB
Glasgow University Department of Neurology, Institute of Neurological Sciences, Southern General Hospital, Glasgow G51 4TF.

Dr. Jamal graduated MBChB from Baghdad University in 1977 with First Class Honours in all subjects, for which he was awarded the prestigious President of Iraq Prize. He continued his studies at Glasgow University completing his PhD Medical Sciences and MD and was the winner of the Cormie Prize. Dr. Jamal returned to Baghdad University as Lecturer of Neurology in 1980 but one year later accepted the position of Research Fellow in the Department of Neurology at Glasgow University. From 1986 to 1988, he became Senior Registrar in the Department of Neurology at St. Bartholomew's Medical School, London University. Dr. Jamal has held his present position as Consultant and Clinical Senior Lecturer in the Department of Neurology at Glasgow University since 1988.

Summary

A variety of neurophysiological studies were performed on a total of 40 patients with the post viral fatigue syndrome (PVFS) who were identified following scrutinised criteria for case definition to maximise accuracy of diagnosis. Among 20 patients examined with EEG, 85% showed modest changes of discrete nature without constant focal features similar to those seen in multiple sclerosis. The EEG changes suggest a patchy disturbance of cerebral function with variable intensity and distribution.

Conventional EMG and nerve conduction studies in 40 patients failed to demonstrate any significant neurogenic or myopathic abnormality. Testing of the small fibre pathway in 30 patients showed normal results.

Single fibre EMG jitter studies in 40 patients produced abnormal values in 75% of the patients. High jitter values were not associated with impulse or concomitant blocking. The organisation of the motor unit was studied in 10 patients with very high jitter values using fibre density estimation method of the Single Fibre EMG technique and these showed normal results suggesting the absence of any remodelling of the motor units in these patients. These findings provide solid evidence of an organic disturbance in the peripheral part of the motor unit. The abnormalities are thought to be primarily due to disturbance of muscle fibre propagation.

The neurophysiological findings provide valuable information concerning transmission of impulses in the peripheral part of the motor unit. The findings accord with a variety of other histological, biochemical and neurobiological abnormalities in muscles of these patients and with other previously reported neurophysiological changes which occur during the acute phase of viral infection.

Introduction

Though muscle fatigue and myalgia are the hallmark of the post viral fatigue syndrome (PVFS), there is a clear absence of conspicuous muscle cell damage when investigated by traditional neurophysiological, biochemical and histological methods. However, when more sophisticated techniques are used, an undisputed evidence of muscle involvement is present (Arnold et al 1984, 1985; Jamal and Hansen 1985, 1989; Archard et al 1988). The possibility of a persistent viral infection as the underlying cause of the PVFS has been raised in recent studies (Behan et al 1985; Yousef et al 1988; Archard et al 1988).

The reported neurophysiological findings in this paper are from patients whose selection were very well scrutinised according to structured criteria for case definition. The criteria highlight the central positive features of the syndrome but are restricted by intention to maximise the accuracy of diagnosis.

Patients included had fulfilled all of the following four major criteria:

Diagnostic Criteria

1. Persistent or relapsing muscle fatiguability and myalgia of at least 6 months duration, present at rest but made worse with a little exercise, accompanied by **negative** neurological examination and, in particular, absent evidence of muscle weakness.

2. All patients were subjected to assessment through careful clinical history, physical examination, conventional EMG and nerve conduction studies and more than 20 laboratory examinations to exclude any other cause for muscle fatigue. Special emphasis was put on excluding cervical radiculopathy, generalised neuropathy, nerve trauma, known myopathies, diabetes mellitus or other endocrine diseases, chronic pulmonary, cardiac, hepatic, renal and haematological disorders, chronic psychiatric illnesses or any other concurrent problem in the neuromuscular system. Patients with excessive alcohol ingestion or those on any neurotoxic drug were also excluded. Defects in neuromuscular junction were excluded in all patients by repetitive studies and acetyle choline receptor antibody measurement.

3. All patients had clear evidence of a recent viral infection at or before the beginning of their illness, by laboratory methods.

4. All patients had two or more of the following abnormalities: in vitro lymphocyte function, lymphocyte subset examination, helper/inducer lymphocyte ratio, immune complex and compliment studies and ultra-structural abnormalities in their muscle biopsy. Muscle biopsy studies also served to exclude any neurogenic or myopathic disorders in these patients.

Concentric Needle EMG and Nerve Conduction Studies

Motor and sensory nerve conduction studies are normal in all cases of PVFS (Richardson 1956; Jamal and Hansen 1985, 1988, 1989). Concentric needle EMG shows no evidence of neurogenic changes or muscle fibre degeneration (Jamal and Hansen

1985, 1988, 1989). Occasional irregular fasciculations have been reported, especially during the early stages of the disease (Richardson 1956) but examination of 40 patients with the PVFS in our laboratory did not show any spontaneous activity (Jamal and Hansen 1985). Disturbances of volition have been reported in the form of grouping of motor unit potentials where they occur in groups interrupted by periods of relative silence in between, particularly during the recovery phase of the illness (Richardson 1956). Such disturbances however are not necessarily organic in nature (McEvedey and Beard 1970; Jamal and Hansen 1985; Thomas 1987). Disturbances of recruitment were seen in half of the 40 patients in our laboratory and in one quarter of these the phenomenon of motor unit potentials grouping was observed (Jamal and Hansen 1985). Individual motor units within these groups had all their parameters entirely normal (Jamal and Hansen 1985). These disturbances of interference patterns are fully restored to normal upon recovery of the patient (Jamal and Hansen 1985). Thomas (1987) reported that the muscle weakness in patients with the PVFS was associated with a low firing rate on maximal volition and this was accompanied by grouping of motor unit activity. Simultaneous activation of agonist and antagonist muscles was reported, thus raising the possibility of simulation of symptoms (Thomas 1987). In a small number of patients on whom we have performed these studies, we have been unable to demonstrate these phenomena. The vast majority of patients are capable of maintaining a steady firing rate in the individual motor unit during the examination with single fibre EMG. We have therefore been unable to reproduce the findings of Thomas (1987) in the patients whom we have selected according to our criteria of case definition.

Concentric needle EMG and nerve conduction studies are therefore normal in patients with the PVFS and only show some changes which are not necessarily organic. They must be performed in every case with the PVFS to exclude neurogenic and or muscular causes of fatigue. The conventional needle EMG provides a good overall picture of the structure and function of individual motor units and the concerted action of these units at a given effort. It does not however discriminate between potentials from different muscle fibres within the motor unit all of which fire almost synchronously. These conventional studies may not be sensitive enough to detect a low grade dysfunction of the motor unit or to identify disturbances in the individual muscle fibres. A variety of methods are available to study the individual muscle fibre physiology, the most valuable of which is the technique of single fibre electromyography (SF-EMG). This technique is valuable not only to study the pathophysiology of the motor unit at individual muscle fibre level but also to provide accurate sensitive quantification of the function of the motor unit in general (Jamal 1989).

Table 1			
Thermal Threshold Values in 30 Patients with PVFS Using the Technique of Jamal et al 1985			
	HT	P	CT	P
Wrist PVFS	0.22 + 0.08	} NS	0.15 +0.06	} NS
cont	0.23 + 0.06		0.15 + 0.05	
F. Arm PVFS	0.24 + 0.07	} NS	0.14 + 0.08	} NS
cont	0.24 + 0.06		0.15 + 0.05	
Ankle PVFS	1.38 + 0.66	} NS	0.14 + 0.08	} NS
	1.35 + 0.73		0.17 + 0.06	
Thigh PVFS	0.24 + 0.05	} NS	0.15 + 0.08	} NS
	0.23 + 0.06		0. 15 + 0.05	

Single Fibre Electromyography

This technique is designed to investigate the motor unit and its components in a much more sensitive way than the conventional neurophysiological methods. It has proved to be useful for the detection of abnormalities and characterisation of the functional status of the motor unit and for assessing the degree of stability of the neuromuscular junction (Jamal 1989). The following parameters of function have been measured in patients with the PVFS.

Jitter

This is the variability of the interpotential interval of

two single muscle fibre potentials which belong to the same motor unit. An impulse which activates the two muscle fibres of the same unit is propagated along the neuron and axon of that unit. It then splits along the individual intramuscular axonal branches to each of the muscle fibres before crossing the neuromuscular junction and travelling along the muscle fibres to reach the point of detection by the SF-EMG electrode. Therefore, jitter can only arise distal to the point where the initially single discharge follows two different pathways to reach the point of recording. The part of the motor unit proximal to the branching of the motor axon does not contribute to the production of the jitter. The source of jitter is from one or more of the following components of the peripheral part of the motor unit; the intramuscular axonal branches, the neuromuscular junction or the muscle fibre (Stalberg and Trontelj 1979; Jamal 1989).

Despite the application of very strict criteria to identify abnormalities of jitter, 75% of 40 patients with the PVFS produced abnormal values (Jamal and Hansen 1985, 1989). Jitter values were as high as 400-500 microseconds in some cases (ULN = 55 microseconds).

Impulse Blocking

If the delay of the second potential is long enough, then it may fail to appear altogether, a phenomenon called blocking (Stalberg and Trontelj 1979; Jamal 1989). This is usually due to inadequate neurotransmitter release and is therefore commonly seen in defects of neuromuscular junction transmission where blocking usually occurs when jitter values exceed 80-100 microseconds (Stalberg and Trontelj 1979). In the two studies that we have performed, no impulse blocking was observed in any of the patients examined despite very high jitter values, sometimes reaching 5 or 6 times this threshold level (Jamal and Hansen 1985, 1989). The phenomenon of **concomitant or paired blocking**, where two or more single fibre potentials always block and reappear simultaneously, is neurogenic in origin (Stalberg and Trontelj 1979, Jamal 1989). This may happen when recording is made from 3 or more single muscle fibres where the block occurs in an axonal branch which is common to the muscle fibres, the potentials of which block simultaneously. Concomitant blocking has not been observed in any

of the patients that we have examined (Jamal and Hansen 1985, 1988, 1989).

Fibre Density

This is a measure of the mean number of single muscle fibre potentials of a motor unit detected simultaneously from within the uptake area of the SF-EMG electrode and is highly correlated to the number of single muscle fibres contained in the motor unit (Stalberg and Trontelj 1979; Jamal 1989). To achieve this measurement, the electrode is randomly inserted in the muscle and the needle is manipulated so that a single fibre potential is optimally recorded and maximised. The number of simultaneously occurring time-locked single fibre potentials for a time interval of at least 5 milliseconds is then counted. At least twenty such estimates are made from different recording sites and the average of these is taken as the fibre density (Stalberg and Trontelj 1979; Jamal 1989). In most muscles the normal mean fibre density ranges from 1.3 - 1.8 (Stalberg and Trontelj 1979). The measurement of fibre density provides a useful indirect assessment of remodelling of the motor unit as a result of denervation and reinnervation process or rearrangement of muscle fibres within the motor unit following myopathic changes (Stalberg and Trontelj 1979; Jamal 1989). Fibre density has been found to be normal in all the patients with PVFS that we have examined, even in those patients with very high jitter values (Jamal and Hansen 1989). Moreover, no significant correlation was found between the fibre density values and the mean overall jitter measurements (Jamal and Hansen 1989).

Assessment of Small Fibre Pathway

The usual stimulation techniques used to record conduction velocity and somatosensory evoked potentials in the afferent fibres bypass the receptors and only investigate the fastest afferent fibre pathway in the neuraxis (Jamal et al 1987). These conventional techniques do not allow us to examine smaller afferent pathways and are therefore insensitive to changes involving these small fibre populations. A specially designed system which provides a very sensitive objective assessment of the unmyelinated and thinly myelinated nerve fibres and their central pathways has been introduced for clinical use (Jamal et al 1985 a,b). This technique was applied in 30 patients with the PVFS who had abnormal jitter values from our first study (Jamal and Hansen 1985). Heat and cold threshold measurements were performed at a distal and proximal site of each of the right upper and lower limbs as described previously (Jamal et al 1985). None of the patients had abnormal values and comparison of the groups of patients and normal subjects did not show significant differences (Table 1). The results therefore rule out any evidence of a neurogenic lesion in the small nerve fibre populations or their central pathways.

Electroencephalography

A standard electroencephalography has been performed in 20 patients with the PVFS identified according to the criteria outlined earlier. This showed modest changes in 85% of the patients of a discrete nature. The changes comprised an excess of irregular slow wave activity with patchy distribution appearing in one or the other side of the brain without any constant focal features. No sharp waves, spikes or complexes were seen at any stage of the disease nor during recovery. The changes described are very similar to those reported by Pampiglion et al (1978). The changes described in these patients are not dissimilar to those seen in some cases of multiple sclerosis. The severity, distribution and character of the EEG changes bear no similarity to those seen in cases of acute encephalitis or encephalopathies of metabolic, endocrine or toxic aetiologies. The severity and extent of EEG changes in PVFS appears to be unrelated to the severity of symptoms (Pampiglion et al 1978).

Discussion

The abnormality of jitter measurement in patients with PVFS provides solid evidence of an organic disturbance in the peripheral part of the motor unit. Increased jitter outside the normal range is an indicator of abnormal conduction in the peripheral part of the motor unit, either the intramuscular axonal branches, the neuromuscular junction or the muscle fibres. Even in the minority of patients who had their values within the normal range, the mean overall jitter has always been higher than the normal mean of a controlled population (Jamal and

Hansen 1985). This abnormality of jitter values (up to 500 microseconds in some instances) without impulse blockings makes the neuromuscular junction an unlikely site of involvement as blockings are expected to occur frequently with jitter values above 100 microseconds in cases of neuromuscular junctional defects (Stalberg and Trontelj 1979; Jamal 1989).

Similarly, absence of concomitant blocking in any of the patients would make the intramuscular axons an unlikely site for the increased jitter values in PVFS patients. Increased fibre density occurs in neurogenic and myopathic disorders in which there is a rearrangement and/or an increase in the number of muscle fibres contained in the motor unit. Fibre density is a very sensitive index of muscle fibre splitting, of general muscular atrophy with shrinkage of muscle fibres and of collateral sprouting (Stalberg et al 1975, Stalberg and Trontelj 1979, Jamal 1989). Normal FD suggests lack of collateral sprouting or muscle fibre splitting in this syndrome. Therefore abnormalities of muscle fibre propagation are the most likely cause of increased jitter in these patients.

It must be remembered that the techniques of SF-EMG jitter do **not** measure the absolute values of conduction in the individual muscle fibres. It rather measures the degree of discrepancy and loss of synergism of muscle fibre conduction within the same motor unit and it is possible that this degree of dys-synergism becomes more excessive as exercise proceeds. This may be far much more important in the pathophysiology of muscle fatigue in the PVFS rather than the overall average conduction of muscle fibres of the same or different motor units. Nonetheless, it will be interesting to see whether or not surface measurement of averaged muscle fibre conduction will show any abnormality since some individual jitter values are high. Such techniques must be applied to a relatively large number of patients and well matched controls to be able to detect any minor trend of abnormality. It is not known yet whether or not there is an additional impairment of excitation/contraction coupling in the T-tubules or sarcoplasmic reticulum in patients with PVFS. Failure of impulse propagation within the T-tubules will not necessarily be detected using SF-EMG jitter measurement which records from the surface of muscle fibres.

The muscle fibre abnormality in the SF-EMG studies is supported by several non neurophysiological findings. Muscle biopsies in patients with PVFS show a variety of non specific changes including subtle and patchy muscle fibre necrosis, scattered atrophic fibres and abnormality of type II muscle fibres (Behan et al 1985). Electron microscopic studies show intramuscular tubular aggregates and mitochondrial abnormalities in some patients (Behan et al 1985; Archard et al 1988).

Examination of patients by the 31p-NMR technique shows evidence of an abnormal early intramuscular acidosis following exercise which is out of proportion to the associated changes in high energy phosphates (Arnold et al 1984, 1985; Grosse et al 1988; Miller et al 1988). This is believed to represent excessive lactic acid formation arising from a disorder of regulation of muscle metabolism involving the relative contributions of aerobic versus anaerobic processes. It is believed that this abnormality is related to ultrastructual damage of the muscle fibre and may be responsible for the muscle fibre membrane disorder. These changes are probably related to the symptom of fatigue. Miller and Milner-Brown (1984) found evidence of impairment of impulse propagation along the muscle fibre membrane following fatigue in healthy individuals. The magnitude of this impairment depended on the degree and duration of fatigue as well as on the intrinsic properties of individual muscles. It remains to be seen whether the muscle propagation abnormalities in patients with PVFS would become even more pronounced following exercise in a much more excessive way to that seen in normal individuals.

Abnormalities of neuromuscular transmission have been reported to occur in patients with acute viral infection even when they do not have associated myalgia (Friman et al 1977, Schiller et al 1977). These changes are transient and disappear after the acute phase is over (Friman et al 1977). More fulminant cases of myositis have been reported following documented viral infection both in children (Ruff and Secrist 1982) and adults (Schwartz al 1978) with rather similar albeit more severe neurophysiological findings to those seen in the PVFS. A variety of muscle enzyme abnormalities and subtle ultrastructural mitochondrial damage have also been reported following viral infections (Astrom et al 1976).

Myalgia which is a frequent feature of acute viral infection may be intense for several days and serum creatine kinase concentration may be slightly raised during this time (Middleton et al 1970, Friman 1976). The literature is not short on reports of severe muscle involvement complicating viral infections (Chou and Gutman 1970; Mejlszenkier et al 1973; Fukuyama et al 1977; Schwartz et al 1978). Severe neurophysiological abnormalities are usually present in these patients (Schwartz et al 1978).

Are the neurophysiological, ultrastructural and metabolic abnormalities described in these patients enough to explain the symptom of excessive fatigue? High energy phosphate compounds which are the main source of energy in the muscle are provided mainly by the aerobic metabolism of glucose while the anaerobic breakdown of this compound is less efficient in this respect. The disturbance of the relevant contribution of anaerobic versus aerobic processes to the provision of muscle energy is therefore likely to affect the amount of high energy phosphate compounds available and this disturbance is likely to escalate with exercise (Edwards 1978; Bigland-Ritchie 1988).

In addition to this a quick accumulation of lactate occurs as the exercise continues and this will change the optimal biochemical surrounding in an adverse fashion and cause further compromisation of the availability of high energy compounds (Sahlin 1986). Energy provision is of paramount importance to maintain all complex cellular functions including the chemical synthesis of materials, the transport of nutrients, the generation and propagation of electrical impulses and therefore for the contraction of the muscle fibres (Luttgua 1965). Therefore, fatigue in PVFS patients is probably multi-factorial (a) due to direct lack of high energy phosphate compounds, (b) lack of optimal surrounding due to the quick accumulation of lactic acid and other metabolites (c) failure of co-ordination and synergism of the contraction of individual muscle fibres of the same motor unit. The effects of these factors are likely to escalate very quickly as exercise continues. It remains to be seen whether there is in addition any failure in the excitation-contraction coupling in the T-tubules or the sarcoplasmic reticulum.

Recent studies have shown a clear evidence of a

persistent virus infection, mainly the entero viruses in muscles of the PVFS patients, using both immunological virus isolation techniques (Yousef et al 1988) and nuclear RNA virus probing (Archard et al 1988). The same techniques demonstrated evidence of persistent entero virus infections in dilated cardiomyopathy, a subject which was extensively reviewed in a recent symposium (Schultheiss 1988). In murine myocarditis (induced by coxsackie viruses) immunological processes including virus specification cross reactive antibodies and immune reactions are associated with severe disease (Bendinelli and Friedman 1988). In human coxsackie viral myocarditis and cardiomyopathy, antibodies that cross react with coxsackie B viruses are present (Schultheiss 1988, Bowles et al 1986). Antibodies that cross react with cardiac B adreno-receptors, with mitochondrial ADT/ATP carriers and with cell surface protein of the muscle causing an overload of the myosites and a consequent dysfunction is emerging as a complex pathogenetic mechanism to explain dilated cardiomyopathy (Schultheiss 1988). This entity was formerly regarded as idiopathic but now is accepted increasingly as a late sequel of infection with entero viruses especially the coxsackie B group (Schultheiss 1988; Caforio et al 1990). It is therefore possible that similar immunological and metabolic disturbances may result from chronic persistent virus infection providing the organic basis of the muscle dysfunction in patients with the PVFS.

A persistent viral infection exerts limited effect where it impairs the specialised functions of cells and decrease synthesis of specific products e.g. of heavy and light myosin chains, hormones, melanin... etc and disturbed immunological functions (Southern and Oldstone 1988). Increased level of (2-5) - oligo - adenylate synthesis, a cellular enzyme specifically induced by interferon have been demonstrated in patients with persistent Epstein-Barr infection (Scott 1983; Morag et al 1982). There is a striking degree of similarity between symptoms of patients with the Post Viral Fatigue Syndrome and the side effect of treatment with Lymphokines such as interferon (MacDonald et al 1987). Low grade persistent intracellular infection may therefore induce a lymphokine response by activated immune cells (T cells and macrophages) with interferon and other factors being episodically or continuously released (Strauss 1985; Ho Yen et al 1988). Such a local lymphokine response may underlie the electro-physiological and NMR abnormalities. Lymphokines have been shown to induce alterations to skeletal muscle - cell membrane potentials and to induce altered cellular energy metabolism both in vitro and in vivo (Morag et al 1982; Tracey et al 1986).

A persistent virus infecting cells may not be killed but may exert limited effect where the infected cell becomes unable to perform specialised function (Southern and Oldstone 1986; Hayward 1986). The infected cell may interfere with the function of immunocompetent cells of the host to avoid the host immune system in order to survive, resulting in specific or non-specific immuno-suppression. This may explain the changes observed in these patients with regards to the immuno regulatory subsets, the abnormal mitogene response and the presence of immune complexes (Tosato et al 1985; Strauss et al 1985; Byrne et al 1985: Caligiuri et al 1987). This is also in accordance with absent minimal cell damage noted in the Post Viral Fatigue Syndrome (Archard et al 1988).

Conclusion

In a critical reappraisal of the syndrome and various studies performed in the PVFS, David et al (1988) stated that the SF-EMG neurophysiological findings are "the most persuasive evidence for muscle dysfunction in this syndrome to date". Although the neurophysiological findings reported here do not form characteristic patterns to provide specific diagnosis of the syndrome, they provide valuable information concerning transmission of impulses in the peripheral part of the motor unit. The changes tend to illustrate the functional disturbances and the possible associated ultrastructual morphological changes in the muscle fibres. These neurophysiological studies should, therefore, play an important role in any case definition criteria for the PVFS. Conventional EMG studies are also essential to exclude other neurogenic or myopathic causes of fatigue. The EEG changes in the PVFS suggest a discrete and patchy disturbance of cerebral function with variable intensity and distribution. These changes though definite, are non specific in nature and are of little help in the diagnosis of the syndrome.

Acknowledgement
The secretarial assistance of Miss Elizabeth Jackson is greatly appreciated.

References

Archard, L.C.; Bowles, N.E.; Behan, P.O. et al (1988) Post Viral Fatigue Syndrome: Persistence of enterovirus RNA in muscle and elevated creatine kinase. J. Roy, Soc. Med., **81**, 326 - 329.

Arnold, D.L.; Bore P.J.; Radda G.K. et al (1985) Enhanced intramuscular acidosis during exercise by patients with post viral exhaustion/fatigue syndrome. Neurology (Cleveland), 35 (Suppl.1), 165.

Arnold, D.L.; Radda, G.K.; Bore, P.J.; et al (1984) Excessive intracellular acidosis of skeletal muscles on exercise in a patient with a post viral exhaustion/fatigue syndrome. Lancet, 1, 1367 - 1369.

Astrom, E.; Friman, G.; Pilstrom, L.; (1976) Effects of viral and mycoplasma infections on ultrastructure and enzyme activities in human skeletal muscle. Acta. Patholog. Microbiol. Scand,; 84, 113.

Behan, P.O.; Behan. W.M.H.; Bell E.J/ (1985) The Post Viral Fatigue Syndrome: An analysis of the findings in 50 cases. J. Infect., 10,211-222.

Bendinelli, M.; Friedman, H. (1988) **Coxsackievuruses, A General Update Plenum**, New York.

Bigland-Ritchie B (1988) Motor Control and neuromuscular fatigue. **AAEE Monograph, Rochester Minnesota: AAEE**, 9-14.

Bowles, N.E.; Richardson, P.J; Olsen E.C.J.; Archard, L.C. (1986) Detection of Coxsackie Virus-Specific from patients with myocarditis and dilated cardiomyopathy. Lancet, i. 1120-1123.

Byrne E., Trounce I., Dennett X. (1985) Chronic relapsing myalgia (Post Vrial): Clinical, hisotological and biochemical studies. Aust. N. Z. J. Med, **15**, 305-308.

Caforio, A.L.P.; Stewart, J.T.; McKenna, W.J. (1990) Idiopathic dilated cardiomyopathy. Br Med J., **300**, 890-891.

Chou, S.M.; Gutman, L.; (1970) Picornavirus - like crystals in subacute polymyositis. **Neurology (New York), 20**, 205 - 213.

David, A.S.; Wessley, S.; Pelosi, A. (1988) Post viral fatigue syndrome: time for a new approach. Br Med J., **296** 696-699.

Edwards, R.H.T. (1978) Physiological Analysis of Skeletal Muslce Fatigue and Weakness. Clin Sci Mol Med; **54**, 463-470.

Friman, G. (1976) Serum creatine phosphokinase in epidemic influenza. Scand. J. Inf. Dis., **8**, 13 - 20.

Friman, G. (1977) Effect of acute infectious disease on isometric muscle strength. Scand. J. Clin. Lab. Invest., **37**, 303 - 308.

Friman, F.; Schiller, H.; Schwartz, M. (1977) Disturbed neuromuscular transmission in viral infections. Scan J. Infect. Dis, **9**, 99 - 103.

Fukuyama, Y.; Ando, T.; Yokota, J. (1977) Acute fulminant myoglobinuric polymyositis with picornavirus - like crystals. J. Neurol. Neurosurg. Psychiat., **40,** 775 - 781.

Galiguiris, M.,; Murray, G.; Buchwald, D et al. (1987) Phenotypic and functional deficiency of natural killer cells in patients with chronic fatigue syndrome. J. Immunol., **139**, 3306-3313.

Grosse, B.; Glasberg, M.; Kensora, T.; Smith, M.B.; Welch, K.M.A.; (1988) 31P   NMR spectroscopy and histochemical study of benign myalgic and fatigue syndrome. **Neurology (New York), 38** (Suppl. 1), 410.

Hayward, A.M. (1986) Patterns of persistent viral infection . Engal. J. Med., **315**, 939-948.

Jamal, G.A.; (1989) Update: Singe fibre electromyography. Principles and applications. **J. Electrophysiol. Technol 15**, 5-16.

Jamal, G.A.; Hansen, S.; (1985) Electrophysiological studies in the post viral fatigue syndrome. J. Neurol. Neurosurg. Psychiat, **48**, 691 - 694.

Jamal, G.A.; Hansen, S.; (1988) Post viral fatigue syndrome. Br. Med. J., **296**, 1067 - 1068.

Jamal, G.A.; Hansen, S.; (1989) Post viral fatigue syndrome: Evidence for underlying organic disturbance in the muscle fibre. Eur. Neurol., **29**, 273 - 276.

Jamal, G.A.; Hansen, S.; Weir, A.I.; Ballantyne, J.P. (1985) An improved automated method for the measurement of thermal thresholds. 1. Normal subjects. J. Neurol. Neurosurg. Psychiat. **48**, 354 - 360o:6.

Jamal, G.A.; Weir, A.I.; Hansen S.; Ballantyne, J.P. (1985) An Improved Automated method for the Measurement of Thermal Thrsholds. 2 patients with peripheral neuropathy. J. Neurol. Neurosurg. Psychiat. **48,** 361-366.

Jamal, G.A.; Hansen, S.; Weir, A.I.; Ballantyne, J.P.; (1987) The neurophysiologic investigation of small fiber neuropathies. Muscle and Nerve, **10,** 537 - 545.

Lattgau H.C. (1965) The Effect of Metabolic Inhibitors of Fatigue of the Action Potentials in Single Muscle Fibres. J. Phsyiol. (Lond.); **178**, 45-67.

McDonald, E.M; Mann, A.H.; Thomas, H.C. (1987) Interferons as mediators of psychiatric morbidity. An investigation in a trial of remominant x-interferon in hepatitis-B carriers. Lancet, ii, 1175-1177.

McEvedy, C.P.; Beard, P.W. (1970) Royal Free epidemic of 1956: a reconsideration. Br. Med. J., 1, 7 - 11.

Mejlszenkier, J.D., Safran, A.P.; Healy, J.J.; Embree, L.; Oullette, E.M. (1973) The myotosis of influenza. Arch. Neurol., 29, 441 - 443.

Middleton, P.H.; Alexander, R.M.; Szymanski, M.T. (1970) Severe myotosis during recovery from influenza. Lancet, 2, 533 - 535.

Miller, R.G.; Boska, M.D.; Moussari, R.S.; Carson, P.J.; Weiner, M.W. (1988) 31p nuclear magnetic resonance studies of high energy phosphates and pH in human muscle fatigue. J. Clin. Invest., 81, 1190 - 1196.

Miller, R.G.; Milner-Brown, S.; (1984) Impulse propagation along the muscle membrane is impaired during muscle fatigue. Neurology (Cleveland), 34, (Suppl. 1), 131.

Morag, A.; Tobi, M.; Ravid, Z.; Revel, M.; Schattner, A. (1982) Increased (2'-5') Oligo-A-Synthetase activity in patients with prolonged illness associated with serological evidence of persistent Epstein-Barr virus infection. Lancet, 1, 744.

Mukherjee, T.M.; Smith, K.; Marcos, K. (1987) Abnormal red blood cell morphology in myalgic encephalomyelitis. Lancet, 2, 328 - 329.

Pampiglione, G.; Harris, R.; Kennedy, J. (1978) Electroencephalographic investigations in myalgic encephalomyelitis. Postgrad. Med. J., 54 752 - 754.

Richardson, A.T. (1956) Some aspects of the Royal Free Hospital epidemic. Ann. Phys. Med., 3, 81 - 89.

Ruff, R.L.; Secrist, D. (1982) Viral studies in benign acute childhood myositis. Arch. Neurol. 39, 261-253.

Sahlin, K (1986) Muscle Fatigue and Lactic Acid Accumulation. Acta Physiol. Scand.; 128, 83-91.

Schiller, H.H,; Schwartz, M.S.; Friman, G. (1977) Disturbed neuromuscular transimssion in viral infection. New Engl. J. Med., 296, 884.

Schwartz, M.; Swash, M.; Gross, M. (1978) Benign postinfection polymyositis. Br. Med. J., 2, 1256 - 1257.

Stalberg, E.; Schwartz, M.S.; Trontelji, J.V. (1975) Single fibre electromyography in various processes affecting the anterior horn cell. J. Neurol. Sci., 24, 403 - 415.

Stalberg, E.; Trontelji, J.V.; (1979) **Single Fibre Electromyography**, Mirvalle Press, Old Woking.

Strauss, S.; Josato, C.; Armstrong, C.; et al (1985) Persisting illness and fatigue in adults with evidence of Epstein Barr virus infection. Ann. Intern. Med, 102, 7 - 16.

Sultheiss, H.P. (1988) **New Concepts in Viral Heart Disease**. Springer, Berlin.

Thomas, P.K.; (1987) Post viral fatigue syndrome. Lancet, 1, 218 - 219.

Tosato, G.; Strauss, S.; Henle, W.; Pike, S.E.; Blaese, R.M. (1985) Characteristic T-cell dusfunction in patients with chronic active Epstein Barr viral infection. J. Immunol., 134, 3082-3088.

Tracey, K.; Lawry, S.; Beutler, B.; et al (1986) Cahchetin tumor necrosis factor mediates changes of skeletal muscle membrane potential. J. Exp. Med., 164, 1368 - 1373.

Wakefield, D.; Lloyd, A.; (1987) Pathophysiology of myalgic encephalomyelitis. Lancet, i, 125.

Yousef, G.E.; Bell, E.J.; Mann, G.F.; et al (1988) Chronic enterovirus infection in patients with post viral fatigue syndrome. Lancet, 1, 146 - 150.

M.E. / CFS and Central Nervous System Injury

Chapter 48

Magnetic Resonance in the Diagnosis of M.E./CFS, A Review

Byron Hyde, M.D., with the kind assistance of Royce Biddle, M.D. and Thomas McNamara, M.D.

Two very different magnetic resonance tools are technically available to the M.E. / CFS researcher. The least known is spectrography. Magnetic resonance spectrography (MRS) is used to examine the subcellular metabolic properties of intact, living cells. The second and better known technique is imaging. Magnetic resonance imaging (MRI), in this case, investigates gross brain anatomy for pathological or space occupying anomalies. It has the advantage over CT scanning of being technologically better at delineating soft tissue variations.

(Please see Chapter 5 for Dr. Hyde's photograph and curriculum vitae.)

Magnetic Resonance Spectrography (MRS)

When researchers Arnold and Radda published their much quoted paper *"Excessive intracellular acidosis of skeletal muscle on exercise in a patient with a post-viral exhaustion / fatigue syndrome"* in *The Lancet* in 1984[1], there was great excitement that one of the fundamental causes in dysfunction in M.E./CFS had been discovered. The conclusion to their paper was that:

"...muscles demonstrated abnormal early intracellular acidosis for the exercise performed. This was out of proportion to the associated changes in high energy phosphates and may represent excessive lactic acid formation resulting from a disorder of metabolic regulation."[2]

This paper fostered the impression that a key M.E./CFS discovery may have been made. However, no series of similar findings in other M.E./CFS patients were noted and corroborating subsequent publications have not been forthcoming. Why?

In retrospect, the Arnold, Radda paper represented the abnormal findings in a single patient. According to the publication, this was a 30 year old general practitioner, who at the age of 26, had been seriously disabled with chickenpox *"which was accompanied by a confusional state"*.[2] He had demonstrated an EEG anomaly or dysfunction in both the left frontal temporal region and the cerebellar regions. An injury to the left frontal temporal region would be capable of creating problems of rational judgement and an injury to the cerebellum could create ataxia. However, the term confusional state, to my knowledge, is used nowhere in the M.E./CFS literature. It is a term

that is frequently used to describe a psychotic state. Psychosis can occur in M.E./CFS, but is rare.[3]

Adult chicken pox/varicella on the other hand is a highly dangerous and well-known illness that frequently results in death, CNS and/or cardiac injury. It is usually accompanied by severe exhaustion. This is definitely a post-viral injury, but it stretches the imagination to term this patient, post-viral fatigue syndrome. I have no criticism of the spectrographic findings but I do of the diagnosis of M.E./CFS in this patient. The failure to have published similar findings in multiple M.E./CFS patients is suspect.

In 1986, I went to the Radcliffe Infirmary in Oxford and spoke to Dr. Simon Frostick, who was one of the researchers at that time. Dr. Frostick stated that very few of the M.E. /CFS subjects who had been referred to their laboratory had been found to have a reproducible intracellular metabolic dysregulation.

It would appear that this reported 30 year old physician did have demonstrable brain changes and did have muscle metabolism abnormalities, but the MRS findings were not consistent with the majority of other M.E./CFS patients. In all likelihood, I could only conclude that the physician with chickenpox did not have M.E./CFS.

To my knowledge, since 1984, no further supporting papers on the subject have been published from the Radcliffe Infirmary in Oxford. However, in Professor Behan's speech in Hamilton in September 1991, he stated that he had 40 PVFS patients that demonstrated MRS dysfunction. Also, in *Neurology* [13] in

1988, Gross et al. in 23 "Benign Myalgic and Fatigue Syndrome" patients, several pathological intracellular findings were noted.

In another paper[14], Miller et al using NMRS to examine human muscle fatigue in normal patients make many useful observations suggesting that acidosis cannot be the only cause of muscle fatigue, and they suggest other metabolities. They also suggest that "it might be argued that accumulation of It+ is associated with muscle pain, producing a secondary decrease in central activation of the muscle in question...though this might be negligible". They conclude by suggesting that manoeuvres designed to prevent intracellular acidification might lead to decreased muscle fatigue."

In conclusion, NMRS will probably continue to produce useful information on M.E./CFS, however, present publications are insufficient to make statements of any certitude.

Dr. Andrew Penn at the University of Alberta, using similar software and MR spectrography is soon to publish a paper that might clarify this question of M.E./CFS and magnetic resonance spectrography.

Magnetic Resonance Imaging (MRI)

In the same Summer that Arnold and Radda published their intracellular acidosis paper, the now legendary Lake Tahoe epidemic occurred at Incline Village, Nevada. One of the first to study that epidemic using MRI was Dr. Royce Biddle, an MRI specialist at the nearby Reno Diagnostic Center. In the Autumn of 1987, I fortunately came across an unpublished copy of an excellent omnibus paper by Buchwald, Cheney, Peterson, Biddle et al that described the various scientific aspects of the Lake Tahoe epidemic. Their paper was finally published four years later in January 1992.[4]

In 1987 I contacted Dr. Biddle for more details on his magnetic resonance scanner instrument, his technique and findings. At that time, Dr. Biddle felt that his series were not conclusive and that he did not have sufficient controls to clearly make a scientifically acceptable statement.

Dr. Biddle, who then moved to California, referred me to Dr. Frank Jolesz at Brigham and Women's Hospital, Harvard University. Dr. Jolesz had studied a significant series of M.E./CFS patients along with controls. At that time it was felt that the findings of Dr. Jolesz indicated significant CNS abnormalities or small punctuate lesions in the patients with M.E./CFS not seen to the same degree in a comparative group of controls.

However, when I finally did speak with Dr. Jolesz, there had been a significant change in their interpretation of these UBOs. The report on the previous page from Dr. Biddle further clarifies the issue and is also consistent with the opinions of Dr. Jolesz.

The following MRI technical information was supplied by Dr. Biddle:

MRI Technical Information

Scanner

His MRI instrument was a 1.5 Tesla, Superconducting Signa Magnetic Resonance Scanner manufactured by General Electric Corp.

Protocol

His protocol was as follows: Spin echo scans were made. The first series included T1 weighted and proton density weighted sagittal scans. The second echo series were T2 weighted transaxial spin echo scans of the brain. These axial M.R. scans were obtained at 5 mm intervals from the foramen magnum to the vertex, with a skip of 1.2 mm. A repetition time (TR) between 2000 and 2500 m.sec. was utilized as well as an echo delay time (T.E.) between 20-30m.sec. for the first echo and 50-80m.sec. for the second echo. These were obtained with multiecho, multi slice technique.

Anomalies

The anomalies, then identified as UBOs (unidentified bright objects), are very tiny and can be seen only in the second echo, the most T2 weighted scan. That increased signal on a T2 weighted scan basically refers to a focal area of water accumulation.

The Present Consensus on MRI in M.E./CFS

Royce J. Biddle, M.D., Stockton, California

In late 1985, I had the privilege of supervising the start-up of Nevada's first MRI Scanner in Reno, Nevada - a G.E. 1.5 Tesla Signa Scanner. By coincidence, this occurred with the outbreak of an unusual debilitating viral illness in Lake Tahoe which has become known as the Chronic Fatigue Syndrome. These patients were seen by Drs. Dan Peterson and Paul Cheney in their Internal Medicine practice in Incline Village, Nevada. From 1985 through 1988 we performed hundreds of MRI Scans on these patients which showed tiny foci of increased signal intensity in the subcortical white matter on T2-weighted images. I presented these findings at the Annual Meeting of the Western Neuro-Radiological Society in Scottsdale, Arizona in October of 1987. My presentation received a mixed response in keeping with the controversial nature of this disease.

In conjunction with Drs. Peterson and Cheney, Dr. Buchwald and Drs. Komaroff and Jolesz of Harvard, and others, we instituted a review of the MR Scans on 142 of these patients, as well as, a controlled study. We found that the areas of increased signal intensity in the white matter occurred in 79% of the patients with Chronic Fatigue Syndrome and in 21% of the controls. However, the two groups were scanned on two different, though otherwise identical, scanners and, therefore, a truly blinded study was unable to be carried out. The differences between the two groups were statistically significant.

At the 1988 Annual Meeting of the American Society of Neuro-Radiology, several papers were presented stating that the tiny foci of increased signal intensity in the white matter tracts of the brain were Virchow-Robin spaces. These are tiny CSF - containing spaces surrounding the penetrating arterioles of the white matter and other deep structures of the brain and are normal structures. These findings were supported by anatomical-pathological specimens. Currently, most Neuro-Radiologists and MRI Specialists concur and consider these findings to be normal.

The perivascular spaces are known to be the site where lymphocytes and other white blood cells pass from the vascular system to the brain parenchyma. This raises the question as to whether these tiny spaces may be abnormal in patients with Chronic Fatigue Syndrome. The following hypothesis is raised: that the lymphocytes in the Chronic Fatigue Syndrome congregate in the perivascular (Virchow-Robin) spaces of the brain and this explains the more frequent occurrence of the spaces in patients with Chronic Fatigue Syndrome. This hypothesis has not been disproven but requires pathologic proof.

In conclusion, the MRI findings in the Chronic Fatigue Syndrome cannot be used to separate patients with that disease from normal patients. These findings are not thought to be abnormal by most MRI specialists and are highly controversial. These findings do suggest that the disease may involve the perivascular spaces of the brain. Proving or disproving this hypothesis would require pathologic proof which is unlikely to be forthcoming.

End of Dr. Biddle's paper.

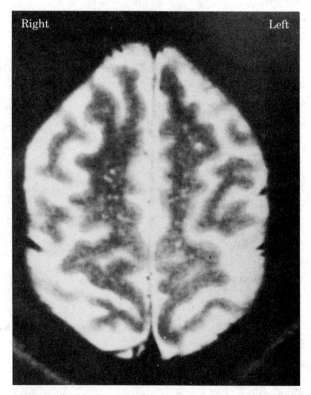

MRI supplied by Dr. Dan Peterson. Note the multiple small patchy UBOs distributed in the white matter of both hemispheres. This MRI has had the UBOs intensified by photographic process, however, they still were clearly visible in the original emulsion.

Further Observations

Another view of these initial studies of the Lake Tahoe group were discussed by Dr. Thomas McNamara at the Third Annual Symposium on Chronic Fatigue Syndrome and the Brain in Los Angeles in 1992.

Dr. McNamara noted the following MRI features of Chronic Fatigue Syndrome.

(1) Low resolution MRI scans gave no indication of UBOs.

(2) No UBOs were detectable in the patients immediately after they fell ill with M.E./CFS but lesions did develop over the first few months. There was a tendency for the lesions to clear with time.

(3) Utilizing a 1.5 tesla resolution, punctate high signal abnormalities were demonstrated. They were referred to as UBOs, unidentified bright objects.

(4) The location of the findings were diverse but UBOs were located primarily in the frontal and parietal lobes just below the grey matter margin. They were located only in the white matter. (It should be noted that the white matter in an MRI appears as grey and thus the white UBOs are quite visible. The grey matter on MRI appears as white and it may be that the white artifacts are simply not visible.) The locations of these lesions were rarely periventricular.

The locations in one study could be subdivided as follows:

white matter	100%
sub cortical	90%
frontal and parietal	70%
occipital	20%
deep	4%
periventricular	2%
brain stem	2%
cerebellum	2%

(5) In the majority of cases there was no correlation between symptom and location.

(6) The UBOs were round or oval in shape, occasionally patchy. They were subdivided into the following groups:

small punctate	86%
larger round	10%
linear	4%

(7) In an initial study utilizing MRI they were able to demonstrate abnormal findings in 36 of 60 M.E./CFS patients, or 60%.

(8) A further study by Drs Biddle and Jolesz was then done to compare MRI findings in normal healthy patients with that of M.E./CFS patients. The findings were as follows:

	tested	UBOs located	Percentage positive
Normal persons	47	10	21%
CFS patients	144	113	78%

(9) It was felt by Dr McNamara that the UBOs represented focal oedema, probably in the perivascular, Virchow Robin spaces. They might also represent areas of demyelination.

Pathological Supporting Evidence

Is there any pathological support for the MRI findings in the literature? What would one look for?

(1) Dilatation of the Virchow Robin spaces would suggest either increased ventricular or spinal fluid pressure.

(2) It could also suggest intracranial arterial or periarterial pathology. In particular, Dr. Biddle suggests that one would expect to find a congregation of lymphocytes in the perivascular spaces around the CNS arteries. Is there evidence of this?

(3) Also it is both my impression and that of Dr. Biddle in earlier conversations that these congested Virchow Robin spaces tend to become more apparent shortly after the illness and tend to decrease in size and sometimes disappear after one year.

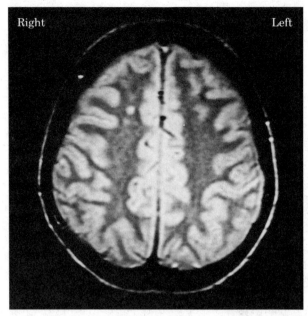

Both MRIs courtesy of Dr. Paul Cheney. Note the very large round UBO in the right frontal lobe with a smaller UBO immediately below it. (The left side of this photograph as it appears, is actually right.)

Note three UBOs, two in the left and right anterior lobes, in the left hemisphere (right side of photograph), there are two UBOs, one in the anterior lobe and the other at the base of what may be the right central gyrus. It is not clearly visible, but there appears to be a string of smaller UBOs between these two larger lesions.

The Literature

Discussion

There is ample evidence that M.E./CFS follows an acute infectious episode, so much so that the British researchers call this illness Post-viral Fatigue Syndrome. This initial acute illness concept is discussed in the cardiovascular review and also in the chapter on the natural history of M.E./CFS Thus, one would anticipate findings to be more apparent in the early days or weeks of the illness.

Evidence of Increased Ventricular or Spinal Fluid (CFS) Pressure

Although the spinal fluid was frequently examined in numerous epidemics, only in a few of the incidences was the CSF pressure recorded. Findings of increased pressure are variable. In the 1934 epidemic, Gilliam states[5] *"Nearly all cases in which the spinal fluid pressure was recorded showed the fluid to be under an increased pressure"*. Pellew[6] states there was no increase in CSF pressure. Lyle[7] states that two subjects had increased CSF pressure but does not state the size of his series. It appears to be small. Fog notes increased CSF pressure in the Danish epidemic[8]

Obviously this area has not been well recorded in the numerous epidemics, however enough data exists to suggest that increased CSF pressure may exist.

Evidence of intracranial arterial pathology

Cumberland Epidemic

There is one M.E./CFS death in the literature that has revealed an artifact that is in an anatomical position similar to that suggested by MRI studies. The report is recorded by Dr. Wallis who refers to the findings of Dr. Klein in his study of the pathology of the 1955 Cumberland epidemic.[9]

The report of Dr. R. Klein of the Crichton Royal, Dumfries states: *"There are in the entire dienencephalon, particularly round the third ventricle numerous small haemorrhages, which extend into the adjacent parts of the mid-brain. Similar haemorrhages can be seen in the corpora mamillare and the supra-mammillary nucleus, the haemorrhages are mostly around small vessels, but some are also to be seen in the free tissue"*[10].

It should be noted that the lesions around the third ventricle could be consistent with the location of pathological Virchow-Robin spaces.

Los Angeles Hospital Epidemic, Animal Experiments

The report on the 1934 epidemic also includes data on experiments in which human M.E./CFS sera was infused into monkeys who, in turn, fell ill. These pathological MRI lesions noted by Dr. Biddle are perhaps consistent with the monkey findings.

"The blood vessels throughout the nervous system were distended with red blood cells....The most characteristic change was the infiltration of the blood vessel walls. This varied from a few round cells to a complete ring. In more advanced cases, the perivascular spaces were packed with cells."[11]

Nightingale Research Foundation Observations

We have now examined approximately 15 patients with the MRI at either the Ottawa General Hospital, the Montreal Neurological Institute or in the United States. There were rarely obvious changes that we could note on these scans that could with confidence be related to M.E./CFS with the exception of one patient with a lesion adjacent to the lateral ventricle.[3] We did find other pathology that allowed us to diagnose two missed cases of M.S., at least one malignancy and a possible post concussion injury. It was of particular interest that each of these four patients had been diagnosed by very competent physicians as anxiety neurosis and the possible M.E./CFS patient as schizophrenic.

Conclusions

Magnetic Resonance Spectrography

From published information, it is not possible to make a case for magnetic resonance spectrography as having demonstrated cellular metabolic changes in a series of M.E./CFS patients. Further publications may alter that view.

Magnetic Resonance Imaging

All patients suspected of being afflicted with M.E./CFS should receive the benefit of an immediate MRI examination to rule out potentially treatable pathology and to maximize pathological findings that peak in the early stages of disease.

There appear to have been statistically significant anatomical changes in MRI's of patients with M.E./CFS.

These are either dilated Virchow-Robin spaces or small CNS lesions, termed UBOs, and they are more common in M.E./CFS patients than in normal controls.

Peer pressure in a disease met with considerable peer skepticism and lack of any supportive (or contrary) publications may be contributing to the scientific caution of Dr. Biddle and Dr. Jolesz.

A negative MRI report may be related to (a) a low tesla resolution machine; (b) a high tesla machine running below its normal resolution. this can be done by rapidly running the patient through the machine resulting in a decreased resolution but a higher payload for the machine, (c) to further economize by decreasing the size of the emulsion image and again losing resolution.

Though MRI may be statistically significant in a series of M.E./CFS patients, and particularly in the first year of disease, it is not at present seen as a useful tool in the diagnosis of individual M.E./CFS patients. It is a useful tool in the field of M.E./CFS research.

A recent announcement by HEM research[12] equates improvement of M.E./CFS patients with the use of Ampligen. Those patients who were found to have most improvement with treatment were those with observed MRI lesions.

M.E./CFS is a disease that elicits incredible positive and negative emotional attitudes in both patients and physicians. If a radiologist does not believe that M.E./CFS exists as a valid diagnosis, he may well overlook the indications of this disorder. Correct technique in a scanner of high resolution is essential in the examination of M.E./CFS patients.

Neuroradiologists tend to look for sclerotic plaques, malignancies and stroke anomalies in MRI scans. When the MRIs of M.E./CFS patients are examined,

UBOs and small sclerotic plaques are quite insignificant in the scale of things and these scans are routinely called normal. This is not a criticism of radiologists but an MRI reported as normal may actually contain pathology and the monitor or negatives should always be examined by the treating physician.

Neuroradiologists who read from the emulsion and not from the monitor, are not likely to take advantage of the available technology inherent in the MRI scanner.

Those few institutions that have MRI (anatomy) and PET (function) technology connected in tandem, are those most likely to resolve the problem of the role of the MRI in the diagnosis of M.E./CFS. At present, magnetic resonance is not a technology of choice in the diagnosis of M.E./CFS Larger and well funded studies are apparently in progress and will hopefully further clarify the role of magnetic resonance in M.E./CFS patients.

References

1. Arnold D.L., Radda G.K., Bore P.J. Styles P. Taylor D.J. Excessive intracellular acidosis of skeletal muscle on exercise in a patient with a post-viral exhaustion/fatigue syndrome" The Lancet, Saturday 23, 1984, pg 1367-1369.

2. Arnold D. Idem (1) page 1367

3. Patient D. M. a university student who attended Nightingale clinic with an intital diagnosis of Schizophrenia following a viral infection. This 23 year old patient demonstrated a .5 by 1.0 cm plaque in the area of the lateral ventricle on MRI his M.E./CFS and schizophrenia resolved completely within 8 months. He returned to university, graduated and has been well for the past three years.

4. Paper published by Buchwald D., Cheney P.,Peterson D., Henry B., Wormsley S., Geiger A., Ablashi D., Salahuddin S., Saxinger C., Biddle R., Kikinis R., Jolesz F., Folks T., Balachandran N., Peter J., Gallo R., and Komaroff A. A Chronic Illness Characterized by Fatigue, Neurologic and Immunologic Disorders, and Active Human Herpesvirus Type 6 Infection, Annals of Internal Medicine, pg 103-113Vol 116, No 2. Jan 15, 1992.

5. Gilliam, A.G., **Epidemiological Study of an Epidemic, Diagnosed as Poliomyelitis, Occurring Among the Personnel of The Los Angeles County General Hospital During The Summer of 1934,** Public Health Bulletin No. 240, April 1938, The United States Public Health Service, page 33.

6. Pellew RAA. Clinical description of disease resembling poliomyelitis, seen in Adelaide, 1949-1951, (1951) Med.J.Australia, I, 944-946.

7. Lyle W.H. An Outbreak of Disease Believed to Have Been Caused by EDHO 9 Virus, Vol 5, No. 2, pg 248-269.

8. Fog, T. Neuritis Vegetativa Epidemica, Ugeskrift for Laeger, Vol. 115, Jul. Sept. 1953, pp. 1244 1250.

9. Wallis A.L. An **Investigation into an unusual disease seen in epidemic and sporadic form in a general practice in Cumberland in 1955 and subsequent years,** Doctoral Thesis, University of Edinburgh (1957).

10. Wallis A.L. idem(9) pages 46-48.

11. Van Wart R. Courville C. Hall E.M. 1934 Epidemic of Poliomyelitis in Los Angeles, American Journal of Public Health, Vol 24, Number 12 pg 1207-1209.

12. HEM presentation, Chicago 1991 These results apparently originate from and will be published by the Lake Tahoe group.

13. Gross B., Glasberg M. et al, 31-P NMR Spectroscopy and Histochemical Study of Benign Myalgic and Fatigue Syndrome, Neurology, (New York) March 1988, 38 (Supplement 1) 410.

14. Miller R., Boska M., et al, Nuclear Magnetic Resonance in Human Muscle Fatigue, The Journal of Clinical Investigation, vol 81, April 1988, 1190-1196.

Chapter 49

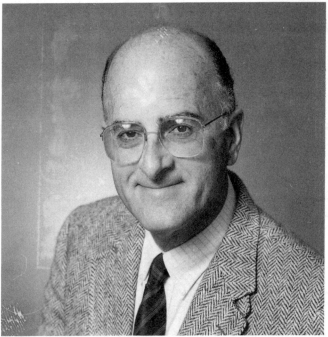

Ismael Mena

Study of Cerebral Perfusion by NeuroSPECT in Patients with Chronic Fatigue Syndrome

Ismael Mena, MD and Javier Villanueva-Meyer, MD Harbor-UCLA Medical Center, Torrance, California, U.S.A.

Dr. Ismael Mena is a diplomat of the American Board of Nuclear Medicine and one of the foremost experts in his field worldwide. His speaking engagements span the globe and he has contributed over 200 abstracts, papers and book chapters. Among his many awards, he has received the Norman Poe Memorial Award of the Society of Nuclear Medicine, the American Cancer Society Award of Merit, and the Distinguished Scientist Award of the Western Chapter of the Society of Nuclear Medicine.

NeuroSPECT, by means of a dedicated brain imaging device, generates both quantitative measurements of rCBF with ^{133}Xe and high resolution images of distribution of cerebral perfusion in gray matter and basal ganglia by means of ^{99m}Tc-HMPAO. Quantitative measurements of rCBF with ^{133}Xe are displayed in a color coded functional image calibrated in ml/min/100g of tissue. ^{133}Xe rCBF is measured by sequential 1 minute acquisition of transaxial cuts of the brain during a 5 minute acquisition. rCBF is calculated from the washout of ^{133}Xe by means of the Kety-Schmidt equation. Immediately after the completion of the ^{133}Xe rCBF measurements, 20 mCi of HMPAO ^{99m}Tc are injected intravenously and imaging begins 1 hour later during a 30 minute period. Twelve 1.6 cm thick transaxial

adjacent cuts of the brain are gathered and displayed in a color scale for visual comparison. These studies are qualitative, and the analysis reports a comparison with adjacent and opposite side lobes. We report on findings of cerebral perfusion in 46 patients with chronic fatigue syndrome.

Results: 46 patients with chronic fatigue syndrome, 30 females age 43 ± 11 years and 16 males 41 ± 9 years are compared with 10 normal individuals. rCBF with ^{133}Xe demonstrates a mean of the right temporal lobe of 59 ± 14 ml/min/100g in the CFS group versus 69 ± 3 ml/min/100g in normal controls ($p < 0.05$). Left temporal, parietal and frontal relative hypoperfusion is not significantly different from values observed in the normal controls. Differences of rCBF are assessed between both temporal lobes and were found to be 22% ± 16 in the CFS group the normal controls (p < 0.001). Asymmetry of perfusion in parietal and frontal lobe was found to be nonsignificantly different from normal controls. 71% of patients had either unilateral temporal hypoperfusion (65%) or bilateral temporal hypoperfusion in (6%).

> It is concluded that the high percentage of patients with chronic fatigue syndrome present with cerebral cortical hypoperfusion in the temporal lobes, most frequently unilaterally and in 6% of the patients bilaterally.

The purpose of this report is to evaluate regional cerebral blood flow in patients with chronic fatigue syndrome. The advent of nuclear medicine single photon emission computed tomography (SPECT) with brain dedicated imaging devices lends itself to quantitative analysis of rCBF and high resolution qualitative evaluation of CBF in the brain cortex.

> The accuracy and reproducibility of these measurements are justification to evaluate possible cerebral perfusion abnormalities in patients with chronic fatigue syndrome. The hypothesis is that most probably temporal lobe perfusion defects may fingerprint primary inflammatory changes or secondary vascular impairment in these patients.

Materials and methods.

Brain SPECT

Instrumentation

Dedicated brain imaging device

The dedicated brain imaging devices are the equipment of choice for high resolution imaging and even more important to obtain ^{133}Xe SPECT rCBF quantitative images.

We have extensive clinical experience with a multiring system that allows sequential performance of both [133]Xe rCBF SPECT and [^{99m}Tc]HMPAO SPECT in each patient[19]. For [133]Xe rCBF measurements, a high sensitivity fan beam collimator is used. The acquisition process consists of movements of the collimator and the detector ring. Three slices are gathered simultaneously, the first 2 cm above the orbitomeatal line with 2 cm interslice spacing. Sequential 1 minute images each are gathered for the 3 slices during 6 minutes. Display of the rCBF images is achieved using a color scale that is coded to ml/100g/min.

Imaging of [^{99m}Tc]HMPAO distribution in cerebral cortex follows using high resolution collimation. Simultaneously, 3 brain slices 16 mm thick and separated by 3.2 cm. are gathered. By means of bed shifts, the blind interslice area is covered and 12 slices are acquired in 30 minutes. A resolution of 8 mm in the periphery and 9.6 mm at the level of the basal ganglia is achieved and compares favorably to the 15 mm resolution of the rotating gamma camera. Coronal and sagittal reconstructions complement the transaxial slices. The coronal slices are particularly useful to evaluate the temporal lobes while the sagittal slices evaluate the frontal lobes.

Radiopharmaceuticals

Single Photon Brain Radiopharmaceuticals

[133]Xe regional cerebral blood flow (rCBF) was developed by Lassen[3]. This technique is quantitative but has low resolution (22mm), and needs in many instances to be complemented with high resolution ^{99m}Tc radiopharmaceutical imaging. Absolute regional blood flow quantification has been achieved and extensive work has been reported by Raynaud[22], and Lassen, et al.[3]

Iodoamphetamines. The production of ^{123}I by (p,5n) reaction, free of [124]I contamination, has improved significantly the quality and reproducibility of brain imaging, while development of a special collimator system has contributed to improvement in imaging. These amines distribute in brain as a function of perfusion and there is an apparent redistribution phenomenon due to the slower washout in the areas of underperfusion, thus these areas appear better perfused in late images three to four hours after the injection. There are also, however, other interpretations of this phenomenon[22].

Cyclic amines. [99mTc] propylene amine oxime (PNAO) and hexamethylpropylene amine oxime (HMPAO) were developed about three years ago, and more recently [99mTc] ethyl cysteinate dimer (ECD) was investigated. These agents, in particular HMPAO, provide excellent images of gray matter and basal ganglia as they distribute in the brain, as a function of brain perfusion. The uptake in brain is completed in 5 to 15 minutes, and there is significant stability of the images during the next two to three hours. This stability may be related to chemical or optical changes in HMPAO forms. The great advantage is the labeling with [99mTc]; it is optimal to image and offers economic advantages over [123I][12, 13].

Receptor binding agents. A muscarinic acetylcholine receptor imaging radiopharmaceutical (MACHR) labeled with [123I] was developed by Eckelman, et al. It is a forerunner of receptor specific binding for SPECT imaging. All other receptor binding agents have been developed using Carbon 11 or Fluorine 18 positron emitters.

[133Xe] rCBF measurements are gathered after inhalation of 30 mCi of this radioactive gas. Quantitative measurements of rCBF with [133Xe] are displayed in a color coded functional image calibrated in ml/min/100g of tissue. [133Xe] is measured by sequential 1 minute acquisition of transaxial cuts of the brain during a 5 minute acquisition. rCBF is calculated from the washout of [133Xe] applied on a pixel by pixel basis by means of the Kety-Schmidt equation[1]. Normal values for adults, age less than 50 years, fluctuate between 60-80 ml/100g/min. of gray matter.

Immediately after the completion of the [133Xe] rCBF measurement, 20 mCi of HMPAO [99mTc] are injected intravenously and imaging begins 1 hour later during a 30 minute period. Twelve 1.6 cm thick transaxial adjacent cuts of the brain are gathered and displayed in a color scale for visual comparison. These studies are qualitative, and the analysis reports a comparison with adjacent and opposite side lobes.

Patient population.

46 patients suffering of different degrees of chronic fatigue syndrome (kindly referred by Jay Goldstein, M.D.) were studied in a blind fashion. 30 were females ages 43 ± 11 years (mean $\pm$ S.D.) and 16 were males 41 ± 9 years. They were compared with 10 normal individuals. 3 were females ages 47-55 years, and 7 were males ages 22-51. Normal individuals had negative medical history, negative physical examination, negative neurological and psychiatric examinations.

Table 1					
	Chronic Fatigue S		Normal controls		
	mean	SD	mean	SD	p
R temp	59.3	14.1	69.2	3.2	.043
L temp	59	16	68.1	3.1	.098
R pariet	48.8	11.1	54.4	10.4	.160
L pariet	47.3	10.9	50.5	7.7	.400
R front	58.1	16.4	61	13.9	.622
L front	54.1	17.6	61	13.9	.273

Data analysis

We report on quantitative data gathered with ^{133}Xe. ^{133}Xe was calculated for each cerebral lobe, differences among contralateral lobes were calculated and a comparison with ^{133}Xe in chronic fatigue syndrome and normals was established for both categories. The results are reported as mean ± SD.

Results

rCBF lobar comparison

Table 1 demonstrates a mean difference of 10 ml/min/100g in the right temporal lobe in comparison with normal population, significant at 0.043 level. All other areas analyzed were not statistically different, and a display of the actual data is done in figures 1, 2 and 3.

Figure 3

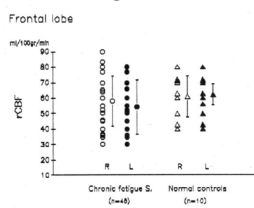

Figure 1

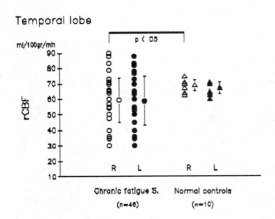

Figures 4, 5 and 6 depict differences of temporal, parietal and frontal lobe pairs expressed in ml/min/100g. Differences in temporal lobes are significant p < 0.001 level. 30 of 46 patients showed significant differences while an additional 3 patients presented with bilateral temporal hypoperfusion. Of the unilateral hypoperfusion group, 15 patients presented with right temporal hypoperfusion and 15 patients with left temporal hypoperfusion. Therefore 71% of patients exhibited with unilateral or bilateral hypoperfusion. The frequency of temporal hypoperfusion was not sex related, 21% ± 17 in 30 females and 25% ± 15 in 16 males. Differences from parietal and frontal lobes were not significantly different. Qualitative high resolution studies with ^{99m}Tc HMPAO confirmed the ^{133}Xe rCBF observations.

Figure 2

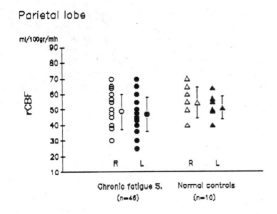

Figure 4

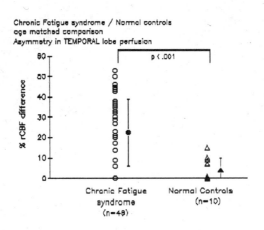

Figure 5

Figure 6

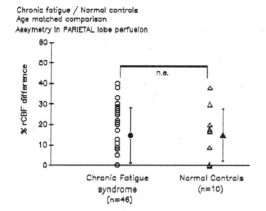

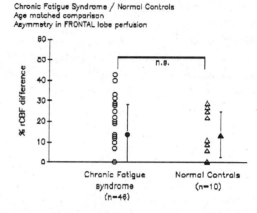

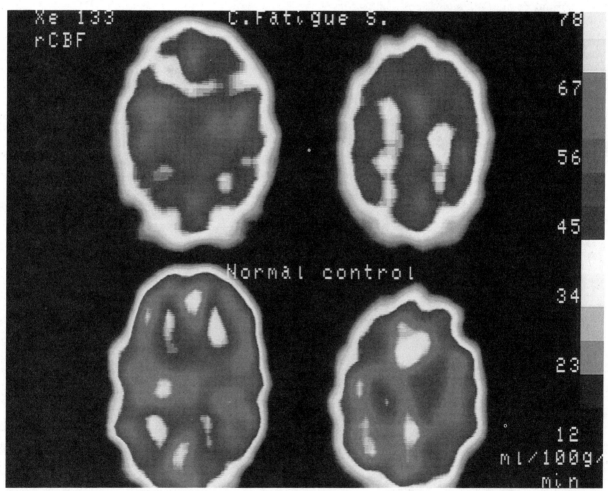

Functional transaxial images of rCBF in a patient with chronic fatigue syndrome and a normal control. The images denote frontal lobe perfusion in the top, occipital lobe in the bottom, left and right are demarcated. Color scale is calibrated in ml/min/100g, with a maximum of 79 ml/min/100g, (normal 60-80 ml/min/100g). The 2 top images demonstrate hypoperfusion at the 35 ml/min/100g level in both anterior temporal lobes and posteroparietal lobes. The maximum appears at 68 ml/min/100g. The control patient demonstrates blood flow fluctuating between 46 ml/min/100g and a maximum of 79 ml/min/100g, with the majority of the areas of the brain perfused at 55-70 ml/min/100g.

Discussion

Quantitative analysis of regional cerebral blood flow (rCBF) in patients of chronic fatigue syndrome (CFS) has demonstrated a heterogeneous population, with 71% of patients presenting with unilateral or bilateral temporal lobe hypoperfusion, with the interlobar differences at a level of diminution of 25% versus a difference of 4% in normal individuals.

This presentation refers to quantitative low resolution studies gathered with a brain dedicated imaging device and a radioactive gas ^{133}Xe, complemented by high resolution studies performed by means of ^{99m}Tc HMPAO, a lipophilic oxime. The resolution of the latter radiopharmaceutical provides images with resolution of 8 mm in the cortex and 9.5 mm in the basal ganglia.

Quantitative measurements with ^{133}Xe are a function of (a) cerebral blood flow, and (b) hypothetically on the cellular lipid content. Lipids are capable of trapping ^{133}Xe as they are highly lipophilic, therefore rendering the washout of the gas from the intracellular space slower. The effect of this phenomenon may be a diminution of rCBF values calculated from the intracerebral washout slopes. On the other hand, studies of cerebral perfusion with HMPAO are more difficult to interpret as the diminished uptake of this oxime can be interpreted as due to: (a) diminished rCBF, (b) inflammatory regional changes, (c) focal cerebral edema, (d) changes in blood brain barrier, (e) cellular hypoperfusion or cellular death.

Temporal lobe hypoperfusion is not sex related as values of 21% $\pm$ 17 were recorded in females and 25% $\pm$ 15 in man.

A very significant percentage of patients studied with this diagnosis (71%) present with unilateral or bilateral pattern of hypoperfusion in the temporal lobes. The etiology of this phenomenon is a matter of further study, and requires clinical psychometric and EEG mapping correlations.

Acknowledgement

The author acknowledges with thanks the referral of the patients with chronic fatigue syndrome by Dr. Jay Goldstein.

References

1. Kety SS. Theory and applications of the exchange of inert gas at the lungs and tissues. Pharmacol Rev 1951; 3:1-41.

2. Obrist WD, Thompson HK, Wang HS, Wilkinson WE. Regional cerebral blood flow estimated by 133Xenon inhalation. Stroke 1975; 6:245-256.

3. Kanno I, Lassen NA. Two methods for calculating regional cerebral blood flow from emission computed tomography of inert gas concentrations. J Comp Assist Tomogr 1979; 3:71-76.

4. Celsis P, Goldman T, Henriksen L, et al. A method for calculating regional cerebral blood flow from emission computed tomography of inert gas concentration. J Comp Assist Tomogr 1981; 5:641-645.

5. Atkins HL, Robertson JS, Croft BY, et al. Estimates of radiation absorbed doses from radioxenons in lung imaging. J Nuc Med 1980; 21:459-465.

6. Sharp PF, Smith FW, Gemmell HG, et al. Technetium-99m HM-PAO stereoisomers as potential agents for imaging regional cerebral blood flow: human volunteer studies. J Nuc Med 1986; 27:171-177.

7. Anderson AR, Friberg H, Knudsen KBM, et al. Extraction of [^{99m}Tc]-d,l-HMPAO across the blood-brain barrier. J of Cerebral Blood Flow and Metabolism 1988; 8:S44-S51.

8. De Jong BM, Van Royen EA. Uptake of SPECT radiopharmaceuticals in neocortical brain cultures. Eur J Nucl Med 1989; 15:16-20.

9. Villanueva-Meyer J, Thompson D, Mena I, Marcus CS. Lacrimal gland dosimetry with [^{99m}Tc]HMPAO. J Nuc Med 1990; in press.

10. Amersham Corporation. Package insert. Ceretec™ kit for the preparation of technetium ^{99m}Tc exametazime injection. Code N.159Z.

11. Walovitch RC, Hill TC, Garrity S et al. Characterization of Technetium-99m-L,L,-ECD for brain perfusion imaging, Part 1: Pharmacology of technetium-99m ECD in nonhuman primates. J Nuc Med 1989; 30:1892-1901.

12. Leveile J, Demonceau G, De Roo M, et al. Characterization of Technetium-99m-L,L,-ECD for brain perfusion imaging, Part 2: Biodistribution and brain imaging in humans. J Nuc Med 1989; 30:1902-1910.

13. Holman BL, Hellman RS, Goldsmith SJ, et al. Biodistribution, dosimetry and clinical evaluation of technetium-99m ethyl cysteinate dimer in normal subjects and in patients with chronic cerebral infarction. J Nuc Med 1989; 30:1018-1024.

14. Winchell HS, Baldwin RM, Lin TH. Development of 123-labelled amines for brain studies: Localization of 123-iodophenylalkyl amines in rat brain. J Nucl Med 1980; 21:940-946.

15. Baldwin RM, Wu JL. In vivo chemistry of iofetamine HCL iodine-123 (IMP). J Nucl Med 1988 29:122-124.

16. Obrist WD, Thompson HK, King CH, Wang HS. Determination of regional cerebral blood flow by inhalation of 133Xenon. Circ Res 1967; 20:124-135.

17. Hagstadius S, Risberg J. Regional cerebral blood flow characteristics and variations with age in resting normal subjects. Brain and cognition 1989; 10:28-43.

18. Lavy S, Melamed E, Bentin S, Cooper G, Rinot Y. Bihemispheric decreases in regional cerebral blood flow in dementia: correlation with age-matched normal controls. Ann Neurol 1978; 4:445-450.

19. Hirose Y, Ikeda Y, Higashi K, Koga K, Hattori H. A hybrid emission CT - Headtome II. IEEE Transactions on Nuclear Science 1982; NS-29:1:520-523.

20. Haxby JV. Evidence of metabolic heterogeneity from positron emission tomography studies, pp 300-302. In Friedland RP, moderator. Alzheimer disease: clinical and biological heterogeneity. Ann Intern Med 1988; 109:298-311.

21. Chollet F, Celsis P, Clanet M, Guiraud-Chaumeil B, Rascol A, Marc-Verges JP. SPECT study of cerebral blood flow reactivity after acetazolamide in patients with transient ischemic attacks. Stroke 1989; 20:458-464.

22. Raynaud C, Rancurel Y, Samson JC et al. Pathophysiologic study of chronic infarcts with I-123 isopropyl iodo-amphetamine (IMP): The importance of the periinfarct area. Stroke 1987; 18:21-29.

23. Raynaud C, Rancurel G, Tzourio N, et al. SPECT analysis of recent cerebral infarction. Stroke 1989; 20:192-204.

24. Mountz JM, Modell JG, Foster NL, et al. Prognostication of recovery following stroke using the comparison of CT and technetium-99m HM-PAO SPECT. J Nucl Med 1990; 31:61-66.

25. Chang Chui H. Dementia. A review emphasizing clinicopathologic correlation and brain-behavior relationships. Arch Neurol 1989; 46:806-814.

26. Hachinsky VC, Iliff LD, Zilhka E, et al. Cerebral blood flow in dementia. Arch Neurol 1975; 32:632-637.

27. Thompson CJ, Mena F J, Villanueva-Meyer J, Mena I. Method of quantitative analysis of [^{99m}Tc]HMPAO SPECT studies in patients with Alzheimer's disease. J Nuc Med 1989; 30:806.

28. Marciano DM, Black K, Phelps ME, Hawkins RA. Evaluation of brain tumors with ^{201}Tl SPECT studies: Correlation with histological results. Clin Nuc Med 1988; 95:10

Chapter 50

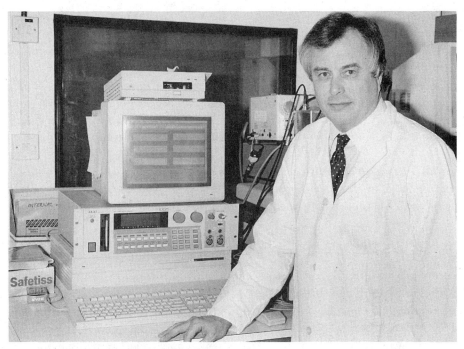

Leslie Findley

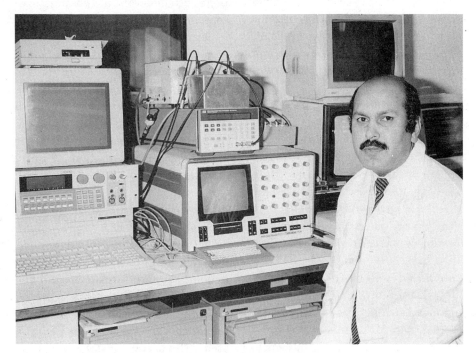

Deepak Prasher

Multi-modality Sensory and Auditory Cognitive Event-related Potentials in Myalgic Encephalomyelitis and Multiple Sclerosis

Deepak Prasher, MD and Leslie Findley, MD

Medical Research Council, Human Movement and Balance Unit, Section of Neuro-Otology, National Hospital Queen Square, London UK

and

Regional Centre for Neurology and Neurosurgery, Oldchurch Hospital, Romford, Essex UK

Dr. Findley is a Consultant Neurologist at the Regional Centre for Neurology and Neurosurgery at Oldchurch Hospital and Senior Lecturer in Neurology in the MRC Human Movement and Balance Unit, The National Hospital for Nervous Diseases, Queen Square, London. In addition, he is Consultant Neurologist to the Queen Elizabeth Military Hospital in Woolwich. Dr. Findley's research interest includes Movement disorders, with particular emphasis on tremor. In the MRC Human Movement and Balance Unit with Dr. Deepak Prasher, his research has been concerned with the evaluation of cognitive evoked potentials (P300) in all subjects and in patients with diffuse and focal brain disorders. In the last two years, he has made a specific comparative study on cognitive evoked potentials, sensory evoked potentials in fatigue syndromes, including M.E.

Dr. Prasher is a PhD Research Scientist with the Medical Research Council. The Human Movement and Balance Unit is interested in clinical neurophysiology and is at present engaged in research in cognitive processing of auditory information processing in normal subjects and patients with central nervous system disorders.

Introduction

Myalgic Encephalomyelitis (M.E.) is a form of chronic post-viral fatigue syndrome which has in the past occurred in epidemic form in several places and has been variously referred to as Royal Free disease, Iceland disease, epidemic neuromyasthenia, and Akureyri disease.[1-3] With its occurrence in epidemic form, absence of any abnormalities on clinical examination, normal routine laboratory investigations and concurrent neuropsychiatric symptoms, doubt was cast upon its organic basis.[4,5]

However, the 1978 international symposium on M.E. at the Royal Society of Medicine[3] concluded that this was a specific disease of viral origin with little evidence of it being a hysterical phenomenon. More recently, the use of the term post infection fatigue syndrome or chronic fatigue syndrome have been suggested[6,7] with several reports [8-10] linking this syndrome with evidence of recent infection by many viruses including Coxsackie A and B, varicella, influenza, and Epstein-Barr. Behan et al.[11] have found antibodies to Coxsackie virus in 70% of their 50 cases and Calder et al.[8] found 46% in their 140 cases compared with 25% in controls. McCartney et al.[12] found specific immunoglobulin (IgM) Coxsackie antibodies in 31% of 118 patients. Yousef et al.[13] reported an enterovirus-group-specific monoclonal antibody which detected enteroviral antigen in the circulation in 51% of their 87 cases. These studies suggest that there are a group of symptoms which are associated with evidence of persistent infection and immunological dysfunction.[11,14,15]

The characteristic features of M.E. are fluctuating fatiguability and myalgia even after minor physical effort. Other symptoms vary from episode to episode in an individual and across patients [6,7] Symptoms which may reflect central nervous system dysfunction are common and include muscle weakness, headache, sensory disturbances, poor short term memory, impairment of concentration and sleep disorders.

Standard electromyography (EMG) has failed to show any definite abnormalities in M.E. However, abnormally increased jitter potentials have been reported[16] with single-fibre EMG but without any impulse blocking which, according to Lloyd et al[17], would not account for the symptom of muscle fatigue in this disorder.

In view of the fact that many patients with M.E. experience some sensory and cognitive disturbances, we decided to examine objectively for evidence of this by using multi-modality sensory evoked potentials and auditory event-related cognitive potentials and comparing these responses to patients with early but definite multiple sclerosis (MS). These potentials result from the synchronous neural activity associated with a particular stimulus or process. Electrical activity time locked and influenced primarily by the physical characteristics of the eliciting stimulus is referred to as the exogenous sensory potentials. By providing information regarding the functional state of the specific pathways stimulated, auditory brainstem, somatosensory and visual evoked potentials have become extremely useful in clinical diagnosis especially in the separation of peripheral from central nervous system disorders, detection of space occupying lesions and demyelination (for reviews see Chiappa[18] and Halliday[19]).

The electrical responses which are primarily affected by the cognitive processes associated with task demands rather than the physical attributes of the stimulus allow inferences to be made regarding the sequence and timing of stimulus evaluation and response selection and execution.[20] Tasks which readily yield a cognitive potential consist of identifying a particular stimulus (target) in a series of randomly presented stimuli which differ in some form or dimension and classifying each according to a defined criterion.

The psychological processes involved in the identification and classification of a specific stimulus or event lead to the appearance of a characteristic response wave in the target average and is usually referred to by its polarity and modal latency as P300 or simply P3 (event related potential [ERP]). It has been linked with memory mechanisms[21,22] and its latency is affected by task complexity[23], aging[24] and has been shown to be prolonged in patients with dementia.[25,26]

Both global and focal cognitive impairment is common in MS but the cognitive ERPs have been neglected as a possible method for the evaluation of these deficits. Because of the similarities in the initial symptoms of some patients with MS and those with M.E. and in view of the neuro-psychological disturbances in these patients, this study examined cognitive potentials, reaction time and performance measures to ascertain the patients' ability to conduct discrimination tasks of varying difficulty.

Methods
Patients

The control group consisted of 68 (35 female) subjects with a mean age of 40 (SD=14) years and the patient groups comprised of 37 (28 female) ME patients (25 with enteroviral antigen (VP1) positive) with a mean age of 39 (SD=13) years, and 40 MS patients (35 MRI positive) with a mean age of 40 (SD=9) years.

Diagnostic criteria

ME: Symptomatic for more than six months (mean duration 60 months)

Preceding febrile illness (presumed viral)

Persistent or relapsing debilitating fatigue
Myalgia which increases following exercise
Poor concentration and memory
Other general or neurological disorders excluded by full clinical examination and haematological, biochemical and immunological screening.

MS: Diagnosed clinically by the presence of relapsing and remitting lesions in the central nervous system white matter separated in space and time. All patients had been referred to the neurological clinic at a district general hospital (Harold Wood Hospital, Romford, Essex) and were untreated at the time of testing.

The evoked potential testing was carried out independently (DKP) at the National Hospital without reference to a diagnosis (blind assessment).

Procedure

Brainstem, visual and somatosensory potentials were recorded using a Medelec Mistral EP system. Silver/silver chloride EEG electrodes were attached to the scalp with collodion and on the mastoids with double sided adhesive discs. Electrode impedance was reduced by slight abrasion of the skin with a blunt needle such that the impedance was below 3000 ohms.

Brainstem Potentials were recorded using alternating polarity click stimulation at a repetition rate of 10Hz from Cz-A1 and Cz-A2 electrode positions with forehead as ground. Responses were amplified (50000 times) and filtered (100-3000 Hz) before 1024 sweeps were averaged for both right and left ear stimulation. Response window was 10 ms with a cursor latency resolution of 0.02ms per point.

Visual Potentials were recorded from three electrodes placed 5cm on either side of a midline electrode 2 cm above the inion. All occipital (01, Oz and O2) electrodes were referred to a midfrontal electrode with mastoid acting as ground. A checkerboard pattern reversal stimulus generated by the Mistral system was used to elicit the responses. The subject viewed the pattern (checksize=20mm, reversal rate 1 Hz) from a distance of one metre. Brightness and contrast were kept constant. Responses were filtered such that the bandpass was 1-125 Hz. Analysis time was set to 300ms and 64 sweeps were averaged for

Figure 1a

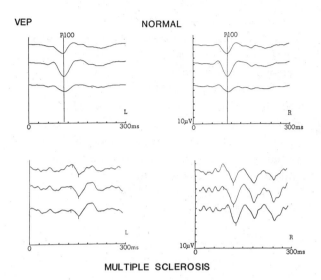

Representative a) pattern reversal visual

each response. Latencies were measured under cursor control with a time resolution of 0.6ms.

Somatosensory potentials were recorded to median nerve stimulation from cervical spine at Cv2 and 2cm posterior to C3 and C4 electrode positions in the 10-20 system. All electrodes were referred to Fz with an earth strap attached proximal to the stimulation at the wrist on the arm being stimulated. Constant current electrical stimulation at a repetition rate of 2Hz with a pulse duration of 0.3ms at an intensity just above motor threshold was used to record the responses. Filter bandpass was set at 30-3000 Hz and an analysis window of 30 ms. 256 sweeps were averaged for each response. Latencies quoted were measured with a time revolution of 0.1ms.

Cognitive Potentials

Two auditory discrimination tasks were used to elicit cognitive potentials.
1. Frequency discrimination: 1.0kHz versus 1.5kHz tone burst of 100ms.
2. Duration discrimination: 200ms versus 100ms tone burst of 1.0kHz.

Subjects were seated in a comfortable chair and listened through headphones (TDH39) to a sequence of tone bursts presented at a rate of one every 3 seconds and their task was to press a response button

as quickly as possible only when the target tone was heard. Reaction time from the onset of tone burst to the button press was recorded. The target for the frequency task was the higher frequency tone burst and for the duration task, the shorter duration burst. The discrimination of duration was judged by a majority of the subjects to be more difficult than the frequency discrimination task. For each task a total of 100 stimuli were presented binaurally at 60dBHL in a random sequence with a ratio of targets to non targets of 30/70. Subjects' performance in terms of the number of targets correctly identified and the number missed and wrongly identified as targets was monitored. Reaction Time (RT) was recorded with a resolution of 0.1 ms.

Electrical activity was recorded from three electrode sites in the International 10:20 system, namely Fz, Cz, Pz with reference to mastoid. Responses were amplified (50000 times), filtered (0.3Hz-32Hz) and averaged using HP9836 computer. 768 points were sampled at a rate of 1kHz giving a window of 768 ms. Latencies quoted are those taken from the Pz electrode position.

Figure 1b

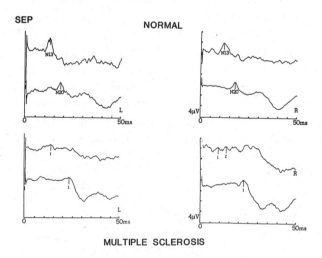

b) median nerve somatosensory

Results
Sensory Potentials

Mean and standard deviation of the latencies of brainstem, visual and somatosensory potentials are

Table 1			
Mean (SD) of latencies of major components of sensory potentials in normals and patients with MS and ME			
	Normals	MS	ME	t-test Sig. Prob. Normals vs MS
Number of subjects	70	40	37	
Age	40.5 (14.4)	40.1 (8.8)	39.4 (13.1)	0.854
VEP P100	96.1 (7.4)	110.8 (19.2)	94.6 (7.3)	0.0001*
AEP Wave I	1.65 (0.16)	1.66 (0.22)	1.60 (0.14)	0.983
AEP Wave III	3.78 (0.18)	3.81 (0.28)	3.78 (0.21)	0.965
AEP Wave V	5.73 (0.19)	6.04 (0.51)	5.70 (0.22)	0.009*
SEP N13	13.0 (1.02)	13.7 (1.03)	13.05 (1.1)	0.009*
SEP N20	18.55 (1.3)	20.3 (3.2)	18.65 (1.3)	0.001*

Normals vs ME: No significant difference.

shown in Table 1 for both control subjects and patients with M.E. and MS. No significant differences in the major component latencies for any of the sensory potentials were found between controls and

Figure 1c

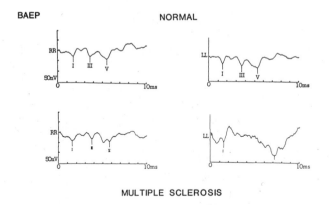

c) auditory brainstem potentials from a normal subject and a patient with MS.

patients with M.E. either with VP1 positive or negative. None of the responses recorded from the patients lay outside the two standard deviation limit from the normal mean. In contrast, the mean difference between the controls and patients with MS in all the major components of the sensory potentials was significant (Table 1). Representative brainstem, visual and somatosensory potential recordings from a control subject and a patient with MS are shown in Figure 1. 31 (78%) of the 40 MS patients had at least one sensory potential abnormal whilst 9 (22.5%) had all three modalities abnormal.

Cognitive Potentials: M.E.

Cognitive event-related potential latencies for each component for both frequency and duration discrimination tasks for controls and patients with M.E. and MS are shown in Table 2. In contrast to the sensory potentials, significant differences in the mean latencies of the cognitive potential N2 (p<.05) and P3 (p<0.001) were found between controls and patients with M.E. for the more difficult duration discrimination task but not for the standard "oddball" frequency discrimination task. Reaction time for both frequency and duration discrimination tasks were significantly (p<0.001) prolonged in comparison with the control subjects. Performance measures in terms of errors in identification of correct target or misclassifying a target (omission and commission) were not significantly increased for either frequency or duration tasks. A statistical comparison between the mean latencies of the major components of the cognitive potentials, reaction time and performance on the basis of the VP1 test showed no significant difference in any of the parameters with respect to the VP1 test. Cognitive potential recordings of frequency discrimination tasks with their associated reaction time and error performance for all patients with M.E. (VP1 positive) are shown in Figure 2 and those for the duration discrimination task in Figure 3. A normal response is shown at the top of the respective figures for comparison. It can be seen that the more difficult duration task elicits a P3 with a longer latency than that obtained with the frequency task. All patients show a similar result. Mean and upper limit of normal P3 latency and reaction time are marked with vertical lines so that the responses falling outside the normal range can be clearly seen

for both tasks. Analysis of individual responses for abnormality on the basis of response presence or absence and latency of P3 and RT (or errors in performance) being within the two standard deviation upper limit from the normal mean shows asignificant proportion of patients to be outside the normal upper limit (Table 3). 20 (80%) of the 25 patients with VP1 positive had either P3, RT or performance abnormal on the duration task and 16(64%) on the frequency task. 13 (52%) of the patients had an abnormality of P3, 12 (48%) of RT and 8 (32%) of performance on either task. 9 (75%) of the 12 patients with VP1 negative had either P3, RT or performance abnormal on the duration task and 8 (67%) on the frequency task. Abnormalities of the P3, RT and performance are considered further for the VP1 positive patients only.

Cognitive Potentials: MS

Mean latencies of P3 were significantly prolonged for patients with MS in comparison with a group of normals for both the frequency and duration tasks.

Table 2

Mean (SD) of latencies of major components of cognitive potentials in normals and patients with MS

Cogntive Components	M.E.	Normals	MS	t-test Sig. Prob. Normals vs MS	t-test Sig. Prob. Normals vs M.E.
N1F	110±14	104 (17)	109 (24)	0.218	.610
N2F	239±35	228 (30)	236 (51)	0.413	.490
P3F	345±51	332 (28)	359 (75)	0.042*	.170
RTF	425±101	358 (62)	395 (132)	0.106	.002*
PerF	2.9 (6.1)	0.76 (1.1)	3.00 (6.0)	0.029*	.096
N1D	109±13	106 (15)	103 (29)	0.540	.610
N2D	288±51	276 (48)	298 (55)	0.061	.032*
P3D	450±49	412 (46)	446 (49)	0.002*	.001*
RTD	513±89	464 (64)	497 (90)	0.056	.001*
PerD	3.6±5.8	2.1 (2.3)	4.5 (6.1)	0.032*	.063

Figure 2

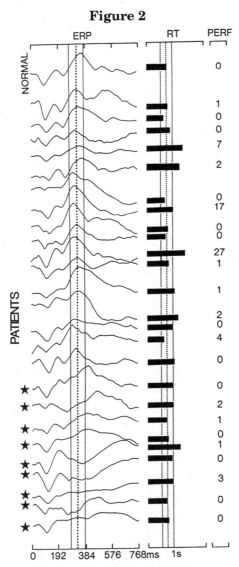

Frequency Task: Cognitive Event-related Potentials to target stimuli recorded from Pz, reaction time (RT) and Performance (Perf) for all 25 patients with ME with a normal response at the top for comparison. Those marked with an asterisk were considered abnormal either in terms of amplitude or latency. Vertical lines indicate normal mean and 2SD limits

Figure 3

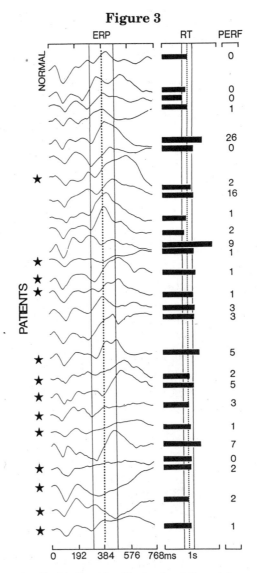

Duration Task: Cognitive Event-related Potentials to target stimuli recorded from Pz, reaction time (RT) and Performance (Perf) for all 25 patients with ME with a normal response at the top for comparison. Those marked with an asterisk were considered abnormal either in terms of amplitude or latency. Vertical lines indicate normal mean and 2SD limits.

Performance on both tasks was also significantly affected in the patients. In contrast to the M.E. group, no significant changes in RT were observed in patients with MS. 30% of the patients had abnormally prolonged P3 in the frequency or duration task and 20% had prolonged RT. Performance was also adversely affected in 20% of the patients. (Table 3).

Discussion

The sensory potentials of the visual, auditory brainstem, and median nerve somatosensory systems remain unaffected in M.E. This is in contrast to the abnormalities of evoked potentials observed in multiple sclerosis (MS) a disorder with known structural and functional abnormalities of the central nervous system. In the early stages of MS, symptoms may be similar to those associated with M.E. which may pose a problem of differential diagnosis. Clearly sensory potentials provide a means of separating the two groups.

Table 3				
% Number of patients with abnormal results				
	Frequency ME (VP1+)	Task MS	Duration ME (VP1+)	Task MS
P3 absent / delayed	20	33	24	30
RT	28	20	48	23
Performance	20	20	24	20

In contrast to the normal sensory potentials, there is clear objective evidence from this study that endogeneous event-related potential, P3, is absent or significantly delayed in patients with M.E. and MS. It is recognised that patients with MS commonly undergo cognitive decline with progression of disease.[27,28,29] Indeed, even patients with isolated lesions as demonstrated on MRI have been shown to have impaired cognitive function.[30] Thus P3 provides a means of evaluating the extent of auditory information processing abnormalities in these patients.

Abnormality of P3 in patients with M.E. is consistent with the universal complaint of these patients of impairment of cognitive functioning in the form of disturbances of memory and concentration. Furthermore, the extent of cognitive potential abnormalities in the 12 patients who were VP1 test negative was not significantly different from those who were VP1 test positive. The psychological processes involved in the type of cognitive tasks used in this study require encoding of stimulus features, detection of relevant signal by comparison with memory and execution of response. The amplitude of P3 provides an indication of attentional capacity devoted to the task and its indication of attentional capacity devoted to the task and its latency provides a measure of the speed of target detection[20]. In the M.E. group, P3 was delayed in some patients whilst in others the amplitude was diminished, sometimes to an extent that the response was labelled as "P3 absent". This implies two subgroups, one with attentional deficits and other with slower speed of information processing.

Those with "P3 absent" had normal performance and

reaction time suggesting that the effect on P3 was not due to a diffuse effect on arousal or due to general fatigue. It is interesting, in this regard, to note that similar effects on P3 have been noticed with administration of scopolamine, a centrally active cholinergic blocking agent which has a detrimental effect on recent memory and attention.[31] Hammond et al.[32] showed that scopolamine abolishes P3 without affecting performance although the subject reported difficulty in maintaining attention. In a number of M.E. patients, this precise effect was observed. In the study of Hammond et al.[30], alteration in P3 also correlated with poor scores on tests of recent memory and at the end of the recording session, P3 and memory scores were restored to their original values indicating that the observed effects on P3 were not due to fatigue.

In terms of accuracy of performance there was no statistical difference in the error scores between the control and M.E. group. At most, 24% of the M.E. patients had impaired performance but this was not always associated with an abnormality of P3. Normal task performance with normal N1 and P2 peaks but absence of P3 suggests that each stimulus is correctly categorised, and in terms of the response, it appears to be appropriately encoded as shown by N1/P2. Normal task performance also indicated accurate detection and categorisation processes but under these circumstances absence of P3 implies that these processes may not be occurring at the same time on each stimulus occurrence to generate a synchronous neural electrical field for generation of a P3.

Several studies have shown that specific psychological processes associated with the P3 component are

Figure 4

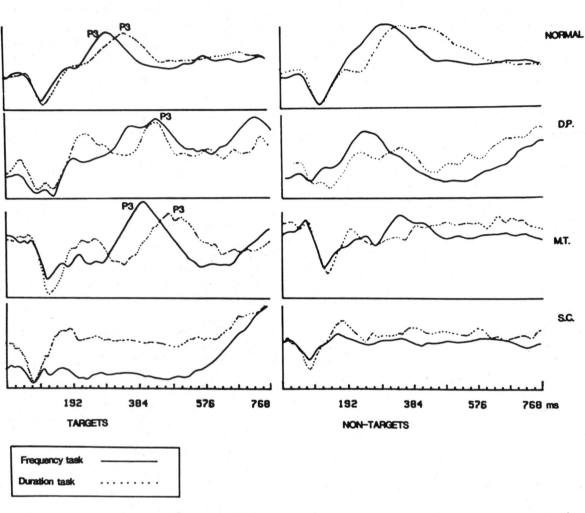

Cognitive event-related potentials to frequency and duration discrimination tasks from a normal subject at the top and three multiple sclerosis patients with 3 (DP), 2 (MT), and 1 (SC) sensory potential abnormality respectively. Reaction time and performance were within normal limits for all patients.

attention[33,34], stimulus evaluation[32], and memory.[36,37]

Thus, it appears that abnormalities of P3 reflect clearly the subjective difficulties of concentration and memory described by patients with M.E. and indeed provides corroborative evidence of deficiencies in the psychological processes involved. It has been suggested that symptoms associated with M.E. such as profound fatigue on physical and mental exertion can also be due to an affective disorder such as depression.[38-40] In this regard, it is significant that Pfefferbaum[39], in his review of studies[42-45] evaluating abnormalities of P3 in mental disorders, concluded that "for depressed patients there are almost no reports of significant changes in P3 latency, while

amplitude reduction is a variable finding". Further studies[46-50] have confirmed that P3 is normal in patients with depression. Thus, it would appear, at least on the basis of the cognitive potentials, that depression is not a factor responsible for the abnormalities detected in patients with M.E.

From the relationship of P3 abnormality, RT prolongation and task performance, it is clear that if general fatigue was a factor of importance in determining the abnormalities then all three parameters (P3, RT and Performance) should have been affected much more in association with one another than they actually were. Although RT was significantly prolonged in patients with M.E. in comparison with normal controls, RT prolongation was not always associated with prolongation or absence of P3 and in fact the correlation between P3 latency and RT in M.E. was much lower than in normals. There was a greater correlation of RT with performance than with P3 or of performance with P3. This implies that accuracy of performance is a factor of influence for RT but not for P3. It suggests further that although both P3 and RT are affected in patients with M.E., they reflect separate processes. At its simplest, it may be argued that stimulus evaluation stages are affected in patients with an abnormal P3 but normal RT, whilst response activation and execution stages may be affected in those in whom RT was prolonged but P3 was normal as the influence of one parameter on the other appears to be minimal.

References

1. Parish JG Early outbreaks of 'epidemic neuromyasthenia'. Postgrad Med J 1978; 54: 711-717.

2. Ramsay AM 'Epidemic neuromyasthenia'. Postgrad Med J 1978; 54: 718-721.

3. Lyle WH and Chamberlain RN Epidemic neuromyasthenia 1934-1977: current approaches. General discussion. Postgrad Med J 1978; 54: 773-774.

4. McEvedy CP and Beard AW Concept of benign myalgic encephalomyelitis. Br Med J 1970; 1: 11-15.

5. Wessely S, David A, Butler S and Chalder T Management of chronic (post viral) fatigue syndrome. J R Coll Gen Pract 1989; 9: 26-29.

6. Holmes GP, Kaplan JE, Gantz NM et al. Chronic fatigue Syndrome: A Working Case Definition. Annals of Internal Medicine 1988; 108: 387-389.

7. Lloyd A R, Wakefield D, Broughton C, Dwyer and J What is myalgic encephalomyelitis?. The Lancet 1988; 1: 1286-1287.

8. Calder BD, Warnock PJ, McCartney RA and Bell EJ Coxsackie B viruses and the post viral syndrome: a prospective study in general practice. J R Coll Gen Pract 1987; 37: 11-14.

9. Bell EJ, McCartney RA and Riding MH Coxsackie B viruses and Myalgic Encephalomyelitis. J. Royal Society of Medicine 1988; 81: 329-331.

10. Archard LC, Bowles NE, Behan PO, Bell EJ and Doyle D Postviral fatigue syndrome: persistence of enterovirus RNA in muscle and elevated creatine kinase. J. Royal Society of Medicine 1988; 81: 26-329.

11. Behan PO, Behan WMH and Bell JB The postviral fatigue syndrome-an analysis of the findings in 50 cases. J Infect 1985; 10: 211-222.

12. McCartney RA, Banatvala JE and Bell EJ Routine use of mu-antibody-capture ELISA for the serological diagnosis of Coxsackie B virus infections. J Med Virol1986; 19: 205-212.

13. Yousef GE, Bell EJ, Mann GF et al., Chronic enterovirus infection in patients with postviral fatigue syndrome. The Lancet 1988; : 146-150.

14. Straus SE, Tosato G, Armstrong G Persisting illness and fatigue in adults with evidence of Epstein-Barr virus infection. Ann Intern Med. 1985; 102: 7-16.

15. Caliguiri M, Murray C, Buchwald D Phenotypic and functional deficiency of natural killer cells in patients with chronic fatigue syndrome. J Immunol 1987; 139: 3306-3313.

16. Jamal GA, Hansen S Electrophysiological studies in postviral fatigue syndrome. J. Neurol. Neurosurg. Psychiat. 1985; 48: 691-694.

17. Lloyd AR, Hales JP, Gandevia SC Muscle strength, endurance and recovery in the post-infection fatigue syndrome. J. Neurol. Neurosurg. Psychiat. 1988; 51: 1316-1322.

18. Chiappa KH Evoked potentials in clinical medicine. 1983 Raven Press New York.

19. Halliday AM (Ed) Evoked Potentials in Clinical Testing. 1982 Churchill Livingstone. Edinburgh.

20. Donchin E Cognitive Psychophysiology: Event-related potentials and the study of Cognition 1984 vol. 1 Erlbaum, Hillsdale, NJ.

21. Gazzaniga MS Advances in cognitive neurosciences: The problem of information storage in the human brain. In: Neurobiology of learning and memory (Eds) Lynch G, McGaugh JL, Weinberger NM. 1984 Guilford Press New York.

22. Johnson RE, Pfefferbaum A and Kopell BS P300 and long term memory: Latency predicts recognition performance. Psychophysiology 1985; 22: 497-507.

23. Kutas M, McCarthy G and Donchin E Augmenting mental chronometry: the P300 as a measure of stimulus evaluation time. Science 1977; 197: 792-795.

24. Pfefferbaum A, Wenegrat BG, Ford JM, Roth WT and Kopell BS Clinical application of the P3 component of Event-Related Potentials. II Dementia, Depression and Schizophrenia. Electroenceph. Clin. Neurophysiol. 1984; 59: 104-124.

25. Goodin DS, Squires KC and Starr A Long latency event related components of the auditory evoked potentials in dementia. Brain 1978; 101: 635-648.

26. Syndulko K, Hansch EC, Cohen SN, Pearce JW, Goldberb Z, Montan B, Tourtellotte WW, Potvin AR Long latency event elated potentials in normal aging and dementia In: Courjon J, Maguiere F, Revol MI eds. Clinical Applications of Evoked Potentials in Neurology. 1982 New York: Raven Press, 279- 285.

27. Charcot JM Lectures on the diseases of the nervous system delivered at la Salpetriere. 1877 London New Sydenham Society.

28. Ivnik RJ Neuropsychological stability in multiple sclerosis Journal of Consulting and Clinical Psychology 1978; 46: 913-923.

29. Rao Sm, Hammeke TA, McQuillen MP, Kharti BO, Lloyd D Memory disturbance in chronic progressive multiple sclerosis. Arch. Neurol. 1984; 41: 625-631.

30. Callanan MM, Logsdail SJ, Ron MA, Warrington EK Cognitive impairment in patients with clinically isolated lesions of the type seen in multiple sclerosis: A psychometric and MRI study. Brain 1989; 112: 361-374.

31. Drachman DA Memory and cognitive function in man: Does the cholinergic system have a specific role? Neurology 1977; 27: 783-790.

32. Hammond Edward J, Meador KJ, Aung-Din R and Wilder BJ Cholinergic modulation of human P3 event-related potentials. Neurology 1987; 37: 346-350.

33. Hillyard S Event-related potentials in selective attention. In: E Donchin (Ed). Cognitive Psychophysiology: Event-related Potentials.

34. Donald M (1983) Neural selectivity in auditory attention. In: Tutorials in Event-related Potential Research: Endogenous components. Elsevaier Amsterdam pp 37-77.

35. McCarthy G and Donchin E (1983) Chronometric analysis of human information processing In: Tutorials in ERP research: Endogenous components. AWK Gaillard and W Ritter (Eds) North Holding Publishing Co.

36. Mulder G (1986) Memory search paradigms and practice effects In: Cerebral Psychophysically: Studies in event-related potentials (EEG Suppl. 38) Eds W C MacCallum, R Zappoli and F Denoth. Elsevier. Amsterdam.

37. Starr A and Barrett G Disordered short term memory in man and event-related potentials. Brain 1987; 110: 935-959.

38. Baker M, Dorzab J, Winokur G and Cadoret R Depressive disease; classification and clinical characteristics. Compr Psychiatry 1971; 12: 354-365.

39. Matthew R, Weinman M and Mirabi M Physical symptoms of depression. Br J Psychiatry 1981; 139: 293-6.

40. Wessely S Myalgic Encephalomyelitis-a warning: discussion paper. J. Royal Soc. Med. 1989; 82: 215-216.

41. Pfefferbaum A (1986) P3 latency and amplitude abnormalities in mental disorders. In: Cerebral Psychophysiology: Studies in Event-Related potentials (EEG Suppl. 38) Eds. W.C. McCallum, R. Zappoli and F. Denoth. Elsevier. Amsterdam.

42. Levit RA, Sutton S and Zubin J Evoked Potential correlates of information processing in psychiatric patients. Psychol. Med. 1973; 3: 487-494.

43. Verleger R and Cohen R Effects of certainty, modality shift and uess outcome on evoked potentials and reaction times in chronic schizophrenia. Psychol. Med. 1978; 8: 81-93.

44. Roth WT, Pfefferbaum A, Kelly AF, Berger PA and Koppel BS Auditory event-related potentials in schizophrenia and depression. Psychiat. Res. 1981; 4: 199-212.

45. Pfefferbaum A, Ford JM, Wenegrat BG, Roth WT and Koppel BS Clinical application of the P3 component of event related potentials: I: Normal Aging. Electroenceph. Clin. Neurophysiol. 1984; 59: 85-103.

46. Shagass C Evoked brain potentials in psychiatry. 1972 Plenum. New York.

47. Teuting P and Levit RA (1979) Long-term changes of Event- related Potentials in Normals, Depressives and Schizophrenics. In: Cognitive components in Cerebral Event-related Potentials and Selective attention. Prog. Clin. Neurophysiol. vol. 6 Ed J E Desmdt pp265-79 Karger Basel.

48. Giedke H, Thier P and Bolz J The relationship between P3 latency and reaction time in depression. Biol. Psychology 1981; 13: 31-49.

49. El Massioui F and Leserve N Attention impairment and psychomotor retardation in depressed patients: an event-related study. Electroenceph. Clin. Neurophysiol. 1988; 70:46-55.

50. Patterson JV, Michalewski HJ and Starr A Latency variability of the components of auditory event-related potentials to infrequent stimuli in aging, Alzheimer-type dementia, and depression. Electroenceph. Clin. Neurophysiol. 1988; 71: 450- 460.

Acknowledgements

We would like to thank The Gebbie Foundation of USA for their support.

Neuropsychological Changes in M.E. / CFS

Chapter 51

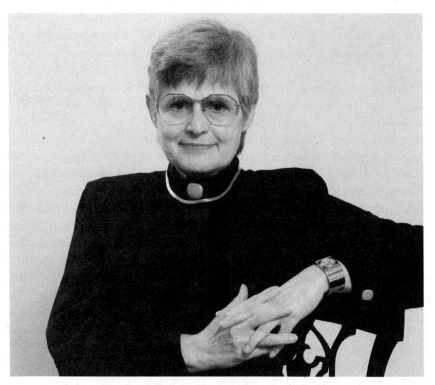

Sheila Bastien

Patterns of Neuropsychological Abnormalities and Cognitive Impairment in Adults and Children

Sheila Bastien, PhD
Psychological Corporation, 2126 Los Angeles Avenue Berkeley, CA 94707 USA

Dr. Sheila Bastien obtained her BA in Psychology from the University of California at Berkeley in 1969, and her MA and PhD in Psychology from West Virginia University in 1974. Dr. Bastien has been involved in Neuropsychology for 20 years and Chronic Fatigue Syndrome research for six years.

Background

Neuropsychometric research is a specific way of documenting brain disorder associated with myalgic encephalomyelitis (ME) / chronic fatigue syndrome (CFS). Eighty-one patients* diagnosed with chronic fatigue syndrome (CFS) from the clinical practice of physicians, Daniel Peterson and Paul Cheney in Incline Village, Nevada were evaluated. The patients were all from northern Nevada and nearby communities. A common cluster of clinical and laboratory features[1] is associated with the illness. All of these patients have met the Centers for Disease Control (CDC) criteria for CFS[2]. Eighty-one patients with an onset of acute respiratory or influenza-like symptoms and fatigue in 1984 did not recover and continued to experience symptoms, often in a cyclical pattern[2].

Neurological Abnormalities

These patients had neurologic abnormalities noted on clinical evaluations, MRI scans, and neuropsychometric testing. Neuropsychometric evaluations exhibit highly significant dysfunction among the patients. Deterioration of IQ** levels, as well as cognitive and motor dysfunction in these patients, suggest a pathological process in the brain. SPECT scans, which measure the brain's blood flow, reveal hypoperfusion in other ME/CFS patients[3]. BEAM scans and PET scans display abnormalities in ME/CFS patients[4,5]. The pattern of focal and lateral

* The medical parameters of these patients have been described in a research article in the Annals of Internal Medicine in collaboration with Peterson, Cheney, Komaroff, et. al., 1992

** Intelligence Quotient

impairments is consistent with patients who have this particular neurologic dysfunction. These results cannot be explained by anxiety or depression alone.

The impairment pattern is consistent across the study group, although impairment levels may vary[2]. This pattern is not seen in other diseases or injuries, such as Alzheimer's, stroke, head injuries, multiple sclerosis, systemic lupus erythematosis, personality disorders, depression, psychosis, malingering, anxiety or panic disorders, somatization disorders, or situational stress disorders[1].

Study Population

Eighty-one patients comprised the sample, ranging in age from 16 to 62; 71 percent were women and 29 percent were male; women between the ages of 30 and 45 were most at risk. Of the sample, 77 percent were college educated; 57 percent were either professionals or had high-level business or management positions. Patients engaged in blue collar employment represented only 8 percent. Blue collar workers were under-represented.

The majority of the patients were highly motivated, successful, and busy individuals prior to their illness.

Overall there was no significant premorbid psychiatric history, including depression or anxiety disorders. Most of these individuals were quite active physically prior to their illness.

Symptoms

The patient sample had the following neuropsychological impairments: word-finding problems; subtle problems with receptive and expressive aphasia, including intermittent dysnomias; decreased concentration; distractability, problems in recall, verbal more than visual, including a remote memory disturbance; dyscalculia (for example, over 50 percent of these patients could not accurately subtract $6.50 from $17.00); both gross and fine motor problems; spatial-perceptual dysfunction, including losing their way while driving; some abstract reasoning disturbance, primarily non-verbal; decreased visual discrimination; and problems in sequencing. In addition, the patients had trouble making decisions and planning. Many of the patients had a personality

change from a previously even-tempered individual, to someone easily frustrated, irritable, impulsive, angry, and sometimes verbally out of control.

Emotional Parameters and Diagnostic Criteria

The Minnesota Multiphasic Personality Inventory (MMPI), was administered to these patients. The mean MMPI profile reveals acute psychological disturbance related to their illness. The profile resembles an individual with a chronic illness. The most prominent features are: an awareness of somatic and sensory difficulties, marked depression, social withdrawal and anxiety, pessimism, and extreme concern for their well-being. There are no indications of malingering, conversion, or of a thought disorder[1]. The validity scales indicate valid profiles. Low self-esteem is evident and most likely secondary to their illness.

These patients also had an impulsiveness not part of their premorbid personality. Over half answered a question in an impulsive manner, that suggests organicity. Previously high functioning and controlled individuals would respond "Yell fire!" to the question, "What should you do if you were the first person in a large crowded room to see smoke and fire?" This kind of response is often found in neurologically compromised patients, and probably represents frontal lobe disinhibition.

Many of the patients met the DSM-III-R diagnostic criteria for an Organic Personality Syndrome with emotional lability, or had an Organic Mood Disorder, Depressed. All of the patients met the DSM-III-R criteria for Dementia, mild[5].

Neuropsychological Tests

The following tests were given: Wechsler Adult Intelligence Scale - Revised (WAIS-R), Wechsler Memory Scale (WMS) (Logical Memory, Visual Reproduction), Knox Cubes, Diagnostic Interview, Minnesota Multiphasic Personality Inventory (MMPI), and Draw-a-Person. In addition, the following tests from the Halstead-Reitan Neuropsychological Battery (HRNB) were administered: The Booklet Category Test (BCT), the Tactual Performance Test (TPT), Finger Oscillation Test, Dynamometer, Trailmaking A and B, Speech-sounds

Perception Test, and Seashore Rhythm Test.

Significant Tests	
Tests	Percentage of Patients Impaired*
Imm. Ver. Recall (WMS)	85%
Del. Ver. Recall (WMS)	80%
TPT N- Dom. (HRNB)	59%
TAP Dom. (HRNB)	54%
Category (HRNB)	54%
Del. Vis. Recall (WMS)	53%
Grip Dom. (HRNB)	46%
Grip N-Dom. (HRNB)	39%
TAP N-Dom. (HRNB)	39%
Imm. Vis. Recall (WMS)	39%
TPT Dom. (HRNB)	30%

* Using Halstead-Reitan cutoffs where appropriate

Knox Cubes, a visual-motor sequencing task, was significantly worse, with 68 patients out of 81 impaired.

Trailmaking A and B are not significant. Seashore Rhythms was significantly better than the normal population.

The Booklet Category Test was significantly worse than the norm. All of the patients were impaired compared to the norms for the general population*, suggesting non-verbal abstract reasoning problems, and difficulty in shifting sets. On this test, 54 percent were impaired indicating a loss of cognitive flexibility, and diminished ability to problem solve.**

Findings - Memory

On the Wechsler Memory Scale (WMS) almost all of the 81 patients (80 to 85 percent) were impaired on immediate and delayed verbal recall. Visual memory was far less impaired, 39 percent (immediate) to 53 percent (delayed). The difference between visual and verbal memory was highly significant. Although these results implicate the temporal lobes bilaterally, (WMS dysfunction is highly correlated to temporal lobe dysfunction) statistical analysis using

*   Instead of Halstead-Reitan absolute cut-off scores
** Using Halstead-Reitan cut-off scores

Cochran's Q test[7], demonstrated significantly more impairment in the left temporal lobe. Left temporal lobe dysfunction is associated with decreased ability to process, encode, and retrieve auditory information. Right temporal lobe dysfunction is associated with depression, irritability, and impaired visual memory.

A word of caution is necessary regarding the localizing of memory. Memory is a complex process involving many areas of the brain. ME/CFS may disrupt networks of distant neurons; even subcortical dysfunction may be present. The same cautionary stance needs to be taken in regards to all localization suggested in this paper. For example, an infectious inflammatory process may well affect distant neuronal networks. Subcortical tracts may well be affected, disrupting cortical processes. (MRI abnormalities are typically found in subcortical white matter.)

Findings - Tactual Perception

Tactual perception (Tactual Performance Test) was impaired in 59 percent of those patients on the non-dominant hand and 39 percent on the dominant hand. (This test correlates with parietal lobe dysfunction.) Although there appeared to be bilateral parietal lobe dysfunction in many patients, the difference between the right and left hand was significant (Cochran's Q), indicating worse right parietal lobe impairment, which is often associated with a decrease in visual-spatial perception.

Findings - Motor Dysfunction

Motor test scores were impaired bilaterally. However, there were significant differences which could possibly point to a focal area of greater dysfunction in the left frontal lobe motor strip. Tapping in the dominant right hand was significantly more impaired than the left. Therefore, the left frontal motor area may be dysfunctional in some way, in the absence of peripheral injury or other peripheral problems. PET scans have confirmed this in some ME/CFS patients.

Pattern of Impairments

The pattern of impairment is one of focal and lateral deficits, consistent with a multi-focal organic brain syndrome. Tests suggest that the most impaired focal areas are the left temporal, right parietal, and left frontal lobes; although there are lesser bilateral impairments in the opposite lobes as well.

Figure Drawings

Right parietal lobe dysfunction is further demonstrated by the spatial-perceptual difficulties patients have on the Draw-a-Person Test. In research, the Draw-a-person Test is not always valid for emotional indicators, but is likely more valid as an organic indicator. The organic signs for the Draw-a-Person results are as follows: gross immaturity of drawing, poor integration of parts, emptiness of facial expression, lack of details, omission of parts - especially the neck, transparent or absent clothing, flattened heads, displacement of the extremities, petal-like or scribbled fingers and toes[8], disproportionately large head, and poor proportionality of parts.

The figure drawings by the 81 CFS/ME patients often had notable differences between the right and left sides of the body. Many patients' drawings would indicate the side of the body more affected by their illness. The eyes in their drawings often lacked pupils. These patients frequently drew themselves as sticks, segmented balloons, puppets, or squared-off robots. Sometimes the figure drawings of CFS/ME patients lean to one side. In summary, most of the organic indicators for these patients are contained in their drawings.

The drawings reflect moderate to severe dysfunction in visual-spatial perception. They are different from those of Alzheimer's patients, where perceptual misplacement is more evident and distortions are far worse. The quality of the drawings is different from dyslexic adults. Many of the figures look like children's drawings and/or reflect a regression to an earlier level of functioning. However, the most notable features are the organic ones; the drawings look like those of patients with neurologic dysfunction.

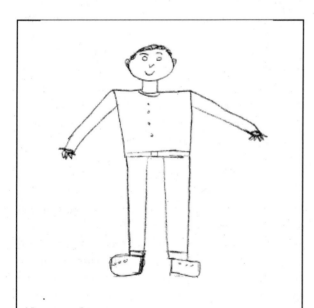

Abnormal

Age: 55
Sex: Female
Upper middle class housewife; B.A. degree
- Squared off, robot-like figure
- Scribbled fingers
- No pupils
- Legs attached to box-like torso

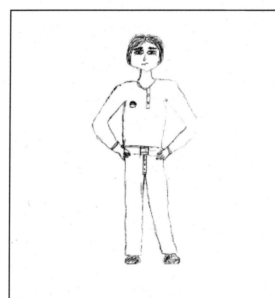

Normal

Age: 27
Sex: Male
Graduate student
- Nice balance and detail
- Appropriate facial expression
- Clothing well integrated

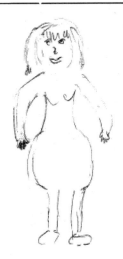

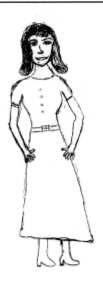

Abnormal

Age: 33
Sex: Female
Homemaker; average height, average weight, accounting work
- Odd proportions
- Figure appears hunched
- Lower half looks like a segmented balloon
- Clothing appears absent

Normal

Age: 30
Sex: Female
Graduate student
-Clothing, facial expression, and proportions are all within normal limits

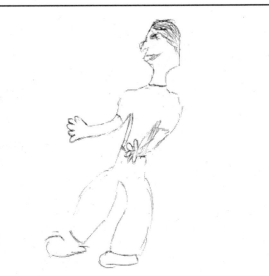

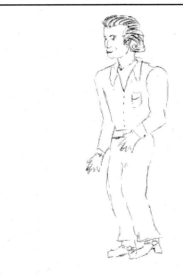

Abnormal

Age: 34
Sex: Female
Real Estate Agent, Body Builder
- Body appears tilted as if falling backwards
- Proportions are off
- One arm appears deformed
- Petal-like fingers

Normal

Age: 35
Sex: Male
Graduate Student
- Excellent details
- Good integration of parts
- Appropriately clothed

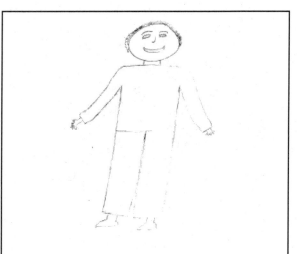

Abnormal

Age: 39
Sex: Female
Gifted student, B.A. in economics from University of California
- Immaturity of drawing
- Figure squared off and almost robot-like
- Enlarged head and scribbled fingers
- Figure tilted, off balance

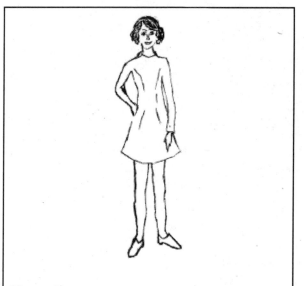

Normal

Age: 17
Sex: Female
From textbook
- Perfectly proportioned
- Appropriately clothed
- Balanced stance

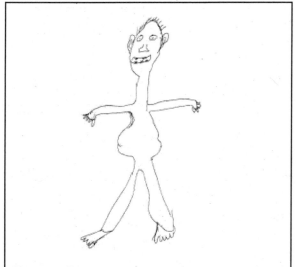

Abnormal

Age: 44
Sex: Male
Pit Boss; disabled since 1985
- Head and neck enlarged
- Displacement of extremities
- Petal-like / scribbled fingers and toes
- Gross immaturity of drawing
- Clothing absent

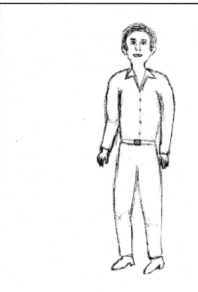

Normal

Age: 36
Sex: Male
Graduate Student
- Good proportion with clothing
- Head not enlarged
- Normal stance

WAIS-R: Verbal IQ, Performance IQ, Full Scale IQ and Subscales

The majority of patients have suffered a decrease in IQ; some of these losses are catastrophic. This loss is revealed in three ways: 1. The degree of scatter between the subtests; 2. The discrepancy between VIQ/PIQ; 3. Intra-subtest scatter (where patients miss simple items and get more difficult ones indicating higher premorbid functioning). Most of these patients were high functioning and successful individuals prior to their illness. Now they have IQ scores in the average range. Performance IQ is significantly lower than Verbal IQ in most of these patients, probably indicating greater right hemisphere dysfunction.

The WAIS-R subtests, Information, Vocabulary, Comprehension and Similarities (all good estimates of premorbid IQ) were all significantly above the mean for the average population using Signed Rank non-parametric statistics. The Verbal IQ scores of this patient population were significantly better than average; the Full Scale IQ was also significantly better than average. These patients were obviously quite intelligent premorbidly. We know this, for after successful treatment, repeated IQ results have increased as much as 40 points.

The Performance IQ scores were lower than average. In this sample of patients, the Performance IQ is clearly worse than the Verbal IQ. This depressed Performance IQ likely reflects greater overall impairment in the right hemisphere. Their Performance scores are significantly worse on Picture Completion, a visual discrimination and visual scanning task. They are not significantly impaired on Picture Arrangement; this is usually one of their highest performance subtest scores. Block Design and Object Assembly are significantly impaired compared to the norms, indicating problems in visual-spatial perception. On Digit Symbol, an eye-hand coordination and visual-motor speed test, patient scores were very impaired compared to the norms, indicating difficulty in shifting sets, and poor clerical speed and accuracy.

Memory and Norms

On the Wechsler Memory Scale, the verbal, immediate and delayed scores were significantly worse in our sample compared to the normal population. Visual memory was not significantly different from population norms. Therefore, there is more lateralization to the left temporal lobe.

Tactual Performance Test and Norms

On the Tactual Performance Test (TPT), the dominant hand, non-dominant hand, and total time are all significantly worse in our sample compared to the normal population. Memory and localization are also significantly worse. The parietal lobes seem to be affected in this disorder.

Tapping scores, both dominant and non-dominant hand were not significantly different than the normal population; however, grip strength was significantly worse bilaterally. The patients report weakness, which is shown in these results. One does not usually see this pattern of weakness in anxiety or depression.

Dyslexia

The CFS patients do not present a classic dyslexia. Dyslexics are abnormal on the Speech/Sounds Perception Test; they have trouble with phonemes. However, the Speech/Sounds Perceptions Test is significantly better in this patient sample than in the normal population. Patients with ME/CFS are never abnormal on this test. Since the onset of their illness, these patients have had problems in language, spelling, and math, but they are not classically dyslexic.

Physician-Case Study

In one CFS/ME case, a 43-year-old female physician had a Verbal IQ of 113, a Performance IQ of 92, and a Full Scale IQ of 103. One would expect a person to have at least an IQ of 120 to be able to get into medical school. We know her Verbal IQ is impaired but her Performance IQ is even more impaired with a significant 21 point VIQ/PIQ difference. Her deficits suggest a deteriorating dementia. In fact, in this particular case, serial testing revealed deteriorating scores over time.

Children

The neuropsychological deficits in children had a

different pattern, depending on age. Dr. David Bell initiated the children's study Daniel Peterson, M.D. and Paul Cheney, M.D. are collaborating.

Most of these children are from the Lyndonville, New York outbreak. The older children seem to follow the same deficit pattern as the adults, in terms of the pattern of impairment. Their Verbal IQ is typically higher than their performance IQ; both are impaired, but the Performance IQ is more impaired.

One particular child, from an upper middle class family and previously an A student, is now functioning with a VIQ of 98, a PIQ 74, and a Full-Scale IQ of only 85.

Another child, a 13-year-old female, who became ill approximately five or six years ago, has a different pattern: a VIQ of 100, a PIQ of 108, and a full scale IQ of 103. The children who became ill at a younger age have their Verbal IQ lower than their performance IQ. This disorder seems to affect their language functioning when they become ill early in their formative years, resulting in lowered VIQ scores compared to PIQ scores.

In summary, younger children have their language function (verbal IQ) more impaired than older children and adults. Adults and older children have their performance skills (PIQ) more affected.

If we identify a specific neuropsychometric CFS pattern and background history, we can establish that these combined impairments are different from depression, anxiety, or other neurologic disorders. In so doing, we can rule out certain etiological factors, a well as establish risk factors.

Neuropsychometric testing is very useful for establishing private disability, workers' compensation, and social security cases for patients who are put through a bewildering maze of bureaucracy, and often misdiagnosed. Documenting the neurological dysfunction helps both clinicians and patients in validating the illness.

References

1. Sandra A. Dougherty, Berch E. Henry, Daniel L. Peterson, Raymond L. Swarts, Sheila Bastien and Robert S. Thomas. Chronic Fatigue Syndrome in Northern Nevada. Reviews of Infectious Diseases, **1991**; 13: S39-44.

2. Gary P. Holmes, M.D.; Johnathan E. Kaplan, M.D.; Nelson M. Gantz, M.D.; Anthony L. Komaroff, M.D.; Lawrence B. Schonberger, M.D.; Stephen E. Straus, M.D.; James F. Jones, M.D.; Richard E. Dubois, M.D.; Charlotte Cunningham-Rundles, M.D.; Savita Pahwa, M.D.; Giovanna Tosato, M.D.; Leonard S. Zegans, M.D.; David T. Purtilo, M.D.; Nathaniel Brown, M.D.; Robert T. Schooley, M.D.; and Irena Brus, M.D. Chronic Fatigue Syndrome: A Working Case Definition. Annals of Internal Medicine, **1988**; 108: 387-389.

3. Ismael Mena, M.D. Study of Cerebral Perfusion by NeuroSPECT in Patients with Chronic Fatigue Syndrome. The Cambridge Symposium on Myalgic Encephalomyelitis (ME), **1990**; 1:21-22.

4. Marshall Handleman, M.D. Neurological Substrates of Behavior: Brain Mapping and the Chronic Fatigue Patient. The Cambridge Symposium on Myalgic Encephalomyelitis (ME), **1990**; 1: 13.

5. Steven Lottenberg, M.D. Positron Emission Tomography in Chronic Fatigue Syndrome. The Cambridge Symposium on Myalgic Encephalomyelitis (ME), **1990**; 1:20.

6. Diagnostic and Statistical Manual of Mental Disorders. Third Edition — Revised. American Psychiatric Association. (Washington D.C.: **1987**)

7. Joseph L. Fleiss. *Statistical Methods For Rates and Proportions.* John Wiley and Sons: New York, **1981**, 128.

8. Mollie S. Schildkrout, M.D.; I. Ronald Schenker, M.D.; Marsha Sonnenblick, M.S. *Human Figure Drawings in Adolescence.* Brunner/Mazel: New York, **1972**.

9. Ian Hickie; Andrew Lloyd; Denis Wakefield and Gordon Parker. "The Psychiatric Status of Patients with the Chronic Fatigue Syndrome." British Journal of Psychiatry. **1990**, 156, 534-540.

Chapter 52

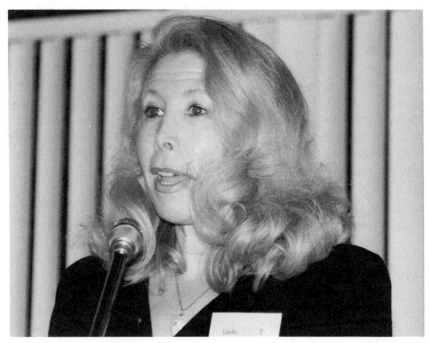

Linda Iger

The MMPI as an Aid to Chronic Fatigue Syndrome Diagnosis

Linda Iger PhD, Neuropsychologist, 75 South Peak Road, Laguna Niguel, CA 92677 USA

(Please see also Addendum II.)

Dr. Iger holds two doctoral degrees, one in counselling psychology and one in clinical psychology. Dr. Iger is the director of psychological services at the Chronic Fatigue Institute where she has participated in research and clinical work with Jay A. Goldstein, M.D. She is a pioneer in identifying many of the commonalities among CFIDS patients. Dr. Iger is responsible for development of the first profile of CFIDS patients using the MMPI. Dr. Iger is trained in biofeedback and cognitive rehabilitations using the learning theory. She is a member of the American board of medical psychotherapists. Dr. Iger is a frequent contributor to the CFIDS Chronicle.

This paper's figures are reproduced with the kind permission of The CFIDS Chronicle, Spring / Summer 1990, pages 37-8.

The Chronic Fatigue Syndrome patient has been referred in increasing numbers to psychologists and psychiatrists. Concomitant with the physiological symptoms, Chronic Fatigue Syndrome patients are experiencing memory loss, depression and anxiety. Most of the Chronic Fatigue Syndrome patients have been ill for years. Many have gone from physician to physician. Some have been labelled as hypochondriacs, malingerers and depressive by their physicians. Psychological referrals based on these misdiagnoses were equally frustrating for both the patient and therapist. Psychologists and psychiatrists seeing Chronic Fatigue Syndrome patients have had little research to help them in their diagnosis and treatment of the patient population.

The Minnesota Multiphasic Personality Inventory (MMPI) is a highly reliable and valid assessment instrument that is frequently being used to screen pathology and delineate between diagnostic categories. The MMPI was developed by Hathaway and McKinley out of the University of Minnesota in 1943. The MMPI is a 567 item, self-report, assessment instrument organized into four validity and ten clinical scales. It has a myriad of uses in both clinical and non-clinical settings. It is used to screen policemen and also, in most penal institutions, to test inmates. It is used to pick firemen, air traffic controllers and pilots. It is used to assess in-patient psychiatric patients and it is also frequently used to select psychologists and psychiatrists. Several of the Fortune 500 companies use it to screen their top executives.

The MMPI has four validity scales that answer the question, "How open and honest was this person in answering the questions?" Because of these four validity scales and its high level of reliability, it is frequently requested by Social Security to aid in determining eligibility for disability benefits. There are no other similar testing instruments available with these validity scales. Because of its ability to screen pathology and delineate between diagnostic categories, the MMPI was thought to hold the potential to be an effective tool to differentiate CFS patients from the established profile for normals, hypochondriacs, depressives, malingering, and other chronic illnesses.

In order to establish the relationship between Chronic Fatigue Syndrome and the MMPI, sixty patients who had been medically diagnosed with CFS were tested with the MMPI. The profiles for the Chronic Fatigue Syndrome patients were then compared to established, commonly used profiles for Hypochondriasis, Depression, Malingering, Chronic Illness, as well the original MMPI normative group.

Sixty subjects, fifty females (N=50) and ten (N=10) males, diagnosed with Chronic Fatigue Syndrome were administered the MMPI. The ratio of women to men of 5:1 closely approximated the ratio (4:1) found in the general population of Chronic Fatigue Syndrome Patients. Demographic data was gathered

about the age of the patients. The range for the sample was 18-69. The mean age for the sample was 40.38 with a standard deviation of 9.1.

The sample of Chronic Fatigue Syndrome patients was divided into females and males consistent with statistical interpretive profiles for the normative sample. The mean and standard deviations were found for the four validity and ten clinical scales. Raw scores were converted to T scores, separate T score conversions were used for males and females. T scores are based upon a mean of 50 and a standard deviation of 10. Two standard deviations are considered clinically significant. For clinical purposes, following standardized procedures, K corrections were made (figure 1).

A profile for female Chronic Fatigue Syndrome patients was created. Clinical significance was achieved on six clinical scales: Scales 1 (Hypochondriasis), 2 (Depression), 3 (Hysteria), 4 (Psychopathic Deviate), 7 (Psychasthenia) and 8 (Schizophrenia). (Figure 2) Using the same procedure a profile for the male Chronic Fatigue Syndrome patients was created. Clinical significance was achieved on the same Scales 1 (Hypochondriasis), 2 (Depression), 3 (Hysteria), 4 (Psychopathic Deviate), 7 (Psychasthenia) and 8 (Schizophrenia) as for the female patients. (Figure 3)

Figure 1

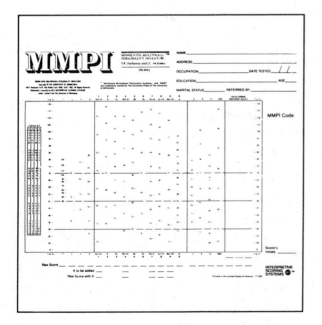

Figure 2

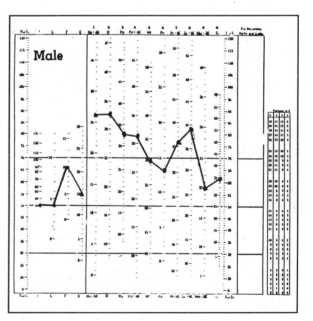

Figure 3

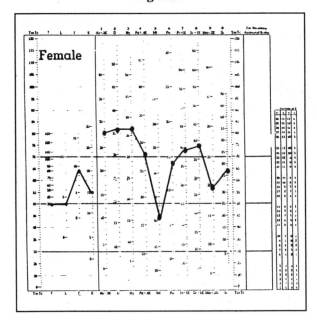

The mean of each of the clinical scales for both male and female Chronic Fatigue Syndrome patients is large with relatively small standard deviations suggesting that a large number of the sample endorsed each of the clinical scales at about the same level. Overlaying the two profiles demonstrates how similar they are (Figure 4).

Figure 4

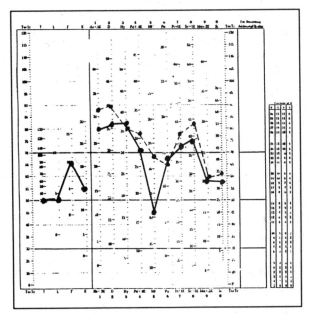

The Chronic Fatigue Syndrome profile was then compared with established profiles for: 1) Normals,

the original normative group of Hathaway and McKinley, 2) Hypochondriasis (Lashar, 1974), 3) Depression (Lashar, 1974), Malingering (Dahlstrom, Welch, & Dahlstrom, 1972), and Chronic Illness (Nabiloff, Cohen, & Yellin, 1982).

Based upon a qualitative and quantitative analysis, using the standardized statistical procedures of means and standard deviations, the sample of Chronic Fatigue Syndrome patients was compared with established, commonly used profiles for Hypochondriasis, Depression, Malingering and Chronic Illness.

Figure 5

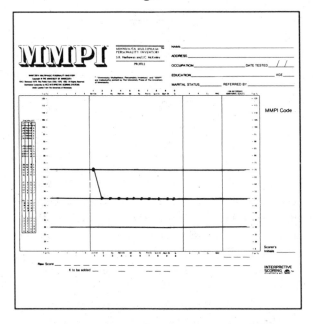

In comparing the profile for Hypochondriasis, The Chronic Fatigue Syndrome sample, while elevated to clinical significance on scale 1 (Hypochondriasis) as is Hypochondriasis, was also elevated two standard deviations on Scales 2 (Depression), 3 (Hysteria), 4 (Psychopathic Deviate), 7 (Psychasthenia) and 8 (Schizophrenia). The profile for Hypochondriasis is not elevated to clinical significance on Scales 2, 3, 4, 7, and 8. (Figure 5)

In the profile for Depression, while both the Chronic Fatigue Syndrome MMPI profile and the Depression profile are elevated to clinical significance on Scale 2, the Chronic Fatigue Syndrome MMPI profile is also elevated to clinical significance on Scale 1 (Hypochondriasis). Scale 3 (Hysteria), Scale 4 (Psychopathic Deviate), Scale 7 (Psychasthenia) and

Scale 8 (Schizophrenia), while the Depression profile is not elevated to clinical significance on Scales 1, 3, 4, 7 and 8. (Figure 6)

Figure 6

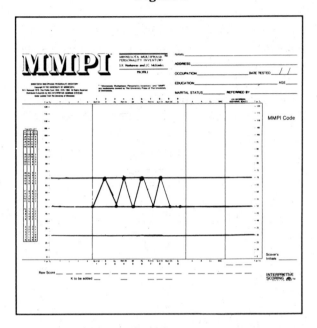

Figure 7

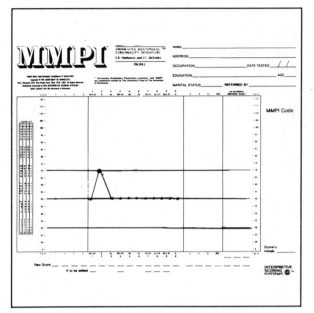

Figure 8

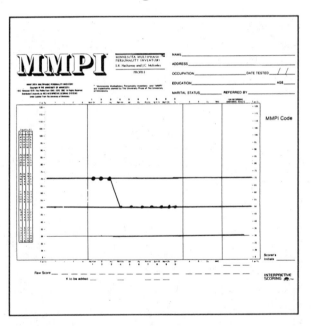

In comparison to the profile for Malingering which is elevated to clinical significance on Scale 2 (Depression), Scale 4 (Psychopathic Deviate), Scale 6 (Paranoia), and Scale 8 (Schizophrenia), this differs from the Chronic Fatigue Syndrome MMPI profile which is elevated to clinical significance on Scale 1 (Hypochondriasis), Scale 2 (Depression), Scale 3 (Hysteria), Scale 4 (Psychopathic Deviate), Scale 7 (Psychasthenia) and Scale 8 (Schizophrenia). (Figure 7)

In comparing the Chronic Fatigue Syndrome MMPI profile with that of Chronic Illness, while both are elevated to clinical significance on Scale 1 (Hypochondriasis), Scale 2 (Depression) and Scale 3 (Hysteria), the Chronic Fatigue Syndrome MMPI profile is also elevated to clinical significance on Scale 4 (Psychopathic Deviate), Scale 7 (Psychasthenia) and Scale 8 (Schizophrenia). (Figure 8)

The Chronic Fatigue Syndrome patient's MMPI profile with its elevations of clinical significance on Scales 1 (Hypochondriasis), 2 (Depression), 3 (Hysteria), 4 (Psychopathic Deviate), 7 (Psychasthenia), and 8 (Schizophrenia) appears to be a new profile. Its meanings and implications for those suffering from the illness are clear. This MMPI profile can help physicians and therapists to differentiate between CFS and normals, hypochondriasis, depression, malingering and other chronic illnesses.

Since hypochondriasis, malingering and depression were the major reasons for referrals to psychotherapists from physicians for undiagnosed Chronic Fatigue Syndrome in the past, this new Chronic Fatigue Syndrome MMPI profile should be a useful diagnostic tool. The Chronic Fatigue Syndrome MMPI profile with its unique configuration will also help therapists and physicians to differentiate Chronic Fatigue Syndrome from other chronic illnesses.

Addendum

Given the configuration of the female Chronic Fatigue Syndrome patient profile, a clinician might expect the following behaviours, issues and concerns associated with these MMPI scores: The testing results indicate that the composite female patient approached the MMPI in an open manner while endorsing a high level of intrapersonal distress and/ or unusual, deviant thoughts, with a possible plea for help. The patient is probably unable to handle confrontation at this time. The Goldberg Index of 37 is consistent with neurotic but not psychotic processes. The profile is probably an accurate and valid sample of behaviour.

This profile is consistent with chronic illness. Testing results indicate a significant level of distress and concern about bodily processes and physical health. Patients with profiles like this are more often seen on medical rather than psychiatric services although there is indication of a significant level of depression. The patient may see the depression as secondary to her somatic complaints. Suicidal ideation must be ruled out.

The patient may have deep concerns and even fearfulness about the possibility of a complete physiological breakdown. Others with profiles similar to this do experience physiological breakdown in middle to late age as a result of consistent autonomic nervous system arousal which may be the result of processing stress physiologically rather than through the emotions. The patient probably is in constant states of tension and anxiety.

The patient favours traditional female defenses of repression and denial and when these fail probably feels overwhelmed. The emotional swing between denial and feeling overwhelmed may be disconcerting to the patient. Testing results indicate the use of obsessive-compulsive defenses which aid by restricting behaviours and utilizing repetitive problem solving strategies even when they are no longer working.

As evidenced by testing, the patient is experiencing difficulty concentrating, memory loss, difficulty maintaining attention and may, at times, feel confused with a possible blurring reality and fantasy. Testing results indicate the patient may be withdrawing from others and restricting activities.

The female patient appears to have traditional values with a high emphasis on home and family, yet there is indication of unexpressed anger and chaotic interpersonal relationships and impulsivity. There may be some level of suspiciousness of the motives of others and difficulty with authority figures.

In summarizing the Chronic Fatigue Syndrome patient profile, it is consistent with chronic illness with memory and concentration losses. A patient with this profile is probably fearful of a total physiological collapse. As evidenced by testing results, the female patient is experiencing a clinically significant level of depression which she may see as secondary to her somatic complaints.

Given the strong similarities in the male and female Chronic Fatigue Syndrome patient MMPI profile and clinical significance on the same Scales 1, 2, 3, 4, 7 and 8, we will focus on the differences between the male and female MMPI profile for the Chronic Fatigue Syndrome patients. The composite male patient is probably experiencing more psychological distress about his health, his fears and concerns about a physiological breakdown are more magnified. The depressive symptoms are experienced at a higher level. Suicidal ideation must be carefully explored. The typical male patient may feel a greater loss of sense of control and have concerns about his masculinity. His self concept and sense of manliness may be shaken. He probably expresses anger more directly and is less suspicious of the motives of others than the female Chronic Fatigue Syndrome patient. The male patient tends to be more tense and more locked in his behaviour pattern. He may obsess and ruminate about his illness and loss of health. Memory, concentration and attentional losses are endorsed at a higher level and he may feel he is losing touch with reality.

References

1. Lashar, D. (1974). *The MMPI: Clinical Assessment and Automated Interpretation.* Los Angeles: Western Psychological Services

2. Dahlstrom, W.G., Welch, G.S., & Dahlstrom, L.E. (1972). *An MMPI handbook: Volume 1. Clinical Interpretation.* Minneapolis: University of Minnesota Press.

3. Naliboff, B.D., Cohen, M.J., & Yellin, A.N. (1982). Does the MMPI differentiate chronic illness from chronic pain? *Pain.* 13(4), 333-341.

Chapter 53

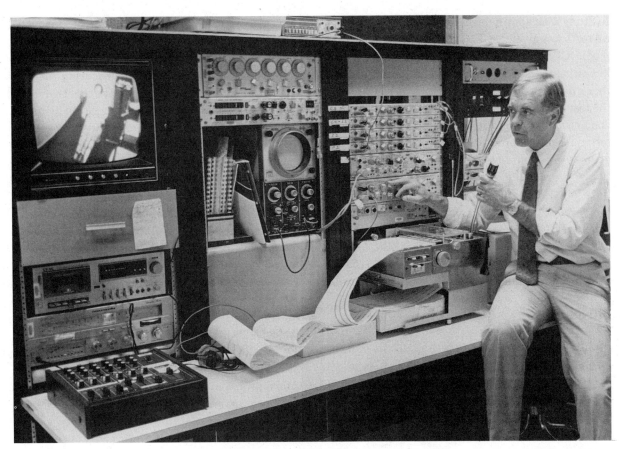

Curt A. Sandman

Is There a Chronic Fatigue Syndrome (CFS) Dementia?

Curt A. Sandman, PhD

Jennifer L. Barron, Ph.D., Karen A. Nackoul, Ph.D., Penny L. Fidler, M.A., Jay Goldstein, M.D.
Memory and Neuropsychological Center, 366 San Miguel, Suite 210, Newport Beach, California, University of California, Irvine, State Developmental Research Institute

Acknowledgements: *The assistance of Lisa Richards is appreciated.*

Dr. Sandman received his PhD in Psychology in 1971 and practiced as Professor of Psychology at Ohio State University from 1972 to 1978. He has held his present positions as Professor of Psychiatry at the University of California at Irvine and Director of Research at the State Development Research Institute, Fairview for 11 years. Dr. Sandman has published over 150 papers and has presented scientific lectures world-wide.

Abstract

Three studies investigated the relationship between chronic fatigue syndrome (CFS) and cognitive function. In Study 1, thirty-nine patients diagnosed with CFS, 23 depressed patients and 129 normals were compared on the Irvine Memory Battery (IMB). Patients with chronic fatigue performed significantly worse on tests of recall as context increased, made more errors when rehearsal was prevented when compared to the depressed patients and controls, and had a significant delay in memory scanning as memory load increased when compared to both groups.

In Study 2, an additional battery of neuropsychological tests was given to CFS and fibromyalgia patients (FM). CFS patients had significantly more visual impairment than the fibromyalgia group, but neither group was in the impaired range compared to the test norms. These results argue against a frank dementia associated with CFS but revealed a characteristic cognitive profile that was distinguished from depressed patients.

In Study 3, measures of immunocompetence were compared with memory performance. Factors associated with CFS dementia were related to numbers of T4 and T8 cells and positivity for EBV. These preliminary results support the relationship of CFS dementia to specific immune influences on the brain.

Introduction

Chronic Fatigue Syndrome (CFS) has been related to unusual profiles of antibodies to Epstein Barr Virus, but the cause of the disorder and its symptoms is unknown (Tobi, Morag, Rivid, et al, 1982; Straus, Tosato, Armstrong et al, 1985). A recent study (Kruesi, Dale and Straus, 1989) suggested that patients with CFS had a higher rate of psychiatric illness preceding their disease than control populations. Among the psychiatric complaints, depression and dysthymia were the most prominent. This retrospective study suggested that psychiatric illness contributes to the pathogenesis of CFS, although not completely explaining it.

Recently Bastien (1989) reported that CFS patients were below the mean of normative populations on nearly every test given in a four hour neuropsychological battery. Among the most distinctive results were that the CFS group had lower IQ than expected from educational achievement. Performance decrements were profound in tests of visual, spatial and motor abilities, and in tests of visual sequencing (Trails A and B). General memory functioning (WMS-R) was below the mean, and verbal memory was especially impaired. These data suggest a general and pervasive "dementia" associated with CFS.

We report here the results of three separate studies. The first study compared memory functioning in CFS and depressed patients and normal control subjects, with a computerized neuropsychological assessment procedure (Willhardt and Sandman, 1988). These computerized tests evaluated efficiency of information processing by measuring memory consolidation (making memories), retrieval of memories, metamemory (expectation about memory), interference (effects of rehearsal and competitive information on memory), memory load (effects of amount of information on recall), semantic memory (old or long-term memory), attention (input) and motor (output) abilities. If psychiatric illness and especially depression shared commonality with CFS, cognitive similarities would be expected between the groups.

The second study compared the CFS sample with a group of patients with similar symptoms [fibromyalgia (FM) patients] on a larger battery of neuropsychological tests. The FM patients were chosen to test the specificity and sensitivity of cognitive profiles for CFS dementia. In addition, the CFS group was informally compared with the published norms for these tests.

In the third study, preliminary measures of immunocompetence were related to computerized assessment of learning and memory. The purpose of this study was to determine if CFS dementia was selectively associated with immunological studies.

Study 1

Methods

SUBJECTS

CFS Patients. Thirty-nine patients referred for neuropsychological testing had the diagnosis of CFS established by ruling out other disorders that might mimic CFS in some respects and fulfilling the case definition published by Holmes, et al, (1988). Duration of illness varied from 6 months to 8+ years. In addition, CFS patients rated cognitive dysfunction as significant on a 10-point symptom checklist. The elements of the cognitive dysfunction symptoms included attention deficit, dyscalculia, memory disturbance, spatial disorientation and dysnomia. The patients had a physical examination that generally was normal except for the detection of tender points characteristic of fibromyalgia in 70%, and an occasional positive Romberg test. Immunological parameters measured included, alpha interferon, detectable in 10%, interleukin-2, elevated in 40% and Raji cell assays, elevated or borderline in 75%. There was no history in any of the patients of hospitalization for mental illness including depression.

Depressed Patients. Twenty-three depressed patients were obtained from the University of California, Irvine, psychiatric inpatient service. All patients were diagnosed by Research Diagnostic Criteria and DSM IIIR by a psychiatrist. Criteria were satisfied for a Major Depressive Episode. All patients entered the hospital medication free for several weeks and were observed to be medication free for at least two days before testing.

Normal Volunteers. Asymptomatic subjects (N=129) were recruited from the student population at the University of California, Irvine and from the staff of Fairview Developmental Center. Subjects were selected for inclusion in the analysis to match the age range of the patient groups.

Procedures

Recall. The Recall subtests consist of a metacognitive estimate, free recall, paired associates, recognition and letter-priming subtests. The metacognitive score is the patient's estimate of the number of words out of 10 they will remember on the free recall test. For free recall, 10 words were presented one at a time and the patient was asked to recall as many as he or she could. The paired-associates tests prompted recall of 10 words by the stem word of a previously presented word pair. The recognition test presented 10 word pairs but recall was a forced choice from four alternatives presented on the screen. Letter priming also was presentation of 10 paired associates, but recall was cued by the stem word and the first letters of the word to be remembered. These tests assess encoding, memory consolidation and retrieval. Increasing structure or context (paired associates, recognition and priming) increases the probability of recalling the information (Craik, 1984). A retrieval slope, determined from the first free recall test, paired-associates and recognition (Willhardt and Sandman, 1988), was calculated by determining the rate of improvement with increased context. A steep retrieval slope may reflect a relative retrieval deficit, indicating that information is processed but is not easily re-

called without cuing. A flat slope in the presence of poor free recall is evidence of an encoding or memory consolidation deficit. A relationship between expected and actual performance was determined by calculating the ratio of estimated free recall and actual recall (META/RECALL). This index is an important guide to the validity of the patient's self-appraisal.

Proactive Inhibition (PI)

The test of Proactive Inhibition (PI) requires the patient to briefly retain three items in memory. Three items to-be-remembered (numbers, letters or words) were presented on the computer screen for 1200ms and then a video game was presented for 10 seconds for the patient to play. The primary purpose of the game was to distract the patient and discourage active rehearsal of the three items. In addition, distraction through manipulation of the semantic similarity of the memory set is achieved. Triads of the three items are very similar (i.e. sets of numbers, letters or related words). The fourth presentation of three items was different than the triad (release from proactive inhibition). Thus, if the first triad of three items were sets of numbers, the fourth set of items was letters. When rehearsal is prevented, previously learned information may be confused with current information and distort memory (error). Furthermore, if the information to be recalled is similar to previous information, the probability of distortion is greater (PI error). Release from PI occurred when a new domain of information was introduced (fourth set of items) and memory of the new information is enhanced. This test allows assessment of interference on memory and specifically: 1) the decay in memory when rehearsal is discouraged and 2) the organization of memory when similar information is presented.

Item Recognition. This test was adapted from Sternberg (1969) to assess the effects on memory of mental load. Load was controlled by asking the patient to remember on each trial either 1, 2 or 4 items (memory set) presented on the computer screen for 800-1200ms. After a 1200ms, a probe appeared on the computer screen and the patient pressed one hand held key if the probe was one of the items in the memory set (matched to dominant hand) and a second key (nondominant hand) if it was not. Half the probes were in the memory set and half were not. The time required to press the key (reaction time, RT) became slower as the number of items in the memory set increased. The slope of this function (RT over mental load) was the memory scanning time and reflected the efficiency of visual memory. The intercept of this function reflected the time required to encode the probe (attention) and to initiate a motor response. The modification of this test involved surrounding the number probe with distracting letters. Efficient performance required that the patient disregard the irrelevant information (letters) and respond only to the number probe.

Semantic Memory Test. This test (SMT) examined the patient's ability to access information stored over the course of their lives. Common categories (e.g. Fabrics) were presented one at a time for 1200ms, followed by words that were (e.g. wool) or were not (e.g. desk) exemplars. Patients made successive retrievals from the same semantic categories so, for instance, "Fabric" was presented twice but was followed with different exemplars (e.g. wool and then silk). Patients depressed one hand-held button (Reaction–Time-RT) as fast as possible if the exemplar was related to the category and a second key if it was not.

Typically, a second successive retrieval from the same semantic category was accomplished faster (i.e. faster RT) than the first retrieval (priming). Strength of the priming effect was controlled by imposing a lag of 0, 1 or 2 items between the first and second category-exemplar pairs. Lags of 0 yielded the fastest RTs and lags of 2 items resulted in the slowest RTs. Absence of RT facilitation suggests delays in semantic activation of old memories and may reveal general inefficiency in the organization of memory.

Results

The CFS patients were compared with the asymptomatic controls and depressed patients in two separate ways. First, Student t-tests of significance were computed. Second, multivariate modelling of the differences of the three groups was done with stepwise discriminant function analysis (SWDA).

Results from the tests of recall are presented in Figure 1. There were no significant differences between CFS compared separately with depressed and controls on their metacognitive estimate or on free recall. However, on tests of increasing context, paired

associates and recognition, the CFS patients did significantly worse ($p < .01$) than both controls and depressed patients. CFS patients had a significantly flatter retrieval slope than controls, reflecting a relative inability to benefit from cuing and context. CFS patients slightly overestimated the efficiency of their memory that was significantly ($p < .01$) different from the characteristic of depressed patients to underestimate their performance. There were no differences between controls and depressed patients.

CFS patients were dramatically impaired on the interference test (Figure 2). Compared to controls and depressed patients, the CFS group made significantly ($p < .001$) more errors in memory when rehearsal was prevented. No differences were detected in the number of proactive interference errors.

Mental scanning (memory) was significantly delayed in the CFS patients compared to the depressed patients ($p < .001$) in the NO condition and to the controls in both the YES and NO conditions ($p < .05$). There were no differences between CFS patients and controls in the intercept (encoding-motor output) but the depressed patients were significantly slower than CFS and controls in the NO intercept (Figure 3). As illustrated in Figure 4, there were no differences for any measures in semantic memory. Because this is a stable memory system, not vulnerable to dementia, it is not surprising there were no differences.

Multivariate equations were constructed that combined the variables to maximize the separation of the patient groups. Variables are selected in stepwise order that contribute to the separation of the groups. After the first variable is selected, subsequent variables are chosen that contribute uniquely to the separation (functionally covariance analysis). The final combination is weighted, and the equation sorts patients into the groups based on similarity of memory profile. A "jackknifed" classification is performed that tests each case against a "first pass" equation, essentially validating the equation. Three comparisons were tested; all three groups, depressed vs. CFS, and normal controls vs CFS. Comparison of three groups yielded equations that significantly ($p < .0001$) distinguished the groups. A total of 68% (33% is chance) of the subjects were classified in their groups accurately based solely on memory performance. Only 2 of the depressed subjects were misclassified as CFS patients. The order of the variables responsible for the separation were interference errors, PI errors and mental scanning efficiency. Two-way contrasts of depressed and CFS yielded 82% classification (50% is chance), which was highly significant (p<.001). Interference errors, input/output response speed, paired associates and estimation of performance cooperated to distinguish the groups. Two-way comparison of control subjects and CFS patients yielded 90% classification (50% is chance). This highly significant result (p<.00001) was due primarily to the accurate classification of normals. The CFS profile was distinctive and rarely, (only 4%), was a normal patient mis-identified as a CFS patient. The same variables (interference, PI errors, input/output response speed and paired associates) contributed to the separation.

Discussion

Several important differences in memory emerged between CFS patients and age-matched normal controls and depressed patients. Unlike findings from the literature (Craik, 1984) and the behaviour of the control and depressed groups, CFS patients performed worse on recall tests as the context increased. Performance on the free recall test was equivalent among groups. However as cuing or context was added, making the test easier, for instance by prompting recall with previously associated words or providing alternatives (recognition), performance in the CFS patients declined. Context improved the performance of the control and the depressed groups. This pattern was reflected in the flat retrieval slope for CFS patients (Willhardt and Sandman, 1988). The inability of CFS patients to profit from added information (i.e. flat slope), but to perform normally on free recall, reflects memory consolidation deficits. They appear to retrieve efficiently but they suffer from a deficit in making memories. Thus, they do as well with context as they do in a free recall situation. It is possible that extra information, even helpful information, is distracting and only a finite amount of data can be processed.

The recall results were supported by the dramatic effects of interference on the memory of CFS patients. They lost the ability to retain simple, three-item lists, when a 10 second task was interposed between the items and recall. It appeared that even simple temporal or informational distraction disrupted the memory trace and the efficiency of information processing deteriorated.

Consistent with this pattern was the delay in memory scanning in CFS patients with increasing memory load. Although the CFS patients were slightly slower than controls on input/output measures, the effects were not significant and they were faster than depressed patients. Indeed the profile of slowing for depressed and CFS patients was different. There was no evidence of mental slowing because of mental load on the depressed patients, but they did evidence retardation in the input/output function (intercept). For CFS patients, the primary defect was the inability to search efficiently through recent memory to match an event in the environment. They were accurate, but the increasing information produced a disproportionate strain on the scanning system.

It is clear from these findings that depressed and CFS patients have distinctly different cognitive/memory profiles. For the most part, the depressed patients do not have a primary loss of memory. They have a significant loss in confidence (underestimate performance META/RECALL) and slowing in the input/output function of an RT task. As discussed above, CFS patients have clear and consistent deficits in memory consolidation, perhaps related to distraction or capacity limitations.

Study 2

Patients

The same sample of 39 CFS patients was included and compared with 7 FM patients. The FM patients were chosen because they resembled the CFS patients except for the absence of cognitive complaints and the greater incidence of tender points.

Methods

Mini-Mental State Examination (MMSE) . The Mini-Mental State Examination is a brief test of several cognitive functions. The scale is a reliable and valid screening instrument for detecting cognitive impairment. It assesses a client's orientation to time and place, instantaneous recall, short-term memory, and ability to perform serial subtractions or reverse spelling. The MMSE also measures constructional ability (the capacity to copy a design) and the use of language. Test-retest reliability of the MMSE in samples of neurologic and psychiatric patients has been .89 and above. Inter-rater reliability has been .82 and above.

Research on the sensitivity and specificity of the instrument has suggested that the MMSE provides a valuable initial screen for cognitive impairment. A score of 23 points or less by an individual with more than 8 years of education may be considered evidence of cognitive impairment.

Wechsler Adult Intelligence Scale-Revised (Wais-R) The WAIS-R is applicable for individuals aged 16 years through 75 years. The test contains 11 subtests, six of which form the Verbal Scale (Information, Comprehension, Arithmetic, Similarities, Vocabulary, and Digit Span) and five of which form the Performance Scale (Picture Completion, Picture Arrangement, Block Design, Object Assembly, and Digit Symbol).

The WAIS-R was standardized on 1800 individuals distributed over nine age levels (ages 16-75). The sample characteristics approximated the 1970 census in terms of educational and occupational levels, geographic region, urban-rural ratio, and race. The WAIS-R yields a deviation IQ that is obtained by comparing each examinee's scores with the scores earned by a representative sample of his/her own age group. The deviation IQ is a standard score with a mean of 100 and a standard deviation of 15 at each age level. Reliability and validity studies provide continued support for the WAIS-R as a reliable instrument for the normal, emotionally disturbed, and neurologically impaired.

Wechsler Memory Scale-Revised (WMS-R) The Wechsler Memory Scale-Revised (WMS-R) is an individually administered, standardized clinical tool for assessing major dimensions of memory functions in clients between the ages of 16 and 74 years. The scale is designed to be used as a diagnostic screening device to assess memory function. Memory for verbal and figural stimuli, meaningful and abstract material, and delayed and immediate recall are the clinically significant functions that are assessed.

Factor analytic studies revealed three factors among subtests: (1) Logical memory, visual reproduction, associate learning (or learning and repetition); (2) Mental control, digit span (or attention and concentration); (3) Personal and current information, orientation (or general orientation). In addition, five composite indexes are obtained: Verbal Memory, Visual Memory, General Memory, Attention/Concentration, and Delayed Recall.

Wisconsin Card Sort Test (WCST) The WCST was devised to study abstract behavior and ability to shift sets. The client must determine principles involved in organizing symbols into categories by deducing the principle from the examiner's responses. For instance, the symbols may be categorized by color, shape, or number. The examiner says "correct" when the patient selects the organizing principle. After 10 correct responses in succession, the correct category is changed by the examiner and the patient must determine the new organizing principle. The test continues until 6 categories are completed or until 120 cards have been presented. Poor performance on this test can result from a variety of cognitive deficits, including impaired capacity for forming abstract concepts, preservation and ability to maintain learning set. This test is sensitive to anterior brain damage, schizophrenia, and alcohol abuse.

Trail-Making Test (TMT). The Trail-Making Test (TMT) has been widely used as an easily administered test of visual-conceptual and visual-motor tracking. Like most other tests that have a large attentional component, it is highly sensitive to the effects of brain injury. It is given in 2 parts, A and B. In Part A, lines are drawn connecting consecutively numbered circles on one worksheet. In Part B, the client must connect consecutively numbered and lettered circles on another worksheet by alternating between letters and numbers. The time required and the number of errors made are recorded, however, and patient errors are corrected. When the time taken to complete Part A is far less than that needed to complete Part B, it is likely that the patient has difficulty in complex conceptual tracking or sequencing.

Boston Naming Test (BNT). The Boston Naming Test was developed as a screening instrument for anomia. A naming test is useful for sorting pure

Figure 1

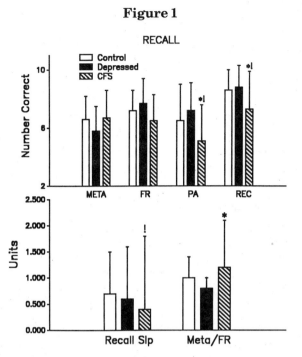

*Top Panel presents number correct for metamemory estimate (META), Free Recall (FR), Paired Associates (PA) and Recognition (REC). Bottom Panel is recall slope illustrating rate of improvement with increasing context and ratio of META and FR. (! =difference between controls and CFS; * = difference between CFS and depressed).*

memory problems from language deficits. A formal quantitative method, which includes many low frequency object names (protractor, trellis) will often reveal impairment that is missed by casual exam. Word-finding difficulty and confrontation-naming deficits have been recognized as common in dementia. The norms include adults age 25 through 85 years.

Irvine Memory Battery (IMB). The Irvine Memory test was described in Study 1.

Luria Nebraska Neuropsychological Battery (LNNB). The LNNB assesses a broad range of neuropsychological functions. It is used to diagnose general and specific cerebral dysfunction, including lateralization and localization of focal brain impairments, and to aid in the planning and evaluation of rehabilitation programs. The LNNB scales are grouped into four major areas, however, only the Visual-Function scale (C4) was used in the present analysis.

Results

The results of demographic data and screening tests are presented in Figure 1. The groups are most significantly different in age or education, though the CFS group have higher mean achievement, and women dominate both samples. The groups are equivalent on almost all tests and compare favorably with the published norms for all of the tests. The only difference between the CFS and FM patients is in the critical level of the LNNB, Visual-Perceptual test. CFS patients perform significantly more impaired than the FM patients but neither is in the organic range.

Figure 2

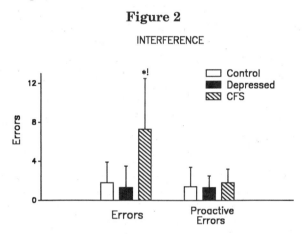

Number of errors due to distraction and proactive errors related to semantic similarity in test of interference.

The results of the Full scale, Verbal and Performance WAIS-R, IQ tests are presented in Figures 2 and 3. The CFS patients are significantly lower on performance IQ than the FM patients. Both groups are within the normal range for all measures of IQ (Figure 2). The CFS patients have lower IQ's (102) than expected given the achieved level of education (3 years of college).

Detailed analysis of WAIS-R test performance is presented in Figure 3. The data are presented as age-corrected scaled scores. A score of 10 is average. Only two differences were detected between the groups.

First, the CFS patients were significantly better on tests of Comprehension than the FM group. Second, the CFS group was lower on Object Assembly. Neither group was dramatically different from the published normative samples. However both groups, but especially the CFS group, performed lower than

Figure 3

ITEM RECOGNITION

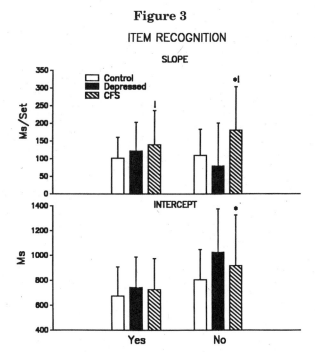

Top Panel is the slope (mental scanning speed) for the yes (match) and no (mismatch) trials. Bottom Panel is the intercept (input / output speed) for yes and no trials.

expected on tests related to educational level (for instance store of information=11).

Results of the WMS-R are presented in Figure 4. These are standard scores with 100 equal to the population average. Each increment of 15 reflects a standard deviation. There are no differences be-

Figure 4

SEMANTIC MEMORY

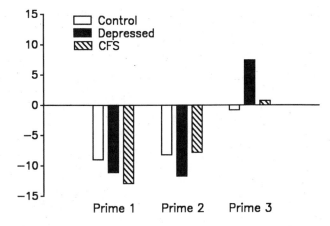

Savings score (improvement in reaction time) as a function of temporal displacement between category-exemplar pairs.

tween the groups for any measure of memory. These scores are comparable to the WAIS-R values and discrepancies suggest particular areas of deficit. However, for both groups, the WMS-R and WAIS-R are equivalent. Moreover, the scores for both groups on all tests are within normal limits. As with the WAIS-R, the values are lower than expected by educational achievement. The only difference between CFS and FM patients on the IMB was increased errors by CFS patients on the test of interference.

Discussion

These results complement the findings in Study 1, and indicate that CFS patients do not have frank dementia reflected by disorientation for time and place, dysnomia, dyscalculia, or dyspraxia. There was evidence of compromised performance in the Trails A and B tests, reflecting visual sequencing deficits and cognitive rigidity. Results of all the standardized tests were within 2 standard deviations of published norms. Thus IQ was within normal limits. However, IQ in the CFS group at the time of testing was lower than expected from educational achievement. Although it is difficult to prove, it is likely that some loss in IQ was evident in the CFS, and perhaps the FM, groups. Except for the results on the Trails Tests, these findings contrast sharply with those of Bastien, (1989), who reported pervasive losses in the CFS group.

As expected, only marginal differences distinguished CFS and FM patients. Since the symptoms are similar, it was surprising that any differences were discovered. The most notable difference was interference errors in the CFS group. In addition, CFS patients had higher comprehension (perhaps reflecting higher premorbid IQ and education) but lower object assembly. Thus CFS patients retained "common" sense but lost the ability to solve puzzles, which may relate to their tendency to be distracted by environmental disorganization.

Study 3

Patients

In this preliminary study, measures of immunocompetence were taken from the same group of 39 chronic fatigue patients.

Methods

Humoral markers (IGG), cellular markers (T4,T8) and mediators (IL2, alpha interferon) of immune function were measured. However, all immune function measures were not available for all patients. The tests of memory and intelligence described above were administered.

Results

Inspection of the scatter plots indicates that most patients were within normal limits on the measures. However, for each marker, several patients had clinically significant findings. Typically, the measures were not highly intercorrelated. The central interest was the relationship of the immune markers to memory.

Figure 5

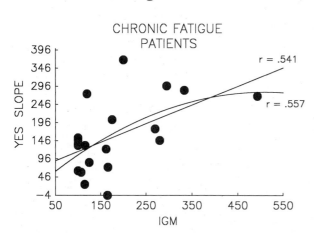

Scatter plot of the relationship between IGM and slope of reaction time (increase as function of increased memory load). Both linear and quadratic functions are plotted and are significant (p<.05).

Humoral Markers

As illustrated in Figure 5, level of IGM was significantly associated (p<.05) with mental scanning speed.

Although most patients clustered in the normal range of IGM, higher values were related to slower mental scanning speed.

Levels of IgG were used to determine positivity for EBV. Only 6 patients in this group tested positive. Comparison of the positive and negative patients is presented in Figures 6 and 7. Patients positive for

EBV had significantly lower (F 1,25 = 6.85, p <.05) free recall performance than patients with negative EBV. Further, the positive EBV patients significantly (F 1,25 = 7.74, p <.01) overestimated their performance and demonstrated a significant (F 1,25 = 6.16 p <.02) deficit in retrieval. Figure 7 illustrates that patients with positive EBV were significantly (F 1, 28 = 4.48, p <.05) less efficient in the scanning test memory as mental load increased.

Figure 6a

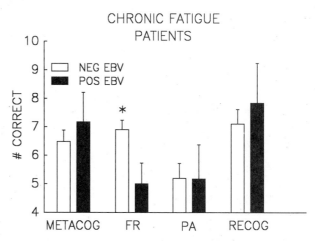

Left panel is recall measures for patients either positive or negative for EBV.

Figure 6b

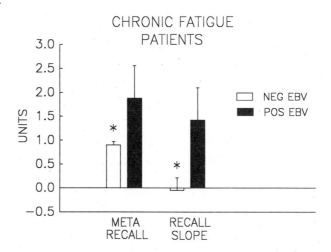

Right panel is the ratio of metamemory estimate and free recall and the recall slope for patients positive or negative for EBV.

Figure 7

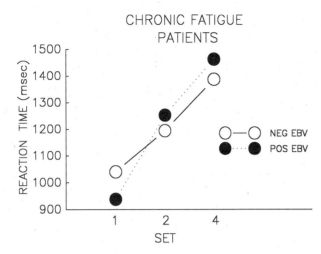

Reaction time for memory set (load) of 1, 2 or 4 items in patients positive and negative for EBV. Slope of RT was steeper (load more disturbing) for patients with positive EBV.

Cellular Markers.

Figure 8 presents the relationship between number of T4 cells and recognition memory. Both linear and quadratic plots are presented. The bottom illustration is the same data with the very extreme patient (2360 T cell count) deleted. It is clear from these figures that performance of recognition memory declines significantly (p<.01) as the number of T4 cells increases. The improved curvilinear relationship in the top figure is due to only 1 patient. Thus, roughly 40% of the variance in a recognition memory task can be predicted by the number of T4 cells in these patients.

Errors in the interference test were correlated with number of T8 cells and are presented in figure 9. The bottom figure is the same data with the two extreme

Figure 8

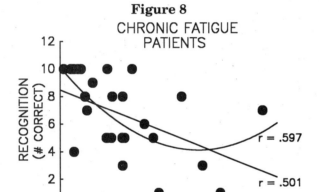

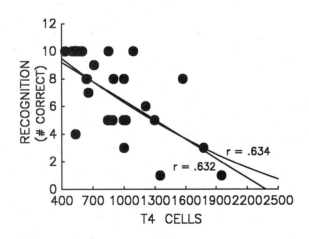

Scatter plot (linear and quadratic) of number of T4 cells and number of items correct on recognition memory. Top panel is with all patients and bottom panel are data with extreme patient (T4) removed.

Figure 9

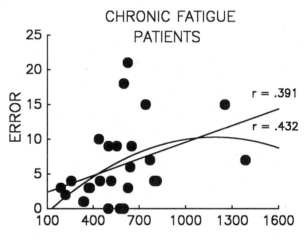

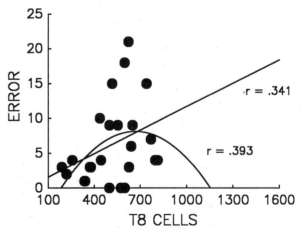

Number of errors in interference test plotted with number of T8 cells. Bottom panel is plotted with 2 extreme patients (T8) removed.

subjects removed, but the correlations do not change significantly. There is a significant (p < .05) relationship between the number of errors made on this test of memory and the number of T8 cells. Number of T8 cells also correlated significantly (p <.01) with the intercept of the item recognition test indicating that input/output speed was slower in patients with more T8 cells (Figure 10). This relationship was even stronger in the patients with values in the normal range (bottom figure). Number of T8 cells also was correlated with the benefits of semantic priming (Figure 11; extreme subjects removed in bottom graph).

Figure 11

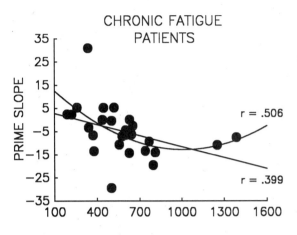

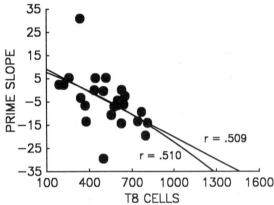

Scatter plot of rate of priming effects and number of T8 cells.

Figure 10

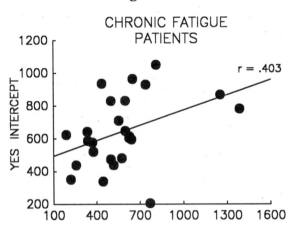

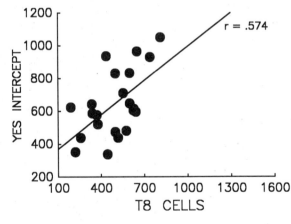

Reaction time intercept (input/output speed) plotted against the number of T8 cells. Bottom panel is plotted with 2 extreme patients (T8) removed.

Mediators

Inability to benefit from semantic priming was apparent in patients with positive alpha interferon values (n=5). There were no significant relationships between memory and IL2.

Attempts to develop multivariate models of the relationship between the immune system and memory were not successful. We assumed that several immune markers may predict memory better than any one measure, but this assumption was not valid. This indicates that the immune markers are largely independent (as the correlations revealed) and do not cooperate in explaining central nervous system functioning. Measures of IQ were not related to immune status, suggesting the effects are mostly on the memory system.

Discussion

These findings are considered very preliminary but suggest strong relationships between the immune system and memory. To our knowledge, this is the first report of immune status and tests of memory in chronic fatigue patients and perhaps any population. In an earlier report (Kelley, Vayuvegula, Sandman, Crinella, Isenhart and Gupta, 1989) we found

Figure 12

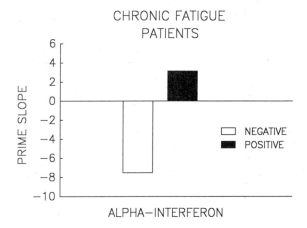

CHRONIC FATIGUE
PATIENTS

ALPHA-INTERFERON

Priming slope shows normal savings in patients with negative alpha interferon but no savings are apparent in patients with positive markers.

a relationship between CD4-CD8 and computerized measures of the EEG. However, our review of the literature suggests that the results of this study are unique.

The results indicate that distinctive deficits were associated with specific markers. EBV and T8 cells had the most pervasive influence on performance. Patients positive for EBV had poor recall and inefficient scanning when challenged with increasing memory load. Patients with elevated T8 cells were susceptible to interference and had slower input/output speed.

The profile for the CFS dementia appeared to be shared by EBV, T4 and T8 cells. Susceptibility to interference was the primary component of CFS dementia and was predicted best (and significantly) by number of T8 cells. Deficits in recognition memory, (memory consolidation) were associated with increased T4 cell populations. Inefficient memory scanning in the presence of informational load, was exacerbated in patients positive for EBV. It is difficult to offer conclusions for CFS from these data because the majority of patients were within normal limits on most measures. The degree of relationship

between immune markers and memory was best among patients in the normal range. It is tempting to conclude that CFS dementia is the result of a number of immune disturbances expressing unique contributions to the syndrome.

Conclusion

Highly significant deficits in memory were detected in patients diagnosed with CFS when compared with normal controls and a depressed patient group. The deficits in CFS patients were characterized by weak memory trace, an inability to make memories and an attention/concentration factor. In addition, CFS patients were extremely vulnerable to interference, suggesting that the memory network was inefficient and disorganized. Significant slowing in mental, but not input/output (motor) speed also distinguished the CFS group. The CFS profile was unique and unlike that of control subjects and depressed patients.

A battery of standardized tests in a controlled comparison with FM, yielded two major findings. First, minimal differences existed between these two related groups. Only vulnerability to interference, improved comprehension and deficient object assembly characterized the CFS group. Second, there was no evidence for pervasive cognitive decline in the CFS group, contrary to the report of Bastien, (1989). It could be argued that the CFS group had lower IQ than expected from educational achievement, but that is difficult to prove.

Finally, Study 3 generated preliminary evidence that unique cognitive deficits were associated with specific immune states. This surprising result, with no apparent precedent, suggested that CFS dementia maybe the result of expression of a variety of immune "conditions". This possibility must be muted by the fact that few CFS patients exceeded the normal range of the immune markers measured. Nevertheless, these results are promising leads for future studies.

Bibliography

Bastien, S. (1989). Neuropsychological deficits in Chronic Fatigue Syndrome. The CFIDS Chronicle, Summer/Fall, 24-25.

Craik, F. I. M. (1984). Age differences in remembering. in L. R. Squire, & N. Butlers (eds.), **Neuropsychology of memory**. (pp. 3-12). New York: Guilford Press.

Holmes, G. P., Kaplan, J. E., Gantz, N. M., & et al. (1988). Chronic Fatigue Syndrome: A working case definition. Annals of Internal Medicine, 387-389.

Kelley, M. J., Vayurequla, B., Sandman, C. A., Crinella, F., Isenhart, R., & Gupta, S. (October 23-27, 1989). Auditory evoked potentials and dual CD4 + CD8 + T cells in normal elderly individuals. **Sixth International Symposium on Neurological Control of Bodily Functions: Basic and Clinical Aspects** [presented]. Irvine, CA.

Kruesi, M. J., Dale, J., & Straus, S. E. (1989). Psychiatric Diagnoses in Patients who have chronic fatigue syndrome. Journal of Clinical Psychiatry , **50**(2), 53-56.

Sternberg, S. (1969). Memory-scanning:Mental processes revealed by reaction-time experiments. **American Scientist, 57**, 421-457.

Straus, S. E., Tosato, G., Armstrong, G., & et al. (1985). Persisting illness and fatigue in adults with evidence of Epstein-Barr virus infection. Annals of Internal Medicine, **102**, 7-16.

Tobi, M., Morag, A., Ravid, Z., & et al. (1982). Prolonged atypical illness associated with serological evidence of persistent Epstein-Barr virus infection. Lancet, **1**, 64-64.

Wilhardt, L., & Sandman, C. A. (1988). Performance of nondisabled adults and adults with learning disabilities on a computerized multiphasic cognitive memory battery. Journal of Learning Disabilities**21**(3), 179-185.

Chapter 54

Physical and Psychosocial Functioning in Chronic Fatigue Syndrome

Diane L. Cookfair, PhD, 1, 2, Diane Heimback, BA, 1, 2, Karl Wende, MS, 1,2, David Bell, MD, 3, and Carolyn Warner, MD, 3, 4

1) Department of Social and Preventive Medicine, State University of New York at Buffalo

2) Roswell Park Cancer Institute, Buffalo, NY.

3) Department of Neurology, State University of New York at Buffalo

4) Dent Neurologic Institute, Buffalo, NY.

Address all correspondence to:

Diane L. Cookfair, Ph.D Department of Social and Preventive Medicine State University of New York at Buffalo 2211 Main Street, Building A Buffalo, New York 14214

Dr. Diane Cookfair has an extensive background in cancer epidemiology and cancer education. Her past research includes studies assessing the long-term health effects of radiation therapy among cancer patients, and she also has conducted research concerning quality of life in cancer patients. Currently, Dr. Cookfair provides design consultation, and coordinates data management and statistical analyses for several clinical research studies. She is an Associate Research Professor at the University of Buffalo, State University of New York, and an Assistant Professor of Social and Preventive Medicine.

Abstract

Patients with CFS often report problems with physical and psychosocial functioning. However, little quantitative data are available concerning the type and level of impairment associated with this disease. We studied physical and psychosocial functioning in 79 CFS patients using the Sickness Impact Profile (SIP). The SIP is a performance-oriented health status measure which has been used to assess functional impairment in a variety of chronic disease populations. Mean scores suggestive of impairment were found for 11 of 12 categories of the SIP. The highest levels of impairment were reported for Alertness Behavior, Recreation Activities and Work function; 22% of respondents indicated that they were unable to work as a result of their illness. Ability to carry out routine household and home management activities was also significantly affected. Our results indicate that CFS patients experience significant levels of disability as a result of their illness. They also suggest that patient education and social and rehabilitative services may be useful in reducing functional impairment and improving quality of life.

Key Words: Chronic Fatigue Syndrome, Sickness Impact Profile, Physical Functioning, Psychosocial Functioning, Quality of Life

Introduction

Patients with Chronic Fatigue Syndrome (CFS) often report problems with physical, cognitive and psychosocial functioning[1,2]. In the United States, chronic disabling fatigue and generalized weakness are among the symptoms most commonly associated with CFS, and the CFS diagnostic criteria established by the Centers for Disease Control (CDC) requires that a patient should have experienced a 50% or greater reduction in activity as a result of fatigue for at least 6 months before they receive a diagnosis of CFS[3]. Despite the common nature of these symptoms, little data are available on the type and level of functional impairment associated with CFS, or the impact of CFS on the patient's quality of life.

Such data are extremely important to the management of a chronic disease, where the goal of treatment is often limitation of symptoms and preservation of function, rather than cure. The goals of our study were to provide quantitative data on physical and psychosocial functioning in CFS and information on quality of life among CFS patients.

Methods

Study Subjects: Patients were recruited from the practice of one physician specializing in the diagnosis and treatment of CFS. Ninety (90) CFS patients who had been seen over a one-year period were contacted by mail, asked to complete the enclosed questionnaires and return them in the postage paid, pre-addressed envelope which was provided. Follow up telephone calls were made to all non-responders. A total of 79 patients completed and returned questionnaires, a response rate of 89%. All patients satisfied the CDC diagnostic criteria for Chronic Fatigue Syndrome[3].

Table 1 provides information on the demographic characteristics of the study population. Patients ranged in age from 14 to 56, with a mean age of 35 years. All subjects were white, and the majority were female, with a female to male sex ratio of approximately 3 to 1. Seventy per cent (70%) had completed one or more years of college at the time of the study. Nine percent (9%) had not completed high school; however, this group included 3 high school students. Eighteen percent (18%) of the study subjects held a high school diploma, but had never attended college.

Length of illness ranged from 7 months to 22 years, with a mean illness duration of 4.8 years. Fifty-seven percent (57%) of the subjects were married, and approximately half had children living at home.

Table 1		
Demographic Characteristics of the Study Population		
Characteristic	Number*	Percent
Sex		
Female	58	73
Male	21	27
Marital Status		
Single	23	29
Married	45	57
Divorced	8	10
Separated	1	1
Unknown	2	3
Education		
Some High School	7	9
High School Diploma	14	18
Some College (<4 yrs)	28	35
Bachelor's Degree	11	14
Grad/Prof Degree	17	21
Unknown	2	3

	Mean	Median	Range
Age (yrs)	35	35	14-56
Duration of Illness (yrs)	4.8	2.6	7 mos-22 yrs

*N = 79

Assessment Procedures: Our working definition of quality of life was that of McSweeney et al[4], which includes the following dimensions: 1) Emotional functioning; 2) Social role functioning, including employment, home management, and social and family relationships; 3) Daily living activities such as self-care skills and mobility; and 4) Ability to engage in enjoyable hobbies, and other recreational pastimes. Quality of life was measured using a work history questionnaire and certain categories of the Sickness Impact Profile. Patients also completed a general information questionnaire and a brief illness history form. Physical and psychosocial functioning were measured using the Sickness Impact Profile.

The Sickness Impact Profile, or SIP, (see following page) is a performance-oriented health status measure of documented reliability and validity[5-8]. It provides information on the impact of illness for a broad range of activities of daily living, and has been found to correlate well with other health status and physiologic measures of disease severity in several chronic disease populations[9-11].

The SIP contains 136 items organized into 12 different functional categories. Each item describes a particular dysfunctional behavior, and patients are asked to check only those statements that describe them today and are related to their health. Table 2 provides sample items from each of the 12 categories[5]. In addition to the category scores, the SIP also provides dimension scores for physical functioning, psychosocial functioning, and a score for overall functioning.

Physical Dimension score is calculated using the items from 3 categories: Ambulation; Mobility; and Body Care and Movement. Psychosocial Dimension score is calculated using the items from four categories: Social Interaction; Communication; Alertness Behavior; and Emotional Behavior. Category and dimension scores are derived by summing the predetermined weights for every item checked from the relevant subscale, dividing by the total sum possible for that subscale, and multiplying by 100[5]. This results in a score which is expressed as percentage dysfunction. Possible scores range from 0 to 100, with higher scores reflecting worse function. The Overall per cent score is calculated in the same manner, using all of the items checked in the entire SIP.

Statistical Analyses: Data were analyzed and tested for statistical significance using Spearman's rank correlation coefficients and Kruskal-Wallis' Analysis of Variance by Ranks test[12].

Results

Table 3 presents the mean SIP scores and standard deviations for CFS patients as well as the maximum value recorded for each dimension and category. Minimum scores recorded for each dimension/category were all zero. Mean SIP scores from a previous study of 624 general population subjects[8] are also provided for purposes of comparison, along with mean SIP scores for four other patient populations, including patients with Rheumatoid Arthritis[13], Head Injury patients 2-4 years post-injury[14], and Myocardial Infarction patients 8 and a half months post event[15].

Mean Overall, Physical and Psychosocial Dimension scores were all elevated for CFS patients, with a mean Overall score of 18.5 (see Table 3 on following page). Mean scores also were elevated for every individual category except Eating Behavior, with the highest scores reported for Alertness Behavior (mean=46.3), Recreation and Pastimes (mean=36.2) and Work (mean=30.3).

The Mean Overall SIP score for CFS patients was similar to that reported for Rheumatoid Arthritis patients[13]. Mean physical score was higher for CFS patients than either Head Injury[14] or Myocardial Infarction[15] patients, and mean psychosocial scores were higher for CFS patients than for any other group included in the table. CFS patients also had higher Alertness Behavior scores than any other group including Head Injury patients.

Comparison of mean dimension scores for CFS patients by sex, age and education, revealed no significant differences in SIP score by sex or age. There were significant differences in Overall SIP score by level of Education (p≤.03), with scores highest in the least educated (some high school) and most educated groups (BA or Grad/Prof Degree). Length of illness showed moderate positive correlations with Overall (r=.361, p≤.001), Physical (r=.263, p≤.05) and Psychosocial scores (r=.358, p≤.001), and Physical and Psychosocial scores were positively correlated with each other (r=.673, p≥.001).

In addition to determining mean SIP scores, the percentage of CFS patients experiencing functional impairment was also calculated for each dimension and category. For these analyses, we chose a SIP Score of 10 or greater as a conservative cut-point for defining impairment. Table 4 (see opposite page) summarizes the percentage of CFS patients reporting no impairment (SIP score=0) vs. the percentage reporting impairment (SIP score of 10 or more).

Only 5% of CFS patients reported no functional impairment of any kind at the time of the survey (Overall SIP score=0). A sizable minority (25%) reported impairment (SIP score ≤10) in physical functioning, and the majority of CFS patients (75%) reported impairment in psychosocial functioning. Over 81% of the study population reported impairment in Alertness Behavior, an important component of psychosocial functioning.

In terms of the parameters used to define quality of life, from 20 to 30% of patients reported impairment (SIP score ≥10) in Daily Living Activities (Ambulation: 30.4%; Mobility: 25.3%; Body Care and Movement: 21.5%). Approximately half of all CFS patients reported impairment in Emotional functioning, and the majority also reported impairment in Recreation and Pastimes as a result of their illness (85% SIP score ≥10). Social role functioning was impaired in a variety of areas including Social Interaction (69.0% SIP score ≥10); Home Management (63.3% SIP score ≥10); and employment (67.1% Work SIP score ≥10).

Further information concerning the impact of illness on employment status is provided in Table 5. Prior to illness onset, approximately 16% of our subjects were students, and 14% were housewives. Excluding housewives, none of the adult subjects was unemployed. Only 8.9% held pre-illness positions of executive or professional status; 15.2% held positions as minor professionals or administrators, 5% were employed as unskilled or menial workers and the remainder were employed in skilled labor, clerical, sales or technical positions. As a result of their illness, sixteen percent (16%) of patients reported changing jobs, and twenty-two percent (22%) were no longer working. Fifty-seven percent (57%) were in the same jobs they held prior to illness onset, although some individuals indicated that they could now only work part time. Four subjects began work-

Table 2

Categories and Sample Items from the Sickness Impact Profile*

Category	Sample Item**
Sleep and Rest	I sit during much of the day I sleep or nap during the day
Eating	I am eating no food at all, nutrition is taken through tubes or intravenous fluids I am eating special or different food
Work	I am not working at all I often act irritable toward my work associates
Home management	I am not doing any of the maintenance or repair work around the house that I usually do I am not doing heavy work around the house
Recreation and Pastimes	I am going out for entertainment less I am not doing any of my usual physical recreation or activities
Ambulation	I walk shorter distances or stop to rest often I do not walk at all
Mobility	I stay within one room I stay away from home for only for brief periods of time
Body Care and Movement	I do not bathe myself at all, but am bathed by someone else I am very clumsy in body movements
Social interaction	I am doing fewer social activities with groups of people I isolate myself as much as I can from the rest of the family
Alertness Behavior	I have difficulty reasoning and solving problems, for example, making plans, making decisions, learning new things I sometimes behave as if I were confused or disoriented in place or time, for example, where I am, who is around, directions, what day it is
Emotional Behavior	I laugh or cry suddenly I act irritable and impatient with myself, for example, talk badly about myself, swear at myself, blame myself for things that happen
Communication	I am having trouble writing or typing I do not speak clearly when I am under stress

*Source: Reference (5).
**Items describe a behavior related to the category listed to their left (2 items are provided per category).

Table 3

SIP Scores in Patients with Chronic Fatigue Syndrome and Comparison Populations*

Dimension or Category	CFS Mean (SD)	Max**	GP Mean	RA Mean	HI Mean	MI Mean
Overall Score	18.5 (13.9)	67.8	3.6	15.6	9.6	6.9
Physical Dimension	6.5 (8.4)	38.2	***	14.0	3.9	4.0
Psychosocial Dimension	25.9 (19.0)	76.1	***	11.3	11.1	5.6
Physical						
Ambulation	7.8 (10.2)	50.0	3.1	21.0	7.2	7.7
Mobility	7.1 (13.2)	67.5	2.7	10.4	3.4	4.2
Body Care and Movement	6.1 (9.0)	46.3	1.0	12.7	3.3	2.4
Psychosocial						
Social Interaction	25.0 (20.2)	89.0	5.2	11.7	8.6	6.3
Communication	10.9 (16.8)	85.9	1.1	6.9	6.8	2.9
Alertness Behavior	46.3 (34.9)	100	4.0	13.0	15.7	6.5
Emotional Behavior	20.3 (22.5)	100	3.8	13.2	9.5	6.1
Independent Categories						
Sleep and Rest	27.7 (22.7)	90.2	7.2	17.6	8.4	11.5
Eating	2.7 (5.1)	18.7	1.6	3.5	1.0	6.8
Household Management	20.6 (19.1)	100.0	5.4	26.3	5.9	12.1
Recreation & Pastimes	6.2 (22.4)	100.0	10.2	26.7	11.1	15.2
Work	30.3 (27.4)	70.1	8.5	46.5	15.4	17.0
Number Studied	79		624	79	78	308

*GP= General Population; These individuals were a randomized sample from a prepaid health plan (8). Males and females were equally represented, as were 3 age groups (18 to 44 yrs, 45 to 64 yrs and 65 to 74 yrs); RA= Rheumatoid Arthritis Patients (13); HI= Head Injury Patients, 2 to 4 yrs. post-injury (14); MI= Myocardial Infarction Patients 8.5 mos. post-event (15)

**Max= Maximum Value Recorded for that dimension or category.

***These scores were not available for this population.

ing after illness onset; all had been students at the time they became ill.

We conducted further analyses to determine whether any variables were predictive of Work Score. There was no difference in mean Work Score by sex, age, or length of illness. Work score varied significantly by Education; least educated (Some HS), and most educated (BA, Grad/Prof) had the highest scores. Work score was positively correlated with Physical score (r=.507, p≤.001), Psychosocial score (r=.669, p≤.001) and Overall score (r=.738, p≤.001). Work score also showed a strong positive correlation with Alertness Behavior (r=.810, p≤.001).

Discussion

Our data indicate that CFS patients may experience significant levels of disability as a result of their illness, and that CFS has a pervasive negative impact on quality of life. Functional impairment was reported for a wide range of daily activities and behaviors. Social role functioning was impaired in several areas for the majority of patients studied, as was ability to engage in enjoyable hobbies and recreational activities. These data suggest a need for patient education programs, greater use of counselling, and increased use of social and rehabilitative services in order to reduce functional impairment associated with CFS.

Data concerning Alertness Behavior suggest that most patients experienced some impairment in this area of functioning. Alertness Behavior score was positively correlated with Emotional Behavior score (p≤.05), and it is possible that some of the problems patients reported with concentration and attention may be associated with emotional distress. However, the two categories were not perfectly correlated, and several patients with high Alertness Behavior scores reported little or no emotional impairment. These data suggest that some patients should receive formal neuropsychological assessment.

Length of illness was positively correlated with Overall, Physical and Psychosocial scores. While this finding appears to suggest a progressive worsening in function over time, it may also be due to the cross-sectional nature of study. It is possible that patients whose disease does not resolve in a short period of time are more ill to begin with, and would have been equally impaired had they been studied at an earlier point in their illness.

Both Work score and Overall score differed by level of education; however, Work score and Overall score were highly correlated. Furthermore, the relationship between Work score and level of education was not clear cut, with both the least educated and most educated groups showing high levels of impairment. As such, these data must be interpreted with caution. Further research will be necessary to determine whether this is a meaningful finding.

The SIP has been administered to a variety of patient groups, and data for a limited number of control populations have also been reported. Some of these data are provided in Table 3 in order to make it easier to interpret the SIP data for CFS patients. The data provided in Table 3 demonstrate that CFS patients may experience levels of functional impairment that are not unlike those reported by other types of chronic disease patients, and suggest that CFS patients experience overall levels of functional impairment similar to those of patients with Rheumatoid Arthritis.

Normative data from a large general population (N=624) are also provided in Table 3. Mean category scores for this group ranged from 1.0 to 10.2, with a mean Overall score of 3.6. This population was a stratified random sample of members from a prepaid health plan. The majority of the general population sample were older than the CFS patients we studied; healthy controls in the age range of our CFS patients might be expected to have slightly lower mean SIP scores than those reported for this general population sample. In a study conducted by McLean et al, 101 healthy male controls ranging in age from 15 to 60 (mean=24.5 yrs) were reported to have median scores of 0 for all 12 categories of the SIP[16].

With the exception of Head Injury patients, the patient comparison populations included in Table 3 (Rheumatoid Arthritis, Myocardial Infection) also tended to be older than the CFS patients we studied, and all included a greater percentage of male study subjects. The majority of the Rheumatoid Arthritis patients were ARA Class II; Head injury patients were studied 2 to 4 years post-injury. At the time of their original injury, 60.3% sustained mild head injury (Glasgow coma scale scores 11 to 14), and

Table 4

Percentage of CFS Patients* Reporting No Impairment Vs The Percentage Reporting Impairment+

Dimension or Category	No Impairment+		Reporting Impairment+	
	Number	Percent	Number	Percent
Overall Score	4	5.1	58	73.4
Physical Dimension	24	30.4	20	25.3
Psychosocial Dimension	9	11.4	59	74.7
Physical				
Ambulation	38	48.1	24	30.4
Mobility	52	65.8	20	25.3
Body Care and Movement	34	43.0	17	21.5
Psychosocial				
Social Interaction	10	12.7	55	69.6
Communication	40	50.6	38	48.1
Alertness Behavior	13	16.5	64	81.0
Emotional Behavior	22	27.8	40	50.6
Independent Categories				
Sleep and Rest	12	15.2	62	78.5
Eating	57	72.2	11	13.9
Household Management	14	17.7	50	63.3
Recreation & Pastimes	8	10.1	67	84.8
Work	22	27.8	53	67.1

+ No impairment = SIP score of 0;

Reporting impairment = SIP score of 10 or greater;

*N = 79; Percentage of individuals with SIP scores ranging from 1 to 9 on any individual dimension or category may be calculated by adding the total of the two percentages presented for that category/dimension and subtracting from 100.

another 29.5% sustained more severe injury (scores≤7); the remainder had scores ranging from 8 to 10. Three quarters of the Head Injury patients had sustained injury to other body areas. These factors should be considered when comparing CFS scores with scores for the other populations included in Table 3.

When interpreting the data presented in this report, it must also be kept in mind that this was an exploratory, descriptive study. The data were collected at one point in time on patients who had been sick for periods ranging from 7 months to 22 years; the patients represented individuals from one geographic region who sought out the care of a specialist. Therefore, although the mean age and sex ratios for our study population were similar to those reported for other series of CFS patients[1,2] the results of our study may not be generalizable to all CFS patients.

There was no physiologic measure of disease available which could be compared with the SIP scores to determine how well SIP scores reported by patients actually correlated with disease severity. However, the SIP is a quantitative measure of documented reliability and validity which has been found to correlate well with other health status and phsyiologic measures of disease severity in several chronic disease populations other than CFS patients[5-8, 9-11].

We did not study the effects of patient illness on family members. However, the age, and marital/family status of our study population suggest that the functional impairment experienced by CFS patients may also have a significant impact on other

family members, and this is a topic that should be considered in future studies. Further study is also necessary to determine the extent to which our data are generalizable to other CFS patients, to determine changes in functional status over time, and to determine other factors which may be associated with individual differences in functioning.

Quality of life and functional status measures are being used with increasing frequency as important outcome measures in clinical research involving other chronic diseases. Health status measures such as the SIP may be useful in studies concerning the management and treatment of CFS, and to measure individual responses to therapy.

Table 5		
Impact of Illness On Employment Status		
Change in Status	Number*	Percent
No change	45	57
Began working after illness onset	4	5
Change in Jobs as result of illness	13	16
No Longer Working as result of Illness	17	22

*N=79

References

1. Komaroff A: Chronic Fatigue Syndromes: Relationship to chronic viral infections. J Virol Meth 1988; 21: 3-10.

2. Jones JF and Straus SE: Chronic Epstein-Barr Virus Infection. Ann Rev Med 1987; 38: 195-209.

3. Holmes GP, Kaplan JE, Gantz NM et al: Chronic Fatigue Syndrome: A Working Case Definition. Ann Intern Med 1988; 108: 387-389.

4. McSweeney AJ, Grant I, Heaton RK, Adams KM and Timms RM: Life Quality of Patients with Chronic Obstructive Pulmonary Disease. Arch Inten Med 1982; 142: 473-478.

5. Bergner M, Bobbitt RA, Carter WB et al: The Sickness Impact Profile: Development and final revision of a health status measure. Med Care 1981; 19: 787-805.

6. Bergner M, Bobbitt RA, Pollard WE et al: The Sickness Impact Profile: Validation of a Health Status Measure. Med Care 1976; 14: 56-67.

7. Pollard WE, Bobbitt RA, Bergner N et al: The Sickness Impact Profile: Reliability of a Heath Status Measure. Med Care 1976; 14: 146-155.

8. Gilson BS, Bergner M, Bobbitt RA et al: "The Sickness Impact Profile: Final Development and Testing, 1975-1978." Seattle, Department of Health Services, School of Public Health and Community Medicine, University of Washington, 1979.

9. Read JL, Quinn RJ and Hoeffer MA: Measuring Overall Health: An Evaluation of Three Important Approaches. J Chron Dis 1987; 40, Suppl 1: 7S-21S.

10. Follick MJ, Smith TW and Ahern DK: The Sickness Impact Profile: a Global Measure of Disability in Chronic Low Back Pain. Pain 1985; 21: 67-76.

11. Deyo RA, Inui TS, Leininger JD and Overman SS: Measuring Functional Outcomes in Chronic Disease: A Comparison of Traditional Scales and a Self-Administered Health Status Questionnaire in Patients with Rheumatoid Arthritis. Med Care 1983; 21: 181-192.

12. SPSS Inc., SPSS Data Analysis System: SPSS-X User's Guide. Chicago, IL: SPSS Inc., 1988.

13. Deyo RA, Inui TS, Leininger J and Overman S: Physical and Psychosocial Function in Rheumatoid Arthritis: Clinical use of a self-administered health status instrument. Arch Intern Med 1982; 142: 879-882.

14. Klonoff PS, Snow WG and Costa LD: Quality of Life in Patients 2 to 4 Years After Closed Head Injury. Neurosurg 1986; 19: 735-743.

15. Bergner L, Hallstrom AP, Bergner M et al. Health Status of Survivors of Cardiac Arrest and Myocardial Infarction Controls. Amer J Pub Health 1985; 75: 1321-1323.

16. Mclean AL, Dikmen S, Temkin N, Wyler AR, and Gale JL: Psychosocial Functioning at 1 Month after Head Injury. Neurosurg 1984; 14: 393-399.

Psychiatry in M.E. / CFS

Chapter 55

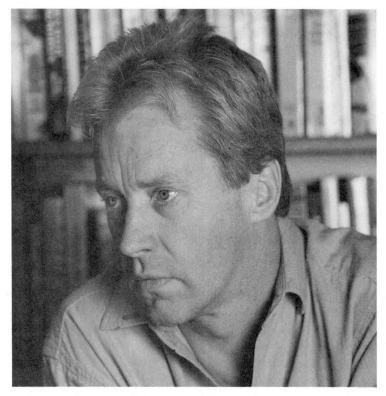

Donald Dutton

Depression\Somatization Explanations for the Chronic Fatigue Syndrome: A Critical Review

Donald G. Dutton, PhD, Department of Psychology, University of British Columbia

Donald Dutton is a Professor of Social Psychology at the University of British Columbia. Social psychology has traditionally been interested in the development of belief systems or ideologies, or what some people describe as paradigms. Dr. Dutton conducts research in this area, particularly as it relates to family violence issues.

Abstract

Empirical studies of the psychiatric status of chronic fatigue syndrome (CFS) patients have, for the most part, operated within the depression/somatization paradigm. According to this paradigm, CFS is attributed to:
1) immune suppression caused by depression;
2) a constitutional neural weakness of which a prior Major Depressive Episode is an indicator; or
3) a tendency for the patient to somatize depression through the symptoms of CFS.

This review examines both theoretical and empirical studies of the relationship between depression and chronic fatigue syndrome. These empirical studies have tended to conclude that chronic fatigue syndrome patients have higher than normal prevalence rates of psychiatric disturbance, typically depression or somatization. However, these studies have tended to confuse post hoc depression with premorbid depression, to confuse chronic fatigue patients with chronic fatigue syndrome patients, and to cluster prior episodes of depression that distally preceded the onset of chronic fatigue syndrome with those that occurred just prior to CFS. Hence, the perceived causal role of depression has been inflated by research in this paradigm. Some suggestions are made for a study of a variety of potential causal factors that have been overlooked by the narrow focus on depression/somatization.

The Kuhnian description of the tendency of a scientific paradigm (in this case the depression\ somatization paradigm) to direct scientific attention is discussed. The question is raised as to whether viral explanations for chronic fatigue syndrome, and possibly the very existence of the disorder, have been obscured by a paradigmatic perspective. Some research questions of potential importance are outlined and a suggestion is made for a multivariate research approach that examines a broader spectrum of psychosocial factors.

History and Definition of Chronic Fatigue Syndrome

Pre-modern epidemiologic thinking tended to emphasize the pathogenicity of a disease agent rather than those host or environmental factors that contributed to the degree of host resistance (Cassel, 1990). Dubos (1965) has argued that this perspective developed because early diseases of interest (e.g., bubonic plague, cholera, typhoid, smallpox) were of such extreme pathogenicity that host factors were overwhelmed. In contrast, most contemporary pathogens are microorganisms that are "ubiquitous in the environment, persist in the body without causing obvious harm under ordinary circumstances, and exert pathological effects only when the infected person is under conditions of physiological stress" (Cassel, p. 32). Although the pathogenicity of some contemporary viruses seems to be quite high, even in the case of HIV there have been reports of infected persons who have not developed AIDS decades after the HIV was recorded (Marvin Ross, Globe & Mail, May 11, 1991). Consequently, current epidemiologic research tends to focus on host factors that are believed to have substantial causal weight in the process of symptom development.

Chronic fatigue syndrome (CFS) is an example of a symptom set of indeterminate causal origin. The objective of this review is not to attempt an etiological clarification, but rather to examine the way evidence bearing on the etiology of CFS has been adduced. Our interest lies in the way the enterprise of discovery has proceeded: the questions that have been asked, the

questions that have been unasked, assumptions that guide the empirical studies, and the combination of data sets that have been used to imply causation.

Since 1985 numerous articles have been published about what is known, inter alia, as myalgic encephalomyelitis (M.E.) in England, low natural killer cell disease in Japan, and chronic fatigue syndrome (CFS) or chronic fatigue-immunity disorder syndrome (CFIDS) in the USA. (In this review we will use the term "CFS.") Although the symptomatology of this disease suggests that it has several historical antecedents, including neurasthenia[1] (Straus, 1991) and neuromyasthenia (Taerk et al., 1987), the prevalence of the disorder does seem to be greater in recent times. Considerable debate has surrounded CFS, turning on issues such as whether it has a viral cause, is merely depression, is a constitutional neurological weakness, or is the result of immunosuppression caused by depression (see Taerk, Toner, Salit, Garfinkel & Ozersky, 1987; Kruesi, Dale & Straus, 1988; Hickie, Lloyd, Wakefield & Parker, 1990; Abbey & Garfinkel, 1991; Katon, Buchwald, Simon, Russo & Mease [in press]).

Chronic fatigue (CF) and chronic fatigue syndrome (CFS) are recognized as two different diagnoses. Chronic fatigue is simply "feeling tired at least half the time for at least the preceding month" (Manu, Mathew & Lane, 1988a, p. 2214). The (U.S.) Center for Disease Control (CDC) "working case definition" for what they call chronic fatigue syndrome has as its major criterion "new and persistent or relapsing, debilitating fatigue or easy fatigability in a person who has no history of similar symptoms, that does not resolve with bed rest, and that is severe enough to reduce or impair average daily activity below 50% of the patient's premorbid activity level for a period of at least six months" (Holmes et al., 1988, p. 388). In addition, there are several minor criteria for symptoms that began at the onset of the fatigue and have persisted or recurred for 6 months. These include mild fever, sore throat, painful lymph nodes, unexplained muscle weakness, myalgia, prolonged fatigue after exercise that would have been easily tolerated in the patient's premorbid state, generalized headaches, arthralgia, sleep disturbance, and neuropsychologic complaints (inability to concentrate, confusion, photophobia, transient visual scotoma, difficulty thinking, forgetfulness, irritability and depression). Physical criteria must be documented by a physician on at least two occasions at least one month apart and include low grade fever, nonexudative pharyngitis and tender lymph nodes.

The CDC definition states that before the diagnosis is given, "other clinical conditions that may produce similar symptoms must be excluded by thorough evaluation." It then lists 46 possible alternative diagnoses, including "chronic psychiatric disease" such as endogenous depression, "chronic use of major tranquilizers...or antidepressive medications" and "autoimmune disease" (op. cit., p. 388). Since, as we shall see below, several studies argue that CFS is an autoimmune disease (Klimas, Salvato, Morgan & Fletcher, 1990), a problem exists with its exclusion. Similarly, a problem exists in excluding endogenous depression. The DSM-III-R (American Psychiatric Association, 1987) definition of a Major Depressive Episode (MDE) includes "fatigue or loss of energy" as well as sleep disorder and inability to concentrate. An MDE is characterized by an alteration of the patient's previous level of functioning as well as at least five of the following nine symptoms, which must include either of the first two: (1) depressed mood; (2) markedly diminished interest or pleasure in all, or almost all, activities; (3) significant weight loss or gain or decrease or increase in appetite; (4) insomnia or hypersomnia; (5) psychomotor agitation or retardation that is observable by other people; (6) fatigue or loss of energy; (7) feelings of worthlessness or excessive or inappropriate guilt; (8) diminished ability to think or concentrate or indecisiveness; (9) recurrent thoughts of death or suicidal ideation or attempts. To establish a diagnosis of MDE, these symptoms must persist for 2 weeks (compared to 6 months for CFS) and the diagnosis is excluded if an organic factor is the cause. Clearly, the commonality of symptoms for depression and CFS sets the stage for diagnostic confusion. In fact, some researchers have argued (e.g., Katon et al., 1982a; Katon et al., in press) that somatized depression can encompass virtually all symptoms of CFS. Other researchers (e.g., Klimas et al., 1990) suggest that depression is an affliction that **follows** onset of CFS.

Perhaps because evidence for a viral cause of CFS has been evasive[2], the tendency of medical researchers to emphasize a role for depression in CFS has increased. The evidence for these relationships takes the form of assessments for both presence of depression and CFS and their temporal relationship.

Depression as a Cause of CFS: The Empirical Studies

Given the theoretical rationale for assessing the causal role of depression in CFS, one might expect some well designed research to examine this possibility. However, when we turn to empirical studies of the role of depression in CFS we find that several definitional and methodological problems have obscured any definitive results.

In general, the strategy of this research is to look for inflated prevalence rates of premorbid psychiatric problems in CFS patients. The presumed etiologic implications of this search are that patients with premorbid depression have immunosuppression as a result of the depression, have a constitutional neurologic weakness from which both depression and chronic fatigue syndrome arise, or have a tendency to somatize psychological problems and the chronic fatigue syndrome represents another manifestation of that somatization (Abbey & Garfinkel, 1991; Katon et al., in press). We examine these assumptions below.

Problems arise in these studies from a variety of sources: chronic fatigue patients are not distinguished from CFS patients, although the theoretical overlap of depression with chronic fatigue (which has one symptom) is greater than the overlap of depression with the entire constellation of specific symptoms constituting CFS. In addition, psychological problems that are sequelae of the CFS are not clearly differentiated from premorbid problems[3]. The effect size of depression is rarely accurately estimated, although this could easily be done by estimating its increased likelihood in CFS populations over controls. Finally, the temporal relationship of depression to CFS is not clearly specified; psychological events that proximally preceded CFS onset and more distant psychological events are inappropriately lumped together, even though they may have quite different theoretical significance in determining the etiology of CFS. These findings are typically coupled with evidence of immunologic suppression by depression based on research that measured this suppression **at the time of the depression, not years after the depression** (see, for example, Abbey and Garfinkel,

		Table 1			
		Empirical studies of depression in CFS patients			
Study	Subjects	CF/CFS Distinction	Pre-Post Distinction	Distal/Proximal Distinction	Conclusion
Taerk et al. (1987)	CFS vs. Hospital Staff	Yes	Yes	No	50% of CFS had premorbid MDE
Manu et al. (1988a)	100 patients with fatigue	No	No	No	36% had depression 15% had somatization
Kruesi et al. (1989)	28 CFS patients	Yes	Yes	No	only 2/28 had premorbid MDE CFS not attributable to depression
Wessely & Powell (1989)	47 patients with PVFS vs. depressives, neuromuscular disease patients	No	Yes	No	47% had prior depression
Hickie et al. (1990)	48 CFS patients 48 depressed patients	Yes	Yes	No	24% of CFS group had premorbid depression (not significantly different from general population rate)
Katon et al. (1991)	98 CF patients 31 with rheumatoid arthritis	Not for data	No	No	67.3% chronic fatigue patients had "lifetime" diagnosis of depression premorbid not reported

1991; Katon et al., in press). The net effect is to convey the impression that depression may play a greater causal (presumably immunosuppressive) role in CFS than is warranted by the data. I am not aware of any studies that investigated immunosuppression at an extended time lag after depression[4] or that would claim that the mere presence of a prior MDE was sufficient basis for inferring immunosuppression. Most of the studies of depression and immune suppression used patients who were hospitalized for depression (see, for example, O'Leary 1990).

A review of research on depression and CFS is reported by Abbey and Garfinkel (1991).[5] No references are made in that review to the methodological problems I cite here. Instead, the authors frequently repeat, in an uncritical manner, many of the misleading conclusions of the original studies and, in many cases, drop qualifying statements by the original authors. I shall quote extensively from these papers

and from Abbey and Garfinkel in order to give the reader a sense of the language of interpretation found in the depression/somatization paradigm. A summary of these studies is presented in Table 1.

Taerk et al. (1987) conducted the first reported systematic investigation of the prevalence of psychiatric symptoms, including depression, in a group of patients who presented with CFS. These patients and a matched comparison of volunteers (who were students or were recruited from the hospital staff) were evaluated by means of a psychiatric interview, the Diagnostic Interview Schedule (which provides diagnoses of psychiatric disorders in accordance with DSM-III, an older version of the DSM-III-R), and a self-reported evaluation of depressive symptomatology (the Beck Depression Inventory [BDI]). As Taerk et al. reported and Abbey and Garfinkel (1991) cited in their review of the literature, the study revealed a significantly higher lifetime prevalence of affective disorders in patients with CFS (major depression in 67%, dysthymia in 25%) than in controls. On the basis of the DIS, 50% of the patients in the CFS sample had a history of an MDE before the development of neuromyasthenia (CFS). According to the BDI data, 67% of the CFS group and 17% of the controls reported experiencing depression, and 46% of the CFS group and none of the controls reported this depression as moderate to severe.

However, as Hickie, Lloyd, Wakefield and Parker (1990) point out, the premorbid prevalence rate for the CFS group (12\24) was not significantly higher than that of the controls (7\24) and the application of DSM-III criteria (as opposed to the more restrictive DSM-III-R criteria) produced high prevalence rates of all psychiatric disorders in both the patients and the healthy controls. These criticisms were not mentioned by Abbey and Garfinkel. Furthermore, the BDI data were all post CFS and consequently have no causal weight (Abbey and Garfinkel reported the data but not the fact that they were post hoc). And for the 12 of 24 CFS patients who reported premorbid depression, no report is made of whether this depression was temporally proximal or distal to the onset of CFS. Despite these methodological shortcomings, Taerk et al. concluded that "the syndrome likely represents the result of an interplay between psychological and organic factors in a susceptible individual...the development of chronicity could be related to a particular response to the illness and its associated debilitation, which triggers a depressive syndrome. Evidence for this occurring in vulnerable people is the extremely high rate of major depression in our group, antedating viral illness" (op. cit., p. 54). By implication, these were people who were vulnerable to depression, which accounts for the chronicity of the problem. Below we will consider whether depression in response to CFS requires any prior "vulnerability" to depression, or whether such reasoning underestimates the psychosocial impact of the illness.

Manu

Manu et al. (1988a) undertook a study "to determine the psychiatric morbidity of patients complaining of chronic fatigue" (op. cit., p. 2213). In this study 100 patients who felt tired at least half the time for at least the preceding month were given a comprehen-sive medical examination and the 1981 version of the DIS which makes psychiatric diagnoses in accordance with DSM-III (an older version of the current DSM-III-R and one that tends to inflate prevalence rates). No clear description is given of how the authors determined which psychiatric problems were premorbid except to say that "prospective rules were established" (op. cit., p. 2214). Sixty-six patients had one or more psychiatric disorders that were considered a major cause of their fatigue (47 had mood disorders [36 were depression], 15 had somatization disorder, and 9 had anxiety disorder). The temporal relationships between these psychiatric diagnoses and the physical fatigue symptoms that (presumably) followed are not reported. The authors conclude "our results suggest that chronic fatigue is an expression of somatization...(and)...that major depression was the most common cause of somatization expressed as chronic fatigue" (op. cit., p. 2216).

Chronic Fatigue vs. Chronic Fatigue Syndrome

This paper exemplifies problems arising when chronic fatigue is not differentiated from chronic fatigue syndrome and when clear rules for the temporal ordering of psychiatric and physical symptoms are not made explicit. Depression and chronic fatigue have great symptom overlap; such may not be the case with the complex symptomology of CFS. It is therefore important not to mix chronic fatigue with chronic fatigue syndrome patients in this research, especially since references to original studies do not always make the distinction clear (e.g., Grafman, Johnson & Scheffers [1991] and Abbey & Garfinkel [1991] both refer to the Manu et al. (1988a) study as though it examined chronic fatigue syndrome).

In another paper, Manu, Lane and Mathews (1988b) established that CFS was present in only 6 of 135 patients with chronic fatigue; 91 other patients were ruled out because they had "psychiatric disorders that were clinically active" (op. cit., p. 555). As no differentiation was made between premorbid depression and depression as a sequela of CFS, patients experiencing depression as a consequence of CFS (as 80% of patients do, see Klimas et al., 1990) were ruled out as having CFS. This paper makes clear the problems with the exclusionary clause in the CDC definition of CFS.

Kruesi

Kruesi, Dale and Straus (1989) studied 28 patients with CFS who were enrolled in placebo-controlled clinical trials for acyclovir, who had been ill for an average of 6.8 years and had been extensively investigated to exclude other possible disorders (with the exception of current or past psychiatric diagnoses which did not exclude them from these drug treatment trials). The revised DIS was used to make psychiatric diagnoses in accordance with DSM-III-R. Abbey and Garfinkel report "a high lifetime prevalence of affective disorder was found—55% in women and 25% in men" (op. cit., p. s74), but this includes post-CFS depression, which Abbey and Garfinkel do not make clear. At the time of assessment, only 40% of the patients who had a lifetime history of affective disorder reported that they were experiencing dysphoric affect. The depression usually occurred concurrently with, or following the onset of, CFS. High premorbid rates were not found for depression (only 2/28 had prior MDE) or for somatization (only 2/28 met these criteria). Kruesi et al. concluded "many of the physical and immunologic features of the chronic fatigue syndrome are not clearly attributable to psychiatric illness" (op. cit., p. 55).

Wessely and Powell (1989) studied 47 patients diagnosed with "post viral fatigue syndrome" (PVFS) and compared them to patients who had peripheral muscular disease characterized by depression and to psychiatric patients with major depression. Fatigue was excluded as a symptom of depression when psychiatric diagnoses were made. Psychiatric disorders were identified in a significantly greater percentage of patients with PVFS (72%) than controls with peripheral neuromuscular disease (36%). Without counting fatigue as a diagnostic for depression, 47% of the PVFS group were still diagnosed as having had a prior depression. Abbey and Garfinkel (1991) state that "the principal difference between the patients with PVFS and the patients with major depression was in the attribution by the patients who had PVFS of a physical cause for their difficulties" (p. s74). However, Wessely and Powell report that 72% of the PVFS group had been exposed to viruses compared to only 21% of the depressed group. The authors dismiss the possibility that affective changes are a result of chronic ill health, as both PVFS and neuromuscular disease controls had been ill for equivalent lengths of time. Their own data, however, suggest that the PVFS group was more completely disabled than the control group, with higher scores on physical fatigue, mental fatigue, and the General Health Questionnaire, and their measure of "psychiatric status" was unrelated to patients' reports of fatigue on mental effort.

Hickie et al.

Hickie et al. (1990) examined 48 patients with CFS as determined by an extensive physical evaluation. The criteria for inclusion were essentially the same as the CDC definition and exclusionary assessments were made to rule out other causes of fatigue. Control subjects were 48 patients with non-endogenous depression selected from the psychiatric services. Subjects were interviewed by a psychiatrist using SCID-P to assess for DSM-III-R diagnoses. Patients' self-reports were corroborated by a relative. Assessments were also made for depression, personality disorders and attitudes toward illness. Hickie et al. concluded that "when compared to non-endogenously depressed controls, our CFS patients did not have a similar premorbid rate of psychiatric disorder, were significantly less neurotic and, when unwell, neither clinically resembled nor had the psychometric profile of non-endogenous depressive patients seen in psychiatric settings" (op. cit., p. 537). The estimated premorbid lifetime rate of psychiatric disorder in the CFS group was 24%. The lifetime prevalences for psychiatric disorder in the general population estimated by three surveys ranged from 24.9% to 26.2%. (Robins et al., 1984). The premorbid lifetime rate for major depression in the CFS group was 12.5%, compared to 18 to 25% reported for the general population in three large scale epidemiological studies using the same test material (Weissman, Myers & Harding, 1978; Reich, Rice, Andreasen et al. (sic) 1980; Bromet et al., 1986). Hence the CFS group did not appear to have rates of either psychiatric disturbance in general, or depression in particular, that exceeded those of the general population. As the authors put it, "our results suggest that CFS patients are no more psychologically disturbed before the onset of their illness than members of the general population" (op. cit., p. 538) and "there is no evidence from our well-defined sample to support the hypothesis that CFS is a somatic presentation of an underlying psychological disorder. In particular, there is no evidence that CFS is a variant or expression of a depressive disorder. Instead, our study supports the hypothesis that the current psychological symptoms of patients with CFS are a consequence of the disorder, rather than evidence of antecedent vulnerability" (op. cit., p. 539).[6]

The Katon Study

A recent study by Katon et al. (in press) has attempted to address several methodological problems in the studies cited above. Katon et al. have improved on these problems by selecting as a control group patients who also have a chronic disease (rheumatoid arthritis) which fits the same gender ratio (females more common than males) as CFS. As the authors put it, "we hypothesized that if psychiatric illness was secondary to the burden of medical illness, then patients with rheumatoid arthritis should have similar rates of psychiatric illness as patients with chronic fatigue...a higher prevalence of psychiatric illness in patients with chronic fatigue, especially psychiatric illness that preceded the fatigue, would provide evidence of a psychiatric etiology" (op. cit., p.6). (Note that such reasoning assumes that both illnesses should be equally depressing, but the lessened ability of CFS patients to get a diagnosis may heighten the rate of depression for CFS.)

Subjects were drawn from a chronic fatigue clinic and were administered, inter alia, the DIS. Chronic fatigue patients were divided into those who met the CDC criteria for CFS and those who did not. The latter are referred to as the chronic fatigue group, the former as the CFS group. All subjects underwent an extensive review of their medical history, a physical examination, laboratory studies, a psychiatric examination and completed various self-report measures. Using the DIS, interviewers ascertained from the subjects the date, month and year of each positive psychiatric diagnosis and the onset of chronic fatigue. (Although it is theoretically possible to affix exact dates to onsets of physical symptoms and/or depressive episodes using the DIS, the vagaries of human memory and the practicalities of data reduction generate the practice of using three temporal categories: during the last month, one to six months ago, and prior to six months ago. The determination of precise temporal ordering within a category thus becomes problematic.) In another advance over prior

studies, Katon et al. scored depression both with and without the symptom of fatigue, and somatization with and without the seven symptoms that overlapped with CFS (headaches, arthralgias, myalgias, periods of muscle weakness, having to leave work or take time off due to unexplained illness, problems with walking, crying spells). The authors state that *"patients were classified as having a current DSM-III-R diagnosis when they met criteria within one month. Lifetime diagnoses were also recorded"* (op. cit., p. 9).

For the two groups reported, chronic fatigue patients had a higher lifetime prevalence of major depression and somatization disorder than the rheumatoid arthritic patients. However, it is not clear that the authors' operational definition of lifetime prevalence is clearly premorbid. If lifetime includes all symptoms occurring prior to the last month (which is defined as current), then many chronic fatigue patients would have experienced fatigue prior to the psychiatric diagnosis, since it would be rare to present at a specialized clinic within one month of disease onset. These elevated lifetime diagnoses dropped when the overlapping symptoms with chronic fatigue were eliminated. With somatization, the lifetime prevalence for chronic fatigue patients dropped from 45.9% to 20.4%; with depression it dropped from 76.5% to 67.3%. What we still do not know is what the premorbid rates were for chronic fatigue syndrome patients in this study. Knowing these rates would be a step toward making some assessment of the causal role of depression and somatization, although we would still like to know the time lag between these diagnoses and the onset of fatigue.

Hence, the Katon et al. study is still inconclusive. The authors themselves, however, conclude that their results are consistent with the notion of affective disease (alone or in combination with a "triggering insult") leading to changes in immune function or with the notion of affective illness being the main cause of the patient's distress (i.e., somatization). As they put it, "...as in our sample of patients with chronic fatigue, patients with chronic pain often have episodes of major depression that have preceded by a number of years the history of chronic pain and have significantly more symptoms of psychological distress...this hypothesis would explain fatigue and other physical complaints as 'somatized' expressions of psychological distress or, alternatively, the biologic effects of depression on multiple bodily systems" (p. 21). Here we have a succinct expression of the depression\somatization paradigm offered with little in the way of confirmatory empirical evidence.

Depression

A critical reading of the above literature leads to the conclusion that consistent evidence for inflated rates of premorbid depression in chronic fatigue syndrome (as opposed to chronic fatigue) patients has not been demonstrated. Of the three studies that differentiated CFS from chronic fatigue patients, two concluded that premorbid depression was not abnormally high in the CFS group; the other used a criterion of depression that inflates its prevalence. An MDE is a risk factor because it suppresses immune function itself, because it is an indicator of a pre-existing (possibly constitutional) neurological weakness, or because it is an indicator of a tendency to be depressive and hence to somatize. In the next section we will examine the premises that initially directed this search.

Depression, CFS and Immune Suppression

As Abbey and Garfinkel (1991) put it, "any argument that CFS is no more than an atypical presentation of MDE (Major Depressive Episode) would have to account for the altered immune function that has been reported in patients with CFS" (op. cit., p. s77). Abbey and Garfinkel report studies that found immune abnormalities in patients with CFS including: reduction in the absolute number of T lymphocytes, including CD2 (total number), CD4 (helper\inducer) and CD8 (suppressor\cytotoxic) subsets; increased T-cell mediated suppression; decreased natural-killer cell activity and cytotoxicity; decreased in vitro antibody synthesis following mitogen stimulation; partial hypogammaglobulinemia; decreased in vitro production of interferon and interferon-2; and other autoimmune phenomena. However, the authors state *"the type and prevalence of abnormal findings have varied widely across studies and have not appeared to correlate with severity of symptoms"* (op. cit., p. s77). Yet Klimas et al., based on their study of 30 patients with CFS and their review of the literature, concluded that *"CFS was a form of acquired autoimmuno-*

deficiency...present in all the subjects that we studied. It has several manifestations, with NK cell dysfunction being the most consistent abnormality" (op. cit., p. 1408). In general, and despite the variability described by Abbey and Garfinkel, all empirical studies of immune function in CFS patients have found some form of altered immune response.

Although MDE is associated with increased risk for illnesses that are associated with altered immune competence (such as changes in neuroendocrine parameters and neurotransmitters that modulate the immune system), direct examination of altered immune response in patients with MDE is far less compelling than the studies of CFS patients. Studies of lymphocyte function in patients with MDE have produced mixed results. Natural killer cell activity has been found to be decreased in individuals with major depression, undergoing bereavement or experiencing high levels of life stress. Yet, in what Abbey and Garfinkel describe as the most comprehensive study to date, Schleifer, Keller, Bond, Cohen and Stein (1989) found no mean differences in mitogen-induced lymphocyte proliferation, lymphocyte subsets and natural killer cell activity between patients with MDE and controls. They ascribe the variability in previous findings to a variety of uncontrolled factors in the research ranging from demographic differences between depressed and control samples, to characteristics of the depressive syndrome itself. As this research currently stands, it is safe to conclude that some immune irregularities are found some of the time in some depressed people while they are depressed. Schleifer et al. drew the conclusion that altered immunity *"does not appear to be a specific biologic correlate of major depressive disorder but may occur in subgroups of depressed patients"* (Abbey and Garfinkel, op. cit., p. s78).

In other words, the case for depression consistently producing immunosuppression is weak, even when the immunosuppression is measured **during** the depression. In some of the studies of premorbid tendencies toward depression that we reviewed, the implication was made that depression occurring at any time prior to the onset of CFS might be serving some immunosuppressive function. Clearly the research on depression and immune suppression does not support such a claim.

Depression, CFS and Neurological Weakness

When depression occurs prior to CFS onset, an alternative interpretation to immunosuppression is that both the depression and the CFS are produced by constitutional neurological weaknesses. Straus (1991), for example, argues that CFS was once neurasthenia and was used to *"signify the lack of strength of the nerves"* (op. cit., p. s2). Abbey and Garfinkel concluded, on the basis of the Schleifer et al. study, that while MDE *"may not be the primary etiologic agent underlying the onset of CFS, it may be the causal factor in the ongoing cycle of disability and distress in patients with CFS"* (op. cit., p. s78). This argument posits that CFS *"reflects the interplay between organic and psychological factors in psychologically vulnerable individuals with a depressive diathesis"* (op. cit., p. s78). In other words, there is an inherited or constitutional tendency to react to illness with depression, and the depression prolongs the recovery period.

If constitutional weaknesses existed in CFS patients, one should expect to see family histories of depression in CFS patients or that subgroups of CFS patients with a longer recovery period would differ from those with a shorter recovery period in their family history of depression. No such research with CFS patients has been reported. There is some frequently cited evidence to implicate depression as a determinant of recovery time from influenza (Imboden, Canter & Cluff, 1961), although that was a small sample of 26 subjects, the main effect for depressive personality was confounded with age and the study has not been replicated.[7] In research assessing the prior existence of MDEs in CFS patients, no attempt is made to determine whether the prior MDE was caused by an illness. If not, the evidence for a depressive reaction to illness that differentiates this population from other patients does not exist. Again, the evidence is weak for a constitutional tendency to react to illness with depression that prolongs the illness. Furthermore, it is not clear how the existence of one two-week episode of depression provides evidence for a constitutional neural weakness, as is implied by depression/somatization research. This being the case, one wonders what having a distal premorbid MDE adds to the explanation of CFS.

Somatization

A third premise of the search for inflated prevalence rates for premorbid depression is the assumption that CFS represents a type of somatization (Katon et al., in press). This interpretation seems a priori self-contradictory since, as we shall see below, people who experience depression affectively and report an MDE are less likely to somatize (Katon et al., 1981). The DSM-III-R defines somatiform disorders as those having physical symptoms where the specific pathophysiologic processes are not demonstrable or understandable by existing laboratory procedures and are conceptualized most clearly by means of psychological constructs. In order to be classified as a somatization disorder one must demonstrate 1) a history of many physical complaints or a belief that one is sickly, beginning before the age of 30 and persisting for several years, and 2) at least 13 from a list of 35 physical symptoms where a) no organic pathology or pathophysiologic mechanism to account for the symptom exists, b) the symptoms have not occurred only during a panic attack, and c) the symptoms have caused the person to take a medicine, see a doctor or alter their lifestyle. The DSM-III-R lists age of onset for somatization in the teen years or, rarely, in the 20's, and that the disorder is typically presented by females. The course of the disorder is described as chronic, with a year seldom passing without some medical attention. Hence, somatization is viewed by the DSM-III-R perspective as a chronic pattern of dealing with psychological problems. It would tend to show up early and would not tend to present as a response to a problem experienced later in life.

The depression\somatization paradigm

Katon, Kleinman and Rosen (1982a) have argued that depression can be somatized by people who: 1) lack an emotional vocabulary; 2) exist in a culture or subculture with sanctions against talking about or perceiving emotional states (like depression); or 3) where there are culturally provided explanations for affective states. They cite cross-cultural studies of depression which show that while a core of vegetative symptoms exist in all cultures, both the affective expression of depression and the cognitive expressions such as guilt and self-deprecation are particular to Western culture. In many other cultures and in Western working class culture, somatic symptoms dominate. Furthermore, families that do not develop psychological language for articulating unpleasant emotions are most likely to focus on somatic manifestations of depression. Katon et al. cite a study by Kreitman, Sainsbury, Pearce and Costain (1965) which showed that patients who presented with persistent somatic symptoms and were eventually recognized as depressed (with the classic vegetative symptoms of sleep disturbance, decreased libido and appetite, weight loss, plus their response to antidepressants) differed from patients who presented primarily with depression, in that significantly more mothers of those in the former group had identical somatic symptoms.[8] Furthermore, in a study of 51 MDE patients, Mathew, Weinman and Mirabi (1981) found the following rates of symptom reporting: impaired concentration, 86%; weakness, 82%; daytime drowsiness, 76.5%; dizziness 65%. Clearly these symptoms are the same as some reported by CFS patients, suggesting that CFS may be a form of somatized depression.

A corollary to the depression\somatization paradigm is the notion that physicians themselves overlook depression because of their orientation to the physical. As Katon, Kleinman and Rosen (1982b) put it, *"the effect on the patient's perception of his illness of the physician's narrow somatic model is that hypochondriacal patterns are reinforced by medical concern and substantial workups. The physician's somatic focus helps externalize the patient's subjective dysphoria as an objective bodily complaint, which often is more palatable to the patient than a diagnosis of depression that may have moral connotations"* (op. cit., p. 243). Hence, this paradigm not only purports to account for the explanation of symptoms, but also the patient's objection to being diagnosed as depressed.

There are some problems with the view that CFS is somatized depression. As mentioned above, somatization disorder, according to the DSM-III-R, involves a history of physical complaints or a belief that one is sickly, beginning before the age of 30. Age of onset is described as usually in the teen years. By contrast, the average age of CFS onset in the empirical studies reported is 37, often with no prior medical history suggesting somatization (Komaroff & Buchwald, 1991). Katon et al.'s (1982a) notion that somatization presents more in people who lack the vocabulary for emotion would lead to the prediction that it would be more prevalent in males, since socialization for that gender includes acquired

alexythymia (Fasteau, 1974; Mosher & Tompkins, 1988), but according to the DSM-III-R, the disorder is rarely diagnosed in males. Also, if patients who somatize do not experience the affective or cognitive aspects of depression, they would be less likely to be diagnosed as having had an MDE on the DIS (Diagnostic Interview Schedule) yet, as we have seen, the empirical thrust of research connecting depression to CFS has been to demonstrate a heightened likelihood of prior MDE in CFS patients. A contrary perspective to Katon et al.'s notion that physicians overlook psychological factors is that when symptoms are presented by patients that are apparently inexplicable through conventional physical diagnosis, a tendency exists to "write off" the symptoms as psychological in origin. A variety of "lifestyle" causes are presented to the patient (such as work stress), at least one of which will apply to most patients. When negative events occur in our lives, we tend to blame ourselves for their occurrence, presumably to find a way of controlling and preventing their recurrence (Wortman, 1976). Hence, when a psychological "solution" is offered, many patients will accept it, until subsequent events disconfirm this analysis.

An empirical question as yet unanswered is whether subjects in studies indicating a viral presence for CFS had any prior history of depression or somatization. Further, it is unclear as to why the particular syndrome of symptoms as described by CFS patients would stand out against the variable patterns of 35 symptoms which are criteria for somatization. CFS patients describe the location of myalgias (e.g., in the trapezius muscle) with greater consistency than should occur from somatization alone.

Secondary Gain, Secondary Loss

Indicative of the circularity in the perspective of depression-somatization is the notion of secondary gain which, according to Katon et al. (1982a), *"...commonly takes the form of disability payments and change in family systems that enable patients to avoid stressful situations like work and to fulfil dependency needs by becoming passive recipients of care by others. Other secondary gains include the sanctioning of failure, "addiction" to the health care system for social support and the manipulation of social relationships"* (op. cit., p.129). Hence, it is assumed that the patient may have some unconscious need to be passive and dependent that is fulfilled and sanctioned by the illness. This assumption is made despite an absence of independent evidence for the existence of these dependency strivings in the identified population. Nowhere in this literature is the concept of secondary **loss** considered, despite CFS patients' reports of inability to work, to have normal social lives, experience choice about dependence-independence, and have a sense of efficacy and control in their lives. These secondary losses may greatly outweigh some vague need for dependence.

Abbey and Garfinkel state that *"there may be a heightened susceptibility to depression in the population with CFS, given the clinical descriptions of the personality characteristics of those patients"* (op. cit., p. s79) and refer to the depression as an *"adjustment disorder."*[9] It has been reported that patients with CFS are achievement-oriented, goal-driven individuals who have been exceptionally active socially, occupationally and physically (Salit, 1985). Arieti and Bemporad (1978) and Beck (1983) describe depressive vulnerability in individuals who are driven toward achievement as a means of stabilizing self-esteem and experiencing pleasure. *"In individuals who are premorbidly characterized by high or overachievement...the experience of incapacitation secondary to a severe or protracted viral illness would result in the loss of the ability to participate....thus rendering them vulnerable to depression"* (Abbey & Garfinkel, 1991, p. s79).

On the one hand it is implied that CFS allows individuals to satisfy previously denied dependency needs, presumably reducing depression; on the other hand it is suggested that low self-esteem drives these individuals into an active life and undermines their capacity to adjust to the restrictions of CFS, thus increasing depression. Both these contradictory theories are without support. As Abbey and Garfinkel note, all personality descriptions of CFS patients are anecdotal. The Salit study cited by Abbey and Garfinkel simply reported demographic characteristics of patients, showing them to be predominantly college graduates whose employment was either professional or managerial. Despite the fact that there is no empirical evidence to support these assumptions, they represent cornerstones of the depression\somatization paradigm that posits psychological traits as the cause of CFS and, as we have

seen, influences the conduct and interpretation of empirical studies. No empirical study of CFS patients has assessed whether they are, in fact, "driven" people or overachievers. Furthermore, there is no evidence that depression plays an immunosuppressive function long after its occurrence, nor is there evidence that depression indicates a neurological weakness. Finally, even if psychosocial factors were prevalent, it would not preclude a search for a viral agent. As Ray (1991) puts it, *"psychological and social factors which enhance vulnerability to disease...are seen as neither necessary nor sufficient prerequisites...and few would wish to argue that conditions such as cancer or tuberculosis should be regarded as psychological disorders"* (op. cit. p. 3).

Depression and CFS: Cause or Consequence?

Is severe and incapacitating physical impairment that occurs without explanation or prognosis sufficient to cause depression regardless of a depressive diathesis? Below we shall argue that psychological sequelae of CFS have been underestimated by medical researches, leading them to make the *"fundamental attribution error"* (Nisbett & Ross, 1980), whereby effects are erroneously attributed to personality traits because of an insufficient appraisal of the power of the situation (or illness).

Studies by Klimas et al. and others demonstrate that depression is a common (i.e., 80%) reaction in CFS patients. Could it not be that aspects of the experience of CFS itself are a sufficient explanation for a reactive depression? As has been described, CFS can be a highly incapacitating disease that renders work activity, concentration and social life difficult if not impossible (Zala, 1989). It has an uncertain duration and prognosis, it recurs cyclically and unpredictably, and is often met with skepticism by physicians and others. Such effects would seem sufficient to explain the depression that CFS patients experience, without recourse to personality explanations.

Prolonged or unpredictable enforced helplessness or loss of control is one definition of psychological trauma (Terr, 1991) and is sufficient to generate depression (Seligman, 1975; Arieti & Bemporad, 1978) and other forms of psychological distress (Ochberg, 1988). Such distress would include alterations of arousal (hyperarousal to hypoarousal), and affective lability alternating with flat affect and generalized irritability. Derogatis and Wise (1989) have argued that depression accompanying prolonged debilitating illness might be more appropriately construed as demoralization or despondency than as a psychiatric disorder. Viewed from this perspective, one wonders about the profile of a patient who does **not** react with depression to this debilitating syndrome. One also wonders about the lack of research attention paid to outlining factors that may predict the post CFS severity of depression. For example, does repeated denial by physicians that the patient is ill or their insistence that the illness is merely somatization increase the patient's distress and depression? Social psychological studies indicate that an absence of validating support about common judgments (Bogdonoff, Kleink, Estes, Shaw, & Back, 1961) produces physiological arousal and a lack of an appropriate label for the arousal increases distress (Maslach, 1979; Marshall & Zimbardo 1979). As Ray (1991) puts it, *"ambiguity is a key determinant of how well people cope with a stressor; it is a difficulty cited by cancer patients, some of whom feel that neither they nor their physicians have a clear understanding of etiology or of the factors that determine outcome (Ray & Baum, 1985). Arguably, this kind of uncertainty is even greater in the case of CFS"* (op. cit., p. 3). Questions concerning iatrogenesis are essentially precluded by the focus of research attention on psychological traits of the patient generated by the depression\somatization paradigm.

CFS as a Discrete Disease

Symptoms not typical of depression

If chronic fatigue syndrome is a discrete disease, it should have some symptoms that are not explicable through the concept of somatization or typically found in somatizers. Symptoms have been reported that appear to differ from symptoms of depression/somatization, including muscle weakness specifically in response to exercise (as opposed to general lethargy associated with depression). As Abbey and Garfinkel put it, *"abnormalities in muscle metabolism remain as one of the most persuasive arguments in favor of the existence of CFS as a bona fide discrete disease"* (op. cit., p. s78). Several studies have demonstrated these abnormalities in CFS patients through, for example, magnetic resonance imaging spectroscopy (Arnold, Radda, Bore, Styles & Taylor,

1984). Although they could initially be caused by a panic reaction to the fatigue, they seem to persist after the panic has passed. Komaroff and Buchwald (1991) reported post exertional malaise in 50 to 60% of 510 patients with chronic fatigue syndrome. As they put it, *"although patients are typically active before the onset of illness (which is usually acute), even modest physical exertion after its onset produces a striking exacerbation of many of their symptoms. Typically, the patient tolerates the physical exertion reasonably well and may even feel energized during and immediately after the exertion. However, 6-24 hours later the patients feel ill, the involved muscle groups feel sore and weak, and 30-70% of patients experience marked worsening of their fatigue, cognitive function, adenopathy, pharyngitis, and fevers. In our experience, this post exertional malaise is unusual in healthy individuals or in those with diseases that have some clinical similarity to CFS"* (op. cit., p. s9-10). I might add that nowhere in the literature describing physical symptoms of depression does one find this specific pattern of muscle fatigue (see, for example, Matthew, Weinman & Mirabi, 1981; Katon & Russo 1989; Escobar et al. 1987).

Several studies have found that complaints of cognitive impairment are frequent in a CFS population. The Klimas et al. study found inability to concentrate, forgetfulness and confusion reported by 90% of their CFS patients (who met CDC criteria). Daugherty et al. (1991) studied 20 patients with severe CFS who reported a symptom syndrome consistent with the CDC criteria. Aggregate scores for this group were significantly below demographic norms for I.Q., attention, problem solving and kinesthetic performance and verbal memory. It is difficult to know the extent to which these impairments are produced by motivational deficits generated by the depression that follows chronic fatigue syndrome. To date no studies have examined depressed and non-depressed chronic fatigue syndrome patients separately. Information processing deficits include reports of CFS patients being unable to function socially because of a sense of information overload in social groups, leading many to the reclusive existence that frequently accompanies the disease (Iger, 1991). Iger also found that, unlike depressed patients, CFS patients could handle dyadic interaction but not group interaction that required constant switching of attention. She described a unique cognitive pattern, unlike anything described in the depression literature.

Iger (1991) has demonstrated an MMPI profile for CFS patients that is quite distinct from those of depressives, hypochondriacs and malingerers. The CFS profile shows elevations in MMPI scales that assess hypochondriasis, depression, hysteria, asocial tendencies, difficulties in concentrating and social withdrawal. Iger emphasizes that these are post hoc profiles and indicate the extensive severity of the psychological reaction to a physically debilitating disease with unknown prognosis. Other aspects of CFS reported by patients (Klimas et al., 1990) that are not reported as sequelae of depression include the ability to date the onset of the illness and photosensitivity.

Daugherty et al. (1991) reported MRI scans on CFS patients that showed two patterns of abnormality. The more common pattern showed tiny punctuate foci with abnormally increased signal intensity in the upper centrum semiovale and bilaterally in the high parasagittal convolutional white-matter tracts. The second, less common pattern, showed multiple bilateral patchy areas of abnormally increased signal intensity in the deep frontal white matter.

Lottenberg (1991) has reported decreased glucose metabolism and decreased blood flow in the precentral gyrus, middle frontal gyrus and caudate nucleus in CFS patients, but not in depressed patients. These deficits correlate with neuropsychological testing (e.g., intelligence tests). Lottenberg's conclusion is that PET scanning presents clearer differences between CFS and control groups because it demonstrates brain function as opposed to structure, and CFS has functional deficits as an objective marker which are quite distinct from depression.

Ray (1991) has developed a working model of CFS that attempts to account for the diversity of symptoms described above. Her working model views CFS as multiply determined by both somatic and psychological causes and involving an alteration in function of the hypothalamic-pituitary-adrenal axis. The hypothalamus regulates many of the functions which characterize the somatic features of both CFS and depression.

Epidemics

If CFS is merely somatized depression, the evidence on epidemics of CFS become difficult to explain, unless one depicts them as hysterical contagions. Curiously, not much attention has been paid to the problem of explaining these epidemics. Salit (1985) cites studies indicating 30 outbreaks of "epidemic neuromyasthenia" (CFS) between 1934 and 1977. Detailed examinations of patients from Incline Village, Nevada (where an outbreak of CFS affected over 400 people from 1984-1988) indicated that the clinical signs of the epidemic illness were indistinguishable from non-epidemic cases (Daugherty et al., 1991). On the assumption that many of the afflicted did not know that others had been affected, the evidence for a hysterical contagion is slight (Colligan, Pennebaker & Murphy, 1982). Long lasting immune dysfunction and neurological impairment has been reported with this group (Daugherty et al., 1991). No reports of their premorbid psychological state have been published. As Kruesi et al. (1989) remarked, epidemic outbreaks of depression\somatization have not been reported. The existence of CFS epidemics points toward an infectious agent and away from psychological traits in individuals when considering the cause of CFS.

The Depression Paradigm Revisited

Ray (1991) has described how a variety of medical disorders have been conceived in terms of a psychological model which has been subsequently abandoned when an organic cause has been unearthed. Further, several kinds of medical illnesses elicit symptoms that are also symptoms of psychological disorders *"where these are a direct result of the underlying physical condition. In neurological disorders, such as Parkinson's disease and multiple sclerosis, patients may present with symptoms of a depressive syndrome; the same applies to some endocrine, metabolic and nutritional disorders and even to some neoplastic disorders"* (op. cit. p. 3). Ray cites the example of patients with thyroid disorders, a proportion of whom meet the criteria for depressive or anxiety disorders, whose psychological symptoms abate when the hypothyroidism is effectively managed. She also points out that mood changes are commonly associated with infection, as are fatigue and malaise, and can occur before other symptoms and last into the convalescent period. For these reasons, she cautions against assigning a causal role to psychological variables in the etiology of CFS.

It is easy to see how the notion that CFS was caused by depression was seductive for medical practitioners. Somatization is one of the most common and troublesome problems faced by primary care physicians. Katon et al. (1982a) cite studies that indicate *"as many as 50% of patients utilizing primary care clinics actually have psychosocial precipitants as opposed to biomedical ones as the main cause of their clinic visits"* (op. cit., p. 128), leading them to conclude that mental disorders commonly present as physical disorders in primary care. Many primary care physicians, mindful of this, are wary of new physical diseases that may have psychosomatic or somatiform bases. Furthermore, CFS symptomatology is the perfect candidate for a psychosocial basis, with considerable symptom overlap with depression. Hence, it is understandable how research on CFS, with its depresso-mimetic qualities, was subsumed under the depression\somatization paradigm.

Kuhn (1962) described a scientific paradigm as a shared reality or lens through which scientific problems were viewed by researchers. As such, a paradigm not only influences the interpretation of studies but dictates what problems will be studied and how they will be studied. By focusing attention on these appropriate problems, other questions are ignored. Paradigms are only challenged when small groups of determined researchers present phenomena that are inexplicable under the old paradigm. Such was the case when Freud and Charcot demonstrated that hysterical symptoms had no organic basis. From that demonstration the recognition of the influence of psychological issues on physical symptoms was developed and has to this day added much to our understanding of previously inexplicable symptoms. The inherent danger of this approach, however, is that when a persuasive paradigm is overextended, especially to symptom syndromes that mimic the substance of the paradigm, the research focus is narrowed and data are interpreted uncritically because the assumptions of the paradigm are not questioned.

The time has arrived for a serious mutivariate examination of the variety of factors that may affect onset of CFS. These would include potential host resistance influences such as constitutional (or genetic-immune) and lifestyle factors, presence of acute and chronic stressors, social isolation, marital disruption or discord, use of recreational drugs, prior viral infections, trait anxiety, need for achievement, and "Type A" personality. A substantial literature now exists to implicate this much broader array of psychosocial factors in immune suppression (O'Leary, 1990; Kiecolt-Glaser, Kennedy, Malkoff, Fisher, Speicher & Glaser, 1988; Verbrugge, 1979; Cohen & Williamson, 1991), and many of these factors have a much greater effect size on immunosuppression than anything reported in the depression/somatization literature. For example, Kiecolt-Glaser et al. report a tenfold increase in HSV-1 antibody titers for separated/divorced men compared to married men. In their study, the divorce could have occurred any time in the last three years, suggesting a more durable form of immunosuppression than reported in the depression literature. These studies have been overlooked by depression/somatization paradigm research and are not cited by authors operating within that paradigm, providing further evidence of how a paradigm focuses research attention away from potentially important factors.

Studies should also evaluate post onset factors that may contribute to symptom severity and duration such as social support and validating-invalidating reactions of friends and physicians (cf. Ray and Baum, 1985). Social withdrawal is a common symptom of CFS for reasons that have to do, in part, with altered information processing capabilities (Iger 1990). This isolation could, in itself, contribute to prolonged immunosuppressive difficulties (Glaser, Kiecolt-Glaser, Speicher & Holliday 1985). Finally, an inevitable question is whether changes in broad system factors such as economic or environmental factors have led to increases in a variety of autoimmune health problems. Such a study would do away with the narrow and questionable univariate focus of depression\somatization and the tendency to view the causal origins of the problem as residing exclusively within the patient.

Footnotes

1 Neurasthenia was named by the neurologist Beard in 1867 and attributed to "exhaustion of nerve cells through depletion of their stored nutriment" (Kendell, 1991). By the 1940's neurasthenia was believed to be caused primarily by psychological factors rather than overwork of endotoxins and now is rarely diagnosed. It does, however, survive as a form of neurotic illness in the International Classification of Mental Disorders. In the DSM-III-R index it is used as a synonym for dysthymia, which is a form of prolonged depression (>2 years) with low energy, poor appetite and poor concentration (inter alia).

2 A variety of potential viral causes for CFS have been reported in the literature including Epstein Barr virus, human herpes virus type 6, Coxsackie B virus and, most recently, a type of retrovirus HTLV-2 (DeFreitas et al., 1990). In the case of the latter, using criteria for positivity to both "gag" and "env" gene products, 41% of CFS patients were positive compared to 6% of healthy controls. This finding must be replicated and found to persist. Prior findings of elevated viral levels have not been found to be persistent (see Kendell, 1991). Also, the **extent** of the elevation over population norms and the likelihood of symptoms given the virus all constitute measurement issues in contemporary immunology.

3 Confusions of depression as a reaction with depression as a cause is not restricted to CFS research. Stark, Flitcraft and Frazier (1979) described how depression resulting from being a victim of spousal assault was "constructed" into a battering syndrome whereby depression became the cause of the violence. The diagnostic problem originates because *"no apparent physiological event links one injury to another...as it becomes clear that neither the women, nor their injuries, on the aggregate will respond to treatment, their problems are reaggregated as symptoms of particular social or psychopathologies, alcoholism, depression, for example. At this point the woman herself, rather than her assailant, appears as a legitimate object of medical control"* (op. cit., p. 470). *"The secondary problems the abused woman has developed in the course of her 'treatment' provide medicine with labels they can use to organize a history of otherwise unrelated 'accidents.' She is, after all,...suffering from one of a myriad of such 'female disorders' as depression, hysteria, hypochondrias, etc. And this explains not only why she has had so many injuries but also why she occasionally appears to have had 'fights' or why she has a poor self image. In other words, she is hurt because this is what happens when persons use drugs or alcohol, or are emotionally unstable"* (op. cit., p. 473).

4 Schaeffer et al. (1985) did show changes in endocrine and immune function several years after a major stressor (Three Mile Island).

5 I cite the Abbey and Garfinkel report here because it is important to see which aspects of the original studies are being emphasized in the literature. The Abbey and Garfinkel review is the most comprehensive to date on the relationship of depression to chronic fatigue syndrome.

6 Abbey and Garfinkel criticize the Hickie et al. study because the sample of CFS patients was derived from a larger sample of 200 patients *"and it is unclear how the patients who were studied compared with the larger group of patients and whether their inclusion in the study was randomly determined. Second, 15 (31.3%) were interviewed after the completion of the trial of immunoglobulin therapy, and it is unclear how this may have affected the results"* (op. cit., p. s75). Regarding the first point, all subject samples in all studies are self-selected; it is unethical to force participation. Therefore, no samples are random. What is more important is that the subjects selected in the Hickie et al. study fit rigorous criteria for CFS. The second point that Abbey and Garfinkel raise is even more curious. How might immunoglobulin therapy affect retrospective reports of physical and psychiatric problems? If we believed this were possible we would have to concede that current depression experienced by the majority of patients with CFS might also affect retrospective reports in such a way as to exaggerate past episodes of depression. In any event, this would be an empirical question easily checked by Hickie et al., comparing the 15 patients who were interviewed post-treatment with the remainder of the group. What is more significant, it seems to me, is Abbey and Garfinkel's uneven application of methodological criticism to studies that confirm and disconfirm the depression-CFS link.

7 The Imboden et al. study is highly cited by researchers in the depression\somatization paradigm. It is clearly an influential study. What is emphasized in the Imboden study is that subjects with a premorbid personality pattern of depression (as measured by the MMPI) had a delayed recovery to influenza. To put this in perspective, however, the study was of 600 subjects of whom only 26 developed influenza. The personality contribution was based on this small sample, subdivided into those who recovered within 15 days (and had depression t scores of 51.5) and those who took longer than 3 weeks (whose t score for depression was 61.0. These scores were significantly different (p<.025). No differences between groups existed on hysteria, hypochondria or other MMPI subscales. The authors pointed out that since the subjects in the group who took longer to recover were eight years older, on average, than those in the other group, age could also have been a factor in recovery rates. It is interesting to compare the tenuousness of the original findings with the weight they are given in citation, as well as the general failure to cite limitations, alternative interpretations, etc. Furthermore, no replications of this 30 year old study are reported by those who cite it although failure to reliably replicate findings of viral antibody titres is a frequent criticism made of viral explanations for CFS (e.g. Abbey & Garfinkel, 1991; Kendell 1991). This epistemological double standard is another indicator of the operation of paradigmatic thinking.

8 Nevertheless, the DSM-III-R cites only female relatives of females with somatization disorder as being more at risk for the disorder. Male relatives are more at risk for Antisocial Personality or Psychoactive Substance Use Disorders.

9 The diagnosis of Adjustment Disorder in DSM-III-R again exemplifies the potential for the fundamental attribution error. Adjustment disorder is diagnosed when "symptoms are in excess of a normal and expectable reaction to stressors." To the extent that the extreme impairment generated in some cases by CFS goes unrecognized by diagnosing physicians, the patient's reaction is more likely to be seen as "in excess.".

References

Abbey, S.E. & Garfinkel, P.E. (1991). Chronic fatigue syndrome and depression: Cause, effect or covariate? Reviews of Infectious Diseases, 13(Suppl 1), S73-83.

American Psychiatric Association (1987). **Diagnostic and statistical manual of mental disorders** (third edition). Washington, DC: American Psychiatric Association.

Arieti, S., and Bemporad, J. (1978). **Severe and mild depression:The psychotherapeutic approach.** New York: Basic Books

Arnold, D.L., Radda, G.K., Bore, P.J., Styles, P., and Taylor, D.J. (1984). Excessive intracellular acidosis of skeletal muscle on exercise on a patient with post-viral exhaustion/fatigue syndrome. A ^{31}P nuclear magnetic resonance study. The Lancet, 1, 1367-9.

Bastien, S. (1989). Neuropsychological deficits in chronic fatigue syndrome. Presented at International Conference "Epstein-Barr": The first 25 years. Oxford University, April.

Beck, A.T. (1983). Cognitive therapy for depression: New perspectives. In: Clayton, P.J.,and Barrett, J.E., (Eds.) Treatment of depression: Old controversies and new approaches (pp. 265-290), New York: Raven Press.

Bogdonoff,, M.D., Kleink R.F., Estes, E.H. Jr., Shaw, D.M. & Back, K.W. (1961). The modifying effect of conforming behavior upon lipid responses accompanying CIS arousal. Clinical Research, 9, 135.

Bromet, E.J., Dunn, L.O., Connell, M.M., et al (sic) (1986). Longterm reliabilty of diagnosing lifetime major depression in a community sample. Archives of General Psychiatry, 43, 435-440.

Cassel, J. (1990). Societal contributions to host resistance. In. R. Ornstein & C. Swencionis (Eds.) **The Healing Brain.** New York: The Guilford Press.

Cohen, S., & Williamson, G.M. (1991). Stress and infectious disease. Psychological Bulletin, 109(1), 5-24.

Colligan, M.J., Pennebaker, J.W., & Murphy, L.R. (1982). **Mass psychogenic illness:A social psychological analysis**. Erlbaum: Hillsdale, N.J..

Daugherty, S.A., Henry, B.E., Peterson, D.L., Swarts, R.L., Bastien, S., & Thomas, R.S. (1991). Chronic Fatigue Syndrome in Northern Nevada. Reviews of Infectious Diseases, 13(Suppl 1), s39-44.

DeFreitas E., Hilliard, B., Cheney, P., Bell, D., Kiggundu, E., Sankey, D., Wroblewska, Z., & Koprowski, H. (1990). **Evidence of retrovirus in patients with chronic fatigue immune dysfunction syndrome.** 11th International Congress of Neuropathology, Kyoto, Japan.

Derogatis, L.R., & Wise, T.N. (1989). **Anxiety and depressive disorders in the medical patient.** Washington, DC: American Psychiatric Press.

Dubos, R. (1965). **Man adapting.** New Haven, CT: Yale University Press.

Escobar, J.I. Burnam, A. Karno, M. Forsythe, A., & Golding, J.M. (1987). Somatization in the community. Arch. Gen. Psychiatry, 44, 713-718.

Fasteau, M.F. (1974). **The male machine**. McGraw-Hill: New York.

Glaser, R., Kiecolt-Glaser, J. Speicher, C.E. & Holliday, J.E. (1985) Stress, loneliness and changes in herpes virus latency. Journal of Behavioral Medicine, 8, 249-260.

Grafman, J., Johnson, R. Jr., & Scheffers, M. (1991). Cognitive and mood state changes in patients with chronic fatigue syndrome. Reviews of Infectious Disease, 13(Suppl.), s45-52.

Hickie, I., Lloyd, A., Wakefield, D., & Parker, G. (1990). The psychiatric status of patients with the chronic fatigue syndrome. British Journal of Psychiatry, 156, 534-540.

Holmes, G.P., Kaplan, J.E., Gantz, N.M., Komaroff, A.L., Schonberger, L.B., Straus, S.E., Jones, J.J., Dubois, R.E., Cunningham-Rundles, C., Pahwa, S., Tosato, G., Zegans, L.S., Purtilo, D.T., Brown, N., Schooley, R.T., & Brus, I. (1988). Chronic fatigue syndrome: A working case definition. Annals of Internal Medicine, 108, 387-389.

Iger, L. M. (1990, July) Chronic Epstein-Barr Virus and its Relationship to the Minnesota Multiphasic Personality Inventory. Dissertation Abstracts International 51 (1-B), 415.

Imboden, J.B., Canter, A., & Cluff, L. (1961). Convalescence from influenza: a study of the psychological and clinical determinants. Archives of Internal Medicine, 108, 393-399.

Katon, W. & Russo, J. (1989). Somatic symptoms and depression. The Journal of Family Practice, 29(1), 65-69.

Katon, W., Kleinman, A., & Rosen, G. (1982a, January). Depression and somatization: A review. Part I. The American Journal of Medicine, 72, 127-135.

Katon, W., Kleinman, A., & Rosen, G. (1982b, February). Depression and somatization: A review. Part II. The American Journal of Medicine, 72, 241-247.

Katon, W.J., Buchwald, D.S., Simon, G.E., Russo, J.E. & Mease, P.J. (in press). Psychiatric illness in patients with chronic fatigue and rheumatoid arthritis.

Kendell, R.E. (1991). Chronic fatigue, viruses and depression. The Lancet, 337, 160 -162.

Kiecolt-Glaser, J.K., Kennedy, S., Malkoff, S., Fisher, B.A., Speicher, C.E. & Glaser, R. (1988). Marital discord and immunity in males. Psychosomatic Medicine, 50, 213-229.

Klimas, N.G., Salvato, F.R., Morgan, R. & Fletcher, M.A. (1990, June). Immunologic abnormalities in chronic fatigue syndrome. Journal of Clinical Microbiology, 1403-1410.

Komaroff, A.L. & Buchwald, D. (1991). Symptoms and signs of chronic fatigue syndrome, Reviews of Infectious Disease, 13(Suppl 1), s8-11.

Kreitman, N., Sainsbury, P., Pearce, K., & Costain, W.R. (1965). Hypochondriasis and depression in out-patients at a general hospital. British Journal of Psychiatry, 111, 607-615.

Kruesi, M.J.P., Dale, J., and Straus, S.E. (1989). Psychiatric diagnoses in patients who have chronic fatigue syndrome. Journal of Clinical Psychiatry, 50, 53-56.

Kuhn, T.S. (1965). **Structure of scientific revolutions**. Chicago: University of Chicago Press.

Lottenberg, S. (1991, April). **Brain functional analysis of chronic fatigue syndrome**. Paper given at the Southeastern Medical Association Conference, New Orleans, LA.

Manu, P., Mathew, S.A., & Lane, T.J. (1988a). The mental health of patients with a chief complaint of chronic fatigue: A prospective evaluation and follow-up. Archives of Internal Medicine, 148, 2213-7.

Manu, P., Lane, T.J., & Mathews, D.A. (1988b). The frequency of the chronic fatigue syndrome in patients with symptoms of persistent fatigue. Annals of Internal Medicine, 109, 554-556.

Marshall, G.D. & Zimbardo, P.G. (1979). Affective consequences of inadequately explained physiological arousal. **Journal of Personality and Social Psychology, 37, 970-988.**

Maslach, C. (1979). Negative emotional biasing of unexplained arousal. Journal of Personality and Social Psychology, 37, 953-969.

Mathew, R.J., Weinman, M.L., and Mirabi, M. (1981). Physical symptoms of depression. British Journal of Psychiatry, 139, 293-296.

Mosher, D.L. & Tompkins, S.S. (1988). Scripting the macho man: Hypermasculine socialization and enculturation. Journal of Sex Research, 25(1), 60-84

Nisbett, R.E., & Ross, L. (1980). **Human inference: Strategies and shortcomings of social judgment**. Englewood Cliffs, N.J.: Prentice Hall.

Ochberg, F.M. (1988). **Post-traumatic therapy and victims of violence**. New York, NY: Brunner/Mazel.

O'Leary, A. (1990). Stress, emotion and human immune function. Psychological Bulletin, 108(3), 363-382.

Ray, C. (1991). Chronic fatigue syndrome and depression: Conceptual and methodological ambiguities. Psychological Medicine, 21, 1-9.

Ray, C., & Baum, M. (1985). **Psychological aspects of early breast cancer.** New York: Springer-Verlag.

Reich, T., Rice, J., Andreasen, N., et al (sic) (1980). A preliminary analysis of the segregation distribution of primary major depressive disorder. Psychological Bulletin, 16, 34-36.

Robins, L.N., Helzer, J.E., Weissman, M.M., Orvaschel, H., Grunberg, E., Burke, J.D. Jr, & Regier, D.A. (1984). Lifetime prevalence of specific psychiatric disorders in three sites. Arch. Gen. Psychiatry, 41, 949-958.

Ross, M. (1991, May 11). Is HIV the only factor? The Globe and Mail.

Salit, I.E. (1985). Sporadic postinfectious neuromyasthenia. Canadian Medical Association Journal, 133, 659-663.

Schaeffer, M.A., McKinnon, W., Baum. A., Reynolds, C.P., Rikli, P., Davidson, L.M. & Fleming, I. (1985). Immune status as a function of chronic stress at Three Mile Island. Psychosomatic Medicine, 47, 85.

Schleifer, S.J., Keller, S.E., Bond, R.N., Cohen, J., & Stein, M. (1989). Major depressive disorder and immunity: Role of age, sex, severity and hospitalization. Arch. Gen. Psychiatry, 46, 81-87.

Seligman, M. E. (1975). **On depression, development and death**. San Francisco: Freeman.

Stark, E., Flitcraft, A., & Frazier, W. (1979). Medicine and patriarchal violence: The social construction of a private event. International Journal of Health Services, 9(3), 461-493.

Straus, S.E. (1991). History of Chronic Fatigue Syndrome. Reviews of Infectious Diseases, 13(supp 1), s2-7.

Taerk, G.S., Toner, B.B., Salit, I.E., Garfinkel, P.E. & Ozersky, S. (1987). Depression in patients with neuromyasthenia (benign myalgic encephalomyelitis). International Journal of Psychiatry in Medicine, 17: 49-56.

Terr, L. (1991). Childhood traumas: An outline and overview. American Journal of Psychiatry, 148 (1), 10-20.

Verbrugge, L.M. (1979, May). Marital status and health. **Journal of Marriage and the Family**, 267-285.

Weissman, M.M., Myers, J.K., & Harding, P.S. (1978). Psychiatric disorders in a US urban community: 1975-76. American Journal of Psychiatry, 135, 459-462.

Wessely, S., & Powell, R. (1989). Fatigue syndrome: A comparison of 'postviral' fatigue with neuromuscular and affective disorder. Journal of Neurology, Neurosurgery and Psychiatry, 52, 940-948.

Wortman, C. (1976). Causal attributions and personal control. New Directions in Attribution Research, 1, 23-52.

Zala, J. (1980). Diagnosing myalgic encephalomyelitis. The Practitioner, 233, 916-919.

Chapter 56

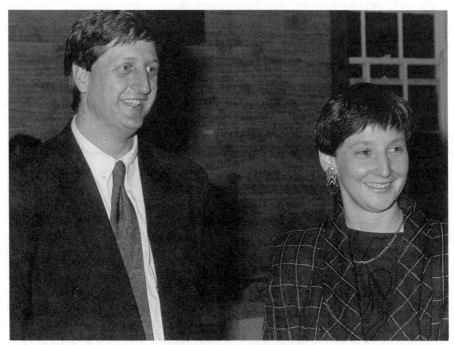

Drs Ian and Catherine Hickie

Photograph courtesy of the Department of Medical Illustration, University of NSW and Teaching Hospitals, ref. 52858.

This article is reprinted with the kind permission of The Royal College of Psychiatrists, The British Journal of Psychiatry, "The Psychiatric Status of Patients with the Chronic Fatigue Syndrome", Ian Hickie, et al., April, 1990, 156, 534-40. The same or similar material was presented at the Cambridge Symposium.

The Psychiatric Status of Patients with the Chronic Fatigue Syndrome

Ian Hickie, FRANZCP, Research Fellow in Psychiatry, Mood Disorders Unit, Division of Psychiatry, Prince Henry Hospital, Sydney, 2036 Australia, Andrew Lloyd, FRACP, NHMRC, Research Fellow, School of Pathology, University of New South Wales, Kensington, NSW, Australia, Denis Wakefield, MD, FRACP, Associate Professor of Pathology, University of New South Wales, Kensington NSW, Australia, Gordon Parker, MD, PhD, FRANZCP, Professor of Psychiatry, School of Psychiatry (University of New South Wales), Prince Henry Hospital, Sydney, Australia

Dr. Hickie presently holds the position of Staff Specialist in Psychiatry at the Prince Henry Hospital and Conjoint Lecturer in Psychiatry, School of Psychiatry, University of New South Wales. His principle research interests have been in the psychiatric assessment and treatment of patients with Chronic Fatigue Syndrome and in the immunological correlates of depressive disorders. Dr. Hickie is a member of the Mood Disorders Unit at the Prince Henry Hospital which has been established to investigate the classification and treatment of depressive disorders.

The prevalence of psychiatric disorder in 48 patients with Chronic Fatigue Syndrome (CFS) was determined. Twenty-two had had a major depressive (non-endogenous) episode during the course of their illness, while 7 had a current major (non-endogenous) depression. The pre-morbid prevalence of major depression (12.5%) and of total psychiatric disorder (24.5%) was no higher than general community estimates. The pattern of psychiatric symptoms in the CFS patients was significantly different to that of 48 patients with non-endogenous depression, but was comparable with that observed in other medical disorders. Patients with CFS were not excessively hypochondriacal. We conclude that psychological disturbance is likely to be a consequence of, rather than an antecedent risk factor to the syndrome.

> *"Acquired neurasthenia is characterised by a diminished power of attention, distractibility, defective mental application, difficulty of thinking, an increased susceptibility to fatigue, increased emotional irritability, and a greater variety of physical symptoms, mostly subjective, including hypocondriasis"*
> (Emil Kraepelin, 1981, first published 1907)

The Chronic Fatigue Syndrome (also termed myalgic encephalomyelitis, Royal Free Disease, post-viral fatigue syndrome), recently defined by the Centers for Disease Control in Atlanta, Georgia (Holmes et al, 1988), has been subject to ongoing controversy (Dawson, 1987; David et al, 1988; Swartz, 1988). Psychological features have often been noted (David et al, 1988), leading some physicians to regard CFS as a psychiatric disorder (McEvedy and Beard, 1973). The demonstration of persistent infection (Yousef et al, 1988) and immunological abnormalities (Behan et al, 1985; Straus et al, 1985; Caliguri et al, 1987; Lloyd et al, 1989), however, have supported alternative hypotheses (e.g. that of Wakefield and Lloyd, 1987) that highlight the role of biological factors in the condition.

Straus (1988) stated that "ultimately, any hypothesis regarding the cause of the chronic fatigue syndrome must incorporate the psychopathology that accompanies and, in some cases, precedes it", emphasising the importance of assessing psychopathology both pre-morbidly and during the illness.

The frequency of neuropsychiatric and depressive symptoms in these patients (David et al, 1988; Straus, 1988) suggested the specific hypothesis that CFS occurs in individuals with a pre-morbid vulnerability to depression. A case-control study of 24 subjects by Taerk et al (1987) supported this notion but may be challenged as controls were healthy hospital personnel, and no attempt was made to validate prevalence estimates. Similarly, Kruesi et al (1989) have reported an increased lifetime prevalence of depressive and anxiety disorders in patients with CFS.

In this paper we record the prevalence of psychiatric morbidity in patients with CFS both during and before the illness episode to determine whether the syndrome is associated with an increase in psychological disturbance, and whether subjects had a higher pre-morbid rate of psychiatric disturbance. We included a control group of patients with non-endog-enous depression to assess whether CFS patients resembled patients with depression, either during the illness episode or on pre-morbid measures.

The non-specific nature of the key symptom of fatigue has necessitated the development of strict criteria for CFS (Holmes et al, 1988; Lloyd et al, 1988a, b). The Centers for Disease Control (CDC) criteria (Holmes et al, 1988) specifically exclude patients with a number of psychiatric disorders and those taking psychotrophic medication, effectively preventing accurate quantification of psychological symptoms in patients with CFS. The difficulty created by those criteria is exemplified by the study of Manu et al, (1988) who reported that 95% of 135 consecutive patients who had attended a fatigue clinic in a university hospital, with at least a six-month history of debilitating fatigue, failed to meet CDC criteria. The overwhelming reason for exclusion was current psychiatric disorder (91/135) and the most prevalent psychiatric diagnosis was "major depression" (67/91). Such concurrent psychiatric morbidity was assumed to be "a *major cause* of these patients' fatigue" (italics added). The criteria used in the present study, however, do not make this assumption, and thereby avoid the limitation of excluding subjects on the basis of psychological symptoms.

Method

We studied 48 subjects with marked and persistent fatigue who met the following operational criteria for CFS (Lloyd et al, 1988a):

To fulfil the criteria a patient must have chronic, persistent or relapsing fatigue of a generalised nature, causing major disruption of usual daily activities, present for more than six months, plus two major or one major and three minor criteria (symptoms, signs, or assessments):

a) **Symptoms**: Persisting at least six months continuously, or relapsing on three or more occasions with a similar pattern over six months or more:

i) Major
Concentration/
memory impairment

ii) Minor
Myalgia
Arthralgia
Depression
Tinnitus
Paraesthesia
Headaches

b) Signs: Present on at least one occasion subsequent to the initial illness:

i) Major
Lymphadenopathy

ii) Minor
Pharyngitis
Muscle tenderness

c) Immunologic Assessment:

i) Major
Cutaneous anergy
T4 or T8 lymphopenia

ii) Minor
Hypoergy

The criteria that we have recommended since are a simplification of those original criteria (Lloyd et al, 1988b). Both of our sets of criteria emphasise the importance of a characteristic pattern of physical and neuropsychological impairment and the demonstration of impaired cell-mediated immunity.

All patients had been referred by their general practitioner to the immunology or infectious diseases' department of a university teaching hospital for evaluation of their chronic fatigue. Patients referred to this service typically had been extensively investigated by their own practitioners and/or other consultant physicians. Additionally, many had been assessed previously by a psychiatrist. The patients in this report were drawn from a previously described sample of 200 patients (Lloyd et al 1988b) who had been assessed rigorously to exclude other possible physical causes of fatigue (infectious diseases or thyroid, neurological, haematological, hepatic, renal, or autoimmune dysfunction). Although the CDC criteria were not established at the time our patients were enrolled, the process of physical evaluation and investigation we used was as extensive as that recommended by Holmes et al (1988).

Twenty-nine of the 48 patients had developed their persistent fatigue immediately after an acute infectious illness. Five of these illnesses had been documented serologically (four Epstein-Barr virus infections, one toxoplasmosis). Patients were approached to progress to a treatment trial on the basis of the persistence of their symptoms and their willingness to give informed consent to participate in a double-blind, placebo-controlled, treatment trial of intravenous immunoglobulin therapy (to be reported elsewhere). The extensive process of physical evaluation within a tertiary referral service, the application of strict clinical and laboratory criteria, and the delay between initial contact with the clinic and inclusion in the treatment trial, all limited the clinical heterogeneity that one might expect within such a sample.

Initially, each subject was asked by the psychiatrist (IH) to describe their 'key symptoms'. The interviewer recorded the frequency with which psychological and neuropsychological symptoms were reported spontaneously before administering a standardised psychiatric interview schedule (SCID-P; Spitzer & Williams, 1985) which generated DSM-III-R (American Psychiatric Association, 1987) diagnostic data. A relative of each patient was interviewed independently to corroborate the patient's report. Because of a delay in the commencement of the psychiatrist's involvement in the trial, 33 patients were interviewed before treatment, and the remaining 15 patients after completion of immunoglobulin infusions.

All subjects completed a number of psychometric measures, including the 30-item General Health Questionnaire (GHQ; Goldberg, 1979), the Zung Self-Rating Depression Scale (Zung, 1965), the Eysenck Personality Inventory (Eysenck and Eysenck, 1964), and the Illness Behaviour Questionnaire (Pilowsky and Spence, 1983). The latter scale generates scores on seven dimensions which indicate the subject's attitudes towards the illness. The 17-item Hamilton Rating Scale for Depression (Hamilton, 1960), and the Newcastle Depression Scale (Carney et al, 1965), used to identify patients with endogenous depression, were administered by the psychiatrist.

Forty-eight patients with non-endogenous depression (Newcastle Depression Scale score less than five) were selected from the inpatient and outpatient psychiatric services of the same hospital for comparison with the patients with CFS.

Results

The mean age of the patients was 36 (range 15-63) years, and there were equal numbers of men and women. The mean duration of illness was 56 (median 46, range 12-156) months. The sample therefore contained patients with chronic illness with little prospect of spontaneous remission.

The control subjects suffering from non-endogenous depression were matched exactly for sex, and similarly for age (36.1 v. 37.8 years, t=1.56, NS) and social class (mean Congalton (1969) score: 3.69 v. 3.89, t= 1.01, NS). Of the 48 control patients, 28 met DSM-III-R criteria for major depression, while the remaining 20 had minor depressive disorders. None of these control patients had been depressed continuously for two years, so that there were no cases of dysthymic disorder. Nineteen were inpatients of a general hospital psychiatry unit, while 29 were from outpatient and liaison psychiatry clinics.

Of the 48 patients with CFS, 19 spontaneously reported psychological and 29 reported neuropsychological complaints among their key symptoms (Table 1).

Twenty-four warranted a psychiatric diagnosis during the course of their illness. The commonest disorder was major (non-endogenous) depression (8 men, 14 women). Six of these 22 depressed patients with CFS also experienced panic attacks, although these were frequent enough in only one case to justify an additional diagnosis of panic disorder. In addition, three non-depressed patients had experienced at least one panic attack, and two of these subjects met criteria for panic disorder. Only one patient, who also met criteria for major depression, fulfilled criteria for somatisation disorder (Briquet's hysteria). There were no cases of generalised anxiety disorder and, although a number of patients reported simple phobias, none was associated with avoidant behaviour leading to significant impairment of daily functioning.

The overall concordance of subject/witness reports was very high (kappa=0.87), with relatives reporting a psychiatric diagnosis in 23 of the patients, strongly supporting the accuracy of our estimate. In the 33 patients assessed before treatment, the prevalence rate of psychiatric disorder in the preceding month was 21% (7/33), all having major (non-endogenous) depression.

The GHQ scores of the 33 subjects assessed immediately before treatment established that 15 had a score of five or above, generally suggestive of psychiatric morbidity (Goldberg, 1979). In patients with known medical disorders, however, significant physical symptoms inevitably lead to positive responses on more of the GHQ items. Zung depression scores for the 33 subjects assessed before treatment showed that 19 scored above the recommended cut-off point of 40 (Zung, 1972) for identifying mild depression in community settings. As with the GHQ, the raw Zung score is known to be significantly elevated in medical patients (Zung et al, 1983). It is possible to overcome this effect, in part, by comparing the number of patients and depressive controls assigned to at least the moderately depressed range (48 or above) on the Zung scale. Using this higher cut-off point, a highly significant difference (X^2=22.06, P<0.001) remained between the number of patients with CFS (8/33) in comparison to the number of depressive controls (37/48). This established that depressive disorders of clinical severity were rare in the CFS sample. Table 2 shows patients' mean scores on the Zung items.

Table 1
Frequency of spontaneous reports of neuropsychological or psychological symptoms as 'key' features by patients with CFS (n=48)

Spontaneous symptoms	Number of patients	Percentage of patients
Neuropsychological impairments:		
-concentration / attention	25	52%
-short-term memory	13	27%
-dysphasia	4	8%
-planning tasks	2	4%
Total = 29		60%
Psychological symptoms:		
-depression	18	38%
-irritability	8	17%
-anxiety / worry / tension	4	8%
Total = 19		40%
Total (neuropsychological and / or psychological)	38	80%

Table 2			
Mean scores from the Zung Self-Rating Depression Scale (n=33)			
Most frequently reported Zung items		Least frequently reported Zung items	
Item No	Mean	Item No.	Mean
12. Not easy to do things	3.5	19. Suicidal	1.1
10. Tiredness	3.4	7. Weight loss	1.2
2. Worse in a.m.	2.8	3. Tearful	1.4
11. Mind not clear	2.8	13. Restless	1.5
16. Indecisive	2.4	9. Palpitations	1.5

This distinction was supported by the significant differences between the mean scores of the CFS patients and depressive controls on the Hamilton (10.6 v. 19.0, t=8.92, P<0.001) and Zung (40.7 v. 55.2, t=7.67, P<0.001) scales. Importantly, patients with CFS also reported significantly lower levels of neuroticism (7.3 v. 15.8, t=7.71, P<0.001). This suggested that any psychiatric morbidity in the CFS sample was less severe, in addition to being less prevalent, than in depressed patients.

Table 3 records the patients', their relatives' and the depressives' estimates of prior psychological morbidity. Again there was substantial agreement between the patients' and relatives' estimates of overall premorbid psychiatric morbidity in the CFS group (kappa=0.81). Thirty of the 48 depressive controls had had a previous episode that met DSM-III-R criteria for major depression, compared with 6 of the 48 CFS patients (X^2=25.6, P<0.001).

The scores of the patients with CFS on the seven dimensions of the Illness Behaviour Questionnaire are shown in Table 4. Comparison of these data with previously reported Australian general practice samples (Pilowsky and Spence, 1983) and patients with Briquet's hysteria (Singer et al, 1988) suggests that the illness behaviour of patients with CFS is characterised by the strong conviction that they are physically ill (i.e. high scores on 'disease conviction': "an attitude of determined certainty as to the presence of disease, and a resistance to reassurance" (Pilowsky, 1988) and low scores on 'psychological v. somatic concern', which is said to be indicative of "somatic focusing" (Pilowsky, 1988)).

Table 3			
Numbers of patients and relatives reporting psychiatric morbidity before onset of CFS (n=48), and controls (n=48) before onset of depression			
	Patients		
DSM-III-R diagnosis	Self-report	Relatives' report	Depressive controls
Major depression	6 (12.5%)	6 (12.5%)	30 (62%)
Panic disorder	1 (2%)	1 (2%)	3 (6%)
Alcohol dependence	4 (8%)	4 (8%)	18 (38%)
Benzodiazepine dependence	——	——	5 (10%)
Psychotic episode	1 (2%)	1 (2%)	——
Total previous morbidity	12 (24.5%)	12 (24.5%)	43 (90%)

In contrast to patients with Briquet's Hysteria, who typically present their psychological concerns in a somatic form, patients with CFS are not hypochondriacal and are not inhibited in their expression of affectively laden topics. *(A high score on 'affective inhibition' is said to indicate "a reluctance to communicate inner feelings to others, particularly those of hostility" and is felt to be related to the notions of "introspection and ...alexithymia" (Pilowsky, 1988).)* Patients with CFS do differ from general practice patients, however, principally in terms of their reluctance to accept psychological interpretations of their somatic symptoms. Further, they have somewhat higher scores on the 'denial' subscale, which purports to measure "the tendency to regard illness as the sole problem, whose resolution would result in a circumstance devoid of difficulties" and "the tendency to displace attention from psychosocial stressors onto physical problems" (Pilowsky, 1988).

Table 4			
Mean scores on dimensions of illness behaviour of patients with CFS as measured by the Illness Behaviour Questionnaire (IBQ)			
IBQ subscale	CFS Patients (n=44) mean (s.d.)	General Practice[1] (n=147) mean	Briquet's Syndrome[2] (n=17) mean
General hypochondriasis (range = 0-9)	1.96 (1.9)	1.44	4.0
Disease conviction (range = 0-6)	4.25 (1.2)	1.59	4.0
Psychological vs. somatic focusing (range = 0-5)	0.45 (0.8)	1.99	1.0
Affective inhibition (range = 0-5)	1.98 (1.7)	2.46	4.0
Dysphoria (range = 0-5)	2.00 (1.7)	2.31	5.0
Denial (range = 0-5)	3.43 (1.6)	2.93	2.0
Irritability (range = 0-6)	2.93 (1.8)	2.45	3.0

[1] Pilowsky and Spence (1983).   [2] Singer et al (1988).

Discussion

Eighty per cent of patients with CFS spontaneously reported that neuropsychological and / or psychological difficulties were among their key complaints, confirming that such symptoms are common components of the CFS syndrome. Half had a psychiatric diagnosis (usually major depression) during the course of the illness, and 21% met criteria for major (non-endogenous) depression at the start of treatment.

The existence of significant psychological morbidity during the illness raises the question as to whether CFS is a mislabelled depressive disorder or a depressive equivalent. As early as 1907 Kraepelin noted that "acquired neurasthenia" needed to be carefully differentiated from melancholia. If CFS is a form of depressive disorder, a similar pattern of current symptoms and past psychiatric disorder might be expected in CFS patients to that observed in depressed psychiatric patients. Our findings do not support that proposition.

The estimated prevalence of pre-morbid lifetime psychiatric disorder in our CFS subjects (24%) is comparable with that reported in three sites of the Epidemiological Catchment Area Survey (ECA), where the lifetime prevalences of psychiatric disorder (excluding phobic disorders) were 24.9%, 23.9% and 26.2% respectively (Robins et al, 1984). Previous large epidemiological studies have indicated a lifetime prevalence rate for major depression of 18-25% (Weissman et al, 1978; Reich et al, 1980; Bromet et al, 1986), larger than our estimate of a 12.5% pre-morbid prevalence rate of depression in CFS patients. Corroborative data from relatives were highly consistent with reports by the subjects and offer strong support for the validity of our data.

When compared with non-endogenously depressed controls, our CFS patients did not have a similar high pre-morbid rate of psychiatric disorder, were significantly less neurotic, and when unwell, neither clinically resembled nor had the psychometric profile of non-endogenous depressive patients seen in psychiatric settings. The percentage of subjects with non-specific psychiatric symptomatology as determined by the GHQ in our sample is consistent with previous findings in general medical (Goldberg & Blackwell, 1970; Maguire et al, 1974) and neurological settings (Bridges & Goldberg, 1984).

The interviewing psychiatrist was not blind to the clinical diagnosis of the patients with CFS or depressive disorders, and so it is important to consider whether a systematic bias may have been introduced in the evaluation of prevalence rates of pre-morbid psychiatric disorder. Given the important differences in the type of symptoms reported by patients with CFS as compared with patients with depressive disorders, it is doubtful that a truly "blind" investigation is possible. We sought, however, to avoid any potential bias by using a highly structured interviewing technique. Further, we corroborated our data in the CFS patients with prevalence results reported by relatives, and we established high levels of agreement. Neither the interviewees nor the relatives were reluctant to report recent psychiatric morbidity. It is unlikely, therefore, that the low pre-morbid rates of disorder can be attributed to systematic under-recording of psychiatric morbidity. It is possible, however, that a recall bias may have been operating, such that past psychiatric morbidity was not remembered by either patients or their relatives as readily as that morbidity associated with their current protracted illness.

Our findings do not confirm those of Taerk et al (1987), who suggested a much higher pre-morbid risk of depressive disorder in patients with CFS. The patients in that study were not as extensively evaluated as the patients in this study or that of Kruesi et al (1989), so that it is likely that their sample was less homogeneous. In their study, however, if one compares the pre-morbid prevalence rate of major depression in the patients (12/24), rather than the total lifetime prevalence rates (67%, which includes the period of the current illness), with the lifetime prevalence rate in the 'healthy' controls (7/24), then there is only a non-significant trend (X^2=2.2, NS) towards higher affective disorder in the patient group. Further, the use of the criteria from the Diagnostic Interview Schedule (DIS) and DSM-III in that study produced high prevalence rates of all psychiatric disorders in both the patients and the "healthy controls", suggesting that the actual threshold for psychiatric diagnosis was low.

Although Taerk et al (1987) did not suggest that depression alone was the cause of their subjects' illnesses, they did suggest that "sporadic neuromyasthenia may be the result of an organic illness in psychologically susceptible (i.e. premorbidly depressed) individuals". By contrast, our results suggest that CFS patients are no more psychologically disturbed before the onset of their illness than members of the general population. Taerk et al used DSM-

III criteria for major depression, whereas we used the more strict criteria of DSM-III-R, and so we would expect lower prevalence rates for this disorder in our study.

Kruesi et al (1989) studied 28 patients who were said to have met CDC criteria for CFS. The patients were interviewed with the DIS to assess lifetime prevalence rates of psychiatric disorder. Patients in that study had been ill for a mean of 6.8 years and had been extensively investigated to exclude other possible disorders, thereby creating a sample quite similar to our own. Contrary to the actual CDC criteria, however, the presence of a current or past psychiatric diagnosis did not exclude those patients from participation in a treatment trial of acyclovir, an antiviral therapy. Lifetime depressive disorders were identified in 54% (15/28) of their patients (13 cases of major depression), while 21% (6/28) were currently depressed. These depressive diagnoses, however, were closely related in time to the onset or course of the fatigue syndrome. Simple phobia was reported as clinically significant in eight patients (29%), a remarkably high proportion. Only two of their patients met criteria for somatisation disorder, while other significant anxiety disorders were rare (one case of panic disorder and no case of generalised anxiety disorder).

Examination of the pre-morbid prevalence rates suggested that eight of their patients had simple phobia, one had panic disorder/agoraphobia and only two had a major depressive disorder. Attaching surprising importance, however, to the pre-morbid diagnoses of simple phobia, the authors concluded that "psychiatric disorders more often preceded the chronic fatigue than followed it". Robins et al, (1984) have noted the high inter-site variation in the prevalence of the diagnosis of simple phobia using the DIS and DSM-III criteria, and reported their lifetime prevalence data for all disorders both with and without this diagnostic category. The high rate of simple phobia reported by Kruesi et al (1989) is therefore likely to be a result of the interview method and is unlikely to be of psychopathological significance in patients with CFS.

If one limits evaluation of their cases to those with axis I diagnoses, but excludes simple phobia, then there are important similarities between their findings and ours. The pre-morbid rate of psychiatric disorder was low, 18% (5/28), (one patient with agoraphobia, two with major depression, and two cases of alcohol abuse, allowing that each diagnosis was actually for a different individual), comparable with our pre-morbid rate of 25%. Depressive disorders were common in association with the fatigue syndrome (54% as compared with our rate of 46%), with a currently depressed case rate of 21%, which is identical to our figure.

Our method of case selection involved the enrolment of individuals who had been extensively evaluated within a tertiary referral service and who had often experienced considerable delay between confirmation of the diagnosis and participation in the treatment trial. This process may have decreased the rate of current psychiatric symptoms. No active psychiatric screening was undertaken by the hospital medical staff before inclusion in the trial, but our patients cannot be considered comparable with patients presenting for the first time complaining of fatigue in general medical settings. Establishing the pattern of pre-morbid and current psychopathology in a group of patients who clearly meet strict clinical and immunological criteria for the disorder is essential, however, before progressing to the evaluation of patients who may share only the symptom of fatigue in common.

The pattern of illness behaviour recorded in our patients was not similar to that previously described in patients with defined Briquet's hysteria (Singer et al, 1988), as patients with CFS were not particularly hypochondriacal, affectively inhibited, or dysphoric. If patients with CFS were dealing principally with psychological distress by the process of somatisation, one might have expected higher scores on those relevant subscales.

Our patients differed from those in Australian general practice, principally in terms of their conviction that they were physically ill. Given the controversy surrounding this disorder, the referral of these patients to a tertiary assessment service and their participation in a pharmacological treatment trial, the firmness with which they held this belief and rejected psychological interpretations of the cause of their illness is not surprising. It may be of considerable clinical importance, however, as conflict may quickly arise between such patients and medical practitioners who are openly sceptical about the disorder.

In conclusion, we have demonstrated that while depression and anxiety are common symptoms in patients suffering from CFS, there is no evidence from our well-defined sample to support the hypothesis that CFS is a somatic presentation of an underlying psychological disorder. In particular, there is no evidence that CFS is a variant or expression of a depressive disorder. Instead, our study supports the hypothesis that the current psychological symptoms of patients with CFS are a consequence of the disorder, rather than evidence of antecedent vulnerability. We are unable to say whether the psychological symptoms occur purely as a result of the fatigue, or as an integral symptom of the disease process. Comparisons between patients with CFS and patients who have fatigue on a peripheral basis (e.g. myasthenia gravis) or on a central basis (e.g. multiple sclerosis (Krupp et al, 1988)) will be undertaken to clarify this issue further.

It is possible that the chronic production of cytokines, such as interferon, which is released by lymphocytes in response to viral infections, may account for the morbidity reported by these patients. These soluble products of lymphocytes may precipitate fatigue and neuropsychiatric syndromes in humans (Denicoff et al, 1987; McDonald et al, 1987) and, therefore, ongoing localised production of these substances within the central nervous system of patients with CFS constitutes a possible explanation for the diverse physical, neuropsychiatric and psychological symptoms encountered in patients with this syndrome (Wakefield and Lloyd, 1987).

Acknowledgements:

Dr. Hickie is funded by the NSW Institute of Psychiatry, and Dr. Lloyd by the National Health and Medical Research Council of Australia.

References

American Psychiatric Association (1987) **Diagnostic and Statistical Manual of Mental Disorders** (Third Edition - Revised). Washington, DC.:APA.

Behan, P. O., Behan, W. M. H. & Bell, E .J. (1985) The postviral fatigue syndrome - analysis of the findings in 50 cases. Journal of Infection, 10, 211-222.

Bridges, K. W. & Goldberg, D. P. (1984) Psychiatric illness in inpatients with neurological disorders: patients' views on discussion of emotional problems with neurologists. British Medical Journal, 289, 656-658.

Bromet, E. J., Dunn, L. O., Connell, M. M., et al. (1986) Long-term reliability of diagnosing lifetime major depression in a community sample. Archives of General Psychiatry, 43, 435-440.

Caligiuri, M., Murray, C., Buchwald, D., et al. (1987) Phenotypic and functional deficiency of natural killer cells in patients with chronic fatigue syndrome. Journal of Immunology, 139, 3306-3313.

Carney, M. W. P., Roth, M. & Garside, R. F. (1965) The diagnosis of depressive symptoms and the prediction of ECT response. British Journal of Psychiatry, 111, 659-674.

Congalton, A. A. (1969) **Status and Prestige in Australia**. Melbourne: F. W. Cheshire Publishing Pty Ltd.

David, A. S., Wessly, S. & Pelosi, A. J. (1988) Postviral fatigue syndrome: time for a new approach. British Medical Journal, 296, 696- 699.

Dawson, J. (1987) Royal Free disease: perplexity continues (editorial). British Medical Journal, 294, 327-328.

Denicoff, K. D., Rubinow, D. R., Papa, M. Z., et al. (1987) The neuropsychiatric effects of treatment with interleukin-2 and lymphokine-activated killer cells. Annals of Internal Medicine, 107, 293-300.

Eysenck, H. J. & Eysenck, S. B. (1964) **Manual of the Eysenck Personality Inventory**. London: Hodder & Stoughton.

Goldberg, D. P. (1979) **Manual of the General Health Questionnaire**. Windsor: NFER Publishing Co.

Goldberg, D. & Blackwell, B. (1970) Psychiatric illness in general medical practice. British Medical Journal, ii, 439-443.

Hamilton, M. (1960) A rating scale for depression. Journal of Neurology, Neurosurgery and Psychiatry, 23, 56-62.

Holmes, G. P., Kaplan, J. E., Gantz, N. M., et al. (1988) Chronic fatigue syndrome: A working case definition. Annals of Internal Medicine, 108, 387-389.

Krepelin, E. (1981) Clinical Psychiatry. (ed. R. I. Watson) New York: Scholars' Facsimiles & Reprints.

Kruesu, M. J. P., Dale, J. & Straus, S.E. (1989) Psychiatric diagnoses in patients who have Chronic Fatigue Syndrome. Journal of Clinical Psychiatry, 50, 53-56.

Krupp, L. B., Alvarez, L. A., LaRocca, N. G. et al. (1988) Fatigue in multiple sclerosis. **Archives of Neurology**, 45, 435-437.

Lloyd, A. R., Hales, J. P. & Gandevia, S. C. (1988a) Muscle strength, endurance and recovery in the post-infection fatigue syndrome. Journal of Neurology, Neurosurgery, and Psychiatry, 51: 1316-1322.

Lloyd, A.R., Wakefield, D., Boughton, C., et al. (1988b) What is myalgic encephalomyelitis? Lancet, i, 1286-1287.

Lloyd, A.R., Wakefield, D., Boughton, C., et al. (1989) Immunological abnormalities in the Chronic Fatigue Syndrome. Medical Journal of Australia, 151, 122-24.

Maguire, G. P., Julier, D. L., Hawton, K. E. et al. (1974) Psychiatric morbidity and referral on two general medical wards. British Medical Journal, i, 268-70.

Manu, P., Lane, T. J. & Matthews, D. A. (1988) The frequency of the Chronic Fatigue Syndrome in patients with symptoms of persistent fatigue. Annals of Internal Medicine, 109, 554-556.

McDonald, E. M., Mann, A. H. & Thomas, H. C. (1987) Interferons as mediators of psychiatric morbidity. An investigation in a trial of recombinant α-interferon in hepatitis-B carriers. Lancet, ii, 1175-1177.

McEvedy, C. P. & Beard, A. W. (1973) A controlled follow-up of cases involved in an epidemic of benign myalgic encephalomyelitis. British Journal of Psychiatry, 122, 141-150.

Pilowsky, I. (1988) Abnormal illness behaviour. In **Handbook of Social Psychiatry** (eds. A. S. Henderson & G. Burrows) Amsterdam: Elsevier Science Publishers.

Pilowsky, I. & Spence, N. D. (1983) **Manual for the Illness Behaviour Questionnaire (IBQ) (Second Edition)**. Adelaide: University of Adelaide.

Reich, T., Rice, J., Andreasen, N. et al. (1980) A preliminary analysis of the segregation distribution of primary major depressive disorder. Psychological Bulletin, 16, 34-36.

Robins, L. N., Helzer, J. E., Weissman, M. M., et al. (1984) Lifetime prevalence of specific psychiatric disorders in three sites. Archives of General Psychiatry, 41, 949-958.

Singer, A., Thompson, S., Kraiuhin, C., et al. (1988) An investigation of patients presenting with multiple physical complaints using the Illness Behaviour Questionnaire. Psychotherapy and Psychosomatics, 47, 181-189.

Spitzer, R. L. & Williams, J. B. W. (1985) **Structured Clinical Interview for DSM-III-R, Patient Version**. (SCID-P, 7/1/85). New York: Biometrics Research Dept., Psychiatric Institute.

Straus, S.E. (1988) The chronic mononucleosis syndrome. Journal of Infectious Diseases, 157, 405-412.

Straus, S. E., Tosato, G., Armstrong, G., et al. (1985) Persisting fatigue and illness in adults with evidence of persisting Epstein-Barr virus infection. Annals of Internal Medicine, 102, 7-16.

Swartz, M. N. (1988) The chronic fatigue syndrome - one entity or many (editorial)? New England Journal of Medicine, 319, 1726- 1728.

Taerk, G. S., Toner, B. B., Salit, I. E., et al. (1987) Depression in patients with neuromyasthenia (benign myalgic encephalomyelitis). International Journal of Psychiatry in Medicine, 17, 49-56.

Wakefield, D. & Lloyd, A. (1987) Pathophysiology of myalgic encephalomyelitis. Lancet, ii, 918-919.

Weissman, M. M., Myers, J. K. & Harding, P.S. (1978) Psychiatric disorders in a US urban community: 1975-76. American Journal of Psychiatry, 135, 459-462.

Yousef, G. E., Bell, E. J., Mann, G. F., et al. (1988) Chronic enterovirus infection in patients with postviral fatigue syndrome. Lancet, i, 146-149.

Zung, W. W. K. (1965) A self-rating depression scale. Archives of General Psychiatry, 12, 63- 70.

Zung, W.W.K. (1972) How normal is depression? **Psychosomatics**, 12, 174-178.

Zung, W. W. K., Magill, M., Moore, J. T. et al. (1983) Recognition and treatment of depression in a family medicine practice. Journal of Clinical Psychiatry, 44, 3-6.

Food Intolerance in M.E. / CFS

Chapter 57

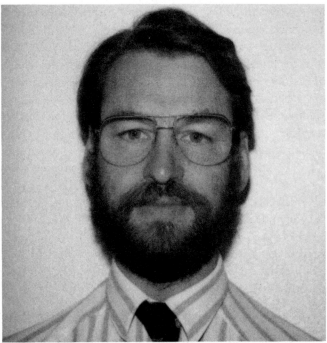

Robert H. Loblay

The Role of Food Intolerance in Chronic Fatigue Syndrome

Robert H. Loblay, MD, PhD[1] and Anne R. Swain, PhD[2]

[1]Senior Lecturer in Immunology, University of Sydney and Director, Allergy Service, Department of Clinical Immunology, Royal Prince Alfred Hospital
[2]Research Dietitian, Allergy Service, Royal Prince Alfred Hospital, Sydney, Australia

Dr. Loblay has been investigating patients with M.E./CFS for the past ten years and has maintained a close association with the New South Wales M.E. Society in Australia. His clinical research interests focus on food allergy and food intolerance. Dr. Loblay's laboratory research interests are T cell regulation of immune responses, tolerance and autoimmunity.

Adverse reactions to foods can be a significant cause of symptoms in some patients with chronic fatigue syndrome, although the contribution of diet is not always easy to recognize. In order to understand why this is so, the problem of food intolerance must first be viewed in a broader perspective. For several decades, food "allergy" has been one of the most confused and controversial areas of clinical medicine. Only in recent years have advances in immunology, pharmacology and food science made it possible to begin understanding the diverse manifestations of food reactions and their underlying pathophysiology.[1,2] It is now becoming clear that although foods can have adverse effects for a variety of reasons, the vast majority of those encountered in clinical practice fall into two broad categories: ***food allergy***, mediated by immunological mechanisms involving IgE antibodies, and non-immunological ***food intolerances***, mediated by sensitivity to the pharmacological effects of various food substances.

Food Allergy

Allergies mostly occur in atopic individuals, i.e. those who are genetically predisposed to make exaggerated IgE antibody responses against many environmental substances, including, in some cases, certain food proteins. Clinically, food allergies exhibit a characteristic pattern.[3] They usually begin in infancy, against an atopic family background, and are most commonly manifested by eczema and/or gastrointestinal symptoms. Typically, children react to just one or two specific foods, with eggs, milk, wheat, peanuts and fish, accounting for more than 90% of cases. Acute reactions can begin within minutes of ingestion with itching and urticaria around the mouth and lips, followed later by vomiting, abdominal cramps and diarrhoea, or an exacerbation of atopic eczema. Rarely, acute asthma, generalized urticaria or anaphylaxis can occur.

In acute cases the diagnosis is usually obvious from the history alone. If there is any doubt, testing for specific IgE by skin prick test or RAST can be performed. A strongly positive result may strengthen a clinical suspicion, but it must be borne in mind that atopic individuals often have IgE antibodies to foods which cause them no clinical symptoms whatsoever. A negative test result therefore has more diagnostic significance than a positive one. In children with chronic symptoms the most reliable means of diagnosis is to withdraw the suspected foods for several days or weeks, allow the symptoms to subside, and then cautiously reintroduce foods one-by-one as oral challenges under close supervision.

The mainstay of treatment is avoidance. Most children "grow out" of their food allergies before puberty, particularly those involving eggs, milk or wheat. Cautious challenges can be carried out every 6 to 12 months, and once symptoms no longer occur the food can be gradually reintroduced into the child's diet. Allergies to peanut and fish are more likely to be severe and persistent, so that lifelong avoidance may be necessary.

Food Intolerance

The symptoms provoked by non-immunological food reactions are more varied and fluctuating than those caused by food allergy.[4] Although in some cases reactions are clinically clear-cut, in others they can be vague or non-specific, and their cause is often obscure. When a relationship between symptoms and diet is recognized, many foods may be suspected, but the variability of responses can be misleading. The reason for this is that reactions are caused by a variety of chemical substances, each common to many foods, and symptoms fluctuate according to the cumulative doses ingested.

Food chemicals

Although much attention has been paid in recent years to the adverse effects of food additives, naturally occurring food chemicals are a more insidious and more common cause of problems. Natural chemicals play a central role in the complex symbiotic relationship between animals and plants which has developed as a result of co-evolution.[5] Plants are known to be capable of synthesizing an enormous range of substances important for their own survival and reproduction. Amongst these are a variety of anti-microbial and anti-parasitic agents, as well as chemicals which can modify the feeding behaviour of insects and higher animals. Not surprisingly, some of these substances can be toxic to humans if ingested in significant quantities.

For their part, higher animals have developed elaborate sensory, metabolic and excretory mechanisms for the avoidance, detoxification and elimination, respectively, of potentially toxic plant chemicals. In addition, through agriculture and selective breeding over thousands of years, the human diet has evolved in such a way as to avoid the more dangerous of these substances. Of course, not all natural chemicals are harmful, at least in the amounts normally consumed. Indeed, some are essential nutrients (vitamins). Others are responsible for the distinctive flavours, aromas and psychophysiological effects which make many foods and drinks so pleasurable. Still others have been exploited for their medicinal properties. In many cases, however, adverse effects can become apparent when higher than usual doses are ingested. Furthermore, within any population there is a distribution of individual responsiveness to such substances. Thus, many commonly eaten foods, especially those derived from plants, contain chemicals which, though of generally low toxicity, can nevertheless have significant adverse effects in susceptible individuals.

Adverse reactions

The most carefully studied natural chemicals known to be capable of provoking adverse reactions are salicylates, biogenic amines, and glutamate. In general, the strength of flavour and aroma of foods is a good guide to the concentration of these substances.

Salicylates, along with many other benzoic acid derivatives, are found in varying concentrations in most fruits and vegetables, nuts, herbs and spices, jams, honey, tea, coffee, wines and many other plant-derived foods and drinks.[6] We have estimated that an average Western diet may contain between 10 and 100 milligrams per day of natural salicylates alone.

Biogenic amines are present in chocolate, cheese, fish products, aged or processed meats, bananas, oranges, avocados, tomatoes, wines and beer, amongst other foods.[7]

Free glutamate (i.e. non-protein-bound) is present naturally in many strongly flavoured foods such as tomatoes, mushrooms, tasty cheeses, gravies, sauces, stock cubes, meat extracts and yeast extracts;[8] its purified sodium salt (MSG) is also used as a flavour enhancer and has achieved notoriety for causing the "Chinese Restaurant" syndrome.

From this brief description it will be clear that not only is each substance found in many foods, but also that a given food may contain several offending chemicals. To further complicate the picture, intolerances are highly idiosyncratic, both in relation to the provoking agents and the symptoms provoked. Affected individuals are frequently sensitive to several substances, including both natural food chemicals and additives, the particular symptoms provoked depending on target organ susceptibility.[4]

The underlying causes of most food intolerances are unknown, but clinical observations suggest that they are likely to have a pharmacological basis. Reactions are dose-dependent, and it is common to observe withdrawal effects, tachyphylaxis and super-persensitivity when intake is modified. The range of symptoms is very similar to those seen as a result of drug side-effects and, indeed, it is common for food-sensitive patients to react adversely to various drugs as well. Not surprisingly, there appears to be a genetic predisposition. A positive family history is very common, and there is a tendency for specific sensitivities to cluster within affected families. In addition, women are affected two to three times more frequently than men, and can sometimes date the onset of symptoms to menarche, pregnancy or the taking of oral contraceptives, suggesting that hormonal factors may play a part.

Table 1
Clinical manifestations of food intolerance

Major syndromes *	Associated symptoms *
urticaria/angioedema	mouth ulceration
migraine	vaginal, bladder irritation
irritable bowel	nasal & sinus congestion
	irritability, depression
	'hyperactive' behaviour
	constitutional symptoms
	(fatigue, malaise, myalgia,
	headache, etc)

* Subdivisions refer to the most common presentations. However, in some cases symptoms listed in the 'associated' column may be the dominant clinical problem.

Clinical manifestations

The most common clinical manifestations of food intolerance are listed in Table 1. Reactions can begin at any age, the peak incidence being in the third and fourth decades. Symptoms often begin insidiously, but about one third of patients date the onset to a severe viral infection or other illness, an adverse drug reaction, a sudden change of diet, or some combination of these events. Chronic or recurrent urticaria and angioedema, irritable bowel syndrome (IBS), or migraine may be isolated presenting syndromes, or may occur in association with one or more of the other symptoms listed. In some cases, constitutional symptoms such as malaise, fatigue, headache, and flu-like aches and pains can dominate the clinical picture, occasionally leading patients to the mistaken belief that they are harbouring a "chronic virus infection" if food intolerance is unrecognized. In children, recurrent headaches, abdominal and limb pains are not uncommon, and may be associated with lassitude, irritability or 'hyperactive' behaviour.

In atopic patients the picture can be complex, since allergies and intolerances sometimes co-exist. In our experience, about one third of food-sensitive children with eczema have a clinically significant food allergy, whereas over 90% have demonstrable chemical intolerances. Food-sensitive asthmatics commonly react to sulphite preservatives, less often to salicylates and/or glutamate, and rarely to true food allergens.

Patient evaluation

In patients presenting with known or suspected food reactions, initial assessment should be aimed at determining whether symptoms are likely to be due to an allergy or to chemical intolerances, since this will determine subsequent investigation and management. Four aspects of the history are particularly important: (i) age of onset, (ii) a personal or family history of atopy, (iii) the pattern and nature of symptoms thought to be provoked by foods, and (iv) the specific foods known or suspected to be involved. Psychological aversions to specific foods can sometimes complicate the picture, but can usually be distinguished with a careful history and systematic testing.

Food reactions in children may be due to allergy, intolerances, or both, but those which first begin in adolescence or adult life can be assumed to be intolerances until proven otherwise. Similarly, symptoms such as recurrent urticaria, angioedema and mouth ulceration have a high probability of being due to food intolerance, even though the patient may be unaware of a relationship with diet. On the other hand, headaches, irritable bowel and most of the other associated symptoms listed in Table 1 are less specific. Even when food intolerance is known to be involved, it may be only one of several factors, both physical and emotional, capable of triggering the same symptoms in a susceptible individual. In these circumstances dietary investigation can be a very useful tool since these other factors are much easier to evaluate once the dietary variables have been eliminated.

The diet history is the least reliable. Whilst it is often

Figure 1

Cumulative effects of food chemicals

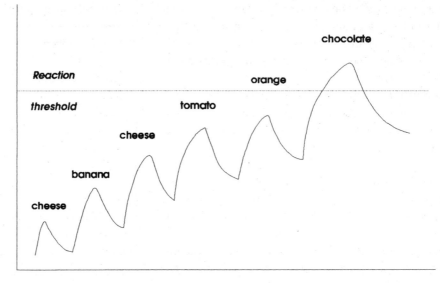

A variety of foods which share a common chemical component, eaten over several days, can contribute to the development of symptoms once the cumulative dose has exceeded the individual's reaction threshold. In this example, cheese, bananas, tomatoes, oranges and chocolate all contain biogenic amines, but the patient is likely only to incriminate the chocolate. On a different occasion, however, the same amount of chocolate in the absence of these other contributing foods may not reach threshold levels and might not provoke any symptoms.

possible to identify a food allergy from the history alone, intolerances are much more difficult to pinpoint in this way. Unlike allergies, reactions to food chemicals are typically delayed, usually by some hours, but by as much as a day or two in some cases. Acute reactions from a particular food can occur if the individual's dose threshold is exceeded, but this depends on what other foods have been eaten over the previous few days (Figure 1). More often, chronic or recurrent symptoms are provoked by the cumulative effects of several chemicals present in many different foods in the daily diet. Thus, it is not surprising that only about 50% of patients are aware of any connection at all between diet and their symptoms, and that fewer still are able to accurately identify the specific foods involved.

Clinically obvious reactions are most likely to occur with foods containing high concentrations and/or combinations of the relevant chemicals (e.g. highly flavoured or spicy foods, processed foods, confectionery, wines, etc.) and the experienced practitioner may then be able to make an educated guess about which substances are likely to be responsible. However, in most cases a definitive diagnosis cannot be made without systematic dietary testing. In general, patients who present with a belief that their symptoms are diet-related usually prove to be correct, but they can easily reach the wrong conclusions about which specific foods are involved.

Investigation and management

In the absence of any suitable diagnostic tests for food intolerance, the only reliable method of investigation is by elimination and challenge testing. The principle behind this approach is first to remove all the suspected foods and food substances from the patient's daily diet and then, if and when symptoms subside, to reintroduce them one by one as "challenges", preferably administered double-blind.

The details of this approach vary considerably between different centres. Within Australia most teaching hospitals have now adopted procedures based on the elimination diet and challenge protocols developed at Royal Prince Alfred Hospital over the past decade. Patients are placed on a stringent diet free of natural salicylates, amines, glutamate and food additives for a period of two to six weeks, depending on clinical response. Milk, wheat, and/or eggs may also be eliminated, depending on the circumstances, and can be reintroduced later as open challenges. Patients whose symptoms subside are given a battery of chemical challenge capsules containing graded doses of purified food substances and placebos, administered in a random order at 48-hour intervals. Symptoms are recorded in a diary, and once the challenges are completed the code is broken for each patient and the results interpreted. In most cases, investigation can be carried out on an outpatient basis, but if there is a history of anaphylactoid reactions, laryngeal oedema or moderate to severe asthma, challenges are performed under careful supervision in hospital. In our hands, symptomatic improvement with dietary elimination occurs in approximately two-thirds of patients with recurrent urticaria, and 40-50% of those presenting with headaches or irritable bowel syndrome. To illustrate the usual reaction pattern, results of challenge tests in these groups are shown in Table 2.

Once the substances responsible for provoking symptoms have been identified in each case, an individu-

ally tailored diet can be prescribed for long-term management. Total abstinence is rarely necessary. After 4-6 weeks of strict adherence, patients are instructed to begin gradual dietary liberalization to determine their individual reaction threshold with foods grouped according to chemical content. Often, regular ingestion of small amounts leads to an increase in tolerance over a period of weeks or months, and some patients may eventually be able to return to a relatively normal diet. In other cases, symptoms can recur insidiously, indicating a need for more stringent avoidance.

Successful dietary management requires the involvement of an experienced dietitian. Attention to seemingly minor details is crucial, and compliance is enhanced greatly by the provision of practical advice about shopping, preparation of meals, social occasions, etc., as well as telephone access to clarify uncertainties as they arise.

Table 2

Double-blind challenge responses (%)*

Challenges	Presentation Urticaria	Migraine	I.B.S.
Active:			
salicylates	61	51	62
amines	29	52	39
glutamate (MSG)	33	54	48
preservatives	47	51	39
antioxidants	29	33	38
propionate	19	32	37
nitrates	38	58	47
tartrazine	34	43	36
erythrosine	35	31	40
brewers yeast	30	40	32
gluten	2	7	16
lactose	7	11	18
placebos:			
starch	5	8	8
sucrose	2	7	5

* Response rates refer only to provocation of main presenting symptoms. Various other symptoms were provoked by each challenge in an additional 0-14% of cases. Numbers of patients challenged in each group were: urticaria 614; migraine 109; irritable bowel 159.

DIET AND CHRONIC FATIGUE SYNDROME

As outlined above, in some patients with food intolerance, constitutional symptoms can dominate the clinical picture, or can be the sole manifestations. They include fatigue, headache, musculo-skeletal aches and pains, malaise, and a variety of neuropsychiatric symptoms such as irritability, depression, impaired memory and concentration, sensory and visual disturbances. Indeed, patients may present with a clinical picture typical of "chronic fatigue syndrome".[9] It should be stressed, however, that the clinical spectrum of food intolerance is such that individual patients can experience any combination of symptoms, with varying degrees of severity, so that precise categorization can be somewhat arbitrary at times.

Challenge test results

We have investigated a total of 966 patients presenting with constitutional symptoms at Royal Prince Alfred Hospital over a nine year period (Table 3), representing about 20% of all patients referred to our clinic for dietary evaluation. Of the 966, approximately one third would satisfy criteria for the diagnosis of chronic fatigue syndrome, although as implied above, the dividing line is not always clear. Ages ranged from 5 to 85 years, with more than 50% falling between 20 and 45 years, and females outnumbered males by 3:1. All patients were initially offered a strict elimination diet to screen for possible food intolerance. Overall, 656 patients reported subjective improvement, and of these 497 underwent formal double-blind, placebo-controlled challenge testing. The remaining 159 were prescribed an empirically modified diet based on open food challenges.

Table 3	
Patients presenting for dietary testing: constitutional symptoms	
	No. of patients
Challenged	497
Empirical diet	159
In progress	34
No improvement	79
Lost to follow-up	197
Total	966

The proportion of patients reacting to each of the double-blind chemical challenges is shown in Table 4. Several points are worthy of note. To begin with, the hierarchy of responses is very similar to that seen in other patient groups presenting with recurrent urticaria, migraine and irritable bowel syndrome (Table 2). Salicylates were the single most common challenge to provoke reactions, followed by preservatives, glutamate, amines and the various other food additives. Brewers yeast contains a complex mixture of phenolic substances, and is most likely to provoke reactions in patients who are sensitive to both salicylates and amines. Gluten and lactose reactions were the least common, and when they did occur there was a tendency for them to provoke mainly gastrointestinal symptoms. The overall placebo reaction rate was low, at around 10%, a result we attribute to the reduction of "background noise" by maintenance of stringent dietary restriction throughout the challenge period.

It is noteworthy that each challenge is capable of provoking any or all of the symptoms, the pattern being highly idiosyncratic but reproducible in each individual. Moreover, by adding the percentages in each column it will be clear that most individuals reacted to several different challenges, the mean being around six, and that each substance was capable of eliciting several symptoms. Overall, it has been our clinical observation that of all patients with food intolerance, those with fatigue and other constitutional symptoms are the most sensitive, reacting to a broader range of challenge substances, with lower dose thresholds and more prolonged symptoms.

Clinical outcome

The long-term benefits of dietary modification in patients with chronic fatigue syndrome are more subjective and difficult to quantify. Nevertheless, we have recently conducted a retrospective survey (follow-up period 12 months to 8 years) in an attempt to gain some insight into this question. Altogether, 225 contactable patients who satisfied our criteria for a diagnosis of chronic fatigue syndrome, were sent a questionnaire by mail. Of these, 153 had undergone dietary investigation. At the time of writing, 102 replies had been received. Patients were first asked to give a global, qualitative assessment of their response to the elimination diet during initial testing

	Table 4					
Symptoms (%) provoked by challenges (495 patients)						
CHALLENGES	Total Reactions (%)	fatigue	aches & pains	CNS & mood	headache	G.I. Tract
Salicylate	75	24	16	27	33	41
Amines	65	23	13	17	33	27
Glutamate (MSG)	66	24	14	21	33	32
Preservatives	67	23	13	21	32	32
Antioxidants	55	19	11	17	24	25
Nitrates	64	20	13	16	33	33
Propionate	53	17	9	16	22	29
Tartrazine	57	20	12	18	27	24
Brewers yeast	46	17	11	13	23	20
Gluten	22	9	5	6	9	11
Lactose	23	8	4	5	11	13
Starch (placebo)	12	5	3	4	6	5
Sucrose (placebo)	9	3	2	3	5	4

(Table 5). A little over one third of the respondents considered themselves to have been "much better" or "completely well", whilst nearly two thirds recalled having felt "no better at all" or only "a little better".

Table 5	
Symptomatic response to elimination diet	
Global response	No. of patients
"No better at all"	38
"A little better"	25
"Much better"	32
"Completely well"	7
TOTAL	102

Patients were next asked whether they were still restricting their diet at the time of follow up, and if so, to what degree. The responses are shown in Table 6. Not unexpectedly, those who initially felt "much

better" or "completely well" had continued to restrict their diet, in most cases stringently. Interestingly, however, more than half of those who recalled feeling "no better at all" on the initial elimination diet had also continued with significant long-term restriction.

Table 6		
Maintenance of long-term dietary restriction		
Initial response	Degree of restriction	
	Any degree	Moderate / severe
'No better'	65%	51%
'A little better'	88%	71%
'Much better'	100%	84%
'Completely well'	100%	83%

At first sight this is a puzzling result. However, our clinical experience has been that even though a patient's global state may not be significantly improved, specific symptoms can respond to dietary modification, sometimes dramatically, with recurrence when the offending substances are reintroduced. The converse is also true, in that patients whose global state is significantly improved may nevertheless find that certain symptoms persist, regardless of the extent to which their diet is restricted.

These clinical impressions were confirmed by responses to the follow-up questionnaire. Patients were asked to subjectively rate the percent improvement in each of their major symptoms as a result of long-term dietary restriction. The results amongst those who had originally considered themselves "much better" or "completely well" on the test diet are summarized in Figure 2. On average, all symptoms remained substantially reduced in this group, headaches showing the most consistent benefit overall. More detailed analysis of responses, however, showed significant individual variability, with no reproducible pattern. Not surprisingly, patients who felt little or no better on the initial elimination diet reported little or no long-term improvement either, on average (Figure 3).

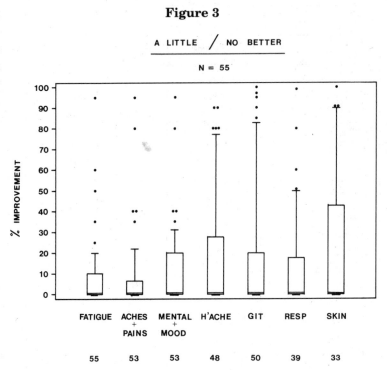

Figure 3

A LITTLE / NO BETTER
N = 55
% IMPROVEMENT
FATIGUE
ACHES + PAINS
MENTAL + MOOD
H'ACHE
GIT
RESP
SKIN
55
53
53
48
50
39
33

Figures 2 & 3 *Boxes show 25th, 50th and 75th percentiles; bars indicate 90th percentiles; closed circles are remaining outliers.*

Nevertheless, individual patients did sometimes obtain significant relief from specific symptoms, most notably headaches, gastrointestinal and skin reactions.

Selection of patients for dietary investigation

Figure 2

FATIGUE
ACHES + PAINS
MENTAL + MOOD
H'ACHE
GIT
RESP
SKIN
% IMPROVEMENT
34
28
32
28
24
23
9
MUCH BETTER / COMPLETELY WELL
(N=34)

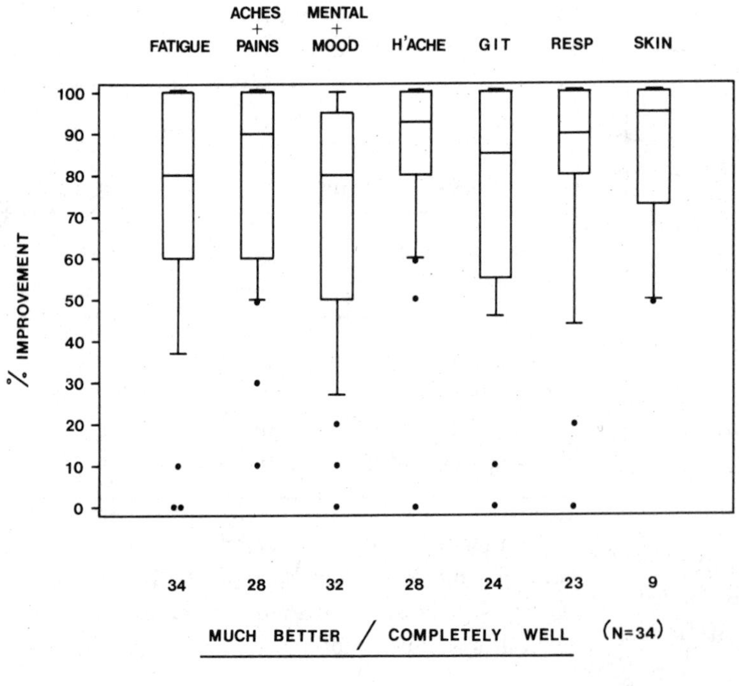

Clearly, not all patients with chronic fatigue can or should undergo the kind of time-consuming dietary investigation outlined above. The elimination diet itself is demanding, inconvenient, socially restrictive and, above all, boring. On top of this the challenges are intended to provoke symptoms which may be distressing and usually continue for several hours or days (even two or three weeks in rare cases). The whole process usually takes between two and three months, and although some patients benefit, many do not. On the other hand, when patients do benefit they can sometimes obtain dramatic relief of long-standing, debilitating symptoms. Even when improvement is less dramatic it can lead to a significant improvement in quality of life and return to productivity for the

chronically ill. In such cases, even a major change of diet may be considered a small price to pay.

Is dietary investigation warranted?

How, then, can the doctor and patient decide whether dietary investigation is warranted? The main factors to be weighed are: the severity of the symptoms, the motivation of the patient, and the probability of success. Severity is very subjective, but can be judged to some extent according to how badly the individual's daily life is disrupted, including work, family life, leisure and recreation. Motivation depends not only on the patient's degree of distress and desire to improve, but also on attitude to food and willingness to sustain the necessary inconveniences during testing.

Before making a final decision, most patients ask about the probability of success. The true prevalence of food intolerance in chronic fatigue syndrome is difficult to determine with confidence. Our estimate is that it is a significant factor in 20-30%, and may be the principal trigger in perhaps 5-10%, though we hasten to add that these figures are subject to an unquantifiable selection bias.

Clinical Clues

There are several clues in the history which may increase the clinician's index of suspicion that food intolerance is a factor: (a) recurrent urticaria, angioedema, and/or mouth ulceration (past or present); (b) associated gastrointestinal symptoms and/or migraine; (c) known food reactions; (d) aspirin or other drug intolerances; (e) a strong family history of food intolerance.

Overview

It is evident from the above observations that the relationship between food intolerance and chronic fatigue syndrome is a complex one. Thus, within the clinical spectrum of food intolerance, we find that pathological fatigue, in varying degrees of severity, is a common symptom. At one end of this spectrum is a sub-group of patients with typical chronic fatigue syndrome, with or without other food-associated

symptoms. Conversely, looking from the perspective of patients presenting with chronic fatigue syndrome, we find that food intolerance can assume varying degrees of significance. In some cases, food plays no discernible part whatsoever in triggering symptoms, whilst in others, symptoms can resolve completely when the diet is suitably modified, with all grades in-between.

The role of viruses is also complex. In agreement with other reports, 35% of patients presenting to our clinic with chronic fatigue syndrome had a clinically evident acute viral infection at the onset of their illness. Two thirds of these were documented EBV infections, but a number of other organisms were implicated in specific cases e.g. influenza, hepatitis B, varicella, rubella, herpes simplex. Enteric infections acquired whilst travelling appeared to be the trigger in several patients, though the responsible organisms were rarely identified. Interestingly, there was no difference in the incidence or distribution of infections between those who proved to have significant food intolerance and those who did not. It is relevant to note that a careful history will implicate a viral infection at the onset of the disorder in some 20 to 30% of all patients with food intolerance, regardless of the clinical manifestations. Thus, chronic fatigue syndrome should not be regarded as unique from this point of view.

It should also be emphasized that infection itself may not always be directly to blame for triggering symptoms. Careful questioning often reveals concurrent events whose significance may only become apparent in retrospect, after dietary testing. For example, many of our patients who suffered an acute viral illness at the outset stopped eating regular meals, consuming instead large amounts of preserved soft drinks, citrus fruit, tea, soups, broths etc. At the same time they often took various medications such as aspirin or other anti-inflammatory and analgesic preparations, proprietary cold and 'flu remedies, cough suppressants, coloured and flavoured lozenges or syrups, antihistamines, sympathomimetics and/or antibiotics. In patients with a sensitive constitution this combination of dietary and pharmaceutical stimuli can be a major insult, particularly when coming on top of an acute systemic inflammatory reaction. Once established, overt food intolerance can then become a self-perpetuating problem, producing recurrent flu-like symptoms which are easily mistaken for a "chronic virus infection".

PATHOGENESIS

Clinically, there are several striking features of chronic fatigue syndrome: the severity of the symptoms compared with the paucity of physical signs; the absence of significant immunopathology; the fluctuating course (short-term and long-term); the occurrence of spontaneous remissions (occasionally full recovery) even after prolonged illness; and the lack of long-term progression in most cases. In particular, patients do not exhibit persistent fever, lymphadenopathy, splenomegaly, leukocytosis, or other signs of a chronic inflammatory process. Indeed, persistent changes in acute phase reactants, serological abnormalities, or evidence of tissue pathology are so rare that, when evident, they suggest the presence of some other undiagnosed disease. Since, in general, the symptoms of viral infections are mostly attributable to the host response, these features themselves, do not support the theory that chronic fatigue syndrome is due to a "chronic active" viral infection.

Immune competence is also typically normal in patients with chronic fatigue syndrome, as judged by their ability to clear intercurrent infections efficiently, and by the absence of repeated or progressive infections with specific organisms, opportunistic or otherwise. Although we do not routinely test immunological function in our own patients, we have done so in selected cases and generally find the results to be within the normal range. In our view, the findings reported by others are non-specific and likely to be of a secondary nature.

Hypothesis

On the basis of the above arguments, the evidence that chronic fatigue syndrome is caused by a chronic viral infection or a primary immunological disorder seems unconvincing, pointing to the need for a fresh approach in attempting to understand this puzzling condition. Similarly, the mechanisms of most adverse food reactions are poorly understood, with no satisfactory explanation for their diverse clinical manifestations. The relationship described here between food intolerance and chronic fatigue syndrome

thus provides us with an opportunity to formulate a unifying hypotheses by which to try and comprehend both problems.

> We propose that both food intolerances and chronic fatigue syndrome are manifestations of primary (perhaps heterogeneous) disorders of neuroregulation, involving abnormalities in the function of one or more receptor families which regulate synaptic transmission.

This hypothesis is based on two separate lines of evidence. The first derives from the clinical associations described here between migraine, irritable bowel syndrome, recurrent urticaria and chronic fatigue syndrome. In each case, an argument can be made that neuroregulatory mechanisms are involved in pathogenesis. The second line of evidence arises from the observation that food intolerance can trigger symptoms in each of these apparently diverse conditions, suggesting that there may be common mechanisms linking them. Considering the nature of the chemical triggers in such patients, and their response characteristics, it is likely that receptor-mediated abnormalities of synaptic transmission and/or neuromodulation are involved.

Clinical associations

Migraine and irritable bowel syndrome are relatively easy to comprehend as neurogenic disorders. In migraine, premonitory and prodromal symptoms preceding headache point clearly to central nervous system (CNS) involvement, although whether this reflects a primary neurogenic event or is secondary to vascular changes remains a subject of debate. Over the past three decades much interest has focused on abnormalities of serotonin release as the basis of the vascular changes in migraine.[12,13] Pain is thought to be mediated by perivascular nerve fibres which contain the sensory neuropeptides substance P (SP) and calcitonin gene-related peptide (CGRP) along with vasoactive intestinal polypeptide (VIP) and neuropeptide Y (NPY),[14] and both SP and CGRP have been shown to be released during headache.[15,16] Although it is generally agreed that these mechanisms are activated in migraine, attention has increasingly shifted towards possible primary CNS abnormalities. Evidence is accumulating that a phenomenon analogous to the spreading depression of Leao[17] may be involved, and it has been suggested that this may be mediated by abnormalities of excitatory (glutamate) or inhibitory (gamma aminobutyric acid, GABA) neurotransmitter function.[18] There has also been considerable interest in the central serotoninergic system, but its pathophysiological role remains to be determined.[19]

Irritable bowel syndrome is characterized by abnormalities in motility of the small and large intestine and abnormal responsiveness to various neurohumoral stimuli,[20] consistent with an abnormality of neuroregulation.[21] In recent years it has become evident that the enteric nervous system is comparable to the spinal cord in terms of the number of neurons present and their structural and neurochemical complexity.[22] In addition to classical neurotransmitters, enteric neurons produce at least 14 neuropeptides, including VIP, SP, NPY, CGRP, cholecystokinin (CCK), enkephalin, dynorphin, and peptide histidine-isoleucine (PHI).[22] Furthermore, peptides released in the CNS have been shown to influence gastrointestinal motility, including CCK, NPY, SP, thyrotropin-releasing hormone (TRH), corticotropin-releasing factor (CRF), neurotensin, oxytocin and somatostatin.[23] Although specific abnormalities have not yet been identified, it is interesting to note that increased irritability has also been found in other organs in patients with irritable bowel syndrome.[24,25,26]

In recurrent urticaria and angioedema the role of neural mechanisms is at first sight more difficult to discern. Drugs, chemicals, foods and physical stimuli are generally believed to release histamine and other mediators from mast cells by pathways not involving IgE, but precise mechanisms have not been delineated in most cases.[27,28] However, there are some tantalizing clinical clues which suggest that neurogenic pathways are involved: the anatomical distribution of lesions; the occurrence of a localized sensory prodrome in some patients; and the common tendency for pressure and other physical stimuli to trigger lesions. It is interesting to note, therefore, that in normal human skin peptides such as SP, VIP, somatostatin, neurotensin, and certain endorphins are capable of stimulating mast cell degranulation.[29] "Neurogenic inflammation" and the axon reflex are thought to be mediated by the release of SP from sensory C-type fibres in the skin, causing release of histamine from nearby mast cells.[30-33] Recently, peptidergic nerve fibres have been observed making direct contact with mast cells in various tissues, providing a structural basis for this interaction.[34-36] Taken together, this evidence has led us[4] and others[37,38] to speculate that recurrent "idiopathic" urticaria and its physical variants might involve an abnormality in the neural regulation of mast cell function.

> Thus, we would argue that the common thread linking migraine, irritable bowel syndrome and recurrent urticaria in patients with food intolerance is an abnormality of neuroregulation.

From here, it does not take a large leap of imagination to suppose that chronic fatigue syndrome might also have a similar basis. Involvement of the CNS would explain many of the bizarre neurological and psychological manifestations of the condition, and could also account for the gastrointestinal and other autonomic symptoms which can be prominent in some patients. Furthermore, it then becomes easy to comprehend the increased sensitivity of such patients to diverse pharmacological stimuli (drugs, alcohol, food chemicals, smells and fumes) and to endogenous factors (stress, exercise, hormonal changes). Finally, on this view, viruses would be seen as triggering clinical symptoms via the exaggerated central effects of inflammatory mediators and lymphokines.[39,40]

Chemical stimuli

The next question is, can we be more specific in considering the nature of such putative neuroregulatory abnormalities? To examine this, we turn to the various stimuli capable of triggering symptoms in different individuals, in particular, the food chemicals described above. The first point to note is that reactions to these substances are highly specific in each individual, even amongst chemicals which are closely related structurally such as the various benzoic acid derivatives, with no predictable pattern. Once established, idiosyncrasies remain fixed over time even though the reaction threshold can vary. Secondly, reactions to these substances exhibit dose-dependence, tachyphylaxis, tolerance, withdrawal reactions, and supersensitivity with chronic ingestion or after abstinence. These phenomena, taken together, are highly characteristic of receptor mediated alterations in synaptic transmission.[41]

The specificities of such receptors, and their possible locations are open to speculation. However, the enormous complexity of neuroregulatory mechanisms now emerging[42,43] should caution us against over-simplification. In addition to the "classical" neurotransmitters there are now over 40 known peptide and other neurotransmitters, each with their own family of receptors, and the number is still growing. Co-localization of several transmitters in a single neuron has become the rule rather than the exception, with some cells containing as many as five. Almost any combination is possible. They can be released together or separately, and their physiological effects can be enormously varied depending on the target cell types and receptors expressed.[42] One interesting feature of neuropeptides is the distinction between their direct actions as effectors of neurotransmission, and their indirect actions in modulating the actions of other transmitters.[43] These are independent properties mediated by different mechanisms. Both can be highly specific (implying action through receptors or other binding sites), but neuromodulation is characterized by slow onset and long duration, slow desensitization, and in some cases multiple actions contributing to a coordinated physiological or behavioural effect.[43]

What inferences can we make, then, from a closer examination of adverse food reactions? One likelihood is that food chemicals act by altering neuromodulation rather than direct neurotransmission, since reactions are typically delayed in onset, and can last for hours or days. Another is that they can probably act through a multiplicity of receptor subtypes, given the structural diversity of the substances involved, and their protean clinical manifestations. However, the fact that several apparently unrelated substances can cause the same set of symptoms in a given individual suggests that there may be convergence of different pathways onto particular target cells and/or 'cross-talk' amongst the different receptors involved.[44] This is supported by our clinical observation of cross-desensitization and cross-tolerance between different substances to which a given individual may be sensitive.

Regarding the actions of specific food chemicals, it is plausible (but perhaps too simplistic) to imagine, for example, that foods containing biogenic amines might act via one or more monoamine receptors. Similarly,

the fact that glutamate is physiologically an excitatory neurotransmitter makes it tempting to speculate that abnormally functioning endogenous receptors might be at fault in MSG-sensitive patients.[45] Although there are now well established examples of 'excitotoxic' amino acids causing neuropsychiatric disorders via NMDA receptors,[46] it should be borne in mind that such cases involve neuronal cell death and irreversible structural pathology, unlike the conditions we are considering here.

Since salicylates are the most common of our challenge substances to elicit reactions, it is of considerable interest to examine their possible mechanism of action. There are four main hypotheses to explain aspirin idiosyncrasy as a cause of urticaria and/or asthma:

(1) cyclooxygenase blockade with diversion of arachidonate into the lipoxygenase pathway,

(2) "direct" mast cell degranulation,

(3) activation of the complement cascade,

(4) activation of the contact system with excess kinin formation.[47]

Of these, the first is the most widely accepted,[48] but detailed review of the evidence has led to the conclusion that the true mechanisms remain unknown.[49] Our own finding of cross-sensitivity between sodium salicylate, acetylsalicylic acid, sodium benzoate, 4OH-benzoate and amines, as well as structurally unrelated compounds such as metabisulphite, tartrazine and MSG, also argues strongly against a primary disturbance of arachidonic acid metabolism. What of other known actions of salicylates such as uncoupling of oxidative phosphorylation or free radical scavenging?[50] At present there is no clinical or laboratory evidence to implicate them, and the cross-sensitivities above argue against the possibility. More informative, perhaps, are the well-known clinical manifestations of chronic salicylate intoxication: headache, nausea, vomiting, diarrhoea, blurred vision, tinnitus, vertigo, and CNS symptoms such as lassitude, drowsiness, confusion, restlessness, excitement, tremor, progressing in severe cases to hallucinations, delirium, convulsions, and eventually coma. Although some of these toxic effects may be secondary to metabolic changes, many of the CNS manifestations are thought to be due to the direct effects of salicylates on neuronal function. The latter include alterations in GABA and serotonin production, altered membrane permeability and reduced synaptic transmission.[50]

Finally, given the clinical evidence of a strong familial predisposition to the various clinical disorders associated with food intolerance, the question arises as to what might be the molecular and genetic basis of the proposed neuroregulatory abnormalities discussed above.

> A possibility we find particularly attractive is that there may be allelic heterogeneity within the population at receptor gene loci.

Although such polymorphisms have not yet been demonstrated in receptor molecules, there is ample biological precedent for this suggestion. Thus, if minor variations in amino acid sequence were located near a transmitter binding site, allosteric sites or other conformationally sensitive parts of the molecule, it would be easy to envisage subtle changes in molecular function. This could include altered affinity for endogenous and exogenous agonists and/or antagonists, changes in receptor turnover and numbers, or alterations in signal transduction mechanisms. Functionally significant allelic variation could also occur in ion channels linked to receptors, or in one or more of the growing family of regulatory G proteins.[51]

We do not consider these various possibilities to be mutually exclusive; indeed, clinical expression of chemical idiosyncrasies might well require the presence of more than one such abnormality. Moreover, even if our speculations about neuroregulation prove correct, additional genetic polymorphisms in detoxification enzymes may lower the threshold for developing chemical intolerances in certain cases. For example, reduced phenolsulphotransferase activity has been demonstrated in some patients with dietary migraine,[52] and low pulmonary sulphite oxidase levels have been reported in asthmatics sensitive to sulphite preservatives.[53] However, this is unlikely to be the rule. We have studied salicylate pharmacodynamics in 26 patients with aspirin-sensitive urticaria and found them to be no different from normal controls (unpublished observations). The significance of other

changes such as altered intestinal permeability remain to be determined.[54]

CONCLUSIONS

Is it "psychosomatic"?

This is a question which frequently arises in relation to all of the conditions discussed above, and which therefore deserves careful consideration. Clinical experience in patients with food intolerance reveals a complex relationship with psychological stress. On the one hand, certain individuals find that acutely stressful situations can aggravate or precipitate symptoms, and during periods of chronic stress the threshold for food reactions may be lowered. This phenomenon is most likely to occur in patients presenting with constitutional symptoms, less so in those with uncomplicated headaches or irritable bowel syndrome, and is rare in those with isolated urticaria. Conversely, patients can experience neuropsychiatric symptoms in response to food chemicals, and in these circumstances they often perceive a given situation as more stressful than it would otherwise have been. Thus, in the sense that psychological and physical symptoms can interact, we could consider the disorders involved as being "psychosomatic", at least in some individuals.

However, it is worth dwelling for a moment on the meaning of this term. In a thoughtful review, Lipowski[55] has drawn a semantic and philosophical distinction between what he regards as the now obsolete idea of psychogenesis, and the more holistic view of biopsychosocial relationships in health and disease. He criticizes application of the term *psychosomatic disorder* to "...any somatic disease or dysfunction in which psychologic factors are postulated to play a necessary or sufficient causal role", suggesting that this has given rise to pointless and misleading polemics. He regards the term as being "...incompatible with the doctrine of multicausality which constitutes a core assumption in the field of psychosomatic medicine" and advocates that it be discarded.

Although this view is reasonably widely accepted nowadays, it remains problematic. Leaving aside the trivial truism that "biopsychosocial" relationships exist in all disease, the doctrine of multicausality does not distinguish between primary causation (sine qua non) and other factors, and it introduces the likelihood that non-causal associations will be mistakenly accorded aetiological status.[56] Witness the confusion surrounding the role of personality factors in pathogenesis of irritable bowel syndrome,[20] where it is now clear that psychosocial variables correlate with health care seeking behaviour rather than with the disease itself.[57] Moreover, multicausality still retains the dualist notion of psychogenesis in that states of mind, even though they may not be considered necessary or sufficient, are nonetheless imagined to contribute in some more-or-less direct way to the development of physical disease. Though popular, this notion must be regarded as speculative, at best.[58,59]

In individual cases, the idea of multicausality encourages practitioners to extract post hoc clinical evidence to support the belief that "stress" is an aetiological factor. Consequently, if a patient admits to neuropsychiatric symptoms and a perception of stress, it becomes an easy matter to confuse correlation with causation,[56,57] or to diagnose primary psychiatric disease where none exists.[60,61] On the other hand, if a patient denies any significant emotional symptoms, this in itself may be taken as evidence of deep-seated psychopathology. Finally, obscuring the fact that the evidence cannot always be made to fit the theory, vague diagnostic labels such as "masked depression" are applied.

What should the "diagnosis" be?

Diagnostic labeling can serve many useful purposes for both patients and doctors, including socio-cultural, conceptual, prognostic and therapeutic ones. However, it can also serve as a cloak for ignorance, prejudice or misguided belief.[62] Nowhere, perhaps, is this more evident than in patients with chronic fatigue and food intolerance, where the diagnostic label used generally reflects the biases of the observer rather than any real understanding of the underlying pathophysiology (Table 7).[63-75]

Kendell[76] argues that "chronic fatigue syndrome" is often a misdiagnosis in patients who, in reality, have an unrecognized depressive illness which would benefit from appropriate treatment. Our clinical experience does not bear this out, being more in line with the view that when depression is evident it is usually

secondary.[77] Many of our patients have, in fact, had a trial of antidepressant therapy at some stage, either before or after referral for dietary investigation, but a favourable response is very much the exception rather than the rule. Indeed, as with most drugs acting on the CNS, such patients often experience exaggerated side-effects and may be forced to abandon treatment as a result. Whilst we share Kendell's general view that there is probably no fundamental distinction between depressive illness and other kinds of "organic" illness,[76] forcing patients with vaguely similar neuropsychiatric symptoms, but no primary mood change, into the same diagnostic category seems more hindrance than help, both from a conceptual and a practical point of view.

Table 7	
Practitioner	Diagnosis
Microbiologist	Post-viral fatigue syndrome Chronic EBV infection
Immunologist	Immune dysfunction syndrome
Rheumatologist	Fibromyalgia syndrome
Internist	Chronic hyperventilation
General Practitioner	Bored housewife syndrome Yuppie Flu
Psychiatrist	Somatization disorder Depression
Neurologist	Myalgic encephalomyelitis Hysteria
Allergist	Food allergy / intolerance
Clinical ecologist	20th century syndrome
Orthomolecular	Hypoglycaemia Vitamin deficiency
Naturopath	Candida hypersensitivity

Another psychiatric designation sometimes applied to patients with chronic fatigue syndrome[78] is "somatoform disorder", one of the subtypes of what used to be called hysteria. Here there exist even greater conceptual problems. Lipowski[79] defines somatization as "...a tendency to experience and communicate somatic distress and symptoms unaccounted for by pathological findings, to attribute them to physical illness, and to seek medical help for them. It is usually assumed that this tendency becomes manifest in response to psychosocial stress brought about by life events and situations." Central to the definition is the patient's persistent search for a medical diagnosis and treatment "...despite doctors' reassurances that physical illness cannot account for their symptoms."[79]

> Thus, the entire concept of somatization is based on the false premise that biomedical science has now reached the point where all physical causes of illness are known, and can be excluded with certainty by a competent physician.[80]

Failure to appreciate the extent of our collective limitations in this regard can lead to false value judgements about illness behaviour[81] and about the legitimacy (or otherwise) of the sick role. To quote Lipowski again: "Somatization ... involves both mind and body, and, as a mimicry of 'real' diseases, is a state of being that is neither wellness nor 'legitimate' sickness."[79] From our own perspective, a hint of the underlying fallacy can be discerned in the findings of one series where nearly 50% of patients judged to have a chronic somatoform disorder reported "food intolerances" amongst their symptoms.[63]

We are often asked by our own patients with chronic fatigue, in whom food intolerance is found to be a significant factor, "What do I really have, doctor, 'food intolerance' or 'chronic fatigue syn-

drome'?" Whilst recognizing the importance of supplying patients with a 'diagnosis' for ease of communication with doctors, employers, family and friends, we nevertheless prefer to offer an operational description where possible. In doing so, we try to convey the idea that neither food intolerance nor chronic fatigue syndrome should be considered disease entities.[82] Rather, we regard food chemicals (like drugs, hormones, viruses, stress) as one of many possible exogenous or endogenous triggers capable of provoking symptoms; and we regard chronic fatigue syndrome as a cluster of neurological symptoms which can arise in response to one or more such stimuli in predisposed people, as illustrated below. Delineation of more meaningful diagnostic terminology must await a deeper understanding of the underlying molecular pathology.

GENETIC PREDISPOSITION

(receptor polymorphisms?)

ENDOGENOUS TRIGGERS

hormones

exertion

stress

inflammatory mediators (viruses etc)

NERVOUS SYSTEM

EXOGENOUS TRIGGERS

food chemicals

drugs

environmental chemicals (smells & fumes)

SYMPTOMS

References

1. Lessof MH. 'Clinical reactions to food'. John Wiley & Sons, Chichester, 1983.

2. Lessof MH, Gray JR, Hoffenberg R, et al. Food intolerance and food aversion. J Roy Coll Physicians Lond 1984;18:83-123.

3. Sampson HA. IgE-mediated food intolerance. J Allergy Clin Immunol 1988;81:495-504.

4. Loblay RH, Swain AR. Food intolerance. In: 'Recent Advances in Clinical Nutrition'. Eds. Wahlqvist ML and Truswell AS, John Libbey, London, Vol. 2, 1986. pp 169-177.

5. Johns T. 'With bitter herbs they shall eat it: Chemical ecology and the origins of human diet and medicine'. University of Arizona Press, Tucson, 1990.

6. Swain AR, Dutton S, Truswell AS. Salicylates in food. J Am Diet Ass 1985;85:950-60.

7. Maga JA. Amines in foods. CRC Crit Rev Food Sci Nutr 1978;10:373-403.

8. Filer LJ, Garattini S, Kane MR, Reynolds WA, Wurtman RJ. Glutamic acid: Advances in biochemistry and physiology. Raven Press, New York, 1979.

9. Holmes GP, Kaplan JE, Gantz NM, et al. Chronic fatigue syndrome: a working case definition. Ann Int Med 1988;108:387-9.

10. Behan PO, Behan WMH, Bell EJ. The postviral fatigue syndrome — an analysis of the findings in 50 cases. J infection 1985;10:211-22.

11. Lloyd A, Wakefield D, Boughton C, Dwyer J. Immunological abnormalities in the chronic fatigue syndrome. Med J Aust 1989;151:122-4.

12. Lance JW, Lambert GA, Goadsby PJ, Zagami AS. 5-Hydroxytryptamine and its putative aetiological involvement in migraine. Cephalalgia 1989;9(suppl 9):7-13.

13. Ribiero CAF, Cotrim MD, Morgadinho MT, Ramos MI, Santos ES, de Macedo TdRA. Migraine, serum serotonin and platelet 5-HT2 receptors. Cephalalgia 1990;10:213-9.

14. Moskowitz MA. Basic mechanisms in vascular headache. Neurology Clinics of North America 1990;4:801-15.

15. Edvinsson L, Goadsby PG, Jansen I, Udman R. Perivascular peptide transmitters: Innervation and release in migraine. Cephalalgia 1989;9(suppl 10):15-6.

16. Nicolodi M, Bianco ED. Sensory neuropeptides (substance P, calcitonin gene-related peptide) and vasoactive intestinal polypeptide in human saliva: their pattern in migraine and cluster headache. Cephalalgia 1990;10:39-50.

17. Leao AAP. Spreading depression of activity in the cerebral cortex. J Neurophysiol 1944;7:379-90.

18. Welch KMA, D'Andrea G, Tepley N, Barkley G, Ramadan NM. The concept of migraine as a state of central neuronal hyperexcitability. Neurology Clinics of North America 1990;8:817-28.

19. Malmgren R. The central serotoninergic system. Cephalalgia 1990;10:199-204.

20. Kellow JE, Langeluddecke PM. Advances in the understanding and management of the irritable bowel syndrome. Med J Aust 1989;151:92-9.

21. Fox JET. Control of gastrointestinal motility be peptides: Old peptides, new tricks — new peptides, old tricks. Gastroenterology Clinics of North America 1989;18:163-77.

22. Sternini C. Structural and chemical organization of the myenteric plexus. Ann Rev Physiol 1988;50:81-93.

23. Tache Y, Garrick T, Raybould H. Central nervous system action of peptides to influence gastrointestinal motor function. Gastroenterology 1990;98:517-28.

24. Whorwell PJ, Lupton EW, Erduran D, et al. Bladder smooth muscle dysfunction in patients with irritable bowel syndrome. Gut 1986;27:1014-47.

25. White A, Upton A, Collins SM. Is irritable bowel syndrome the asthma of the gut? Gastroenterology 1988;94:A494.

26. Kellow JE, Miller LJ, Phillips SF et al. Altered sensitivity of the gall bladder to cholecystokinin octapeptide in irritable bowel syndrome. Gut 1988;29:1236-43.

27. Lemanske RF, Sampson HA. Adverse reactions to foods and their relationship to skin diseases in children. Adv Pediatr 1988;35:189-218.

28. Wasserman SI. Chronic urticaria — a frustrating but increasingly understandable disorder. West J Med 1990;152:292-3.

29. Church MK, Lowman MA, Rees PM et al. Mast cells, neuropeptides and inflammation. Agents Actions 1989;27:8-16.

30. Lembeck F, Holzer P. Substance P as neurogenic mediator of antidromic vasodilatation and neurogenic plasma extravasation. Arch Pharmacol 1979;310:175-83.

31. Foreman JC. Substance P and calcitonin gene-related peptide: effects on mast cells and in human skin. Int Archs Allergy Appl Immunol 1987;82:366-71.

32. Pearce FL, Kassessinoff TA, Liu WL. Characteristics of histamine secretion induced by neuropeptides: implications for the relevance of peptide-mast cell interactions in allergy and inflammation. Int Arch Allergy Appl Immunol 1989;88:129-31.

33. Arzubiaga C, Morrow J, Roberts J, Biaggioni I. Neuropeptide Y, a putative cotransmitter in noradrenergic neurons, induces mast cell degranulation but not prostaglandin D2 release. J Allergy Clin Immunol 1991;87:88-93.

34. Newson B, Dahlstrom A, Enerback L, Ahlman H. Suggestive evidence for a direct innervation of mucosal mast cells. An electron microscopic study. Neuroscience 1983;10:565-70.

35. Skofitsch G, Savitt JM, Jacobovitz DM. Suggestive evidence for a functional unit between mast cells and substance P fibers in the rat diaphragm and mesentery. Histochemistry 1985;82:5-8.

36. Bienenstock J, Tomioka M, Matsuda H, Stead RH, Quinonez G, Simon GT, Coughlin MD, Denburg JA. The role of mast cells in inflammatory processes: Evidence for nerve/mast cell interactions. Int Archs Allergy Appl Immun 1987;82:238-43.

37. Foreman JC. Neuropeptides and the pathogenesis of allergy. Allergy 1987;42:1-11.

38. Church MK, Lowman MA, Robinson C, Holgate ST, Benyon C. Interaction of neuropeptides with human mast cells. Int Arch Allergy Appl Immunol 1989;88:70-8.

39. Smedley H, Katrak M, Sikora K, Wheeler T. Neurological side effects of recombinant human interferon. Br Med J 1983;286:262-4.

40. McDonald EM, Mann AH, Thomas HC. Interferons as mediators of psychiatric morbidity. An investigation in a trial of recombinant alpha interferon in hepatitis B carriers. Lancet 1987;ii:1175-9.

41. Snyder SH. Receptors, neurotransmitters and drug responses. N Engl J Med 1979;300:465-72.

42. Furness JB, Morris JL, Gibbins IL, Costa M. Chemical coding of neurons and plurichemical transmission. Ann Rev Pharmacol Toxicol 1989;29:289-306.

43. Kow L-M, Pfaff DW. Neuromodulatory actions of peptides. Ann Rev Pharmacol Toxicol 1988;28:163-88.

44. Hill SJ, Kendall DA. Cross-talk between different receptor-effector systems in the mammalian CNS. Cellular Signalling 1989;1:135-41.

45. Olney JW. Excitotoxic food additives — relevance of animal studies to human safety. Neurobehav Toxicol Teratol 1984;6:455-62.

46. Olney JW. Excitotoxic amino acids and neuropsychiatric disorders. Ann Rev Pharmacol Toxicol 1990;30:47-71.

47. Stevenson DD. Diagnosis, prevention, and treatment of adverse reactions to aspirin and non-steroidal anti-inflammatory drugs. J Allergy Clin Immunol 1984;74:617-22.

48. Stevenson DD, Lewis RA. Proposed mechanisms of aspirin sensitivity reactions. J Allergy Clin Immun 1987;80:788-90.

49. Slepian IK, Mathews KP, McLean JA. Aspirin-sensitive asthma. Chest 1985;87:386-91.

50. Rainsford KD. 'Aspirin and the salicylates'. Butterworths, London, 1984.

51. Birnmaumer L. G proteins in signal transduction. Annu Rev Pharmacol Toxicol 1990;30:675-705.

52. Glover V, Littlewood J, Sandler M, Peatfield R, Petty R, Rose FC. Biochemical predisposition to dietary migraine: the role of phenolsulphotransferase. Headache 1983;23:53-8.

53. Jacobsen DW, Simon RA, Singh M. Sulfite-oxidase deficiency and cobalamin protection in sulfite-sensitive asthmatics. J Allergy Clin Immunol 1984;73:135.

54. Paganelli R, Fagiolo U, Cancian M, Sturniolo GC, Scala E, D'Offizi GP. Intestinal permeability in irritable bowel syndrome. Effect of diet and sodium cromoglycate administration. Ann Allergy 1990;64:377-80.

55. Lipowski ZJ. What does the word "psychosomatic" really mean? A historical and semantic inquiry. Psychosomatic Med 1984;46:153-71.

56. Stehbens WE. The concept of cause in disease. J Chron Dis 1985;38:947-50.

57. Smith RC, Greenbaum DS, Vancouver JB, Henry RC, Reinhart MA, Greenbaum RB, Dean HA, Mayle JE. Psychosocial factors are associated with health care seeking rather than diagnosis in irritable bowel syndrome. Gastroenterology 1990;88:293-301.

58. Angell M. Disease as a reflection of the psyche. N Engl J Med 1985;312:1570-2.

59. Hall JG. Emotion and immunity. Lancet 1985;ii:326-7.

60. Nicholson GA, Wilby J, Tennant C. Myasthenia gravis: the problem of a "psychiatric" misdiagnosis. Med J Aust 1986;144:632-8.

61. Rosenhan DL. On being sane in insane places. Science 1973;179:250-8.

62. Skrabanek P, McCormick J. 'Follies and fallacies in medicine'. Prometheus Books, Buffalo, NY, 1990.

63. Woodruff RA, Goodwin DW, Guze SB. Hysteria (Briquet's syndrome). In "Hysteria", ed A Roy, John Wiley, New York, 1982; pp 117-29.

64. Jones JE, Ray CG, Minnich LL, et al. Evidence for active Epstein-Barr virus infection in patients with persistent unexplained illnesses: Elevated anti-early antigen antibodies. Ann Intern Med 1985;102:1-7.

65. Tobi M, Straus SE. Chronic Epstein-Barr virus disease. Ann Intern Med 1985;103:951-3.

66. Buchwald D, Goldenberg DL, Sullivan JL, Komaroff AL. The "chronic active Epstein-Barr virus infection" syndrome and primary fibromyalgia. Arthritis Rheum 1987;30:1132-6.

67. Goldenberg DL, Simms RW, Geiger A, Komaroff AL. High frequency of fibromyalgia in patients with chronic fatigue syndrome seen in primary care practice. Arthritis Rheum. 1990;33:381-7.

68. Wessely S. Old wine in new bottles: neurasthenia and ME. Psychol Med 1990;20:35-53.

69. Pearson DJ, Rix KJB, Bentley SJ. Food allergy: How much in the mind? A clinical and psychiatric study of suspected food hypersensitivity. Lancet 1983;i:1259-61.

70. Stewart DE, Raskin J. Psychiatric assessment of patients with "20th century disease" ("total allergy syndrome"). Can Med Assoc J 1985;133:1001-6.

71. Terr AI. Clinical ecology. J Allergy Clin Immunol 1987;79:423-6.

72. Ferguson A. Food sensitivity or self-deception? N Engl J Med 1990;323:476-8.

73. Hofeldt FD, Adler RA, Herman RH. Postprandial hypoglycemia. Fact or fiction? J Am Med Ass 1975;233:1309.

74. Best JD. Reactive hypoglycemia in perspective. Patient Management 1984;8:113-21.

75. Crook WG. 'The yeast connection'. Professional Books, Jackson, Tennessee. 2nd ed, 1984.

76. Kendell RE. Chronic fatigue, viruses and depression. Lancet 1991;337:160-3.

77. Hickie I, Lloyd A, Wakefield D, Parker G. The psychiatric status of patients with chronic fatigue syndrome. Br J Psychiatry 1990;156:534-40.

78. Kruesi MJP, Dale J, Straus SE. Psychiatric diagnoses in patients who have chronic fatigue syndrome. J Clin Psychiatry 1989;50:53-6.

79. Lipowski ZJ. Somatization: the concept and its application. Am J Psychiatry 1988;145:1358-68.

80. McIntyre N, Popper K. The critical attitude in medicine: the need for a new ethics. Br Med J 1983;287:1919-23.

81. Pilowski I. Abnormal illness behaviours and their treatments. Med J Aust 1990;153:346-8.

82. Jennings D. The confusion between disease and illness in clinical medicine. Can Med Assoc J 1986;135:865-70.

Immunology

Chapter 58

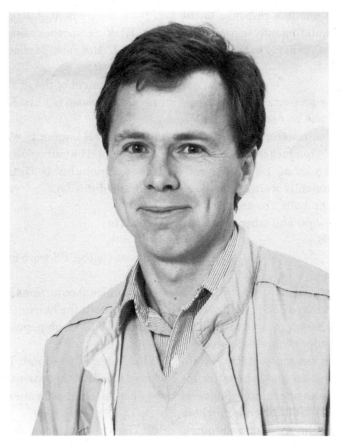

Andrew Lloyd

Immunological Abnormalities in Patients with Chronic Fatigue Syndrome

Andrew Lloyd, MD, FRACP, Denis Wakefield, MD, FRACP, Clem Boughton, MD and John Dwyer, PhD, FRACP, Departments of Infectious Diseases and Immunology, The Prince Henry Hospital, Little Bay, Sydney, Australia.

Dr. Lloyd has recently completed a postgraduate research degree (MD) at the University of New South Wales, Sydney, Australia, on the topic of "The pathogenesis of Chronic Fatigue Syndrome", Dr. Lloyd was funded during this period by a scholarship from the National Health and Medical Research Council of Australia and a grant from the NSW ME Association. The research focused on an immunological hypothesis of the pathogenesis of CFS, but covered diverse aspects including studies of neurophysiology, epidemiology, psychiatry, genetics and immunological therapy. His other areas of current research include the immune dysfunction associated with psychiatric disorders particularly depression and schizophrenia. He has recently commenced a period of research in the Laboratory of Molecular Immunoregulation, National Cancer Institute, USA.

Introduction

Persistence of a virus or viral antigen has been proposed to be central to the pathogenesis of chronic fatigue syndrome (Wakefield and Lloyd, 1987). This hypothesis has been supported not only by the detection of enteroviral RNA in the muscles of patients with the syndrome (Archard *et al*, 1988), but also by the demonstration of persistent enteroviral antigen in their serum (Yousef *et al*, 1988). If these data are valid, disturbance of the immune response to the enterovirus or other precipitating infection (thereby allowing antigen to persist), is likely to be crucial to the development of CFS.

The conflicting data on the presence of immunological abnormalities which may be necessary to allow the antigen to escape mechanisms for its clearance in patients with CFS led us to conduct controlled studies to clarify the issue (Lloyd *et al*, 1989). Both cell-mediated and humoral immunity were assessed using standard measures, as both are essential for effective resolution of the viral and other infections thought to precipitate CFS.

Subjects and methods

Patients were considered to have CFS if: (i) they gave a history of marked exercise-aggravated muscle fatigue, of at least six months duration, associated with typical constitutional and neuropsychiatric symptoms; (ii) physical examination and exhaustive investigation did not provide an alternative diagnosis (Lloyd *et al*, 1988). One hundred patients in whom CFS was producing significant morbidity, frequent medical consultation, and considerable time lost from work were studied. They were compared as a group to 100 healthy control subjects, who were recruited from the hospital and laboratory staff. Blood samples were collected in the early to mid-morning period from all subjects to avoid the effect of diurnal variation in T cell numbers and function (Ritchie *et al*, 1983). None of the patients or control subjects was receiving medications known to produce immune deficiency.

The degree of disability produced by CFS was evaluated by questionnaire assessing the ability to participate in work, recreation and social activities during the illness in comparison to the pre-morbid situation. For the purposes of this study, a score was generated from this questionnaire to provide a continuous measure of the severity of symptoms.

Assessment of cell-mediated immunity (CMI) was completed by:

(1) peripheral blood T cell subset analysis using flow cytometry;

(2) measurement of delayed-type hypersensitivity (DTH) skin responses using a commercially-available kit (*CMI Multitest*, Merieux, France); and by:

(3) assessment of the *in vitro* lymphocyte proliferation in response to phytohaemagglutinin (PHA).

(4) Humoral immunity was evaluated by measurement of total immunoglobulins by nephelometry and immunoglobulin G (IgG) subclasses by radial immuno-diffusion.

Results

Patients with CFS were found to have:

(1) significant reductions in the absolute lymphocyte count in both the helper (CD4) and the suppressor/cytotoxic (CD8) sub-populations.

(2) Abnormally reduced DTH skin responses were found in 88% of the patients, with 54% having absent responses (cutaneous anergy).

(3) The lymphocyte response to PHA was significantly lower in patients with CFS than in healthy control subjects.

(4) Although total serum immunoglobulin levels were normal, reduction in the levels of IgG1 and IgG3 subclasses was noted in the patients with CFS.

Thirty-nine of the patients (39%) reported in the questionnaire that they were severely disabled (i.e. completely unable to participate) in at least two of the three aspects of daily activity (work, recreation and social life), because of CFS. Eighty-four percent of the patients rated the degree of disability as moderate or severe in all three aspects. All patients reported a moderate reduction in their ability to participate in at least one aspect of daily activity.

Regression analysis did not demonstrate that any clinical variables (age, sex, disease duration or disease severity) predicted the abnormal measures of cellular immunity.

Discussion

This study evaluated the immunity of a large number

of carefully-defined patients with CFS. The patients had a predominantly long-standing disorder which was causing major disruption of their usual daily lives. The abnormal cellular and humoral immunity documented, supports the hypothesis that an immunological disturbance may be central to the pathogenesis of CFS. The abnormalities demonstrated may represent a "marker" of an underlying disruption of the regulation of the immune response to a precipitating infection in patients with CFS.

The finding of reduced DTH responses in the majority of the patients provides the strongest evidence reported of disordered CMI in patients with CFS. One percent of healthy Australian adults demonstrate cutaneous anergy using this test system (Frazer et al, 1985), and such values have previously been shown to fall below the fifth percentile in studies of healthy adults in the US (Kniker et al, 1984). Acute viral infection, such as with CMV or EBV is associated with the development of reduced or absent DTH responses including responses to unrelated antigens (Haider et al, 1973). Both a-IFN and g-IFN modulate DTH and have been shown to variably affect the response in man (Toy, 1983). Abnormal DTH skin responses in patients with CFS have also been reported by Murdoch, (1988).

The T cell lymphopenia documented in the patients with CFS also suggests disturbed CMI. In previous studies quantitating peripheral blood T cells in patients with CFS (Behan et al, 1985; Straus et al, 1985;

Jones et al, 1985), the subsets were reported as percentages rather than as an absolute number of circulating cells, giving results of uncertain significance as the actual value may vary widely, depending upon the total lymphocyte count. T cell lymphopenia is common in acute viral infection (Rouse and Horohov, 1986). In this context, T cell lymphopenia may occur as a result of lysis or functional impairment of the lymphocytes after their direct invasion by a virus such as HIV, or it may result from the activity of soluble factors of viral or host origin, including cytokines such as g-IFN (Schattner et al, 1983).

The demonstration of impaired lymphocyte proliferation in response to PHA in patients with CFS, provides further evidence of abnormal immune function in patients with this syndrome. The reduction in the response was mild (characteristically 1SD or less from the mean of the response in normal subjects) and hence, the results indicate immune dysfunction rather than clinically significant immunodeficiency. Lymphocyte proliferative responses to mitogen are characteristically reduced during acute viral infection (Haider et al, 1973; Rouse and Horohov, 1986) and are also reduced in association with administered a-IFN (Einhorn et al; 1983).

These data demonstrate that CFS is associated with disordered cellular and humoral immunity in a pattern similar to that seen transiently in acute viral infection. This disturbance may potentially be important in the pathogenesis of the syndrome.

References

Archard LC, Bowles NE, Behan PO, Bell EJ, Doyle D. Postviral fatigue syndrome: persistence of enterovirus RNA in muscle and elevated creatine kinase. J Royal Soc Med 1988; 81: 326-329.

Behan P, Behan W, Bell E. The postviral fatigue syndrome - an analysis of the findings in 50 cases. J Infect 1985; 10: 211-222.

Einhorn S, Blomgren H, Einhorn N, Strander H. In vitro and in vivo effects of interferon on the response of human lymphocytes to mitogens. Clin Exp Immunol 1983; 51: 369-377.

Frazer I, Collins E, Fox J, Jones B, Oliphant R, Mackay I. Assessment of delayed-type hypersensitivity in man: A comparison of the "Multitest" and conventional intradermal injection of six antigens. Clin Imm Immunopathol 1985; 35: 182-190.

Haider S, Coutinho M de L, Emond RTD, et al. Tuberculin anergy and infectious mononucleosis. Lancet 1973; 2: 74.

Jones JF, Ray CG, Minnich LL, Hicks MJ, Kibler R, Lucas DO. Evidence for active Epstein-Barr virus infection in patients with persistent, unexplained illnesses: elevated early antigen antibodies. Ann Intern Med 1985; 102: 1-7.

Kniker W, Anderson C, McBryde J, Roumiantzeff M, Lesourd B. Multitest CMI for standardised measurement of delayed cutaneous hypersensitivity and cell-mediated immunity. Normal values and proposed scoring system for healthy adults in the USA. Ann Allergy 1984; 52: 75-82.

Lloyd A, Wakefield D, Boughton C, Dwyer J. What is myalgic encephalomyelitis? Lancet 1988; i: 1286-1287.

Lloyd A, Wakefield D, Boughton C, Dwyer J. Immunological abnormalities in the chronic fatigue syndrome. Med J Aust 1989; 151: 122-124.

Murdoch JC. Cell-mediated immunity in patients with myalgic encephalomyelitis syndrome. NZ Med J 1988; 101: 511-512.

Rouse B, Horohov D. Immunosuppression in viral infections. Rev Infect Dis 1986; 8: 850-873.

Straus SE, Tosato G, Armstrong G, *et al*. Persisting illness and fatigue in adults with evidence of Epstein-Barr virus infection. Ann Intern Med 1985; 102: 7-16.

Toy JL. The interferons. Clin Exp Immunol 1983; 54: 1-13.

Wakefield D, Lloyd A. Pathophysiology of myalgic encephalomyelitis. Lancet 1987; ii: 918-919.

Yousef GE, Mann GF, Smith DG, Bell EJ, Murugesan V, McCartney RA, Mowbray JF. Chronic enterovirus infection in patients with postviral fatigue syndrome. Lancet 1988; i: 146-149.

Chapter 59

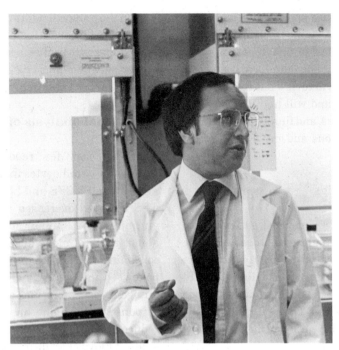

Sudhir Gupta

Recent Developments in Immunological Aspects of Chronic Fatigue Syndrome

Sudhir Gupta MD, PhD

Division of Basic and Clinical Immunology, California College of Medicine, University of California, Irvine, CA 92717, USA

Correspondence: Professor Sudhir Gupta, Medical Sciences I, C-264A, University of California at Irvine, Irvine, CA 92717 USA

Dr. Gupta is an internationally known immunologist with expertise in the field of research related to immunodeficiency disorders. He has published more than 300 scientific papers and edited 7 books. He has served on the Allergy, Immunology, and Transplantation subcommitee of the National Institutes of Health. He serves on the Editorial Board of Thymus and Journal of Allergy and Immunology, and is an Advisory Board member of Life Sciences (AIDS Section), Modern Medicine, and Advances in Immunity and Cancer Therapy. He is also the inaugural and current Editor-in-Chief of the Journal of Clinical Immunology. He is also a member of the Advisory panel (medical devices) of the Food and Drug Administration. Dr. Gupta is involved in the basic research and clinical management of patients with Chronic Fatigue Syndrome.

Introduction

Chronic fatigue syndrome (CFS) is a poorly-defined, recently recognized CDC (Center for Disease Control)-defined disorder that is comprised of a group of signs and symptoms complex with no definitive laboratory diagnostic test(s). The most common symptom of CFS is a debilitating muscle fatigue of 6 months and longer duration. Prior to the CDC-definition[1] of this syndrome, it was termed as chronic EBV syndrome, chronic infectious mononucleosis, encephalomyalgic syndrome etc. Recently CDC has reinforced the idea that CFS is indeed a real entity rather than the common belief within some of the medical community that it is a psychological disease. This syndrome appears to have several etiologic agents, including Epstein-Barr virus (EBV), human herpes virus-6 (HHV-6), and a newly reported retrovirus. However, no cause and effect relationship has been established. A number of investigators have studied immunological profile in patients with chronic fatigue and conflicting data have been accumulated. In this paper I will review our results in the context of other reports and will highlight the reasons for such discrepancies, and finally propose some new areas of investigations and my own thoughts about this syndrome.

Patient Characteristics

Our study included 20 CDC-defined patients with CFS and 20 healthy age and sex-matched controls. These patients had a Karnofsky Performance Score (KPS) of 80-90. The mean duration of illness was 14 months (range 8-28 months). Each group comprised of 15 females and 5 males. The age range in the patient group was 21-39 years and in the control group between 20-46 years.

Results and Discussion

Quantitative analysis of T and B Lymphocytes

The data on monoclonal antibody-defined T cell subsets are conflicting. In non-CDC-defined acute post-viral chronic fatigue syndrome (PVCFS), Behan et al[2] reported decreased proportions of CD3+ and CD8+ T cells. These patients were positive for coxsackie virus antibodies. Straus et al[3] observed normal proportions of T cell subsets in patients with positive EBV serology. In CDC-defined CFS patients Subira et al[4] reported decreased proportions of CD3+ T cells but the normal proportions of CD5+ and CD2+ total T cells, CD4+, CD8+ T cell subsets and M3+ monocytes. This observation is intriguing and can be explained by the presence of very low density of CD3 molecules since T cells defined by other antigens (CD2 and CD5) are normal. We[5] reported normal proportions and numbers of CD3+, CD4+ and CD8+ T cell subsets. The reports of normal proportions/numbers of total T cells and T cell subsets in CFS reported by Subira et al[4] and Gupta and Vayuvegula[5] are in contrast to decreased numbers of CD2+, CD4+, CD8+ T cells reported by Lloyd et al[6]. The reduced numbers of these subsets of T cells appears to be due to severe lymphopenia in their cases; no data were given for the proportions of T cells and T cell subsets, but it appears that there was no significant differ-

ence in the proportions of any of these subpopulations. The reason for severe lymphopenia reported by Lloyd et al[6] appears to be due to the marked severity and of longer duration of the disease. In our study CD20+ B cells were normal in proportions and numbers[5].

Functional analysis of T lymphocytes:

There are very few reports regarding functional analysis of lymphocytes in this syndrome. Behan et al[2] in acute PVCFS and Lloyd et al[6] in CDC-defined CFS reported decreased response to phytohemagglutinin (PHA). In our study we have observed no abnormality of mononuclear cell response to PHA, concanavalin A (both T cell specific mitogens), or pokeweed mitogen (T helper cell-dependent B cell mitogen), except in one patient who had reduced response to PHA and an another patient who had reduced response to all the three mitogens[5]. In the study of Lloyd et al[6] decreased PHA response is most likely due to severe lymphopenia. If a correction for T cell number had been made in mononuclear cell cultures, most likely, on a cell per cell basis, the responses would have been normal. In the study of Behan et al[2] decreased PHA response could be due to the direct effect of the coxsackie virus.

There are no studies for T cell responses to soluble recall antigens in CFS. The precursor frequency of antigen responsive cells is much smaller than those responding to mitogens. Therefore, tests for antigen response are much more sensitive than those of mitogen response, especially in defining T cell defects in early stages of disease or where there are subtle immune defects. In our study, we observed significantly reduced DNA synthesis in response to soluble antigens, particularly to E. coli and mumps antigens[5]. This observation of normal mitogen response and depressed antigen response is not surprising, as has been observed in patients with HIV infection[7,8]. The mechanism(s) for reduced antigen response remains to be defined. This could be due to any or a combination of mechanisms including, depletion of small proportions of antigen responsive cells, reduced IL-2 production, IL-2 receptor expression, binding of IL-2 to its receptors, and/or response to IL-2.

Straus et al[3] reported normal delayed type hypersensitivity (DTH) reaction in patients with chronic EBV syndrome. Lloyd et al[6] reported anergy

Figure 1

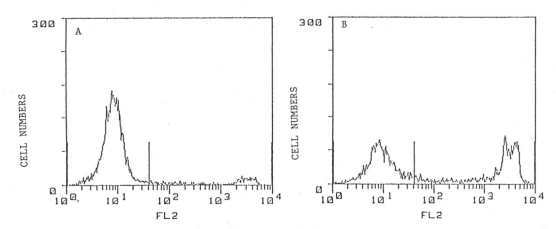

A representative experiment of natural killer activity in control (A) and patient with CFS (B). The data are expressed as percent of target K-562 cells killed by mononuclear effector cells at a ration of 1:5. Patients had markedly reduced NK activity (10.1%) as compared to control (48.0%).

or hypoanergy to recall antigens in 88% of patients with CFS. This figure is as severe as in patients with HIV infection. It appears that very different spectrum immunological defects exist in patients with CFS in Australia, who are severely ill and perhaps might have different etiological agent(s) for CFS, as compared to other countries.

Quantitative and qualitative analysis of natural killer cells:

A deficiency of natural killer (NK) activity has been reported in chronic EBV syndrome[9], that was associated with reduced gamma-IFN (gamma interferon). Caliguri et al[10] reported decreased proportions of NK cells as defined by CD3-CD16+ cells. They also showed decreased NK functional activity that was not reconstituted by IL-2. In our study we found decreased proportions and numbers of NK cells as defined by three different monoclonal antibodies, CD16, CD56, and CD57[5]. In addition, we also observed a functional abnormality of NK functions as evaluated by a newly developed flow cytometry technique (Figure 1). This is perhaps the single most common abnormality that is observed in patients with CFS.

Cell adhesion molecules:

Cell adhesion between T lymphocytes and other cells, including macrophages is an essential early event in generating effective immune response. In addition, cell adhesion molecules appear to play an important role in migration, homing and recirculation of lymphocytes. Recently, a number of cell adhesion molecules that enhance T lymphocyte functions have been defined and termed as lymphocyte function-associated or LFA antigens[11,12]. LFA-1, CD2, CD4, and CD8 antigens appear to function as adhesion molecules for T cell responses. More recently, ligands for a number of adhesion molecules have been defined[12,13]. These include, intercellular adhesion molecule 1 (ICAM-1), a ligand for LFA-1, major histocompatibility complex (MHC) class I and class II antigens, ligands for CD8 and CD4 respectively and LFA-3 a ligand for CD2. LFA-1 is present on thymocytes, T and B lymphocytes, large granular lymphocytes, monocytes, activated macrophages and neutrophils. ICAM-1 is widely distributed on leucocytes, fibroblasts, epithelial cells and endothelial cells and its expression is regulated by various cytokines. Adhesion molecules also play an important role in the generation of specific cytolytic T cells.

Gregory et al[14] showed that during the progression of EBV+ Burkitt's lymphoma (cell line that shows restricted expression of EBV-latent gene) to a cell surface phenotype characteristic of EBV transformed B lymphoblastoid cell line (associated with broader pattern of EBV latent gene expression) is associated with upregulation of the ICAM-1 and LFA-1.

We examined the expression of LFA-1 and ICAM-1 on lymphocytes and monocytes from 20 patients with CDC-defined CFS who had no evidence of chronic

EBV syndrome as evident by negative serology for early antigens and compared them with age and sex matched healthy controls. We show an enhanced expression of ICAM-1 and LFA-1 on CD4+ T cells from patients with CFS as compared with controls[5,15].

No significant difference was observed in the expression of LFA-1 and ICAM-1 on CD8+ T cells between CFS and normal controls. This observation is in contrast with the findings in patients with multiple sclerosis in which increased expression of ICAM-1 is found on CD8+ T cells[16]. The density of ICAM-1 and LFA-1 expression on monocytes from the patients with CFS was greater than that of normal controls. Gamma-IFN is known to induce/increase the expression of ICAM-1 and LFA-1 in a number of cell types[17,18]. In our study we observed a blunted response of recombinant gamma-IFN on the expression of LFA-1 and ICAM-1 on monocytes from patients with CFS as compared to controls[5]. We suggest that an enhanced expression of ICAM-1 and LFA-1 on CD4+ T cells and monocytes play a role in the pathogenesis of CFS. The relationship of these changes with the presence of HHV-6 is currently under investigation.

Cytokines in Chronic Fatigue syndrome:

There are very few studies of cytokine production in CFS. Kibler et al[9] reported decreased production of IL-2 by mononuclear cells from patients with chronic EBV with chronic fatigue. In contrast, Cheney et al[19] reported increased serum levels of IL-2 in patients with CFS. In their study IL-2 measurements were done by a commercial laboratory. These results need to be confirmed in research laboratories by both bioassay and immunoassays. The data pooled from 4 different studies suggest the presence of IFN in 2% of patients with CFS[20]. Lever et al[21] reported increased circulating levels of IFN-alpha in CFS. Kibler et al[9] reported decreased gamma-IFN production by mononuclear cells from patients with active chronic fatigue syndrome. Interleukin 6 (IL-6) is a newly described cytokine that has immunoregulatory and inflammatory properties[22]. We have recently examined the production of IL-6 from T cells and macrophages from peripheral blood of patients with CDC-defined CFS. Data are shown in Figure 2 for T cell and in Figure 3 for macrophage produced IL-6. IL-6 produced by PHA-activated T cells from CFS was comparable to that of controls (measured by ELISA

assay). In contrast, lipopolysaccharide-induced macrophage produced IL-6 was increased in CFS. It would be of interest to examine other cytokines, like IL-1 and tumor necrosis factor (TNF) in CFS, since they also share many immunoregulatory and inflammatory properties with IL-6.

Figure 2

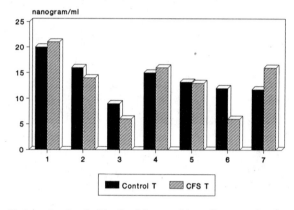

INTERLEUKIN 6 PRODUCTION BY T CELLS IN CHRONIC FATIGUE SYNDROME

IL-6 production by T cells. Mononuclear cells were stimulated with 5 mg/ml of PHA for 48 hours, supernatants collected, filtered and analyzed by ELISA. Data are expressed for 7 different patients and paired controls.

Serum immunoglobulins and specific antibody response in CFS:

Serum immunoglobulins in CFS are generally normal. However, several investigators have reported decreased levels of IgG subclasses[23-25]. There is no single subclass in which deficiency has been observed. It is likely that many if not all of these patients have a primary deficiency of IgG subclasses and should, therefore, be excluded from the CFS category. Lloyd et al[6] described high frequency of IgM and IgA in their patient population. It remains to be determined whether these deficiencies were primary or secondary to the disease process. Only prospective studies will be able to address these questions.

There are no published reports on the analysis of specific antibody response in CFS. We have recently examined the specific antibody response against diptheria-tetanus (as an example of protein antigens) and pneumococcus vaccine (as an example of polysaccharide antigens). No abnormality of specific antibody response to diphtheria/tetanus antigens was observed. However, response to several serotypes of pneumococcus was decreased[5]. Therefore, it appears that the patients with CFS demonstrate defective specific antibody response to polysaccharide antigens.

Autoantibodies in CFS:

A large number of autoantibodies have been reported in patients with CFS[3,9,26]. None of these antibodies are in high titers that may be associated with autoimmune diseases. We have observed consistently negative antibodies to double stranded DNA, sm and RNP antigens, thus excluding any possibility of lupus erythematosus. The antinuclear antibody (ANA) was the most common autoantibody observed (30%) in our patients with CFS[5]. The presence of autoantibodies in CFS suggests a dysregulated immune system.

Figure 3

INTERLEUKIN-6 PRODUCTION BY MONOCYTES IN CHRONIC FATIGUE SYNDROME

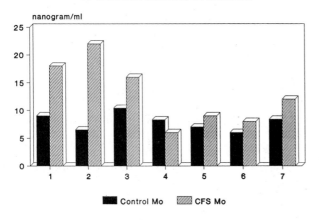

IL-6 production by monocytes. Monocytes were prepared by plastic adherence and then stimulated with lipopolysaccharide for 18 hours, supernatants collected and filtered, and analyzed by ELISA assay. Data are expressed for the same 7 patients and 7 controls as in Figure 2.

Human herpes virus 6 antigen and antibodies:

Recently HHV-6 (formerly termed as human B lymphotropic virus [HBLV]) has been implicated in the etiology of CFS. Krueger et al[27] observed the presence of HHV-6 antibodies in a patient with EBV negative CFS. HHV-6 antibodies are present in general population, albeit in low titers ($\leq 1/40$), but high titers are present in a number of malignant, viral and autoimmune disorders[28]. HHV-6 virus has been isolated from blood of patients with a variety of disorders, including CFS[28]. In our study we observed increased levels of anti-HHV-6 antibody titers ($\geq 1/80$) in the majority of patients with CFS[5]. Interestingly, when we examined the presence of HHV-6 antigen (using PHA-activated T cells and monoclonal antibodies against HHV-6 kindly provided by Dr. D. Ablashi, National Cancer Institute, NIH, Bethesda, MD), we found no correlation between titers of HHV-6 antibodies and HHV-6 antigens. Because HHV-6 infects and kills CD4+ T cells[29], it is tempting to speculate that HHV-6 might be responsible for the depletion/dysfunction of the very small antigen responsive CD4+ T cells responsible for blunted antigen specific responses in CFS as observed by us.

Summary and Some Thoughts:

Chronic Fatigue syndrome is a heterogeneous disorder with variable immune defects. The most consistent and frequent abnormality is a quantitative and qualitative defect of NK cells. However, this test cannot be considered diagnostic of CFS since these abnormalities are observed in a variety of human diseases. The mechanism of reduced NK activity remains to be determined both at the level of precursor frequency and at the level of the regulation by cytokines (upregulation and downregulation).

It is also apparent that many etiological agents are responsible for this syndrome. I strongly believe that in order to further the knowledge about the etiopathogenesis of CFS, studies of cytokines, particularly of IL-1, IL-6, and TNF should be done. In addition, analyses of T cell responses to recall soluble antigens and of B cell response to polysaccharide antigens (e.g. pneumovax and H. influenza B) should be routinely done on all cases of CFS. More importantly, serial sequential studies are crucial to differentiate between preexisting and secondary immune defects.

Furthermore, more detailed information regarding Karnofsky Performance Score and duration of illness should be recorded and provided in any publication of data in CFS.

It is also important that attempts be made to isolate

virus and/or demonstrate virus antigens in cultured leucocytes from these patients and then stratify their immunological profile based upon the type of virus infection. Molecular approaches should be used to define the presence of virus infection, wherever virus isolation is not possible. It is through a concerted effort on the part of investigators and clinicians, to approach these patients in a uniform manner, that we will be able to better define this disorder and understand its etiopathogenesis.

References:

1. Holmes G.P., Kaplan J.E., Gantz N.M. et al. Ann. Int. Med. 108: 387, 1988.

2. Behan P.O., Behan W.M. and Bell E.J. J. Infect. 10: 210, 1985.

3. Straus S.E., Tosato G., Armstrong G., Lawley T. et al. Ann. Int. Med. 102: 7, 1985.

4. Subira M.L., Castilla A., Civeira M-P., and Prieto J. J. Infect. Dis. 160: 165, 1989.

5. Gupta S. and Vayuvegula B. Scand. J. Immunol. Vol 33, 319, 1991.

6. Lloyd (&A.R., Wakefield D., Boughton C.R., and Dwyer J.M. Med. J. Austr. 151: 122, 1989.

7. Lane H.C., Depper J.M., Greene W.C. et al. New Eng. J. Med. 313: 79, 1985.

8. Gupta S. and Safai B. J. Clin. Invest. 71: 296, 1983.

9. Kibler R., Lucas D.O., Hicks M.J. et al. J. Clin. Immunol. 5: 46, 1985.

10. Caliguri M., Murray C., Buchwald D. et al. J. Immunol. 139: 3306, 1987.

11. Springer T.A., Dustin M.L., Kishimoto T.K., and Marlin S.D. Ann. Rev. Immunol. 5: 223, 1987

12. Bierer B.E. and Burakoff S.J. FASEB J. 2: 2584, 1988

13. Makagoba M.W., Sanders M.E., Ginther Luce G.E. et al. Nature 331: 86, 1988

14. Gregory C.D., Murray R.J., Edwards C.F. and Richardson A.B. J. Exp. Med. 167: 1811, 1988

15. Gupta S. in: Epstein-Barr Virus and Human Diseases (Eds. D.V. Ablashi, A. Faggioni, G.R.F. Krueger, J.S. Pagano, G.R. Pearson). Humana Press, Clifton, NJ. pp 405, 1989.

16. Frohman T.C., Frohman E.M., van den Noort S. and Gupta S. (submitted)

17. Dustin M.L., Singer K.H., Tuck D.T., and Springer T.A. J. Exp.Med. 167: 1323, 1988.

18. Frohman E.M., Frohman T.C., Dustin M.L., Vayuvegula B. et al. J. Neuroimmunol. 23: 117, 1989.

19. Cheney P.R., Dorman S.E. and Bell D.S. Ann. Int. Med. 110: 321, 1989.

20. Levine P.H., Grueger G.R.F., Kaplan M. et al. in: Epstein-Barr virus and Human Diseases. (Eds. D.V. Ablashi, A. Faggioni, G.R.F. Krueger, J.S. Pagano and G.R. Pearson). Humana Press, CliftonN.J. pp.405, 1989.

21. Lever A.M.L., Lewis D.M., Bannister B.A. et al. Lancet 2: 101, 1988.

22. Gupta S. Scand. J. Rheumatol. S76: 189-201, 1988.

23. Linde A., Hammerstrom L. and Smith C.I.E. Lancet 1: 885, 1988.

24. Komaroff A.L., Geiger A.M., and Wormsley S. Lancet 1:1288, 1988.

25. Read R., Spickett G., Harvey J., Edwards A.J. and Larson H.E. Lancet 1: 241, 1988.

26. Jones J.F., Ray C.G., Minnich L.L. et al. Ann. Int. Med. 102: 1, 1985.

27. Krueger G.F.R., Koch B. and Ablashi D.V. Lancet 2: 36, 1987.

28. Ablashi D.V., Zompetta C., Lease C et al. in Proceedings of the Chronic Fatigue Syndrome Workshop. Central Health Lab. Publish., Toronto (in press)

29. Ablashi D.V., Josephs S.F., Buchbinder A. et al. J. Virol. Methods 21: 29, 1988.

Chapter 60

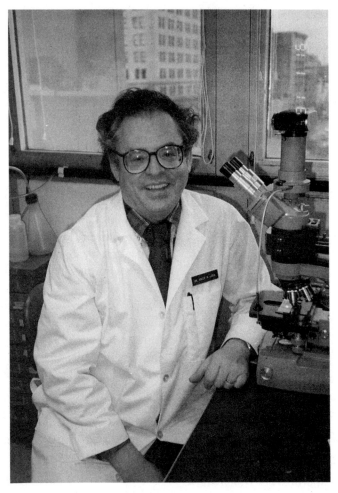

Roger M. Loria

Host Factors Affecting the Course and Outcome of Viral Disease

Roger M. Loria, PhD

Departments of Microbiology, Immunology and Pathology, Virginia Commonwealth University, Schools of Basic Health Sciences and Medicine, Medical College of Virginia, Richmond VA 23298-0678.

Mailing address: Dr. Roger M. Loria, Professor, Microbiology, Immunology and Pathology, Medical College of Virginia, Richmond, VA 23298-0678

Dr. Loria is a tenured Professor of Microbiology, Immunology and Pathology at the Schools of Basic Health Sciences and Medicine. His area of expertise is host virus interactions. He has broad multi-disciplinary training in the areas of Medical Sciences with formal training in clinical microbiology, clinical biochemistry, mammalian physiology, histology and pharmacology. Dr. Loria was the first to demonstrate the synergistic interaction between dietary cholesterol and a human cardiotropic coxsackievirus, and subsequently he reported on the unique and specific interaction between a host with a known genetic predisposition for diabetes and a human diabetogenic virus. His recent studies have shown that it is feasible to achieve protection against lethal infection by upregulating the host immune response.

1. Introduction

The goal of this review will be to focus on **host factors** which influence the outcome and severity of viral infections. The term host factor will be used throughout this report to connote physiological, metabolic, genetic, and pathophysiological conditions which influence the host response to viral and bacterial infections. Humoral or cellular immune responses to infection will be considered only when pertinent to the understanding of the effects of host factors on infection. Because several other chapters in this text discuss topics which also focus on particular host conditions, such subjects will be discussed only briefly in order to maintain continuity.

Host factors determine the outcome of infections with many different viruses, however, for the sake of brevity and clarity most of the results presented here will be derived from our work with human group B coxsackieviruses (CVB). As members of the picornaviridae family, these small RNA viruses infect humans primarily by the oral route and have been classified as enteroviruses and consist of approximately 70 different agents. These include the Polio, group A and B coxsackie, and the ECHO viruses. These agents are resistant to inactivation by the low PH of stomach acid; properties which allows them to infect the gastrointestinal tract. Some enteroviruses cause myositis, and focal necrosis, both of which are associated with considerable disturbance in the Na+ and K+ content of the infected muscle cells resulting in muscle fatigue[1]. Since these viruses also infect the CNS, an imbalance of the Na+ and K+ levels in the neurons may be associated with slower re-polarization of infected neurons and, thus, fatigue.

The clinical syndromes associated with enterovirus infections are listed in Table 1. The wide range of clinical syndromes caused by this group of viruses illustrates their opportunistic nature. This may be an indication that other factors, particularly, host factors may contribute to the heterogeneity of the clinical syndromes caused by the enteric viruses.

Viral pathogenesis is caused by acute, chronic, latent, oncogenic and unconventional virus infections. In all cases, cause and effect can be proven in accordance with Koch's hypothesis or as a modification thereof, by Evans[2]. Accordingly, the presence of the agent or

its genetic material is a requirement for the pathogenic process to evolve. A relatively new and different category of virus induced pathogenesis, primarily dependent on host factors, is now recognized. In this situation, the virus essentially functions as a trigger, and host factors determine pathogenesis.

In the article entitled **Virus disease without virus**, Huppert and Wild[5] advanced the hypothesis that certain virus infections cause disease by a "hit and run" mechanism. Accordingly, virus would infect, cause initial damage, and subsequently be cleared from the host having no direct role in the ensuing pathogenic process. Therefore, host conditions would be the major determinant in the development and progression of disease. Indeed, Loria, et al[6] suggested that CVB4 might be a triggering agent in the host with a genetic predisposition to diabetes mellitus; host conditions, in this case, genetics, would determine the type of response to infection. Similarly, host conditions, such as nutrition and levels of dietary lipids[7] are major host factors which influence the outcome of cardiovascular disease and atherosclerosis. Additionally, hormones have the ability to increase host susceptibility or resistance to a wide range of lethal infections[8].

The influence of host genetics on susceptibility and on the nature of the interaction with the infecting virus has been documented by many investigators[9-12]. Host-virus interaction is a complex phenomenon in which the host genetic component is polygenic in nature. Factors associated with the major histocompatibility complex (MHC, H-2 in the mouse) are only one facet of this system. Therefore, MHC and other host factors as determined by genetic predisposition are an important aspect of the host-virus interaction.

2. Diabetes Mellitus

It is generally accepted that there is a hereditary predisposition to diabetes mellitus (DM)[13]. However, its mode of inheritance and the mechanisms by which a particular diabetic genotype is expressed as a diabetic phenotype remain unknown[14]. Studies with identical twins who developed insulin-dependent diabetes mellitus (IDDM) suggest, at most, a 50% genetic predisposition. Furthermore, since a variety of environmental factors were shown to influence the

---

Table 1

*Clinical Syndromes Associated with Enterovirus Infection[a]

Polioviruses, Types 1-3

Paralysis (complete/slight muscle weakness)
Aseptic meningitis
Undifferentiated febrile illness

Coxsackieviruses, Group A, Types 1-24[b]

Acute Hemorrhagic conjunctivitis (type 24)
Acute lymphatic or nodular pharyngitis (type 10)
Aseptic meningitis (types 1-11, 14, 16-18, 22, 24)
"Common cold" (types 21,24)
Exanthem (types 4-7, 9, 16)
Encephalitis (types 2, 5-7, 9)
Epidemic myalgia (types 4, 6, 10)
Hand-foot-and-Mouth disease (types 5,10,16)
Hepatitis (types 4,9)
Herpangina (types 1-6, 8, 10, 22)
Infantile diarrhea (types 18, 20-22, 24)
Paralysis (infrequently (types 4, 7, 9))
Pneumonitis of Infants (types 9, 16)
Upper respiratory illness (types 10, 21, 24)

Coxsackieviruses, Group B, types 1-6

Aseptic meningitis (types 1-6)
Encephalitis (types 1-3, 5)
Epidemic myalgia (types 1-5)
Hepatitis (type 5)
Paralysis (infrequently) (types 2-5)
Pericarditis myocarditis (types 1-5)
Pleurodynia (types 1-5)
Rash (type 5)
Severe systemic infection in infants
Meningoencephalitis and myocarditis (types 1-5)
Undifferentiated febrile illness (types 1-6)
Upper respiratory illness and pneumonia (types 4, 5)

Echoviruses, Types 1-34

Aseptic meningitis (all except 12, 24, 26, 29, 32-34)
Paralysis (types 2,, 4, 6, 9, 11, 30)
Encephalitis, ataxia, or Guillain-Barré syndrome
(types 2, 6, 9, 19, possibly 3, 4, 7, 11, 14, 18, 22)
Exanthem (types 2, 4, 6, 9, 11, 16, 18)
Respiratory disease (types 1-4, 6-9, 11, 16, 19, 20, 22, 25)
Others: Diarrhea (different types)
        Epidemic myalgia (types 1, 6, 9)
        Pericarditis and myocarditis (types 1, 6, 9, 19)
        Hepatic disturbances (types 4, 9)

Enterovirus, types 68-72[c]

Acute hemorrhagic conjunctivitis (type 70)
Hand-foot-and-mouth disease (type 71)
Hepatitis (type 72)
Meningoencephalitis (types 70, 71)
Paralysis (types 70, 71)
Pneumonia and bronchiolitis (type 68)

[a] Adapted from Kibrick S.[3], and Melnick J. L.[4] [b] Coxsackievirus 23 was never formally accepted as a new type. It was found to be identical with the previously described echovirus 9. [c] Since 1969, new enterovirus types have been assigned enterovirus type numbers rather than being subclassified as coxsackieviruses or echoviruses. The vernacular names of the previously identified enteroviruses have been retained.

---

onset of DM, a multifactorial etiology was proposed. Dietary intake, gross obesity[15], pregnancy, elevated estrogen levels[16] and infectious agents, particularly group B coxsackieviruses[17-23], are some of the environmental factors implicated in IDDM onset.

Experimentally, it has been possible to demonstrate the influence of host genetics in situations where a particular mutation or host condition is associated with an increased susceptibility to virus infection. One such host condition is the genetic predisposition to diabetes mellitus. We have used the inbred mouse C57BL/KsJ, with the diabetes mutation, **db+/db+**, as a model to determine the influence of a given diabetic genotype on the host response to infection with human CVB4. The viral agent used in these studies was isolated by Kibrick and Bernirschke[24] from the myocardial tissue of an infant with generalized disease including focal necrosis and inflammation of the pancreas. Both endocrine and exocrine involvement of the pancreas were evident in this case. A detailed passage history and protocol for preparation of virus pools for experimentation has previously been reported[6].

Table 2

Susceptibility of the inbred C57BL/KsJ diabetic mutant to Coxsackievirus B4

Dose[1] Coxsackie B4	db/db	C57BL/KsJ Genotype db/+	+/+
		Mortality %	
10^4	100	10	10
10^6	100	50	10
10^8	100	100	50

[1] Plaque forming units/animal; 124 animals in this experiment.
Adapted from Loria[30].

The diabetic mutant mouse is hyperphagic, obese, and develops spontaneous diabetes mellitus when fed ad libitum (AL). During the early stages of the disease hyperinsulinemia is evident, but during later stages hyperinsulinemia is insufficient, and necrosis of islet cells and death occurs[25,26]. In order to separate between the pathophysiological effects of diabetes and the influence of genetic predisposition to the disease, the dietary intake of the homozygote **db+/db+**

Figure 1

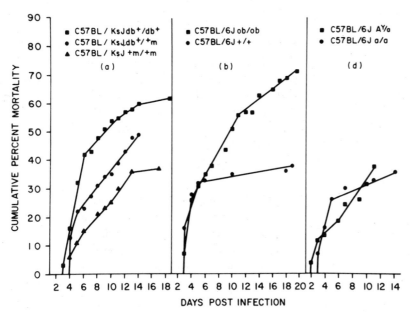

animal was restricted (R) to limit the effects of hyperphagia. This was achieved by pair feeding with the control which subsequently resulted in prevention of the spontaneous onset of diabetes[27-29]. All experiments were performed with male mice of the three genotypes in the inbred C57BL/KsJ mouse strain (**db/db**, **db/+**, and **+/+**). Each was challenged with CVB4. The results in Table 2 show that genetic predisposition to diabetes was associated with an increase in susceptibility to CVB4.

As evident from histopathological, virus mediated pancreatic pathology was shown to be influenced by the diabetic mutation. Coxsackievirus B4 infection of the homozygote C57BL/KsJ **db+/db+** mice resulted in both acinar and islet cells destruction, while in the heterozygote db/+, only acinar cell damage was evident. In normal C57BL/KsJ **+/+** mice, infected with CVB4, pancreatitis was the prominent histopathological observation. Because there were no significant differences in CVB4 titers in the pancreas, liver, heart, or spleen of these genetic variants, it was concluded that virus-induced pathology was determined by host factors and was independent of

virus tissue titers[6]. Furthermore, we also reported that CVB4 infection of the heterozygote **db/+**, which does not spontaneously develop diabetes, results in a pattern of glucose intolerance consistent with diabetes mellitus[31].

Loria et al[6], reported that the diabetes mutation **db**, on chromosome 4 in the inbred C57BL/KsJ mouse exerted a specific influence on host response to CVB4 infection as determined by LD$_{50}$ studies and percent cumulative mortality responses. This host influence was specific since two other diabetes mutations, the yellow-obese, **A^y/a** on chromosome 2 or the obese-diabetes, **ob/ob** on chromosome 6, did not have the same effect. Mice with the misty coat color mutation, **m/m** located one centimorgan from the diabetes mutation db on the same chromosome, also had a different LD$_{50}$ and cumulative mortality response than that of the diabetic mutant mice. This clearly illustrates the influence of a particular diabetes mutation at a specific chromosome loci on host susceptibility to viral infection.

Table 3

Pancreatic titers of Coxsackievirus B4[a] in diabetic and non diabetic mice

Host	Genotype	Host Phenotype	Infecting Dose[b]	Pancreatic Titer[c]
C57BL/KsJ	db+/db+	diabetes	1	9.56
C57BL/KsJ	db+/+m	none	1	9.88
C57BL/KsJ	+m/+m	misty coat	3	9.55
C57BL/6J	ob/ob	obese-diabetes	1	9.27
C57BL/6J	+/+	control	1	9.04
C57BL/6J	A^y/a	yellow-obese	3	9.80
C57BL/6J	a/a	control	2	9.24

Mean titer ± S.D. 9.50 ± 0.10

[a] Adapted from Loria[6]. [b] Dose is in log PFU/animal rounded to the closest integer. Performed 3 days after I.P. infection. [c] Titer of virus is expressed as log PFU/gr tissue.

All values are the mean of 3 independent titrations, each done in duplicate.

As previously stated, virus titers in the pancreas of all genotypes and their inbred controls were essentially identical (9.50 +/- 0.1 log PFU/gr tissue) irrespective of the difference in the inoculating dose, Table 3. These results illustrate that viral genotype dictates the level of virus replication in the target tissue, while host genetics determine the susceptibility and rate of interaction between the host and infecting virus.

The influence of genetic predisposition to diabetes without the complications of the pathophysiological changes of the disease on the immune response was also tested. Neutralization antibodies to CVB4 were not produced in **db+/db+** mice without diabetes following infection with 1/2 a CVB4 LD$_{50}$ dose. However, the same homozygous **db+/db+** mice allowed to overeat developed overt diabetes. When challenged with CVB4 these animals produced neutralizing antibodies after a lag period[33], Table 4 and Figure 2.

Table 4

Coxsackievirus B4 Serum Neutralization Levels[a]

| | | Genotypes | | |
Days	+m/+m	db+/+m	db+/db + **AL**[c]	db+/db+**R**
7	1280	1280	< 10[b]	< 10
14	1280	160	< 10	< 10
21	1280	< 10	< 10	< 10
56	Not Done	320	< 10	< 10
74	Not Done	320	160	< 10
112	Not Done	320	160	< 10
140	Not Done	160	>1280	< 10

[a] Levels represent the reciprocal of serum dilution at which 50% plaque reduction was observed.

[b] If < 10, 50% reduction was not achieved at any dilution.

[c] AL = With overt disease, R = genetically predisposed, but phenotypically normal.

These findings demonstrate that host factors as characterized by genetic predisposition and the resulting phenotypic expression in the form of diabetes have a marked and significantly distinct influence on the course of CVB4 infection including the ability to develop neutralizing antibodies. In order to estab-

lish the effects of the diabetic genotype and phenotype on the number of spleen antibody forming cells (AFC), ten days after CVB4 infection animals were immunized with sheep red blood cells. Prior to virus infection, the heterozygote **db+/+m** had a significantly higher number of spleen AFC at 234.4 per million cells. Furthermore, both the misty coat color control **+m/+m**, and the **db+/db+ AL** mutant with diabetes had a higher number of spleen AFC than the **db+/db+ R** genotype without disease[29], whose level was approximately 1.5 that of the **db+/+m** heterozygote (P <0.05) Figure 3. Following virus infection AFC counts of the misty controls, the **db+/+m** heterozygote and the **db+/db+ R** homozygote without disease were, respectively, 1/11, 1/2, and 1/3 the level of the **db+/db+ AL** with overt disease. This elevation seen with the phenotypically diabetic mouse was significant at P<0.05.

Figure 2

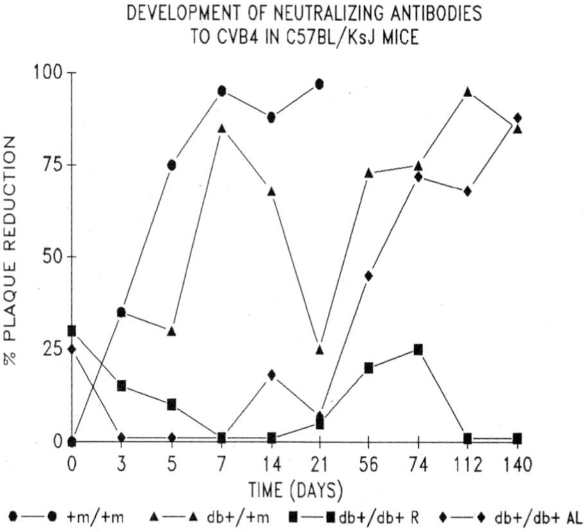

DEVELOPMENT OF NEUTRALIZING ANTIBODIES TO CVB4 IN C57BL/KsJ MICE

Efforts were undertaken to determine whether these differences in the immune response were the consequence of the altered diabetic metabolic environment or the result of an inherent cellular defect. Therefore the results from **in vivo** immunization with SRBC were compared to **in vitro** SRBC priming of spleen cells taken from uninfected or virus infected mice. The **db+/db+** mice expressing overt diabetes showed a greatly increased response to **in vivo** SRBC immunization following CB4 infection but did not mimic this pattern when priming was performed **in vitro**. Instead, the response was similar to that observed in uninfected animals. The similarity between **in vivo** and **in vitro** data in all groups except the **db+/**

db+ mutants with diabetes mellitus suggests that the methodological differences between the two immunization protocols was not a factor. In this context, the diabetic microenvironment was of great consequence to the altered immune responses seen in the **db+/db+ AL** with the diabetic phenotype when compared to the genetically identical, non diabetic **db+/db+ R** mice[34].

Figure 3

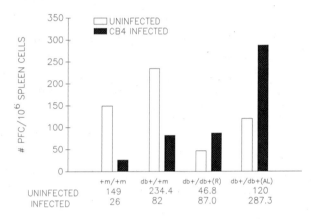

	+m/+m	db+/+m	db+/db+(R)	db+/db+(AL)
UNINFECTED	149	234.4	46.8	120
INFECTED	26	82	87.0	287.3

Adapted from Montgomery et al [29]

A comparison of these experimental animal observations with results obtained by other investigators with human studies reveals that there is a considerable degree of analogy between the animal studies and human studies. Banatvala, et al[35] reported that 4 IDDM patients, all of whom were Austrian, tested negative for CVB specific IgM at the onset of illness but were positive when tested approximately 3 months after onset of IDDM. They further commented that they had frequently observed several patients with acute CVB in whom specific IgM responses did not appear until some weeks after the onset of symptoms. The specificity of the interaction between the human with a genetic predisposition to diabetes and CVB is also illustrated in a previous study by King, et al[36]. They found a positive IgM to CVB types 1-6 as measured by ELISA in 11 of 28 (39%) children 3-14 years of age, in whom IDDM developed during the same year. A homotypic response to CVB4 was evident in 5/11 (45%) and 1/11 (9%) to CVB5. Islet cell cytoplasmic antibodies (IgG) and complement fixing islet cell antibodies were detected only in 6 which were positive for CVB specific IgM, suggesting that

these antibodies do not cross react. CVB specific IgM responses were present in only 16/290 (5.5%) of age matched, non diabetic children from London whose sera was collected during the same time period. Banatvala, et al[35] confirmed and extended these observations. Recently diagnosed IDDM patients from England, Austria and Australia and their matched controls were tested for IgM responses to CVB types 1-5. Thirty percent, 37/122, had a positive IgM response at age <15, while only 15/204 (6%) of their matched controls were positive,(P< 0.005). Schernthaner, et al[37] extended these findings by showing that 96% of patients with positive CVB4 specific IgM response had at least one of the HLA genes associated with the genetic predisposition for diabetes. In an independent study of a CVB4 outbreak, Niklasson, et al[38] reported that the only individual to develop diabetes was found to have the HLA-DR phenotypes 3 and 4 which is associated with IDDM. All 22 CVB positive individuals were tested for Islet Cell Cytoplasmic Antibodies and islet surface antibodies and found negative. In their study, Frisk et al[39], found evidence of an acute infection within 2 months of IDDM diagnosis in 13 out of 24 (54%) children. CVB specific IgM responses were detected by reverse RIA in 16 out of 24 (67%) patients on the day of IDDM diagnosis. Age matched controls (non-diabetic) during the same period did not have CVB specific antibodies.

In conclusion, these observations demonstrate that in the host with a genetic predisposition for diabetes mellitus it is evident that prior to the expression of diabetes, the host has considerable immunodeficiencies. This compromised immune system renders the host unable to respond adequately to an infection by a human diabetogenic virus. Such infections may then trigger a series of events which are primarily determined by host factors and thus determine the outcome and severity of the disease.

3. Nutrition and Hyperlipidemia

Severe malnutrition in the form of marasmus reduces the normal body weight by 60%, causing a drastic increase in susceptibility to CVB3. Graded undernutrition, which reduced body weights by only 34%, did not cause such an effect[40,41]. Restoration of marasmic mice to normal food intake on the day of the infection resulted in no deaths six days later.

Figure 4

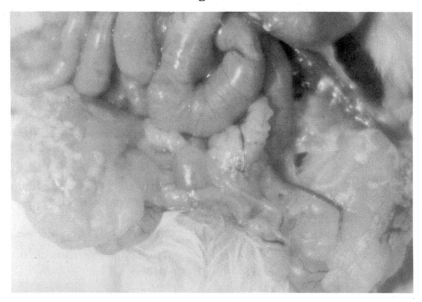

Woodruff[40,41] showed that marasmus was associated with increased CVB3 titers in tissues, gross cardiac lesions, and massive hepatic necrosis. Starvation caused lymphocytopenia, marked depression of the mononuclear cell inflammatory response, and severe atrophy of the lymphoid tissues.

Feigin, et al[42] showed that infection with CVB3 in mice was associated with a decrease in the total concentration of blood amino acids, particularly the amino acids necessary for the **de novo** synthesis of proteins. Loria, et al[43] perorally infected mice with CVB5 and measured intestinal absorption; **in-vivo** intestinal perfusion, 3 days after infection, was associated with increases in glucose (26.5%) and leucine (17%) absorption. These results suggest that host nutrients and their reserves are being taxed during virus infection. The host nutritional condition may contribute markedly in the competition with the virus for specific nutrients.

As mentioned previously, some human enteroviruses display a tropism for adipose tissue which is clearly illustrated in Figure 4. Necrosis of the abdominal adipose tissue following infection with a human coxsackievirus B5 isolate in the CD-1 outbred mouse is evident. The selective nature of the enteroviruses for adipose tissue, and the influence of the genetic predisposition is further manifested in the example provided in Figure 5. The inbred diabetic-obese mouse, C57BL/6J **ob/ob**, with the obese mutation on chromosome 6, is markedly more obese and hyperinsulinemic than the diabetic **db+/db+** mouse. Following infection of the ob/ob mouse with CVB5, the degree of adipose tissue necrosis is similar to the one observed in the diabetic mutant mouse db+/db+, infected with a 10 fold higher virus inoculum[32].

Furthermore, dietary hypercholesteremia induced hepatic fatty changes are sufficient to markedly increase the degree and extent of CVB5 induced hepatic necrosis, as evident in Figure 6[32]. It can be concluded that both genetic and environmental factors such as dietary hyperlipidemia markedly increase the degree of adipose tissue necrosis by lipotropic viruses.

Overnutrition, in the form of excessive caloric or lipid intake can also be a form of malnutrition. Loria, et

Figure 5

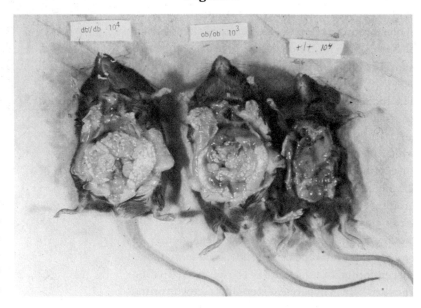

Figure 6

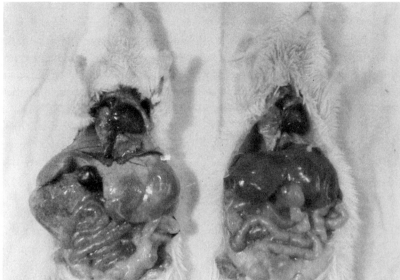

al[44] reported that dietary induced hypercholesteremia in both outbred and inbred mice was associated with a 100% increase in susceptibility to CVB5. Infection of hypercholesteremic animals was associated with leukopenia, severe fatty metamorphosis, focal necrosis of the liver and paralytic ileus, cardiomyolysis, and lack of inflammatory response. The synergistic effect of hypercholesteremia and CVB5 infection was further documented by Campbell et al[45] which showed increased replication and persistence of virus in tissues, particularly the aorta. There was a distinct augmentation of CVB5 mediated cardiopathy, resulting in persistent cardiomyolysis, which was not evident in normocholesteremic animals. Hypercholesteremia associated pathological change in the aorta of CVB5 infected mice became evident several months after acute infection. Figures 7, 8, and 9.

The increased susceptibility to CVB5 was shown to be associated with physiological changes, particularly the accumulation of intrahepatic cholesterol which leads to altered host resistance. Maximum susceptibility to CVB5 was shown to coincide with a 2.5 fold increase in the ratio of hepatic cholesterol to protein. This metabolic imbalance led to reduced virus clearance from the blood and liver. These dietary conditions were shown to independently impair the host immune response leading to increased susceptibility to infection[46]. The decreased resistance to CVB5 in hypercholesteremic mice was prima-

rily mediated by a defect in the nonspecific immune responses of macrophages and monocytes[47]. In summary, human lipotropic and cardiotropic viruses have the ability to cause necrosis of adipose tissue and heart muscle — a characteristic dependent in part on host genetic predisposition and various environmental factors, particularly those leading to increased hypercholesteremia and lipid deposition in the target organs.

4. Effect of Hormones on Infection

Gelfand, et al[48] found significantly higher enterovirus infections among males than among females during population surveillance studies for polio and coxsackieviruses. Indeed, several investigators have demonstrated a relationship between sex hormones and susceptibility to CVB1 in male mice[49, 50]. Aibender, et al[51] reported that females' IgA response to Polio virus was significantly higher than the males'. Huber et al[52] and Lynden and Huber[53], however, showed that administration of progesterone to female and castrated mice prior to virus inoculation resulted in increased cellular and

Figure 7

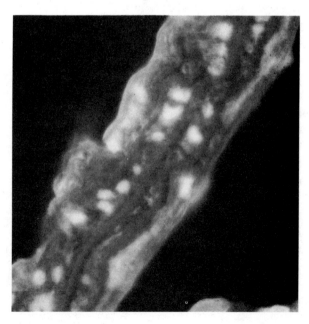

humoral CVB specific immune response, which, in this case, led to a more severe myocarditis. The authors proposed that progesterone may directly increase virus replication or independently enhance both virus replication and T cell responses.

Figure 8

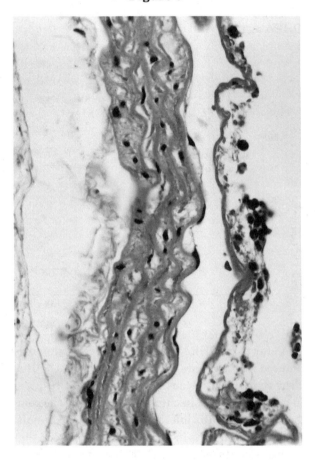

Other hormones such as cortisone were shown to increase the susceptibility of adult mice to CVB infection[54]. Rytel[55] suggested that cortisone related susceptibility to CVB infection was mediated by a decrease in the level of interferon. Virus titers, however, were increased in cortisone treated mice, as was the interferon level. Consequently, it appears that interferon levels may be determined by the degree of viral replication, rather than interferon itself limiting CVB replication. Indeed, it was reported that interferon may have only a limited role in CVB infections. Gatmaitan, et al[56] showed that when CVB3 infected mice were forced to swim in a warm pool, the virulence of CVB3 was drastically augmented by 530 fold over control. Reyes, et al[57] reported that this severe exercise induced stress may

Figure 9

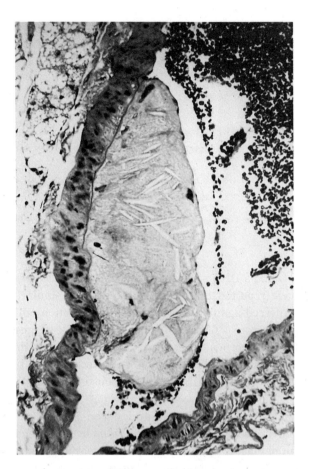

be mediated by host hormonal conditions. Using Swiss ICR mice infected with CVB3, they report that exercise is associated with the release into the plasma of catecholamines, epinephrine and norepinephrine. Accordingly, these neurohormones regulate intracellular concentrations of cyclic AMP and GMP which modulate humoral and cellular immune responses as well as inflammation leading to the increase in viral susceptibility. Recently, Jamal and Hansen[58] reported that abnormal single fiber electromyography was evident in 40 patients with postviral fatigue syndrome, 35 of the 40 patients had a CVB infection.

4.(b) Dehydroepiandrosterone Experiments

Recently, we reported that the administration of the steroid hormone dehydroepiandrosterone (DHEA) mediates a facilitation and upregulation of the specific host immune response resulting in host protection from acute lethal virus infection[59,60]. In addition to protecting against an RNA virus (coxsackievirus

Figure 10

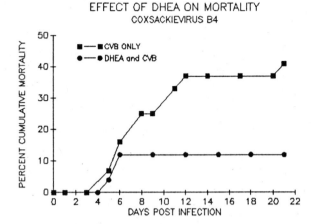

EFFECT OF DHEA ON MORTALITY
COXSACKIEVIRUS B4

B4) and a DNA virus (herpes virus type 2), we also have reported that DHEA protection is similarly conferred against a lethal bacterial infection with Streptococcus faecalis. The present results suggest that this hormone does not have a direct effect on the infectious agent but mediates its protective effect by facilitating the host immune response.[59]

DHEA (3ß-Hydroxy-5-androsten-17-one, or dehydroiso-androsterone) is sulfated by an adrenal sulfokinase to DHEA sulfate and thereby excreted in the urine in humans, and likewise, but to a lesser extent, in rodents[61]. This hormone is quantitatively one of the major adrenal cortical steroid hormones in humans and other mammals and its level begins to decline in the second decade of life, reaching 5% of the original level in the elderly[62]. Although DHEA appears to serve as an intermediary in gonadal steroid synthesis, the primary physiological function of this hormone is unclear. It is relevant to also mention that DHEA has been shown to have an effect on plasma lipid levels, both in humans[63] and rodents[64], and has an effect as an anticancer agent[65,66]. It also has an effect in stimulating neurite formation and growth[67].

The effects that 1 g/kg DHEA injected subcutaneously (s.c.) has on viral mediated mortality due to CVB4 and HSV-2 infection are presented in Figures 10 and 11, respectively. The results show that the percent cumulative mortality of animals following CVB4 infection was close to 42% in the control group that did not receive DHEA. In sharp contrast to this,

only 12% of animals in the DHEA treated group died. This is a significant reduction from the control (P<0.03). Similar observations were made with reference to animals infected with HSV2. Again 42% of the control population not receiving DHEA died, whereas only 8% of those treated with DHEA died, (P<0.03). These statistically significant observations explicitly illustrate the protective effects of DHEA against viral disease.

Figure 11

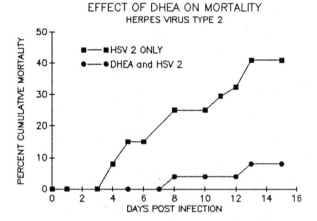

EFFECT OF DHEA ON MORTALITY
HERPES VIRUS TYPE 2

The effects of DHEA on **Streptococcus faecalis** induced mortality are presented in Figure 12. It is clear that subcutaneous DHEA treatment resulted in a 50% reduction in cumulative mortality as compared to **S. faecalis** infected and untreated animals. Based on the results in Figure 12 it is apparent that in this case the effects of DHEA are early since its protective effects are manifested within the first 24 hours following infection.

Our results show that, when compared to untreated CVB4 infected animals, administration of DHEA to CVB4 infected animals resulted in a marked increase in the number and size of the splenic germinal centers, suggesting hyperplasia of the B lymphocytes. There was also a marked increase in the hemopoietic activity in the spleen red pulp areas[8]. Finally, we have evidence that there is a significant protection of the target tissues, i.e. the heart and the pancreas from virus mediated necrosis in animals treated with DHEA.

Preliminary results of two clinical studies where DHEA was administered to patients with advanced multiple sclerosis (MS)[68, 69] indicate a beneficial effect in humans. In the first study done at the Medical College of Virginia, 17 patients were treated with DHEA at 40 mg/kg/day. While in the second study at the City of Hope, 21 patients were treated with 90mg/day. Both studies reported a striking increase in patient energy and mood in one third of this MS population.

Figure 12

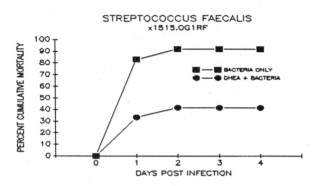

In conclusion, DHEA which is a natural steroid hormone, is thought to function by activation of host factors which then effectively confer resistance to infection. Moreover, its other physiological properties including effects on lipid levels, neurite growth and diabetes, make it a good candidate for the treatment of virus mediated disease including chronic fatigue syndrome.

5. Other Agents

Various agents have been shown to markedly influence host response to group CV infections. Rezkalla and Khatib[70] showed that nonsteroidal anti-inflammatory agents, such as salicylates and indomethacin may adversely affect the course of acute CVB3 murine myocarditis. The use of these anti-inflammatory agents for the relief of aches or fever during CVB3 myocarditis may essentially aggravate the disease process. Andrews, et al[71] illustrated that botulinum toxin increases the replication of Coxsackie Virus (CVA) in the skeletal muscle of mice. The effects of the toxin on the muscle were similar to the effects of surgical denervation, suggesting that synaptic

transmission may have a role in regulating the susceptibility of muscle to CVA. Treatment with gold salts was done experimentally in CVB3 infected mice and was shown to markedly increase mortality and virus replication presumably by inhibition of RES function[72]. Other factors such as psychological stress[73], and X-radiation[74, 75] also may influence the outcome of CV infection.

6. Summary

This report has emphasized the role of genetic predisposition, host factors and endocrine conditions on the consequences of the infectious process. It is evident that host factors exert a marked influence over the entire spectrum of host-virus interactions. The common belief that the unimmunized host is essentially a passive or inactive partner in such interaction is clearly incorrect.

Figure 13

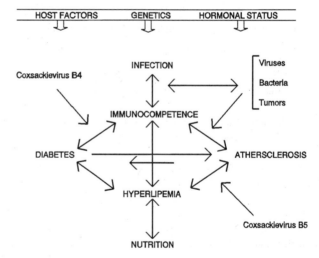

As illustrated in Figure 13, the host with a genetic predisposition for diabetes mellitus, (with the diabetic genotype, but without its phenotypic expression) has considerable immunodeficiencies which lead to a greater susceptibility to infections. Infection with a diabetogenic virus triggers a series of events which are host directed and, subsequently, determine the outcome and severity of the disease. Similarly, Figure 13 depicts the influence of both genetic and environmental factors, such as dietary hyperlipidemia on the degree of adipose tissue necrosis by lipotropic viruses. These factors independently compromise the host immune response leading to increased pathology, the development of cardiovascular disease, and atherosclerosis.

The relationship between diabetes and atherosclerosis has been well documented[75]. As illustrated in Figure 13, host factors, genetic predisposition and hormonal status are major factors in determining the outcome and severity of these syndromes. Furthermore, it becomes apparent that lipid levels, immunity and response to viral infection as determined by host

factors are common denominators of these syndromes. Endocrine status, in addition to its now accepted physiological effects, can either aggravate the severity or result in protection of the host from disease. In conclusion, the non-immune host has a remarkably active role in determining the outcome of the infectious process and the extent of virus mediated pathogenicity.

Acknowledgement:

The assistance of Mr. David Padgett in preparation of this manuscript is acknowledge and greatly appreciated.

References

1. Dalldorf G., Melnick J.L., and Curnen E., The coxsackie virus group. In **"Viral and Rickettsial Infections of Man"** Rivers T. M., and Horsfall Jr. F. L. eds. (J. B. Lippincott Comp. Philadelphia, Montreal) 1959. pp 519-546

2. Rothschild H. and Cohen J. C., Viruses and Cancer. In **Virology in Medicine**. Eds. Rothschild H. and Cohen J. C., (Oxford University Press. New York, Oxford) 1986, pp 241-242.

3. Kibrick, S., Current status of coxsackie and Echo virusese in human disease. Progr. Med. Virol. 6: 27-70, 1964.

4. Melnick, J. L., Chapter 33 in **Virology** B. N. Fields, et al. eds (Raven Press, New York, N.Y.) 1985. pp 739-794.

5. Huppert J. and Wild T. F., Virus Disease without a virus. Annal. De Virol. 135: 327-333, 1984.

6. Loria, R. M., Montgomery, L. B., Corey, L.A. and Chincilli, V., Coxsackie virus B4 infection in animals with diabetes-mellitus genotype. Arch Virology, 81: 251-262. 1984.

7. Loria, R. M., Coxsackievirus B, Lipids and Immunity as common denominators in diabetes and atherosclerosis in **"Lessons from Animal Diabetes"**, Shafrir, L., and Renold A. E, Eds. (John Libbey & Company Limited Publisher, London, Great Britain.) 1984, pp 573-578.

8. Loria, R. M., Inge, T. H., Cook, S., Szakal A., and Regelson, W., Protection against acute lethal viral infections with the native steroid dehydroepiandrosterone (DHEA). J. Med. Virology 26: 301-314, 1988.

9. Medrano, I., and Green, H. 1973, Picornavirus receptors and picornavirus multiplication in human-mouse hybrid cell lines. Virology 54: 515-524, 1973.

10. Coullin, P., Bone A., Relourcet, R., Van-Cog, N., Permissivite' de clone cellulaire hybride hommesouris a trois enterovirus: Polio II, Coxsackie B3. et Echo II. Pathol. Biol. (Paris) 24: 195, 1976.

11. Gerald P.S., and Bruns, G. A., Genetic determinants of viral susceptibility. **Birth Defects** XIV: 1-7. 1978.

12. Miller D.A., Miller, O.J., Dev, V. G., et al., Human chromosome 19 carries a poliovirus receptor gene. Cell 1: 167, 1974.

13. Foster, D. W., Goldstein, J. L., Brown, M. S., et al., (eds.) "Diabetes Mellitus" in **The Metabolic Basis of Inherited Disease.** (McGraw Hill Pub., N.Y.) 1983, p. 99-117.

14. Rotter J. I., and Rimoin, D. L., "Genetics", in **Handbook of Diabetes Mellitus, Vol 1: Etiology/Hormone Physiology.** Brownlee, M., ed. (Garland Pub. Inc., N. Y.) 1981, p. 3-94.

15. Soeldner, J. S., Sonksen, P. H. and Gleason, R. E., in **Early Diabetes**, Camerini-Davalos, Ragael A. and Cole, Harold S. eds. (Academic Press, New York,) 1970.

16. O'Sullivan, J. B. In **Early Diabetes**, Camerini-Davalos, Ragael A. and Cole, Harold S. eds. (Academic Press, New York,) 1970.

17. Maugh, T. H., Diabetes: model systems indicate viruses a cause. Science 188: 436-438, 1975.

18. Gamble, D. R., and Taylor K. W. Coxsackie B virus and diabetes. Brit. Med. J. I. 289, 1973.

19. Coleman, T. J., Taylor, K. W. and Gamble, D. R. The development of diabetes following coxsackie B virus infection in mice. Diabetologia 10: 755-759, 1974.

20. Report of the National Commission on Diabetes on the Congress of the United States, Dec. 10, 1975 (Summary). Diabetes Forecast, Vol. 28. Supplement No. 1, 60 pp., Dec. 1975 (Summary). Diabetes Forecast, Vol. 28. Supplement No. 1, 60 pp., Dec. 1975. Amer Diabetes Assoc., Inc.

21. Fajans, S. S. and Freinkel, N., In **Diabetes Mellitus**, S. S. Fajans ed., (DHEW Publ. No. 76-854 NIH), 1976, p. 1-7.

22. Craighead, J. E. The role of viruses in the pathogenesis of pancreatic disease and diabetes mellitus. Prog. Med. Virol. 19: 161-214, 1975.

23. Gamble, D. R. The epidemiology of insulin dependent diabetes, with particular reference to the relationship of virus infection to its etiology. Epidemiol. Rev. 2: 49-70, 1980.

24. Kibrick, S. and Benirscke, K., Severe generalised disease (encephaloheptomyocarditis) occurring in the newborn period due to infection with coxsackie virus group B. Pediat. 22: 857-875, 1958.

25. Wyse B. M., Dulin W. E., The influence of age and dietary conditions on diabetes in the db mouse. Diabetologia 6: 267-273, 1970.

26. Hummel, K. P., Dickie, M. M. and Coleman, D. L. Diabetes, a new mutation in the mouse. Science 153: 1127-1128, 1966.

27. Chick L. W., Like A. A., Effects of diet on pancreatic beta cell replication in mice with herediatary diabetes. Am J. Path. 221: 202-208, 1971.

28. Webb, S. R., Loria, R. M., Madge, G. E., and Kibrick, S. Susceptibility of mice to group B coxsackievirus is influenced by the diabetic gene. J. Exp. Med. 143: 1239-1248, 1976.

29. Montgomery, L. B. and Loria, R. M., Humoral Immunity in Hereditary and Overt Diabetes Mellitus. Med. Virology. 12: 255-268, 1986.

30. Loria, R. M., Virological and Immunological aspects of coxsackievirus B4 Infection in Diabetic Mutant mice., in **"Lessons From Animal Diabetes"**, Shafrir, L. and Renold A.E., Eds. p. 284-289, John Libbey &Company Limited Publisher, London, Great Britain, 1984.

31. Webb, S.A., Loria, R. M., Madge, G.E., and Kibrick, S. Coxsackievirus B infection in the mouse: effects associated with the diabetic gene db. Current Microbiol. 3: 15-19, 1979.

32. Loria, R.M., Viruses as Functional Probes of Hereditary Diabetes and Obesity. Nutrition 4: 459-463, 1988.

33. Loria, R.M., Montgomery, L.B., and Tuttle- Fuller, N. and Gregg, H.M., Genetic predisposition to diabetes mellitus is associated with impaired humoral immunity to coxsackievirus B4. Diabetes Res. and Clin. Practice 2: 91-96, 1986.

34. Montgomery, L.B., Loria, R.M., and Chincilli, V. Immunodeficiency as Primary Phenotype of Diabetes Mutation db: Studies with Coxsackievirus B4. Diabetes 39: 675-683, 1990.

35. Banatvala, J.E., Bryant, J., Schernthaner, G., et al, Coxsackie B, Mumps Rubella, and Cytomegalovirus specific IgM responses in Patients with Juvenile-onset insulin-depend-ent diabetes mellitus in Britain, Austria, and Australia. The Lancet 1: 1409-1411, 1985.

36. King, M.L., Shaikh, A., Bidwell, et al., Coxsackie-B-virus-specific IgM responses in children with insulin-dependent (juvenile-onset; type I) diabetes mellitus. Lancet 1:1397-9, 1983.

37. Schernthaner, G., Banatvala, J. E., Scherbaum W., et al., Coxsackie B virus specific IgM responses, complement fixing islet cell antibodies, HLA Dr antigens and C peptide secretion in insulin dependent diabetes mellitus. The Lancet 2: 630-632, 1985.

38. Niklasson, B. S., Dobersen, M. J., Peters, C. J., et al., An outbreak of coxsackievirus B infection followed by one case of diabetes mellitus. Scand. J. Infect. Dis. 17:15-18, 1985.

39. Frisk, G., Fohlman, J., Kobbah, M., et al., High frequency of Coxsackie-B-virus-specific IgM in children developing type I diabetes during a period of high diabetes morbidity. J. Med. Virol. 17: 219-27, 1985.

40. Woodruff, J. F., The influence of quantitative post - weaning under nutrition on coxsackievirus B-3 infection of adult mice. I. Viral persistence and increased in severity of lesions. J. Inf. Dis. 121: 137-163, 1970.

41. Woodruff, J. F., The influence of quantitative post - weaning under nutrition on coxsackievirus B-3 infection of adult mice. II. Alteration of host defenses mechanisms. J. Inf. Dis. 121: 164-181, 1970.

42. Feignin, R. D., Middelkamp, J. N., and Reed, C.A., Murine myocarditis due to coxsackie B3 virus: Blood amino acid, virologic and histopathologic correlates. J. Inf. Dis. 126: 574-584, 1972.

43. Loria, R. M., Kibrick, S., and Broitman, S. A., Pathophysiological aspects of coxsackievirus B intestinal infection. Am J. Clin. Nutrition. 30: 1876-1879, 1977.

44. Loria, R. M., Kibrick, S., Madge, G., Infection in hypercholesteremic mice with coxsackievirus b. J. Inf. Dis. 133: 655-662, 1976.

45. Campbell, A. E., Loria, R. M., and Madge, G. E., Coxsackievirus B cardiopathy and angiopathy in the hypercholesteremic host. Atherosclerosis. 31: 295-306.

46. Campbell, A. E., Loria, R. M., Madge, G. E., and Kaplan, A.M., Suppression of immunity of coxsackievirus by dietary hypercholesteremia. Infect. and Immunity. 37: 307-317.

47. Kos, W. L., Loria, R. M., Snodgrass, M. J., et al., Inhibition of host resistance by nutritional hypercholesteremia. Infect. Immun. 26: 658-667, 1979.

48. Gelfand, H. M., The occurrence in nature of the coxsackie and EHO viruses. Prog. Med. Virology 3: 193-244, 1961.

49. Berkovich S., and Ressel, M., Effect of gonadectomy on susceptibility of the adult mouse to coxsackie B1 virus infection. Proc. Soc. Exp. Biol. Med. 119: 690-694, 1965.

50. Berkovich S., and Ressel, M., Effect of sex on susceptibility of adult mice to coxsackie B1 virus infection. Archiv Fur die Gesamte Virusforsch. 22: 246-251, 1967.

51. Ainbender, E., Weisinger, R. B., Hevizy, M., and Hodes, H. L., Differences in the immunoglobulin classes of polio antibody in the serum of men and women. J. Immunol. 101: 92-98, 1968.

52. Huber, S. A., Job, L. P. and Woodruff, J. F., Sex-related differences in the pattern of coxsackievirus B-3-induced immune spleen cell cytotoxicity against virus-infected myofibers. Infect. Immun. 32: 8-73, 1981.

53. Lynden, D. L., and Huber, S. A., Aggravation of coxsackievirus, group B, type 3 induced myocarditis and increase in cellular immunity to myocyte antigens in pregnant Balb/c mice and animals treated with progesterone. Cellular Immunol. 87: 462-472, 1984.

54. Kilbourne, E. D., and Horsfall, F. L., Jr., Lethal Infection with Coxsackievirus of Adult Mice given Cortisone. Proc. Soc. Exp. Biol. Med. 77: 135-138, 1951.

55. Rytel, M. W., Interferon Response During Coxsackie B-3 Infection in Mice. I. the effect of cortisone. J. Infect. Dis. 120: 379-382, 1969.

56. Gatmaitan, B. G., Chason, J. L., and Lerner A. M., Augmentation of virulence of murine coxsackievirus B3 myocaridopathy by exercise. J. Exp. Med. 131: 121-1136, 1970.

57. Reyes, M. P., Thomas, J. A., Smith, F. E., and Lerner A. M., Elevated thymocytes norepinephrine and cyclic guanosine 3'5' monophosphate in T-lymphocytes from exercised mice with coxsackievirus V3 myocarditis. Biochem. Biophys. Res. Comm. 109: 704-708, 1982.

58. Jamal, G. A., and Hansen, S., Electrophysiological studies in the post-viral fatigue syndrome. J. Neurol. Neurosurg. Psychiatry. 48: 691-4, 1985.

59. Loria, R. M., Inge, T. H., Cook, S., et al., Protection against acute lethal viral infections with the native steroid dehydroepiandrosterone (DHEA). J. Med. Virology 26: 301-314, 1988.

60. Loria, R. M., Regelson W., and Padgett D. A., Immune Response facilitation and resistance to virus and bacterial infections with dehydroepiandrosterone (DHEA). In "The Biologic Role of Dehydroepiandrosterone (DHEA)". Kalimi and Regelson Eds. (Walter De Gruyter & Co. Publ.) 1990 pp. 107-130.

61. J. B. Tyrell, and P. H. Forshan. In: Basic and Clinical endocrinology, F. S. Greespan, P. H. Forsham, eds. (Los Altos California, Lange Medical Publications.) 1983, pp. 258-294.

62. E. Barrett-Connor, K. T. Khaw, and S. S. Yen. A prospective study of dehydroepiandrosterone sulfate, mortality, and cardiovascular disease. N. E. J. M. 315: 1519-1524, 1986.

63. J. E. Nestler, C. O. Barlascini, J. N. Clore, and W. G. Blackard. Dehydroepiandrosterone reduces serum low density lipoprotein levels and body fat but does not alter insulin sensitivity in normal men. J. Clinical Endocrinology and Metabolism 66: 57-61, 1988.

64. T. T. Yen, J. A. Allan, D. V. Pearson, and J. M. Acton. Prevention of obesity in mice by Dehydroepiandrosterone. Lipids 12: 409, 1977.

65. A. Schwartz, in: Molecular biology of aging, A. D. Woodhead, ed. Vol 35. (Plenum Pub. Co. New York) 1985, pp. 181-191.

66. Gordon G. B., Shantz L. M., and Talalay P., in Advances in Enzyme Regulation. Weber G., ed. vol. 26 (Pergamon Press, New York) 1987, pp. 355-382.

67. Roberts E., Bologa L., and Flood J. F., et al, Effects of DHEA and its sulphate on brain tissue in culture and memory in mice. Brain Research 406: 357-362, 1987.

68. Kalabrese, V. T., Issac E. and Regelson W., in "**The Biologic Role of Dehydroepiandrosterone (DHEA)**". Kalimi and Regelson Eds. (Walter De Gruyter & Co. Publ.) 1990 pp. 95-100.

69. Roberts E., in Treatment Development strategies for Alzheimer Disease. T. Crook, et al., eds. (Mark Powwley and Assocites.) 173-219 1986.

70. Rezkella, S., Khatib, G., and Khatib, R., Coxsackievirus B 3 murine myocarditis: deleterious effects of nonsterodial anti-inflammatory agents. J. Lab. Clin. Med. 107: 393-5, 1986.

71. Andrews, C. G., Drachman, D.B., Pestronck, A., and Narayan, O., Susceptibility of skeletal muscle to coxsackie A2 virus infection: effects of Botulinum toxin and denervation. Science 223: 714-716, 1984.

72. Kabiri, M., Basiri, E., and Kadivar, D., Potentiation of coxsackievirus B3 infection in adult mice pretreated with gold salt. J Med. Virology. 3: 125-136, 1978.

73. Friedman, S. B., Alder, R., and Glasgow, L. A., Effects of Psychological Stress in Adult Mice Inoculated with Coxsackie B viruses Psychosom. Med. 27: 361-368.

74. Schneck, L., and Berkovich, S., Effects of X-Irradiation on the Susceptibility of Neonatal Rat Brain and Muscle to Coxsackie B1 Virus Infection. Proc. Soc. Exp. Biol. Med. 118: 658-661, 1965.

75. Reaven, G. M., and Steiner G., eds: Proceedings of a conference on diabetes and artherosclerosis. Diabetes 30 Suppl. 2, 1981.

Chapter 61

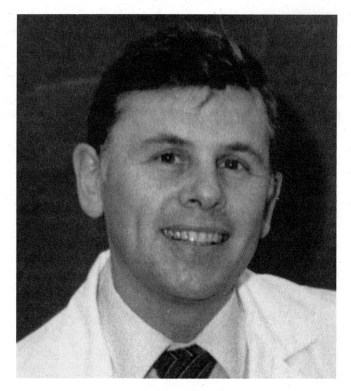

Hugh F. Pross

Abnormalities of Natural Killer (NK) Cell Numbers and Function in Patients with Chronic Fatigue Immune Dysfunction Syndrome (CFIDS)

Hugh F. Pross MD, PhD, FRCPC, Department of Microbiology and Immunology
Queen's University, Kingston, Ont., Canada, K7L 3N6

Dr. Hugh Pross received his MD degree at Queen's University in 1968 and subsequently interned in medicine at Duke University. He then obtained his PhD degree in Immunology at Queen's (1972) and studied tumor biology at the Karolinska Institute in Stockholm. He has been a member of the Faculty of Medicine at Queen's University since 1974 and was Head of the Department of Microbiology and Immunology from 1986-1990. He is currently Professor of Microbiology and Immunology and of Oncology, and is the Associate Dean of Undergraduate Medical Education.

Abstract

In this paper, the literature on chronic fatigue and immune dysfunction is briefly reviewed. The effects of this disease on the immune system are myriad, and the laboratory results vary from patient to patient and from report to report. The results of a small study of natural killer (NK) cell function and markers in CFIDS patients are reported. These data confirm 3 main points in the literature - 1) NK activity is significantly lower than normal controls, 2) total CD56+ cells are increased, and 3) the proportion of CD3-CD56+ cells is decreased. It can also be seen that by expressing NK activity as lytic units/CD56+

cells, the difference between normal and CFIDS patients is further exaggerated. We conclude that, unlike a number of laboratory tests studied in this disease, mean NK cell markers and function (for the group as a whole) have been shown to be abnormal in a sufficient number of reports to warrant further investigation, not only in large cohorts of patients with the disease, but also in the appropriate controls.

Chronic fatigue and immune dysfunction syndrome (CFIDS) is a term used to describe a condition characterized by long-term, debilitating fatigue and loss of energy in association with a variety of non-specific signs and symptoms. As reviewed elsewhere in this book, the condition has been termed chronic fatigue syndrome (CFS), post-viral syndrome, post-viral fatigue syndrome, chronic infectious mononucleosis, chronic Epstein-Barr disease, myalgic encephalomyelitis (M.E.), neurasthenia, primary fibromyalgia syndrome, and so on. CFIDS is usually characterized by a relatively sudden onset of extreme fatigue in a previously vigorous and healthy adult. By definition (see below) the fatigue is severe enough to reduce daily activity to 50% or less of the premorbid level. In some cases it is possible to identify a recent specific viral illness and the diagnosis of post-viral or chronic EBV disease is quite appropriate. In many cases, the cause is not identifiable. CFIDS affects an estimated several thousand people in North America, and is seen in both the pediatric and adult population. The mean age within the adult population is about 37 years, with three quarters of the patients being female[1].

Typical complaints include subjective fever, sore throat, painful axillary and/or cervical lymph nodes, muscle weakness and aching, pressure-like headaches, joint pains without swelling or redness, forgetfulness, confusion, difficulty thinking, inability to concentrate, changes in sleep pattern, numbness and tingling of the extremities, transient visual scotomata and an aversion to light. Patients have also noted medication sensitivities and alcohol intolerance.

In an attempt to standardize the diagnostic criteria for this syndrome, a group of physicians from the Division of Viral Diseases, Centers for Disease Control in Atlanta, and a number of other U.S. medical centers, proposed a working case definition in which 2 major criteria must be fulfilled - 1)

persistent fatigue as described above, and 2) exclusion of a long list of conditions ranging from malignancy to HIV infection, which could lead to similar symptoms[2]. Other symptoms were defined as minor criteria, with a requirement that 8/11 be present or recurrent over a 6 month period. The required number of minor criteria were reduced to 6/11 if physical examination included two or more of low grade fever on 2 occasions, at least one month apart, nonexudative pharyngitis and palpable or tender axillary or cervical lymph nodes. Thus, this diagnosis is primarily one of exclusion to ensure that the patient is not suffering from some other serious, possibly treatable, illness. The publication of the working case definition gave this group of patients a degree of credibility that they did not have before, but there has still been some controversy over the exclusions and acceptable criteria. However, the case definition has served as a common reference point for clinical investigators trying to identify the cause(s) and laboratory characteristics of this condition.

Laboratory abnormalities in CFIDS

The lack of laboratory diagnostic tests for CFIDS has hampered research in this area considerably. It is possible that no single causative agent is responsible for the condition, but rather that the disease is the result of any one of a number of chronic viral infections and/or an inappropriate immunological response to a viral infection. Antibody titres against EBV proteins have been documented in numerous studies, with several early reports showing moderately increased titres of IgG antibody to EBV early antigen (EA) and capsid antigen (VCA) and, occasionally low titres of EBNA ab or IgM anti-VCA[3,4], suggesting reactivation of an EBV infection. Subsequent studies have shown that such titres are not uncommon in the normal population and are not necessarily associated with CFIDS[5]. Bell **et al.**[6] have published findings showing elevated titres against Coxsackie B virus in patients with "postviral fatigue syndrome". This may be unique to a particular outbreak since it was not confirmed in a larger study by the same group[7]. Further, it is apparent that CFIDS patients frequently have elevated tires against a number of common viruses such as CMV, HSV and measles, suggesting an underlying immune dysfunction[2].

Recently a study of spontaneous EBV-induced lymphocyte transformation was conducted by Jones **et al.**[8] CFS patients with 2 years illness were subdivided into 3 groups based on EA titre ≥ 80, < 80 and negative. These were compared with controls who were seropositive with or without a history of infectious mononucleosis (IM). Patients who were seropositive had lymphocyte spontaneous transformation rates **in vitro** of 32 and 27%, compared with seropositive normal rates of 11 (IM+) and 5% (IM-). Lymphocytes from 1/9 seronegative CFIDS patients spontaneously transformed. Of 250 consecutive CFIDS patients, lymphocytes from 30% showed transformation compared with 5% of normals. These data suggest that lack of control of EBV outgrowth **in vitro** is correlated with antibody evidence of EBV infection **in vivo** in some patients with CFIDS. Although these studies suggest a role for EBV in some CFIDS patients, there appears to be general agreement that this cannot be the only cause of the syndrome. Elevated antibody titres against EBV antigens are common in healthy controls and, conversely, not all CFIDS patients have evidence of EBV infection[3-5].

Interest in CFIDS was heightened last year with the announcement by DeFreitas that more than 50% of samples from 31 CFIDS patients from a broad area of eastern USA were positive by Western blotting for antibodies against human T lymphotrophic virus (HTLV)[9]. Twenty non-contact controls were negative. To distinguish between HTLV-I and II, specific regions of the proviral DNA were amplified by PCR, followed by Southern blotting. None of the blood samples contained detectable HTLV-I **gag** sequences, but DNA positive for the HTLV-II **gag** subregion was detected in the blood of 83% of the adult and 72% of the pediatric CFIDS patients. 7/10 PCR positive samples had HTLV-II **gag** mRNA by **in situ** hybridization, indicating the gene was functional. However, the HTLV-II **tax** region was not detected. There was a high, but not invariable, association of ab to HTLV with detectable HTLV-II-like **gag** DNA. Although the virus may be a secondary infection in patients with a basic immune dysfunction, it is unlikely that it represents reactivation of a latent virus, since seropositivity in healthy non-contact controls is virtually non-existent. These studies await confirmation by others and have been accepted with caution because of the exquisite sensitivity of the polymerase chain reaction, raising the possibility of contamination.

Another virus which has received considerable attention recently for its association with CFIDS is human herpes virus 6[10-13]. HHV6 infects B and T cells and, as with EBV, most adults have been infected with HHV6. Typically, in the U.S., primary infection occurs very early with little morbidity[14]. It is also associated with atypical polyclonal lymphoproliferation (APL), a benign lymphoproliferative syndrome[15,16] and with atypical mononucleosis[16,17] which is in many ways analogous to EBV. Elevated titres against HHV6 are seen in many viral, autoimmune and malignant disorders[10]. Ablashi **et al.**[10] have reported that CFIDS patients have higher ab titres than controls, especially those patients with neurological involvement. Interestingly, cultures of lymphocytes from CFIDS patients showed signs of spontaneous activation of HHV6 infection - increase in cell size, overgrowth, cytopathic changes and cell death - similar to that seen when normal lymphocytes are infected **in vitro** with HHV6. The enlarged cells stained positively for HHV6 and **in situ** hybridization showed HHV6 specific RNA. It is suggested that in CFIDS the viral infection is not causative, but reactivated from the latent state in association with, or perhaps due to, compromised immunity.

Immunological studies in CFIDS

Numerous studies have reported immunological abnormalities associated with CFIDS (reviewed in[18,19]). Cell mediated immunity is reported to be low by some authors[20,21], with a high proportion of patients showing anergy on Multitest skin testing. This was not observed in studies by others[4]. Lower than normal results were found with phytohemagglutinin (PHA) responses[21,22] (**cf.**, however,[12]), soluble antigen response[12], specific antibody response to pneumococcus vaccine[12], natural killer cell activity[23-26], (**cf.**, however,[27]), NK proportions[12,23,24] and CD3 proportions[22,28] (**cf.**, however,[12]). Lloyd **et al.**[21] reported decreased proportions of CD4 and CD8 cells, but this was not observed by other groups[3,4,12,28]. Various Ig deficiencies[4,21,29,30] and increased levels of immune complexes have also been reported[4,31]. Again, others have reported normal values for these parameters[12,29]. Increased levels of cytokines such as alpha interferon (IFN)[21,32], and interleukin-2[33] (**cf.**, however,[4,34]) could indicate a state of chronic viral infection and immune activation, including decreased, "exhausted" NK cell function. Lloyd **et al.**[21] reported increased MHC Class II expression by peripheral blood mononuclear cells (PBMC) from patients with CFIDS, also suggesting immune activation. In response to these reports, Strauss **et al.**[35] assessed serum IFN's-alpha, and gamma, IL-1 beta, IL-2 and tumour necrosis factor (TNF). Although there were wide ranges in activity, the levels were not significantly different from age and sex-matched control subjects. No increase in serum IFN-alpha was seen in a group of patients with primary fibromyalgia[34], but Lever **et al.**[32] showed that PBMC from a group of individuals with well-defined post-viral (Coxsackie B4) fatigue syndrome produced significantly more IFN-alpha than controls. Chao **et al.**[36] assessed 3 markers of cell activation - neopterin (produced by activated monocytes), beta-2-microglobulin, and IL-6. Beta-2-microglobulin levels were not different from normal, but both neopterin and IL-6 were elevated in about 30% of CFS patients, suggesting that there may be "chronic perturbation" of mononuclear phagocytes due to persistent viral infection.

A frequent observation in CFIDS studies has been the presence of some type of NK cell defect. Kibler **et al.**[24] reported reduced NK activity and decreased IFN-gamma production in patients with chronic active EBV syndrome. An actual decrease in NK function has been documented by Aoki **et al.**[26], Caligiuri **et al.**[23], and Klimas **et al.**[25] Each had a fairly homogeneous population of patients. Caligiuri **et al.** demonstrated that CFIDS patients have normal numbers of CD56+ cells with a relative deficit in the CD56+CD3- (NK) population. Blocking with anti-CD3 antisera showed that the CD3+CD56+ population was responsible for much of the residual non-MHC-restricted activity. The activity could be enhanced by IL-2, but IL-2-induced cytotoxicity against EBV infected lines was lower than normal. Subsequent to this report, three other groups have documented changes in CD56+ cells. Gupta **et al.**[12] showed a significant decrease in CD16, CD56 and CD57+ cells, while Klimas **et al.**[25] and Morrison **et al.**[37] reported an **increase** in CD56+ cells. In the Morrison study, CD16+ (Fc gamma) cells were decreased and CD3+CD56+ cells were increased in proportion to CD3-CD56+ cells, supporting the Caligiuri observations to some extent. The authors also found significantly increased CD56+CD25+(IL-2R) and CD56+CD71+ (transferrin receptor) cells. A higher proportion of the CD56+ cells were "Bright+"

compared to normals. Taken together, these observations are compatible with a chronic viral activation syndrome resulting in an alteration in the relative proportions of T and NK non-MHC-restricted cytotoxic cells. In some patients, this is sufficient to result in diminished functional NK activity. The literature is difficult to evaluate, however, because of the frequent use of "NK" to describe both CD3+ and CD3- non-MHC-restricted killing, and the frequent equating of phenotype (e.g. CD56) with NK cells and NK function. There are also differences in the methods used to perform and analyze the NK assays. Caligiuri **et al.**[23] report data at a high E/T ratio, making assessment of the effect of IL-2 levels at the plateau difficult to evaluate. Klimas **et al.**[25] carried out NK assays on whole blood and expressed their data as lytic units (LU)/CD56+ cells, which tends to emphasize the NK defect. A more difficult problem which has not been addressed is the fact that many healthy donors have low NK activity[38], making NK assays on individuals of limited use as a diagnostic tool. It is also unknown whether the phenotypic and functional characteristics of the cytotoxic cells are similar or different between low NK normals and low NK CFIDS patients. The fact that patients suffering from major depression (not CFIDS-related) have reduced NK activity, possibly due to a related, unknown, mechanism[39], is also a potentially confounding variable since some element of depression can be associated with CFIDS.

It is obvious from this brief literature review that there are a myriad of conflicting reports with little evidence of a common causative agent in CFIDS. To some extent, this is due to different definitions of the syndromes - some requiring evidence of specific viral infection, others excluding such cases as being of known etiology. The recent working definition may decrease the heterogeneity to some extent. In spite of the disparate reports, there is certainly a subset of patients who are either "post-viral" or who show evidence of reactivation of latent viral infection. In view of the relationship between NK activity and anti-viral defence, the frequent reports of abnormalities of NK function and frequency in CFIDS patients merit further investigation.

Several previous reports are compatible with a role for NK cells in CFIDS. 1) NK cells are stimulated by IFN released early in viral infection, but an excess of

IFN or IL-2 may lead to inhibition of activity[40], 2) "pure" congenital defects in NK function lead to life-threatening herpes virus infections[41,42], 3) virally-infected targets, including EBV-transformed cells, are more susceptible to NK lysis than uninfected cells and may be controlled by NK cells[43,44], and, 4) transformation of B cells by EBV can be shown to be regulated by NK cells **in vitro** (Menezes, personal communication).

The studies reporting NK cell abnormalities in CFIDS patients do not address the mechanism of the defect and, in some instances, it is apparent the authors are referring to marker-bearing cells (e.g. CD56+) as NK cells, regardless of the CD3 status of the cells and the published reports that both T cells and NK cells may express increased levels of CD56 on activation **in vitro**[45,46].

We have recently completed studies using lymphocytes from patients in the Kingston CFIDS community. The objective was twofold: 1) to establish links with the CFIDS community so as to assess the feasibility of conducting studies on their blood, and 2) to determine if we could reproduce results published in the literature on NK cells. Our first project was an assessment of herbal remedies in a small group of 6 patients (Leyton and Pross, submitted for publication). As expected, no statistically significant alterations in NK function or markers were observed either in the patients or the normal controls as a result of the treatment. However, it was observed that NK activity was lower in these patients than the normal range. The study was intended as a pre/post therapy comparison and the normal controls were not intended to be compared with the patient population. Recently, we have examined CD markers and NK activity in 19 CFIDS patients (15 female, 4 male, CDC defined), each tested several times in

comparison with 4 normal controls (3 female, 1 male) of similar age range. The controls were chosen because they included a range of NK activity from 0.4 to 2.2 times normal (95% confidence limits in previous studies)[38,47]. The following results were obtained in a 4 hour assay, using K562 as the prototype NK cell target[47-49]. The data are expressed as mean ± standard error.

Group	n	LU/10^6	CD16	CD3-CD16+	CD56	CD3-CD56+
Normal	4	70.7±3.9	19.7±3.1	15.6±1.5	12.3±2.8	13.3±1.4
CFIDS	19	33.6±3.9	18.9±1.2	11.2±.9	17.4±1.5	7.8±.8

These data confirm 3 main points in the literature - 1) NK activity is significantly lower than controls, 2) total CD56+ cells are increased, and 3) the proportion of CD3-CD56+ cells is decreased. It can also be seen that by expressing the data as lytic units (LU)/CD56+ cells, the difference between normal and CFIDS patients would be further exaggerated. The biological significance of these observations await further investigation. We conclude, however, that, unlike a number of laboratory tests studied in this disease, mean NK cell markers and function (for the group as a whole) have been shown to be abnormal in a sufficient number of reports to warrant further investigation. These investigations should address the basic mechanism of the abnormality, as well as establishing the range of normal values in the appropriate control groups.

Acknowledgements

I thank Mrs. P. Bandy-Dafoe and Mrs. G. Lawrance for excellent technical assistance. I would also like to thank Dr. Mary Maxwell and the members of the M.E. Association of Kingston for their generous donation of time and peripheral blood samples. The work was supported in part by grants from National Cancer Institute of Canada, and the Medical Research Council of Canada.

References

1. Komaroff AL, Buchwald D: Signs and symptoms of chronic fatigue syndrome. Rev Infect Dis 13 Suppl. 1:S8-S11, 1991.

2. Holmes GP, Kaplan JE, Gantz NM, et al: Chronic fatigue syndrome: a working case definition. Ann Intern Med 108:387-389, 1988.

3. Jones JF, Ray CG, Minnich LL, et al: Evidence for active Epstein-Barr Virus infection in patients with persistent, unexplained illnesses:elevated anti-early antigen antibodies. Ann Int Med 102:1-7, 1985

4. Straus SE, Tosato G, Armstrong G, et al: Persisting illness and fatigue in adults with evidence of Epstein-Barr virus infection. Ann Intern Med 102:7-16, 1985.

5. Sumaya CV: Serologic and virologic epidemiology of Epstein-Barr virus: Relevance to chronic fatigue syndrome. RID 13 Suppl. 1:S19-S25, 1991.

6. Bell EJ, Irvine KG, Gardiner AJS, et al: Coxsackie B infection in a general medical unit. Scott Med J 28:157-159, 1983.

7. Miller NA, Carmichael HA, Calder BD, et al: Antibody to coxsackie B virus in diagnosing postviral fatigue syndrome. Br Med J 302:140- 143, 1991.

8. Jones JF, Streib J, Baker S, et al: Chronic fatigue syndrome: I. Epstein-Barr virus immune response and molecular epidemiology. J Med Virol 33:151-158, 1991.

9. DeFreitas E, Hilliard B, Cheney PR, et al: Retroviral sequences related to human T-lymphotropic virus type II in patients with chronic fatigue immune dysfunction syndrome. Proc Natl Acad Sci (USA) 88:2922-2926, 1991.

10. Ablashi DV, Zompetta C, Lease C, et al: Human herpes virus-6 (HHV- 6) and chronic fatigue syndrome (CFS), in Proc. Chronic Fatigue Syndrome Workshop. Toronto, Central Health Laboratory, 1990.

11. Krueger GRF, Koch B, Ablashi DV: Persistent fatigue and depression in patient with antibody to human B-lymphotrophic virus. Lancet 2:36, 1987.

12. Gupta S, Vayuvegula B: A comprehensive immunological analysis in chronic fatigue syndrome. Scand J Immunol 33:319-327, 1991.

13. Buchwald D, Freedman AS, Ablashi DV, et al: A chronic postinfectious fatigue syndrome associated with benign lymphoproliferation, B-cell proliferation, and active replication of human herpesvirus-6. J Clin Immunol 10:335-344, 1990.

14. Saxinger C, Polesky H, Eby N, et al: Antibody reactivity with HBLV (HHV-6) in U.S. populations. J Virol Meth 21:199-208, 1988.

15. Krueger GRF, Manak M, Bourgeois N, et al: Persistent active herpes virus infection associated with atypical polyclonal lymphoproliferation (APL) and malignant lymphoma. Anticancer Res 9:1457-1476, 1989.

16. Steeper TA, Horwitz CA, Ablashi DV, et al: The spectrum of clinical and laboratory findings due to human herpesvirus-6 (HHV-6) in patients with mononucleosis-like illnesses not due to EBV or CMV. Am J Clin Pathol 93:776-783, 1990.

17. Irving WL, Cunningham AL: Serological diagnosis of infection with human herpes virus type 6. Br Med J 300:156-159, 1990.

18. Gin W, Christiansen FT, Peter JB: Immune function and the chronic fatigue syndrome. Med J Australia 151:117-118, 1989.

19. Buchwald D, Komaroff AL: Review of laboratory findings for patients with chronic fatigue syndrome. RID 13 Suppl. 1:S12-S18, 1991.

20. Murdoch JC: Cell-mediated immunity in patients with myalgic encephalomyelitis syndrome. NZ Med J 101:511-512, 1988.

21. Lloyd AR, Wakefield D, Boughton CR, et al: Immunological abnormalities in the chronic fatigue syndrome. Med J Australia 151:122-124, 1989.

22. Behan PO, Behan WM, Bell EJ: The postviral fatigue syndrome. An analysis of the findings in 50 cases. J Infect 10:210, 1985.

23. Caligiuri M, Murray C, Buchwald D, et al: Phenotypic and functional deficiency of natural killer cells in patients with chronic fatigue syndrome. J Immunol 139:3306-3313, 1987.

24. Kibler R, Lucas DO, Hicks MJ, et al: Immune function in chronic active Epstein-Barr virus infection. J Clin Immunol 5:46-54, 1985.

25. Klimas NG, Salvato FR, Morgan R, et al: Immunologic abnormalities in chronic fatigue syndrome. J Clin Microbiol 28:1403-1410, 1990.

26. Aoki T, Usuda Y, Miyakoshi H, et al: Low natural killer syndrome: clinical and immunologic features. Nat Immun Cell Growth Regul 6:116-128, 1987.

27. Gold D, Bowden R, Sixbey J, et al: Chronic fatigue. A prospective clinical and virologic study. JAMA 264:48-53, 1990.

28. Subira ML, Castilla A, Civeira MP, et al: Deficient display of CD3 on lymphocytes of patients with chronic fatigue syndrome. J Infect Dis 160:165-166, 1989.

29. Read R, Spickett G, Harvey J: IgG1 subclass deficiency in patients with chronic fatigue syndrome. Lancet 1:241-242, 1988.

30. Komaroff AL, Geiger AM, Wormsley S: IgG subclass deficiencies in chronic fatigue syndrome. Lancet 1:1288-1289, 1988.

31. Behan PO, Behan WM, Bell EJ: The postviral fatigue syndrome - an analysis of the findings in 50 cases. Ann Intern Med 10:211-222, 1985.

32. Lever AML, Lewis DM, Bannister BA, et al: Interferon production in postviral fatigue syndrome. Lancet 2:101, 1988.

33. Cheney PR, Dorman SE, Bell DS: Interleukin 2 and chronic fatigue syndrome. Ann Int Med 110:321, 1989.

34. Wallace DJ, Bowman RL, Wormsley SB, et al: Cytokines and immune regulation in the primary fibromyalgia (fibrositis) syndrome. Arthritis Rheum 32:1334-1335, 1989.

35. Straus SE, Dale JK, Peter JB, et al: Circulating lymphokine levels in the chronic fatigue syndrome. J Infect Dis 160:1085-1086, 1989.

36. Chao CC, Gallagher M, Phair J, et al: Serum neopterin and interleukin-6 levels in chronic fatigue syndrome. J Infect Dis 162:1412-1413, 1990.

37. Morrison LJ, Behan WH, Behan PO: Changes in natural killer cell phenotype in patients with post-viral fatigue syndrome. Clin Exp Immunol 83:441-446, 1991.

38. Pross HF, Baines MG: Studies of human natural killer cells. I. In vivo parameters affecting normal cytotoxic function. Int J Cancer 29:383-390, 1982.

39. Irwin M, Smith TL, Gillin JC: Low natural killer cytotoxicity in major depression. Life Sci 41:2127-2133, 1987.

40. Maluish AE, Ortaldo JR, Conlon JC, et al: Depression of natural killer cytotoxicity after in vivo administration of recombinant leukocyte interferon. J Immunol 131:503-507, 1983.

41. Fleisher G, Koven N, Kamiya H, et al: A non-X-linked syndrome with susceptibility to severe Epstein-Barr virus infections. J Pediatrics 100:727-736, 1982.

42. Biron CA, Byron KS, Sullivan JL: Severe herpes virus infections in an adolescent without natural killer cells. N Engl J Med 320:1731-1735, 1989.

43. Santoli D, Trinchieri G, Koprowski H: Cell-mediated cytotoxicity against virus-infected target cells in humans. II. Interferon induction and activation of natural killer cells. J Immunol 121:532- 538, 1978.

44. Bishop GA, Glorioso JC, Schwartz SA: Relationship between expression of herpes simplex virus glycoproteins and susceptibility of target cells to human natural killer activity. J Exp Med 157:1544-1561, 1983.

45. Perussia B, Ramoni C, Anegon I, et al: Preferential proliferation of natural killer cells among peripheral blood mononuclear cells cocultured with B lymphoblastoid cell lines. Nat Immun Cell Growth Regul 6:171-188, 1987.

46. Lanier LL, Le AM, Civin CI, et al: The relationship of CD16 (Leu-11) and Leu-19 (NKH-1) antigen expression on human peripheral blood NK cells and cytotoxic T lymphocytes. J Immunol 136:4480-4486, 1986.

47. Pross HF, Maroun JA: The standardization of NK cell assays for use in studies of biological response modifiers. J Immunol Meth 68:235-249, 1984.

48. Jondal M, Pross HF: Surface markers on human B- and T-lymphocytes. VI Cytotoxicity against cell lines as a functional marker for lymphocyte subpopulations. Int J Cancer 15:596-605, 1975.

49. Pross HF, Baines MG, Rubin P, et al: Spontaneous human lymphocyte-mediated cytotoxicity against tumour target cells. IX. Quantitation of natural killer cell activity. J Clinical Immunol 1:51-63, 1981.

Blood Cell Changes

Chapter 62

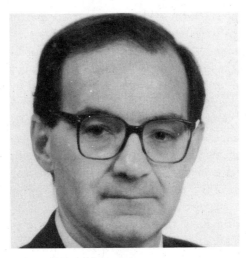

Jesus Prieto

Opioid-Mediated Monocyte Dysfunction in the Chronic Fatigue Syndrome

J. Prieto, MD, J. Camps-Bansell, A. Castilla, Department of Internal Medicine, University Clinic, Pamplona, Spain.

Dr. Prieto has held his present position as Director of the Department of Medicine at the University of Navarra, Spain since 1979. He began his career as Research fellow and honourary Clinical Assistant in the Academic Department of Medicine of the Royal Free Hospital in 1972 and has held numerous other senior positions at the University of Santiago de Compostela, the General Hospital of Galicia, the University of Oviedo and the University of Valladolid. Dr. Prieto specializes in the area of immunology of viral diseases.

Abstract

The chronic fatigue syndrome (CFS) is characterized by persistent or recurrent fatigability, and frequently by other symptoms like low-grade fever, myalgias, headache, painful lymphadenopathies and neuropsychiatric symptoms. Viral, neuroimmunologic, psychogenic and other etiopathogenic hypotheses have been proposed. Recent studies have confirmed the close connections among the psychological, neuroendocrinological and immunological spheres. Thus, it has been demonstrated that B-endorphin and enkephalins, which are liberated during the stress response, have important actions on the immune system. Many studies using animal and human models have shown that stress can alter immunity, giving rise to an increased risk of infections and apparition of tumors. Experiments performed by Shavit et al showed that NK cell activity suppression in rats during stress was mediated by opioid peptides. This effect could be blocked by an opioid antagonist, naltrexone, and reproduced with morphine. Diverse immunological alterations and serological positivity to various viruses have been demonstrated in patients with CFS.

We evaluated the action of B-endorphin, met-enkephalin and leu-enkephalin on the in vitro expression of immunoreactive vimentin filaments (ir-VF) by monocytes. We simultaneously examined their effects on phagocytosis of Candida albicans and on the expression of membrane molecules. The 3 peptides at concentrations of 10^{-6}, 10^{-8} and 10^{-10} M, markedly reduced phagocytosis and the expression of both ir-VF, and HLA-DR molecules. Those effects were reversible with naloxone 10^{-8} M. The intravenous administration of fentanyl, a synthetic opiate agonist, to patients subjected to coronary surgery, induced similar monocyte changes. The expression of ir-VF was directly correlated with the HLA-DR, CR3 molecules and with phagocytic activity.

We also studied the monocyte function in 35 consecutive patients with CFS and in 25 healthy controls. In 85% of the patients with CFS, we found a monocyte dysfunction characterized by a marked reduction in the number of monocytes positive for ir-VF, a decreased index of phagocytosis and a reduced expression of HLA-DR antigens. These values markedly increased after incubation of monocytes with naloxons. A decrease in the blastogenic response of lymphocytes and in the number of monocytes expressing receptors for the Fc portion of IgG and C3b was also observed. These findings suggest that an increased opioid activity acting through a classic receptor mechanism is present in a high percentage of patients with CFS.

The chronic fatigue syndrome (CFS) is characterized by the presence of persistent or recurrent muscular fatigability (for a duration of 6 months or more) that causes a 50% decrease in the performance of daily activities. Patients suffering from this syndrome present, with great frequency, other symptoms such as low grade fever, myalgias, painful lymphadenopathies, gastrointestinal complaints and headache. Likewise, the great majority of them have neuropsychiatric symptoms such as difficulty in concentration, insomnia, anxiety and depressive traits. To arrive at a diagnosis of this syndrome, it is necessary to exclude other pathologies that can also give rise to similar symptomatology[1-4].

Viral[5-13], neuroimmunologic[14-17], psychogenic[18-19] and other hypotheses have been proposed to explain the etiopathogenesis of CFS. However, it seems difficult to support a single etiology for this condition. Most probably, the symptomatology - low-grade fever, asthenia, myalgias, neuropsychiatric alterations, etc. - correspond to unspecific manifestations of several causative agents[20].

During the past few years, significant advances have been achieved with regard to the pathophysiology of the stress response to cognitive (emotional, etc.) and non-cognitive stimulus (infections, physical exercise, surgery, etc.)[21-24]. As a result of these developments, a new area of science, which has been named psychoneuroimmunology, is emerging. The explanation for this development lies fundamentally upon studies which have confirmed close connections among the psychic, neuroendocrinologic and immunologic "compartments"[21,23]. It can be assumed that the central nervous system (CNS) orchestrates the response to possible threats to the organism. This is made possible by the nerve endings and humoral factors acting at a distance. The higher centers of the CNS receive and process the cognitive stimulus and act on the hypothalamus so that it can produce corticotropin releasing hormone (CRH). The latter in turn induces the anterior hypophysis to produce proopiomelanocortin (POMC). The POMC is a polyprotein that gives rise to various biologically active peptides by enzymatic fragmentation[25-28]. Among these peptides are ACTH and beta-endorphin. ACTH is known to act on the suprarenal cortex which liberates cortisol. Until now, beta-endorphin that is liberated equimolarly with ACTH by the hypophysis, does not have an identified target organ nor a known dominant action. Recent evidences suggest that beta-endorphin has a role in immunomodulation at the peripheral level[29-33]. In the CNS, beta-endorphin and its derivatives, alpha and gamma-endorphin, have important actions on behavioral homeostasis, notably in the response to stress. The hypothalamus also controls the autonomic nervous system, which in turn, governs the liberation of catecholamines and enkephalins by the suprarenal medulla as a response to stress[34]. The enkephalins (met and leu-enkephalin) are peptide opioids made up of 5 aminoacids that derive from the gene of the preproenkephalin which is phylogenetically related to the POMC. The enkephalins do not have a target organ. "In vitro" and "in vivo" studies have demonstrated that they have important actions on immunocompetent cells[35-38]. Thus, the stress axis, in addition to liberating cortisol and catecholamines by the suprarenal cortex and medulla respectively, has another pathway. This recently recognized pathway originates in the anterior hypophysis with the liberation of beta-endorphin and in the suprarenal medulla with the release of enkephalins (Figure 1). This pathway exerts potent actions on the immune system.

Many studies using human and animal models have shown that stress can alter immunity, in some cases giving rise to the appearance of infections, or the reactivation or appearance "de novo" of tumors[39-47]. Thus, it has been shown that there is a decrease in the proliferative response of lymphocytes to mitogens

Figure 1

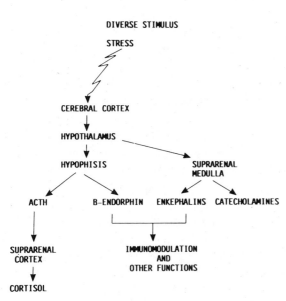

The stress axis.

in subjects during bereavement[39]. Other studies have demonstrated that such effects on the immune system depend on one's capacity to accept or handle the stressful situation. Women, for example, who have suffered a miscarriage and who have not accepted this event, present a significant reduction in the response of their T lymphocytes to mitogens, while those who are capable of accepting this situation do not present the same alterations[48]. Experiments in rats with avoidable and non-avoidable painful stimulus have provided similar results[47]. A complete agreement among the various authors does not exist as to the possible CNS mediators that produce this immunomodulation in response to stress. It is known that lymphocytes possess receptors for diverse neurotransmitters and hormones[49-54]. The experiments of Shavit and co-workers[32] published in 1984 showed that the observed suppression of the natural killer (NK) cell activity in rats subjected to a non-avoidable painful stimulus was mediated by peptide opioids. In addition, it was shown that the suppression could be blocked by an opioid antagonist, naltrexone, and could be reproduced with the administration of morphine. From this work, it can be deduced that it may be possible for the opioid peptides liberated endogenously during stress to induce the supression of NK cell activity by acting on the receptors on the surface of the lymphocytes. Other pieces of work have shown the various actions that the opioid peptides have "in vitro" on the diverse functions and cellular subtypes of the immune system[37,38,55-57]. Divergent results, however, have been communicated and it seems possible that there exists more than one receptor for the opioid peptides on the surface of the immunocompetent cells: mu and delta. In addition, it appears that a peptide like beta-endorphin, which is made up of 31 aminoacids can act on one or another receptor depending on the side of the molecule which couples to the receptor. It is also possible that the cellular condition (non-activated or activated) may influence these effects.

It has been observed that immunocompetent cells produce, under diverse stimulus, hormones and peptide opioids[58-62]. At the same time, lymphokines produced during the activation of the immune system may act on the hypothalamus, activating the stress axis[63,64]. These findings thus complete the connections between the nervous and the immune system[21].

Diverse immunological alterations have been demonstrated in subjects with CFS. In those patients, serological positivities to various viruses (Epstein-Barr, herpes simplex, cytomegalovirus, coxsackie, human herpes virus-6) have also been found[6-8,10,11,65]. However, the available evidence indicates that none of these viruses could be implicated as a single causative agent of CFS. Therefore, it is tempting to speculate that immunological alterations can favor their activation or chronification of viral infections. Interestingly, the same patients suspected of suffering viral infections, exhibit psychic disorders such as anxiety, insomnia and depression which constitute a situation of marked stress, that in turn might induce immunosuppression.

All these data suggest that opioid peptides can play a role in immune disorders. They may also be secondarily involved in the activation of viral infections in patients with CFS.

We thus studied several immunologic parameters in patients with CFS. We specifically concentrated our study on the monocyte because it is a key cell in the immune system[66-69]. Monocytes are responsible for the presentation of antigens to lymphocytes during the development of specific immunity. They act as accessory cells, in part, through the liberation of soluble factors. They also participate in defence against infections through the phagocytosis and destruction of invasive organisms and the release of a great amount of factors involved in immunity and inflammation (Figure 2). It has also been proven that they possess antitumoral activity. Monocytes and macrophages exhibit a dense skeleton of intermediate filaments composed of vimentin monomer[70,71]. The intermediate filaments establish functional connections between the plasmalemma and the nucleolemma. It is believed that they are important in cellular motility[72]. The coupling and organization of the intermediate filaments depend on the phosphorylation of vimentin[73], a process that is subject to hormonal regulation[74-75].

examined their effects on the phagocytosis of Candida albicans and on the expression of membrane molecules[76]. The three opioid peptides at concentrations of 10^{-6}, 10^{-8} and 10^{-10} M, markedly reduced the expression of ir-vimentin filaments, the phagocytic activity and the surface expression of molecules HLA-DR (Figure 3). On the other hand, the intravenous administration of fentanyl, a synthetic opiate agonist, to patients subjected to coronary surgery, induced similar changes on the monocytes. In other experiments, beta-endorphin at a concentration of 10^{-8} M decreased the expression of CR3 molecules but did not influence the expression of CD13, a surface protein whose function is not known. The expression of vimentin filaments was directly correlated with that of HLA-DR and CR3 molecules, and with the phagocytic activity.

Figure 2

Figure 3a

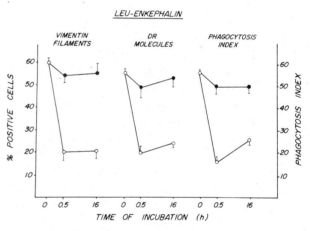

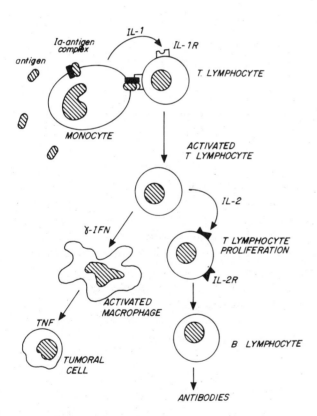

Monocyte functions in the immune response.

Figure 3b

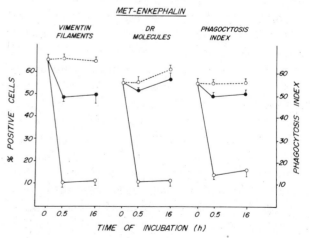

In an earlier study, we evaluated "in vitro" the action of beta-endorphin, met-enkephalin and leu-enkephalin on the expression of the immunoreactive cytoskeletal vimentin filaments by monocytes using immunofluorescence technique. We simultaneously

These results indicate that these opioid peptides and the opiates depress the phagocytic activity of the monocytes, as well as the expression of the intermediate vimentin filaments and the surface molecules such as HLA-DR and CR3. As the mentioned effects are blocked by naloxone, it is postulated that these actions take place through a mechanism mediated by an opioid receptor. It is known that monocytes present opioid receptors mu and delta. The maximum effect of met-enkephalin and leu-enkephalin is reached between 30 and 90 minutes, while that of beta-endorphin takes place after 16 hours. This may mean that they act on distinct receptors. The enkephalins have a greater affinity for receptors delta, while the beta-endorphin acts more at the mu. In addition, naloxone only partially blocks the actions of beta-endorphin. This suggests that it simultaneously acts on a receptor that is not a classic opioid receptor. Hazum and co-workers reported that lymphocytes possess non-opioid specific receptors for beta-endorphin[52].

Since the intermediate filaments play a very important role in the expression of membrane molecules and receptors, this probably explains the close cor-

relation between the expression of ir-vimentin filaments, the phagocytic activity and the expression of HLA-DR and CR3 molecules. In fact, it has been demonstrated at the level of the neuromuscular junction that the cytoskeleton is important in the maintenance of receptors in the post synaptic membrane[77]. The exact mechanisms by which the opioids can act on the coupling and uncoupling of the vimentin filaments are not yet known. They might act on vimentin phosphorylation, a reaction that is very sensitive to humoral influences. Since vimentin kinase, which is responsible for phosphorylation of vimentin, is identical to neurofilament kinase[78], it might be speculated that the actions of opioids on the CNS might also implicate cytoskeletal changes. The opioid concentrations which have been used in our experiments can be found in physiological situations such as in response to stress. This may indicate that our findings have more than just pharmacological implications.

At least some cases of CFS are possibly due to chronic viral infections. It is also possible that stress could have contributed to the development of this clinical condition. We thus studied the possible existence of an immunological disregulation in these patients. As we have commented before, stress is known to be capable of inducing immunodepression that can reactivate viral infections and facilitate the appearance of tumors[41].

We studied the monocyte function in 35 consecutive patients with CFS, diagnosed in our center, and in 25 healthy controls[16]. In 85% of the patients with CFS, we found a monocyte dysfunction characterized by a marked reduction in the number of monocytes that express ir-vimentin filaments, a decreased index of phagocytosis and a reduced expression of HLA-DR antigens. These values markedly increased after the incubation of the monocytes with naloxone (Figure 4). We also observed other immunological alterations in these patients such as a decrease in the blastogenic response of the lymphocytes and a decrease in the number of monocytes expressing receptors for the Fc portion of IgG (FcR) and the C3b (CR1). These findings suggest that an increased opioid activity acting through a classic receptor mechanism is present in a high percentage of patients with CFS. As we have seen opioid peptides are capable of producing similar

Figure 3c

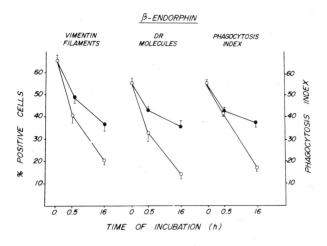

Leu-enkephalin (Fig. 3a), met-enkephalin (Fig. 3b) and beta-endorphin (Fig. 3c) reduce the expression of vimentin filaments, the phagocytic activity and the display of DR molecules in monocytes. The figures reflect the results after 0,5 and 16 h. of incubation with the opioid peptide at 10⁻⁸ M concentration with (darkened circles) or without (empty circles) addition of 10⁻⁸ M naloxone. None of the variables was significantly modified in the control suspensions of monocytes (empty circles connected by broken line in Fig. 3a).

Figure 4

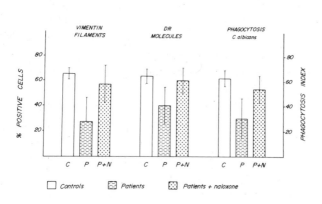

Naloxone-reversible monocyte dysfunction in CFS. Differ-ences are statistically significant (p< 0,001) between controls and patients for all parameters. Studies were done using suspensions of purified monocytes from healthy controls and patients, in the presence or absence of naloxone. Naloxone induced in patients a significant elevation of all monocyte parameters.

Table 1

Symptoms	Number of Patients	(%)
Chronic fatigue	30	100
Painful muscle tension	30	100
(tension headache and/or backache		
Sleep disorders	27	90
Difficulty in concentration	27	90
Resltessness, anxiety	24	80
Abdominal pain	22	73.3
Depression	21	70
Myalgia	20	66.6
Constipation	16	53.3
Migraine	16	50
Low-grade fever	15	50
Arthralgia	15	50
Sore throat	12	40
Frequent sensation of cold	12	40
Recurrent oral aphthous ulcers	9	30
Painful lymph nodes		
(cervical or axillar region)	5	16.6
Recurrent herpes infection	3	10

actions" in vitro". The circulating levels of ir-beta-endorphin in patients with CFS were similar to those of the healthy group. However, the liberation of beta-endorphin follows a circadian rhythm. Thus, it cannot be excluded that these patients exhibit an increase in the total quantity of beta-endorphin liberated within 24 hours. Likewise, it cannot be excluded that the effects observed "in vivo" can be mediated by enkephalins or by the autocrine or paracrine action of the opioid peptides released by the monocytes and lymphocytes themselves. In fact, it has been shown that some viruses act as stimulus for the production of opioid peptides by the lym-phocytes and monocytes[62]. Perhaps, the infection of immunocompetent cells in patients with CFS by some viruses (Epstein-Barr, human herpesvirus-6) may play a role in these alterations[79,80]. As mono-cytes have important antiviral actions and play a crucial role in the activation of lymphocytes, the monocyte dysfunction mediated by opioids can be responsible for the diminution in blastogenesis and facilitate the reactivation of latent viral infections. In a group of 44 patients meeting criteria for CFS[1], we found a prevalence of seropositivities for human herpes virus-6 significantly elevated as compared to controls. In this same study, we failed

to observe differences in serologic titers against Epstein-Barr virus capsid antigen between CFS patients and controls. It is thus possible that herpes virus-6, a new member of the herpes family, might be implicated in the pathogenesis of CFS[81]. In fact, many of the symptoms observed in our patients with CFS have been described in patients with chronic infections by a variety of viruses. On the other hand, the presence of patients with recurrent herpes zoster, herpes labialis and oral ulcers in our series (Table 1) suggests that the reactivation of latent viral infections may play a role in the patho-genesis of CFS.

We have also described a monocyte dysfunction in patients with major unipolar depression which was similarly reversible with naloxone[82]. It is well known that immunologic alterations exist in some patients with depression[43]. An increase in the levels of beta-endorphin has also been described in these patients[83]. This could also explain the alterations in the activation of T lymphocytes in this syndrome.

The immunologic alterations induced by opioid pep-tides in patients with CFS suggest that various factors can be implicated in the etiopathogenesis of

Figure 5

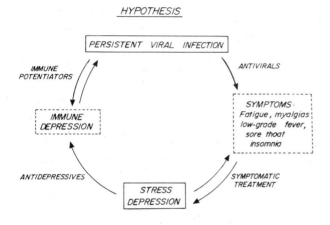

Unifying hypothesis of the CFS.

this syndrome. This has led us to develop an integrated hypothesis that is reflected in Figure 5.

In our hypothesis, psychophysical stress may initiate the CFS in a considerable number of cases. We propose that there are two possible efferent pathways of the stress (Figure 6). The first one, or pathway "A", may be initiated when the stressful situation is perceived as avoidable. In this case the neuroendocrine response would mainly involve the production of ACTH-cortisol and cathecolamines. This biologic response is orientated to activity, locomotion and fighting, and the pathological consequence would be coronary artery disease. The second pathway, or pathway "B", would occur when the stressor setting is perceived as unavoidable. In this case the neuroendocrine reaction would mainly include beta-endorphin and enkephalins production. The result would be immunosuppression, infections and depression, with the pathological consequence being CFS. Probably the naloxone-reversible monocyte dysfunction reflects this last stress reaction pathway.

Figure 6

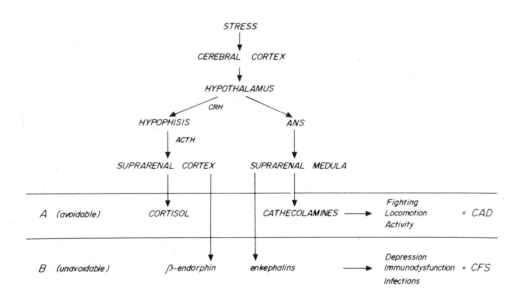

Types of stress response. Type A: Stress perceived as avoidable involves ACTH, cortisol and cathecolamines, and is oriented to fighting and activity. Its pathological consequence would be coronary artery disease (CAD). Type B: Stress perceived as unavoidable involves beta-endorphin and enkephalins. The result of this response would be depression, immunosuppression and infections. The pathological consequence would be the CFS and its biological and diagnostic marker the naloxone-reversible monocyte dysfunction.

References

1. Holmes GP, Kaplan JE, Gantz NM, et al. Chronic fatigue syndrome: a working case definition. Ann Intern Med 1988;108:387.

2. Lloyd AR, Wakefield D, Boughton C, Dwyer J. What is myalgic encephalomyelitis? Lancet 1988;i:1286.

3. Manu P, Lane TJ, Matthews DA. The frequency of the chronic fatigue syndrome in patients with symptoms of persistent fatigue. Ann Intern Med 1988;109:554.

4. Kroenke K, Wood DR, Mangelsclorff AD, et al. Chronic fatigue in primary care. Prevalence, patient characteristics and outcome. JAMA 1988;260:929.

5. Straus SE. The chronic mononucleosis syndrome. J Infect Dis 1988;157:405.

6. Straus SE. EB or not EB. That is the question. JAMA 1987;257:2335.

7. Bell EJ, McCartney RA, Riding MH, et al. Coxsackie B viruses and myalgic encephalomyelitis. J R Soc Med 1988;81:329.

8. Kneger GRF, Koch B, Ablashi DV. Persistent fatigue and depression in a patient with antibody to human B lymphotropic virus. Lancet 1987;ii:36.

9. Behan P, Behan W, Bell E. The postviral fatigue syndrome: an analysis of the findings in 50 cases. J Infec 1985;10:211.

10. Holmes GP, Kaplan JE, Stewart JA, Hunt B, Pinsky PF, Schonberger LB. A cluster of patients with a chronic mononucleosis-like syndrome: is Epstein-Barr virus the cause? JAMA 1987;257:2297.

11. Jones JF, Ray CG, Minnich LL, Hicks MJ, Kibler R, Lucas DO. Evidence for active Epstein-Barr virus infection in patients with persistent, unexplained illnesses: elevated anti-early antigen antibodies. Ann Intern Med 1985;102:1.

12. Straus SE, Tosato G, Armstrong G, et al. Persisting illness and fatigue in adults with evidence of Epstein-Barr virus infection. Ann Intern Med 1985;102:7.

13. Tobi M, Morag A, Ravid Z, et al. Prolonged atypical illness associated with serological evidence of persistent Epstein-Barr virus infection. Lancet 1982;i:61.

14. Tosato G, Straus S, Heule HE, et al. Characteristic T cell dysfunction in patients with chronic active Epstein-Barr virus infection (chronic infectious mononucleosis). J Immunol 1985;134:3082.

15. Subirá ML, Castilla A, Civeira MP, Prieto J. Deficient display of CD3 on lymphocytes of patients with chronic fatigue syndrome. J Infect Dis 1989;160:165.

16. Prieto J, Subirá ML, Castilla A, Serrano M. Naloxone-reversible monocyte dysfunction in patients with chronic fatigue syndrome. Scand J Immunol 1989;30:13.

17. Caligiuri M, Murray C, Buchwald D, et al. Phenotypic and functional deficiency of natural killer cells in patients with chronic fatigue syndrome. J Immunol 1987;139:3306.

18. Schindler BA. Stress, affective disorders, and immune function. Med Clin North Am 1985;69:585.

19. Stein M, Keller SE, Schleifer SJ. Stress and immunomodulation: the role of depression and neuroendocrine function. J Immunol 1985;135(2):827s.

20. Prieto J, Camps J, Castilla A. El síndrome de astenia crónica. In **Avances en medicina interna**. Pp:159-178 Aran Eds. 1989.

21. Blalock JE, Smith EM. A complete regulatory loop between the immune and neuroendocrine systems. Fed Proc 1985;44:108.

22. Ballieux RE, Heijnen CJ. Brain and immune system: a one-way conversation or a genuine dialogue?. In Progress in brain research. Vol 72. De Kloet ER, Wiegant VM, De Wied D Eds. 1987. Elsevier Science Publishers BV.

23. Blalock JE, Smith EM. The immune system: our mobile brain? Immunol Today 1985;6:115.

24. Blalock JE, Smith EM, Meyer III WJ. The pituitary-adrenocortical axis and the immune system. Clin Endocrinol Metab 1985;14:1021.

25. Lynch DR, Snyder SH. Neuropeptides: multiple molecular forms, metabolic pathways and receptors. Ann Rev Biochem 1986;55:773.

26. Cotman CW, Brinton RE, Galaburda A, McEwen B, Schneider DM. **The neuro-immune-endocrine connection**. 1st edn. Raven Press. New York. 1987.

27. Fraioli F, Moretti C, Paolucci D, Alicicco E, Crescenzi F, Fortunio G. Physical exercise stimulates marked concomitant release of beta-endorphin and adrenocorticotrophic hormone (ACTH) in peripheral blood in man. Experientia 1980;36:987.

28. Guillemin R, Vargo J, Rossier J, et al. Beta-endorphin and adreno-corticotrophin are secreted concomitantly by the pituitary gland. Science 1977;197:1367.

29. Brown SL, Van Epps DE. Supression of T lymphocyte chemotactic factor production by the opioid peptides beta-endorphin and met-enkephalin. J Immunol 1985;134:3384.

30. Chang K-J. Opioid peptides have actions on the immune system. Trends Neurosci 1984;7:234.

31. Shavit Y, Terman GW, Martin FC, Lewis JW, Liebeskind JC, Gale RP. Stress, opioid peptides, the immune system, and cancer. J Immunol 1985;135:834.

32. Shavit Y, Lewis JW, Terman GW, Gale RP, Liebeskind JC. Opioid peptides mediate the suppressive effect of stress on natural killer cell cytotoxicity. Science 1984;223:188.

33. McCain HW, Lamster IB, Bozzone JM, Grbic JT. Beta-endorphin modulates human immune activity via non-opiate receptor mechanisms. Life Sci 1982;31:1619.

34. Lewis JW, Tordoff MG, Sherman JE, Liebeskind JC. Adrenal medullary enkephalin-like peptides may mediate stress analgesia. Science 1982;217:557.

35. Miller GC, Murgo AJ, Plotnikoff NP. The influence of leucine and methionine enkephalins on immune mechanisms. Int J Immunopharmacol 1982;4:367.

36. Plotnikoff NP, Faith RE, Murgo AJ, Good RA. Enkephalins and endorphins. **Stress and the immune system.** 1st edn. Plenum Press. New York. 1986.

37. Plotnikoff NP, Murgo AJ, Miller GC, Corder CN, Faith RE. Enkephalins: immunomodulators. Fed Proc 1985;44:118.

38. Wybran J. Enkephalins and endorphins as modifiers of the immune system: present and future. Fed Proc 1985;44:92.

39. Bartrop RW, Lazarus L, Lockhurst E, et al. Depressed lymphocyte function after bereavement. Lancet 1977;i:834.

40. Jemmot JB, Borysenko M, Chapman R, et al. Academic stress, power motivation, and decrease in secretion rate of salivary secretory immunoglobulin A. Lancet 1983;i:1400.

41. Editorial. Depression, stress and immunity. Lancet 1987;i:1467.

42. Jones DR, Goldblatt PO, Leon DA. Bereavement and cancer. Br Med J 1984;289:461.

43. Kronfol Z, Silva J, Greden J, et al. Impaired lymphocyte function in depressive illness. Life Sci 1983;33:241.

44. Tecoma ES, Huey LY. Psychic distress and the immune response. Life Sci 1985;36:1799.

45. Riley V. Psychoneuroendocrine influences on immunocompetence and neoplasia. Science 1981;212:1100.

46. Lewis JW, Shavit Y, Terman GW, Nelson LR, Gale RP, Liebeskind JC. Apparent involvement of opioid peptides in stress induced enhancement of tumor growth. Peptides 1983;4:635.

47. Visintainer MA, Volpicelli JR, Seligman ME. Tumor rejection in rats after inescapable or escapable shock. Science 1982;216:437.

48. Samuel D, Naor S, Pecht M, Trainin N. Bereavement and the immune system: the effect of the loss of an unborn child on mitogenic stimulation of T cells. Proc International workshop on neuroimmunomodulation. Dubrovnik. June 1986.

49. Lopker A, Abood LG, Hoss W, Lionetti FJ. Steroselective muscarinic acetylcholine and opiate receptors in human phagocytic leukocytes. Biochem Pharmacol 1980;29:1361.

50. Wybran J, Appelbloom T, Famely J-F, Govaerts A. Suggestive evidence for receptors for morphine and methionine-enkephalin on normal human blood T lymphocytes. J Immunol 1979;123:1068.

51. Carr DJJ, Kim CH, De Costa B, Jacobson AE, Rice KC, Blalock JE. Evidence for delta-class opioid receptors on cells of the immune system. Cell Immunol 1988;116:44.

52. Hazum E, Chang K-J, Cuatrecasas P. Specific non-opiate receptors for beta-endorphin. Science 1979;205:1033.

53. Blalock JE, Harbour-McMenamin D, Smith EM. Peptide hormones shared by the neuroendocrine and immunologic systems. J Immunol 1985;135:858.

54. McDonough RJ, Madden JJ, Falek A, et al. Alteration of T and null lymphocyte frequencies in the peripheral blood of human opiate addicts; in vivo evidence for opiate receptor sites on T lymphocytes. J Immunol 1980;125:2539.

55. Peterson PK, Sharp B, Gekker G, Brummitt C, Keane WF. Opioid-mediated suppression of interferon-gamma production by cultured peripheral blood mononuclear cells. J Clin Invest 1987;80:824.

56. Sharp BM, Keane WF, Suh HJ, Gekker G, Tsukayama D, Peterson PK. Opioid peptides rapidly stimulate superoxide production by human polymorphonuclear leucocytes and macrophages. Endocrinology 1985;117:793.

57. Brown SL, Van Epps DE. Opioid peptides modulate production of interferon-gamma by human mononuclear cells. Cell Immunol 1986;103:19.

58. Lolait SJ, Clements JA, Markwick AJ, et al. Proopiomelanocortin messenger ribonucleic acid and posttranslational processing of beta-endorphin in spleen macrophages. J Clin Invest 1986;77:1776.

59. Lolait SJ, Lim ATW, Toh BH, Funder JW. Immunoreactive beta-endorphin in a subpopulation of mouse spleen macrophages. J Clin Invest 1984;73:277.

60. Smith EM, Blalock JE. Human lymphocyte production of corticotropin and endorphin-like substances: association with leukocyte interferon. Proc Natl Acad Sci USA 1981;78:7530.

61. Harbour-McMenamin D, Smith EM, Blalock JE. B lymphocyte enriched populations produce immunoreactive endorphin that binds to delta opiate receptors and may play a role in endotoxic shock. In Puett D, Ahmad F, Black S, Lopez DM, Meiner MH, Scott WA, Whelan WJ Eds. Advances in gene technology: molecular biology of the endocrine system. 1st edn. Pp:378-379. Cambridge University Press. Cambridge 1986.

62. Westly HJ, Kleiss AJ, Kelley KW, Wong PKY, Yuen P-H. Newcastle disease virus-infected splenocytes express the proopiomelanocortin gene. J Exp Med 1986;163:1589.

63. Woloski BMRNJ, Smith EM, Meyer III WJ, et al. Corticotropin-releasing activity of monokines. Science 1985;230:1035.

64. Oppenheim JJ, Gery I. Interleukin 1 is more than an interleukin. Immunol Today 1982;3:113.

65. Yousef GE, Bell EJ, Mann GP, et al. Chronic enterovirus infection in patients with postviral fatigue syndrome. Lancet 1988;i:146.

66. Unanue ER, Allen PM. The basis for the immunoregulatory role of macrophages and other accessory cells. Science 1987;236:551.

67. Morahan PS, Connor JR, Leary KR. Viruses and the versatile macrophage. Br Med Bull 1985;41:15.

68. Johnston RB. Monocytes and macrophages. N Engl J Med 1988;318:747.

69. Shevach EM. Macrophages and other accessory cells. In Paul WE Ed. Fundamental immunology. Pp:71-107. Raven Press. New York 1984.

70. Lazarides E. Intermediate filaments as mechanical integrators of cellular space. Nature 1980;283:249.

71. Geiger B. Intermediate filaments. Looking for a function. Nature 1987;329:392.

72. Wang E, Michel J, Pfeffer LM, Silverstein SC, Tamm I. Interferon suppresses pinocytosis but stimulates phagocytosis in mouse peritoneal macrophages: related changes in cytoskeletal organization. J Cell Biol 1984;98:1328.

73. Inagaki M, Nishi Y, Nishizawa K, Matsuyana M, Sato C. Site-specific phosphorylation induces disassembly of vimentin filaments in vitro. Nature 1987;328:649.

74. Coca-Prados M. Regulation of protein phosphorylation of the intermediate-sized filament vimentin in the ciliary epithelium of the mammalian eye. J Biol Chem 1985;260:10332.

75. Browning ET, Sanders MM. Vimentin: a phosphoprotein under hormonal regulation. J Cell Biol 1981;90:803.

76. Prieto J, Subirá ML, Castilla A, Arroyo JL, Serrano M. Opioid peptides modulate the organization of vimentin filaments, phagocytic activity and expression of surface molecules in monocytes. Scand J Immunol 1989;29:391.

77. Frochner SC. The role of the postsynaptic cytoskeleton in AchR organization. Trends Neurosci 1986;9:37.

78. Toru-Delbauffe D, Pierre M, Osty J, Chantoux F, Francon J. Properties of neurofilament protein kinase. Biochem J 1986;235:283.

79. Prieto J, Castilla A, Subirá ML, Serrano M, Morte S, Civeira MP. Cytoskeletal organization and functional changes in monocytes from patients with chronic hepatitis B: relationship with viral replication. Hepatology 1989;9:720.

80. Chen M, Goorha R, Murti G. Interaction of frog virus 3 with the cytomatrix: IV. Phosphorylation of vimentin precedes the reorganization of intermediate filaments aroud the virus assembly sites. J Gen Virol 1986;67:915.

81. Cuende JI, Civeira MP, Riezu-Boj JI, Castilla A, Prieto J. Virus herpes humano tipo 6 y síndrome de astenia crónica. Med Clin (Barc) 1990 (in press).

82. Castilla A, Subirá ML, Camps J, et al. Disfunción monocitaria inducida por opioides en pacientes con depresión y ansiedad. An Med Intern (Madrid) 1988; suppl III:132.

83. Genezzani AR, Petralgia F, Sinforani E, et al. Dysregulation of plasma pro-opiomelanocortin-related peptides in neurotic depression. Acta Endocrinol 1986;112:1.

Chapter 63

Paired Age, Sex and Ethnically Matched Studies of Peripheral Blood Leucocyte Profiles in Early Chronic Fatigue Syndrome.

Michael J. Holmes, MD

Christopher J. Chapman, Alistair J. Young, John P. Cross, PhD and Brian E. Niven

University of Otago Dunedin NEW ZEALAND. Correspondence to: Dr. M. J. Holmes, Senior Lecturer, Department of Microbiology, University of Otago Medical School P.O. Box 56, Dunedin, New Zealand.

(Please see Chapter 33 for Dr. Holmes' photograph and curriculum vitae.)

Summary

Peripheral blood leucocytes from 30 'early' CFS patients paired, and age, sex and ethnically matched with healthy controls were phenotyped using a range of enzyme and fluorescein-conjugated monoclonal antibodies. Differential white cell counts using a Technicon H6000/C analyser and FACScan analyses revealed depleted basophil and T helper cell populations and increased numbers of large unstained cells (LUC) (including activated lymphocytes) and natural killer cell (HNK) in CFS patients. Reversed T helper/inducer : suppressor/cytotoxic ratios were present in 60% of subjects. Correlations were established between severity of symptoms and depletion of HNK cells, and the augmentation of LUC's, activated macrophages, total lymphocytes and T cells. In a second group of 20 CFS patients with a wider range of duration of symptoms, a positive correlation was established between recovery of T helper cell numbers and time.

Introduction

The aetiology of chronic fatigue syndrome (CFS) is still obscure and studies which have concentrated on implicating microbes isolated from sufferers as a direct cause of the condition have proved less than satisfactory. Isolates from different outbreaks differ widely and usually it has been difficult to match their known characteristics with observed symptoms[1-5]. These isolates do have one thing in common however; they all fall broadly into the category of 'opportunistic infections'. Furthermore, a significant portion of CFS cases develop following an acute virus infection[6]. It has also been pointed out that the symptoms of CFS bear a startling resemblance to those of interferon poisoning[7,8] and a high proportion of patients suffer bowel allergies.

The circumstantial evidence therefore suggests an underlying immune disturbance and this has been borne out by a number of cytological and serological studies[8-15]. Until recently, however, many of them have offered anecdotal and often conflicting evidence of immune disequilibria. Some of the differences can be reconciled if it is accepted that the immunocytological profile of CFS changes and develops during the course of the disease and the situation would be further improved if the various investigating teams agreed on matching terms of reference. But major inconsistencies remain.

It has been our experience that the presentation of CFS findings generates a more opinionated response than in any other field we have studied. Every report in the literature appears to have its detractors, seeking to discredit the work on grounds of observer bias and inadequate or mismatched control groups. This is not altogether surprising. The observed changes are minimal and, while means may differ significantly between study and control groups, the majority of values tend to lie within physiological limits. In addition, the criteria upon which a clinical diagnosis is based are by no means universal. Finally, the nature of the disease is such that there is an ever-present risk of the findings being distorted by misdiagnosed patients taking part in clinical studies.

Before any work is likely to be accepted as definitive it is therefore essential, in view of these constraints, that the most extreme precautions are taken in experimental design. Inevitably, studies dealing with human volunteer subjects will fall short of this ideal but this paper represents an attempt to observe the immunocytology of 'early' CFS with minimised bias and using the closest matching feasible in the control group.

Materials and Methods
Subjects

Group 1

Thirty subjects with CFS, 20 female and 10 male, were selected from a pool of 76 volunteers living in the district of Otago, New Zealand. All had either been diagnosed as cases of CFS by their general practitioner or had been referred to us via the Department of General Practice of the Otago Medical School. Ages ranged from 13 to 51 with a mean of 28.6 years. The study group was selected primarily on the basis of a relatively short history of disease (mean duration 1.92 years), however, it included 4 patients who had suffered from the condition for between 3 and 5 years and who had reported recent exacerbations. Cases were ranked in apparent order of clinical severity. Although in 3 cases the clinical diagnosis was felt to be in doubt, the subjects were still accepted to avoid compromising the criterion of an 'external' diagnosis of CFS as the qualifying requirement. The criteria used for clinical ranking within the study group include most of those proposed by Holmes[16] but with variations in emphasis, notably in our assignation of a primary role to muscle fatigue. In this respect we favour the clinical definition of Ramsay[17].

Healthy control subjects were recruited from amongst the students and staff (or their families) of the University of Otago. Pairing was randomised by allotting control subjects in each age and sex-cohort to patients in chronological order of sampling. The majority of pairs were matched to within 1 year and in no case did the age difference exceed 4 years.

Group 2

A second group of 20 volunteers, 12 female and 8 male, from the same pool of patients, took part in an earlier phase of these studies. Duration of symptoms ranged from 6 months to 6 years with a mean of 3.2 years. Ages ranged from 14 to 52 with a mean of 31 years. This group was not paired, but compared with a group of 10 healthy controls, half of whom were female and whose ages ranged from 20 to 46 with a mean of 26 years.

Cell Samples

Group 1

Two 5 ml peripheral venous blood samples were taken from the antecubital vein between 11 am and midday to minimise circadian variations[18]. The first was reserved for a full blood count, carried out using a Technicon H6000/C analyser at Dunedin Public Hospital. Nine 100 µl aliquots of whole blood were dispensed from the second sample, the erythrocytes flash-lysed and the leucocytes pelleted and washed twice in Fluorescent Activated Cell Sorter (FACScan) diluent (0.1% BSA, 0.1% sodium azide in isotonic PBS). Each aliquot was then incubated in the dark for 30 minutes with 1 of 9 antiphenotypic mouse anti-human monoclonal antibodies (table 1), washed and subsequently labelled with fluorescein isothiocyanate (FITC) tagged rabbit anti-mouse antibody for 30 minutes. Specimens were then washed and fixed in 0.6% paraformaldehyde, coded, randomised, stored at 4°C in the dark and analysed by FACScan within 2 weeks of preparation. Preparation of FACScan specimens was carried out by observers who had no access to the clinical histories.

FACScan Analysis

All specimens were analysed by 5000 event dot-plots, gated either for lymphocytes or macrophages. Negative controls for the samples from each subject were provided by a mouse anti-rat peritoneal macrophage antibody (1644). Results were expressed as number of cells 10^9/l. The FACScan analyses were carried out blind in a random sequence of control and clinical subjects by a separate observer.

Group 2

Peripheral blood leucocytes from subjects in the pilot group were identified by immunoperoxidase labelling since the FACS was not then available. The same battery of monoclonal antibodies were used but in this case tagged with 1:300 peroxidase-conjugated F(ab') rabbit-anti-mouse immunoglobulin (Dako). Mononuclear cells were separated on Ficoll-Conray interfaces, cytocentrifuged on to glass slides, then prepared and stained according to the method of Moir and colleagues[19].

Figure 1

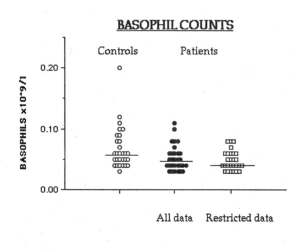

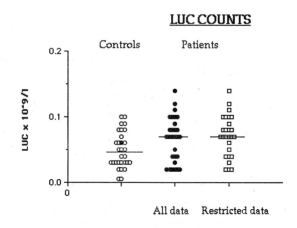

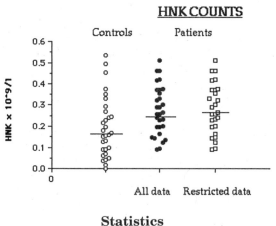

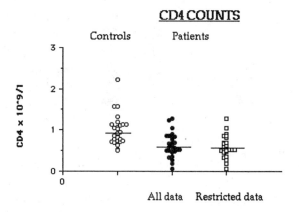

Statistics

Group 1

Paired data were analysed using the Wilcoxon signed-rank test. Two data sets were considered, the full study group and a second set in which the 3 clinically aberrant cases were omitted. As a cross-check and an indication of whether age and sex were relevant variables, an unpaired analysis was carried out using the Mann-Whitney U-test. In addition, Spearman Rank correlation coefficients were established for age, duration of symptoms and perceived clinical severity against the full range of cytological data for males and females in the control and patient groups.

Group 2

The pilot data were analysed by the Mann-Whitney U-test and a Spearman Rank correlation coefficient was established for the duration of symptoms against T helper/T cytotoxic suppressor (CD_4/CD_8) cell ratios.

Group 1

Total Counts. Control group values corresponded well with accepted physiological ranges. No significant differences were observed between patient and control groups in numbers of total leucocytes, neutrophils, total lymphocytes, monocytes or eosinophils.

Two significant differences were observed, namely a decrease in basophils ($p = 0.0126$) and an increase in 'large unstained cells' (LUC) ($p = 0.0457$) in the CFS group. The degree of significance was accentuated in both cases when the 3 clinically aberrant subjects were omitted ($p = 0.0036$ and 0.0159), and even by unpaired analysis the differences were still significant ($p = 0.011$ in both cases) (Figs. 1 and 2).

Mononuclear Cells. No significant differences were observed between groups for total T cells, (CD_2) mature T cells, (CD_3) cytotoxic/suppressor (CD_8) cells,

Figure 2A & 2B

WILCOXON SIGNED RANK TESTS

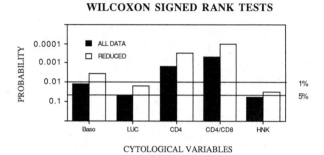

Figure 3

DEPRESSION OF THE CD4/CD8 RATIO

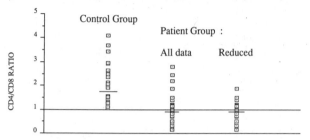

Fig. 2B

MANN-WHITNEY U-TESTS

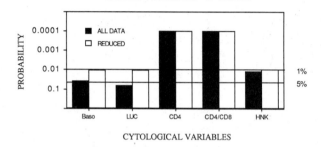

Spearman Rank coefficients

No relationships significant at the 5% level emerged in the control group between age or sex and any of the 18 cytological criteria. Including both patient groups, a total of 19 out of 228 rank coefficients were significant at the 5% level when age, sex or severity of symptoms were compared with each of the cytological criteria.

Correlations with Age: In the full study group, males tended to have reduced numbers of neutrophils (p = 0.0108) and monocytes (p = 0.0163) and also fewer activated (DR+) lymphocytes (p = 0.0245) and DR+ Mø (p = 0.033) with increasing age, although their HNK numbers tended to be higher (p = 0.0417). These relationships were not sustained amongst female patients, where only the eosinophil counts appeared to decrease with age (p = 0.045), When the 3 aberrant cases were omitted, the relationship of increasing age in males with reduced numbers of neutrophils was sustained (p = 0.028) and so were those of DR+ lymphocytes (p = 0.0149) and DR+ Mø (p = 0.0208). Two new correlations also appeared, an increase in B cell numbers (p = 0.0149) and a decrease in monocytes (p = 0.0138). Neither of these was reflected in the female patients. (Fig. 4).

Correlations with Duration of Symptoms: There were no correlations between any data set and duration of symptoms. The relative uniformity of the group did not, however, lend itself easily to demonstrating relationships of this type.

Correlations with Severity of Symptoms: This group contained the correlates most likely to be of clinical significance. In the full study group, males

activated lymphocytes carrying HLA-DR markers, B cells, macrophages (Mø) or activated macrophages (DR+Mø). Only one significant difference was observed in the full study group, namely a decrease in T helper (CD$_4$) cells (p = 0.0015). This was accentuated by removal of the 3 aberrant cases (p = 0.0003) and further accentuated in unpaired testing (p = 0.0001). When the 3 clinically aberrant cases were omitted, however, a trend towards an increase in Natural Killer (HNK) cells in the CFS group (p = 0.0545) also became significant at the 5% level (p = 0.0306). The increase was also significant by unpaired testing (p = 0.0122 and 0.0098) (Figs. 1 and 2). A B cell deficiency earlier noted in the pilot study group could not be confirmed (data not shown). The CD$_4$/CD$_8$ - cell ratios were significantly lower in CFS patients in both sets by paired (p = 0.0005 and 0.0001) and unpaired (p = 0.0001 in both cases) testing and the ratio was reversed in 60% of cases (Fig. 3).

Overall, paired and unpaired results agreed closely.

Figure 4 & 5

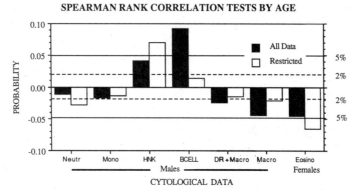

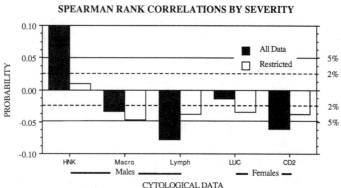

Fig. 5

ratios. A B cell deficiency was also recorded (p = 0.001), but this was not confirmed in group 1.

The major finding was a positive Spearman rank correlation between patients with low CD_4/CD_8 ratios and a shorter duration of symptoms (p = 0.02) (Fig. 6). This relationship was also not confirmed by the group 1 results.

tended to have more DR+ Mø with more severe symptoms (p = 0.033) and this was sustained in the group without aberrant cases (p = 0.0465). The latter group also had fewer HNK cells in the more severe cases (p = 0.0102). Females in the full study group had more LUC's with more severe symptoms (p = 0.0128) and this was reflected in the reduced study group (p = 0.0348), in which there was also a positive correlation between LUC's and DR+ lymphocytes (p = 0.0261). A trend towards increased total lymphocyte numbers in more severe disease (p = 0.0772) reached significant proportions in the reduced group (p = 0.0374) and could have been due to an overall increase in T cell numbers (p = 0.0372) (Fig. 5).

Group 2

The results of the pilot study are not presented here in detail. It is noteworthy, however, that a T-helper cell deficiency was also present in this group (p= 0.001) and 40% of patients had reversed CD_4/CD_8

Discussion

Although a number of apparent differences between patient and control groups emerged in this study, any interpretation of the results, and, indeed, the results themselves must be viewed with caution. The T helper cell deficiencies and natural killer cell fluctuations and the low or inverted CD_4/CD_8 ratios are probably genuine and certainly imply the likelihood of a functional immune deficiency. In both cases, our findings complement those of Behan and colleagues[6] and, more recently, Lloyd and colleagues[8] and Caligiuri and colleagues[9] although the recovery of T helper cell numbers with time seems to conflict with the results of Behan's group, who recorded persistently low T helper cell values in a sample of 5 patients followed over 2 years. Behan did not, however, specify how long these patients had been afflicted before the surveillance period began and this group could correspond to subjects amongst those in the present study with a relatively short history of illness. This is an important point to resolve. If T helper cell deficiencies are linked to clinical manifestations of CFS, their tendency to be replenished with time implies both the prospect of recovery and the presence of a prognostic marker for the condition. Although this trend was observed only in the pilot group, it is nevertheless likely to be a genuine observation, since the duration of symptoms in the main group was so much more uniform that relationships of this type would not be apparent.

Figure 6

CD4/CD8 RATIO RELATED TO LENGTH OF ILLNESS

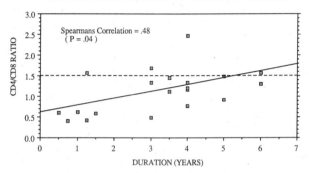

The other two differences, namely the decrease in basophils and the increase in LUC's amongst the patients both accord well with the clinical picture. A reduction in basophils corresponds appropriately with the high percentage of patients suffering food or other allergies. The LUC's are likely to include activated lymphocytes and the validity of this observation is greatly enhanced by the positive correlation with DR+ lymphocytes measured by FACScan. It is entirely consistent with a chronic infectious process and further weight is added by the positive correlation between increased LUC numbers and severity of symptoms in the female patients.

The B cell deficiency recorded in the pilot group would also accord with reports of immunoglobulin deficiencies[8, 11,13]. These seem to be more evident in long-standing cases[8], so it is, in any case, unlikely that a B cell deficiency would have been evident in the main study group.

The Spearman rank correlations, however, may include a number of spuriously significant results. Although the control group contained no correlations whatsoever at the 5% level, up to 10 or more could be expected on a random basis out of almost 230. Cor-

relations above the 1% level are therefore suspect. Those most likely to be genuine are the correlates with severity of symptoms where a significant difference in phenotype numbers also exists between patients and controls. In this category, the depletion of HNK cells and the increased number of LUC's in patients with more severe symptoms are probably genuine although the increase of DR positive Mø and increased total lymphocyte and T cell numbers with increased severity of symptoms would also fit the clinical picture. Our findings are largely consistent with the literature although much less florid than those of the recent Australian study by Lloyd and colleagues[8]. Our cases were all ambulant, however, whereas Lloyd describes theirs as 'predominantly long-standing and severe'. The subjects in our study group probably approximate more closely to the average ranges of clinical severity when first seen by general practitioners, which is important if cytological criteria can be established as a diagnostic aid. We believe that this is possible and are currently attempting to develop a multifactorial test to give a characteristic cytological profile independent of abnormal cytological values or alterations in lymphocyte circulation kinetics[20]. This is desirable since, despite the depletion of T helper cells and basophils and increases in activated lymphocyte natural killer cells in the group means, the majority of values lie within physiological limits[21]. The correlations with the age of patients are less dramatic but clinically consistent with the more chronic and relapsing pattern of CFS seen with increasing age of onset.

In conclusion, while we are confident that our findings represent evidence of immune dysfunction in CFS, we do not claim that they provide anything like a complete picture. The available evidence suggests that cytological changes continue and develop during the course of the disease and the majority of them remain to be accurately delineated.

Acknowledgements

The authors wish to record their appreciation to the Australia-New Zealand Myalgic Encephalomyelitis Society (New Zealand) Inc., who supported this work, and to the human volunteers who took part in the clinical study.

References

1. Bell, E. S., McCartney, R. A. and Riding, M. H. (1988). "Coxsackie -B viruses and Myalgic Encephalomyelitis." J. Royal Soc. Med. **81**: 329-331.

2. Dale, J. K., Straus, S. E., Ablashi, D. V., Salahuddin, Z. S., Gallo, R. C., Nishibe, Y. and Inoue, Y. K. (1989). "The Inoue-Melnick virus, Human Herpesvirus Type 6 and the Chronic Fatigue Syndrome." Ann. Int. Med. **110** (1): 92-93

3. Holmes, G. F., Kaplan, J. E., Stewart, J. A., Hunt, B., Pinsky, P. F. and Schonberger, L. B. (1987). "A cluster of patients with a chronic mononucleosis-like syndrome: Is Epstein-Barr virus the cause?" J.A.M.A. **257**: 2297-2302.

4. Odds, F. C. (1988) *in* "Candida and Candidosis." Baillière and Tindall. London. Chapter 24 pp. 233-234

5. Yousel, G. E., Bell, E. J., Mann, G. F., Murugeson, V., Smith, D. G., McCartney, R. A. and Mowbray, J. F. (1988). "Chronic enterovirus infection in patients with Postviral Fatigue Syndrome." Lancet. **1**: 146-150.

6. Behan, P. O., Behan, W. M. H. and Bell, E. J. (1985). "The post-viral fatigue syndrome: an analysis of the findings in 50 cases." J. Infect. **10**: 211-222.

7. Wakefield, D. and Lloyd, A. R. (1987). "Pathophysiology of Myalgic Encephalomyelitis." Lancet. **2**: 918-919.

8. Lloyd, A. R., Wakefield, D., Boughton, C. R. and Dwyer, J. (1989). "Immunological abnormalities in the chronic fatigue syndrome." Med. J. Aust. **151**: 122-124.

9. Caligiuri, M., Murray, C., Buchwald, D., Levine, H., Cheney, P., Peterson, D., Komaroff, A. L. and Ritz, J. (1987). "Phenotypic and functional deficiency of natural killer cells in patients with chronic fatigue syndrome." J. Immunol. **130**: 3305-3313.

10. Gin, W., Christiansen, F. T. and Peter, J. B. (1989). "Immunological abnormalities in chronic fatigue syndrome." Med. J. Aust. **151**: 117-118.

11. Linde, A., Hammarstrm, L. and Smith, I. G. (1988). "IgG1 subclass deficiency in patients with chronic fatigue syndrome." Lancet. **1**: 241-242.

12. Murdoch, J. C. (1988). "Cell mediated immunity in patients with myalgic encephalomyelitis." N.Z.J.Med. **101**: 511-514.

13. Read, R., Spickett, G., Harvey, J., Edwards, A. J. and Larsen, H. E. (1988). "IgG1 subclass deficiency in patients with chronic fatigue syndrome." Lancet. **1**: 241-242.

14. Straus, S. E., Dale, J. K., Wright, R. and Metcalfe, D. D. (1988). "Allergy and the Chronic Fatigue Syndrome." J. Allergy Clin. Immunol. **81**: 791-795.

15. Tosato, G., Straus, S. E., Henle, W., Pike, S. E. and Blaese, R. M. (1985). "Characteristic T cell dysfunction in patients with chronic active Epstein-Barr virus infection (chronic infectious mononucleosis)." J. Immunol. **134**: 3082-3088.

16. Holmes, G. P., Kaplan, J. E. and Gantz, N. M. (1988). "Chronic Fatigue Syndrome: a working case definition." Ann. Int. Med. **108**: 387-389.

17. Ramsay, A. M. (1988) *in* **"Myalgic Encephalomyelitis and Postviral Fatigue States."** Gower Medical Publishing. London.

18. Ritchie, A. W. S., Ostwald, I., Micklem, H. S., Boyd, J. E., Elton, R. A., Jazwinska, E. and James, K. (1983). "Circadian variations of lymphocyte subpopulations: a study with monoclonal antibodies." Brit. Med. J. **286**: 1773-75.

19. Moir, D. J., Ghosh, A. K., Abdulaziz, A., Knight, P. M. and Mason, D. Y. (1983). "Immunoenzymatic staining of haematological samples with monoclonal antibodies." Brit. J. Haem. **55**: 395-410.

20. Cross, J. P., Baxter, O. J. and Holmes, M. J. (1990). "Working towards a Diagnostic Aid in Chronic Fatigue Syndrome: Analysis of Peripheral Blood Leucocyte Profiles by Radial Plot." (**ME / CFS, The Cambridge Review**).

21. Goff, L.K., Habeshaw, J.A., Rose, M.L., Gracie, J.A. and Gregory, W. (1985) "Normal values for the different classes of venous blood mononuclear cells defined by monoclonal antibodies." J. Clin. Pathol. **38**: 54-59.

Chapter 64

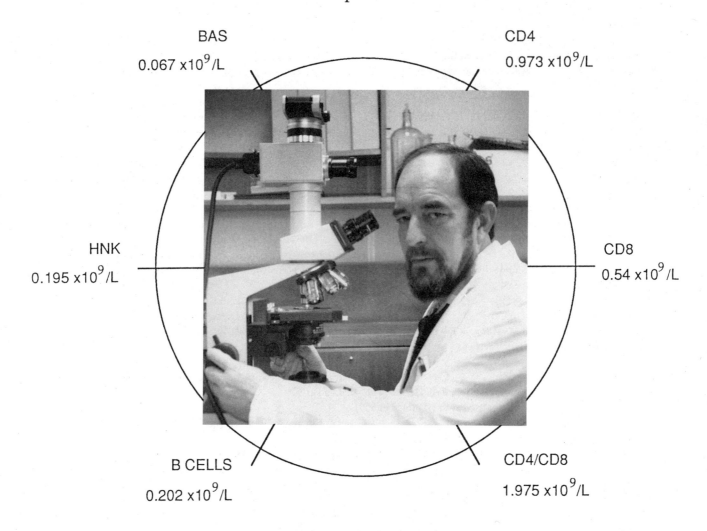

BAS
0.067 x10^9/L

CD4
0.973 x10^9/L

HNK
0.195 x10^9/L

CD8
0.54 x10^9/L

B CELLS
0.202 x10^9/L

CD4/CD8
1.975 x10^9/L

John P. Cross

Working Towards a Diagnostic Aid in Chronic Fatigue Syndrome: Analysis of Peripheral Blood Leucocyte Profiles by Radial Plot

John P. Cross, BSc (Soton), M Med Sci (Haem)., PhD
Owen J. Baxter B.Sc (Otago), Michael J. Holmes MD (L'pool). Correspondence to: Dr. M. J. Holmes, Dept. of Microbiology, University of Otago, P.O. Box 56, Dunedin, New Zealand.

Dr. John Cross is the inventor of the radial plot as a diagnostic tool in M.E. / CFS. This was first presented at Cambridge and has subsequently been taken up by other leading experts such as Dr. Paul Cheney. Dr. Cross qualified as a Fellow of the Institute of Medical Laboratory Science (London) and a BSC (Hons) in Physiology and Biochemistry at Southampton. He obtained an M. Med. Sci. (Haem) degree in South Africa and received his PhD in 1991 while employed as Senior Technical Officer in Microbiology at Otago University, New Zealand. He has worked at Pathology Laboratories in the UK and USA (John Hopkins) and taught Medical Laboratory Science in Eire and Africa.

Summary

Peripheral blood leucocyte profiles from 30 Chronic Fatigue Syndrome (CFS) patients were compared with those of 30 healthy age and sex-matched controls. Six criteria were selected and represented graphically for each subject as hexagons on computer-generated radial plots. The patterns generated by CFS patient data were recognisably different from those of control subjects. A significant statistical relationship was established between the clinical assessments of the patients and the shape of the plots. Four plots were indistinguishable from the control reference set and, of these, 3 belonged to subjects who were clinically ranked as probable misdiagnoses, suggesting the technique may have some predictive capacity. The shape of the plot identified with CFS patients was recognisable even in cases where all results lay within control reference limits.

Introduction

A significant proportion of the public and, indeed, a significant number of clinicians, remain unwilling to accept chronic fatigue syndrome (CFS) as a genuine clinical entity. Some of our patients see the additional burden of misery and even guilt that this attitude generates as their major single problem in coping with the condition. Non-acceptance is not helped by the fact that there is no reliable diagnostic test and that even the clinical diagnosis is made by exclusion. One of our main aims in this laboratory is, therefore, to explore the possibilities of developing such a test. Ideally, it would be made on a single peripheral blood specimen.

Although immunological disequilibria have been reported in CFS with sufficient frequency to suggest 'chronic fatigue immune dysfunction syndrome' as an appropriate, if cumbersome, alternative title, much of the evidence has been conflicting, and only now is a coherent picture emerging (Behan et al. 1985, Caligiuri et al. 1987, Murdoch 1988, Linde et al. 1988, Lloyd et al. 1989, Gin et al. 1989). In the process, two more major problems have become evident. Firstly, the observed differences appear to change during the course of the disease (Behan et al. 1985, Holmes et al., in press). Secondly, and more importantly, the individual values obtained for each cytological criterion are usually within normal limits, although they differ in terms of statistical significance between carefully screened and matched patients and controls.

Our problem is therefore formidable: namely, how to develop a reliable diagnostic test for a condition

where the cytological profiles not only change during the course of the disease, but where they also remain within normal limits.

The concept we offer rests upon the premise that, while individual criteria may remain within normal limits, a number considered together may form a characteristic, recognisable pattern significantly different from those generally seen in healthy persons, and, hopefully, in patients with other chronic and debilitating diseases. The values obtained for each parameter are plotted on separate equidistant radial axes of a circular plot. When these points are joined up, an irregular hexagon is formed whose shape will be determined by the magnitudes of the various values.

This paper describes preliminary efforts to demonstrate a characteristic shape, recognisable at a glance as compatible with the cytological profile of a CFS patient and significantly different from that of a healthy control. The technique is clearly worth further scrutiny, since, even at this stage, we have indications that the patterns generated can be helpful in arriving at a diagnosis of CFS. We wish to stress, however, that our present criteria are not necessarily ideal or even appropriate. Our intention is simply to demonstrate the possibility of developing a reliable diagnostic test for a condition where no single value measured need lie outside the normal physiological range.

Materials and Methods

Subjects. Thirty volunteers from among CFS sufferers in Otago, 20 female and 10 male, were age and sex matched with 30 healthy control subjects. Ages ranged from 13 to 51 with a mean of 28.6 years. Volunteers were either recruited locally or referred via the Department of General Practice of Otago Medical School, as described elsewhere (Holmes et al., in press).

Cell samples. Two 5 ml. peripheral venous blood samples were taken between 11 am and midday to minimise the effect of circadian variation (Ritchie, Ostwald et al. 1983). One specimen was reserved for a full blood count which was carried out using a Technicon H6000/C analyser at Dunedin Public Hospital. After lysing the erythrocytes, the second sample was labelled with fluorescein tagged monoclonal antibodies and counted in a fluorescence activated cell sorter (FACScan) as described elsewhere (Holmes et al., in press). All data were collected blind.

Radial Plots. The radial plot method for displaying laboratory findings was first developed for the PLATO large scale time-sharing computer system (Williams et al. 1977), adapted for the Apple 2 microcomputer (Love 1984), simplified and enhanced in versatility (Cross, unpublished), and finally converted for use on the Macintosh computer (Baxter and Cross, unpublished).

Statistics. The distribution of the data from the controls was checked for normality with Lilliefors' modification of the Kolmogorov-Smirnov test (Lilliefors 1967), using a programme specially written for the Apple 2e computer (Cross, unpublished). Where this was not Gaussian, logarithmic transformation was attempted. If this failed, the reference range was taken as the minimum and maximum observed values, as the best available estimate.

Results

Control reference ranges are shown in Table 1. These values were entered into the radial plot program and the mean of the control values plotted (figure 1). The means of the variates with Gaussian distributions

fall on the centre line, while those with non-Gaussian distributions are off-set.

Table 1		
Interim reference ranges for control group in cells x 10⁹/L.		
Parameter	Lower limit	Upper limit
CD4	0.48	1.77
CD8	0.16	0.92
CD4/CD8	1.041	4.109
B cells	0.021	0.384
HNK cells	0	0.48
Basophils	0.03	0.12

Results from CFS patients were plotted onto the reference set diagram. The means of 20 clinically diagnosed CFS cases were plotted on the same reference set (Figure 2.) For the purposes of this study the resulting plot has been regarded as representative of CFS and used as a standard reference pattern. The radial plot pattern for each patient was then ranked according to the degree of matching with the designated CFS pattern. At the same time, the cases were ranked independently into 'severe', 'moderate', 'mild' and 'probably misdiagnosed' categories. When these ranks were compared using the Kruskal-Wallis procedure they showed evidence of co-incidence (p<0.02). Four plots were identified as having no resemblance

Figure 1

Radial plot diagram of FACScan results from 30 controls

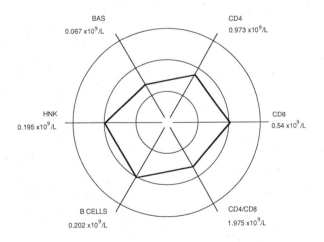

Figure 2

Radial plot diagram of FACScan results from the first 20 clinically ranked Chronic Fatigue Syndrome cases

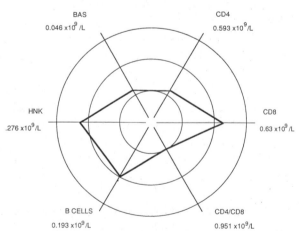

at all to the designated CFS pattern, and 3 of these 4 fell into the 'probably misdiagnosed' clinical ranking.

Further cases are illustrated in Figure 3, and patients P28, P30 and P16 are of particular interest as showing the 'CFS pattern' while none of the results lie outside the control reference range. There were 11 patients who fell into this category.

Discussion

With a view to establishing cytological diagnostic criteria, the study group was recruited from cases as early as possible in the course of the disease. The rationale for this was that, if CFS profiles change with time, then more uniform profiles might be expected in a more uniform group. Furthermore, the earlier the case, the more closely the cytological profiles should correspond to those at the time the patient was first diagnosed. Nevertheless, some of our subjects had suffered from the condition for more than 2 years.

A minority of patients were also accepted into the study group on the grounds that they had been diagnosed as CFS cases by other clinicians, although in 3 cases it was felt that they could have been misdiagnosed. These 3 are of particular interest to this study, since a blind clinical assessment correlated directly with a blind assessment by radial plot. Two of the 3 appeared to be suffering from unrelated chronic, debilitating disease, while the symptoms of the third probably had a functional rather than an organic basis. With so few cases, the evidence can only be regarded as anecdotal, but even so, a certain predictive capacity in the radial plot pattern is implied.

Extension of the control database by collection of more data should strengthen the resulting reference range. In the case of non-Gaussian distributions, the percentile method could then be used (Herrera 1958). The programme as presented by Love was cumbersome to use and adapt to parameters other than those of the original clinical chemistry studies. It was extensively modified in our laboratory to increase the versatility, speed and ease of operation on the Apple 2, and recently converted by us, with further enhancements, to run on a Macintosh microcomputer. The programme uses the familiar Macintosh user interface which makes learning times short. For

instance, all commands are accessible through pull-down menus, and do not have to be memorised. Up to 60 sets of data can be imported from a spreadsheet programme, and a spreadsheet-type format simplifies the use of the radial plot programme itself.

While the more clinically severe CFS cases showed some 'CFS characteristics' in the radial plot pattern, those most obviously different to the controls (e.g. P 23, Figure 3) corresponded more closely to the middle range of clinical severity. In this context it must be borne in mind that the designated CFS reference pattern was derived from a clinical spectrum of 20 cases. The result is therefore to some extent arbitrary and likely to be modified in the light of future experience.

Figure 3

Radial plot patterns of FACScan results of patients clinically diagnosed as Chronic Fatigue Syndrome

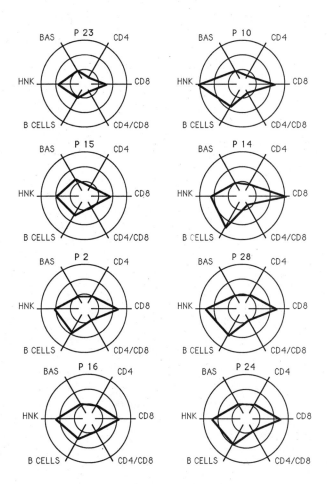

In conclusion, we wish to re-emphasise that our criteria have been abstracted from a single specific cytological study. Therefore, we expect that further developments will utilise other parameters such as IgG$_3$ subclass deficiencies (Lloyd et al. 1989) to provide a broader diagnostic platform.

References

1. Behan, P. O., W. M. H. Behan and E. J. Bell. (1985). "The post-viral fatigue syndrome: an analysis of the findings in 50 cases." J. Infect. **10**: 211-222.

2. Caligiuri, M., C. Murray, D. Buchwald et al. (1987). "Phenotypic and functional deficiency of natural killer cells in patients with chronic fatigue syndrome." J. Immunol. **130**: 3305-3313.

3. Gin, W., F. T. Christiansen and J. B. Peter. (1989). "Immune function and the chronic fatigue syndrome." Med. J. Aust. **151**: 117-118.

4. Herrera, L. (1958). "The precision of percentiles in establishing normal limits in Medicine." J. Lab. Clin. Med. **52**: 34-42.

5. Holmes, M. J., C. J. Chapman, A. J. Young and B. Niven. "Paired Age, Sex and ethnically matched studies of peripheral blood mononuclear lymphoid cell profiles in early chronic fatigue syndrome." **The Nightingle Foundation Review**:Chapter 64.

6. Lilliefors, H. W. (1967). "On the Kolmogorov-Smirnov test for normality with mean and variance unknown." J. Am Statist. Ass. **62**: 399-402.

7. Linde, A., L. Hammarstrom and I. G. Smith. (1988). "IgG1 subclass deficiency in patients with chronic fatigue syndrome." Lancet. **1**: 241-242.

8. Lloyd, A. R., D. Wakefield, C. R. Boughton and J. M. Dwyer. (1989). "Immunological abnormalities in the chronic fatigue syndrome." Med. J. Aust. **151**: 122-124.

9. Love, J. E. (1984). "A computer graphic representation of multivariate laboratory data." J. Med. Tech. **1**: 353-358.

10. Murdoch, J. C. (1988). "Cell mediated immunity in patients with myalgic encephalomyelitis." N.Z.J.Med. **101**: 511-514.

11. Ritchie, A. W. S., I. Ostwald, H. S. Micklem et al. (1983). "Circadian variations of lymphocyte subpopulations: a study with monoclonal antibodies." Brit. Med. J. **286**: 1773-75.

12. Williams, B. T., R. L. Johnson and T. T. Chen. (1977). **PLATO based medical information system overview.** Proc. First Illinois Conf. Med. Information Systems.

Chapter 65

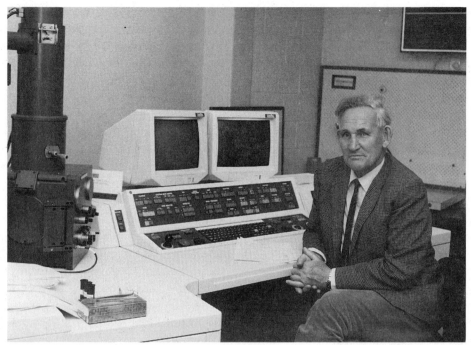

L. O. Simpson

The Role of Nondiscocytic Erythrocytes in the Pathogenesis of Myalgic Encephalomyelitis / Chronic Fatigue Syndrome

L.O. Simpson, PhD

Department of General Practice, Otago University Medical School, Dunedin, New Zealand

Acknowledgement: This study was sustained by grants from the A.N.Z. Myalgic Encephalomyelitis Society (New Zealand) Inc. and the financial support is gratefully acknowledged.

Dr. L. O. Simpson has 25 years experience in experimental pathology working with inbred strains of autoimmune mice with a specific interest in renal pathophysiology. Dr. Simpson developed the concept of basement membrane thixotropy to explain vascular permeability and proteinuria; he has lectured on these topics in America, Asia, Australia and Europe. Latterly, he has been studying various aspects of blood rheology. In addition to this, Dr. Simpson practised as Research Assistant in the Department of Surgery at the Otago Medical School working in the field of tissue transplantation. He also lectured in Biology at the Central Medical School in Fiji for seven years and spent 2 years sheep farming. Dr. Simpson is an Ex-President and the only New Zealand Life Member of the Australian Society for Experimental Pathology. He is also credited with approximately 70 publications.

Abstract

Blood samples from 39 males and 60 females who suffered from chronic tiredness and easy fatiguability due to M.E./CFS were subjected to a scanning electron microscope-based analysis of red cell shape. The results confirmed those of an earlier study of blood samples from 22 males and 80 females which showed the presence of increased percentages of nondiscocytic erythrocytes. The pathophysiological significance of such cells is that they will impair flow in capillaries smaller than the diameter of the cells and may initiate stasis in the smallest capillaries.

The most frequent change involved cup-transformed erythrocytes while a much smaller number of samples had an increased percentage of cells with altered margins. A small minority was characterised by having high percentages of flat cells. The mechanisms involved in the cell shape changes are unknown.

The possibility is explored that chronic tiredness could be due to inadequate oxygen delivery as a consequence of poorly deformable nondiscocytes and for this reason "fatigue" may be an inappropriate term in such circumstances. A pathogenesis is proposed which envisions that when the number of nondiscocytes exceeds some unknown threshold value they may impair capillary blood flow sufficiently for stasis to develop in the smallest capillaries. If the stasis did not resolve, focal lesions of ischaemic necrosis would develop. Multiple causes for chronic tiredness are indicated by the fact that different types of nondiscocytes are increased in the blood of those suffering similar symptoms.

Introduction

The primary assumption behind the reasoning in this paper is that normal tissue function requires normal supplies of oxygen and metabolic substrates which can be achieved only in the presence of normal capillary blood flow. Starling[1] recognised this as early as 1892 when he wrote that "Capillaries may be regarded as the chief part of the circulation," and pointed out that the arteries and veins acted mainly as conduits to and from a pumping organ, the heart. It needs to be emphasised that many capillaries are smaller than the diameter of normal erythrocytes and perfusion of such capillaries requires that erythrocytes change from their normal discocyte form. Erythrocyte deformability is to a major degree determined by the presence of "spare" membrane which exists in the cell concavities and it seems reasonable to assume that the intravascular pressure which causes red cells to deform is the intracapillary pressure associated with normal transudation.

Many physiological and pathological factors reduce red cell deformability either by their influence on red cell shape or by decreasing the fluidity of the cell membrane lipid bilayer. The pathophysiological significance of poorly deformable cells is that they require higher intravascular pressure to induce shape change and the increased pressure will increase transudation, but if an adequate rise in pressure is not forthcoming stasis may occur. Such events are most likely to occur first in the smallest capillaries and on the venous side of the capillary bed where intracapillary pressures are lowest. An estimate of red cell deformability may be obtained by filtering

blood through polycarbonate filters[2] and we found that blood samples from acutely unwell subjects with myalgic encephalomyelitis (M.E.) were less filterable than samples from similarly aged blood donors.[3] After recovery from the acute sickness blood filterablilty was not different from that of the blood donors.

It seemed possible that the reason for reduced blood filterability could be due to loss of discocytic shape. As previous studies had shown that blood filterability decreased with increasing age, scanning electron microscopy of blood samples from healthy elderly men was undertaken and revealed that nondiscocytic red cells were common. Those observations led to the development of a scanning electron microscope-based technique for quantifying the observed shape changes.[4] That technique has been applied to the study of blood samples from subjects with M.E. and the results from the first 102 samples have been published.[5]

This paper describes the findings related to red cell shape in blood samples from a further 99 subjects suffering from chronic tiredness and easy fatiguability. Most were members of the ANZME Society who learned of the test through the Society's journal which had reported the results of the first M.E. samples. Those samples were obtained during a collection of blood samples from subjects with multiple sclerosis from those members of the Gisborne Multiple Sclerosis and Myalgic Encephalomyelitis Society who had M.E. Subsequently members or friends of members of the ANZME Society either telephoned or wrote directly or through their general practitioner to request red cell shape analysis. The results of analyses are used as a basis for a possible pathogenesis based upon impaired capillary blood flow.

Materials and Methods

(a) Participants.

Fifty-six subjects (23 male, 33 female) with symptoms of chronic tiredness and easy fatiguability requested red cell shape analyses either by letter or by telephone while 16 males and 27 females made requests through their general practitioners. The average age of the males was 37.4 years (range 12-59) and of the females was 42 years (range 12-76). A vial containing 5 mls of a 2.5% solution of glutaraldehyde in 0.1M cacodylate buffer at pH 7.4 was sent to all applicants with instructions for obtaining a 3-drop sample of venous blood. In addition a brief questionnaire asked participants to declare their state of health at the time their blood sample was collected, in the range from severely unwell to being well with no symptoms. Because of the efficiency of the fixative[6] it has been possible to examine blood samples from Australia, England and the United States of America. Results were mailed to participants or their doctors.

(b) Preparatory techniques.

As details have been published previously[5] the technique is merely summarised here. Blood samples which had been fixed at room temperature for at least overnight were washed twice in buffer, dehydrated in ascending concentrations of ethanol to absolute, rinsed in 2 changes of pure, dry acetone and suspended in a third change of acetone. One drop of the final suspension was placed on an acetone-washed coverslip fixed to an aluminium stub with double-sided adhesive tape. After air-drying, the preparation was gold coated in a Polaron sputter coater. Cells were photographed at 600 x on fine grain film in an ETEC Autoscan electron microscope at 20kV and enlarged 2 x at printing. All cells identifiable under a 3 x lens were counted and classified as normal red cells, flat cells, cells with surface changes, early cup forms, late cup forms or cells with altered margins, according to published criteria.[5] The proportions of each cell class present were expressed as percentages of the total number of cells counted. The different shape-determined classes of red cells are dynamic rather than static and it seems that flat cells may stand in some sort of transitional relationship to normal red cells. For that reason the two classes are combined to form a class of "discoid" cells which seems to provide a measure of normality. As both early and late cup forms are poorly deformable they have been combined into a single class of "cup forms" which provides a measure of their contribution to impairment of capillary blood flow.

Results:

The data are summarised in Table 1 where they are contrasted with the data from the first 102 M.E. samples analysed and the control data. In terms of the changes in cup forms it seems possible that

females may not only be afflicted more frequently but also more severely than males. The higher female average value for cup forms was due to the influence of 12 cases with very high values and when they were omitted there was no difference between male and female values. If females are more severely affected, then this could explain the disparity between the values for cup forms between the first and second panels as there was a greater proportion (80:22) of females in the first panel. The higher average values for cells with altered margins in this study were due to the influence of a small number of high values including two with more than 40% of this cell type in their blood samples. Seven subjects (5 males, 2 females) had essentially normal blood except for marked increases in the percentage of flat cells.

Table 1				
	Discoid Cells	Cells with surface changes	Cup forms	Cells with altered margins
Data from this study				
Males n=39	56.6% (34.4-78.8)	20.5% (8.7-32.3)	14.6% (0.0-31.2)	8.6% (0.0-27.0)
Females n=60	51.2% (29.2-73.2)	21.9% (8.5-35.3)	21.0% (1.1-40.9)	7.3% (0.0-24.5)
Combined n=99	53.3%* (30.9-75.7)	21.4%* (8.4-34.5)	17.6%* (0.0-37.3)	7.6%* (0.0-25.1)
Previous data from reference 5				
Combined n=102	58.4%* (38.4-78.4)	19.1%* (6.0-25.5)	19.0%* (2.3-35.7)	3.4%* (0.0-11.9)
Controls n=52	71.8% (55.3-88.3)	14.4% (0.9-27.9)	8.9% (2.2-15.6)	4.6% (0.0-11.9)

* = significantly different from controls at 0.05 level.

The results of red cell shape analysis for the 99 subjects in this study contrasted with the results from the first 102 samples studied.

Questionnaires were returned by 36/39 males and 55/60 females and showed that 11.1% of males and 16.3% of females considered they were severely unwell; 33.3% of males and 40.0% of females were moderately unwell; 30.5% of males and 29.1% of females were slightly unwell; 22.2% of males and 14.5% of females were well with slight symptoms. A single male (2.7%) was well with no symptoms at the time his sample was collected. There was no correlation between health status and red cell morphology.

Discussion

Introduction

These results, which are indistinguishable from those reported previously,[5] show that blood from subjects suffering from chronic tiredness and who respond to slight to moderate stress or exertion by becoming physically and/or mentally exhausted, is characterised by the presence of increased numbers of nondiscocytic erythrocytes. In most cases the debility was preceded by a "flu-like" illness. As there were increases in different classes of nondiscocytes it seems likely that different factors may influence red cell shape. At present the mechanisms involved are not understood. Although the presence of different shaped cells in normal human blood was described first in 1972 the utility of quantifying the variously shaped cells has yet to be evaluated.

Does red cell shape analysis provide a diagnostic test for those suffering from chronic tiredness related to M.E.? If so, what is it diagnostic of? In subjects who always feel unwell and tired but who have no abnormal results in the usual laboratory tests the presence of nondiscocytes in greater than usual numbers may be the only evidence of a pathophysiological change. In such conditions the test is indicative of an abnormal state but the state being diagnosed has yet to be given a generally acceptable name. As no blood samples from subjects with defined behavioural disorders or from those meeting the criteria of Holmes et al[7] for the chronic fatigue syndrome (CFS) have been studied, the following observations do not include those disorders although it is possible that the concepts may be relevant and applicable. Manu et al[8] have noted that only a small proportion (6 of 135) of subjects suffering from persistent fatigue (is this synonymous with chronic tiredness?) met the criteria for CFS and later 4 of the 6 were rediagnosed.

Although different opinions have been aired[9,10] the matter of nomenclature remains unresolved. Irrespective of what name is eventually adopted (myalgic encephalomyelitis, chronic fatigue syndrome, post-viral fatigue syndrome, post-infection syndrome) the significance of red cell shape analysis is that it identifies groups of subjects with similar symptoms but with different erythrocyte populations. Therefore by the use of the technique it would be possible to obtain better defined and more homogeneous panels for study in the future.

Is the term "fatigue" appropriate in these conditions? David et al[11] has drawn attention to the problems arising from the use of the term "fatigue" in symptom descriptions and speculated that there may be a need to define a new type of fatigue. Ellis has pointed out that fatigue is not a term used by patients who usually refer to being tired and not feeling well.[12]

The writers of editorials which addressed the physiological aspects of fatigue[13] or the medical perceptions of fatigue[14,15] did not satisfactorily distinguish between "being tired" and "fatigue". As the effects of poorly deformable nondiscocytes in the microcirculation will be to impair oxygen and nutrient delivery, tiredness may merely reflect suboptimal metabolic activity. Ellis noted that rapid falls in haemoglobin are very likely to cause tiredness implying the involvement of reduced oxygen supply to the tissues but without discussing the topic. Similarly an anonymous editorial in *The Lancet* discussed the physiological aspects of fatigue without mentioning that reduced oxygen availability was a possible cause of fatigue.[13] But attention was drawn to the fact that depletion of muscle glycogen stores was closely correlated with the onset of exhaustion and that alteration in the rate of glycogen utilisation (of which oxygen availability is a major factor) will influence exercise capacity.

The pathophysiological significance of nondiscocytic erythrocytes.

Nondiscocytes will be able to traverse capillaries slightly smaller than cell diameter only with difficulty and may not to be able to pass through the smallest capillaries. In order to appreciate the implications of such events the following generalisations should be considered.

1. That the effects of poorly deformable nondiscocytes will be manifested first as impaired capillary blood flow which could lead to small foci of ischaemic necrosis as a consequence of the development of irresolvable stasis in small capillaries.

2.   That impaired capillary blood flow in tissues or organs with secretory functions may result in reduced secretory activity. In those tissues or organs which by chance have smaller than usual or a preponderance of small capillaries, the reduction in function could reach pathological levels.

3.   Individuals with smaller than usual capillaries will be more adversely affected by reduced red cell deformability than subjects with large capillaries and capillary size may be an important determinant of who develops symptoms.

Figure

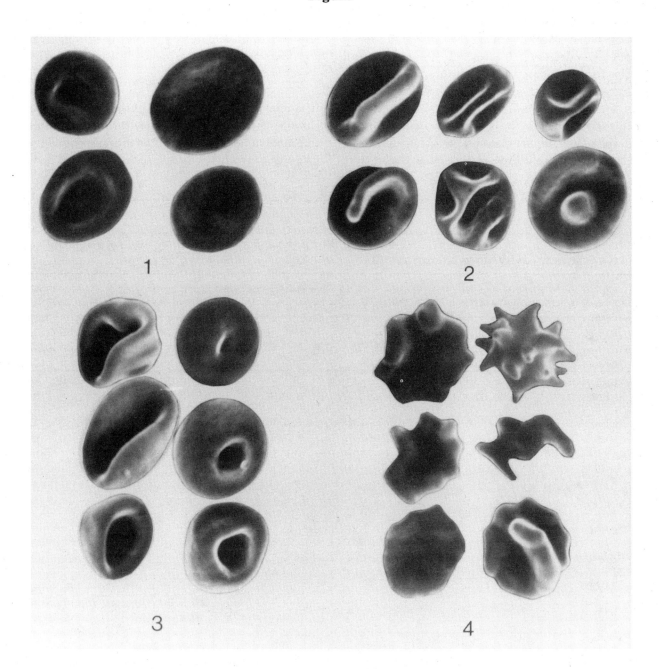

Series of cells to show the characteristics of the cell classes referred to in the text.
1. Discoid cells. 2. Cells with surface changes. 3.   Cup forms. 4. Cells with altered margins. Magnification of the original 600 x. Print magnification 2,520 x.

This latter point could explain why there was no correlation between the percentage of nondiscocytes and health assessment in this study and observations in other studies support the idea. Persistently high levels of cells with altered margins have been observed in repeated samples from 5 subjects. Two symptomless men aged 72 years, who had blood samples taken at monthly intervals over 4 months were found to have respectively 31.9% to 48.7% and 66.0% to 75.4% cells with altered margins. Increased percentages of cells with altered margins, although to a lesser degree (19.0% to 39.3%), were found in all blood samples obtained at monthly intervals for 4 successive months from 3 women with chronic tiredness.

It is speculated that the lack of symptoms in the men despite their higher percentages of nondiscocytes could indicate that their mean capillary diameters were larger than those of the women with symptoms. However it should be noted that non-symptomatic individuals with high percentages of nondiscocytes would be at risk in the event of severe stress or prolonged exertion when catecholamine-induced increases in blood viscosity[16] and decreases in red cell deformability[17] occur.

On the pathogenesis of ME / CFS.*

Note that in this paper CFS is used in the general sense and does not refer to the condition identified by prescribed criteria.[7]

It is proposed that when any of the nondiscocytes shown in the Figure increased beyond some unknown threshold value which will be related to mean capillary diameter, they will impair microcirculatory blood flow.

		Discoid Dells	Cells with surface changes	Cup forms	Cells with altered margins
Table 2					
L.O. Simpson - daily blood sample results					
Details of the results from daily samples of the author's blood. Note that the day after an upper respiratory tract infection the values were normal. After a severe head cold there was an increase in cup forms which took 14 days to return to normal.					
1988 Saturday	September 17	upper respiratory tract infection			
Sunday	September 18	upper respiratory tract infection			
Monday	September 19	71.3%	22.4%	5.3%	1.1%
Sunday	October 2	head cold			
Monday	October 3	56.5%	21.7%	10.7%	11.0%
Tuesday	October 4	51.2%	26.8%	21.0%	1.0%
Wednesday	October 5	54.1%	23.8%	20.8%	1.5%
Thursday	October 6	50.7%	31.9%	15.4%	2.0%
Friday	October 7	52.6%	30.3%	16.1%	0.9%
Monday	October 10	63.9%	24.4%	8.5%	3.2%
Tuesday	October 11	58.2%	28.7%	11.5%	1.5%
Wednesday	October 12	64.8%	20.4%	7.8%	6.9%
Thursday	October 13	76.3%	17.6%	5.8%	0.3%

Their main effect will be to reduce capillary perfusion rate to the extent that an autoregulated vasodilation occurs to restore the flow rate to normal. The resulting rise in intracapillary pressure will enhance transudation and such a mechanism could explain the "endogenous haemoconcentration" which was observed during emotional stress.[16] The slower the rate of capillary blood flow the greater the rate of proximal oxygen extraction and the lower the distal oxygen tension. In stimulated muscle (where small capillaries are common) reduced oxygen availability may lead to lactic acid formation and excessive intracellular acidosis has been demonstrated by magnetic resonance imaging.[18] However to explain their observations the authors opted for "excessive glycolytic activity" rather than "inadequate oxidative metabolism".

Lactic acid at physiological concentrations has been shown by an in vitro technique to reduce blood filterability.[19] Therefore lactic acid release will exacerbate any pre-existing problems of capillary blood flow and in the smallest capillaries stasis may develop as a prelude to focal ischaemic necrosis. While focal necrosis in muscles has been reported in subjects with the post-viral syndrome,[20] it seems possible that in similar conditions focal necrosis might develop in any tissue. Focal necrotic lesions arising in this manner could be associated with the high intensity signals seen by magnetic resonance imaging (MRI) in the white matter of individuals who met the criteria for CFS.[21]

Such signals indicate localised increases in water content and show that the blood brain barrier has been opened focally allowing enhanced transudation. It is suggested that vasoactive substances diffusing from small necrotic lesions could stimulate temporary endothelial cell contraction and breach the blood brain barrier. The MRI white matter signals would persist only until macrophages had removed necrotic tissue, i.e. the source of the vasoactive substances. It is unlikely to be chance alone which is responsible for the occurrence of high intensity white matter signals in conditions which have been found to have increased proportions of nondiscocytic erythrocytes, namely multiple sclerosis, systemic lupus erythematosus, sickle cell anaemia and in the elderly. In two of these conditions (multiple sclerosis and the elderly) it has been shown also that cerebral blood flow was less than in controls.[22]

Considerable research into the antibody profiles and lymphocyte populations in subjects with the symptoms of ME/CFS have shown some unusual patterns. However the reported observations provide no obvious link with symptoms which would help to explain their pathogenesis although it is possible that antibodies may in some way influence red cell shape. A healthy subject responded to one of two viral infections with a temporary increase in cup cells (Table 2). In contrast, subjects with ME/CFS have raised percentages of cup forms which persist for considerable periods. While this could be due to the persistence of the stimulating virus it may also indicate an impaired ability to restore discocyte shape. The best evidence which suggests that cup-transformed erythrocyctes are important in the development of symptoms comes from observations on the blood of individuals before and after an injection of vitamin B_{12}. Subjects whose well being improved after the vitamin injection were found to have reduced numbers of cup forms while there was no change in the red cell population of those who felt no better.

Table 3 shows the details of the red cell shape analyses of pre- and post- B_{12} injection samples from a subject who felt better and from another whose condition was unchanged. So far 14 pairs of pre- and post-B_{12} blood samples have been studied and it seems that the vitamin-induced changes occur in only 50%. This result is much different from the results of Ellis and Nasser[23] who used much larger injections of B_{12} to alleviate chronic tiredness. Their data showed that tiredness was not simply a consequence of vitamin deficiency and the manner in which the B_{12} improved well being was unexplained. However the fact that only 50% of subjects benefited from B_{12} may provide means of subdividing subjects with chronic tiredness and obtaining more homogeneous panels for future study. Because of the number of potentially confounding variables a better understanding of the pathogenesis of chronic tiredness will emerge only from the study of well defined panels.

Conclusion

It is concluded that red cell shape analysis provides a basis for identifying a sub-population of subjects suffering from chronic tiredness believed to have M.E. The reported observations indicate that little is

Table 3				
	Discoid Cells	Cells with surface changes	Cup forms	Cells with altered margins
Female 1				
Pre B_{12}	39.0%	27.9%	32.6%	0.5%
Post B_{12} (24 hrs)	66.2%	15.2%	13.0%	5.6%
Female 2				
Pre B_{12}	39.4%	24.0%	36.6%	0.0%
Post B_{12} (24 hrs)	43.6%	23.5%	32.9%	0.0%
Post B_{12} (72 hrs)	37.6%	24.0%	38.4%	0.0%

Red cell shape analysis results from blood samples obtained before and after an injection of vitamin B_{12}. Female 1 experienced a marked improvement in wellbeing which was accompanied by a reduction in cup forms. Female 2 obtained no benefit from the B_{12} injection and there was no change in the red cell population.

known about the factors which control red cell shape in vivo and question the relevance of views based upon the results of in vitro studies on agents causing changes in red cell shape. As the blood of subjects with chronic tiredness is characterised by raised percentages of nondiscocytes which will impair capillary blood flow, more attention should be paid to means of improving microcirculatory blood flow, to alleviate symptoms.

References

1. Starling E.H. **Elements of Human Physiology.** London, J. & A. Churchill 1892. p.196.

2. Reid H.L., Barnes A.J., Lock P.J., Dormandy J.A., Dormandy T.L. A simple method for measuring erythrocyte deformability. J Clin Path 1976; 29: 855-858.

3. Simpson L.O., Shand B.I., Olds R.J. Blood rheology and myalgic encephalomyelitis: a pilot study. Pathology 1986; 18: 190-192.

4. Simpson L.O. Blood from healthy animals and humans contains nondiscocytic erythrocytes. Br J Haematol 1989; 73:561-564.

5. Simpson L.O. Nondiscocytic erythrocytes in myalgic encephalomyelitis. N Z Med J 1989; 102:126-127.

6. Hayat M.A. Glutaraldehyde: role in electron microscopy. Micron 1986; 17: 115-135.

7. Holmes G.P., Kaplan J.E., Gantz N.M. et al. Chronic fatigue syndrome in patients with persistent fatigue. Ann Intern Med 1988;109: 554-556.

8. Manu P., Lane T.J., Matthews D.A. The frequency of the chronic fatigue syndrome in patients with persistent fatigue. Ann Intern Med 1988; 108:387-389.

9. Lloyd A.R., Wakefield D., Boughton C., Dwyer J. What is myalgic encephalomyelitis? Lancet 1988; i: 1286-1287.

10. Ramsay A.M. Myalgic encephalomyelitis, or what? Lancet 1988; ii: 100.

11. David A.S., Wessely S., Pelosi S.J. Postviral fatigue syndrome: time for a new approach. Br Med J 1988; 296: 696-699.

12. Ellis Sir J. Malaise and fatigue. Symptoms which depress a doctor but which should not. Br J Hosp Med 1984; 32:312-314.

13. Anonymous. Fatigue. Lancet 1988; ii: 546-548.

14. Swartz M.N. The chronic fatigue syndrome - one entity or many? New Engl J Med 1988; 319: 1726-1728.

15. Bass C. Fatigue states. Br J Hosp Med 1989; 41:315.

16. Ehrly A.M. Landgraf H., Hessler J., Saeger-Lorenz K. Influence of video film-induced emotional stress on the flow properties of blood. Angiology 1988; 39: 341-344.

17. Rasmussen H., Lake W., Allen J.E. The effects of catecholamines and prostaglandins upon human and rat erythrocytes. Biochim Biophys Acta 1975; 411: 63-73.

18. Arnold D.R., Bore P.J., Radda G.K., Styles P., Taylor D.J. Excessive intracellular acidosis of skeletal muscle on exercise in a patient with a post-viral exhaustion/fatigue syndrome. Lancet 1984; i: 1367-1369.

19. Shand B.I. Changes in blood rheology induced by lactic acid. Proc Univ Otago Med Sch 1986; 64: 71-72.

20. Behan P.O., Behan W.M.H., Bell E.T. The postviral fatigue syndrome - an analysis of the findings in 50 cases. J. Infection 1985; 10: 211-222.

21. Komaroff A.L. Chronic fatigue syndrome: relationship to chronic viral infections. J Virol Methods 1988; 21: 3-10.

22. Swank R.L., Roth J.G., Woody D.C. Cerebral blood flow and red cell delivery in normal subjects and in multiple sclerosis Neurol Res 1983; 5: 37-39.

23. Ellis F.R., Nasser S. A pilot study of vitamin B_{12} in the treatment of tiredness. Br J. Nutr 1973; 30: 277-283.

Chapter 66

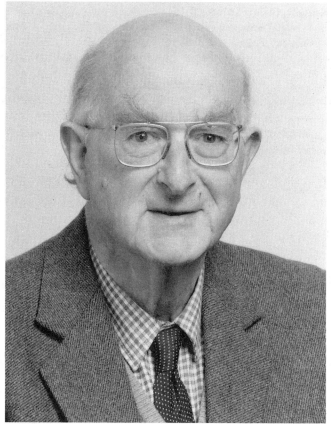

E. J. Field

Differentiation between Multiple Sclerosis (MS) and Myalgic Encephalomyelitis (ME)

E. J. Field, FRCP, London, Naomi Bramson Research Centre, The Science Park, University of Warwick, Coventry CV4 7EZ   England.

Introduction

Multiple Sclerosis and Myalgic Encephalomyelitis are quite different in origin and character. Whilst the latter is infective and has as yet a poorly defined but generalized pathology, MS is seemingly confined to the central nervous system though there is recent evidence of a systemic factor[1].

Each when in typical form has a characteristic and virtually diagnostic history (*"Better a blind neurologist than a deaf one"* - Mumenthaler: Berne) so that clinical differentiation is not difficult. There are, however, patients in whom features of ME are prominent and shared with MS, leading to ready confusion. Thus tiredness coupled with pins and needles or other paraesthesia and some unsteadiness may support a diagnosis of MS. Of course, in the great majority, other symptoms, listed in detail elsewhere in this Conference, nearly always clarify the diagnosis. But for some, an **objective test,** which can show (a) the presence of organic brain destruction which invariably occurs in ME, albeit non-specific or (b) that the patient has an MS **diathesis** (i.e. he has the ability to develop the disease either already or later), is a useful adjunct. The test does **not** show that the patient **has** MS. The value of a test which demonstrates the organic nature of ME in a world where so many believe that "it is all in the mind" needs no emphasis.

Without being drawn into underlying membrane-theory, as yet unclear, the principle of the test depends upon the peculiar charge properties of red blood cells (RBC) in MS; in **O**ther **N**eurological **D**isease (OND) where there is organic destruction of brain tissue from any cause other than MS; and on normal RBC (and those of "carriers" of MS - chiefly women)[2]. The differences are made manifest by changes produced in net charge on RBC by the presence of 0.08 mg/ml linoleic acid (C18:2 n-6). The LA used throughout is made up as follows. 100mg LA (Sigma London Chemical Ltd.) is dissolved in 4ml ethanol and stored under pure nitrogen at 65°C. With 100 mg LA in 4ml i.e. 25 mg/ml, 10μ will contain 0.25 mg and if this is delivered into 3ml of cells the final concentration is 0.08 mg/ml. The method of bringing out charge differences is by cell electrophoresis and this laboratory has always used the Zeiss (Oberkochen) Cytopherometer (whilst Seaman's laboratory[3], which has confirmed the MS diathesis test uses the original Seaman-Bangham "Fish tank" apparatus with equal success).

Laser Test

In this modification of the electrophoresis test for differentiation of MS and ME the procedure is as follows:

Blood obtained by sterile venipuncture is defibrinated with glass beads and red cells suspended in plasma drawn off and washed well three times in sterile saline (1:50 volumes) at 10°C and spun at 3000 g and a fourth time in Hanks' medium 199 with glutamine (Gibco Europe Ltd., Glasgow) and then suspended in the same medium in which all mobility measurements are made. The concentration of cells is measured in a Coulter counter and the volume necessary to make up 20ml of suspension at 2.6×10^6/ml cells/mm^3 calculated. The diluent used is the same Hanks' solution. From the 20ml of cell suspension 6 bijoux bottles each containing 3ml are made and before beginning an experiment are put into a water bath at 25°C.

Method

As control, 10μ of ethanol is added to one 3.0ml bijou of RBC and mobility determined by 20 readings in both directions of the potential field difference. All measurements are recorded by computer which calculates mean mobility +/- SD and percentage SD/mean. Readings which differ by more than 10% in the two directions are recorded but not used in the calculation. The control specimen may be irradiated (as described below) or not, without significant difference in result.

3.0 ml aliquots of the same RBC are exposed to collimated emanation from a He-Ne laser (.5mW Spectra Physics) situated 19 cm above the surface of the suspension, for a given length of time, with a Zeiss UV filter interposed between the radiation source and the specimen. At the end of the chosen exposure time, 10μl of LA giving a final strength of 0.08 mg/ml, is added to the tube, lightly shaken and electrophoretic mobility determined.

The value of the mobility with time of exposure was originally plotted[2] for RBC derived from normal subjects, those with Multiple Sclerosis, those suffering from organic brain lesions other than MS, and from relatives of MS patients. The presence of 0.08 mg/ml LA increased mobility of RBC as compared with the control (alcohol alone) value. RBC from normal individuals show increased mobility and this is maintained when the mixture is exposed to He-Ne UV filtered laser emanation until somewhere between 65 and 70 seconds when suddenly - over an interval of one additional second - the mobility drops to control value and remains so at longer irradiation periods. Red blood cells from normal individuals show mobilities which jump to control value by irradiation of no more than 70 seconds.

Red blood cells from subjects with MS **diathesis** maintain their fast mobility for somewhere near 106 seconds exposure to the He-Ne UV filter beam and then at some point between 104 and 110 seconds revert suddenly to control value. This is characteristic of MS **diathesis** and is not to be regarded as a test for MS. But if the diathesis is **not** present, then whatever disease the patient has got, it cannot be MS. On the other hand if the diathesis is present and the clinical picture is consonant with, or suspicious of, MS the diagnosis is much reinforced. A word of warning must be given here. A man may have an MS diathesis and yet develop another disease e.g. amyotrophic lateral sclerosis, glioma, diabetes or be killed in a traffic accident. His MS diathesis is stamped on his RBC at birth and will take precedence over the next test to be described - that for Other Neurological Disease (OND). If such a person with an inborn MS diathesis develops ME then we have a situation in which the clinical picture is characteristic of ME but the laboratory test shows an MS candidate - the Biblical "voice of Jacob and the hands of Esau". Such patients can present real difficulty, for with diseases as common as MS and ME, they may have ME and either full MS or MS diathesis. Then the MS diathesis alone will be brought out by the test. Furthermore, if the patient is an MS "carrier", then this will take precedence over the ME. But such cases are rare.

To sum up:

When only one disease is present as occurs in the vast majority of cases, either MS or ME, then differentiation is simple by determining the "break point" (75-80 seconds for ME; and 106-110 for MS) as described. If ME develops in an individual with MS diathesis or who is an "MS carrier" then difficulties arise.

Plasma laser method

The practical situation is made easier utilizing the demonstration from Seaman's group at the time when they confirmed the MS phenomenon[3], that plasma[4] contains a factor which is responsible for the specific properties of RBC. They showed that incubating MS-RBC with normal plasma (but **not** serum) induced a normal result from MS RBC; the reverse was also true. The plasma endows any RBC with the properties brought out by the test. Since then, this important observation of Seaman's has been much expanded[5] and we now use the plasma test routinely. This greatly reduces experimental labour. The only drawback is that the active principle in plasma does not survive more than 8 - 10 hours and cannot be preserved by freezing.

Method

A sterile stock suspension of well washed RBC (preferably from a patient with MS long treated with essential fatty acids) suspended in fresh Hanks' medium 199 with glutamine (Gibco Europe, Glasgow) is prepared and stored at 4°C for 3-4 weeks (even longer if the source of the RBC is an Italian). These are the "carrier cells" for plasma derived from the patient to be tested.

3.0 ml of blood from the patient is collected in a Westergren tube and spun at 10°C for 4-5 minutes at 3000g. It is then placed in a 25°C water bath for a few minutes. 3.0ml aliquots of the standard carrier cells are made up in bijoux bottles so that each contains 2.6×10^6 RBC/ml and put into the water bath. One of the 3.0 ml bijoux bottles containing RBC is taken from the 25°C water bath, 10μl of plasma carefully added and the bottle agitated lightly for a second or two. It is then irradiated as before through a Zeiss UV-filter by the laser (which has been allowed to warm up for 15 minutes) for a selected number of seconds (say 78). 10μl of the LA is then added i.e. 0.25 mg put into 3.0 ml of cell suspension giving a concentration of 0.08 mg/ml, and the mobility of the cells measured. (μ/sec/V/.cm at 25°C). The control value with alcohol alone is determined. The time for which irradiation must continue in order to cause the mobility of the coated RBC to change suddenly to control value is determined by direct experiment (the "break point").

If the plasma came from an ME (or an **OND**) then the irradiation time will be 75 - 80 seconds; if from an MS, 106 -110 seconds. The statistical significance of the break which is very sharp (a difference of 1 second producing the effect) is evaluated by the computer into which the Zeiss Cytopherometer readings have all been fed and printed out, is always < .001. Readings are not accepted for calculations, though put in reverse print, if they differ by 10% or more in the two directions of potential difference applied in the apparatus.

All cases of ME give an OND type result **i.e.** they indicate that organic disease of the brain is present and that the patient is not primarily "psychiatric" or "psychological", Of course, feeling as ill as he does, he is depressed about it.

Figures 1 and 2 show typical results plotted out for an OND and an MS. In general, the more severe the ME appears clinically, the higher the "break point" in the 74 -80 second range. For example, a mild case may show a break from fast to control mobility at 75- 76 seconds whilst a severe case is usually about 79 -80 or even 81 seconds, MS cases are well away in the 105 - 110 seconds range. It will be clear that all ME cases are thus tested for MS, something which alleviates a patient's anxiety.

Figure 1, M.E. (or OND)

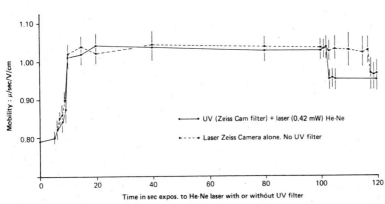

Patient with M.E., or Other Neurological Disease (OND). Ordinate mobility in
μ / sec / V / cm. Abscissa time of irradiaiton.
Zeiss UV-filter over mouth of bijou containing 3.0 ml of washed RBC in Hanks'
medium 199 and 0.08 mg / ml linoleic acid. Note sudden change in mobility in
the OND interval (74-80 seconds) irradiation.

Figure 2, MS

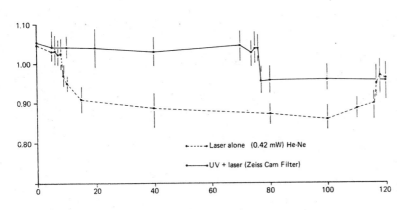

Patient with MS: conditions as in Figure 1.
Note sudden change in mobility in the MS interval (106-110 seconds)
irradiation.
(Published by permisssion of I.R.C.S. Med. Sci., 12, 717-718, 1984).

One more curious fact may be added. Whilst MS results will revert from MS diathesis figures (105 -110 seconds) to normal after about nine months exhibition of essential fatty acids — especially of the long chain C20:5 (w-3) and C22:6 (w-3) acids, similar treatment of ME is without result - the figure remains in the 75 - 80 seconds' range.

The differentiation between MS and ME may be shortened still further. If the 3.0 ml bijou of carrier RBC with 10μl of patient's plasma is irradiated for (say) 90 seconds then this is well above the top ME mobility and an ME case will give a control mobility. At the same time it is well below the MS diathesis minimum (104 seconds). Thus the differentiation between MS and ME can be reduced to a two specimen procedure, measurement of control; and measurement at 90 seconds irradiation from the laser through a Zeiss UV-filter.

My thanks are due to Miss Greta Joyce for her collaboration throughout this work.

References

1. Field, E. J. In: "Multiple Sclerosis: a conceptual reappraisal with heuristic implications. CC Thomas, Springfield, Illinois, 1989.

2. Field, E. J., Joyce, G., and Field, D. Multiple sclerosis: further observations on the effect of light from a He-Ne laser on erythrocytes. I. R. C. S. (Med. Sci.), **12,** 717-718, 1984.

3. Seaman, G. V. F., Swank, R. L., Tamblyn, C. H., and Zukoski, C.F. iv. Simplified red-cell elctrophoretic mobility test for multiple sclerosis. Lancet, **1,** 1138, 1979.

4. Seaman, G. F. V., Swank, R. L., Tamblyn, C. H. Red-cell membrane differences in multiple sclerosis are acquired from plasma. Lancet, **1,** 1139, 1979.

5. Field, E. J., and Joyce, G. Use of plasma for immediate diagnosis of multiple sclerosis (plasma- erythocyte unsaturated fatty acid (E-UFA) test. Neur. Res., **8,** 57-60, 1986.

Dr. Ephraim Joshua Field was born in London on March 20, 1915 and obtained his MB BS in 1938, his MS in 1944, his PhD at Bristol in 1943, his MD at Durham in 1946 and his FRCP at London in 1969. Dr. Field holds such prestigious titles as Professor Emeritus, Experimental Neuropathology, at the University of Newcastle, Honorary Director of the Naomi Bramson Research Centre, Science Park, University of Warwick and is a member of the Pathology Society. He is a past Honorary Director, MRC, Demyelinating Diseases Unit. Dr. Field has authored many articles in leading medical journals with his recent publications focusing on Multiple Sclerosis and Myalgic Encephalomyelitis.

New Investigation Techniques

Chapter 67

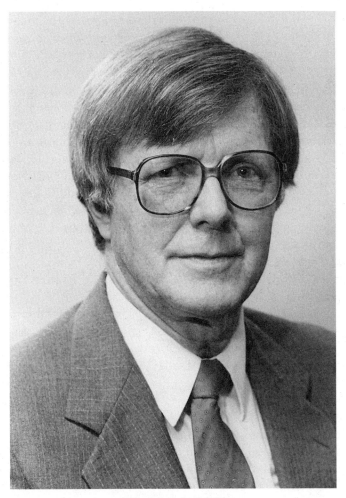

Robert J. Suhadolnik

Biochemical Defects in the 2-5A Synthetase/RNase L Pathway Associated with Chronic Fatigue Syndrome with Encephalopathy

Robert J. Suhadolnik, PhD[1], Nancy L. Reichenbach, BS[1], Robert W. Sobol, MS[1], Richard Hart, Jr., BS[1], Daniel L. Peterson, MD[2], David R. Strayer, MD[3], Berch Henry, PhD[4], Dharam V. Ablashi, DVM[5], David H. Gillespie, PhD[3], and William A. Carter, MD[3]

[1]Temple University School of Medicine, Philadelphia, PA 19140   [2]Incline Village, NV 89450, [3]Hahnemann University, Philadelphia, PA 19102, [4]University of Nevada School of Medicine, Reno 89557, [5]National Cancer Institute, Bethesda, MD 20892

*Dr. Robert J. Suhadolnik is Professor of Biochemistry, Temple University School of Medicine, and has held this position for 14 years. In addition to his academic and teaching responsibilities, Dr. Suhadolnik's research has been focused on the role of structurally and stereochemically modified nucleoside analogs in cellular processes with particular emphasis on the 2'-5'A synthetase / RNase L antiviral and antiproliferative system. In addition to basic research related to the molecular biology of these reactions, Dr. Suhadolnik has interacted clinically in the treatment of patients with various neoplasms and viral infections. Dr. Suhadolnik's research has been published extensively. Dr. Suhadolnik has published two books, **Nucleoside Antibiotics** and **Nucleosides As Biological Probes**.*

Introduction

The 2-5A synthetase/RNase L system is acknowledged to be part of the antiviral defense mechanism in mammalian cells (for review, see Lengyel, 1982). This system may also be important in the regulation of cell growth (Wells and Mallucci, 1985). 2',5'-Oligoadenylates (2-5A) are synthesized from ATP by 2-5A synthetase. 2-5A activates a latent endoribonuclease, RNase L, to degrade cellular and viral RNA.

We had reported earlier on changes in the 2-5A synthetase/ RNase L system as part of cellular regulatory functions in human cancers and HIV-1 infected individuals before and during therapy with mismatched double-stranded RNA [poly(I)-poly(C_{12}U), Ampligen] (Suhadolnik et al., 1983, 1985; Carter et al., 1987; Strayer et al., 1990). Ampligen is a biological response modifier which augments NK cell activity and has been used in long term clinical trials in cancer without toxicity (Carter et al., 1985a,b; Brodsky et al., 1985; Strayer et al., 1990). On the basis of these observations and the possible role of reactivated viruses, including herpes virus 6 (HHV-6) in chronic fatigue syndrome with encephalopathy (CFSE), we reasoned that the clinical and immune manifestations observed in CFSE might involve alterations in the 25A synthetase/RNase L pathway.

Figure 1 (panel A)

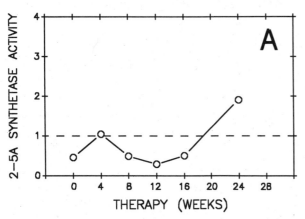

Panel A: Serial latent 2-5A synthetase levels in an individual with CFSE during therapy with Ampligen.

Chronic fatigue syndrome is associated with general viral reactivation, including EBV (Holmes et al., 1987, 1988) and HHV-6 (Ablashi et al., 1989). CFSE is associated with changes in serum levels of lymphokines which, along with chronic virus reactivation, may contribute to the persistent illness and fatigue observed (Straus, 1988). Caliguiri et al. (1987) reported that a majority of patients have low numbers of NKH1[+]T3[-] lymphocytes; this population represents the great majority of NK cells in healthy individuals. In this study, we report additional immunological defects in (i) latent 2-5A synthetase, (ii) bioactive 2-5A and (iii) RNase L in fifteen individuals with CFSE. In addition, we report correction of these immunological/biochemical defects in the 2-5A synthetase/RNase L pathway during therapy with Ampligen.

Figure 1 (panel B)

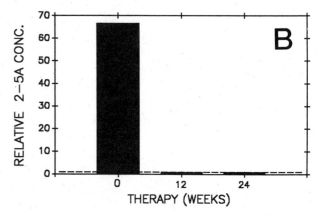

Panel B: Concentration of intracellular bioactive 2-5A as determined in core-cellulose assays. Data points represent mean of triplicate determinations. Average value obtained in assays of normal samples (n = 26) is indicated by dashed line.

Methods

Patients selected for this study, drug regimens, and virus culture methods were as described in a companion paper (Peterson et al., 1990). Heparinized whole blood was obtained from 15 individuals diagnosed as CFSE as well as healthy controls. Isolation of peripheral blood mononuclear cells (PBMC) by Ficoll-Hypaque centrifugation and extract preparation in a NP40 lysis buffer were as described (Suhadolnik et al., 1983).

2-5A synthetase (EC 2.7.7.19) from extracts of fresh PBMC (25 µg protein/assay) was isolated by affinity chromatography on poly(I)-poly(C)-agarose and assayed **in vitro** for its ability to convert [alpha-[32]

P]ATP to 2-5A (Suhadolnik et al., 1983). Products were quantitated by bacterial alkaline phosphatase treatment and thin layer chromatography (Li et al., 1990). 2-5A was isolated from the ethanol-soluble fraction of PBMC extracts and quantitated in core-cellulose assays (Strayer et al., 1990). Activation of RNase L was determined by specific cleavage product (SCP) formation in ribosomal cleavage assays (Strayer et al., 1990).

Results and Discussion

The levels of **latent** 2-5A synthetase (i.e., the 2-5A synthetase **not** bound to its dsRNA activator) were assayed directly in PBMC extracts (without mitogen stimulation) from 15 patients with CFSE. In >80% of the patients studied, the level of the 2-5A synthetase in PBMC extracts in the CFSE patients was abnormally low (30-70% below the level obtained for healthy individuals). Normal individuals converted an average of 20.1 nanomoles of ATP to 2-5A per mg protein. During therapy with Ampligen, there was a transient increase in the latent 2-5A synthetase. The decreased pretherapy level of the 2-5A synthetase in individuals with CFSE suggested that most of the 2-5A synthetase was bound to a dsRNA activator. To test this hypothesis, bioactive 2-5A was isolated from extracts of PBMC from individuals with CFSE. All CFSE patients had markedly elevated concentrations of bioactive 2-5A before therapy; Ampligen therapy resulted in a decline towards normal values in twelve weeks. Figure 1 shows the 2-5A synthetase level (panel A) and the elevated bioactive 2-5A concentration (panel B) in one of these individuals with CFSE.

The activity of RNase L, the key functional enzyme of the antiviral pathway, is dependent on activation by its allosteric modifier, 2-5A (Lengyel, 1982). Therefore, RNase L activity was measured in extracts of PBMC from individuals with CFSE. Before Ampligen therapy, the RNase L was elevated, as determined by disappearance of substrate (28S and 18S rRNA) and specific cleavage products (SCP). The activity of RNase L was restored to normal with administration of Ampligen, as early as 4 weeks after initiation of therapy. Figure 2 presents the rRNA cleavage assay of a representative CFSE patient before and during Ampligen therapy.

Figure 2

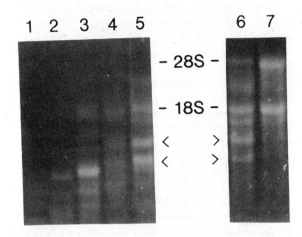

RNase L activity in an individual with CFSE during therapy with Ampligen. Determined by specific cleavage product (SCP) formation in rRNA cleavage assays (Strayer et al., 1990). Lanes 1-5: 0, 4, 8, 12, and 16 weeks of therapy; lane 6, normal control; lane 7, 28S and 18S rRNA control. Arrows indicate location of SCP.

The restoration of the 2-5A synthetase/RNase L pathway occurs in the same time frame as the pronounced and sustained disappearance of HHV-6 antigen-positive cells and clinical improvement (see companion paper, Peterson et al., 1990). The majority of CFSE patients studied had a pretherapy antiviral phenotype as noted in Table 1. Levels of 2-5A synthetase are elevated in individuals with many acute viral infections (Schattner et al., 1981a; Williams et al., 1982) as well as in cancer patients undergoing interferon therapy (Schattner et al., 1981b).

Biochemical defects in the 2-5A synthetase/RNase L antiviral pathway have been observed in PBMC extracts of HIV-infected individuals. Elevated levels of 2-5A synthetase have been reported from several laboratories (Preble et al., 1985; Read et al., 1985; Strayer et al., 1990). In addition, our laboratory has demonstrated low bioactive 2-5A concentrations and low activated RNase L in individuals with LAS, ARC and AIDS which like CFSE are corrected toward normal with Ampligen therapy (Strayer et al., 1990). Because of changes in 2-5A synthetase levels in CFSE patients and because 2-5A synthetase is a key functional enzyme in the antiviral pathway, the direct measurement of 2-5A synthetase levels **in vitro** in HHV-6 infected cells is currently being explored.

**Table 1
Antiviral Phenotype of
CFSE Patients Studied**

low levels of latent 2-5A synthetase

elevated concentrations of bioactive 2-5A

elevated RNase L activity

In summary, we have identified molecular fingerprint(s) which characterize CFSE patients, i.e., markedly reduced latent 2-5A synthetase, elevated bioactive 2-5A and elevated RNase L. This pathway phenotype is that of hyperactivity which suggests that this hyperactivity may result from chronic

overstimulation of blood cells produced as a result of HHV-6 or EBV reactivation. Furthermore, the results described here show that Ampligen is a biologically active drug in CFSE as evidenced by the correction of biochemical defects in the 2-5A synthetase/ RNase L system. This conclusion is supported by clinical improvements as described in a companion paper in this volume (Peterson et al., 1990).

Acknowledgements

These studies were supported in part by U.S. Public Health Service Grant PO1 CA-29545 from the National Cancer Institute and grants from HEM Research, Inc.

References

Ablashi, D.B., Zompetta, C., Lease, C., Josephs, S.F., Balachandran, N., Komaroff, A.L., Krueger, G.R.F., Henry, B., Luka, J., and Salahuddin, S.Z. (1989) Human herpesvirus-6 (HHV-6) and chronic fatigue syndrome (CFS). In Proceedings of the Chronic Fatigue Syndrome Workshop, published by the Central Public Health Laboratory, Toronto, Canada (Sept. 2829, 1989).

Brodsky, I., Strayer, D.R., Krueger, L.J., and Carter, W.A. (1985) Clinical studies with Ampligen (mismatched double-stranded RNA). J. Biol. Response Modif. 4, 699-675.

Caliguiri, M., Murray, C., Buchwald, D., Levine, H., Cheney, P., Peterson, D., Komaroff, A.L., and Ritz, J. (1987) Phenotypic and functional deficiency of natural killer cells in patients with chronic fatigue syndrome. J. Immunol. 139, 3306-3313.

Carter, W.A., Strayer, D.R., Hubbell, H.R., and Brodsky, I. (1985a) Preclinical studies with Ampligen (mismatched double-stranded RNA). J. Biol. Resp. Modif. 4, 495-502.

Carter, W.A., Hubbell, H., Krueger, L., and Strayer, D.R. (1985b) Comparative studies of Ampligen (mismatched double-stranded RNA) and interferons. J. Biol. Resp. Modif. 4, 613-620.

Carter, W.A., Strayer, D.R., Brodsky, I., Lewin, M., Pellegrino, M.G., Einck, L., Henriques, H.F., Simon, G.L., Parenti, D.M., Scheib, R.G., Schulof, R.S., Montefiori, D., Robinson, W.E., Mitchell, W.M., Volsky, D.J., Paul, D., Paxton, H., Meyer, W.A., III, Kariko, K., Reichenbach, N., Suhadolnik, R.J., and Gillespie, D.H. (1987) Clinical, immunological, and virological effects of Ampligen, a mismatched double-stranded RNA, in patients with AIDS or AIDS-related complex. Lancet i, 1286-1292.

Holmes, G.P., Kaplan, J.E., Stewart, J.A., Hunt, B., Pinsky, P.F., and Schonberger, L.B. (1987) A cluster of patients with a chronic mononucleosis-like syndrome: Is Epstein-Barr virus the cause? J. Amer. CMed. Assoc. 257, 2297-2302.

Holmes, G.P., Kaplan, J.E., Glantz, N.M., Komaroff, A.L., Schonberger, L.B., Straus, S.E., Jones, J.F., Dubois, R.E., Cunningham-Rundles, C., Pahwa,, 5., Tosato, G., Zegano, L.S., Purtilo, D.T., Brown, N., Schooley, R.T., and Bris, I. (1988) Chronic fatigue syndrome: a working case definition. Ann. Intern. Med. 108, 387-389.

Krueger, G.R.F., Manak, M., Bourgeois, N., Ablashi, D.V., Salahuddin, S.Z., Josephs, S.F., Buchbinder, A., Gallo, R.C., Berthold, F., and Tesch, H. (1989) Persistent active herpes virus infection associated with atypical polyclonal lymphoproliferation (APL) and malignant lymphoma. Anticancer 9, 1457-1476.

Lengyel, P. (1982) Biochemistry of interferons and their actions. Annu. Review Biochem. 51, 251-282.

Li, S.W., Moskow, J.J., and Suhadolnik, R.J. (1990) 8-Azido doublestranded RNA Photoaffinity Probes. Enzymatic synthesis, characterization, and biological properties of poly(I,8azidoI)-poly(C) and poly(I,8-azidoI)-poly(Cl2U) with 2',5'oligoadenylate synthetase and protein kinase. J. Biol. Chem. 268, 5470-5474.

Peterson, D.L., Strayer, D.R., Bastien, S., Henry, B., Ablashi, D.V., Breaux, E.J., Walters, D.J., Gillespie, D.R., and Carter, W.A. (1990) Clinical improvements obtained with Ampligen in patients with severe chronic fatigue syndrome and associated encephalopathy. [companion paper, this volume]

Preble, O.T., Rook, A.H., Steis, R., Silverman, R.H., Krause, D., Quinnan, G.V., Masur, H., Jacob, J., Longo, D., and Gelmann, E.P. (1985) Interferon-induced 2',5'-oligoadenylate synthetase during interferon- therapy in homosexual men with Kaposi's sarcoma: Marked deficiency in biochemical response to interferon in patients with acquired immunodeficiency syndrome. J. Infectious Dis. **152**, 457-465.

Read, S.E., LeBrocq, F.J., and Williams, B.R.G. (1985) Persistent elevation of 2-5A synthetase and prognosis in the AIDS-related complex (ARC). In **The 2-5A System: Molecular and Clinical Aspects of the Interferon-Regulated Pathway** pp. 405-413, Alan R. Liss, New York.

Salahuddin, S.Z., Ablashi, D.V., Markham, P.D., Josephs, S.F., Sturzenegger, S., Kaplan, M., Halligan, G., Biberfeld, P., Wong-Staal, F., Kramarsky, B., and Gallo, R.C. (1986) Isolation of a new virus, HBLV, in patients with lymphoproliferative disorders. Science **234**, 596-603.

Schattner, A., Wallach, D., Merlin, G., Hahn, T., Levin, S., and Revel, M. (1981a) Assay of an interferon-induced enzyme in white blood cells as a diagnostic aid in viral diseases. Lancet 2, 497-500.

Schattner, A., Merlin, G., Wallach, D., Rosenberg, H., Bino, T., Hahn, T., Levin, S., and Revel, M. (1981b) Monitoring of interferon therapy by assay of (2'-5')oligo-isoadenylate synthetase in human peripheral white blood cells. J. Interferon Res. 1, 587-594.

Straus, S.E. (1988) The Chronic Mononucleosis Syndrome. J. Infect. Dis. **157**, 405-412.

Strayer, D.R., Brodsky, I., Pequignot, E.C., Crilley, P.A., Carter, W.A., Fenning, R., Kariko, K., Reichenbach, N.L., Sobol, R.W., Li, S.W., and Suhadolnik, R.J. (1990) The antitumor activity of Ampligen, a mismatched double-stranded RNA, which modulates the 2-5A synthetase/RNase L pathway in cancer and AIDS. **Advances in the Chemotherapy of AIDS** (Diasio, R.B., and Sommadossi, J.-P., eds.), p. 23-31, Pergamon Press, New York.

Suhadolnik, R.J., Flick, M.B., Mosca, J.D., Sawada, Y., Doetsch, P.W., and Vonderheid, E.C. (1983)   2',5'-0ligoadenylate synthetase from cutaneous T-cell lymphoma: Biosynthesis, identification, quantitation, molecular size of the 2',5'oligoadenylates, and inhibition of protein synthesis. Biochemistry 22, 4153-4158.

Suhadolnik, R.J., Reichenbach, N.L., Lee, C., Strayer, D.R., Brodsky, I., and Carter, W.A. (1985) Ampligen treatment of renal cell carcinoma: Changes in 2-5A synthetase. 2-5A oligomer size and natural killer cell activity associated with antitumor response clinically. In: **The 2-5A System: Molecular and Clinical Aspects of the Interferon-Regulated Pathway**, pp. 449-465 (Williams, B.R.G, and Silverman, R.H., eds.), Alan R. Liss, New York.

Wells, V., and Mallucci, L. (1985) Expression of the 2-5A system during the cell cycle. Exp. Cell Res. **159**, 27-36.

Williams, B.R.G., Read, S.E., Freedman, M.H., Carver, D.H., and Gelfand, E.W. (1982) The assay of 2-5A synthetase as an indicator of interferon activity and virus infection in vivo. In **Interferons** (UCLA symposia on molecular and cellular biology, vol. 25) (Merigan, T.C., and Friedman, R.M., eds.), pp. 253-267, Academic Press, New York.

617

Chapter 68

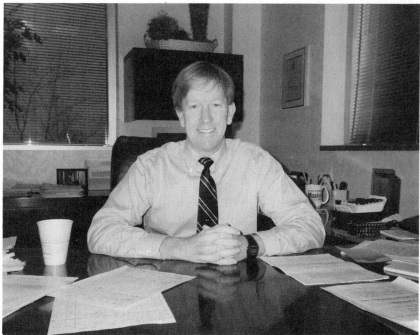

Paul Cheney

Evidence for T-Cell Activation by Soluble IL-2-R and T8-R in the Chronic Fatigue Syndrome

Paul R. Cheney M.D., Ph.D., Mercy General Hospital, 10620 Park Road, Suite 234, Charlotte, North Carolina 28210 USA

Dr. Cheney received a doctorate in physics from Duke University in 1975 and his medical degree from Emory University School of Medicine in 1977. He was a research associate in the Division of Immunology, Centers for Disease Control in Atlanta from 1976 to 1977 and Chief of Medicine (Major USAF MC) at the USAF Hospital in Mt. Home, Idaho from 1980 to 1983. While in the private practice of internal medicine in Incline Village, Nevada from 1983 to 1987, he along with Dr. Daniel Peterson documented a large cluster of cases of Chronic Fatigue Syndrome in the Lake Tahoe region. Since 1987, Dr. Cheney has conducted clinical research in a private practice setting in Charlotte, North Carolina.

Abstract

Immunologic Activation Markers as Correlates of Functional Disability

Chronic Fatigue Syndrome (CFS) relates to a chronic, usually relapsing and often evolving illness of unknown cause. CFS is usually characterized by dysfunctional fatigue but also includes a constellation of other signs and symptoms. Laboratory correlates of the degree of functional disability seen in the Chronic Fatigue syndrome are needed to guide physicians in treatment and disability assessments.

The correlation of various mononuclear cell activation markers, both soluble and membrane bound, with clinical status using the Karnofsky performance scale will be presented. Soluble markers such as the IL-2 receptor and the CDS receptor will be discussed as well as membrane bound markers including the DR antigen and IL-2 receptor. A generic membrane activation marker, MC-540, will also be discussed.

Introduction

Chronic Fatigue Syndrome (CFS) is a chronic, usually relapsing, and often evolving illness characterized by severe fatigue accompanied by other flu-like symptoms and/or neurologic disorders. Different patients may have different constellations of signs and symptoms, but among the most common are debilitating fatigue; low-grade fever and subnormal temperatures; myalgias and arthralgias; headaches; sleep disorder; swollen glands; balance problems; sensitivities to heat, cold, light, sound, or chemicals; and often severe cognitive problems. The cognitive impairment usually develops somewhat later but typically dominates the clinical picture over time. CFS often begins with the abrupt onset of a flu-like or mononucleosis-like illness. However, it may begin with neurologic problems or may develop slowly or insidiously over time. Approximately three out of four CFS patients are women, and most are between the ages of 25 and 45. There are however, significant numbers of children with this syndrome, many of whom are severely disabled.

In the United States, a case definition for CFS developed by the Centers for Disease Control (CDC) has been in use since 1988[1]. It remains uncertain as to whether the clinical entity defined by this case definition is largely one disorder or a multitude of related "post-infectious or post-viral syndromes". It is also uncertain whether the emerging clinical disorder defined by the CDC in 1988 is the same disorder described in the older medical literature by other names such as neurasthenia or myalgic encephalomyelitis (ME).

Recently, there has been a growing impression that CFS is increasing in frequency in the population. The syndrome may be well represented in the 20% of primary care patients who complain of significant and prolonged fatigue of abrupt onset[2]. Half of all patients given the diagnosis of primary fibromyalgia may find the label CFS a better fit [3]. A survey of large numbers of well-defined patients in this clinic suggest a rising case production since the late 1970's and early 1980's (Fig.1).

CFS is a controversial disease. There are important questions of etiology, diagnosis and treatment. There is also compelling evidence that CFS is an organic disease. Many of the signs and symptoms (especially some of the neurologic signs, fevers, and swollen glands, to name a few) are certainly organic. There is also objective laboratory evidence that CFS patients have immune dysfunction. The most common pattern is T-cell activation[4,5], natural killer cell functional deficiency[6,7] and variable B-cell dysfunction[4,5,8].

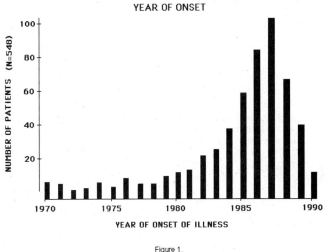

Figure 1.

The Experiment

In this study we investigated two biological markers of T-cell activation, namely, IL-2-R and T8-R in their soluble form in sera. The soluble forms of both these receptors represent partial subunits of more complex membrane bound receptors expressed on T-cells. T-cell activation is mediated by the binding of activating ligands to a variety of specific receptors on the cell surface membrane of circulating T-lymphocytes. The sustained proliferation of such activated T-cells in vitro depends on the presence of membrane bound IL-2 receptors as well as the availability of IL-2[9]. High levels of soluble IL-2-R have been reported in a variety of disorders which collectively might be termed T-cell activation states. They include, but are not limited to, multiple sclerosis[10], lupus erythematosis[11] and other autoimmune disorders[12], AIDS[13] and hematologic malignancies[14,15].

The soluble T8-receptor is a subunit of the membrane bound CD8 receptor which typically resides on suppressor/cytotoxic T-lymphocytes. Soluble T8-R is released during activation of CD8 marked lymphocytes and typically indicates either increased

Figure 2

Karnofsky Performance Scale

Able to carry on normal activity; no special care is needed	100	Normal; no complaints; no evidence of disease.
	90	Able to carry on normal activity; minor signs or symptoms of disease
	80	Normal activity with effort; some signs of symptoms of disease
Unable to work, able to live at home and care for most personal needs; a varying amount of assistance is needed	70	Cares for self, unable to carry on normal activity or to do active work
	60	Requires occasional assistance but is able to care for most of needs
	50	Requires considerable assistance and frequent medical care
Unable to care for self; requires equivalent of institutional or hospital care; disease may be progressing rapidly.	40	Disabled; requires special care and assistance
	30	Severely disabled; hospitalization is indicated although death is not imminent
	20	Very sick; hospitalization necessary; active supportive treatment is necessary
	10	Moribund; fatal processes progressing rapidly
	0	Dead

suppressor or cytotoxic activity[16]. Elevated levels of soluble T8-R have been reported in pediatric lymphomas[17] and AIDS[18].

Patients and Methods

Two overlapping groups of nearly consecutive patients presenting for either their first office visit or a follow-up visit were selected for analysis. One group was analyzed for IL-2-R and the other for T8-R. A majority had blood for both receptors drawn at the same time. Most had been taking some medication for symptom relief on an intermittent basis. A minority were on over-the-counter multivitamins. None were receiving primary immunotherapy or antiviral therapy. To be selected for further analysis, the patient had to meet strict CDC criteria with no confounding medical or psychiatric problem which could plausibly explain his/her symptoms. Each patient meeting the case definition was functionally categorized independently by two clinicians according to the Karnofsky Performance Scale (Fig. 2). Any disagreement between clinicians (there were two disagreements) was resolved before entry into the analysis. Healthy community controls were recruited who generally matched the age (25-45) and sex (three

females to one male) distribution of the patients. Blood was typically drawn between 9 AM and 11 AM.

Serum levels of soluble IL-2-R and T8-R were determined using a T-cell Sciences (Cambridge, MA) EIA kit and measured on a BioMass (Los Angeles, CA) microplate reader using serum collected and stored at -70°F.

Patients from the two groups were run in duplicate on consecutive microplate runs intermixed with controls. The paired t-test was used for statistical comparison between patient categories and controls.

Results

CFS patients had significantly higher levels of these two receptors compared with controls (Fig. 3).

Figure 3			
Patients	**IL-2-R**	**T8-R**	**p-value**
n=63	658+282 U/ml	-	p<0.016
n=79	-	548+223 U/ml	p<0.03
Controls	IL-2-R	T8-R	
n=15	326+64 U/ml	287+59	-

There was correlation between severity of illness as measured by the Karnofsky Performance Scale and soluble receptors for both IL-2-R (Fig.4) and T8-R (Fig.5). The very highest values for both receptors were seen in the most severe clinical categories (Karnofsky < 60). Of note was that patients with low values of IL-2-R in the more severe clinical categories (Karnofsky 60 or below) had in most cases, very high T8-R values suggesting a reciprocal relationship between these receptors among sicker patients. The milder patient categories (Karnofsky >70) were not significantly different than controls.

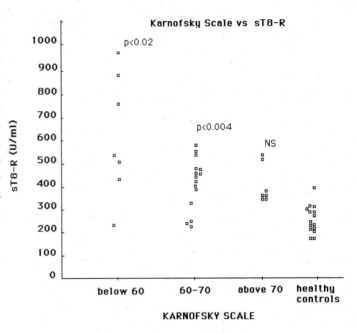

Figure 5.

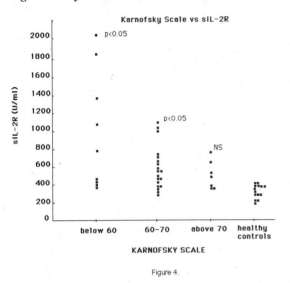

Figure 4.

Discussion

The data presented here strongly suggests that CFS patients belong to a larger group of diverse disorders characterized by T-cell activation. This diverse group of disorders range from autoimmune diseases (SLE) to chronic viral illnesses (AIDS and mononucleosis) to hematologic malignancies (Lymphoma). If forced to choose between these broad categories as the most likely for CFS to belong; a chronic viral illness would best fit the symptoms and evolution of these patients. Given the known systemic effects of exogenously administered cytokines (IL-2[19], IFN-alpha[20]), it is also likely that T-cell activation may itself drive many if not all of the symptoms of CFS. One might also predict rare or even common complications among CFS patients based on chronic T-cell activation, including autoimmune disorders themselves as well as functional or even structural central nervous system injury[21,22] in the susceptible host. The larger issue of what is provoking this degree of T-cell activation is as yet unanswered. The apparent rising case production and notable severity of illness in many of these patients suggests to this author that although there may be technically many potential causes of CFS, it is also[1] possible that a novel cause has entered the scene in the last fifteen years and may be dominating the CFS case production in the last two decades of this century.

References

1. Holmes GP, Kaplan JE, Gantz NM, Komaroff AL, Schonberger LB, Straus SE, Jones JF, Dubois RE, Cunningham-Rundles C, Pahwa S, Tosato G, Zegans LS, Purtilo DT, Brown N, Schooley RT and Brus I. Chronic Fatigue Syndrome: A Working Case Definition. Ann Intern Med. 1988;108:387-9.

2. Buchwald D, Sullivan JL and Komaroff A. Frequency of "chronic activeEpstein-Barr virus infection" in a general medical practice. JAMA 1987;257:2303-8.

3. Buchwald D, Goldenberg DL, Sullivan JL and Komaroff A. The "Chronic Active Epstein-Barr Virus Infection" Syndrome and Primary Fibromyalgia. Arth.Rheum.1987;30:1132.

4. Klimas N, Salvato F, Morgan R and Fletcher M. Immunologic Abnormalities in Chronic Fatigue Syndrome. J. of Clinical Microbiology.1990;28:1403-1410

5. Lloyd AR, Wakefield D, Boughton CR, Dwyer JM. Immunological Abnormalities in The Chronic Fatigue Syndrome. Medical Journal of Australia. 1989;151(3):122-124.

6. Caliguri M, Murray C, Buchwald D, Levine H, Cheney P, Peterson D, Komaroff AL and Ritz J. Phenotypic and Functional Deficiency of Natural Killer Cells in Patients with Chronic Fatigue Syndrome. J. Immunol.1987;139:3306-3313.

7. Aoki T, Usuda Y, Miyakoshi H, Tamura K, Herberman RB. Low Natural Killer Syndrome: Clinical and Immunologic Features. Nat.Immun.Cell Growth Regul.1987;6:116-128.

8. Komaroff AL, Geiger AM, Wormseley S. IgG Subclass Deficiencies in Chronic Fatigue Syndrome. Lancet. 1988;i(8597):1288-89.

9. Dinarello CA, Mier JW. Interleukins. Ann. Rev. Med. 1986.37:173-78

10. Adachi K, Kumamoto T, Araki S. Elevated Soluble IL-2 Receptor Levels in Multiple Sclerosis Patients, Lancet. 1989;Mar:559-60.

11. Wolf RE, et al. Soluble Interleukin-2 Receptors in Systemtic Lupus Erythematosus. Arthritis Rheum. 1988;31:729-735.

12. Campen DH, et al. Serum Levels of Interleukin-2 Receptor and Activity of Rheumatic Diseases Characterized by Immune System Activation. Arthritis Rheum. 1988; 31:1358-1364.

13. Kloster BE, et al. Soluble Interleukin-2 Receptors are Elevated in Patients with AIDS or at Risk of Developing AIDS. Clin. Immunol. and Immunopathol. 1986;45:440.

14. Nelson DL, A Soluble Form of the Human IL-2 Receptor, pp. 13-16. In Green WC, moderator. The Human Interleukin-2 Receptor: Normal and Abnormal Expression in T cells and HTLV-Induced Leukemias. Ann. Intern. Med. 1986.

15. Wagner DK, et al. Soluble Interleukin-2 Receptor Levels in Patients with Undifferentiated and Lymphoblastic Lymphomas: Correlation with Survival. J. Clin. Oncol. 1987;5:1262-1274.

16. Fujimoto J, et al. Spontaneous Release of the Leu-2 (T8-Receptor) Molecule from Human T Cells. J. Exp. Med.1983;159:752-766.

17. Pui CH, Ip SH, Dodge RK, Carrabis S, Brown M, Crist WM, Berard CW, Kung P, Dahl GV and Murphy SB. Serum Levels of CD8 Antigen in Childhood Lymphoid Malignancies: A Possible Indicator of Increased Suppressor Cell Activity in Poor-Risk Patients. **Blood.** 1988;72(3):1015-1021.

18. Walker CM, Moody DW, Stites DP, Levy JA. CD8+ Lymphocytes Can Control HIV Infection in Vitro by Suppressing Virus Replication, **Reports**. 1986;Dec:1563.

19. Denicoff KD, Rubinow DR, Papa MX, et al.The Neuropsychiatric Effects of Treatment with Interleukin-2 and Lymphokine Activated Killer Cells. Ann. Intern. Med.1987;107:293-300.

20. Adams F, Quesada JR, Gutterman JU. Neuropsychiatric Manifestations of Human Leukocyte Interferon Therapy in Patients with Cancer. JAMA. 1984;252(7):938.

21. Daugherty SA, Henry BE, Peterson DL, Swarts RL, Bastien S and Thomas RS. Chronic Fatigue Syndrome in Northern Nevada. Reviews of Infectious Diseases. 1991; 13(Suppl 1):S39-44.

22. Buchwald D, Cheney PR et al. A Chronic Illness Characterized by Fatigue, Neurologic and Immunologic Disorders, and Active Human Herpesvirus-6 Infection. Ann Intern Med. 1992;116(2):103-113.

Treatment

Chapter 69

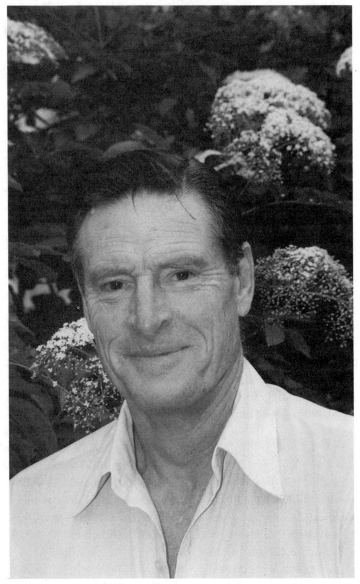

Clem Boughton

(Dr. Boughton is part of the M.E. Sydney, Australia team.)

Intravenous Immunoglobulin Therapy in Patients with Chronic Fatigue Syndrome

Andrew Lloyd, MD, FRACP, NHRMC, Ian Hickie, MD, FRANZCP, Denis Wakefield, MD, FRACP, Clem Boughton, MD and John Dwyer, PhD, FRACP, Departments of Infectious Diseases and Immunology, Division of Medicine and the Mood Disorders Unit, Division of Psychiatry, The Prince Henry Hospital, Little Bay, Sydney, Australia.

(Please see Chapter 58 for Dr. Lloyd's photograph and curriculum vitae.)

Introduction

Evidence has been presented for abnormal cellular and humoral immunity in patients with chronic fatigue syndrome (CFS; Behan *et al*, 1985; Lloyd *et al*, 1989). These findings support the hypothesis that

CFS is associated with a disordered immune response to an antigenic challenge (such as a viral infection), potentially allowing persistence of antigen and stimulation of a continued immune response. Alternatively, the immune response may persist in the absence of residual antigen (Wakefield and Lloyd, 1987).

Immunomodulatory therapy with high dose intravenous immunoglobulin has been demonstrated to be beneficial in a number of diseases featuring disordered immunoregulation (Dwyer, 1987). Consequently, intravenous immunoglobulin was initially administered to patients with CFS, in an uncontrolled trial, on the rationale that improved immunological function following immunoglobulin treatment might correct immunoregulatory disturbances or assist in the clearance of antigen and resolution of the syndrome. In addition, replacement therapy with immunoglobulin may assist in restoring normal humoral immune function. Nineteen of the 29 patients (66%) treated in a preliminary study reported symptomatic benefit from intravenous immunoglobulin. Therefore a randomised, double-blind, placebo-controlled trial was undertaken (Lloyd *et al,* 1990).

Subjects and methods

Forty-nine adult patients with CFS, who had received no previous immunological therapy, were enrolled. The diagnosis of CFS required: (i) a history of marked exercise-aggravated muscle fatigue, of at least six months duration, associated with typical constitutional and neuropsychiatric symptoms and (ii) that CFS was producing frequent medical consultation, and a substantial reduction in the ability to participate in usual daily activities when compared to the subject's pre-morbid status, for example considerable time lost from school or work, and inability to participate in sports (Lloyd *et al,* 1988). All patients had chronic and persisting symptomatology, rather than a relapsing and remitting course sometimes reported for CFS. A physical examination and standardised investigation protocol excluded other chronic infectious or immunodeficiency-related disorders.

Patients were randomly allocated to receive either intravenous immunoglobulin (*Intragam*, Commonwealth Serum Laboratories [CSL], Australia - a product based on the formulation of Gamimune-N, Cutter Laboratories, USA) administered by continuous infusion in a dosage of 2g(IgG)/kg or placebo (10%w/v maltose) in an equivalent volume. Three infusions lasting 24 hours were administered at monthly intervals. The response to therapy three months after the final infusion was chosen as the principal time point for evaluation of outcome.

All subjects were interviewed by a physician (AL) to determine their suitability for the study. At this interview an assessment of the severity of the symptoms and the degree of disability attributable to CFS was made. Specific details of the degree of involvement in work or school, leisure, sporting and social activities were recorded. A standardised psychiatric interview was also conducted by a psychiatrist (IH).

Effectiveness or otherwise of therapy was established at the post-infusion interview by the physician's assessment of symptomatic and functional improvement. These interviews were conducted three months after the final infusion with neither the patient nor the interviewer being aware of the treatment received. In addition, the psychiatrist rated each subject before and after treatment using the detailed Hamilton Depression Scale (Hamilton, 1960). Cell-mediated immunity was assessed by T cell subset analysis, DTH skin testing and by T cell stimulation with phytohemagglutinin (PHA) using standard methods.

Adverse effects were monitored both during and after the infusions by a combination of investigator recordings (of phlebitis) and self-reports (of constitutional symptoms during and after the infusions).

Results

There was no significant difference in the demographic variables (age, sex, disease duration), or entry measures of physical or psychological well-being, or immunity between the treatment groups.

At the completion of the trial, the blinded evaluation of symptoms and disability by the physician demonstrated that 43% of the immunoglobulin recipients and 11% of the placebo recipients had a marked reduction in symptoms and improvement in functional capacity.

All of the subjects designated as "responders" increased their level of participation in work, leisure and social activities. In contrast, the remaining subjects had little or no change in their ability to participate in these activities. The responders also had a reduction in their psychiatric morbidity and a significant improvement in measures of cell-mediated immunity.

Phlebitis and constitutional symptoms including headaches, worsened fatigue and concentration impairment were frequent and occurred more commonly in the immunoglobulin recipients than in the patients who received placebo.

Discussion

The results of this study demonstrate that a significant proportion of patients with well-characterised, severe and long-standing CFS responded to high-dose, intravenous immunoglobulin therapy. This represents the first report of an effective treatment modality for at least some patients with CFS evaluated in a double-blind, placebo-controlled trial. The response to solely immunological therapy adds further evidence to the immunopathological hypothesis of CFS.

The pattern of response to therapy suggested that only some patients achieve benefit from intravenous immunoglobulin using this dosage regimen. The majority of the patients had long-standing disability from CFS, with the not unexpected secondary physical and psychological morbidity associated with chronic illness. These secondary factors may have prevented a satisfactory treatment response in some patients.

The difference in prevalence of adverse effects noted between the immunoglobulin and placebo recipients in this study provided some difficulty with the double-blind aspect of the protocol, as the effects were more common in the group infused with immunoglobulin. However, all of the patients were advised at enrollment that either the immunoglobulin or 10% maltose infusion may be associated with phlebitis, and similarly that either infusion may precipitate a transient exacerbation of the symptoms of the syndrome.

Immunoglobulin may provide symptomatic benefit in patients with CFS, associated with the effect of improving cell-mediated immunity in this disorder. Whether or not this relationship is causal is unknown. Analysis of larger groups of treated patients will be required to detect immunological or other variables which best predict the therapeutic response. Further studies to define the dose-response relationship of immunoglobulin to benefit in the treatment of patients with CFS and the time course of the beneficial effect are underway.

References

Behan P, Behan W, Bell E. The postviral fatigue syndrome - an analysis of the findings in 50 cases. J Infect 1985; 10: 211-222.

Dwyer J. Intravenous therapy with gammaglobulin. Adv Intern Med 1987; 32: 111-136.

Hamilton M. A rating scale for depression. J Neurol Neurosurg Psychiatry 1960; 23: 56-62.

Lloyd A, Wakefield D, Boughton C, Dwyer J. What is myalgic encephalomyelitis? Lancet 1988; i: 1286-1287.

Lloyd A, Wakefield D, Boughton C, Dwyer J. Immunological abnormalities in the chronic fatigue syndrome. Med J Aust 1989; 151: 122-124.

Lloyd A, Hickie I, Wakefield D, Boughton C, Dwyer J. High dose intravenous immunoglobulin therapy in the chronic fatigue syndrome: A double-blind, placebo-controlled trial. Am J Med 1990; 89:561-568.

Wakefield D, Lloyd A. Pathophysiology of myalgic encephalomyelitis. Lancet 1987; ii: 918-919.

Chapter 70

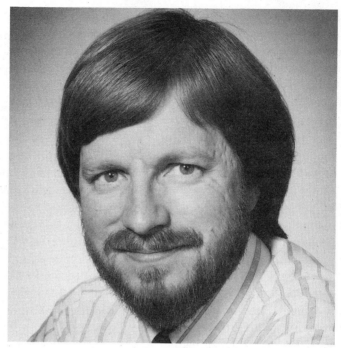

Michael D. Winther

Essential Fatty Acid Therapy for Myalgic Encephalomyelitis

Dr. Michael D. Winther
Head of Preclinical Research, Scotia Pharmaceuticals Ltd., Woodbridge Meadows, Guildford,
Surrey GU1 1BA

Dr. Winther obtained his BA in Biochemistry and Molecular Biology (High Honours) from the University of California at Santa Barbara in 1975. This was followed by studies at the University of Sterling, Scotland, leading to the award of PhD in Biochemistry in 1978. These studies of fungal biochemistry and molecular biology were continued during a postdoctoral position at the University of Essex. Dr. Winther's past employment includes working as a senior scientist in the Department of Molecular Biology, Wellcome Research Laboratories and as head of the department developing and producing experimental vaccines and other proteins derived from recombinant DNA technology. Dr. Winther currently is involved in the study of the role of essential fatty acids in various disease conditions, with an emphasis on postviral illnesses. As head of Preclinical Research, he is also involved with investigating antiviral drugs and other pharmacologically active compounds.

In Search of New Therapies

In recent years, Myalgic Encephalomyelitis has been investigated by researchers from all around the world but still the cause of the illness remains a mystery. A viral origin is suspected but not proven, so the hunt for a causative viral agent continues. However, even demonstrating the occurrence of an acute virus infection that is associated with the onset of symptoms does not establish the existence of a chronic infection or explain the particular group of symptoms common to M.E. sufferers.

Clearly this lack of understanding makes the rational development of any therapy very difficult. Unfortunately, it may take many more years before we have sufficient understanding of M.E. to design new and effective treatments. For those presently suffering from M.E. this may not seem a sufficient response to their medical needs and a more broadly based search for therapies should be supported.

One such approach has grown out of our interest in determining the role of essential fatty acids in human diseases. We are beginning to accumulate evidence that fatty acids also have a role in M.E. and are actively pursuing the scientific and therapeutic opportunities this observation presents.

Essential Fatty Acids

The requirement for certain long chain polyunsaturated fatty acids (PUFA) in the diet was demonstrated in the 1930s[1]. Since then, the pathways have been elucidated in greater detail. Some long chain PUFAs can be synthesised from the precursors palmitic acid and stearic acid which are produced in the body. However, other PUFAs are produced from linoleic acid and gamma-linolenic acid. These precursors cannot be manufactured in the body but must be obtained in the diet, hence they are termed Essential Fatty Acids or EFAs.

The pathways for metabolism of n-6 and n-3 EFAs are shown in Figure 1.

Figure 1

Pathways of Metabolism of EFAs

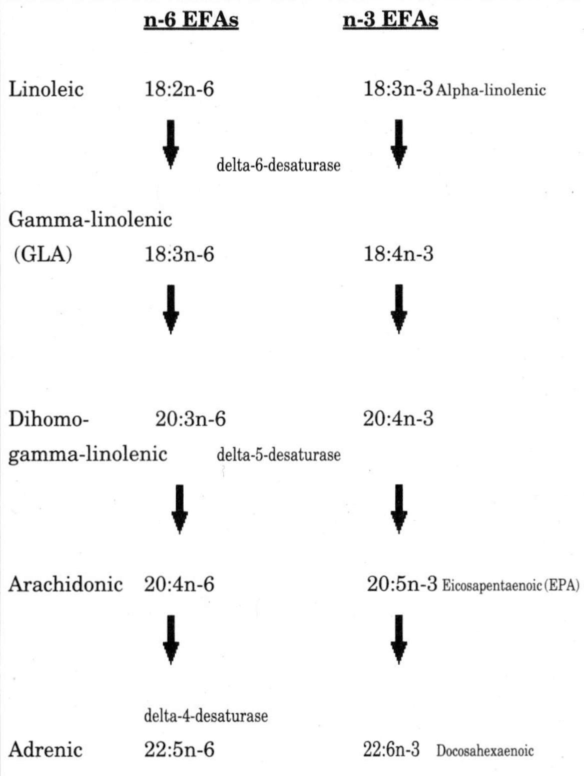

The idea that EFA metabolism may be disturbed in M.E. comes from attempting to relate six relevant clinical observations :

1. there is already a very clear example of a specific illness, atopic eczema, that can be a consequence of low levels of essential fatty acids[2];

2. patients with eczema are highly susceptible to viral infections - not just cutaneous infections due to the fragile nature of the skin barrier, but also to systemic upper respiratory tract infections and EBV[3,4];

3. atopic disorders have been observed to occur after a viral infection in patients with no previous history of such a condition[5];

4. serum EFAs can drop after a viral infection[6,7];

5. carnitine is required for normal transfer of EFAs into cells and carnitine deficiency results in fatigue and myalgia similar to that found in M.E.[8];

6. M.E. frequently occurs after viral infections[9].

In these cases where the enzyme delta-6-desaturase is low or absent, even an abundance of linoleic acid in the diet cannot bring about adequate levels of EFAs. However, supplementation with GLA will bypass the blockage as it enters the metabolic pathway after the blocked step. This strategy is successful with atopic eczema and has resulted in the development of a pharmaceutical product containing GLA in the triglyceride form (under the registered name "Epogam").

The source of GLA must be found in natural products since the complete chemical synthesis of this compound is not practical. The main source of GLA is from oil extracted from the seeds of the Evening Primrose (Oenothera). The GLA is present as part of a mixed triglyceride that is probably broken down to free fatty acids and glycerol during digestion. However, it has been observed that other sources of GLA such as blackcurrant seeds, borage seeds and fungal oil produce a material with a different biological activity. The precise reason for this is not known but may be due to the GLA being present in different triglyceride structures or to interfering factors in the other oils.

Functions of EFAs

The functions of EFAs fall into three distinct categories:-

1. they are structural components of cellular membranes;

2. they are precursors to prostaglandins and leukotrienes; and

3. they function in the transport and oxidation of cholesterol.

The biochemistry and regulation of EFAs is complex and requires further studies. Although prostaglandins and leukotrienes are all specifically metabolised from EFAs, the location and regulation of this is not understood. This is a very important point since prostaglandins act locally and have a very short half-life in the body. Due to this, it is not very accurate (or meaningful) to measure prostaglandin levels in the blood.

Another intriguing observation is that the antiviral activity of interferon may also be dependent on fatty acids. It has been shown that interferon is inactive in cell lines lacking the enzyme cyclo-oxygenase[10]. Since EFAs are substrates for this enzyme, it implies a role in the mechanism of action of interferon. Thus interferon, whether endogenously produced or administered as a drug, may require sufficient levels of EFAs in the body to be effective in eliminating or reducing virus infections.

What would be the clinical implications of a drop in EFA levels? This is not possible to predict for certain because EFA deficiency may show itself in a range of ways. This may depend on the degree of deficiency, the exact nature of the deficiency (e.g. exactly which n-3 and n-6 EFAs are low), the location of the deficiency, which may be restricted to certain parts of the body, and other factors (coincident infections, dietary habits).

EFAs are essential substrates in muscle oxidative phosphorylation and neuronal metabolism. It seems reasonable to suggest that fatigue may be a result of an EFA deficiency in the muscle. Indeed the observation that carnitine deficiency results in fatigue would support this.

Viral Disturbance of EFA Metabolism

While it is not clear what proportion of M.E. is caused or triggered by a virus infection it is clear that fatigue and other symptoms characteristic of M.E. can follow on from a virus infection. This is particularly the case with Epstein-Barr Virus infections which can result in a prolonged recovery time.

In a study carried out amongst college students in Columbus, Ohio, it was clearly shown that patients suffering infectious mononucleosis for three months had abnormal serum fatty acids[7]. Below normal proportions of arachidonic acid and a reversal of the usual serum ratio of linoleic and oleic acids were maximal at this time.

The pattern of EFAs also suggested that the enzymic deficiency was with the desaturase activity rather than chain elongation. Not only did the EFA abnormalities coincide with the symptoms of increased physical malaise, but the persistence of low linoleic acid occurred in all of the students that continued to show clinical symptoms for a year.

There are a variety of ways in which a virus can disturb EFA metabolism. Replicating viruses can directly use host lipids and so alter remaining levels. The virus may also destroy host cells through induction of immunomediators.

There are also possible indirect factors such as decreased dietary intake of fats due to poor appetite, decreased intestinal absorption of fats and an increased rate of host lipolysis. Whatever the cause, the end effect may be similar.

Since the majority of the EFAs in the blood were synthesised in the liver by hepatic microsomes, damage in this area would effect EFA levels throughout the body.

Clinical Studies with EFAs

As there are no recognised laboratory markers for M.E., it is necessary to assess therapeutic benefit solely by the changes to the patients' symptoms. This emphasizes the need to conduct proper double blind studies to allow for placebo effects.

The first controlled trial of essential fatty acids for M.E. was conducted at the Glasgow Southern General Hospital in 1986/7 by Dr. Peter Behan. The results of this study have been reported[11,12] and will only be summarised here.

63 patients with M.E. were entered into the study, taking 8 capsules per day (active or placebo) for a total of 3 months. Baseline analysis of EFA levels in the red cell membrane phospholipids showed a statistically significant drop in the levels of two n-6 fatty acids (arachidonic and adrenic) and trends towards lower levels of n-3 fatty acids (although not reaching statistical significance). The product used for this study, Efamol Marine, contains 80% evening primrose oil and 20% marine oil, so both classes of EFAs will be provided.

After three months therapy the two groups were asked to rate their overall condition relative to that when beginning the trial. The results (Table 1) show a clear benefit from the EFA therapy with over three times as many patients saying they are improved on active therapy (31% vs 9%). Statistical differences between those improved or much improved on active therapy (84%) vs placebo (18%) by a likelihood ratio test gave the result 2 p = <0.0001.

Clinical assessments were made for a range of M.E. symptoms (exhaustion, muscle weakness, aches and pains, lack of concentration, dizziness, vertigo, depression and loss of memory). All of these symptoms showed statistically significant improvements after three months of therapy (Table 2). It is easiest to consider the changes to the global score derived by averaging all of the above symptoms scored on a four point scale (0 = no symptom, 1 = mild, 2 = moderate, 3 = severe).

Table 2			
	Baseline	1 month	3 months
Efamol Marine	1.88	1.25*	0.96**
Placebo	1.78	1.45	1.62

* P = 0.0033 active vs placebo at one month
** P = <0.0001 active vs placebo at one month

It is interesting to note that all patients on Efamol Marine improved steadily over the three months of the trial, eventually finishing with a 50% reduction of their global score. The control patients had a slight improvement over the first month but this was subsequently lost and they finished the trial with their global score being virtually unchanged from the pretrial score.

These changes in clinical conditions were matched by changes in the fatty acid levels as shown in Figure 2. With Efamol Marine there are rises in both n-3 and n-6 EFAs and a drop in saturated and monounsaturated fatty acids.

Due to these encouraging results a much more extensive multicentre trial has been organised with over four hundred patients enrolled in the UK and New Zealand. Since all patients will have their medical histories recorded, this study will also reveal any major differences in the nature of M.E. as it is found in these very different locations. This should enable us to define a group or subset of patients who are most likely to benefit from this therapeutic strategy. Results from this double blind placebo controlled trial will be available late towards the end of 1991 and should begin to establish the role for EFA therapy of post-viral illnesses.

Table 1				
Percentage of Patients Assessed as:				
	much worse	worse	unchanged	improved	much improved
Efamol Marine n=38	0	0	16	53	31
Placebo n=22	0	9	73	9	9

Figure 2
Fatty Acid Concentrations (expressed as mg/100mg lipid)

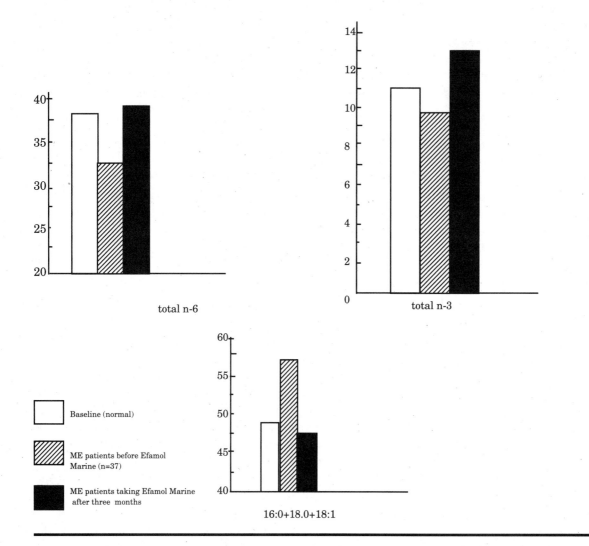

total n-6

total n-3

Baseline (normal)

ME patients before Efamol Marine (n=37)

ME patients taking Efamol Marine after three months

16:0+18.0+18:1

References

1. Sinclair, H M (1990). History of Essential Fatty Acids. In: Omega-6 Essential Fatty Acids: pathophysiology and roles in clinical medicine. D. Horrobin ed., Alan R Liss Inc, p. 1-20.

2. Wright, S (1990). Essential Fatty Acids and Atopic Eczema. Biochemical and immunological studies. In: Omega-6 Essential Fatty Acides: Pathophysiology and roles in clinical medicine. D Horrobin ed., Alan R Liss, New York.

3. Strannegard, O., Strannegard, I-L and Rystedt, I. (1985). Viral infections in atopic dermatitis. Acta Derm Venereol (Stockh); Suppl 114:121-124.

4. Rystedt, I., Strannegard, I-L and Strannegard, O. (1986). Recurrent viral infections in patients with past or present atopic dermatitis. Br J Dermatol, 114:575-582.

5. Barnetson R.S., Hardie, R.A. and Merrett, T.G. (1981). Late onset atopic eczema and multiple food allergies after infectious mononucleosis. Br Med J; 283:1086.

6. Stoessar A.V. (1935). Effect of acute infection on iodine number of serum fatty acids. Proc Soc Exp Biol Med; 32:1326-1327.

7. Williams, L, L., Doody, D.M. and Horrocks, L.A. (1988). Serum fatty acid proportions are altered during the year following acute Epstein-Barr virus infection. Lipids; 23:981-988.

8. Rebouche, C.J. and Engel, A.G. (1983). Carnitine metabolism and deficiency syndromes. Mayo Clin Proc **58**, 533-540.

9. Straus, S.E. (1988). The chronic mononucleosis syndrome. J Infect Dis; 157:405-412.

10. Chandrabose, K.A., Cuatrecasas, P., Pottathil, R. and Lang, D.J. (1981). Interferon-resistant cell line lacks cyclooxygenase activity. Science 212:329-331.

11. Behan, P.O. and Behan, W.M.H. (1990). Essential fatty acids in the treatment of postviral fatigue syndrome. In: Omega-6 Essential Fatty Acids: Pathophysiology and roles in clinical medicine. D Horrobin ed., Alan R Liss Inc, p. 275-282.

12. Behan, P.O., Behan, W.M.H. and Horrobin D (1990). Effect of high doeses of essential fatty acids on the postviral fatigue syndrome. Acta Neurol. Scand 82: 209-216.

Chapter 71

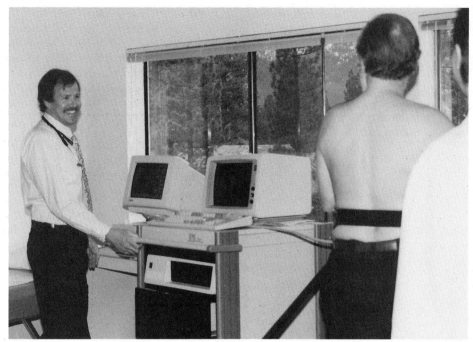

Daniel L. Peterson (see also Chapter 3 for photograph)

Clinical Improvements Obtained with Ampligen in Patients with Severe Chronic Fatigue Syndrome and Associated Encephalopathy

Daniel L. Peterson[1], David R. Strayer[2], Sheila Bastien[3], Berch Henry[4], Dharam V. Ablashi[5], Elizabeth J. Breaux[6], David J. Walters[6], David R. Gillespie[2], and William A. Carter[5,6]

[1]Incline Village, NV 89450, [2]Hahnemann University, Philadelphia, PA 19102, [3]Psychological Corporation, Berkeley, CA 96707, [4]University of Nevada School of Medicine, Reno, NV 89557, [5]National Cancer Institute, Bethesda, MD 20892, [6]HEM Research, Inc., Philadelphia, PA 19103

Dr. Daniel L. Peterson has been active in Chronic Fatigue Syndrome clinical research since 1985 in association with the University of Nevada Reno, National Institutes of Health, CDC in Atlanta, Georgia, and Brigham and Women's Hospital in Boston, Massachusetts.

Introduction

Chronic fatigue syndrome and associated encephalopathy (CFSE) is an illness characterized by persistent, debilitating fatigue and cognitive dysfunction. In order to distinguish CFSE from other diseases, the United States Center for Disease Control has established a working definition which provides a rational basis for diagnosis of patients with chronic fatigue of undetermined cause (Holmes et al., 1988). This syndrome has been associated with a general reactivation of a number of viruses. One such virus is human herpes virus 6 (HHV-6). Antibody to HHV-6 has been reported to be significantly high in CFSE patients as determined by indirect immunofluorescence assay (Ablashi et al., 1989). HHV-6 reactivation was detected in CFSE in patients' peripheral blood lymphocytes in culture using HHV-6 monoclonal antibodies (Balachandran et al., 1988). Presence of HHV-6 specific IgM antibody is further evidence of HHV-6 reactivation. Since the first isolation of HHV-6 in 1986 (Salahuddin et al., 1986), numerous other isolations from various diseases including CFSE have been described (see Ablashi et al., 1989 for review).

Figure 1

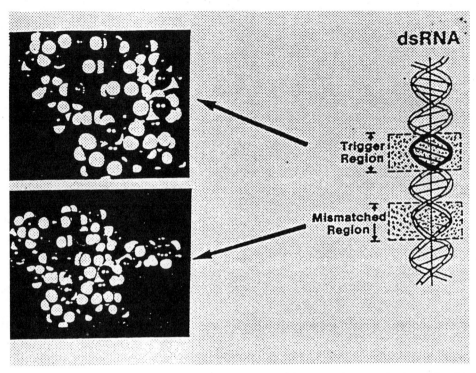

Mismatched dsRNA (Ampligen) preserves the "trigger region" which stimulates interferon production and activates intracellular mediators, while eliminating toxicity.

Because of the viral reactivation in CFSE, an agent with broad antiviral activity is an attractive therapeutic approach. Double-stranded RNAs (dsRNA) are a new class of biological response modifiers with broad spectrum antiviral and immunomodulatory activity (Strayer et al., 1990). The development of physiologically active dsRNAs as either antiviral or antitumor agents has been limited because of **in vivo** toxicity. dsRNAs with periodically mispaired regions retain the lymphokine-inducing potential without having the known dsRNA toxicities (Figure 1). A mismatched dsRNA [Ampligen, poly(I)-poly($C_{12}U$)] has been used in long-term phase I-II clinical trials in cancer patients without evidence of cumulative toxicity (Brodsky et al., 1985; Strayer et al., 1990).

Ampligen also augments natural killer (NK) and monocyte activities and may aid in B-cell maturation (Carter et al., 1985a,b). Ampligen has recently shown marked clinical, immunological and virological effects in patients with HIV-related immunodeficiency (Carter et al., 1987; Strayer et al., 1990). In addition,

several dsRNA-dependent enzymes thought to be related to the interferon-associated natural antiviral pathway are modulated by mismatched dsRNA (Strayer et al., 1990). On the basis of the documented antiviral and immunomodulatory properties of mismatched dsRNA and the evidence that CFSE may involve chronic virus reactivation and immune dysregulation, we reasoned that Ampligen might be a useful therapy for CFSE. In this study, we describe the clinical results and virological changes in fifteen CFSE patients treated with Ampligen.

Methods

Fifteen individuals with persistent debilitating fatigue were identified who met the CDC definition for chronic fatigue syndrome and also showed evidence of encephalopathy (CFSE) by neuropsychological testing and abnormal T2 weighted high white matter changes in MRI brain scans. Patients who were taking other immunomodulatory drugs, pregnant or had other defined disease processes were excluded.

All patients gave informed consent for the study and were treated at Incline Village, Nevada.

Ampligen (HEM Research, Rockville, MD) was administered intravenously twice a week at a dosage level of 200-400 mg to all patients. Ampligen used in this study was formulated in glass bottles as previously described (Carter et al., 1987). Treadmill exercise tolerance, neuropsychological testing, clinical, viral and immunological data were obtained on all patients during Ampligen therapy.

Activity of HHV-6 in Ampligen treated patients was determined by the use of a number of qualitative and quantitative tests which included: (i) an **in vitro** biological test to detect the presence of virus replication in patient lymphocytes (Salahuddin et al., 1986; Josephs et al., 1986), (ii) indirect immunofluorescence assays employing defined high titer polyclonal sera (Goldman, 1968; Josephs et al., 1986; Salahuddin et al., 1986; Sternberger, 1986), (iii) polymerase chain reaction (PCR) assays of patient lymphocytes using an HHV-6 specific probe (generously provided by Dr. Robert Honess) (Erlich, 1989; Innis et al., 1990), (iv) immunofluorescence assays to detect viral antigen expressing cells employing monoclonal antibodies against HHV-6 (Balachandran et al., 1988; Ablashi et al., 1989) and (v) **in situ** hybridization of patient lymphocytes using HHV-6 specific probes (Erlich, 1968; Innis et al., 1990).

Results and Discussion

Patients participated in treadmill testing before and during Ampligen therapy. The length of time the treadmill exercise could be performed and the maximum O_2 consumption during exercise testing were determined. By 24 weeks in the group as a whole, treadmill duration increased by 20% and maximum O_2 consumption during exercise doubled. The majority of the 15 patients entered the study with impaired short term memory, as evidenced by the Wechsler Memory Scale. Wechsler scores improved >50% in these patients during the study. Gains in IQ were also noted. Full scale IQ increased by 12%, from 106 to 119. Performance IQ increased 19% while verbal IQ increased 10%.

To detect virus reactivation, peripheral blood mononuclear cells from all patients were cultured and examined for the presence of giant cells. Virus culture was confirmed by immunofluorescence (Salahuddin et al., 1986). All patient cell cultures were positive for virus at baseline. Virus reactivation was reduced during Ampligen treatment in 13 of 14 patients. The decrease in virus reactivation was further studied in seven of the CFSE patients before and during therapy. Pretherapy, the percent HHV-6 positive cells ranged between 5 and 35%. All seven patients showed a reduction of HHV-6 antigen positive cells with Ampligen therapy.

Historically, Ampligen has been well tolerated, with minimal side effects seen in over 2,500 patient treatment weeks within the dose range 10-300 mg twice weekly (Strayer et al., 1990). Hematological and biochemical parameters during therapy with mismatched dsRNA at the 200-300 mg dose level show no significant toxicities. Cumulative doses of over 50 grams have been administered to several HIV-infected patients without any adverse effects. No dsRNA antibody formation has been observed during prolonged administration of mismatched dsRNA (Brodsky et al., 1985). No CFSE patient required dosage reduction or discontinuation of Ampligen therapy due to toxicity.

These clinical and laboratory findings suggest that Ampligen is a biologically active antiviral drug in CFSE. As with other viral infections, CFSE is associated with changes in serum levels of lymphokines which are essential for bodily defenses. However, a sustained lymphokine burst may exhaust the antigen-driven system and may contribute to the symptoms of the disease. As part of continuing studies in CFSE, we are now measuring cytokines with time during Ampligen therapy to test the hypothesis that one biological role of Ampligen may involve the neutralization of cytokine-associated side effects, as have been well documented with interferon and interleukin-2. Other changes noted during Ampligen therapy of CFSE included restoration of the proper functioning of the antiviral 2-5A synthetase/RNase L pathway (see companion paper, Suhadolnik et al., 1990), at the same time as the pronounced and sustained decrease of HHV-6 culturability. Furthermore, the direct effect of Ampligen on HHV-6 infection and replication **in vitro** is being investigated to strengthen the findings with patients treated with Ampligen.

A problem in the treatment of HIV-1 infected individuals is the control of coinfections with other viruses including HHV-6, HTLV-I, CMV, EBV, etc. As the HIV disease state progresses, HHV-6 antigen-producing cell disappear (Ablashi et al., 1988; Buchbinder et al., 1988). Several viruses commonly found in HIV-1 infected individuals are capable of transactivating the HIV-1 LTR in CD4$^+$ T cell lines (Lusso et al., 1989; Ensoli et al., 1989). Furthermore, **in vitro** CD4$^+$ T cells can be readily infected with HHV-6 (Ablashi et al., 1988). Krueger et al. (1989) showed that in lupus patients CD38 and CD4 cells contain HHV-6 genome and HHV-6 antigens. The coinfection of CD4$^+$ T cells with HIV-1 and HHV-6 leads to accelerated cell death (Ensoli et al., 1989). High HHV-6 titers have also been observed in patients with certain malignancies with the vast majority of the virus carried by CD38 cells (Ablashi et al., 1988; Krueger et al., 1989). Previously, Ampligen has been shown to be active against HIV-1 with demonstrated ability to improve immune function and correct defects in the 2-5A synthetase/RNase L pathway (Carter et al., 1987; Strayer et al., 1990). In this report, we have demonstrated that Ampligen is active against HHV-6 with the ability to correct derangements in the 2-5A synthetase/RNase L pathway. As a biological response modifier, Ampligen appears to have the dual ability to restore immunological function and to control virus replication. As such, Ampligen is a very attractive therapeutic modality for control of multiple virus infections by a single drug.

Acknowledgements

These studies were supported in part by U.S. Public Health Service Grant P01 CA-29545 from the National Cancer Institute and grants from HEM Research, Inc., Sierra Research Foundation, and Medical Research Funding, Inc. We thank Karen O'Brien and Debbie Pilkington, R.N., for research assistance in the preparation of this report.

References

Ablashi, D.V., Josephs, S.F., Buchbinder, A., Hellman, K., Nakamura, S., Llana, T., Lusso, P., Kaplan, M., Dahlberg, J., Memon, S., Imam, F., Ablashi, K.L., Markham, P.D., Kramarsky, B., Krueger, G.R.F., Biberfeld, P., Wong-Staal, F., Salahuddin, and Gallo, R.C. (1988) Human B-lymphotropic virus (human herpesvirus-6). J. Virological Meth. **21**, 29-48.

Ablashi, D.B., Zompetta, C., Lease, C., Josephs, S.F., Balachandran, N., Komaroff, A.L., Krueger, G.R.F., Henry, B., Luka, J., and Salahuddin, S.Z. (1989) Human herpesvirus-6 (HHV-6) and chronic fatigue syndrome (CFS). In Proceedings of the Chronic Fatigue Syndrome Workshop, published by the Central Public Health Laboratory, Toronto, Canada (Sept. 28-29, 1989).

Balachandran, N., Amelse, R.E., Zhou, W.W., and Chang, C.K. (1988) Identification of proteins specific for human herpes virus 6 infected human T cells. J. Virol. **63**, 2385-2840.

Brodsky, I., Strayer, D.R., Krueger, L.J., and Carter, W.A. (1985) Clinical studies with Ampligen (mismatched double-stranded RNA). J. Biol. Response Modif. **4**, 699-675.

Buchbinder, A., Josephs, S.F., Ablashi, D.V., Salahuddin, S.Z., Klotman, M.R., Manak, M., Krueger, G.R.F., Wong-Staal, F., and Gallo, R.C. (1988) Polymerase chain reaction and in situ hybridization for the detection of human B lymphotropic virus. J. Virol. Meth. **21**, 191-197.

Carter, W.A., Strayer, D.R., Hubbell, H.R., and Brodsky, I. (1985a) Preclinical studies with Ampligen (mismatched double-stranded RNA). J. Biol. Resp. Modif. **4**, 495-502.

Carter, W.A., Hubbell, H., Krueger, L., and Strayer, D.R. (1985b) Comparative studies of Ampligen (mismatched double-stranded RNA) and interferons. J. Biol. Resp. Modif. **4**, 613-620.

Carter, W.A., Strayer, D.R., Brodsky, I., Lewin, M., Pellegrino, M.G., Einck, L., Henriques, H.F., Simon, G.L., Parenti, D.M., Scheib, R.G., Schulof, R.S., Montefiori, D.E., Robinson, W.E., Mitchell, W.M., Volsky, D.J., Paul, D., Paxton, H., Meyer, W.A., III, Kariko, K., Reichenbach, N., Suhadolnik, R.J., and Gillespie, D.H. (1987) Clinical, immunological, and virological effects of Ampligen, a mismatched double-stranded RNA, in patients with AIDS or AIDS-related complex. Lancet i, 1286-1292.

Erlich, H.A. (1989) **PCR Technology, Principles and Applications for DNA Amplification**, M. Stockton Press, New York.

Ensoli, B., Lusso, P., Schachter, F., Josephs, S.F., Rappaport, J., Negro, F., Gallo, R.C., and Wong-Staal, F. (1989) Human herpes virus-6 increases HIV-1 expression in co-infected T cells via nuclear factors binding to the HIV-1 enhancer. EMBO J. **8**, 3019-3027.

Goldman, M. (1968) **Fluorescent Antibody Methods**, Academic Press, New York.

Holmes, G.P., Kaplan, J.E., Glantz, N.M., Komaroff, A.L., Schonberger, L.B., Straus, S.E., Jones, J.F., Dubois, R.E., Cunningham-Rundles, C., Pahwa,, S., Tosato, G., Zegano, L.S., Purtilo, D.T., Brown, N., Schooley, R.T., and Bris, I. (1988) Chronic fatigue syndrome: a working case definition. Ann. Intern. Med. **108**, 387-389.

Innis, M.A., Gelfand, D.H., Shinsky, J.J., and White, T.J., eds. (1990) **PCR Protocols, A Guide to Methods and Application**, Academic Press, New York.

Josephs, S.F., Salahuddin, S.Z., Ablashi, D.V., Schachter, F., Wong-Staal, F., and Gallo, R.C. (1986) Genomic analysis of the human B-lymphotropic virus (HBLV). Science **234**, 601-603.

Krown, S.E., Friden, G.B., Khansur, T., Davies, M.E., Oettgen, H.F., and Field, A.K. (1983) Phase I trial with the interferon inducer polyI:polyC/poly-L-lysine (polyICL). J. Interferon Res. **3**, 281-290.

Krueger, G.R.F., Manak, M., Bourgeois, N., Ablashi, D.V., Salahuddin, S.Z., Josephs, S.F., Buchbinder, A., Gallo, R.C., Berthold, F., and Tesch, H. (1989) Persistent active herpes virus infection associated with atypical polyclonal lymphoproliferation (APL) and malignant lymphoma. Anticancer **9**, 1457-1476.

Lusso, P., Ensoli, B., Markham, P.D., Ablashi, D.V., Salahuddin, S.Z., Tschachler, E., Wong-Staal, F., and Gallo, R.C. (1989) Productive dual infection of human CD4[+] T lymphocytes by HIV-1 and HHV-6. Nature **337**, 370-373.

Salahuddin, S.Z., Ablashi, D.V., Markham, P.D., Josephs, S.F., Sturzenegger, S., Kaplan, M., Halligan, G., Biberfeld, P., Wong-Staal, F., Kramarsky, B., and Gallo, R.C. (1986) Isolation of a new virus, HBLV, in patients with lymphoproliferative disorders. Science **234**, 596-603.

Sternberger, L.A. (1986) **Immunocytochemistry**, third edition, Wiley, New York.

Strayer, D.R., Brodsky, I., Pequignot, E.C., Crilley, P.A., Carter, W.A., Fenning, R., Kariko, K., Reichenbach, N.L., Sobol, R.W., Li, S.W., and Suhadolnik, R.J. (1990) The antitumor activity of Ampligen, a mismatched double-stranded RNA, which modulates the 2-5A synthetase/RNase L pathway in cancer and AIDS. **Advances in the Chemotherapy of AIDS** (Diasio, R.B., and Sommadossi, J.-P., eds.), p. 23-31, Pergamon Press, New York.

Suhadolnik, R.J., Reichenbach, N.L., Sobol, R.W., Varnum, J.M., Hart, R., Jr., Peterson, D.L., Strayer, D.R., Henry, B., Ablashi, D.V., Gillespie, D.H., and Carter, W.A. (1990) Biochemical defects in the 2-5A synthetase/RNase L pathway associated with chronic fatigue syndrome with encephalopathy. [companion paper, this volume]

Chapter 72

Immunological Therapy with Transfer Factor in patients with chronic fatigue syndrome - A double-blind, placebo-controlled trial

Andrew Lloyd, FRACP, NHMRC, NH & MRC Research Fellow, School of Pathology, University of New South Wales, Kensington, NSW, Australia, Ian Hickie, MD, FRANZCP, Research Fellow in Psychiatry, Mood Disorders Unit, Division of Psychiatry, Prince Henry Hospital, Sydney, 2036 Australia, Alan Brockman, B. ApplSc, Trials Coordinator, Immunopathology Department, Prince Henry Hospital, Sydney, 2036, Australia, John Dwyer, PhD, FRACP, Professor of Medicine, University of New South Wales, Kensington, NSW, Australia, Denis Wakefield, MD, FRACP, Associate Professor of Pathology, School of Pathology, University of New South Wales, Kensington, NSW, Australia.

(Please see Chapter 58 for Dr. Lloyd's photograph and curriculum vitae.)

Introduction

Transfer factor (TF) is a dialyzable component of leucocytes that is capable of transferring delayed-type hypersensitivity (DTH) in man. It has been used for therapy primarily in patients with disorders in which a defect in cell-mediated immunity has been established such as chronic mucocutaneous candidiasis, or in infectious diseases associated with disordered cell-mediated immunity, such as lepromatous leprosy (for review see Fudenberg & Fudenberg, 1989).

The demonstration of prevalent abnormalities in cell-mediated immunity in patients with CFS, led us to conduct a preliminary, open and uncontrolled study of the efficacy of TF therapy (Dwyer *et al*, 1989). Sixteen of the 22 patients in this initial study had an apparently worthwhile response to therapy with TF. Consequently, we conducted a double-blind and placebo-controlled trial of the benefit of TF in the treatment of patients with CFS.

Subjects and methods

Ninety adult patients (68 females, 22 males) with chronic and disabling fatigue, who fulfilled our diagnostic criteria for CFS (Lloyd *et al,* 1988) were enrolled. Standardised doses of TF were prepared for each patient by sonication, digestion and dialysis of leucocytes (predominantly mononuclear cells) obtained by cytopheresis of a healthy family member whenever possible ("specific TF"), or from unrelated donors ("non-specific TF"). TF prepared using this method in this laboratory was shown to transfer

DTH reactivity to keyhole limpet haemocyanin (KLH).

Patients were randomly allocated to receive 8 injections of TF (specific or non-specific) or placebo (lyophilised normal saline) at fortnightly intervals, after which follow-up was completed for 3 months during which no additional therapy was undertaken.

Before, during and after therapy patients monitored the severity of their physical symptoms and their physical capacity by Quality of Life visual analogue scores and by standardised diaries of daily activities. Psychological symptoms were monitored using the Profile of Mood States (POMS) questionnaire. Cell-mediated immunity was measured by T cell subset analysis and DTH skin testing prior to and at 3 months after the completion of therapy.

Assessment of a second treatment modality - physical/psychological rehabilitation, was combined with the trial of TF by a separate, superimposed randomised code. Patients were randomly allocated to attend rehabilitation as well as receiving TF/placebo or simply to attend the clinic for TF/placebo. In this study design evaluation of efficacy was possible for each treatment (TF and rehabilitation) considered separately or combined. The data from the rehabilitation arm of this study will be reported elsewhere.

Analysis of variance (ANOVA) for repeated measures was used to assess outcome on each of the self-report measures of physical and psychological well-being.

Results

The randomisation code allocated 44 patients to receive placebo injections and 46 to receive TF (25 "specific", 21 "non-specific"). Prior to treatment, there were no significant differences in the age, sex, duration of symptoms, self-report symptom measures or immunological measures between patients who received TF in comparison to those who received placebo injections.

There was no significant difference between the change in the physical, psychological or immunological measures in TF recipients (for "specific" or "non-specific" or combined groups) and placebo recipients during the course of the trial. Approximately one third of each group, including placebo recipients, reported greater than one standard deviation of improvement in the assessments of physical and psychological status over the period of therapy and subsequent follow-up. No significant difference was found in the measurements of cell-mediated immunity taken prior to and 3 months after therapy.

No major adverse effects were noted in either the TF or placebo treatment group. Minor discomfort at the injection site was common with both treatments.

One TF recipient developed a pruritic skin eruption which did not necessitate discontinuation of therapy.

Discussion

Immunological therapy with TF provided no therapeutic benefit over placebo in the patients with CFS in this study. TF prepared from healthy family members, which may potentially confer cell-mediated immunity to a specific antigen possibly implicated in the pathogenesis of the syndrome (such as an enterovirus), also did not produce greater improvement than did placebo.

In this study we have incorporated a large sample size and utilised a blinded and placebo-controlled design, therefore the negative findings provide no evidence to support further treatment of patients with CFS with TF prepared either from unrelated or family member donors.

The finding that a substantial (and similar) number of the patients receiving TF or placebo experienced significant improvement in their physical and psychological well-being, supports the concept of a self-limiting natural history for many patients with CFS, albeit over a prolonged time period.

References

Dwyer J, Lloyd A, Wakefield D. Transfer factor for chronic fatigue syndrome. Proceedings of the Sixth International Workshop on Transfer Factor, Beijing, 1989, Xue Yuan Press, pp 290-293.

Fudenberg H Hugh, Fudenberg H Haskell. Transfer factor: past, present and future. Annu Rev Pharmacol Toxicol 1989; 29: 475-516.

Lloyd A, Wakefield D, Boughton C, Dwyer J. What is myalgic encephalomyelitis? Lancet 1988; i: 1286-1287.

Lloyd A, Wakefield D, Boughton C, Dwyer J. Immunological abnormalities in the chronic fatigue syndrome. Med J Aust 1989; 151: 122-124

Chapter 73

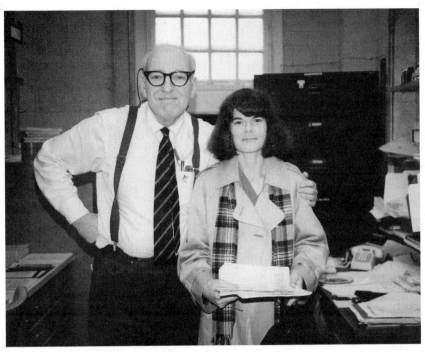

H. Hugh Fudenberg with Sara L. Bard

The Florence Nightingale Disease (FND): A Multisystem Experiment of Nature: A 50 Patient Five Year Analysis

H. Hugh Fudenberg, M.D.
Director of Research, NeuroImmuno Therapeutics Research Foundation, Spartanburg, South Carolina.

Supported in part by the Immunology-Hematology Research and NeuroImmuno Therapeutics Research Foundation.

Professor H. Hugh Fudenberg is one of the pioneers of clinical immunology and one of the most distinguished and original minds in the field of immunology, being internationally known since he was awarded The Medal of the Institut Pasteur at the age of 32 . During his research with immunomodulators and the interaction of the brain and the immune system, Professor Fudenberg became interested in the problems of patients afflicted with ME. He is currently treating patients with this and other diseases with a therapeutic substance derived from human lymphocytes termed Dialyzable Lymphocyte Extract (DLyE) enriched in Transfer Factor.

Florence Nightingale Disease (previously termed Myalgic Encephalomyelitis in British Commonwealth countries and C.F.I.D.S. in the U.S.) appears to be due to immune dysregulation as a result of antigenic stimulation by incomplete, dead (and/or perhaps latent) virus secondary to a defect in antigen presentation and/or processing. In contrast to others who believe that a single virus is the cause of illness in all patients, our evidence indicates that any one of a number of viruses is responsible, probably due to an antigen-selective defect for one virus in a genetically predisposed individual. The chief disabling symptom, cognitive dysfunction, is secondary to aberration in immunologic regulation of the Central Nervous System, probably involving both the memory area of the brain and the hypothalamus. All patients have sub-clinical endocrine deficiency. 50% of FND patients had a chemical or food hypersensitivity. Almost all of 50 severely affected FND patients were normalized by individualized immunotherapy by 18 months, and remain well if on therapy. Six patients taken off therapy at 24 months are well up to 3 1/2 years later.

During the last decade, an increasingly large number of patients have consulted physicians because of symptoms of cognitive dysfunction, severe muscle pain, daily persistent headache and marked hyperfatigability after minimal exercise[1,2]. These symptoms usually occur following a prolonged viral infection or injection with a live virus vaccine or, in rare cases, severe pain and associated stress (e.g., automobile accident)[3]. All the patients have exacerbation of hyperfatigability, not only after mild physical exercise but also often after prolonged intellectual labor (e.g., graduate students studying 15 hours a day for 7 days in preparation for Ph.D. examination)[3]; all also have sleep disorder and anhedonia. A list of other symptoms are presented in Table 1. The disease may occur in either sporadic or epidemic form. The disease was rediscovered in 1985 by Behan, Behan and Bell in Great Britain[4a] and in the United States by Barnes[4b].

The medical profession has remained skeptical as to the existence of such disease, e.g. ref. 5, or whether it is a disease at all and, if it does exist, whether it is one disease or several (severity and incidence of symptoms differ and therefore, terminology varies in Great Britain, Australia, and New Zealand from that used in the U.S.). The disorder appears to be a post-viral disorder and epidemics thereof have been reported in the past, the world over, under a variety of names, e.g., Icelandic Disease, Epidemic Neurasthenia, etc.[5b] The scientists working on this syndrome believe its cause is the same in all patients, and have termed it Chronic Myalgic Encephalomyelitis in Great Britain, Australia and New Zealand[1], and Chronic Fatigue Syndrome in the United States.[2]* The symptoms of CFS and ME are identical but there is considerable variability in the incidence and degree of severity of various symptoms. The data presented in this paper strongly suggest that FND is not due to EBV, but rather to abnormal immune dysregulation due to any one of a large number of enteroviruses or respiratory viruses. When first rediscovered, six to seven years ago, it was initially termed Chronic Epstein-Barr Virus (EBV) Disease[6a,b,c,d] because sera from patients with infectious mononucleosis showed high titers to one EVB antigen[7,8], namely the "early" antigen; it is this antigen[7] to which antibodies are directed early in the course of infectious mononucleosis but the antigen towards which the antibodies were directed was later identified as that present in the early course of EBV disease[9].* This syndrome is only rarely due to Epstein Barr Virus. (In the early 80's, the first

papers on this syndrome included the Henles as co-authors as they performed the EBV serology.[6d] In later papers, anti-EBV titer elevation was significantly less. This discrepancy may be due to the fact that the Henles used EBV cell lines established earlier in culture. During these 30 years, antigenic drift may have occurred.)[10]

Table 1			
1.	Cognitive Functions		
	a.	Intermittent Amnesia	100%
	b.	Shortened Attention Span	100%
	c.	Delayed Response to Questions	100%
	d.	Loss of Reasoning Ability	100%
	e.	Other	100%
2.	Sleep Disorder		100%
	a.	Insomnia	
	b.	Hypersomnia	
	c.	Frequent Waking	
	d.	Unable to fall asleep until 3 or 4 a.m.	
3.	Fatigability		
	a.	Unable to walk four blocks without exacerbation	96%
	b.	Unable to swim 1/2 mile	90%
4.	Anhedonia		90%
5.	Muscle and Joint Pain		50%
6.	Daily Persistent Headache		50%
7.	Depression		50%
8.	Bladder Problem		20%
9.	Unexplained Diarrhea		16%
10.	Photophobia		10%
11.	Low-grade Fever		0%

Further confusion is due to controversy over whether Chronic Fatigue Syndrome (CFS, the term used in the U.S.) and Myalgic Encephalomyelitis (ME, the term used in the British Commonwealth countries) are the same disease, two different disease entities, or two overlapping diseases[1,2,3]. The arguments resemble those advanced from the idea many years ago concerning the identity or non-identity of the so called "collagen diseases" before laboratory tests were developed for differential diagnosis of Lupus Erythematosis and Rheumatoid arthritis. Neither term, Chronic Fatigue Syndrome, Myalgic En-

---

* The term "Chronic Fatigue Syndrome" is an abominable name for this diseases since it is named after only 1 of the many symptoms of FND (and not the most disabling one, namely Cognitive Dysfunction). The British Commonwealth countries refuse to accept this name (Hyde's introduction in reference 1.)

cephalomyelitis, the Yuppie Syndrome[12], nor any other terminology (e.g. Epidemic Neurasthenia) reflect the common most disabling symptom namely, cognitive dysfunction; furthermore, neither term reflects the etiology or pathogenesis. The term "Yuppie Syndrome"[12], was used because the most common age of onset is 30-40. (The patients I have seen have ranged in age from 15 to 65 at the onset of symptoms, but a high occurrence in children has been reported by practitioners who restrict their practice to patients with this disorder.)[13]

The conflicting current terminologies are confusing to both physicians and laymen and, as stated above, describe neither the symptoms, etiology, nor pathogenesis. As noted, the terminologies have lead to continuing conflict as to whether or not this is a single disease entity. As discussed later herein, the pathogenesis of CFS and ME appears to be identical, namely persistent antigenic stimulation by dead, incomplete or latent virus (predominantly rubella and cytomegalovirus and herpes in the U.S.- Table 2) and enteroviruses in British Commonwealth countries. Hence, one term could be used to designate this disorder. I have therefore proposed to use the noncommittal term Florence Nightingale Disease (FND) to describe this disorder[1]. Her letters and biographies indicate a viral infection of unusually long duration late in the Crimean War; she subsequently developed all of the typical symptoms of the postviral disorder[14]. Investigators in Great Britain and countries whose inhabitants are derived from British ancestry (e.g. New Zealand, Australia, and the Province of Ontario in Canada) are enthusiastic about the new terminology. Indeed, the center most heavily involved in handling patients with this disorder, in Ottawa, Canada is called the Nightingale Research Foundation.

As noted above, severe myalgia is present in almost 100% of patients of British descent, and high IgG titers are present to one or another of various enteroviruses (e.g., Coxsackie I, Coxsackie II, polio, etc.); these all share a common enteroviral antigen[15]; "Indeed, IgA antibodies complex to enteroviral antigen have been recovered from the stools of such patients"[16a,b] and enteroviral RNA has been recovered from muscle biopsies of such patients[17a,b] (Coxsackie viruses commonly migrate to skeletal muscle and occasionally to cardiac muscle causing idi-

opathic myocarditis[18a,b], a phenomenon almost unheard of in American patients with FND). In the 50 U.S. patients with severe FND I have studied (completely unable to work or study for at least 2 years - many up to 12 years), myalgia was present in approximately 50% and usually less severe, and cognitive malfunction always present and usually much more severe, than in patients in Great Britain, New Zealand, and Australia. In our patients (See Table 2), elevated IgG titers are not to enteroviruses but to viruses of the herpes group (rubella 50%; cytomegalovirus 25%, herpes 1 and 2 10%). Many patients had elevated IgG titers to many viral antigens (presumably due to polyclonal B-cell activation[19a]) but Table 2 lists only the one to which the titer was the highest. HHV6 is thought by many to be the cause of this syndrome.[19a-e] HHV6 titers were elevated in about 40% of my patients but usually by only 2-3 doubling dilutions, and probably reflect a secondary phenomena due to depressed cell mediated immunity since we have seen moderate elevations in other immunological disorders[3]. In one case I have seen, treated by others with materials suggested by me (the virus isolated by University of California at Davis Veterinary School was Bovine Herpes 3) the patient owned a herd of cows that died of Bovine Herpes 3. She developed severe FND symptoms shortly thereafter. BVH 3 was isolated from the patient's spinal fluid[20] as was an HTLV-2-like virus, a virus erroneously thought by other investigators to be responsible for this disease.[21] Still others have suggested a newly discovered spumavirus is the cause[22]. I believe, as discussed below, that many different viruses can produce the symptoms of this one disorder since the symptoms are not related to the virus per se but to the immunologic dysregulation resulting from virus- induced persistent antigenic stimulation. Immune dysregulation is the cause of cognitive defects. This is due to liberation of cytokines, e.g. interleukin 2, tumor necrosis factor, etc. as a result of persistent antigenic stimulation by dead, incomplete or latent virus.

We and others have evidence that the immune system regulates cognitive and other functions of the Central Nervous System.[23a,b,c] FND probably involves genetic predisposition due to immune response genes coding for deficient cell-mediated immunity (CMI), in T cells, B cells and / or monocytes[24] to one infectious agent or another or to genetic defect

(s) causing abnormalities in antigen presentation and perhaps in secondary processing [26]. (Inbred mice with differing genes respond similarly to lysozyme but do not process peptides thereof in the same way, and in those with poor processing, little immune response occurs.) Indeed, defects in phagocytic cells have been reported in FND.[26]

Table 2
Markedly elevated IgG antiviral antibodies* in fifty consecutive U.S. patients with Florence Nightingale Disease of at least two years duration**.

Virus	Percent
Rubella	50
Cytomegalo Virus	26
Herpes I and/or II	12
Measles	4
Epstein-Barr Virus (early antigen)	4
Coxsackie Virus	2
Rabies	2

* Performed by ELISA for almost all viruses.

** Many patients had marked elevations to several viruses. The one listed was the greatest relative to the normal.

The pathogenesis appears to be the same in both ME and CFIDS, as mentioned previously, namely, persistent antigenic stimulation by dead, incomplete, or latent viruses, provoking a continued, elevated immune response. This is a "post-viral syndrome[4a]", e.g. Coxsackie virus, or one retrovirus or another in muscle[21], dead or latent virus of the Herpes group on lymphocytes and monocytes. Hence the cognitive defects (as noted above), since the regulatory role of CMI cells on the Central Nervous System (CNS) has been shown by many researchers. e.g.23a-c.

FND is not a trivial disease; as noted above, those severely affected have not only marked impairment in quality of life but a greater death rate than normals in the same age range. I have seen several severely affected patients who have had impairment of function of the brain areas connected with their 2nd and 7th and 8th cranial nerves during severe exacerbations[3]. These exacerbations were also accompanied by exacerbations of cognitive defect. Dr. Behan has stated that this disorder is a chief cause of suicide in individuals 34-40 years of age who have been unable to function for 4 to 8 years and who

foresee no effective therapy in the future[27]. A high incidence of suicide in this age group of patients with this disorder has been noticed in this country.[3] Furthermore, B-cell lymphoma in patients with FND of 6 to 10 years duration is far more common than in age-matched controls (estimated to be 1000 times more common in terms of life years at risk than in the normal population[19a,28]). The incidence of other malignancies (e.g., lung, breast, etc.) appears no greater than normal. It is postulated that patients elsewhere with genetically determined immune deficiencies (ataxia telangiectasia, adult onset agammaglobulinemia, etc.) lymphocytes are dividing more rapidly than normal in an attempt to compensate for the immune defect[29]. The more cell divisions, the greater the chance for chromosomal error and the more chromosomal error the greater the chance of malignancy of the tissue involved[30]. It is also possible that failure of normal immune regulation leads to activation of oncogenes or loss of genes that suppress oncogenes. To my knowledge, abnormal oncogenes have not been searched for in this disorder. In those in whom lymphoma developed, clonality was not searched for.

Although many physicians have dismissed FND as a trivial disease, or merely "psychologic" disease, in addition to its clinical importance (see below), it is of considerable interest, since it is a multi-system disease involving the Central Nervous System, the Endocrine System, and the Immune System, and Muscle (often skeletal and occasionally cardiac.) Studies of patients with this experiment of nature should lead to a better understanding of the interrelationships and interregulatory mechanisms between these systems. Further reasons for the accurate diagnosis of FND are listed later herein.

FND is usually misdiagnosed or undiagnosed since no abnormalities are detected on physical examination of patients who have had the disorder for at least two years, and clinical chemistries (SMA 20) show normal liver, cardiac, and kidney functions. Many of our patients saw 6 to 60 physicians before the diagnosis was made (the diagnosis is probably missed in 75-90% of patients). Other reasons that make the correct diagnosis important include but are not limited to the following:

1. Errors in diagnosis may lead to the use of anti-

depressant medications that may cause marked exacerbation of all symptoms.[3,11]

2. Certain medications, e.g. Klonopin, may lead to unnecessary surgery, e.g. for benign prostatic hypertrophy (BPH), (vide infra).

3. In many patients with "idiopathic" myocarditis, Coxsackie virus homing to cardiac muscle may be the primary mechanism.[18a,b] If this is the case, the diagnosis is no longer "idiopathic", perhaps the optimal therapy may be different for this subset myocarditis.

4. The incidence of mitral valve prolapse (MVP) in FND patients is about 50%, and is considerably higher than normal (reason unknown), but in these patients appears to be of no clinical significance. Although prophylactic antibiotics have rarely been used in dental procedures in such patients, sub-acute bacterial endocarditis has not been reported.

5. Emotional costs: About 2/3 of the marriages and 2/3 of the housemates separate permanently, since the mate of the patient has been told by numerous physicians that either the symptoms are merely psychological or that the affected individual is just "merely lazy"[3]. When the patients (and spouses) finally learn that they indeed, have a biological and not psychiatric disease, and are not merely lazy or malingering, their interpersonal relationships usually go back to normal.[3]

6. Economic costs are very high. Canadian data suggest $250 million yearly are lost in income taxes alone[11] because of the inability to work, but in Canada since all medical costs (in terms of physicians' time, medication, hospitalization, laboratory tests, etc.) are covered by the government, there is no way to compare total economic loss (e.g. hospitalizations, insurance, disability payments, and physician fees) in the U.S. Estimates suggest that total cost per patient is at least 10 fold greater in the U.S. than in Canada. Thus, the total cost estimate in the U.S. would range from 5-50 billion dollars yearly.[31]

7. Amplification of Effects of Misdiagnosis

(a) Depression

Patients who first see a psychiatrist, because depression is their first or their predominant symptom, are usually diagnosed as "atypical depression".[32-34] Questions relevant to malfunction of other organ systems are rarely asked. However, ordinary depression is worse in the morning and becomes progressively less severe as the day goes along. In contrast, in my FND patients, questioning has elicited the fact that depression and other symptoms are usually at their worst when CMI is lowest, that is, 1:00 to 3:00 P.M., and in very severe cases will waken at 1:00 to 3:00 A.M.[3] (CMI cycles twice daily)[35a,b]. The majority of our FND patients were seen by at least one psychiatrist (one saw a dozen psychiatrists). Of those who received only "talk therapy", there was no change in severity of symptoms. Diagnosis was either depression, "somatization"[36], laziness or malingering. Various psychotropic drugs were without significant benefit; while most antidepressants had no adverse effects, others (e.g., Nardil, Valium, lithium) caused severe exacerbation of cognitive malfunction[3]. In addition, most psychiatrists advised their depressed patients to get mild exercise every day (e.g., an early morning 2-mile walk). Although this is often helpful in patients with ordinary depression, in the vast majority of our FND patients it caused severe exacerbation of all symptoms, often to an extent requiring confinement to bed for several weeks.[3]

As cited above, this disease is not psychologic in origin. Atypical depression is secondary to the primary cause or is perhaps due to direct action of the Central Nervous System (CNS) Immune Cells on the CNS neuronal cells (glial cells outnumber neuronal cells eight to one). Although until recently many reports concluded that FND is a purely psychologic disorder, recent evidence provided by BEAM Scans, PET Scans and other neuroradiologic procedures have shown characteristic abnormalities in FND patients.[38a,b,c] Further, immunologic abnormalities present in FND have not been seen by us in "other disease controls", i.e. patients with pure depression, pure myalgia, pure recurring headache, etc.[3]

(b) Myalgia

Those FND patients who presented with severe muscle pains as the predominant symptom were initially referred to a rheumatologist and diagnosis of fibromyalgia[37] was commonly made and usually nonsteroid anti-inflammatory medications were prescribed. In FND patients, as noted earlier, such medications can also often cause exacerbation of symptoms[11].

(c) Benign Prostatic Hypertrophy (BPH)

Occasionally patients present to a urologist because of increased urinary frequency and incomplete voiding and no urge to void until the bladder is completely full.

In males over 55, this usually results in a diagnosis of BPH and subsequent unnecessary transurethal resection of the prostate. Furthermore, as stated above, some of the psychotropics used (e.g., Klonopin) will cause an exacerbation of these urologic symptoms and in some instances will cause these symptoms in subjects who had no such symptoms before[3]. Again, a 55-60 year old male FND patient with such symptoms is uniformly diagnosed as BPH and treated by transurethal resection. According to my queries of 20 urologists, half from Academia, half from private practice, only one had heard of this syndrome; all either failed to ask which medications that patient was taking or had not consulted the **Physician's Desk Reference (PDR)** to see whether such medications produce symptoms of prostatic hypertrophy.[3]

Endocrine Abnormalities

All of our patients had endocrine problems although blood hormone values were almost always normal. Eleven patients had histories of viral thyroiditis, thyroid surgery, and/or thyroid antibodies prior to the onset of symptoms of FND. The vast majority of patients lacking these had clinical symptoms of hypothyroidism (e.g., very low first morning pulse and temperature, hypohydrosis, need for more blankets than spouse) despite normal laboratory tests for free T3, free T4, and TSH (perhaps deficiency of an as yet undetected thyroid hormone is responsible). The FND patients have symptoms of abnormal thyroid function despite normal serum thyroid hormones levels because of an overlap in normals with hypothyroid and hyperthyroid levels. Indeed, free T3, free T4 and TSH hormone levels are rarely of value in patients with FND.[3,39] FND patients have impaired adrenal function or impaired adrenal reserve as shown by blood cortisol levels immediately before and one hour after injection of 15mg of ACTH.[3] Two of the 50 we studied had low estrogen levels, but

whether this is primary or secondary to hypothalamic or pituitary defects is still undetermined. Four patients studied before endocrine therapy or immunotherapy, TRF and or CRF were abnormal.[3]

Furthermore, the FND patients did not respond to any form of immunotherapy (see below) unless symptoms of hypothyroidism, and in two cases, adrenal cortical hypofunction abnormalities were first eradicated by administration of small amounts of dessicated thyroid, with gradual increase until first morning pulse and temperature were normalized; (we use Armour's Dessicated Thyroid since it presumably contains the putative as yet undetected thyroid hormones, [e.g. "T19" and/or "T20"]). Indeed, a third type of brain receptor for thyroid hormone has recently been discovered.[40] Three patients who failed to respond to synthyroid and/or levothyroid did respond to dessicated thyroid. Some endocrinologists in California have removed normal thyroid glands from FND patients in hopes that symptoms would disappear; instead, the severity of symptoms increased[41]. Most of the patients had significant diminution in severity of FND symptoms after clinical hypothyroidism was corrected, that is before the initiation of immunotherapy (average time, approximately three months). In 2 patients, 3-3 1/2 grains of thyroid did not correct symptoms, but addition of 5mg of Prednisone did so. (These 2 patients had low adrenal reserve). Indeed correction of endocrine abnormalities usually resulted in decrease in severity of symptoms. Furthermore, the endocrine dysfunction might well be the cause, at least in part, of the pervasive fatigability. It is also necessary to know what other types of endocrine products, if any, are being taken since some patients with subclinical adrenal insufficiency may develop overt Addison's disease when given thyroid.

With regard to the endocrine abnormalities noted above, it is noteworthy that peripheral blood immune cells (PBIC) have CNS equivalents with similar properties and products, and that both PBIC and CNS cells regulate the endocrine system. For example, of 4 subsets of human monocytes[42], one subset has functions identical to microglia in the CNS (i.e., are rich in Fc receptors and phagocytic ability and lack HLA class II antigens), while another monocyte subset, responsible for antigen presentation, is rich in HLA class II antigens, and is identical in function and antigenic profile (with monoclonal antibodies) with one subset of astrocytes[42]. Furthermore, peripheral blood immune cells (PBIC) have receptors for hypothalamic-releasing factors (e.g., cortisol-releasing factor (CRF), thyroid-releasing factor[43]) and, once bound, these ligands and their receptors are internalized with subsequent production of ACTH and TSH that in the test tube are indistinguishable from their pituitary counterparts and that stimulate the adrenal cortex and the thyroid respectively, with subsequent production of their hormones and regulation of the BBIC receptor. To date, these have not been examined in FND, but in Alzheimer's Disease CRF production is low[43] and receptor function is up-regulated[3].

Immunologic Laboratory Data

Immunologic abnormalities were not one of the original CDC criteria for the diagnosis of CFS.[44] Many different immunologic abnormalities have been described in these patients,[45a,b,c] but for each abnormality published, at least one paper has been published refuting that abnormality in FND. Most, but not all, of our FND patients, had mild abnormalities in lymphocyte DNA in response to the PHA, Con-A, and/or Pokeweed mitogens. (Occasionally, dramatic reduction in B cell and/or DNA synthesis in response to Pokeweed was present). However, most had abnormal DNA synthesis in response to anti-CD3 and alpha-1 acid glycoprotein (alpha-1 AGP) which we have discovered to be an immunoregulatory protein.[46] In general, CD4/CD8 ratios were elevated in many but only to a mild degree[3]. In a few IgG$_3$ or IgG$_1$ were deficient.[47] These differences may reflect differences a) in severity and/or duration of disease or indeed b) inaccurate diagnosis since individuals with frank febrile illness at six months may well have a disease other than FND, and most authors include patients with all degrees of severity (mild, moderate or severe) of six months duration, twelve months duration, two years duration, etc. and variable impairment of work capacity. In contrast, our data is based on severely affected patients (symptom severity score average table (SSSA), see Table 3, of greater than 4.2 on a scale of 1-5), who have had severe disease during the two years prior to being seen here and had no unusual febrile episodes during those two years. Furthermore, an immunologic abnormality was originally not considered a criteria for diagnosis

by the CDC.[44,48] More recent authors will not make the diagnosis unless one immunologic parameter is abnormal: but if 20 tests are done, the possibility of one patient having a deficiency in one of the 20 tests is five percent, and with multiple subjects, much greater variations would be expected. Number and/or function of natural killer cells noted by several investigators,[49a,b] was present in about 40% of our patients but this may be secondary to severity and/or duration of disease. Furthermore, we have seen this occur frequently in many other immunologic disorders, most notably in the one patient with Creutzfeldt-Jacob disease I have studied.[3] These patients have immunologic abnormalities such as antibodies to neuron-axon filament proteins.[3] We have studied one patient with this disorder, age 18, in whom the disease was produced because of administration of growth hormone derived from a pool of 10,000 human pituitaries 12 years previously. The patient's NK cells were only 0.1% of total leukocytes. His father and mother, clinically asymptomatic, also only had 0.1% NK cells. This suggests that a genetic deficiency in NK cells may predispose individuals to FND but it does not prove that it is the cause since the parents are asymptomatic. The CDC criteria for diagnosis are grossly inadequate or are no longer held tenable by leaders in the field (reviewed in references 1; 2). Our laboratory results are based on severely affected patients completely incapacitated for at least two years in so far as this study is concerned. None of these patients during the two years prior to the time I first saw them had symptoms severity score average (SSCA) rating greater than 4.2 and each had at least 2 laboratory parameters compatible with immune dysregulation. Again, most authors used the CDC criteria, namely patients with symptoms of six months duration and varying impairment in reduction of work capacity ("up to 50%"). Furthermore, some authors who designated the patient as having FND solely on the basis of one abnormal immunologic test (e.g., in a panel of eight tests), when active viral infection was still present, have failed to consider the possibility of margin for error.

Of considerable interest were FND patients with fibromyalgia; on immunofluorescence examination of skin biopsies using areas exposed to the sun, they often had positive reactions for IgG, IGM and C3. However, they also had positive reactions with control antiserum (anti-albumin) suggesting increased capillary permeability or abnormalities in "tight junction" rather than any autoimmune process.[3] In two patients with severe atypical depression, spinal fluid protein was greatly increased but was almost solely albumin, another finding compatible with increased capillary permeability.[3] Most of our FND patients had abnormal DNA synthesis in response to anti-CD3 and/or alpha-1 acid glycoprotein [a$_1$AGP][50], which we have discovered to be an immunoregulatory protein[46]). Also, most had abnormalities in DNA synthesis by peripheral blood lymphocytes when exposed to a$_1$AGP[51]. Many had increased numbers of activated T cells. (In 18 patients, pretherapy spontaneous DNA synthesis by lymphocytes in the absence of mitogen was increased, there were also abnormal findings compatible with persistent antigenic stimulation.) Most of the patients had significant elevated immune complexes by at least 1 of our 4 standard methods[52] before therapy; these disappeared after therapy, but reappeared during relapses in patients in whom DLyE therapy was discontinued prematurely for one reason or another. Defects in natural killer cells number and/or function exist in all FND patients according to Aoki et. al.[49], but in our patients (again all severe, all incapacitated for at least 2 years prior to testing) were present in only 40%. This defect is probably a secondary phenomena and not the cause of FND. I believe this test reflects presentation of antigen by B cells to T cells. Monocytes defects have also been reported[24] and the defective viral degradation by phagocytes may well be a result of defects in antigen presentation which in turn might be due to defects in cytosol binding protein.

All our patients had a deficiency in function of a subset of B cells which interact with T cells to form a rosette, as measured by the interactive T cell test[53]. I believe this test reflects B cell presentation of antigen in vitro, a phenomenon which some others also believe far more important in vitro than monocyte presentation of antigen T cells (e.g. 25, 54).

It was also noteworthy that fifty percent of our FND patients had food and/or chemical allergy (IgE-mediated) and/or hypersensitivity (non IgE-mediated and no response to antihistamines or cromolyn). True allergy, i.e., an IgE-mediated phenomenon, comprises only about 10-20% of those FND patients whose symptoms are exacerbated following exposure to offending food and/or chemicals (that is, only 5-10% of all FND patients). I postulate that enzymes (e.g. cytochrome P450), phosphosulfotransferase present in normal lymphocytes are diminished in a number in FND patients, not only in PBIC but especially in the gastrointestinal-associated lymphoid tissue (GALT) and the bronchial-associated lymphoid systems (BALT); a deficiency of such enzymes would cause failure of cleavage of the side chains of food proteins and petrochemical derivatives, respectively[55]. Hence, these materials would pass into the circulation without cleavage. Presumably, these undigested materials directly, or through antibody formation to them, will cause precipitation of symptoms, perhaps by binding to immune complexes which attach to the Fc receptors in monocytes and the monocyte-derived cells of the brain (e.g., glial cells)[3,29] and, in preliminary experiments, to the hypothalamus. Again, only about 10-20% of the FND patients with food and/or hypersensitivity have true IgE allergy although medical ecologists have used the term "brain allergy"[56a-d] to describe the symptoms. Since this phenomenon is not IgE-mediated, most physicians, especially allergists, have assumed that the symptoms are purely psychological in origin[57]; they are not, since I have seen deliberate exposure to offending food or chemicals cause marked exacerbation of symptoms in a few patients[58].

Indeed, many authors have published papers strongly suggesting that the symptoms in all these individuals with chemical hypersensitivity are psychological and that no biologic abnormalities exist[61], e.g. As noted above, the medical ecologists use the term "brain allergy", but since, in the vast majority of patients, the symptoms are not an IgE response and do not respond to antihistamines or cromolyn, the rest of the medical profession not only disbelieve the "allergy" but also disbelieve that chemical and/or food exposure can cause such symptoms. This is another reason why correct diagnosis is essential.

However, in 50% of FND patients exposure to diesel oil fumes, oil-based paint, hair spray, perfume, men's deodorant, scented detergents, insecticides, certain inks in glossy magazines, and certain photocopy and computer paper may cause severe exacerbation of symptoms. In some patients, exacerbation occurs immediately; in others, the delay is up to 48 hours, so the patient does not associate prior exposure with the symptoms (e.g., patients come from California to South Carolina and improve while here, on Monday through Thursday; after returning home they develop severe exacerbation of symptoms from being exposed to perfume, hair spray, etc., both in the airplane and in the airport when they are travelling back home on that Saturday or Sunday). The same exacerbation occurs after exposure to the same chemical substances during intermission at concerts, theatre performances, etc. Indeed, it is possible that such hypersensitivity is the cause rather than the result of FND. In two patients, symptoms of FND began after breaking a bottle of benzene, and after severe insecticide exposure respectively.[3]

Among foods, milk and milk product proteins, wheat and wheat product proteins, and substances containing corn syrup are the prime offenders. Many FND patients have seen medical ecologists who treated their symptoms either with marked dietary restriction or with multiple dietary supplements, but without attention to the immunologic abnormalities, the myalgia, or the daily persistent headache.

Therapy

Since all of the patients had immunologic aberration, experimental immunotherapy seemed warranted, especially since no success was achieved by a host of previous treatments. The immunotherapy we selected was Dialyazlable Lymphocyte Extract[59a] (DLyE) prepared from the cells from highly selected donors by lymphopheresis and frozen immediately after collection[59b]. Initial dosage was 12 S.C. units for three days every six weeks for six months* with gradual reduction in amount and frequency as determined by laboratory test of immunologic function. Of the 50 patients accepted in S.C. for study (geographical distribution of the patients was roughly proportional to the population of each state - the greatest number from California, the next greatest from New York, etc.), 34 of 39 patients completely unable to work for two years prior to therapy, who were treated with DLyE enriched in Transfer Factor (TF) derived

---

* Potency of one of S.C. unit equals about ten International Units (material prepared from leucocytes (non-immune cells) of a single donor. With pooled cells of multiple donors, especially with stored blood, potency may be nil, and with stored outdated blood obtained from leucocytes in blood bags designed for red cell transfusion, the final product may be dangerous.

from selected household contacts (HC) and administered in far greater dosage than is usual in other laboratories, were back to normal activities in 18 months. Only 3 of 11 in whom cells were derived from carefully selected non-household contacts (NH) were similarly back at work; in this group, sometimes 3 or 4 donors were necessary before best donor was identified. Of the 34 HC-TF responders, five have been off immunotherapy for 1 1/2 to 3 1/2 years. Four have been completely normal; the other relapsed after 50 injections of an immunosuppressive steroid by a dermatologist for a skin condition.

Our synthetic pyrrolidones and/or inosine-rich compounds (TF is rich in inosine, Ampligen contains one strand of polyinosine) caused marked improvement in four of the six patients to whom they were administered. (Pyrrolidone is a precursor of pyrrolidinone, a substance present in brain and immune cells at five times its concentration in other body cells; its degradation products provide cell energy via entry into the Dickens shunt).[60]

Of additional interest are five female patients not included in the fifty with classic FND, including two sisters and the daughter of one of them from Pennsylvania, and two unrelated patients from South Carolina. From birth to the age of 40, these patients suffered monthly episodes of severe febrile upper respiratory infection (temperature 104° to 106° for five to seven days, with marked cervical lymphadenopathy). They had repeated negative blood, urine and throat cultures with no response to antibiotics. These findings seem to exclude a bacterial cause. The genetics appear to exclude Periodic Disease, either of the Mediterranean or Portuguese variety, so presumably these episodes were viral in origin. I have termed this symptom constellation the Cox Syndrome, after patient Cox, the first such patient encountered.[61]

On DLyE, the five patients remained completely free of febrile episodes. When DLyE was discontinued, the patients passed first through a stage identical with FND in symptoms and, as they relapsed further, lost FND symptoms and again developed the severe febrile episodes. (These seemed to occur prior to ovulation and also prior to menstruation in three patients; in two patients panhysterectomies had been performed.)

When DLyE was reinstituted, patients passed from the febrile episodes to the FND symptoms and then to normal, again, suggestive evidence that a viral infection (presumably aberrant response thereto) is responsible for the symptoms of FND. Again, it is my belief that genetic factors determine which virus will cause the symptoms, and, although many investigators suggested HHV6, HLTV2, spumavirus etc., as the agent solely responsible for the disease in all FND patients, I believe that there is no one single agent. There have been verbal reports of similar findings in animals and in view of very severe FND symptoms in one patient with high IgG titers to bovine herpes 3 who responded well to bovine DLyE made against BVH3 and administered by her California physician after approval by his hospital's Human Experimentation Committee, the possibility that viruses usually affecting only infrahuman species may be responsible, should be explored.

Although such findings in the above patients and in the patient with the Cox Syndrome are rare, they hopefully will stimulate other physicians working with FND to inquire as to whether periodic, severe, febrile episodes, presumably viral, preceded the symptoms of FND and, if so, the interrelationship between the two disorders. The temporal sequence of events provides strong evidence that FND symptoms are secondary to immunologic dysfunction.

Acknowledgement

I am greatly indebted to our Immunologic Science Editor, Ms. Lisa A. Cox for superb editorial assistance and her unceasing labor. The manuscript could not have been completed without her help!

References

1. Hyde, B.M., 1990. Discussion, The First International Symposium on Myalgic Encephalomyelitis (M.E.), Cambridge University, April 9-12, 1990.

2. Goldstein, J. Introduction. First International Symposium on Chronic Fatigue Syndrome, Los Angeles, CA. February 17-19, 1990.

3. Fudenberg, H.H., 1991. Unpublished observations.

4a. Behan, PO, Behan, WM and Bell, EJ, 1985. The Postviral Fatigue Syndrome. J. Inf. 10:210.

4b. Barnes, DM, 1986. Mystery Disease at Lake Tahoe baffles Virologists and Clinicians. Science 234, Oct 7, 1986.

5a. Strauss, S.E., Dale, J.K., Tobi, M., et al., 1988. Acyclovir treatment of the chronic fatigue syndrome: lack of efficacy in a placebo-controlled trial. N. Engl. J. Med. 319:1692-1698.

5b. Strauss, S.E., 1991. History of chronic fatigue syndrome. Rev. Infect. Dis. Jan-Feb 13:S2-7.

6a. Jones, J., and Strauss, S., 1987. Chronic Epstein-Barr virus infection. Ann. Rev. Med. 38:195-209.

6b. Strauss, S.E., Tosato, G., Armstrong, G., et al., 1985. Persisting illness and fatigue in adults with evidence of Epstein-Barr virus infections. Ann. Intern. Med. 102:7-16.

6c. Tobi, M., Morag, A., Ravid, Z., Chowers, I., Feldman-Weiss, V., Michaeli, Y., Ben-chetrit, E., Shalit, M., and Knobler, H., 1982. Prolonged atypical illness associated with serological evidence of persistent Epstein-Barr virus infection. Lancet. 1:61-64.

6d. Tosato, G., Strauss, S., Henle, W., Pike, S.E., and Blaese, R.M., 1985. Characteristic T cell dysfunction in patients with chronic active Epstein-Barr virus infection (chronic infectious mononucleosis). J. Immunol. 134:3082-3088.

7. Hellinger, W.C., Smith, T.F., Van Scoy, R.E., Spitzer, P.G., Forgacs, P., and Edson, R.S., 1988. Chronic fatigue syndrome and the diagnostic utility of antibody to Epstein-Barr virus early antigen. JAMA 260:971-973.

8. Jones J.F., Ray, C.G., Minnich, L.L., Hicks, M.J., Kibler, R., and Locas, D.O., 1985. Evidence of active Epstein-Barr virus infection in patients with persistent, unexplained illnesses: elevated anti-early antigen antibodies. Ann. Intern. Med. 1-2:1-7.

9. Henle, W., Henle, G., Anderson, J., Ernberg, I., Klein, G., Horwitz, C.A., Marklund, G., Rymo, L., Wellinder, C., and Strauss, S.E., 1987. Antibody responses to Epstein-Barr virus-determined nuclear antigen (EBNA)-1 and EBNA-2 in acute and chronic Epstein-Barr virus infection. Proc. Natl. Acad. Sci. USA. 84:570-574.

10. Palese, P, Young, JR. Variation in Influenza A, B and C Viruses. Science 1982, 1468-1439.

11. Hyde, B. Personal communication.

12. Johnson, E. Journey into Fear, Rolling Stones Magazine, Aug;7, 1987.

13. Bell, D.S., 1990. ME/CFIDS in children: a historical overview (abstract). The First International Symposium on Myalgic Encephalomyelitis (M.E.), Cambridge University, April 9-12, 1990, this volume, B. Hyde, Editor, (tentatively) Ottawa University Press.

14. Vicinuss, E.R.V. and Nergaard, H., 1990. Ever Yours, Selected Letters of Florence Nightingale, Harvard University Press.

15. Yousef, G.E., Mann, G.F., Mowbray, J.F., 1987. Clinical and research applications of an enterovirus group reacted monoclonal antibody. Enterovirol. 28:185.

16a. Mowbray, J.F., 1990. Evidence for chronic enterovirus infection in ME (abstract). The First International Symposium on Myalgic Encephalomyelitis (M.E.), Cambridge University, April 9-12, 1990, this volume, B. Hyde, Editor, (tentatively) Ottawa University Press.

16b. Yousef, G.E., Bell, E.J., Mann, G.F., Murugesan, V., Smith, D.G., McCartney, R.A., Mowbray, J.F., 1988. Chronic enterovirus infection in patients with post-viral fatigue syndrome. Lancet. 1:146-150.

17a. Gow, J.W., Behan, W.M., Clements, G.B., Woodall, C., Riding, M., and Behan, P.O., 1991. Enteroviral RNA sequences detected by polymerase chain reaction in muscle of patients with postviral fatigue syndrome. BMJ. March 23, 302:692-696.

17b. Mowbray, J.F., 1991. Personal communication.

18a. Bowles, W.R., Richardson, P.J., Olson, C.J., Archard, L.D., 1981. Coxsackie B virus specific sequence in myocardial biopsies in patients with myocarditis and cardiomyopathy. Lancet. 1:7120-7124.

18b. Koontz, C.H., 1974. The role of Coxsackie virus infection in sporadic myocarditis. Am. Heart Jour. 82:750-758.

19a. Buchwald, D., Freedman, A.S., Ablashi, D.V., Sullivan, J.L., Caligiuri, M., Weinberg, D.S., Hall, C.G., Ahsley, R.L., Saxinger, C., and Balachandran, N., et al., 1990. A chronic "post infectious" fatigue syndrome associated with benign lymphoproliferation, B-cell proliferation, and active replication of human herpesvirus-6. J. Clin. Immuno. Nov. 10:335-344.

19b. Ablashi, D.V., Josephs, S.F., Buchbinder, A., Hellman, K., Nakamura, S., Liana, T., Lusso, P., Kaplan, M., Dahlberg, J.,

Memon, S., Imam, F., Ablashi, K.L., Markham, P.D., Kramarsky, B., Krueger, G.R.F., Biberfield, P., Wong-Stall, F., Salahuddin, S.Z., and Gallo, R.C., 1988. Human B lymphotropic virus (human herpes virus-6). J. Vira. Methods. 21:29.

19c. Josephs, S.F., Henry, B., Balachandran, N., Strayer, D., Peterson, D., Komaroff, A.L., and Ablashi, D.V., 1991. HHV-6 reactivation in chronic fatigue syndrome (letter). Lancet. 337:1346-1347.

19d. Niederman, J., Chun-Ren, L., Kaplan, M., and Brown, N., 1988. Clinical and serological features of human herpesvirus-6 infection in three adults. Lancet ii:817-819.

19e. Salahuddin S.Z., Ablashi, D.V., Markham, P., Josephs, S.F., Sturzenegger, S., Kaplan, M., Halligan, G., Biberfield, P., Wong-Stall, F., Kramarsky, B., and Gallo, R.C., 1986. Isolation of a new HBLV in patients with lymphoproliferative disorders. Science. 234:295.

20. Casttro, D., Goldstein, J. and Fudenberg, H.H. Unpublished observation.

21. DeFrietas, E., Hilliard, B., Cheney, P.R., Bell, D.S., Kiggundu, E., Sankey, D., Wroblewska, Z., Palladino, m., Woodward, J.P., and Koprowski, H., 1991. Retroviral sequences related to human T-lymphotropic virus type II in patients with chronic fatigue immune dysfunction syndrome. Proc. Natl. Acad. Sci. USA. Apr. 88:2922-2926.

22. Martin, W.J. Personal communication.

23a. Singh, V.K. and Fudenberg, H.H., 1986. Can blood 'immunocytes' be used to study neuropsychiatric disorders? (inv. rev) J. Clin. Psychiat. 47:592-595.

23b. Singh, V.K. and Fudenberg, H.H., 1986. Immunologic approach to etiology and therapy of neuropsychiatric disorders. In: Molecular Mechanisms for Pathogenesis of Central Nervous System Disorders (eds. Bignami, Bolis, and Gadjusek). F.E.S.N. 3:120.

23c. Blalock, J.E., Harbour-McMenamin, D., and Smith, E.M., 1985. Peptide hormones shared by the neuroenocrine and immunologic systems. J. Immunol. 135:858s.

24a. Prieto, J., 1990. Moncyte dysfunction (abstract). The First International Symposium on Myalgic Encephalomyelitis (M.E.), Cambridge University, April 9-12, 1990, in press, B. Hyde, Editor, (tentatively) Ottawa University Press.

24b. Prieto, J., Subira, M.S., Castilla, A., and Serrano, M., 1989. Naloxone-reversible monocyte dysfunction in patients with chronic fatigue syndrome. Scand. J. Immunol. 30:13-20.

25. Gontijo, M., and Moller, G., 1991. Antigen processing and presentation by small and large B cells. Scand. J. Immunol. 34:207-213.

26. Antigen Processing: A New Pathway Discovered. Science March 1992, 6:1214-15.

27. Behan, P.J. Personal communication (Cambridge, 199).

28. Grufferman, S., 1991. Discussion. The First International Symposium on Myalgic Encephalomyelitis (M.E.), Cambridge University, April 9-12, 1990.

29. Fudenberg, H.H., 1966. Immunologic deficiency, autoimmune disease and lymphoma: observations, implications, and speculations. (inv. rev.) Arth. Rheum. 9:464-472.

30. Fudenberg, H.H., Stites, D., and Caldwell, J., 1982. Basic and clinical immunology. Lang Press, Los Altos, CA. Third edition.

31. Fudenberg, D.D., and Tirole, J. Game Theory, the MIT Press, Cambridge, Mass, 1991.

32. Kruesi, M.J., Dale, J., and Strauss, S.E., 1989. Psychiatric diagnoses in patients who have chronic fatigue syndrome. J. Clin. Psych. 50:53-56.

33. Millon, C., Salvato, F., Blaney, N., Morgan, R., Mantero-Antienza, E., Klimas, N.G., and Fletcher, M.A., 1989. A psychologic assessment of chronic fatigue syndrome/chronic Epstein-Barr virus patients. Psych. Health. 3:131-141.

34. Strauss, S.E., Tosato, G., Armstrong, G., et al., 1985. Persisting illness and fatigue in adults with evidence of Epstein-Barr virus infections. Ann. Intern. Med. 102:7-16.

35a. Carter, J.B., Barr, G.D., Levin, A.S., Byers, V.S., Ponce, B., Fudenberg, H.H., and German, D.F., 1975. Standardization of tissue culture conditions for spontaneous thymidine-2-14C incorporation by unstimulated normal human peripheral lymphocytes: circadian rhythm of DNA synthesis. J. Allerg. Clin. Immunol. 56:191-205.

35b. Kaplan, M.S., Byers, V.S., Levin, A.S., German, D.F., Fudenberg, H.H., and LeCam, L.N., 1978. Circadian rhythm of stimulated blastogenesis: a 24-hour cycle in the mixed leukocyte culture reaction with SKSD stimulation. J. Allerg. Clin. Immunol. 58:180-189.

36. Katon, W., Berg, A.O., Robins, A.J., and Risse, S., 1986. Depression: medical utilization and somatization. West. J. Med. 144:564-568.

37. Wysenbeck, A.J., Shapira, Y., and Leibovici, L., 1991. Primary fibromyalgia and the chronic fatigue syndrome. Rheumatol-Int. 10:227-229.

38a. Goldstein, J. Detection of Brain Deficiency in CFS by NeuroSpect. First International Symposium on Chronic Fatigue Syndrome, Los Angeles, CA. February 17-19, 1990.

38b. Lottenberg, s. 1990. Positron emission tomography in chronic fatigue syndrome (abstract). The First International Symposium on Myalgic Encephalomyelitis (M.E.), Cambridge University, April 9-12, 1990, this volume, B. Hyde, Editor, (tentatively) Ottawa University Press.

38c. Mena, I., 1990. Study of cerebral perfusion by NeuroSPECT in patients with chronic fatigue syndrome (abstract). The First International Symposium on Myalgic Encephalomyelitis (M.E.), Cambridge University, April 9-12, 1990, this volume, B. Hyde, Editor, (tentatively) Ottawa University Press.

39. Hertogh, C.H., 1991. Personal communication.

40. Thompson, C.C., Weinberger, C., Lebo, R., Evans, R.M. Identification of a novel thyroid hormone receptor expressed in the mammalian central nervous system. Science. 237:1610.

41. Carrigg, N. Personal communication.

42a. Chou, Y., Virella, G., Fudenberg, H.H., 1991. Monocyte subset using monocyte-hepatoma hybrids. Submitted for publication.

42b. Khansari, N. and Fudenberg, H.H., 1984. Functional heterogeneity of human blood monocytes. Scand J. Immunol. 19:337-342.

43. Fudenberg, H.H. and Singh, V.K., 1988. Binding of the CRF to Receptors on Peripheral Blood Immune Cells. In progress, Switzerland: Averlag.

44. Holmes, G.P., Kappling, G., Gantz, Binding. Chronic Fatigue Syndrome - A working Case, 1988. Ann Intern Med 18:s53-55.

45a. Borystewica, L.K., Haworth, S.J., Mundin, J., Ricklouse, A., and Sissons, J.G.P., 1986. Epstein Barr virus specific immune defects in patients with persistent symptoms following infectious mononucleosis. Q.J. Med. New Ser. 58:111-121.

45b. Cheney, P.R., Dorman, S.E., and Bell, D.T., 1989. Interleukin 2 and chronic fatigue syndrome. Ann. Int. Med. 110:321.

45c. Komaroff, A.L., 1990. Myalgic encephalomyelitis/chronic fatigue and immune deficiency syndrome/post-viral fatigue syndrome (ME/CFIDS/PVFS): an overview (abstract). The First International Symposium on Myalgic Encephalomyelitis (M.E.), Cambridge University, April 912, 1990, this volume, B. Hyde, Editor, (tentatively) Ottawa University Press.

45d. Lever, A.M.L., Lewis, D.M., Bannister, B.A., Fry, M. and Berry, N., 1988. Interferon production in postviral chronic fatigue syndrome. Lancet 1:101.

45e. Lloyd, A.R., Wakefield, D., Boughton, C.R., Dwyer, J.M., 1989. Immunological abnormalities in the chronic fatigue syndrome. Med. J. August. 151:122-4.

45f. Subira, M.L., Castilla, A., Civeria, M.P., and Prieto, J., 1989. Deficient display of CD3 on lymphocytes of patients with chronic fatigue syndrome. J. Infect. Dis. 160:165-166.

46. Nel, A.E., Dirienzo, w., Stefanini, G.F., Wooten, M.W., Canonica, G.W., Lattanze, G.R., Stevenson, H.C., Miller, P., Fudenberg, H.H., and Galbraith, R.M., 1986. Inhibitory effect of an antibody against alpha$_1$-acid glycoprotein (alpha$_1$-AGP) on autologous mixed lymphocyte reaction and anti-T3 T lymphocyte activation. Cellular Immunol. 103:65-72.

47a. Komaroff, A.L., Geiger, A.M., and Wormsley, 1988. IgG subclass deficiences in chronic fatigue syndrome [letter]. Lancet. 1:1288-1289.

47b. Linde, A., Hammarstrom, L., and Smith, C.I.E., IgG subclass deficiency and chronic fatigue syndrome [letter]. Lancet. 1:885-886.

47c. Read, R., Spickett, G., Harvey, J., Edwards, A.J., and Larson, H.E., 1988. IgG1 subclass deficiency in patients with chronic fatigue syndrome [letter]. Lancet. 1:241-242.

48. Holmes, G.P., 1991. Defining the chronic fatigue syndrome. Rev. Infect. Dis. Jan-Feb. 13:S53-55.

49a. Aoki, T., Usuda, Y., Miyakoshi, H., Tamura, K., and Herberman, R.B., 1987. Low natural killer syndrome: clinical and immunologic features. Nat. Immun. Cell Growth Regul. 6:116-128.

49b. Caligiuri, M., Murray, C., Buchwald, D., et al., 1987. Pheontypic and functional deficiency of natural killer cells in patients with chronic fatigue syndrome. J. Immunol. 139:3306-3313.

50. Dirienzo, W., Stefanini, G.C., Singh, V.K., Paulling, E.E., Cnonica, G.W., and Fudenberg, H.H., 1986. Does normal lymphocyte DNA synthesis in response to PHA exclude cell-mediated immunodepression? Clin. Immunol. and Immunopathol. 41:227-235.

51. Singh, V.K. and Fudenberg, H.H., 1986. Lymphocyte stimulation in vitro by orosomucoid glycoprotein. Immunol. Let. 14(1):9-13.

52a. Arlen, M., Scherrer, J.W., Fudenberg, H.H., Virella, G., Arlen, P., and Levowitz, B., 1983. IgG immune complexes in patients with progressive tumor growth. Immunomodulation and Thermotherapy in Cancer (eds. Fudenberg, Pontiggia, and Ogier). Acta Medica Press, Rome. 283-292.

52b. Virella, G., Kilpatrick, J.M., Chenais, F., and Fudenberg, H.H., 1981. Isolation of soluble immune complexes from human serum: combined use of polyethylene glycol precipitation, gel filtration, and affinity chromatography on protein 1-sepharose. Methods Enzymol. 74:644-663.

53. Goust, J.M. and Fudenberg, H.H., 1983. T cell binding to lymphoid B cell lines in humans. A marker for T-B cell interaction? J. Immunol. Meth. Vol. 59 pp29-38.

54. Robert A. Good, personal communication.

55. Finn, R. and Cohen H.N., 1978. Food allergy - fact or fiction. Lancet. i:426-428.

56a. Brostoff, J. and Challacombe, S.J. (eds.), 1987. Food allergy and intolerance. Bailliere Tindall. London.

56b. Philpott, W.N. and Kalitus, P.K., 1957. Brain Allergy. Keals Publishing.

56c. Rowe, A.H., 1931. Food allergy. Springfield, IL. Charles C. Thomas.

56d. Springer, T., Dustin, M.L., Kishimoto, T.K., and Marlin, S.D., 1987. The lymphocyte function-associated LFA-1, CD2, and LFA-3 molecules: cell adhesion receptors of the immune system. Ann. Rev. Immunol. 5:223.

57a. Campbell, M.B., 1970. Allergy and epilepsy. Speer, F., ed. Allergy of the nervous system. Springfield, IL: CC Thomas. 59-78.

58. Liebeman, A. 1991. Personal communication.

59a. Fudenberg, H.H., and Fudenberg, H. Transfer Factor: Past, Present and Future. Annual Reviews of Pharmacology and Toxocology, 1989 vol 29:475-516, Annual Reviews, Inc., Palo Alto, CA.

59b. Fudenberg, H.H., and Gross, A. The Effect of Percent of Granular Sites in the Leucocyte Pool and the Effect of Recipient Donor Contact on the Clinical Benefit of Transfer Factor. Submitted for publication.

60. Fudenberg, H.H. and Singh, V.K., 1988. Immune Modulators in Progress In Drug Research.

61. Fudenberg, H.H. The Cox Syndrome Constellation Complex, in preparation.

Chapter 74

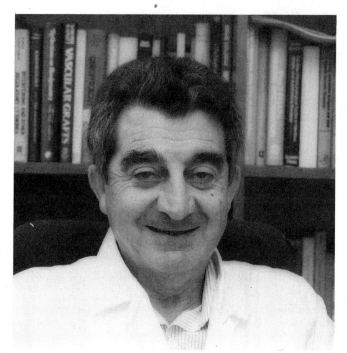

N. Trainin

The Role of Thymic Hormones in Viral Infections

N. Trainin, MD[1], Y. Burstein, PhD[2], M. Pecht, PhD[1], Z.T. Handzel, MD[3] and B. Rager-Zisman, PhD[4]

[1]Department of Cell Biology, [2]Department of Organic Chemistry, The Weizmann Institute of Science, Rehovot, Israel. [3]Ben-Ari Institute of Immunology, Kaplan Hospital, Rehovot, Israel [4]Department of Immunology and Virology, Ben-Gurion University, Beer-Sheva, Israel.

In 1955, Dr. Trainin joined the Department of Experimental Biology at the Weizmann Institute of Science and for five years was involved with the investigation of initiation and promotion of carcinogenesis and leukemogenesis with Prof. I. Berenblum who established this revolutionary concept in cancer. Later, Dr. Trainin devoted his research to immunosurveillance of cancer and the role of the thymus in this framework; in particular, he investigated the hormonal mechanism of thymic function, isolating a hormone, THF, which was synthesized later on and found it active in differentiation and maturation of the lymphoid system.

Introduction

In the past two decades, interactions between viruses and the immune system were extensively studied[1-3]. These investigations revealed that a large repertoire of specific and non-specific mechanisms protect the host against infection, diminish viral spread and promote recovery. Obviously, there is considerable variation in the relative importance of each mechanism, which is strongly dependent on the nature of the virus in question[4].

Virus specific antibodies provide a major immune mechanism to viral infections. They may serve to restrict spread of infection by viral neutralization, limit the extent of viremia which in turn prevents viral dissemination and afford protection against reinfection. Since antibodies do not ordinarily penetrate cells, they are largely ineffective at preventing the cell to cell spread of intracellular virus as it occurs in measles and herpes infections[5,6]. Viruses may also mature at the cell membrane and insert foreign antigens on the cell surface. The concept of immune surveillance of altered somatic cells by cell mediated immunity is derived from the rejection of allografts and tumors. Such mechanisms include specific cytotoxic cells, natural killer cells, macrophages and antibody-mediated cellular cytotoxicity. While these mechanisms are ineffective at preventing virus spread, they promote recognition and elimination of virus infected cells[7,8]. It must be noted that lysis of virus infected cells is effective at controlling infection only if it occurs before virus assembly in the infected cell. Otherwise, cell lysis will promote the release and subsequent spread of mature infectious virus from infected cells and tissues. Therefore, these mechanisms are maximally effective against those viruses such as herpes and influenza, which insert viral proteins into the host cell membrane long before maturation of progeny virions.

Thymus-derived lymphocytes or T cells are pivotal in regulating all cell-mediated immune responses. Cytotoxic T cells are known to play a role in resistance to many virus infections and for the development of an effective cell-mediated cytotoxic response a helper T-cell is required[9]. In addition, most antiviral antibody responses in vivo are thymus-dependent and therefore also require the cooperation of viral antigen-specific helper T cells. Other T cells also contribute indirectly to other anti-viral immune mechanisms. Antigen stimulation of sensitized T cells may result in the synthesis and release of a wide range of soluble factors or lymphokines. For example, gamma-interferon released from these stimulated T cells may serve locally or systemically to limit viral dissemination[9].

One common viral stratagem is the suppression of host effector immune responses[10,11]. Prominent examples, are Measles virus and Cytomegalovirus (CMV) where the second stage of the infection is associated with lymphopenia and a decrease in the circulating T cell pool for as long as two weeks[12] while CMV probably homes directly to T cells[13] as manifested by its cytotoxic effect on this cell population. Lately, with the increasing use of aggressive anti-cancer chemotherapy and radiotherapy, long-term immunosuppression became a common clinical phenomenon. These patients may become easy targets not only to the viruses mentioned above, but also to others which normally cause only minor illness, and evoke life-long specific immunity. The main culprit in this category is Varicella-Zoster, but all Herpes viruses may cause severe infections in these patients[14,15]. Generally all viruses for which an intact cell-mediated immunity (CMI) is required for protection, or for recovery from infection, pose a potential threat to immunocompromised individuals[3]. Thus, fulminant measles pneumonia and encephalitis or incapacitating adenovirus pneumonitis are common challenges in pediatric oncology units.

Therapeutic attempts at interrupting this chain of events can therefore be directed toward either elimination of the offending intruder by anti-viral chemotherapy, or enhancement of the numbers and function of the faltering immunocytes. Thymic hormones are appealing candidates for implementing the latter approach, since some of them have been demonstrated to increase the pool of circulating T cells and their proliferative and effector capacities, as has been described in some detail[16].

Biological properties of Thymic Hormones

Following our original observations that intraperitoneal implantation of thymus tissue inside cell impermeable diffusion chambers led to significant improvement of the anatomic and functional damage produced by neonatal thymectomy in mice[17], we aimed at isolating and characterizing the soluble product of the thymus gland responsible for this hormone-like type of activity. Since then we have found this activity in the extracts of the thymus of mice, rabbits, sheep and calves[18].

Thymic humoral factor gamma 2 (THF-gamma 2) was purified from calf thymus. The purification of THF-gamma 2, monitored in vitro and in vivo in mouse splenocyte proliferation assays, was achieved by gel filtration of low molecular weight thymus extracts followed by ion-exchange chromatography and sequential reversed-phase high performance liquid chromatography. The process yielded 5µg of THF-gamma 2/1000 kg of thymus tissue. The concentration of THF-gamma 2 required for augmentation of lymphocyte proliferation and interleukin 2 production was 5 ng/ml in vitro and 10 ng/kg per mouse in vivo. THF-gamma 2 has the amino acid sequence Leu-Glu-Asp-Gly-Pro-Lys-Phe-Leu. The proposed structure has been confirmed because a peptide was synthesized on the basis of this sequence that showed activity identical with that of the biological molecule. THF-gamma 2 retains essentially all the biological activity of the thymus extract from which it is derived[19]. Amongst the most important biological properties of THF investigated in mice are those shown in Table 1.

Table 1

Biological Activities of THF in mice

1. Promotes hematopoiesis
2. Augments the proliferative response of thymus and spleen cells to T-mitogens.
3. Increases the helper effect of T cells in the production of SRBC antibodies.
4. Raises the competence of T cells to participate in MLC, GVH and CML in allogeneic or xenogeneic systems.
5. Augments T-cell killing effect against syngeneic tumor cells.
6. Increases the secretion of interleukin-2 by T-cells.
7. Abrogates early thymocyte autoreactivity.

On the other hand neither direct B-cell activation nor interleukin-1 production by macrophages have been observed with THF. We thus postulated that in addition to its stimulatory effect on the production and differentiation of T-cells, THF has a modulatory function by which it can bring back the balance of the different T-cell subpopulations to normal, when this balance has been impaired[20]. In addition to THF-gamma 2, the other synthetic products originally obtained from calf thymus and also described as participating in T-cell differentiation and maturation, include Thymosin α_1, and Thymopoietin.

Thymosin α_1 is derived from Thymosin Fraction 5 and consists of 28 amino acids with a mol. wt of 3108 and the N-terminal blocked by acetyl group. Thymosin a_1 has been synthesized by standard techniques[21] and by cloning in bacteria. Tryptic maps and partial sequence indicated that human α_1 from fraction 5 had identity with the bovine preparation[22].

The thymopoietins I and II are closely related polypeptides isolated from bovine thymus[23], composed of 49 amino acid residues each, with a known sequence[24]. The peptides are cross reactive and may be isohormonal variants. Thymopoietin I and II have largely identical sequences. Synthetic thymopoietin II has biological activity similar to that of the native peptide. A pentapeptide TP-5 corresponding to residues 32-36 of thymopoietin II retains the biological activity of thymopoietin II[25].

Bach et al. have isolated from pig serum a factor, FTS, Facteur Thymic Serique which is active on T-cell rosette forming cells. FTS is a neutral nonapeptide. Synthetic FTS exhibited biological activity and displayed identical patterns by chromatographic elution to the native molecule[26]. A compound of FTS with zinc (FTS-Zn) called Thymulin, is apparently more active than the isolated peptide[27].

Although the thymic hormones isolated in various laboratories are all peptidic they differ in chemical structure, in the biochemical mechanism of target-cell triggering and also in the range of cell subsets they specifically activate. All of the them are derived from the thymus including FTS, since its presence in the serum depends apparently on that of the thymus. These hormones, play an essential role in the stepwise process of differentiation and maturation of thymocytes and of T-cells, in the absence of antigenic stimulation. Moreover, some of them seem to act earlier upon the progeny of bone-marrow stem cells, leading them towards lymphoid differentiation and proliferation. Recent data from various laboratories also confer on thymus hormones a role as regulators of differentiation of the various T-cell subsets and thus as contributors to the balance of T-helper, T-cytotoxic and T-suppressor compartments.

Antiviral effect of THF and other thymic hormones

The first experimental evidence of an in-vivo antiviral effect of THF was brought by Rager-Zisman et al.[28]. These authors found a considerable therapeutic effect of THF on mice infected with a potentially lethal dose of Sendai virus administered intranasally. Sendai virus had a striking pathogenic effect in the infected mice expressed as a decrease in total body weight, thymus involution, pneumonia and a low antibody response to the virus. Administration of THF following Sendai virus infection led to a marked improvement in all the parameters studied.

Preliminary suggestion of the clinical use of THF as an antiviral drug was gathered from the effect of this hormone on lymphocytes damaged by previous exposure to different viruses. Varsano et al. reported that lymphocytes of patients suffering from subacute sclerosing panencephalitis (SSPE) were impaired in their cell mediated immunity and that preincubation of their peripheral blood lymphocytes with THF led to an improvement of their performance in the various assays tested[29]. These observations were later confirmed and extended by Handzel et al.[30]. Moreover, THF induced an in vitro increase in proliferation of human peripheral blood lymphocytes in response to a challenge with varicella zoster virus (VZV) antigens[31]. In order to understand the mechanism of this antiviral effect of THF we developed a murine model of immune impairment induced by cytomegalovirus (MCMV) infection.

Systemic treatment of MCMV-infected mice with THF-gamma 2 resulted in reconstitution of the immune competence as manifested in the normalization of T-mitogenic responses, IL-2 secretion and also in the recovery from acute pathologic symptoms such as reduced spleen weight and liver inflammation. The effect of THF-gamma 2 was mainly on the T-cell compartment, whereas NK cells were not involved[32]. Although the specific immunologic pathways and cell types responsible for recovery are not clearly delineated, it seems that CMV-immune T-cells have a pivotal role in local or systemic infections[33]. Thus, we investigated whether in vivo treatment with THF-gamma 2 would enhance the antiviral activity of MCMV-immune spleen cells in an adoptive transfer model. Indeed, recipient mice concomitantly treated with MCMV and cyclophosphamide (CY) were rescued from a fatal infection by THF-gamma 2 treated immune spleen cells (93% survival) in contrast to immune spleen cells alone (38% survival) and 9% survival of CY-treated MCMV-infected group[34]. These experiments provided direct evidence for the antiviral capacity of THF-gamma 2 through its immunomodulatory effect on immune T-cells.

These results opened the way for clinical trials with THF in patients with severe systemic viral infections, either primary or secondary to cancer chemoradiotherapy, associated with T-cell impairments. The first attempt was the administration of THF to patients with severe SSPE and T-cell defects following measles infection. Treatment resulted in an increase in circulating T-cells in all patients some of whom showed no further clinical deterioration.

Herpes and adenovirus infections were commonly encountered secondary to high dose chemotherapy pulses in lymphoma and leukemia. The clinical syndromes afflicting these patients were usually generalized varicella (mainly in children with acute leukemia), severe herpes zoster, pneumonias, and severe encephalitis due to herpes simplex or measles.

Treatment

During THF treatment, the clinical course in these patients was usually characterized by a rapid decline in fever and a regression of the herpetiform and varicella lesions within 3 days, with the appearance of dry crusts, arrest of diarrhea, and disappearance of signs of secondary infections, if present. It is noteworthy that reconstitution of T-cell counts and functions took place gradually during the first or second week of treatment, often after the clinical signs had already regressed. In a series of 6 cases of different types of severe viral encephalitis, with comatose or delirious states, patients regained complete consciousness within three days after the initiation of THF treatment, became afebrile and suffered no neurological sequelae. Concurrenly, lymphocytes and T-cell sub-population counts gradually returned to normal. Cases of pneumonia, mainly of viral origin which had progressed rapidly to the point of requiring intensive care, cleared rapidly while on THF treatment. All of the trials cited so far were performed in an open, uncontrolled protocol, over an extended period of time, and in several clinical centers in Israel[35].

The fact that measles in Africa often tends to be a life-threatening condition, associated with prolonged immune deficiency and additional secondary infections, provided the rationale to conduct a controlled, randomized trial in a group of children with complicated measles in Capetown, South Africa[36]. Twenty patients with severe measles, some requiring intensive care, were randomly divided into two equal and age-matched groups and treated up to two weeks with partially purified THF or placebo. Admissions to intensive care, length of the febrile period and laboratory signs of inflammation were significantly reduced in the THF-treated group when compared to the placebo group.

Since the discovery of HIV an intensive research on

the effect of synthetic thymic hormones in AIDS is being carried out in various medical centers[37,38].

Thymopentin (TP5) has been shown to augment anti Hepatitis B antibody levels in vaccinated volunteers[39]. The effect of TP5 is being presently tested in a wide variety of infectious diseases including those of viral etiology in human[40, 41] and animal models[42].

Conclusion

On the basis of our experience and others', thymic hormones require to be extensively tested in viral diseases with the aim to evaluate their efficacy in single or combined schedules. Moreover, the therapeutic use in association with other antiviral drugs such as AZT, etc. and other biological response modifiers should be considered.

References

1. A.C. Allison. Prog. Med. Vir. 18:15. 1974.

2. D.J. Drutz, and J. Mills. *In*: **Basic and Clinical Immunol.** eds. H.H. Fudenberg, D.P. Stites, K.L. Caldwell, J.V. Wells, p. 228, 1978.

3. C.A. Mims. **The Pathogenesis of Infectious Disease,** Academic Press, p. 204, 1982.

4. A.C. Allison and W.H. Burns, *In*: **Immunogenicity,** ed. F. Borek, p. 154, 1972.

5. R. Rustigian, J. Bacteriol, 92:1792, 1966.

6. J.C. Stevens and M.L. Coole, J. Immunol. 113:1685, 1974.

7. B.R. Bloom and B. Rager-Zisman *In*: **Viral Immunology and Immunopathology,** ed. A.L. Notkins, p. 113, 1975.

8. R.M. Zinkernagel, P.C. Doherty, Contemp. Top. Immunobiol., 7:179, 1977

9. P.A. Neighbour and B.R. Bloom, *In*: **Seminars in infectious Diseases.** Ed. B.N. Field, p. 272, 1981.

10. S.W. Huang and R. Hong, N. Engl. J. Med. 292:1296, 1975.

11. H. Kirchner, Immunobiology of infection with H. Simplex Virus (Monographs in virology, Vol. 13, ed. J.L. Melnick), 1983,

12. H.C. Whittle, J. Dossetor, A. Oduloju, A.D. Bryceson and B.M. Greenwood, J. Clin. Invest. 62:678, 1978.

13. J.D. Hamilton, Cytomegalovirus and Immunity (Monographs in Virology, Vol. 12, ed. J.L. Melnick), 1982.

14. S.W. Feldman, W.T. Hughes and C.B. Daniel, Pediatrics, 56:388, 1975.

15. F. Reboul, S.S. Donaldson and H.S. Kaplan. Cancer 41:95, 1978.

16. N. Trainin, M. Pecht, and Z.T. Handzel, Immunol. Today, 4:16, 1983.

17. N. Trainin, Physiol. Reviews, 54:272, 1974.

18. N. Trainin, A. Bejerano, M. Strahilevitch, D. Goldring and M. Small, Isr. J. Med. Sci, 2:549, 1966.

19. Y. Burstein, V. Buchner, M. Pecht, and N. Trainin, Biochemistry, 27:4066, 1988.

20. B. Shohat, Z. Shapira, C. Servadio and N. Trainin, Transplantation, 35:68, 1983.

21. T.W. Wong and R.B. Merrifield, Biochemistry, 19:3233, 1980

22. T.L.K. Low and A.L. Goldstein, *In*: **The Year in Hematology,** (eds. R. Silber, J. LoBuc and A.S. Gordon) p. 281, 1978.

23. G. Goldstein, Nature (London) 247, 11, 1974.

24. D.H. Schlesinger, G. Goldstein and H.D. Niall, Biochemistry, 14:2214, 1975.

25. G. Goldstein, M.P. Sheid, E.A. Boyse, D.H. Schlesinger and J. Van Wauwe, Science, 204:1309, 1979.

26. J.F. Bach, M.A. Bach, J. Charreire, M. Dardenne and J.M. Pleau, Ann. N.Y. Acad. Sci. 332:23, 1979.

27. D. Kaiserlian, W. Savino and M. Dardenne, Clin. Immunol. Immunopathol. 28:192, 1983.

28. B. Rager-Zisman, Z. Harish, V. Rotter, Y. Yakir and N. Trainin, *In*: **Advances in Allergology and Immunology,** ed. A. Oehling, Pergamon Press Oxford and New York p. 25, 1980.

29. I. Varsano, Y. Danon, L. Jaber, E. Livni, B. Shohat, Y. Yakir, A. Shneyour and N. Trainin, Isr. J. Med. Sci. 12:1168, 1976.

30. Z.T. Handzel, N. Gadot, D. Idar, M. Schlesinger, E. Kahana, R. Dagan, S. Levin and N. Trainin, Brain and Development, 5:29, 1983.

31. N. Trainin, V. Rotter, Y. Yakir, R. Leve, Z.T. Handzel, B. Shohat and R. Zaizov, *In*: **Subcellular Factors in Immunity**, ed. H. Friedman, Ann N.Y. Acad. Sci. 332:9, 1979.

32. E. Katorza, M. Pecht, R.N. Apte, D. Benharroch, Y. Burstein, N. Trainin, B. Rager-Zisman, Clin. Exp. Immunol., 70:268, 1987.

33. M.J. Reddehase, F. Welland, K. Munch, S. Jonijic, A. Luske and U.H. Koszinowski, J. Virol. 61:23, 1985.

34. B. Rager-Zisman, F. Zuckerman, D. Benharroch, M. Pecht, Y. Burstein and N. Trainin, Clin. Exp. Immunol. 79:246, 1990.

35. Z.T. Handzel, Y. Burstein, V. Buchner, M. Pecht, and N. Trainin, J. Biol. Resp. Modifiers , 9: 269,1990.

36. D.W. Beatty, Z.T. Handzel, M. Pecht, C.R. Ryder, J. Hughes, K. McKabe and N. Trainin, Clin. Exp. Immunol. 56:479, 1984.

37. P. Hermans and Clumeck N. Med. Oncol. Tumor Pharmacother., 6:55, 1989.

38. N. Trainin, Nat. Immun. Cell Growth Regulation, 9: 155, 1990.

39. K. Zaruba, M. Rastorfer, P.J. Grob, H. Joller-Jemelka and K. Bolla, Lancet, ii:1245, 1983.

40. J.P. Waymack and J.W. Alexander, Comp. Immunol. Microbiol. Infect. Dis. 9:225, 1986.

41. J.DeMaubeuge, E. Haneke, D. Djawari, K. Wolff, G. Stingl, L. Molin, E. Schöpf, R. Stengel, H. Degreef, E. Panconesi, B. Wüthrich, and K. Bolla, Surv. Immunol. Res. 4 (suppl. 1):30-36, 1985.

42. R. Cappel, F. de Cuyper, K. De Neef, W. Höbel, and K. Bolla, Surv. Immuol. Res. 4 (suppl. 1):48, 1985.

Fibrositis / Fibromyalgia

Chapter 75

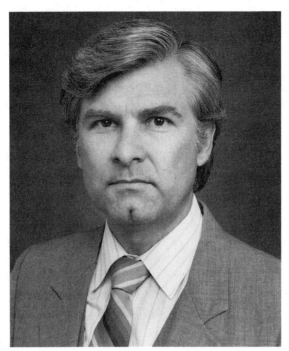

I. Jon Russell

Fibrositis / Fibromyalgia Syndrome

I. Jon Russell, MD, PhD
Associate Professor of Medicine Director, Brady-Green Clinical Research Center The University of Texas
Health Science Center San Antonio, Texas 78284-7874
Sponsored in part by a grant from the Upjohn Company

Since joining the faculty at the University of Texas Health Science Center at San Antonio, Dr. Jon Russell has conducted a number of studies in the immunology, pathogenesis, and management of rheumatic diseases. He directs the Medical School's Advanced Physical Diagnosis course for which he developed the Condition Diagramming method of clinical assessment. Dr. Russell has authored over 50 original medical publications and several chapters in medical textbooks. He travels extensively, speaking to medical audiences about rheumatic disease and medial education issues. He also holds a patent on an acoustic arthrography device which "listens" to joint sounds.

Abstract

Cytokine Abnormalities in Fibrositis/ Fibromyalgia Syndrome

Fibrositis/fibromyalgia Syndrome (FS) is a painful musculoskeletal syndrome affecting predominantly females, who complain of insomnia and exhibit reproducible tenderness to palpation at multiple points about the body. A recent multicentre study conducted in the United States and Canada has identified features of FS that distinguish it from other disorders of non-articular pain. From that data have come highly sensitive and specific criteria for the diagnosis of FS that will be adopted by the American College of Rheumatology. As a result, FS should now be considered and diagnosed in patients who meet clinical criteria, without deference to other medical conditions that may be present. Of course, a more consistent recognition of this disorder by all physicians will naturally increase the pressure on medical care systems to study this epidemiology, pathogenesis and treatment.

The prevalence of FS in the general population is not known, but it was found in more than 5% of patients waiting to see the doctor in a university medical clinic. It is present in about 15% of all patients seeking care from rheumatologists. The initiating cause of FS and the mechanisms which perpetuate it are still elusive, but recent research findings have led to a growing optimism. Sleep abnormalities and psychological aspects of the syndrome continue to receive attention, but structural, immunologic and metabolic aspects of FS are also receiving serious consideration. The compelling evidence for a metabolic defect in FS is providing a more directed basis for investigations into its pathogenesis. Finally, it is hoped that a better understanding of the underlying mechanisms in this disorder will lead to more effective therapy.

"And a woman spoke," saying, "Tell us of pain."

"And he said: 'Your pain is the breaking of the shell that encloses your understanding. And could you keep your heart in wonder of the daily miracles of your life, your pain would not seem less wondrous than your joy.'"

Excerpted from The Prophet by Kahlil Gibran, 1923

I. Introduction

Fibrositis/fibromyalgia syndrome [FS] is a painful musculoskeletal syndrome in which affected individuals, predominately female, complain of insomnia and exhibit reproducible tenderness to palpation at multiple points about the body[1-5]. Reviews of the medical literature[6,7] indicate that such a disorder has existed in Europe for centuries. Despite that, many physicians still question its validity as a clinical entity. Such skepticism is the natural result of confusion regarding its subjective manifestations, the paucity of objective biological markers, the lack of an animal model, and the suspicion that it may be emotively mediated. FS may never achieve confident clinical status unless most, or all, of these vagaries can be scientifically addressed.

Sir Edward Gowers coined the term fibrositis in 1904[8] to describe the inflammation he thought was responsible for the stiffness and pain experienced by a group of non-arthritic patients. Physicians are now critical of that term because it seems to be a misnomer for the disorder it represents[2,9]. A focus of histologically demonstrable inflammation has not been identified in the tissues of patients with FS, so it is currently assumed that there is none[2]. For that reason, it is difficult to justify use of the "-itis" suffix, despite the FS patient's rheumatic-like symptoms. A solution to the dilemma was proposed[2] with the term "fibromyalgia syndrome," which has now become a synonym for "fibrositis syndrome."

In the mid 1940s, Dr. Philip Hench was trying to teach the young physicians in his tutelage at the Mayo Clinic about FS[10]. He would describe how the fibrositic symptoms associated with rheumatoid arthritis were qualitatively different from those seen in hypothyroidism or systemic lupus erythematosus [SLE]. One of Dr. Hench's resident physicians at the time, has since confessed his own inability to fully appreciate such subtle differences, but he is still willing to believe that Dr. Hench could do so.

The concept of FS has undergone a gradual transformation since the days of pioneers like Gowers and Hench[6]. It was, for many years, considered to be a subjective disorder of vague musculoskeletal pains which the physician could not objectively document on a physical examination nor confirm by any laboratory test. When the diagnosis was made, it was usually by exclusion, only after an extensive clinical evaluation had failed to disclose another etiology for the patient's illness. It was perceived to be a benign disorder which, once diagnosed, could be safely ignored thereafter. At the same time, most physicians and their patients harbored the disquieting sense that something important may have been missed.

II. Classification

FS can be classified as one of several non-articular rheumatism disorders. As a group, these disorders are characterized by pain emanating from peri-articular structures located outside of the joint capsule and periosteum. The anatomic structures involved may include ligaments, tendons, fascia, bursae, and muscles, which constrain the bones in a physiologic position and/or facilitate mechanical function. Injuries to these soft tissue structures can accompany an arthritic syndrome or can present as a completely independent process in non-arthritic patients. In either case, the resultant dysfunction can be comparable to that associated with arthritis[13-15]. From a functional perspective, then, the non-articular rheumatism disorders are not benign.

Table 1

Classification of Non-Articular Rheumatism Disorders

Localized Disorders

1. Tenosynovitis	**2. Bursitis**
a. Biceps	a. Subacromial
b. Supraspinatus	b. Olecranon
c. deQuervain's	c. Trochanteric
d. Achilles	d. Prepatellar
e. Trigger Fingers	e. Pes Anserine
	f. Achilles
	g. Last

3. Enthesopathies	**4. Entrapment Syndrome**
a. Epicondylitis	a. Carpal Tunnel
b. Plantar Fascitis	b. Ulnar Tunnel
c. Costochondritis	c. Tarsal Tunnel
d. Pellegrini-Stieda	d. Morton's Neuroma
e. Osgood-Schlatter's	

5. Referred Pain
a. Diaphragm-Shoulder
b. Heart-Left Elbow
c. Hip-Knee

Regionalized Disorders

1. Myofascial Pain Syndrome
2. Myofascial Pain Dysfunction Syndrome

Generalized Disorders

1. Polymyalgia Rheumatica
2. Hypermobility Syndrome
3. Chronic Fatigue Syndrome
4. Psychogenic Rheumatism
5. Fibromyalgia Syndrome

A. Non-Articular Rheumatism

Table 1 shows a proposed classification under the overall heading of "Non-articular Rheumatism" [NAR]. The main subheadings indicate localized,

regionalized and generalized processes. Most of the localized disorders are thought to result from mechanical injury to non-articular tissues, often caused by repetitive use of a poorly conditioned structure. The regionalized disorders may involve more than one body structure, but are still limited in anatomic scope. The generalized disorders seem to be systemic processes which affect the musculoskeletal system in a rather global way.

With only a few exceptions, the "Localized Disorders" are named anatomically and are diagnosed from the exquisite tenderness disclosed by digital palpation of the involved structure. The list is not necessarily all-inclusive, because its intended role is merely to illustrate the concept.

The "Regionalized Disorders" are clearly more diffuse than the localized processes, but involve less of the body than do the "Generalized Disorders."

The myofascial pain syndrome [MPS], as described by physiatrist authors[16-18], is a painful musculoskeletal disorder characterized by the presence of one or more trigger points in a taut band of skeletal muscle near its junction with a ligament or tendon. When palpated vigorously, the trigger point exhibits local tenderness [like a tender point, see below], but also refers pain to one or more distal areas. These referral sites can themselves become "Satellite Trigger Points" as the symptoms spread. Trigger points are thought to be of two types [active and latent] in stages of transition. Active trigger points are symptomatic areas which are locally tender to palpation and also refer pain, while latent trigger points are asymptomatic until palpation discloses that they are involved. When a taut band is snapped by the examining finger or when the trigger point is needled, it is expected to exhibit a reflexic "local twitch response."

The myofascial pain and dysfunction syndrome [MPDS] is a painful disorder of the head and neck usually diagnosed and treated by dentists[19,20]. It was originally thought to result principally from pathology in the temporomandibular joint [TMJ], but many symptomatic patients don't exhibit any definable articular abnormality. Stress, nocturnal myoclonus, dental malocclusion, muscle spasm and excessive catecholamine production are regularly implicated in etiologic subclassification of MPDS. The distinction between MPS and MPDS may be more related to their anatomic location and to the professions required to deal with them than with differences in their underlying pathogenesis. On the other hand, it is suspected that many patients diagnosed as having MPDS also have FS which was not detected because the dentist examines only the head and neck.

The third main category is "Generalized Non-articular Rheumatism." Patients with one of the listed disorders are usually aware of pain affecting multiple areas of their bodies.

Polymyalgia rheumatica [PMR] is a systemic disorder in which elderly patients complain of disabling shoulder and pelvic girdle pain, have elevated sedimentation rates [usually greater than 50 mm/hr], and are at increased risk of having coexistent giant cell [temporal] arteritis[21]. This disorder is clearly generalized, but some might object to its inclusion in a line-up of non-articular disorders, because there is growing evidence to indicate that some PMR patients have an associated arthritis[22].

Hypermobility syndrome [double jointedness] is usually less painful than the other disorders discussed, but certainly can be very troublesome. About 30% of grade school children are asymptomatically hypermobile, but articular laxity is substantially less common [about 5% prevalence] in adults[23]. When symptoms are present, the lower extremities are more severely affected than the upper extremities, even though the ligamentous laxity is more readily demonstrated in the hands, elbows and shoulders. The typical problem in childhood is chronic, recurrent ankle sprains, but the disorder is seldom diagnosed until its persistence into adolescence or adulthood prompts clinical evaluation. It may be a common cause of back pain in adult women[24].

The terms "Chronic Fatigue Syndrome" and "Myalgic Encephalomyelitis" [ME] seem to be synonyms for the same disorder. The chronic fatigue syndrome was defined by a committee of the U.S. Center for Disease Control as a symptomatic disorder exhibiting six months of persistent idiopathic fatigue [allowing a level of function less than 50% of the premorbid state], plus at least six of the following features: recurrent fevers, nonexudative pharyngitis, painful cervical adenopathy, generalized weakness, myalgias,

prolonged fatigue following modest exertion, headaches, arthralgias, sleep disturbances and decreased libido, dizziness, impaired mentation or memory or emotional lability[127]. A study by Goldenberg et al[135] has indicated that the musculoskeletal pain component of this disorder is identical to FS.

Psychogenic rheumatism is defined as a true psychiatric disorder [psychosis or neurosis] in which the patient experiences musculoskeletal symptoms as somatic manifestations[25]. Patients with this disorder may exhibit very bizarre behavior. They have been observed to walk with a dramatically non-physiological gait or to maintain abnormal posturing. If the examiner should abduct the patient's arm, for example, and then release it in process of examining the other extremity, the patient may just hold it there without apparent recognition of the unnecessary effort. Patients with this disorder exhibit an inconsistent musculoskeletal examination from one time to the next or from one patient to the next.

In contrast, patients with FS exhibit a very homogeneous pattern. Their historical and physical features are so similar from one individual to another that they could be medical twins. The findings on musculoskeletal examination of an untreated patient will remain almost constant for extended periods of time[48]. Those observations alone should be convincing evidence that FS is an objective [rather than a subjective] disorder that merits careful study. While there are similarities between FS and ME, there are also substantial definitional differences, so it seems likely that they are distinct disorders with some overlap of symptoms.

B. Old Classification of FS

Table 2 outlines a classification of FS that was reasonably well accepted until recently[9,25]. It is shown here principally to emphasize its fall from favor.

This listing implies that idiopathic fibrositis syndrome is of uncertain etiology, while secondary fibrositis is caused by the associated medical illness. The obvious advantages to this nomenclature scheme are its simplicity and its long-standing entrenchment in medical terminology. Unfortunately, it suffers from several important flaws. Firstly, the term primary FS implies an intrinsic distinction from secondary

FS that has never been clearly demonstrated and probably is incorrect. Secondly, there is no convincing evidence to indicate that the associated medical illnesses are etiologically responsible for the FS symptoms. As a result, there is a contemporary move to develop a more defensible nosology[9] in which FS is always an independent disorder that may coexist with one or more other clinical disorders.

Table 2

An Outdated* Classification of Fibrositis/ Fibromyalgia Syndrome

I. Primary [Idiopathic] FS

II. Secondary FS

      A. Rheumatic Diseases
          1. Systemic lupus erythematosus
          2. Rheumatoid arthritis
          3. Polymyositis/Dermatomyositis
          4. Polymyalgia rheumatica

      B. Chronic Infections
          1. Tuberculosis
          2. Tertiary syphilis
          3. Bacterial endocarditis

      C. Endocrine Disorders
          1. Hypothyroidism
          2. Hyperparathyroidism

      D. Miscellaneous
          1. Trauma
          2. Malignancy

*See text for an explanation

C. The Term "Fibromyalgia"

The term fibromyalgia was proposed by Yunus et al[2,9] as a new name to take the place of fibrositis. The logic was to eliminate the "-itis" while preserving obeisance to the important role of fibrous tissue in the patient's symptoms. The term fibromyalgia also implies that muscle [...my...] is critically involved in the process. While subsequent study has failed to find any characteristic structural abnormality [see below], there is some evidence to indicate a role for abnormal skeletal muscle function in patients with FS. The term fibromyalgia has achieved some literature ac-

---

ceptance, but may not yet be the ideal term. The term fibrositis is still used by most referencing and indexing services.

D. The Term "Fibralgia"

One potential solution to the dilemma of nomenclature would be to establish a new system of reference for all of the disorders with similar or overlapping features. Such a system could be based on a generic term like fibralgia [cf the generic terms arthralgia or arthritis] which could be coupled with a descriptive prefix representing the presumed pathogenesis. It would be given a role in the taxonomy of painful non-articular disorders similar to that of the term "arthritis" for articular disorders.

Table 3 provides a hypothetical nomenclature based on this concept. Since the actual pathogenesis of FS is not yet known, the Table lists a variety of potentially responsible processes. For each numbered entry in the Table, the prefix would be followed by the common generic term fibralgia to indicate musculoskeletal pain with associated tenderness to palpation at multiple discrete soft tissue sites. Terms like rheumatoid arthritis or osteoarthritis would be mimicked with "Primary Fibralgia," meaning primary fibromyalgia/fibrositis syndrome; or "Hypothyroid Fibralgia," referring to fibromyalgia associated with hypothyroidism; or "Post-Viral Fibralgia," referring to the presumed etiology of the "Chronic Fatigue Syndrome/Myalgic Encephalomyelitis"[128].

This taxonomy can be expanded or compressed as indicated by the progress of science and could remain fairly fluid until the pathogenesis of these disorders becomes more clear. In the meantime, the suffix fibralgia would uniformly identify the class of disease referred to.

III. Epidemiology of NAR and FS

Despite the perception that FS must be quite common in the general population, there are no data which directly document its prevalence. Table 4 summarizes the frequency of non-articular rheumatism in several epidemiologic studies. In each case, the inhabitants of a small community were polled for the presence of musculoskeletal pain. When a response was affirmative, the affected individual was examined to establish the rheumatologic diagnosis. From such studies it can be deduced that rheumatoid arthritis [RA] has a prevalence of 0.8% to 3.0%. Osteoarthritis [OA], which exhibits a higher frequency among older individuals, ranges from 6.9% to 15%. In the same communities, non-articular rheumatism occurs in about 10% of the general population.

Table 3

Proposed Etiology-based Nomenclature for Fibralgia (Fibrositis/Fibromyalgia) Syndrome*

I. Medical Conditions

A. Rheumatic diseases	B. Infectious
1. Rheumatoid	1. Tuberculous
2. Lupoid	2. Syphilitic
3. Polymyalgic	3. Endocarditic
4. Spondylitic	4. Viral

C. Endocrine	D. Malignancy
1. Hypothyroid	1. Myelonic
2. Hyperparathyroid	
3. Steroid withdrawal	
4. PMS-induced	

E. Pharmacologic	F. Metabolic
1. Para-chloro-phenyl-alanine-induced	1. Catecolenergic
2. [Medication]-induced	2. Serotonergic
3. Caffeine-induced	3. Hyposerotonergic
4. Xaninene-induced	4. Hypocalcemic

G. Post-Operative
Post-hysterectomy
Post-oophorectomy
Past-pericardiotomy
Muscular
Myopathic
Myoglobinuric
Non-myoglobinuric

II. Examination signs-based	**III. Miscellaneous**
A. Tender point	A. Post-traumatic
B. Trigger point	B. Lithogenous
C. Nodular	C. Hypermobile
	D. Occupational
	E. Adolescent
	F. Childhood

IV. Psychologic
A. Stress-induced
B. Depressive
C. Loss-induced
1. Death
2. Health
3. Self-concept
D. Anxiety-induced
E. Panic-induced
F. Apneic
G. Insomnic
H. Situational

*The terms in the Table would be prefixes to the generic term "fibralgia," eg "rheumatoid fibralgia" or "hypothyroid fibralgia."

Table 4

Epidemiology of Non-articular Rheumatism: The Frequency Of Musculoskeletal Problems In The General Population

Author	Population	N	RA	OA	NAR
Kellgren (1953)	England	3,515	3.0	-	11.2
De Blecourt (1955)	Netherlands	3,378	0.8	6.9	10.3
De Blecourt (1963)	Netherlands	543	1.8	15.2	10.4
Spitzer (1976)	Canada	5,478	2.1	12.0	12.0

References: (121-124)

The question that cannot be answered with data is: What proportion of patients with non-articular rheumatism actually have FS? On the other hand, surveys of several rheumatology practices [Table 5] indicate FS to be the second or third most common disorder prompting patients to seek care from a specialist. The overall frequency of FS in those practices ranged from 15% to 19%.

Table 5

Epidemiology of Fibrositis/Fibromyalgia Syndrome in Rheumatology Practices

Author/ Reference	Number Of New Patients	Percentage With PFS	Percentage With SFS	Relative Frequency Of FS*
Yunus [1981]	285	19%	na	Second
Mazanec [1982]	150	16%	na	Second
Russell [1982]	468	12%	6%	Second
Wolfe [1983]	1,473	4%	11%	Third
Alarcon-segovia [1983]	1,000	15%	na	Third

References: (2,136-139)
Second or third most common condition diagnosed in the investigators' rheumatology practice. PFS, primary fibrositis/fibromyalgia syndrome; SFS, secondary fibrositis/fibromyalgia syndrome; na, not available.

A screening questionnaire was used to identify patients with FS in a large general practice clinic waiting room at the University of Oregon[4]. Forty-two [7%] of the 596 patients who answered the questionnaire met the criteria for possible FS. It was later shown that over 80% of those with a positive questionnaire met more rigid physical examination criteria for FS. Since the questionnaire was substantially more specific than sensitive[39], it has been suggested that the actual prevalence of FS in that waiting room was higher than the reported 5.6%. From these and other projections it has been estimated that FS may occur in up to 5% of the general population.

Another important epidemiologic parameter is the effect of a disorder on society. There is a growing awareness that FS has a major impact on the patient's ability to function in her or his daily environment. Questionnaire measures of pain and activity levels have shown that patients with FS are nearly as disabled as patients with RA[26,27]. [See also "Disability in Patients with FS" below]. Physical measures of musculoskeletal function have shown that the muscles of FS patients exhibit less strength and tend to fatigue more readily than do those of normal controls[28,29].

FS patients lose work days and probably work less efficiently because of their symptoms[26]. The overall magnitude of the loss to the work place caused by FS is unknown, but the cost of RA to the United States economy is estimated in the billions of dollars. If the estimated 5% prevalence of FS is correct, it might exceed RA in cost several-fold. It has been shown[30] that the utilization of health care services by FS patients tends to decrease after the correct diagnosis is made, but continues to be substantially greater than that for the general population of comparable age. Whether indirect costs parallel the direct costs in FS as they do in RA[52] is uncertain.

IV. Clinical Presentation of FS

The typical patient with FS is a middle-aged female who may say to her physician, "Doctor, I hurt all over." She may look fatigued, a little bewildered or even agitated, but usually doesn't appear chronically ill. The symptoms seem to be no respector of persons, so she could be of any ethnic background, socioeconomic status, marital status, and educational level.

A. Sex and Age Distribution of FS

All studies to date have indicated that FS is principally a female disorder affecting women in 70% to 90% of cases. (See Table 6). It is unlikely that all of this gender specificity can be explained by the fact that women are more likely than men to seek medical care.

Table 6
Demographic Characteristics of Adult Patients with Fibrositis/Fibromyalgia Syndrome

Investigators	Date of Report	N	Sex (%F)	Age (Years)	Duration of Symptoms
Yunus et.al.	[1981]	50	86	29	5.0
Campbell et.al.	[1983]	22	73	56	7.6
Wolfe et.al.	[1985]	155	86	50	—
Dinerman et.al.	[1986]	118	86	43	4.9
Felson et.al.	[1986]	39	84	44	4.3
Lessard et.al.	[1989]	973	85	46	—
Russell et.al.	[1989]	78	89	47	8.1
Mean Values			84	45	6.0

References: (2,4,11,33,35,40,140)

Individuals of all ages have been found to have FS. The ages of the majority of patients in most adult studies aggregate around the three decades from 30 to 60 years[2,4,11,33,35,40,140]. On the other hand, clinical experience[33] shows that octogenarians can have symptomatic FS, and 12% of 33 children reported to have FS developed their symptoms before the age of 6[32].

Subjective Complaints in FS

A listing of the patients' most common subjective complaints is shown in Table 7, along with the approximate frequencies of those complaints in the patient populations of several referenced populations[2,4,11,33,40].

Patients consistently complain of pain that they may at first say is related to their joints, but on questioning will localize to non-articular structures such as muscles, bursae and tendons. They usually describe neck pain and illustrate its location by massaging the lateral border of the trapezius at the base of the neck. They may report shoulder pain, but when asked to point with one finger, will identify the distal deltoid and biceps muscle area of the proximal arm. After complaining of elbow pain, they reproducibly point to the proximal forearm near the lateral epicondyle.

Table 7

Subjective Complaints of Patients with Fibrositis/Fibromyalgia Syndrome

Symptom/Trait	Yunus [N=50]	Campbell [N=22]	Wolfe [N=155]	Russell [N=78]	Lessard [N=973]
Aches & Pains	98	100	83	100	100
Poor Sleep	56	100	62	82	60
Fatigue	92	100	75	87	75
A.M. Stiffness	84	91	76	79*	83*
Subj Numbness	26	na	na	64	na
Subj Swelling	32	na	na	68	na
Chr Headache	44	55	na	58	49
Irrit Bowel	34	50	na	40	25
Worse with:					
Weather	92	++	57	85	na
Exertion	62	++	67	86	na
Anxiety	68	na	na	60	25
Better with:					
Moist Heat	92	++	57	73	na
Massage	64	na	na	na	na

Abbreviations: Irrit Bowel=Irritable bowel syndrome, Chr Headache=chronic "tension" cephalgia;
Subj=subjective;
na=data not available
++=very common but % not available
References: (2 ,4 ,11, 3 3 ,40)
* Morning stiffness duration>15 minutes.

FS patients sometimes depict chest pains in such graphic terms that angina is simulated. As a result, many pre-menopausal females have been hospitalized in the cardiac intensive care unit and even subjected to coronary angiography in an attempt to understand the cause of their episodic chest discomfort. Similarly, a description of low back pain that radiates down one or both legs can prompt the unwary physician to perform unnecessary electrodiagnostic or radiographic studies. The seemingly continuous sciatica-like pain, which radiates from the low back

to below the knee, is simulated by three distinct localized components. On examination, the patient may be found to have local tenderness to palpation at the pre-sacral fat pad or gluteus fascia, the trochanteric bursa/tensor fascia lata and the pes anserine bursa inferomedially to the knees. If necessary, any or all of these structures can be anesthetized locally for diagnostic confirmation.

The pain is generally worse in the morning when it is associated with stiffness that typically lasts for one to three hours. In that respect FS resembles RA [AM stiffness>30 minutes] more than it does the non-inflammatory OA [AM stiffness<15 minutes]. The pain and stiffness tend to be most severe on cold, rainy days. By contrast, a warm, balmy day may substantially reduce the level of pain, as does a hot bath or shower. Most patients feel better when they can be up and around, but overexertion one day may cause musculoskeletal pain so severe that the patient must resign herself to bed rest for the subsequent day or two.

Two graphic descriptions of the pain associated with FS are as follows: "It's like constantly having a bad sunburn, a hangover, and soreness in every muscle from doing yard work all weekend," or "It feels like I fell out of a speeding car and got all scraped and bruised from bouncing along the cement pavement."

One of the most frustrating problems for these patients is their inability to achieve normal restorative sleep. They report spending large portions of the night awake, wandering about their homes, trying to read or watch television. They come to envy the man who snores away, oblivious to their frustration. Then, in the morning, they feel even more exhausted than they did the night before. During the day, they understandably feel tired but have difficulty taking naps to make up for their lost sleep. Some patients enter a vicious cycle of taking large quantities of caffeine-containing beverages during the day, which then interfere with any medication that might be used to help them sleep at night.

Chronic headache seems to be a very common problem among patients with FS and becomes almost unbearable for some. The pattern is identical to muscle contraction cephalgia or tension cephalgia as occurs in individuals not affected with FS. Temporary relief can be obtained by neck massage or by a nap while supporting the supine neck with a very small pillow.

Patients often describe numbness or tingling of their hands or lips and a sense of hand or finger swelling. On questioning, however, they will usually acknowledge that the fingers do not really look swollen. This phenomenon resembles the symptoms of hyperventilation syndrome but lacks the respiratory component. Perhaps, the sensation of numbness or dysesthesias of the hands causes them to feel swollen.

Irritable bowel-like symptoms are seen in about 40% of patients with FS[2]. Patients may complain of troublesome constipation or constipation interspersed with intermittent cramping and diarrhea. Usually, the diarrhea is only a minor component. Seldom will the patient have noticed mucous on the surface of the excreted stool typical of mucous colitis/irritable bowel syndrome.

B. Physical Findings in FS

In the past, the major impediment to establishing the diagnosis of FS on a firm clinical and scientific basis was the lack of an objective physical sign. Physicians who hear wheezes, document an exacerbation of asthma, feel pitting edema in support of orthopnea, or see swollen joints in patients with arthritis, have understandably balked at diagnosing FS entirely on the basis of a patient's subjective report of pain. As a result, the diagnosis of FS was made by exclusion. After all other causes of musculoskeletal pain had been objectively excluded, the physician might say hesitantly that the pain might be related to FS.

It is now apparent, however, that the diagnosis can be made objectively and prospectively. It can even be diagnosed concomitantly in a patient who is suffering from another disorder known to cause musculoskeletal pain. The resource responsible for this new-found confidence is the so-called "tender point."

In 1972, Smythe[1,37] made a quantum leap in laying the groundwork for the current use of tender points in the diagnosis of FS. He described the location of 14 sites around the body at which patients with FS were found to have "exaggerated tenderness." The tender point was tender at the site of palpation, but **did not induce referral of pain to a distant site**, thus distinguishing it from the "trigger point" classically found in the MPS. Tender palpable nodules and taut bands which exhibit twitch responses, said to accompany the trigger points in patients with MPS, were not found in FS or, at least, were not considered necessary to its diagnosis.

One problem with attempting to make a clear distinction between MPS and FS may have been that examiners seeking trigger points ignored the failure of a given tender point to refer pain [as required in the definition of a trigger point]. Similarly, examiners seeking tender points may have failed to recognize the referral patterns of trigger points. The distinction between FS and MPS is now made easier by recognizing that MPS is a regional disorder while FS is generalized. Certainly, it is possible that features of both disorders may coexist in some patients, just as hypertension and diabetes mellitus are not mutually exclusive.

Since the original reports by Smythe et al[1], criteria for the diagnosis of FS proposed by other investigators[2-5,38] have variously depended upon the detection of tender points. There is reason to believe that the tenderness identified at the FS tender points is not due to unique pathology at those structures, but rather that those sites simply represent weak links in the sensitivity of musculoskeletal structures to firm palpation.

Support for the latter conclusion comes from the finding that tenderness at the control points parallels at a lower magnitude the tenderness at the designated tender points[40].

C. Diagnosis of FS

In 1987, the American College of Rheumatology Criteria Committee established a Subcommittee to systematically evaluate FS and to propose criteria for the diagnosis of FS that could be universally accepted. A study was undertaken, utilizing the expertise of investigators across the US and Canada, to determine which symptoms and signs would best discriminate FS from normal individuals and from patients with other musculoskeletal disorders. The resultant criteria[39] require a history of musculoskeletal pain involving multiple parts of the body and subjective [1+ on the Severity Scale, see below] tenderness to palpation at 11 of 18 well defined sites about the body, involving the head/neck area, the upper extremities, the lower extremities, and the trunk. The 18 sites are anatomically defined in Table 8. These criteria exhibit a high sensitivity [88.4%] and specificity [81.1%], and have been officially adopted by the ACR.

Table 8
The 1989 Criteria for the Classification of Fibrositis/Fibromyalgia Syndrome

1. From history - widespread musculoskeletal pain.

Definition: Pain is widespread when it is experienced in all of the following locations: in both sides of the body, above and below the waist, in the axial skeleton (eg. cervical spine or anterior chest or thoracic spine or low back). Shoulder and buttock involvement counts for either side of the body. "Low back" is lower segment.

2. From examination - pain induced by palpation at tender points.

Definition: Pain must be present in at least 11 of the following 18 (bilateral) tender point sites:

1, 2.	Occiput: at the suboccipital muscle insertions.
3, 4.	Low cervical: at the anterior aspects of the inter-transverse spaces at C5-C7.
5, 6.	Trapezius: at the midpoint of the upper border.
7, 8.	Supraspinatus: at origins, above the scapula spine near the medial border.
9, 10.	2nd rib: at the second costochondral junctions, just lateral to the junctions on upper surfaces.
11, 12.	Lateral epicondyle: 2 cm distal to the epicondyles.
13, 14.	Gluteal: in upper outer quadrants of buttocks in anterior fold of muscle.
15, 16.	Greater trochanter: posterior to the trochanteric prominence.
17, 18.	Knees: at the medial fat pad proximal to the joint line.

Reference: (39)

D. Quantitating Tenderness with the Tender Point Index (TPI)

The severity of the discomfort induced by palpation pressure at the designated tender points can easily be quantitated to provide additional information about the patient[38,39]. About 4 kg of pressure [the pressure required to blanch the blood from the thumbnail] is induced at each tender point. The patient's verbal and physical responses are then observed and gauged against the severity scale shown in Table 9. The appropriate severity scale value at each site is noted. and a running arithmetic sum is tallied. Once each of the 18 sites has been examined, the recorded total is called the Tender Point Index [TPI].

The TPI can range from 0 to 72, since it comprises 18 components, each scored from 0-4. It is determined from an examination that takes less than a minute of the physician's time. The only equipment it requires is the examiner's thumb. More importantly, it is a reproducible measure of FS disease status at any point in time that is sensitive to changes in the patient's condition as she or he responds to therapy[40].

Table 9
Severity Scale for Quantitating Tenderness induced by Palpation with 4kg Pressure at Tender Points of Patients with Fibrositis/ Fibromyalgia

Severity Scale	Patient Response to Pressure
0	"No, that doesn't hurt."
1 +	"Yes, that hurts." La belle indifference. Not objectively tender.
2 +	"Ouch, that hurts!" plus-a wince, jerk, withdrawal. Objective tenderness.
3 +	Dramatic "Ouch, that hurts!!!" Exaggerated withdrawal, rubs site. Objective tenderness.
4 +	Warning "Don't touch there, too painful!" Untouchable. Beyond objective tenderness.

E. Reliability and Validity of the Tender Point Index (TPI)

Untreated patients will exhibit a very consistent TPI from one time to the next, as evidenced by a study[40] in which 78 FS patients were examined by two physicians on two occasions, two weeks apart. There was no significant difference between the values obtained from the patients at the two different times [p=0.36]. Inter-rater reliability was also high [p=0.80]. The correlation of the TPI values with simultaneously measured dolorimeter values indicated a high level of agreement regarding severity [correlation coefficient = -0.649]. Campbell[4] used a similar approach in support of the tender point concept.

The TPI will increase if the patient's symptoms get worse and will decrease if the symptoms improve. A change of nine units in a patient's TPI scale should indicate a statistically significant [p<0.05] and probably clinically meaningful change in musculoskeletal pain. That number was derived from doubling the one standard deviation value [4.55] derived from the square root of the variance [20.73] for within-subject variation among 78 patients with an average TPI of 25.7 who were examined twice, with a 2-week interval between measurements[40]. In that study, the average TPI of FS patients fell by approximately 11 points, in parallel with a decrease in the patients' self-assessment of pain on the 10-cm visual analog scale.

F. FS Associated with Other Conditions

As noted in Table 10, FS can exist in the presence of other clinical disorders. The precise relationship between FS and disorders like RA, SLE, hypothyroidism or tuberculosis is unclear, but it is apparent that some patients with typical FS also exhibit one or more of those disorders with a frequency that has caught the attention of clinicians. Very few studies have critically evaluated this phenomenon. It is not even certain that the associations are occurring with a frequency greater than would be expected by chance, especially considering how common FS appears to be in the general population.

In San Antonio, between 1980 and 1982, 468 new patients were seen in the author's rheumatology practice. Among them, 82 patients [75 of them women] met the San Antonio criteria for FS. Of the female FS patients, 49 [65%] had no associated clinical disorder and were defined as having only FS. Twenty-six of the 75 [35%] had an associated condition like hypothyroidism [9 patients, 2 of which also had RA], RA [7 patients], SLE [7 patients], tuberculosis [2 patients] or other [1 patient].

Table 10			
Relative Prevalence of Selected Medical Conditions with Fibrositis/Fibromyalgia Syndrome*			
Medical Condition	General Prevalence	Prevalence among FS Patients in: Grand Forks	San Antonio
Number		973	75
Rheumatic Diseases			
Osteoarthritis	37.0%	35.0%	n. t.
Rheumatoid Arthr.	1.5%	9.8%	9.3%
Systemic Lupus	0.02%	1.4 *	9.3%
Ankylosing Spond.	0.15%	0.9%	none
Vasculitis	0.14%	0.2 %	none
Gouty Arthritis	0.8%	0.6%	none
Chronic Infections			
Tuberculosis	0.03%	none	4.0%
Syphilis	0.04%	none	none
Bacterial Endocar.	na	none	none
Endocrinopathy			
Hypothyroidism	1.0%	2.9%	12.0 *
Hyperparathyroid	na	0.2%	none
Malignancy	0.5%	5.6%	none

* Data for General Prevalence from "Current Topics in Rheumatology: Epidemiology of the Rheumatic Diseases, 1984[41]; and from Harrison's Principles of Internal Medicine 6th ed.[42].

* Data for FS populations: Grand Forks[33]; San Antonio[137]

Abbreviations: na=no data available, not tested or not reported; none=was sought in the database population and none were found.

The location of the tender points and the relative severities of the tenderness at those points was not different in FS patients with concomitant RA than in patients with FS alone. In addition, the FS component was as clearly distinguishable from the features of RA on examination as a tender point is from synovitis. Thus, patients with FS and RA exhibited tenderness at the designated locations, while patients with RA alone were not tender at those locations. The same appeared to be true of SLE.

When FS and RA coexist, the FS component appears to be unresponsive to the modalities used to treat RA, so the FS persists even after the active synovitis has been resolved with immunomodulatory therapy. The clinician must, therefore, take care not to treat RA patients with immunosuppressive agents of increasing toxicity potential when the pain demanding more therapy is from the FS component. It is interesting to note that RA patients who have been educated about the difference in manifestations between FS and RA can inform the clinician quite accurately which disorder is responsible for their symptoms at any point in time.

Hypothyroidism is associated with FS about 3 to 12 times more frequently than would be expected from the 1% prevalence of hypothyroidism in the general population. Hypothyroidism should be considered in FS patients because the musculoskeletal symptoms can improve considerably with thyroid replacement[43]. Patients with hypothyroidism exhibited the same pattern of deep sleep deprivation seen in FS but it improved somewhat with thyroid replacement[83]. The relationship between these clinical findings and the discovery of thyrotropin-releasing hormone in the serotonergic axons of experimental animal models[118] will require further study.

G. Clinical Laboratory Findings in FS

The best defense against missing an associated medical illness in patients with FS is to conduct a thorough history and physical examination on all patients with musculoskeletal pain. There are at present no clinical laboratory tests that can be counted on to assure or rule-out a diagnosis of FS. At a risk of being accused of cookbook medicine, the author recommends the inexpensive panel of screening tests shown in Table 11. The cost to the patient is conservative, when one considers many undiagnosed FS patients who come referred after having had an EMG for their hand dysesthesias, a full GI series for their irritable bowel, a CT scan for their muscle contraction headache, three hospital admissions crowned by coronary angiography for their costochondral chest wall pain and psychoanalysis for their reactive depression.

H. Disability In Patients With FS

There is very little information available to indicate how disabling FS may be to patients suffering from it. Two recent publications[29,45] about FS refer to the potential of this disorder to cause disabling symp-

toms. Since they do not support those conclusions with data or references, they infer it to be common knowledge. At present, however, the U.S. Government Social Security Administration does not recognize FS as a disabling condition[30] but Australia [Repetitive Strain Syndrome] and the Ontario Provincial Government of Canada [Fibrositis Syndrome] do[46].

Table 11
Laboratory Tests Which May Help Identify an Associated Medical Illness in Patients with Fibrositis/Fibromyalgia Syndrome

Clinical Disorder	Screening Tests
1. Rheumatic Disease	
a. SLE	ANA + ESR
b. RA (rheumatoid arthritis]	RF + ESR
c. Polymyositis	CPK
2. Chronic Infections	
a. TB	PPD + ESR
b. Syphilis	VDR
c. SBE (subacute bacterial endocarditis)	Culture + ESR
3. Endocrine Disorders	
a. Hypothyroidism	T4 + TSH
b. Hyperparathyroidism	Ca++PTH
4. Miscellaneous	
a. Malignancy	Stool Occult blood

One approach toward establishing prospective has been to compare FS with RA, because the disability status of RA has been fairly well established. In the course of several studies[26,27], FS and RA have been found comparable in their potential to interfere with a patient's function and quality of life. A common lament of FS patients is that they appear to look so well when they feel so miserable. The sense of discomfort they experience is dramatized by the painful terms they use to describe their symptoms[14]. Diffuse, aching musculoskeletal pain is the most important cause of disability in FS patients[48]. Pain is an important contributor to the disability associated with musculoskeletal diseases in general[49], but the pain caused by FS is apparently comparable in severity with that experienced by patients with RA[5,26,27,50,51]. Work testing[26] of patients with RA, patients with FS and normal controls demonstrated that work capacity for both patient groups was clearly compromised relative to the controls, but did not differ significantly from each other.

I. Natural History of FS

The natural outcome of FS over a period of time is to remain nearly the same, despite periodic exacerbations and remissions[48].

V. Pathogenesis of FS

The cause of FS and the mechanisms which perpetuate it are still unknown. There is, however, a growing optimism that current research efforts will improve our understanding of this disorder. Table 12 lists some of the theories relating to possible pathogenic mechanisms. Sleep abnormalities and psychological aspects of the syndrome continue to receive attention, but structural, immunologic and metabolic aspects of FS are also being seriously considered.

Table 12
Proposed Pathogenesis of Fibrositis/Fibromyalgia Syndrome

1.	Abnormal sleep
2.	Idiopathic edema
3.	Psychological pathology
4.	Muscle pathology
5.	Hearing and vestibular pathology
6.	Immunologic abnormalities
7.	Hypoxia
8.	Catecholamines metabolism
9.	Serotonin metabolism
10.	Physical trauma
11.	Endocrinopathy
12.	Chronic infection
13.	Subclinical connective tissue disorder

A. Psychological Pathology

The relevance of psychological parameters to the pathogenesis of FS remains elusive, despite the cumulative efforts of many investigators[4,27,54,61,64,129,141-147] who have tried to clarify it. Twenty years ago, the literature[54-57] was replete with speculations that during times of stress, family trauma, anxiety and war, an excess of new cases of RA developed, while patients with established disease suffered exacerbations. During the past five years, the same kinds of questions have been asked about FS [see Table 13]. There

is now much less discussion about emotional factors in RA, because the emphasis has shifted to swollen joints, synovial tissue, T cells and lymphokines. Perhaps, when the pathogenesis of FS is better understood, there will be less emphasis on emotive factors in it as well. Most likely, the emotional milieu that gave pause to investigators studying RA in the past, are still bothersome to RA patients. They are distressed because they can't be effectual parents, contributing spouses and productive citizens. By analogy, FS patients may also be legitimately frustrated with the limitations imposed upon them by their disease.

Table 13	
Is There a Psychological Disturbance in Fibrositis/Fibromyalgia Syndrome	
Strong Evidence For:	Questionnaire **Instrument Used**
Payne et al 1982	MMPI
Hudson et al 1985	DIS,DSM III,HDS
Some Evidence For:	
Ahles et al 1984	MMPI,LEI,AAS
Ahles et al 1987	MMPI,Zung
Wolfe et al 1984	MMPI
Kirmayer et al 1988	DIS, CES-D,SCL-90
Russell et al 1989	HDS,HAS,NIMH
Bishop et al 1989	HLC
Dailey et al 1989	Hassles,Uplift,LES ISSB,AIMS
No Evidence For:	
Campbell et al 1983	Beck-D,SCL-90,STAI
Clark et al 1985	Beck-D,SCL-90,STAI
References: (4,27,64,129,141-147)	

Two concepts of interest have been identified in psychological assessments of FS patients. A multicenter study of Health Locus of Control[64] among FS compared with matched normal individuals indicated that the FS patients were less confident of control over their own health outcomes and viewed chance as a major factor determining whether they improved or worsened. In another study[12] comparing RA and OA patients with FS patients, it found them to have similar exposures to stressful major life events and had similar resources for emotional support, but the FS patients experienced more stress from everyday hassles than the other two groups[129]. The Hassles Scale scores correlated with the psychological component of the Arthritis Impact Measurement scale, but not with the physical component [pain, limitation in function] of the disease. A lack of correlation between physical and psychological components of FS was noted in a study[40] of 78 FS patients and supports the concept that psychopathology is not the likely cause of FS.

B. Physical Trauma

Physical trauma has been proposed as a cause of FS[1,51,65]. The typical situation is an auto accident or a fall at work. Within two or three months, affected individuals may begin to notice musculoskeletal pain, particularly in the neck. After an examination that is usually limited to the presumably injured part, the physician orders x-rays which are invariably normal. Reassurance that the symptoms will eventually resolve proves incorrect and the patient returns for another explanation.

Eventually, the patient becomes frustrated with unsatisfying diagnoses. The physician, meanwhile, feels threatened by the persistence of the patient's vague complaints, which may be viewed as veiled accusations of the physician's incompetence. When the topic of disability is raised, the physician may suspect the patient of malingering for secondary gain or financial compensation. One argument against malingering as a cause of symptom persistence in FS came from the review of Lessard's patients[33]. In that group of 973 individuals with FS, 19% attributed the onset of their symptoms to antecedent trauma. Nearly half of those were involved in litigation, but none experienced resolution of their symptoms when the claims were settled.

C. Neurosensory Pathology

The fortuitous observation of one FS patient's abnormally high sensitivity to loud speech prompted Gerster and Hadj-Djilani[66] to prospectively evaluate neuro-otological function in FS. A comparison of their findings with those of patients with Meniere's disease identified similarities, but the patterns were not identical[67]. Two studies by a group of Swedish

investigators[68,69] have uncovered evidence suggesting that some FS patients have a previously unsuspected brainstem dysfunction.

D. Immunologic Abnormalities

Suggestions of immune dysfunction in FS come from the finding of IgG_4 deposits at the dermal epidermal junction[70,71] of the skin in some FS patients; an occasional low titer antinuclear antibody[35,72]; increased levels of sub-optimally activated T lymphocytes[73,117]; and lower than normal natural killer cell function[105].

E. Hypoxia

Another hypothesis maintains that there are localized areas of ischemia in the skeletal muscles of FS patients. That concept is supported by the work of Bengtsson et al[78] and of Gidlof et al[79] who showed low transcutaneous oxygen tensions and abnormal capillary perfusion in the area of tender points. This proposed mechanism must be clearly distinguished from claudication of extremities due to arterial insufficiency.

F. Muscle Pathology

For over a century, it has been suspected that the symptoms of FS may be caused by an abnormality in skeletal muscles[17,36]. Evidence for changes in structure or function[2,29,45,74-77] has failed to explain the clinical symptoms. Nuclear magnetic resonance [31P-NMR] studies[29,34] involving muscle examined at rest and after exercise have indicated abnormalities in high energy phosphate metabolism. It is apparent that FS patients have abnormalities in their skeletal muscles, even when the comparison population is poorly conditioned healthy controls. The question remains whether the muscle abnormalities develop first and cause a cascade of symptoms, or the pain causes disuse fiber atrophy and distorted metabolism. The fact that a substantial proportion of FS muscle biopsies [up to 25%] are normal, suggests that skeletal muscle abnormalities may be the result rather than the cause of FS.

G. Idiopathic Edema

Idiopathic edema was suggested[80] as a cause of musculoskeletal pain in some middle-aged women who developed swelling in their hands and ankles associated with carpal tunnel syndrome. The concept was appealing, but this mechanism is clearly not necessary or sufficient to explain the many manifestations of FS.

H. Hypermobility

The finding of ligamentous laxity may be helpful in understanding the symptoms of some patients recognized to have FS[81], because hypermobile individuals experience a variety of mechanical problems which can be averted with education and prophylaxis[24].

I. Abnormal Sleep

The high frequency of insomnia symptoms among patients with FS prompted Moldofsky and colleagues to propose a pathogenic basis for the syndrome[82]. When FS patients were studied in the sleep laboratory and compared with normal controls, the FS patients reported more awakenings, spent more time in the lighter stages of sleep [stage 2 non-REM] and less in the deep stages [stage 4 non-REM] of restorative sleep. There is evidence[132] to indicate that stage 4 non-REM sleep is at least partially devoted to physiologic restoration of musculoskeletal tissues. It was of interest that musculoskeletal symptoms could be induced by deprivation of stage 4 non-REM sleep in healthy individuals[130].

Sleep studies of 50 San Antonio FS patients revealed that 43% had some degree of alpha intrusion in non-REM sleep and 75% had one or more objective sleep abnormalities[133]. Observed among that group of patients was an incidence of about 25% for sleep apnea, 14% for nocturnal bruxism, and 16% for nocturnal myoclonus. It is of interest that the connection between FS and hypothyroidism[83] and even depression[131] may be via effects on deep sleep.

J. Norepinephrine and Epinephrine

Patients with MPDS have difficulty sleeping at night, partly because of nocturnal bruxism. Those with long-standing symptoms usually have associated temporomandibular joint disease, but that is not a prerequisite for the diagnosis. A metabolic study[19] of patients with MPDS examined the severity of the bruxing relative to urinary excretion of epinephrine and norepinephrine. Patients with severe bruxing were found to excrete significantly more of both catecholamines than did normal controls.

A similar study[38], which initially involved 14 FS patients, has been expanded to 20 FS patients[85]. The 24-hour urinary excretions of epinephrine and norepinephrine were measured in untreated FS patients and matched, pain-free, normal controls. Epinephrine excretion by the patients before treatment of their FS was nearly identical to that of the controls. Some of the patients had substantially higher [values more than 2 SD above the control mean] excretion of norepinephrine than the controls, but there was much overlap between the two groups and the means were not significantly different. The only significant correlation of demographic data with the norepinephrine excretion by the FS patients was their self-report of caffeine intake. After treatment for 16 weeks with a combination of alprazolam and ibuprofen, their epinephrine excretion was less than that of the normals and the norepinephrine excretion had normalized.

There is evidence to suggest that norepinephrine and serotonin may exert additive or synergistic functions in modulating the interpretation of painful sensory stimuli[86]. If serotonin is deficient in FS, as will be suggested in the following paragraphs, an increase in norepinephrine production might represent a compensatory response. At this point, the relationship of catecholamine production to the pathogenesis of FS is still unclear, so further study is needed.

K. Serotonin [5-hydroxytryptamine]

In a series of publications, Moldofsky and co-workers[58,87] described the clinical logic behind their investigation of serotonin as an important participant in the pathogenesis of FS. Serotonin was already known to be a neurotransmitter with a role in the regulation of deep restorative sleep and in the interpretation of painful stimuli[88]. They hypothesized that too little serotonin was available in the brain tissues of FS patients. As a result, patients might be expected to sleep poorly and to experience a greater than normal magnitude of pain from a graded stimulus given to the peripheral nervous system. Both of those problems will be recognized as nearly universal clinical features of FS.

In a study of nine FS patients[89], the serum concentration of serotonin was measured. It was found to be significantly lower in the FS patients than in the matched controls. Since serum was used for these assays, there may have been a substantial contribution by serotonin stored in platelets. While the differences in serum serotonin between patients and controls was significant, there was overlap between them. It is certainly possible that the abnormalities seen are characteristic of a subpopulation of FS, but not necessarily present in all.

L. Serotonin Re-uptake Sites on Platelets

Other approaches were needed to further evaluate the hypothetical deficiency of serotonin. A potentially useful method was found in the neurophysiology and psychiatry literatures. It had been known for some time that both the pre-and post-synaptic surfaces of certain intracranial axon terminals have re-uptake sites for serotonin, because of its role as a neurotransmitter[90,91]. Peripheral blood platelets also exhibit high avidity receptors and re-uptake sites for serotonin on their membrane surfaces[92]. The re-uptake sites have the physiologic function of taking up serotonin for re-storage in platelet granules.

Imipramine and a number of other psychotropic drugs apparently bind to the serotonin re-uptake sites, since they effectively compete with serotonin for binding to brain tissue and to platelet membrane fragments[93]. Imipramine has several advantages over serotonin as a ligand for studies of the serotonin re-uptake sites, because it is readily available and is not as easily degraded by circulating enzymes. Radio-labeled imipramine [3H-imipramine] now serves as a marker for serotonin re-uptake sites on platelet membrane fragments.

The utility of measuring imipramine-binding receptors in humans was exemplified by studies of depressed individuals[94,95]. The density of imipramine-binding receptors on the peripheral platelets of depressed patients was significantly lower than that of normal controls [see Table 14]. That difference was apparently not due to a variant receptor, because the affinity of the receptors in patients and controls was the same. These findings were even more meaningful when coupled with the observation that the

imipramine-binding receptor density tends to normalize with clinical resolution of the depressed state[96].

Table 14				
Impramine Binding to Platelets in Depression* and in Fibromyalgia/Fibrositis Syndrome				
Study	Subjects	n	3H-imipramine** binding (fm/mg protein)	Significance
*Previous Report, Briley[94]	Depressed	16	289±28	P<0.0ol
	Controls	21	612±56	
This report	Fibromyalgia	22		
	untreated		836±58	P<0.05+
	treated		679±37	P<0.05#
	Controls	22	694±53	

** Mean ± SEM
+ Compared with normal controls
# Compared with untreated fibromyalgia

The relationship of depression to FS has been controversial. Estimates of its frequency in FS have ranged from "normal" to 72% in different clinical studies[1]. Considering the vagaries in the clinical assessment of depression, it seemed logical to apply the more objective imipramine receptor assay to the study of FS. That was accomplished with 22 sequentially enrolled FS patients, unselected for any psychological characteristic, and an equal number of pain-free, matched controls. The result was a significantly higher [not lower as in depression] receptor density in FS[89].

An interesting postscript to that series of experiments was that patients in the study responded, over a 16-week period, to treatment with a combination of alprazolam and ibuprofen. In the same period of time, there was a complete normalization of the platelet imipramine receptor density, which correlated with changes in several of the clinical measures[89].

The imipramine-binding data raise some interesting questions about the psychological environment of FS. For example, they may help investigators understand why treatment of FS can be successful with doses of an antidepressant [eg. amitriptyline, 10-35 mg/day] that would be sub-therapeutic for patients with true depression[97]. The implication is: what is being called depression in FS may really be something else. The other potential value of these findings is that they strengthen the evidence for aberrant metabolism in the pathogenesis of FS.

M. Tryptophan Levels

Tryptophan is termed an essential amino acid because it cannot be synthesized by the human body. The digestion of dietary proteins in the gut releases tryptophan, which is then actively absorbed into the blood from the small intestine. Some of that tryptophan is removed from the blood during its first pass through the liver. A small portion of the remainder circulates as free plasma tryptophan, while the majority circulates reversibly bound to albumin.

Free plasma tryptophan can be actively transferred across the blood brain barrier into the central nervous system[98]. It is then taken up by serotonergic nuclei like the brain stem's raphe nucleus. The magnitude of tryptophan's effect on brain function can be influenced by its free plasma concentration relative to the concentrations of other amino acids which compete with it for transfer across the blood-brain barrier[99]. An oxidative decarboxylation of tryptophan, catalyzed by the enzyme tryptophan decarboxylase, results in the formation of 5-hydroxytryptamine [5-HT, serotonin, see Figures 1,2]. Further metabolism of 5-HT by monoamine oxidase breaks it down to the inactive 5-hydroxyindole acetic acid, which is then eliminated. As a result, the rate of 5-hydroxyindole acetic acid production may prove to be a useful measure of serotonin turnover[100].

It was predicted[53] that FS patients might exhibit a deficiency of free plasma tryptophan. That was a logical extension of the serotonin-deficiency hypothesis, because tryptophan is the critical metabolic precursor of serotonin. Measuring its concentration in the peripheral blood would not answer the major questions directly, but it might represent a reasonable first step. After all, human brain tissue is not readily accessible for metabolic studies.

The Toronto investigators measured the free plasma tryptophan in a group of nine FS patients and compared that value with each patient's level of musculoskeletal pain[53]. The results indicated a highly significant inverse relationship. The patients with the most severe pain had the lowest free plasma tryptophan levels. Those findings fit perfectly the investigators' hypothesis of a serotonin deficiency in the central nervous systems of FS patients.

An attempt was made to supplement these patients' diets with tryptophan, hoping to increase the plasma levels of tryptophan and reduce the severity of the symptoms[53]. One desirable result from such treatment was a measurable increase in sleep, but the musculoskeletal pain actually worsened.

A more recent study[101] of this question involved 20 FS patients and an equal number of age-, sex-, and race-matched normal controls. Total serum amino acid [free plus protein-bound] levels could be measured by a standard automated analyzer method. The tryptophan concentration was significantly lower in the FS group than the controls. These two studies of tryptophan concentration in FS measured different tryptophan pools, but both supported the concept of a serotonin deficiency. Of interest was the finding that the levels of six other amino acids were significantly lower in FS. The meaning of such a finding is yet unclear, but it could represent an important clue to the pathogenesis of this disease.

N. Substance P

Neurophysiologists have been studying the relationship of substance P to the functions of the central and peripheral nervous systems. It was found to be associated with serotonin in somatic and sympathetic autonomic motoneurons[102]. It appears that normal levels of serotonin exert a dampening effect on substance P-related discharges of sensory nerves, but that control is lacking when serotonin is deficient[103]. The clinical result could be hyperalgesia in serotonin deficiency.

There was an interesting integration of these factors in a study of high frequency transcutaneous nerve stimulation for patients with chronic pain[100]. Patients who responded to the therapy developed increases of endorphins and substance P in their cerebral spinal fluid levels. In addition, early responders exhibited a trend toward decreasing 5-hydroxyindole acetic acid, consistent with a decrease in the catabolism of serotonin. 5-hydroxyindole acetic acid tended to increase in the spinal fluid of non-responders.

It seems likely that substance P is somehow involved in the pathogenesis of FS, because it was found to be elevated in the cerebral spinal fluid of FS patients[104].

One could speculate that normal or even elevated levels of substance P and a serotonin deficiency in the region of peripheral nerves and/or the central nervous system could cause an exaggerated perception of normal sensory stimuli [see Figure 3]. Thus, the two key clinical features of FS [pain and insomnia] may be parallel consequences of serotonin deficiency rather than sequentially related phenomena [eg. chronic insomnia leading to pain intolerance].

Figure 1

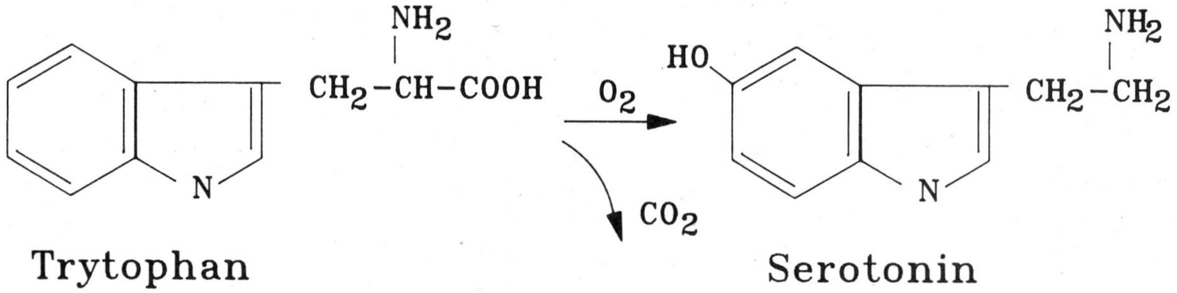

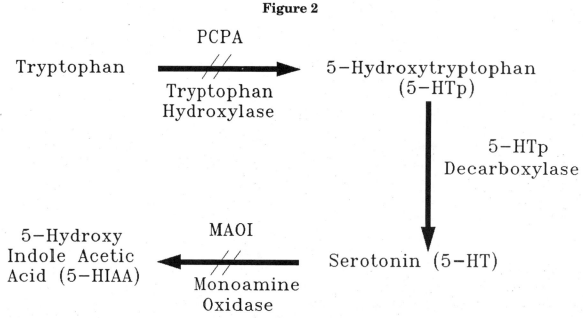

Oxidative decarboxylation of tryptophan to serotonin. An oxidative decarboxylation of tryptophan, catalyzed by the enzyme tryptophan decarboxylase, results in the formation of 5-hydroxytryptamine (5-HT, serotonin).

Figure 2

Tryptophan →[PCPA / Tryptophan Hydroxylase]→ 5-Hydroxytryptophan (5-HTp)

5-Hydroxytryptophan (5-HTp) →[5-HTp Decarboxylase]→ Serotonin (5-HT)

Serotonin (5-HT) →[MAOI / Monoamine Oxidase]→ 5-Hydroxy Indole Acetic Acid (5-HIAA)

Metabolism of tryptophan and serotonin. Tryptophan that crosses the blood-brain barrier is converted to serotonin (5-HT) enzymatically. Metabolism of 5-HT by monoamine oxidase (MAO) converts it to the inactive 5-hydroxyindole acetic acid. Parachlorophenylalanine (PCPA) inhibits the conversion of tryptophan to serotonin. monoamine oxidase inhibitors (MAOI) and tricyclic antidepressants inhibit the inactivation of serotonin. Adapted from Siegel GJ, et al: Basic Neurochemistry, ed 3. Boston, Little Brown, 1981, p. 212.

Figure 3

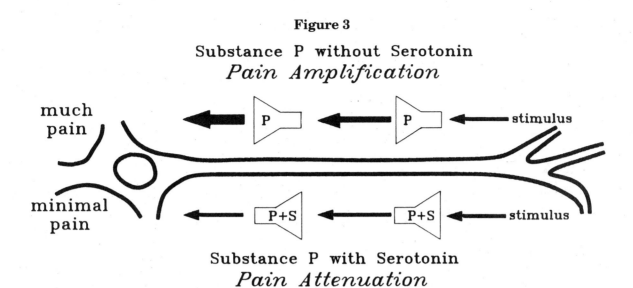

Substance P without Serotonin
Pain Amplification

Substance P with Serotonin
Pain Attenuation

Effects of serotonin and substance P on pain perception. Normal or elevated levels of substance P (P), in the face of a serotonin (S) deficiency (upper half of figure), could cause an exaggerated perception (enlarging arrows) of normal sensory stimuli (smaller arrows). Normal levels of serotonin (P+S, lower half of figure) prevent amplification of pain (small arrows).

0. Natural Killer Cell Activity

Immunologic testing of FS patients can also be seen to support the serotonin deficiency hypothesis. Patients and matched normal controls were tested for the number of phenotypic natural killer cells and for their cytolytic activity against a cultured tumor cell line in vitro[105]. The numbers of natural killer cells in the blood of FS patients, as assessed by specific monoclonal antibody binding, was not different from the controls. The percentage of natural killer cells with surface HLA-DR antigen was only marginally lower than controls. In contrast, the cytolytic activity of natural killer cells in FS was significantly lower than normal for all killer cell:target cell ratios.

Serotonin may influence the function of natural killer cells through its action on monocytes/macrophages. Serotonin affects the function of macrophages in three ways. It inhibits the expression of murine Ia [comparable to HLA-DR in humans]; it augments latex particle phagocytosis, and it stimulates the release of a monokine called "natural killer cell cytotoxicity effector factor"[106,107].

As illustrated in Figure 4, the monokine induces the transition of resting natural killer cells into active, immunopotent natural killer cells, which are quantitated by their ability to destroy cultured tumor cells in vitro. The stimulation with 8-OH DPAT, plus the inhibition experiments with cyproheptadine and ketanserine, simply show that the monocyte receptor for serotonin involved in this response is specific for 5-HT1.

The finding of low natural killer cell activity in FS could be readily integrated with the proposed serotonin deficiency hypothesis. A generalized deficiency of serotonin would theoretically result in decreased production of "natural killer cell activation factor" and the observed decrease in natural killer cell activity.

P. Somatic Smooth Muscle

The recognized effects of serotonin on smooth muscle could possibly be implicated to help explain the observed frequency of Raynaud's phenomenon[97,104] and bowel-related complaints[2,108] among patients with FS.

For example, gastrointestinal stimuli, like a meal or an electrical current administered to the vagus nerve, cause a large increase in circulating serotonin, substance P and gastrin. Both serotonin and substance P are then discharged into the intestinal lumen[109]. It is not yet clear what the missions of those neurotransmitters are in the gut, but they likely have something to do with bowel motility and homeostasis.

Figure 4

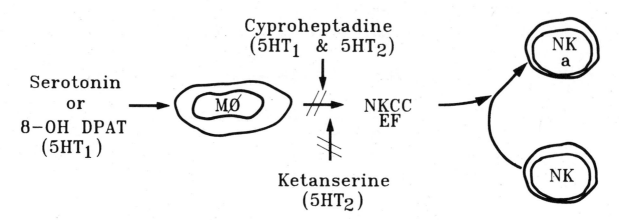

Link between serotonin and natural killer cells. Serotonin induces the transition from resting natural killer cells into active natural killer cells by a monocyte-dependent mechanism of action, illustrated as natural killer cell cytotoxicity enhancing factor. Stimulation with 8-OH DPAT and inhibition by cyproheptadine but not ketanserine imply a 5-HT1 related mechanism.

One can easily imagine that patients lacking normal secretory surges of these factors might experience dysmotilities similar to those reported by many patients with FS. Those with the most prominent irritable bowel symptoms might exhibit blunted surges of serotonin, substance P and gastrin induced by a meal.

Q. Successful Therapies

Table 15 summarizes the responses of FS patients to a variety of medical regimens. The question to be asked of successful therapies should be: "How do they work in FS?" and "What can be learned from their mechanisms that can help clarify the pathogenesis of FS?"

Amitriptyline and cyclobenzaprine probably have a similar mechanism of action in FS. They both have the basic structure characteristic of tricyclic antidepressants. Both inhibit the oxidative metabolism of serotonin to 5-hydroxyindole acetic acid. In doing so, they probably increase the effective concentration of serotonin within the interneural spaces.

Alprazolam is a triazolobenzodiazepine derivative with recognized anxiolytic and antidepressant effects. It is known to inhibit the binding of platelet activating factor to its specific receptor on platelets[110]. It inhibits the action of platelet activating factor on smooth muscle in the ileum and afferent renal arterioles[111,112]. It normalizes the elevated

	Table 15				
	Relative Outcomes of Blinded, Placebo-Controlled Pharmaceutical Therapeutic Studies in Fibrositis/Fibromyalgia Syndrome				
Center	No. Subjects	Drug(s)	Duration	Benefit	Ref
Toronto	7	L-Tryptophan	20 days	+	(87)
	8	Chlorpromazine	20 days	++++	
Portland Ramat	20	Prednisone	14 days	0	(116)
Aviv	20	Imipramine	3 months	0	(67)
Boston	15	Naproxen	6 weeks	+	(97)
	15	Amitriptyline	6 weeks	+++	
	15	Napr. + Amitr.	6 weeks	++++	
New Zealand	35	Amitriptyline	4 weeks	+++	(134)
Toronto	27	Amitriptyline	9 weeks	+++	(125)
Oregon	50	Cyclobenzaprine	12 weeks	+++	(126)
San Antonio	17	Ibuprofen	6 weeks	+	(40)
	17	Alprazolam 6 weeks		+	
	17	Ibu. + Alpraz.	6 weeks	+++	

Figure 5

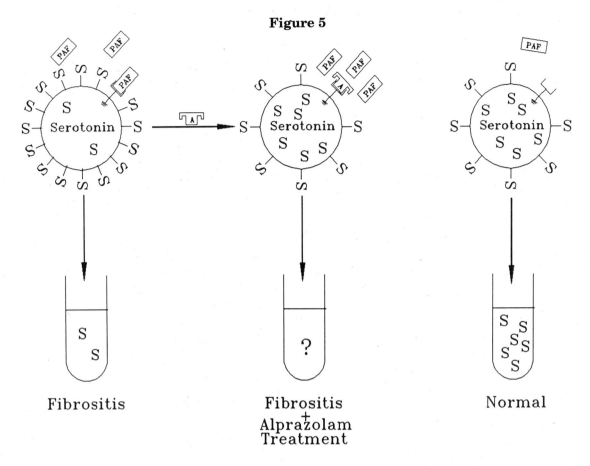

Hypothetical model depicting the proposed involvement of platelet-activating factor in FS. It is speculated that platelet activating factor (PAF, rectangular symbol) has a higher-than-normal activity in FS, or that the platelets (large circular symbols) in FS patients are sensitive to activation by PAD. If that were the case, FS platelets could be chronically depleted of stored serotonin. Since much of the serum serotonin comes from platelets activated during the clotting process, the serum (illustrated in test tubes below) serotonin concentration would be low and the number of serotonin reuptake sites (S symbols surrounding the circles) on the platelet surface would be increased. Alprazolam (A, in the symbol resembling a telephone) apparently binds to the PAF receptor and sterically prevents PAF-induced platelet activation. That might allow a more normal accumulation of serotonin in circulating platelets, and explain the normalization of serotonin reuptake sites on the platelet surfaces with treatment. Serum serotonin has not been measured after alprazolam treatment, so a question mark fills the tube.

plasma levels of platelet factor 4 and beta-thromboglobulin in patients with agoraphobia, indicating an inhibition of the high platelet turnover in that disorder[113]. Finally, it decreases the number of beta-adrenergic (eg. norepinephrine) receptors in the brain[114].

The combination of ibuprofen and alprazolam reduced the severity of painful symptoms in patients with FS[40]. The observations that this combination also increased the number of peripheral platelets and normalized the number of platelet re-uptake sites for serotonin could potentially implicate plate-let activating factor in the pathogenesis of FS [see Figure 5]. It is conceivable that platelet activating factor has a higher than normal activity in FS or that the platelets of FS patients are unduly sensitive to it. As a result, their platelets could be chronically depleted of stored serotonin and low serum serotonin would be found on testing. In this hypothetical scenario, the presence of alprazolam might allow a more normal accumulation of serotonin in circulating platelets, and decrease the need for increased numbers of re-uptake sites on the platelet surfaces.

In the clinical efficacy study of amitriptyline for the

management of FS[97], it was noted that amitriptyline was more effective than naproxen, but the nonsteroidal drug alone was more effective than placebo. The most effective therapy was the combination of both drugs, which gave additive or even synergistic benefit. A similar enhancement by a nonsteroidal anti-inflammatory drug was noted in the study which examined the efficacy of alprazolam and ibuprofen for the treatment of FS[40].

What, then, could be the mechanism of action for the propionic acid, nonsteroidal, anti-inflammatory drugs used in these two studies? Simple pain relief is a possibility, but an effect of such drugs on the tryptophan-serotonin pathway has been postulated. Diclofenac administration has been shown to alter the physical structure of albumin-displacing tryptophan and increasing the level of free plasma tryptophan[115].

The observed benefit associated with administration of both a sedative hypnotic drug and a nonsteroidal anti-inflammatory drug might be explained as follows: If the free plasma tryptophan were rate-limiting, as suggested by Moldofsky & Warsh[53], having a nonsteroidal anti-inflammatory drug present might increase the free plasma tryptophan available for transport. The increased availability of substrate could enhance the effect of simultaneously administering an inhibitor of serotonin catabolism.

VI. Treatment of FS

It will not be the purpose of this monograph to propose treatment for FS. There is clearly no consensus in the United States regarding how to treat it. On an international basis, there is even more diversity of opinion. Despite that, there is continuing research in this area and progress is being made. A statement by Rene Cailliet[119] may be cogent in this setting. He said, "Our ignorance should never lead us to complacency, nor should any patient who complains of disabling musculoskeletal pain be denied a searching mind nor a willingness to explore innovative treatment."

The protocol outlined in Table 16 is the one followed in the author's practice. The multi-disciplinary approach offers the opportunity for a variety of health professionals to contribute to the care of these patients and offers the patients access to a number of personalities with which to interact.

Table 16
A Treatment Protocol for Fibrositis/ Fibromyalgia Syndrome

1.	Test for other medical conditions
2.	Reassurance and explanation
3.	Evaluation of emotional factors
4.	Analgesic drug
5.	Physical Therapy
6.	Soft tissue injection
7.	Sedative antidepressant drug

A patient complaining of musculoskeletal pain should be given a careful medical history and physical examination to determine whether the cause of the pain is articular, non-articular or both. Once the diagnosis of FS is established and the TPI recorded, the data, including appropriate laboratory tests, should be reviewed, seeking evidence for an associated condition requiring separate therapy.

Once the physician has the patient's confidence [often this requires two or more visits], potential emotional factors should be carefully explored. Regular scheduled visits with the physician in the upcoming year should be more frequent than all medical visits in the prior 12 months. This approach has the effect of giving the patient assurance of a support system and thereby reduces telephone calls.

Non-steroidal anti-inflammatory drugs are given because they are effective analgesics. Patients are sent to physical therapy for a comprehensive integrated program of treatment, graded exercise, and education about body mechanics. If, after a month of this therapy, the patient returns with substantial discomfort in a specific area, a local injection may be appropriate[120]. A number of psychotropic agents, including chlorpromazine, amitriptyline, cyclobenzaprine or alprazolam, have been used in low dosage primarily for their sedating properties.

When a patient calls the physician complaining of severe musculoskeletal pain, it is difficult to know how to relieve the acute symptoms that have been called "FS Storm." In that setting it is invaluable to remember the almost magical benefit derivable from total body heat. Advising the patient to take a hot bath for 15-30 minutes and then lie, well covered, in a dark, quiet room until he or she has slept at least one hour, almost never fails to make the symptoms remit to bearable levels.

VII. Summary and Conclusions

The overriding theme of this discussion has been that FS can be prospectively considered and should be diagnosed in patients who meet clinical criteria, without deference to other medical conditions that may be present. Simply making the proper diagnosis may help some patients understand themselves better. Making an informed diagnosis can also avert unnecessary worry, diagnostic tests and doctor-shopping for an answer.

The prevalence of FS in the general population is not known, but it was found in more than 5% of patients waiting to see the doctor in a university medical clinic. It is present in about 15% of all patients seeking care from rheumatologists.

A more consistent recognition of this disorder by all physicians will naturally place increasing pressure on the medical care system to study its epidemiology, pathogenesis and treatment. The initiating cause of FS and the mechanisms which perpetuate it are still elusive, but recent research findings have led to a growing optimism. Sleep abnormalities and psychological aspects of the syndrome continue to receive attention, but structural, immunologic and metabolic aspects of FS are receiving serious consideration. The growing evidence for a defect in the metabolism of serotonin has provided a basis for more directed investigation of its cause. With a more thorough understanding of FS should come better approaches to serving affected individuals.

VIII. References

1. Smythe, H.A. and Moldofsky, H. Two contributions to understanding of the "fibrositis" syndrome. Bull Rheum Dis 28:928, 1977.

2. Yunus, M., Masi, A.T., Calabro, J.J., Miller, K.A. and Feigenbaum, S.L. Primary fibromyalgia (fibrositis): Clinical study of 50 patients with matched normal controls. Semin Arthritis Rheum 11:151, 1981.

3. Simms, R.W., Goldenberg, D.L., Felson, D.T. and Mason, J.H. Tenderness in 75 anatomic sites. Arthritis Rheum 31:182, 1988.

4. Campbell, S.M., Clark, S., Tindall, E.A., Forehand, M.E. and Bennett, R.M. Clinical characteristics of fibrositis. I. A "blinded," controlled study of symptoms and tender points. Arthritis Rheum 26:817, 1983.

5. Wolfe, F. The clinical syndrome of fibrositis. Am J Med 81:7, 1986.

6. Goldenberg, D.L. Fibromyalgia syndrome. An emerging but controversial condition. JAMA 257:2782, 1987.

7. Layfer, L. Fibromyalgia (fibrositis). IMJ 167:131, 1985.

8. Gowers, W.R. Lumbago: Its lessons and analogues. Br Med J 1:117, 1904.

9. Yunus, M.B. Fibromyalgia syndrome: a need for uniform classification [editorial]. J Rheumatol 10:841, 1983.

10. Hench, P.S. Differentiation between "psychogenic rheumatism" and true rheumatic disease. Postgrad Med 460, 1946.

11. Wolfe, F., Hawley, D.J., Cathey, M.A., Caro, X.J. and Russell, I.J. Fibrositis: symptom frequency and criteria for diagnosis. An evaluation of 291 rheumatic disease patients and 58 normal individuals. J Rheumatol 12:1159, 1985.

12. Fisk, J.W. Fibromyalgia [letter]. NZ Med J 95:91, 1982.

13. Boyer, J.T. Non-articular rheumatism. Prim care 11:341, 1984 .

14. Leavitt, F., Katz, R.S., Golden, H.E., Glickman, P.B. and Layfer, L.F. comparison of pain properties in fibromyalgia patients and rheumatoid arthritis patients. Arthritis Rheum 29:775, 1986.

15. Sheon, R.P., Moskowitz, R.W. and Goldberg, V.M. Soft tissue rheumatic pain: Recognition, management, prevention. Philadelphia: Lea & Febiger, Ed. 2, 1987, pp. 1-332.

16. Bonica, J.J. Management of myofascial pain syndromes in general practice. JAMA 164:732, 1957.

17. Simons, D.G. Muscle pain syndromes-part 1. Am J Phys Med 54:289, 1975.

18. Travell, J.G. and Simons, D.G. The Trigger Point Manual. Baltimore: Williams & Wilkins, 1983.

19. Clark, G.T., Rugh, J.D. and Handelman, S.L. Nocturnal masseter muscle activity and urinary catecholamine levels in bruxers. J Dent Res 59:1571, 1980.

20. Evaskus, D.S. and Laskin, D.M. A biochemical measure of stress in patients with myofascial pain-dysfunction syndrome. J Dent Res 51:1464, 1972.

21. Chuang, T., Hunder, G.G., Ilstrup, D.M. and Kurland, L.T. Polymyalgia rheumatica: A lo-year epidemiologic and clinical study. A Int Med 97:672, 1982.

22. Chou, C. and Schumacher, H.R.Jr. Clinical and pathologic studies of synovitis in polymyalgia rheumatica. Arthritis Rheum 27:1107, 1984.

23. Raskin, R.J. and Lawless, O.J. Articular and soft tissue abnormalities in a "normal" population. J Rheumatol 9:284, 1982.

24. Howes, R.G. and Isdale, I.C. The loose back: An unrecognized syndrome. Rheum Phys Med 11:72, 1971.

25. Beethan, W.P., Jr. Diagnosis and management of fibrositis syndrome and psychogenic rheumatism. Med Clin North Am 63:433, 1979.

26. Cathey, M.A., Wolfe, F. and Kleinheksel, S.M. Functional ability and work status in patients with fibromyalgia. Arthritis Care Res 1:85, 1988.

27. Russell, I.J., Fletcher, E.M., Tsui, J. and Michalek, J.E. Comparisons of rheumatoid arthritis and fibrositis/fibromyalgia syndrome using functional and psychological outcome measures. 1989. (UnPub)

28. Clark, S. and Bennett, R.M. Exercise endurance capacity in patients with fibrositis/fibromyalgia, presented at Nonarticular Rheumatism Study Group, American Rheumatism Association meeting, May 25, 1988. (UnPub)

29. Bartels, E.M. and Danneskiold-Samsoe, B. Histological abnormalities in muscle from patients with certain types of fibrositis. Lancet 1:755-757, 1986.

30. Cathey, M.A., Wolfe, F., Kleinheksel, S.M. and Hawley, D.J. socioeconomic impact of fibrositis. Am J Med 81:78, 1986.

31. Travell, J. Identification of myofascial trigger point syndromes: A case of atypical facial neuralgia. Arch Phys Med Rehabil 62:100, 1981.

32. Yunus, M.B. and Masi, A.T. Juvenile primary fibromyalgia syndrome. A clinical study of thirty-three patients and matched normal controls. Arthritis Rheum 28:138, 1985.

33. Lessard, J.A. and Russell, I.J. Fibrositis/fibromyalgia in private rheumatology practice: Systematic analysis of a patient data base. 1989. (UnPub)

34. Mathur, A.K., Schumacher, H.R., Bank, W.J. and Gatter, R.A. Phosphorus nuclear magnetic resonance (31P-NMR) spectroscopy in fibromyalgia. 1989. (UnPub)

35. Dinerman, H., Goldenberg, D.L. and Felson, D.T. A prospective evaluation of 118 patients with the fibromyalgia syndrome: Prevalence of Raynaud's phenomenon, sicca symptoms, ANA, low complement, and Ig deposition at the dermal-epidermal junction. J Rheumatol 13:368, 1986.

36. Simons, D.G. Muscle pain syndrome-part 2. Am J Phys Med 55:15, 1976.

37. Smythe, H.A. Non-articular rheumatism and the "fibrositis" syndrome. In: Arthritis and Allied Conditions, edited by Hollander, J.L. and McCarty, D.J. Philadelphia: Lea & Febiger, 1972, pp. 874-884.

38. Russell, I.J., Vipraio, G.A., Morgan, W.W. and Bowden, C.L. Is there a metabolic basis for the fibrositis syndrome? Am J Med 81:50, 1986.

39. Wolfe, F., Smythe, H.A., Yunus, M.B., et al. Criteria for fibromyalgia. Arthritis Rheum 33:160, 1990.

40. Russell, I.J., Fletcher, E.M., Michalek, J.E., McBroom, P.C. and Hester, G.A. Treatment of primary fibromyalgia/fibrositis syndrome with ibuprofen and alprazolam: A double-blind, placebo-controlled study. Arthritis Rheum 34:552, 1991.

41. Lawrence, C. and Shulman, L.E. Current topics in rheumatology: Epidemiology of the rheumatic diseases, New York: Gower Medical, 1984.

42. Wintrobe, M.M., Thorn, G.W., Adams, R.D., et al. Harrison's Principles of Internal Medicine, New York: McGraw-Hill, 1970.

43. Wilke, W.S., Sheeler, L.R. and Makarowski, W.S. Hypothyroidism with presenting symptoms of fibrositis. J Rheumatol 8:626, 1981.

44. Statistical Abstract of the United States, Bureau of Census: U.S. Department of Commerce, 1984. Ed. 104

45. Kalyan-Raman, U.P., Kalyan-Raman, K., Yunus, M.B. and Masi, A.T. Muscle pathology in primary fibromyalgia syndrome: a light microscopic, histochemical and ultrastructural study. J Rheumatol 11:808, 1984.

46. Littlejohn, G.O. and Miller, M.H. Repetitive strain injury: Divide and conquer. Am Fam Physician 15:409, 1986.

47. Bombardier, C., Ware, J., Russell, I.J., Larson, M., Chalmers, A. and Read, J.L. Auranofin therapy and quality of life in patients with rheumatoid arthritis. Results of a multicenter trial. Am J Med 81:565, 1986.

48. Hawley, D.J., Wolfe, F. and Cathey, M.A. Pain, functional disability, and psychological status: A 12-month study of severity in fibromyalgia. J Rheumatol 15:1551, 1988.

49. Kazis, L.E., Meenan, R.F. and Anderson, J.J. Pain in the rheumatic diseases: Investigation of a key health status component. Arthritis Rheum 26:1017, 1983.

50. Wolfe, F. Non-articular symptoms in fibrositis, rheumatoid arthritis, osteoarthritis and arthralgia syndromes. Arthritis Rheum 25:Sl46, 1982. (Abstract).

51. Weinberger, L.M. Traumatic fibromyositis: A critical review of an enigmatic concept. West J Med 127:99, 1977.

52. Thompson, M.S., Read, J.L., Hutchings, C., Paterson, M. and Harris, E.D., Jr. The cost effectiveness of auranofin: Results of a randomized clinical trial. J Rheumatol 15:35, 1988.

53. Moldofsky, H. and Warsh, J.J. Plasma tryptophan and musculoskeletal pain in nonarticular rheumatism ("fibrositis syndrome"). Pain 5:65, 1978.

54. Moos, R.H. and Solomon, G.F. Minnesota multiphasic personality inventory response patterns in patients with rheumatoid arthritis. J Psychosom Res 8:17, 1964.

55. Nalven, F.B. and O'Brien, J.F. Personality patterns of rheumatoid arthritic patients. Arthritis Rheum 7:18, 1964.

56. Polley, H.F., Swenson, W.M. and Steinhilber, R.M. Personality characteristics of patients with rheumatoid arthritis. Psychosomatics 11:45, 1970.

57. Spergel, P., Ehrlich, G.E. and Glass, D. The rheumatoid arthritic personality: A psychodiagnostic myth. Psychosomatics 19:79, 1978.

58. Moldofsky, H. Rheumatic pain modulation syndrome: The interrelationships between sleep, central nervous system, serotonin and pain. Adv Neurol 33:51, 1982.

59. Zung, W.W.K. and Durham, N.C. A self-rating depression scale. Arch Gen Psych 12:63, 1965.

60. Melzack, R., Stillwell, D.M. and Fox, E.J. Trigger points and acupuncture points for pain: Correlations and implications. Pain 3:3, 1977.

61. Caro, X.J., Kinstad, N.A., Russell, I.J. and Wolfe, F. Increased sensitivity to health related questions in patients with primary fibrositis syndrome. Arthritis Rheum 30:63, 1987. (Abstract).

62. Smythe, H.A. Fibrositis and other diffuse musculoskeletal syndromes. In: Textbook of Rheumatology, edited by Kelley, W.N., Harris, H.D. and Ruddy, S. Philadelphia: Saunders, 1981, pp. 485-493.

63. Wallston, B.S., et al. Development and validation of the Health Locus of Control Scale. J Consul Clin Psychol 44:580, 1976.

64. Russell, I.J., Fletcher, E., Bishop, G., Caro, X. and Wolfe, F. A controlled prospective, multicenter study of Health Locus of Control among fibrositis patients. 1989. (UnPub)

65. Burda, C.D. Immunoglobulin-G deposits at the dermal-epidermal junction in secondary (traumatic) fibromyalgia syndrome [letter]. Clin Exp Rheum 2:195, 1984.

66. Gerster, J.C. and Hadj-Djilani, A. Hearing and vestibular abnormalities in primary fibrositis syndrome. J Rheumatol 11:678, 1984.

67. Heloe, B., Heiberg, A.N. and Krogstad, B.S. A multiprofessional study of patients with myofascial pain-dysfunction syndrome. Acta Odontol Scand 38:109-117, 1980.

68. Rosenhall, U., Johansson, G. and Orndahl, G. Neuroaudiological findings in chronic primary fibromyalgia with dysesthesia. Scand J Rehabil Med 19:147, 1987. (Abstract).

69. Rosenhall, U., Johansson, G. and Orndahl, G. Eye motility dysfunction in chronic primary fibromyalgia with dysesthesia. Scand J Rehabil Med 19:139, 1987. (Abstract).

70. Harrist, T.J. and Mihm, M.C., Jr. The specificity and clinical usefulness of the lupus band test. Arthritis Rheum 23:479, 1980.

71. Caro, X.J., Wolfe, F., Johnston, W.H. and Smith, A.L. A controlled and blinded study of immunoreactant deposition at the dermal-epidermal junction of patients with primary fibrositis syndrome. J Rheumatol 13:1086, 1986.

72. Yunus, M.B. and Masi, A.T. Prevalence of antinuclear antibodies and connective tissue disease symptoms in primary fibromyalgia syndrome. Clin Res 33:924A, 1985. (Abstract).

73. Russell, I.J., Vipraio, G.A., Michalek, J. and Fletcher, E. Abnormal T cell subpopulations in fibrositis syndrome. Arthritis Rheum 31: S98, 1988. (Abstract).

74. Danneskiold-Samsoe, B., Christiansen, E., Lund, B. and Anderson, R.B. Regional muscle tension and pain ("fibrositis"). Scand J Rehab Med 15:17, 1982.

75. Jacobsen, S. and Danneskiold-Samsoe, B. Isometric and isokinetic muscle strength in patients with fibrositis syndrome. New characteristics for a difficult definable category of patients. Scand J Rheumatol 16:61, 1987.

76. Klemp, P., Nielsen, H.V., Korsg'ard, J. and Crone, P. Blood flow in fibromyotic muscles. Scand J Rehabil Med 14:81-82, 1982.

77. Henriksson, K.G., Bengtsson, A., Larsson, J., Lindstrom, F. and Thornell, L.E. Muscle biopsy findings of possible diagnostic importance in primary fibromyalgia (fibrositis, myofascial pain syndrome). Lancet 2:1395, 1982.

78. Bengtsson, A., Henriksson, K.G. and Larsson, J. Reduced high energy phosphate levels in the painful muscles of patients with primary fibromyalgia. Arthritis Rheum 29:817, 1986.

79. Gidlof, A., Hammersen, F., Larsson, J., Lewis, D.H. and Liljedahl, S.O. Is capillary endothelium in human skeletal muscle an ischemic shock tissue. In: symposium on Induced Skeletal Muscle Ischemia in Man, edited by Linkoping, Sweden, 1980, pp. 63-79.

80. Pinals, R.S., Dalakos, T.G. and Streeten, D.H.P. Idiopathic edema as a -cause of nonarticular rheumatism. Arthritis Rheum 22:396, 1979.

81. Goldman, J.A. is fibrositis associated with hypermobility? J Muscul Med 12, 1985.

82. Moldofsky, H. Sleep and musculoskeletal pain. Am J Med

83. Kales, A., Heuser, G., Jacobson, A., et al. All night sleep studies in hypothyroid patients, before and after treatment. J Clin Endocrinol 27:1593, 1967.

84. Mendels, J., Hawkins, D.R. and Hill, C. Sleep and depression. Arch Gen Psychiat 16:344, 1967.

85. Russell, I.J., Vipraio, G.A., Morgan, W.W. and Bowden, C.L. Catecholamine excretion in fibromyalgia syndrome. 1988. (UnPub)

86. Minor, B.G., Post, C. and Archer, T. Blockade of intrathecal 5-hydroxytryptamine-induced antiociception in rats by noradrenaline depletion. Neuroscience Letters 54:39, 1985.

87. Moldofsky, H. and Lue, F.A. The relationship of alpha and delta EEG frequencies to pain and mood in "fibrositis" patients treated with chlorpromazine and L-tryptophan and electroencephalography. Clin Neurophysiol 50:71-80, 1980.

88. Harvey, J.A., Schlosberg, A.J. and Yunger, L.M. Behavioral correlates of serotonin depletion. Fed Proc 34:1796, 1975.

89. Russell, I.J., Bowden, C.L., Michalek, J., Fletcher, E. and Hester, G.A. Imipramine receptor density on platelets of patients with fibrositis syndrome: Correlation with disease severity and response to therapy. Arthritis Rheum 30:S63, 1988. (Abstract) J. Rheum 19:(in press), 1992.

90. Brunello, N., Chuang, D.M. and Costa, E. Different synaptic location of mianserin and imipramine binding sites. science 215:1112, 1982.

91. Sette, M., Raisman, R., Briley, M. and Langer, S.Z. Localization of tricyclic antidepressant binding sites on serotonin nerve terminals. J Neurochem 37:40, 1981.

92. Briley, M.S., Raisman, R. and Langer, S.Z. Human platelets possess high affinity binding sites for 3H-imipramine. Eur J Pharmacol 58:347, 1979.

93. Paul, S.M., Rehavi, M., Rice, K.C., Ittah, Y. and Skolnick, P. Does high affinity [3H]-imipramine binding label serotonin reuptake sites in brain and platelet? Life Sciences 28:2753, 1981.

94. Briley, M.S., Langer, S.Z., Raisman, R., Sechter, D. and Zarifian, E. Tritiated imipramine binding sites are decreased in platelets of untreated depressed patients. Science 209:303, 1980.

95. Paul, S.M., Rehavi, M., Skolnick, P., Ballenger, J.C. and Goodwin, F.K. Depressed patients have decreased binding of tritiated imipramine to platelet serotonin. Arch Gen Psychiatry 38:1315, 1981.

96. Suranyi-Cadotte, B.E., Wood, P.L., Vasavan Nair, N.P. and Schwartz, G. Normalization of platelet [3H] imipramine binding in depressed patients during remission. Eur J Pharmacol 85:357, 1982.

97. Goldenberg, D.L., Felson, D.T. and Dinerman, H. A randomized, controlled trial of amitriptyline and naproxen in the treatment of patients with fibromyalgia. Arthritis Rheum 29:1371, 1986.

98. Gessa, G.L., Biggio, G., Fadda, F., Corsini, G.U. and Tagliamonte, A. Effect of the oral administration of tryptophan-free amino acid mixtures on serum tryptophan, brain tryptophan and serotonin metabolism. J Neurochem 22:869, 1974.

99. Moller, S.E., Kirk, L. and Honore, P. Relationship between plasma ratio of tryptophan to competing amino acids and the response to L-tryptophan treatment in endogenously depressed patients. J Affective Disord 2:47, 1980.

100. Almay, B.G., Johansson, F., Von Knorring, L., Sakurada, T. and Terenius, L. Long-term high frequency transcutaneous electrical nerve stimulation (hi-TNS) in chronic pain. Clinical response and effects on immunoreactivity (SPLI) and pain measures. J Psychosom Res 29:247, 1985.

101. Russell, I.J., Michalek, J., Vipraio, G.A., Fletcher, E. and Wall, K. serum amino acids in fibrositis/fibromyalgia syndrome. J Rheumatol 16:158-163, 1989.

102. Wessendorf, M.W. and Elde, R. The coexistence of serotonin and substance P-like immunoreactivity in the spinal cord of the rat as shown by immunofluorescent double labeling. i Neurosci 7:2352, 1987.

103. Murphy, R.M. and Zemlan, F.P. Differential effects of substance P on serotonin-modulated spinal nociceptive reflexes. Psychopharmacology (Berlin) 93:118, 1987.

104. Vaeroy, H., Helle, R., Forre, O., Kass, E. and Terenius, L. Elevated CSF levels of substance P and high incidence of Raynaud's phenomenon in patients With fibromyalgia: New features for diagnosis. Pain 32:21, 1988.

105. Russell, I.J., Vipraio, G.A., Tovar, Z., Michalek, J. and Fletcher, E. Abnormal natural killer cell activity in fibrositis syndrome is responsive in vitro to IL-2. Arthritis Rheum 31:S24, 1988. (Abstract).

106. Hellstrand, K. and Hermodsson, S. Role of serotonin in the regulation of human natural killer cell cytotoxicity. J Immunology 139:869, 1987.

107. Sternberg, E.M., Trial, J. and Parker, C.W. Effect of serotonin on murine macrophages: suppression of Ia expression by serotonin and its reversal by 5-HT2 serotonergic receptor antagonists. J Immunology 137:276, 1986.

108. Wiley, J. and Owyang, C. Participation of serotonin and substance P in the action of cholecystokinin on colonic motility. Am J Physiol 252:431, 1987.

109. Ferrara, A., Zinner, M.J. and Jaffe, B.M. Intraluminal release of serotonin, substance P and gastrin in the canine small intestine. Dig Dis Sci 32:289, 1987.

110. Chesney, C.M., Pifer, D.D. and Cagen, L.M. Triazolobenzodiazepines competitively inhibit the binding of platelet activating factor (PAF) to human platelets. Biochem Biophys Res Commun 144:359, 1987.

111. Baer, P.G. and Cagen, L.M. Platelet activating factor vasoconstriction of dog kidney. Inhibition by alprazolam. Hypertension 9:253, 1987.

112. Voelkel, N.F., Chang, S.W., Pfeffer, K.D., Worthen, S.G. and McMurtry, I.F. PAF antagonists: Different effects on platelets, neutrophils, guinea pig ileum and PAF-inducted vasodilation in isolated rat lung. Prostaglandis 32:359, 1986.

113. Sheehan, D.V., Coleman, J.H., Greenblatt, D.J., et al. Some biochemical correlates of panic attacks with agoraphobia and their response to a new treatment. J Clin Psych Pharmacol 1:66, 1984.

114. Sethy, V.H. and Hodges, D.H., Jr. Role of beta-adrenergic receptors in the antidepressant activity of alprazolam. Res. Commun Chem Pathol Pharmacol 36:329, 1982.

115. Aylward, M., Fowler, P.D., John, V.A., Maddock, J. and Seldrup, J. The influence of diclofenac in free protein bound and total plasma L-tryptophan in adult healthy male subjects. Rheum Rehab 2S:47, 1979.

116. Clark, S., Tindall, E. and Bennett, R.M. A double blind crossover trial of prednisone versus placebo in the treatment of fibrositis. J Rheumatol 12:980, 1985.

117. Peter, J.B. and Wallace, D.J. Abnormal immune regulation in fibromyalgia. Arthritis Rheum 31:S24, 1988.

118. Bedard, P.J., Tremblay, L.E., Barbeau, H., et al. Action of 5-hydroxytryptamine, substance P, thyrotropin-releasing hormone and clonidine on motoneurone excitability. Can J Neurol Sci 14:506, 1987.

119. Cailliet, R. Low Back Pain Syndrome, Philadelphia: F.A. Davis Company, 1968. Ed. 2.

120. Yunus, M.B. Diagnosis, etiology, and management of fibromyalgia syndrome: An update. Comp Ther 14:8, 1988.

121. Kellgren, J.H., Lawrence, J.S. and Aitken-Swan, J. Rheumatic complaints in urban population. Ann Rheum Dis 12:5-15, 1953.

122. De Blecourt, J.J. Rheumatism and social medicine in Netherlands.Rheumatism 11:83-85, 1955.

123. De Blecourt, J.J. and Westendorp Boerma, F. Population studies of rheumatic diseases on a coastal island. I. Clinical and serologic study. Ann Rheum Dis 22:429-431, 1963.

124. Spitzer, W.O., Harth, M., Goldsmith, C.H. et al. The arthritic complaint in primary care: Prevalence, related disability, and costs. J Rheumatol 3:88-89, 1976.

125. Carette, S., McCain, G.A., Bell, D.A. and Fam, A.G. Evaluation of amitriptyline in primary fibrositis. A double-blind, placebo-controlled study. Arthritis Rheum 29:655, 1986.

126. Bennett, R.M., Gatter, R.A., Campbell, S.M., Andrews, R.P., Clark, S.R., and Scarola J.A. A comparison of cyclobenzaprine and placebo in the management of fibrositis. A double-blind controlled study. Arthritis Rheum 31:1535-42, 1988.

127. Holmes, G.P., Kaplan, J.E., Gantz, N.M., et al. Chronic fatigue syndrome: A working case definition. Ann Intern Med 108:387-389, 1988.

128. Behan, P.O.: Post viral fatigue syndrome. Crit Rev Neurobiol 4 (2) :157-178, 1988.

129. Dailey, P.A., Bishop, G.D., Russell, I.J. and Fletcher, E.M. Psychological stress and the fibrositis/fibromyalgia syndrome. J Rheumatol 17:1380, 1990.

130. Moldofsky, H. and Scarisbrick, P. Induction of neurasthenic musculoskeletal pain syndrome by selective sleep stage deprivation. Psychosomatic Med 38:35-44, 1976.

131. Gresham, S.C., Agnew, M.A. Jr. and Williams, R.L. The sleep of depressed patients: An EEG and eye movement study. Arch Gen Psychiat 13:503-507, 1965.

132. Adam, K. Sleep as a restorative process and a theory to explain why. Progr Brain Res 53:289-305, 1980.

133. Hamm, C., Derman, S. and Russell, I.J. Sleep parameters in fibrositis/fibromyalgia syndrome (FS) . Arthritis Rheum 32:S70, 1989. (Abstract).

134. Treadwell, G.J. Fibromyalgia. NZ Med J Aug:157, 1981.

135. Goldenberg, D.L. Fibromyalgia and other chronic fatigue syndromes. Sem Arthritis Rheum 18:111-120, 1988.

136. Mazanec, D.J. First year of a rheumatologist in private practice [letter]. Arthritis Rheum 25:718-719, 1982.

137. Hester, G., Grant, A.E. and Russell, I.J. Psychological evaluation and behavioral treatment of patients with fibrositis. Arthritis Rheum 25:S148, 1982. (Abstract).

138. Wolfe, F. and Cathey, M.A. Prevalence of primary and secondary fibrositis. J Rheumatol 10:965-968, 1983.

139. Alarcon-Segovia, D., Ramos-Niembro, F. and Gonzalez-Amaro, R.F. One thousand private rheumatology patients in Mexico City [letter]. Arthritis Rheum 26:688-689, 1983.

140. Felson, D.T. and Goldenberg, D.L. The natural history of fibromyalgia. Arthritis Rheum 29:1522-1526, 1986.

141. Payne, T.C., Leavitt, F., Garron, D.C., et al. Fibrositis and psychologic disturbance. Arthritis Rheum 25:213-217, 1982 .

142. Hudson, J.I., Hudson, M.S., Pliner, L.F., et al. Fibromyalgia and major affective disorder: A controlled phenomenology and family history study. Am J Psychiatry 142:441-446, 1985.

143. Ahles, T.A., Yunus, M.B., Riley, S.D., Bradley, J.M. and Masi, A.T. Psychological factors associated with primary fibromyalgia syndrome. Arthritis Rheum 27:1101-1106, 1984.

144. Ahles, T.A., Yunus, M.B. and Masi, A.T. Is chronic pain a variant of depressive disease? The case of primary fibromyalgia syndrome. Pain 29:105-111, 1987.

145. Wolfe, F., Cathey, M.A., Kleinheksel, S.M., et al. Psychological status in primary fibrositis and fibrositis associated with rheumatoid arthritis. J Rheumatol 11:500-506, 1984.

146. Kirmayer, L.J., Robbins, J.M. and Kapusta M.A. Somatization and depression in fibromyalgia syndrome. Am J Psychiatry 145:950-954, 1988.

147. Clark, S., Campbell, S.M. Forehand, M.E., Tindall, E.A. and Bennett, R.M. Clinical characteristics of fibrositis. II. A "blinded," controlled study using standard psychological tests. Arthritis Rheum 28:132-137, 1985.

Conclusions

Summary

Over the past 60 years, the majority of clinicians and researchers whose work appears in this text became involved in the study of this disease due to infectious episodes, usually an epidemic of M.E./CFS. This was true in 1934 in the United States of America, when Assistant Surgeon General, Dr. Alexander Gilliam, started the exploration with his brilliant and detailed investigation of the Los Angeles hospital epidemic. This was still true exactly half a century later when Drs Paul Cheney and Daniel Peterson became the first to awaken the world to the Lake Tahoe epidemic, that was itself an episode of the 1984-1988 North American pandemic. To further underline the infectious basis of this illness, in Great Britain, Professor Behan and many of the British physicians and researchers refer to M.E./CFS as Post-Viral Fatigue Syndrome, implying that this illness starts with and is the result of an infectious disease process.

Yet individuals such as historian Edward Shorter write books that equate M.E./CFS with hysteria, suggesting that this disease process is no more than a psychosomatic illness, a somatization, the modern equivalent of the self-flagellating hysterics of the middle ages. How can such a dichotomy exist amongst supposedly intelligent individuals?

Dr. Shorter answered the question very well when I interviewed him on a Toronto television programme. "You have just written a book that discusses M.E./CFS patients. How many M.E./CFS patients have you actually seen?" I asked. "Why none of course, I am an historian." he replied. Too many reputed "experts" exist who have never seen an M.E./CFS patient. Many "experts" have seen few M.E./CFS patients and have never attempted to investigate seriously the few patients that they have seen.

However, we cannot say that all of those who believe that M.E./CFS is the result of a primary neurotic, depressive or psychotic brain have little or no clinical experience with these patients. Once we reject those physicians who make a lucrative part of their income acting for the insurance industry, once we dismiss those who are merely ridiculous, we are still left with a number of reputable physicians who still doubt the existence of M.E./CFS as a valid disease process. Why?

There are several reasons that immediately come to mind. In the past, the literature has been obscure and difficult to obtain. Even considering Sigurdsson's "six years after study" there has been no well funded assessment of any of the disabling consequences of the some 60 recorded epidemics. Until the very recent development of specific viral probes, polymerase chain reaction and immune marker and receptor technology, there has been no way truly to investigate this fascinating but complex pathophysiological disease process. It is hoped that these remarkable and relatively inexpensive technologies will soon elaborate the viral and immune dysfunction causes of M.E./CFS

Many of these doubting physicians have little time for long case histories and even longer work-ups. Time is money. Multiple tests are expensive to both the patient and the state. Modern physicians tend to feel very insecure without an accurate test to confirm their diagnostic impressions. Even those of us who have seen thousands of M.E./CFS patients live in fear of mistaking a well hidden and treatable malignancy that masquerades as M.E./CFS. Believer and doubter alike, we all want that confirming test. A specific test is as necessary to bring the doubting physicians in from the world of disbelief as it is to rule out many progressive illnesses. In this text, we outline several laboratory techniques to diagnose M.E./CFS. Unfortunately, they are all in their infancy. They tend to be relatively expensive, and sometimes they depend upon serum not easily transportable to the investigating laboratory or technical equipment not available in many communities, or even totally unavailable in some countries. However, the fact is these tests now exist, whereas a few years ago there was only a testing abyss. All of this technology can be expected to improve rapidly and become more available over the next few years.

Whatever the parameters are that will eventually define this illness, there can be no doubt that the primary disabling characteristics of M.E./CFS are those of an acquired physiological brain dysfunction. Dr. Jay Goldstein and his California associates have done much to pioneer these revealing investigative techniques. It is unfortunate for the American patient that the NIH has so far excluded this group (and those others examining the retrovirus findings) from adequate research funding. It is tragic that the entire British Health Service have not found fit to establish a single well equipped M.E./CFS investigation and treatment centre in England. Neither can the health care system in Canada be proud of its denial of basic access to Canadian citizens.

I would like to laud all of the clinicians and researchers who have contributed chapters to this text and who have striven to understand and to help those disabled patients. They are all courageous pioneers and I wish them well.

Finally, it was not our intention in this book simply to explore the disease and forget the patient. However, until now, patients with M.E./CFS and their families have been largely forgotten, not just by the majority of physicians, but above all by the governments that play an increasing role in providing access to reasonable investigation and treatment of illness. This text does not go into the particular educational plight of children, but I know of no state, anywhere in the world, that has adapted a programme to allow these thousands of M.E./CFS disabled children to gain normal access to a reasonable education. Perhaps it will someday be forthcoming.

Byron Hyde, M.D.
Ottawa, Canada
May, 1992

Addendum I

A Model for Dysfunctional CNS Neuroregulatory Pathways

Jay A. Goldstein, M.D.

Director, Chronic Fatigue Syndrome Institute, 500 South Anaheim Hills Road, Suite 206, Anaheim Hills, California 92807 USA

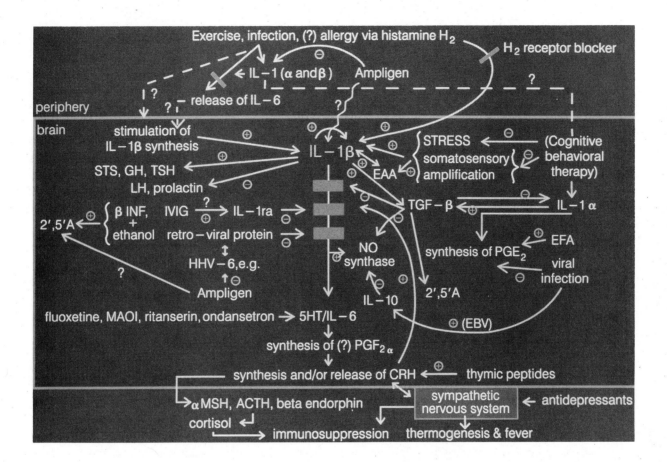

The Role of Interleukin 1 Beta

This flow diagram is used as a model for possible dysfunctional CNS neuroregulatory pathways in CFS. **Stemming from the clinical observation that virtually any type of stress (exercise, emotional, cognitive, infectious, sleep deprivation) makes CFS worse, it postulates that the pleotropic cytokine interleukin-1 beta (IL-1B) has a central role in maintaining homeostasis.**

Through intermediaries such as 5HT, IL-6 and prostaglandins (PG), central IL-1B stimulates, modulates or inhibits the release of numerous neuropeptides and other transmitter substances, and is known to be involved in sleep induction, immunosuppression, hypalgesia, fever, thermogenesis and weight loss through activation of brown fat. Many of its effects occur as a result of increased corticotropin releasing hormone (CRH) production. Other important functions of IL-1B include stimulation of nitric oxide synthase to promote vasodilatation and facilitation of opening of the chloride channel of the GABA receptor.

The neuroanatomic localization of IL-1 mRNA in the dentate gyrus and the dorsal raphe suggest functional results of antagonism of IL-1 effect by various endogenous substances such as transforming growth factor beta (TGF-B), IL-10, an independently regu-

---

Actions of IL-1 In The Brain

1)   Local Effects in Brain: altered EEG and neuronal activity, inhibition of long term potentiation, cortical inhibitory postsynaptic function, neurotransmitter release / turnover, induction of NGF, self-induction (of IL-1ß), astrogliosis, neovascularization and augmentation of $GABA_A$ receptor function.

2)   Metabolic Actions: fever, increased metabolic rate (thermogenesis), sympathetic activation of brown fat, hypophagia, and altered gastric function.

3)   Endocrine Actions: hypothalamic-pituitary hormone release (CRH, GnRH, TSH, ACTH), pituitary-adrenal activation and insulin release.

4)   Behavioral Actions: sleep, and sickness behavior (e.g. reduced exploration), hypalgesia.

5)   Immune Actions: peripheral IL-6 release, decreased peripheral IL-2 production, reduced natural killer cell activity, leukocytosis, and hepatic acute phase protein synthesis.

---

lated cytokine called IL-1ra (receptor antagonist) and viral protein gene products which can interfere with IL-1B signal transduction.

Sudden state changes could be transduced by excitatory amino acids (EAA's) Intero-and exteroceptive stimuli, integrated in paralimbic areas, could undergo faulty processing if a multifactorial limbic encephalopathy producing increased synaptogenesis were present, resulting in somatosensory amplification. Such dysfunction is amenable to cognitive behavioral therapy.

This model predicts that CFS patients would have decreased central biogenic amines, and that production of substances such as cortisol, growth hormone, beta endorphin and catecholamines after a stress

such as exercise would be impaired. It should be difficult to induce a fever in this population, as well, and such patients should not increase, and may even reduce, regional cerebral blood flow after exercise. Anxiety, sleep, weight gain, low blood pressure, and pain disorders should be more prevalent in this population, which may have peripheral immune activation as a result of impaired central immunosuppression.

Although tremendously oversimplified, the model that CFS symptoms are caused by an imbalance between IL-1 beta and its endogenous or multifactorially induced inhibitors can enhance understanding of the disorder and direct efforts toward remediation.

Addendum II

Update to MMPI-1

Dr. Linda Miller Iger
Neuropsychologist
Chronic Fatigue
Syndrome Institute
500 South Anaheim Hills Road,
Suite 206
Anaheim Hills, California 92807
USA

The MMPI-2 has just recently been introduced and come into acceptance. With the advent of the MMPI-2, its developers promised that there would be no significant alterations in the profiles configurations that had been developed for specific populations (such as CFS/ME) using the original MMPI.

Dr. Iger sought to test this hypothesis. In a new study, fifty-three (N=53) patients, forty-one females (N=41) and twelve males (N=12) diagnosed with CFS/ME were administered the MMPI-2. Using comparative analyses, Dr. Iger examined the original MMPI vs. MMPI-2 profiles and determined there was no alteration in the MMPI-2 CFS/ME female profile. There were, however, differences in the male profile. Clinical significance for the MMPI-2 has been lowered from 70T to 65T. Scale 4 for male CFS/ME patients no longer meets that criterion. The MMPI-2 scales 1-2-3 configuration for male CFS/ME patients appears to be internal alteration in the MMPI-2 as profiles scored back from the MMPI-2 to the original MMPI conform to the original MMPI CFS/ME male profile configuration. A replication study has been completed by an independent researcher with the same results.

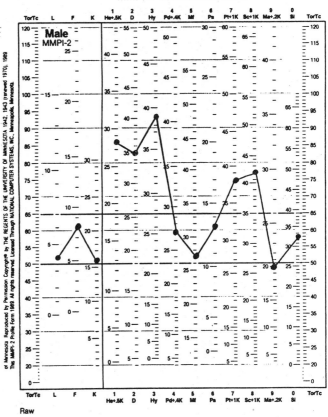

MMPI-2 Basic Scale Profile

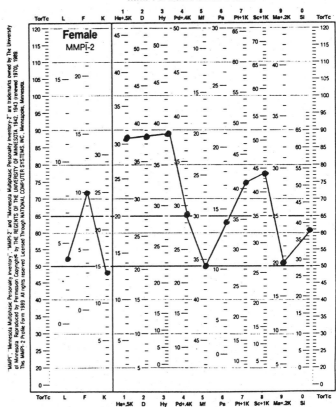

MMPI-2 Basic Scale Profile

Addendum III

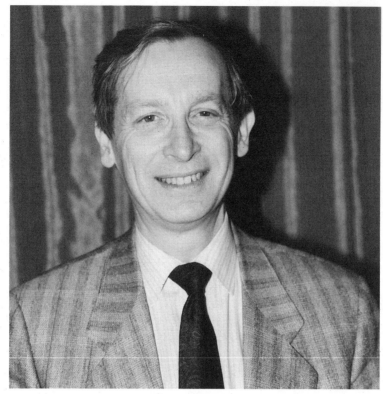

Harvey Moldofsky

Harvey Moldofsky, M.D.
Professor of Psychiatry and Medicine, University of Toronto, 399 Bathurst Street, Toronto, Ontario
M5T 2S8 Canada

From 1979 to 1989, Dr. Moldofsky was Psychiatrist-in-Chief at Toronto Western Hospital, now a division of the Toronto Hospital. From 1966 to 1979, he served on the staff of the Clarke Institute of Psychiatry where he was Chief of the Department of Clinical Neurophysiology and of the Psychosomatic Medicine Unit. He was a research fellow at Langley Porter Neuropsychiatric Institute at the University of California, San Francisco (1970-1971) and has received several awards. He is a fellow of the American Psychiatric Association, Vice-President of the International College of Psychosomatic Medicine and an assistant editor of Psychosomatics. He is the author and co-author of numerous publications on sleep physiology and psychosomatic aspects of rheumatologic disorders.

Abstract

The Significance of Sleep-Wave Physiology and Immune Functions to Chronic Fatigue Syndrome (CFS) and Fibromyalgia

Chronic diffuse musculoskeletal pain, localized areas of tenderness in specific anatomic regions, chronic fatigue, and unrefreshing sleep are shown to be features of both the Chronic Fatigue Syndrome and Fibromyalgia. These symptoms are related to a physiologic arousal disorder within sleep, the alpha EEG sleep anomaly.

Our studies show that aspects of the immune system, i.e., pokeweed mitogen response, NK cell activity, IL-1 and IL-2 are related to sleep-wake physiology. The circadian pattern of these cellular and humoral substances are altered by sleep deprivation. Changes in measures of fatigue, sleepiness, mood and cognitive performance during sleep deprivation are related to changes in mitogen responses. We theorize that disordered chronobiology of aspects of the immune system link nonrestorative sleep physiology to pain and fatigue symptoms.

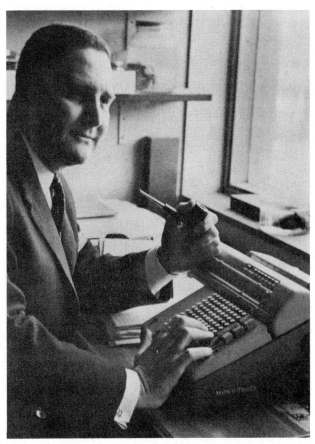

David C. Poskanzer

David C. Poskanzer, M.D., M.P.H.
(1929-1988)

The late David C. Poskanzer, M.D., M.P.H. was born in Albany, New York in 1929. A graduate of Harvard University Medical School, he completed his training in Epidemiology at Harvard University School of Public Health. He did his residency in Neurology at the Massachusetts General Hospital and remained on staff there until 1982. After a brief period of private practice he joined the Division of Cancer Control, National Cancer Institute, National Institutes of Health, where he served as program director until his premature death due to a glioblastoma in 1988.

Dr. Poskanzer was the principal author of the epidemiological study titled **Epidemic Neuromyasthenia, An Outbreak in Punta Gorda, Florida**, NEJM 1957. This was an important study of M.E./CFS and the only one in which a door to door canvass of a municipality was accomplished. This study revealed that, contrary to the findings of many studies in the United States, that may have been unintentionally racially biased, large numbers of blacks were equally affected by M.E./CFS.

Dr. Poskanzer was also co-author of the 1964 JAMA paper, **Epidemic Neuromyasthenia, Outbreak in a Convent in New York State**, a the principal author of "Epidemic Protracted Debility at Punta Gorda, Florida: An Illness Resembling Iceland Disease", which appeared in the Transactions of the American Neurological Association in 1967. He did extensive research into the epidemiology of neurologic disease and in particular multiple sclerosis.

Dr. Poskanzer was also instrumental in studies leading to recognition of the effects of prenatal exposure to stilbestrol.

Addendum V

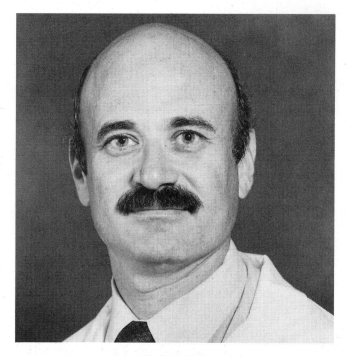

Alfredo A. Sadun

Neuro-ophthalmologic Manifestations of Chronic Fatigue Syndrome

Alfredo A. Sadun, M.D., Ph.D., and Pravin U. Dugel, M.D.
Doheny Eye Institute, USC School of Medicine, 1355 San Pablo Street, Los Angeles, California 90033-1088

Dr. Sadun is professor of ophthalmology and neurosurgery at the USC School of Medicine and a neuro-ophthalmologist at the Doherty Eye Clinic. He is particularly interested in the study of visual function in Chronic Fatigue Syndrome.

Very few ophthalmologists and even fewer neuro-ophthalmologists have addressed the issue of ocular symptomology in chronic fatigue syndrome (CFS) yet the neuro-ophthalmological manifestations of CFS are myriad and common. One major problem in establishing the frequency of ocular signs and symptoms in CFS is that the ophthalmologist only sees a self-selected group of patients with ocular problems severe enough to bring them to the ophthalmologist's office. To avoid this difficulty with self-selection, we made a surprise visit to a CFS support group. Only one organizer of the CFS support group knew of our intentions or ophthalmological interest. The remaining 44 CFS patients in attendance were completely unaware of our interest or expertise. All 44 patients in attendance participated by filling out a questionnaire that elicited a commentary on their ocular status. As each patient exited the room and handed in the questionnaire he or she underwent a simple neuro-ophthalmological examination.

Patient Complaints and Signs

All 44 patients with CFS related some visual or ocular complaint in their questionnaire. The symptoms fell into one of five categories. Almost every patient had at least some **asthenopic symptoms** (the eyes feel tired, sore, dry, watery or weak). Two-thirds of the patients complained of **blurred vision** much greater at near; over half of the patients complained of blurred vision at distance; one quarter of the patients complained of **oscillopsia** (bouncing or jiggling of the visual environment) and one out of seven of the patients complained of binocular **diplopia** (double vision).

Nystagmus

The most obvious objective ophthalmological sign noted among these patients was nystagmus. Twenty-three percent of the patients had a primary horizontal nystagmus; an additional eighteen percent had an obvious lateral gaze nystagmus; two percent of the patients had vertical nystagmus. While lateral gaze nystagmus may be a normal finding in about five percent of the population, the existence of this large amplitude nystagmus in eighteen percent of the population was intriguing. It was even more astonishing that approximately one quarter of the patients had a primary horizontal or vertical nystagmus since such nystagmus is always pathological.

Accomodative Inertia

We had an opportunity to examine a smaller number of CFS patients in much greater detail. This led to a better appreciation of several other more subtle signs. In particular, most patients with CFS were shown to have abnormalities in accommodation. Accommodation is a process by which the curvature of the lens changes, shifting the plane of focus from distance to near. As the lens gets less elastic with age, there is a predictable and remarkably invariant reduction in the range of accommodation which almost inevitably leads to the need for reading glasses (typically at ages 45 or 50). However, the CFS patient describes symptomotology in relationship to accommodative insufficiency which is distinctive as compared to the usual presbyopic symptoms. For example, the CFS patient is far more likely to describe a latency in being able to focus up close as opposed to the usual presbyopic symptoms of not being able to hold objects at a close distance and still in focus. Moreover, the CFS patient is just as likely to complain of a long latency in going from near to distance focus. Hence, it is more appropriate to describe the abnormalities associated with accommodation among CFS patients as "accommodative inertia" as opposed to accommodative insufficiency.

Accommodative inertia could be due to either mechanical factors (decreases in compliance) or neural factors. It is unlikely that these problems can be attributed to either changes in lens elasticity or to muscle weakness since neither addresses the very long latency required for the CFS patient to shift focus.

Duction Limitation

Further studies of several CFS patients also disclose limitations of ductions, and in particular, adduction. This combination of adduction paresis and adduction nystagmus falls under the rubric of intranuclear ophthalmoplegia. Given the frequency with which we see various forms of ophthalmoplegia and nystagmus, it is not surprising that approximately half of all CFS patients describe diplopia and oscillopsia among their symptomology.

Possible Brain Cell Dysfunction

Purely from a neuro-ophthalmological point of view, many of the ocular manifestations of CFS point to one area of the brain. All three classes of problems: accommodative inertia, adduction ophthalmoplegia, and nystagmus, are referrable to the dorsal midline nuclei of the mesencephalon and perhaps slightly more caudally to the mesencephalic pontine juncture. Thus, it is possible that a brainstem encephalitis in this region could produce many of the neuro-ophthalmological manifestations described above.

Treatment Suggestions

In regard to strategies to help the patient, several points need to be made. Many CFS patients describe asthenopic symptoms, in particular, dry eyes which can be alleviated through the copious use of artificial tears (available over the counter). CFS patients, especially those complaining of diplopia, oscillopsia and long latencies in refocusing, should be encouraged not to wear bifocals. Separate glasses should be prescribed for distance and near. Bifocal glasses, especially those that are "blended" make inordinate demands on eye movement control at different focal planes. It is conceivable that, in the future, concentric contact lenses could be prescribed for CFS patients. These lenses take advantage of the fact that the pupils become more myotic at near, hence the near add can be placed centrally in the lens and the distance correction in a peripheral ring. Finally, it should be emphasized that, once CFS patients are made aware of the nature of their neuro-ophthalmological manifestations, they not only derive a certain measure of reassurance, but can apply a variety of common sense strategies to circumvent many of these problems.

Oscillopsia and Glasses

Byron Hyde M.D.

Oscillopsia refers to oscillating vision and is quite rare in the general population. In real terms it refers to the inability of the patient to focus easily on a given non-moving object. The object appears to jiggle. This effect, plus the problems of double vision, makes reading difficult. Also the patient tends to avoid direct eye contact and the resulting faulty implementation of the servo-mechanism by which an individual can make precise judgements concerning distance, movement and speed. It has been suggested by Dr. Sadun that the cause of this phenomenon may be due to a central brainstem encephalitis or a mesencephalic encephalitis and that the location of this defect is in the area of the Edinger-Westphal nucleus and the third or oculomotor nerve.

Dr. Sadun presented slides of this CNS architecture similar to the two figures included in this section.

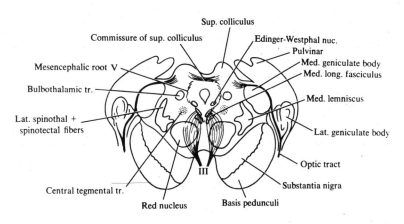

Section through Upper Midbrain indicating position of Edinger-Westphal Nucleus

Reprinted with the kind permission of Ben Pansky, Ph.D., Review of Neuroscience, Second Edition, New York: McGraw-Hill, Inc.,1988:85.

Further Parasympathetic Dysfunction

The CNS area affected may actually be larger than this. We have noted the abnormal and contrary pupillary light reflex common to M.E./CFS. This defect also is related to the Edinger-Westphal nu-

cleus. In this defective light reflex, the retinal pathway through the pretectal nuclei and **the parasympathetic preganglionic neurons** of the midbrain project via the oculomotor nerve to the ciliary ganglion and thence to the constrictor muscles of the iris. This abnormal reflex can be illustrated when a pen light is shone into the patient's eye. In many patients, rather than a rapid **closure** of the pupil, the physician will observe a typical cogwheel **opening** of the pupil. This typical M.E./CFS defect of course gives rise to further problems of accommodation and photophobia. It is of further interest, that these parasympathetic nuclei are approximate to the salivatory and vagus nuclei. M.E./CFS patients routinely complain of loss of normal salivation and sometime in their post-infectious period probably all complain of problems associated with the vagus nerve reflexes to the larynx, heart, oesophagus, and stomach. Ultimately all of these nuclei are regulated from the limbic system through the hypothalamus.

This acquired defect is a common feature of M.E./CFS and according to Dr. Sadun occurs in 27% of the M.E./CFS patients that he has examined. We find that it is even more common in the first year of illness. The problem is frequently compounded when the patient attends an ophthalmologist and receives glasses.

The problem is that the M.E./CFS patient frequently cannot track through a normal reading corridor. The negative effect is dramatic. If the M.E./CFS patient chooses narrow "half glasses", those with a short vertical diameter available at most drugstores, he or she has difficulty in reading since their line of vision continues to move over the vertical borders of the lens. Dr. Sadun has pointed out that this negative effect is further compounded when the patients purchase bifocals and the defective eye coordination allows the the centre of the focusing mechanism to "jiggle" back and forth across two different visual corrections. The slow accommodation rate of these patients plus the oscillopsia makes reading with bifocals impossible. Not understanding the problem, we have seen some patients then purchase the very expensive "progressive" or no-line multifocals that have graduated lenses. This makes matters even worse and the M.E./CFS patient staggers, becomes uncoordinated and disorientated. The correct approach is to purchase two pairs of glasses each with a large and constant accommodative surface area, one for reading and one for more distant vision.

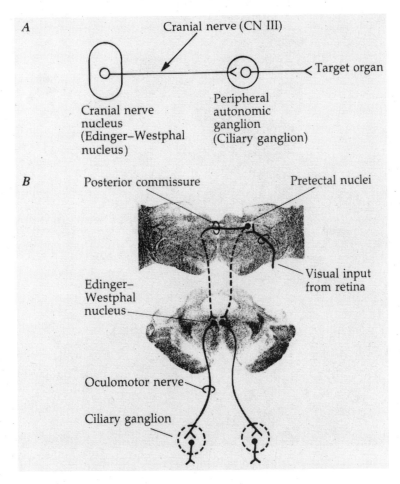

Location of the Edinger-Westphal Nucleus

Reprinted by permission of the publisher from Chapter by John H. Martin, Neuroanatomy, Text and Atlas, pp. 332. Copyright 1989 by Elsevier Science Publishing Co., Inc.

Addendum VI

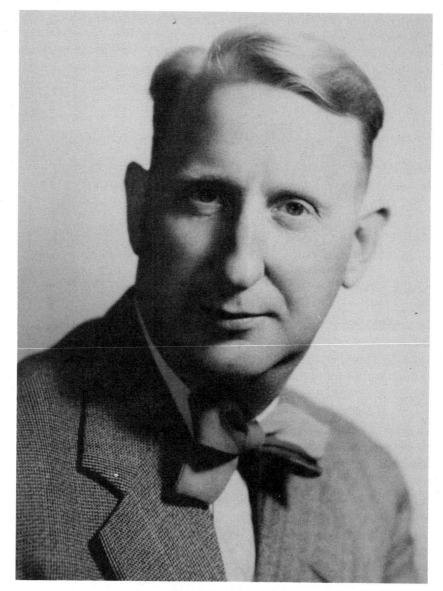

Björn Sigurdsson

Björn Sigurdsson, M.D., Ph.D.

(1913-1959)

Byron Hyde M.D., with the kind assistance of Guömundur Pétursson, M.D., Keldur, Reykjavik

Most physicians involved in the study of M.E./CFS, know Björn Sigurdsson as the scientist who described the most numerically significant epidemic of M.E./CFS, known as Akureyri or Iceland Disease. In this epidemic, that started in one of the principal schools of Akureyri, approximately 1,116 children and adults fell ill. We know him as the first physician scientist to write about the chronic features of the disease. However, like Acheson, who became Chief Medical Officer of England, and Henderson and Shelokov, who achieved equally outstanding positions in the United States, Björn Sigurdsson went on to become one of the leading men of science in his country.

He was born in a small farmhouse on March 3, 1913 in Skagafjordur, in northern Iceland. He left home at the age of 14 to enrol in Grammar School in Reykjavik. He was Chairman of the Students Council in 1935.

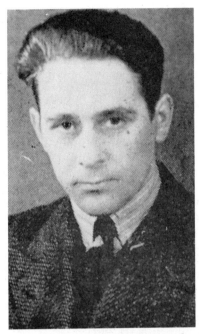

Björn Sigurdsson as a young researcher

He graduated in Medicine at the age of 24, interned in Reykjavik and then sailed to Copenhagen to study at the Carlsberg Fund Institute for Biology and the Danish State Institute for Serology. He was known for his keen sense of humour, his good company, his love of poetry, the arts and music and his quick and frank mind.

He returned to Iceland in 1940 and worked at the University Institute of Pathology. From 1941-3 he attended Princeton, New Jersey, at the Rockefeller Institute where he specialized in animal and plant virology. He then returned to Iceland to the Institute for Pathology and organized the planning and building of a science Institute.

With a matching grant of $200,000 that Björn received from the Rockefeller Foundation to the University of Iceland, and funds from the Icelandic Government, he built the Institute for Experimental Pathology that opened at Keldur just outside Reykjavik in 1948. The only stipulation of the donor was that Björn Sigurdsson become the Scientific Director of the Institute. He presented his doctoral thesis in 1955 on the development of a new vaccine. Dr Sigurdsson devoted all of his time and energy to the scientific

interests of the Institute until his untimely death from kidney cancer at the age of 49 on October 16, 1959. He was survived by his wife Una Johannesdottir and his three children, who all became physicians.

One is amazed by the sheer volume of high quality scientific work that he produced during such a brief career. A pathologist by training, he produced major works on virology, bacteriology, immunology, and epidemiology. He produced his first paper at the age of 23 on the investigation of an outbreak of typhoid fever on a remote island off the northern coast of Iceland. He was one of the scientists who was responsible for the establishment of the WHO World Influenza Center in 1948.

His major scientific work was that of the concept of slow viral infections, demonstrating the transmissibility and progressive course of visna, maedi, rida and pulmonary adenomatosis. He was the first to grow visna virus in vitro. This virus was introduced into Iceland in sheep imported from Germany during the thirties. His important early work is responsible for an important part of our early understanding of retrovirolgy.

Björn Sigurdsson was responsible for the significant work on Akureyri (Iceland) Disease and was the first scientist to lay down the facts concerning the chronicity of M.E./CFS.

As he lay dying in his bed, too weak to write, he dictated to his wife his final communication. It was to a colleague and outlined the similarities between visna (a retrovirus) and multiple sclerosis. Björn Sigurdsson would be excited to learn of the retroviral findings of Michael Holmes, Cheney-Bell-DeFreitas-Terunuma and John Martin in this text. He would be interested equally in the work of Elaine DeFreitas that was the first to draw our attention to an HTLV-like retrovirus associated with an M.S. like illness.

This material was taken from the separate writings of Thorarinn Gudnason M.D., Margrét Gudnadóttir, M.D., and Pall Palsson, M.D. DVM.

Index of Clinicians, Researchers and Associates

Y. Burstein, PhD
Department of Organic Chemistry,
The Weizmann Institute of Science,
Rehovot, Israel

J. Camps-Bansell
Department of Internal Medicine,
University Clinic, Pamplona, Spain

William A. Carter, MD
Hahnemann University,
Philadelphia, Pennsylvania
191402 USA

A. Castilla
Department of Internal Medicine,
University Clinic, Pamplona, Spain

Borys Chabursky
76 Hartfield Road
Islington, Ontario
M9L 3EZ   Canada

Christopher J. Chapman
University of Otago,
P.O. Box 56   Dunedin, New Zealand

Paul Cheney, MD, PhD
Suite 234 10620 Park Road, Charlotte,
North Carolina   28210 USA

Alexander C. Chester III, MD, FACP
Clinical Professor of Medicine,
Georgetown University Medical Center,
Foxhall Internists, PC, Suite 348
3301 New Mexico Ave., NW, Washington, D.C.
20016 USA

Diane Cookfair, PhD
Head, Clinical Epidemiology Consulting
Laboratory, Department of Biomathematics,
Roswell Park Cancer Institute, Buffalo,
New York   14263 USA

John P. Cross, BSc, PhD
Senior Technical Officer
Microbiology Department, University of Otago,
P.O. Box 56, Dunedin, New Zealand

Louise Cunningham, PhD
Department of Biochemistry,
Charing Cross & Westminster Medical School,
St. Dunstans Road, London,
W6 8RF England

Elaine DeFreitas, PhD
Associate Professor
The Wistar Institute
Thirty-Sixth Street at Spruce
Philadelphia, Pennsylvania   19104-4268 USA

Betty Dowsett, MD, ChB
Honorary Consultant Microbiologist
Basildon & Thurrock Health Authority
7 West Park Crescent
Billericay, Essex
CM129ED, UK

David Doyle, RD, MD
Consultant Neuropathologist
Department of Neuropathology,
Institute of Neurological Sciences,
Southern General Hospital,
1345 Govan Road, Glasgow, G51 4TF, Scotland

Pravin U. Dugel, MD
Doheny Eye Institute,
USC School of Medicine
1355 San Pablo Street
Los Angeles, California   90033-1088 USA

Donald G. Dutton, PhD
Professor
The University of British Columbia,
Department of Psychology, 2136 West Mall,
Vancouver, British Columbia
V6T 1Z4   Canada

John Dwyer, PhD, FRACP
Departments of Infectious Diseases and
Immunology, Division of Medicine and the Mood
Disorders Unit, Division of Psychiatry,
The Prince Henry Hospital, Little Bay, Sydney,
Australia

Richard H.T. Edwards, PhD, FRCP
Director of University of Liverpool
Muscle Research and Magnetic Resonance
Research Centres, Professor (Chairman) of
Medicine, University of Liverpool, Senate House,
Abercromby Square, P.O. Box 147 , Liverpool
L69 3BX England

Francine L. Fidler, MA
Memory and Neuropsychological Center,
366 San Miguel, Suite 210, Newport Beach,
California, University of California, Irvine,
State Developmental Research Institute
92717 USA

E.J. Field, FRCP
London, Naomi Bramson Research Centre,
The Science Park, University of Warwick,
Conventry
CV47EZ England

Leslie J. Findley, TD, MD, FRCP
Consultant Neurologist
Regional Centre for Neurology and
Neurosurgery, Oldchurch Hospital, Romford
RM7 0BE England

H. Hugh Fudenberg, MD
Director of Research
Neuro Immune Therapeutics Research
145 North Church Street, Spartansburg,
South Carolina   29301 USA

David H. Gillespie, PhD
Hahnemann University,
Philadelphia, Pennsylvania 191402 USA

Alexander G. Gilliam, MD
deceased

Michael Goldberg, MD
Pediatrics - Adolescents Medicine
18411 Clark St., Suite 103
Tarzana, California   91356 USA

Jay Goldstein, MD
Director, Chronic Fatigue Syndrome Institutes
of Anaheim Hills and Beverly Hills
500 South Anaheim Hills Road, Suite 206
Anaheim Hills, California   92807 USA

Seymour Grufferman, MD, Dr. PH
Chairman
Department of Epidemiology and Preventive
Medicine, School of Medicine,
University of Pittsburgh, M-200 Scaife Hall,
Pittsburgh, Pennsylvania   15261 USA

Sudhir Gupta, MD, PhD
Professor of Medicine, Pathology, Neurology,
and Microbiology and Molecular Genetics
Chief, Division of Basic and Clinical
Immunology, University of California at
Irvine, Irvine, California
92717 USA

D. Halliday, MD
Nutrition Research Group, Clinical Research
Centre, Watford Rd., Harrow
3UJ UK

Z.T. Handzel, MD
Ben-Ari Institute of Immunology,
Kaplan Hospital, Rehovot, Israel

Richard Hart Jr., BS
Temple University School of Medicine,
Philadelphia, Pennsylvania 19140 USA

Reid R. Heffner, Jr., MD
Departments of Neurology and Pathology,
SUNY at Buffalo School of Medicine
Buffalo, New York
14214 USA

Diane Heimback, BA
Department of Social and Preventive Medicine,
State University of New York at Buffalo,
Roswell Park Cancer Institute, Buffalo,
New York   14214 USA

Donald Henderson, MD, MPH
Associate Director for Life Sciences
Office of Science and Technology Policy
Executive Office of the President
Washington, D.C.   20506 USA

Berch Henry, PhD
University of Nevada School of Medicine,
Reno, Nevada   89557 USA

Ian Hickie, MD, FRANZCP
Mood Disorders Unit, Prince Henry Hospital,
Little Bay, N.S.W.   2036 Australia

Gary P. Holmes, MD
Division of Viral Disease
Center for Infectious Diseases
Centers for Disease Control
Atlanta, Georgia   30333USA

Michael J. Holmes, MD
Senior Lecturer
Department of Microbiology, University of Otago,
P.O. Box 56, Dunedin, New Zealand

Byron Hyde, MD
Chairman
The Nightingale Research Foundation,
383 Danforth Avenue, Ottawa, Ontario,
K2A 0E1   Canada

Linda Iger, PhD
Neuropsychologist, Chronic Fatigue Syndrome
Institutes of Anaheim Hills and Beverly Hills
500 South Anaheim Hills Road, Suite 206
Anaheim Hills, California   92807 USA

Anil Jain, MD
Clinical Director
The Nightingale Research Foundation
121 Iona Street, Ottawa, Ontario
K1Y 3M1   Canada

Goran A. Jamal, MD, PhD, MB, ChB
    Consultant and Senior Lecturer
    Institute of Neurological Sciences,
    Southern General Hospital, Glasgow
    G51 4TF, United Kingdom

James Jones, MD
    Associate Professor of Pediatrics
    National Jewish Center for Immunology
    and Respiratory Department of Medicine,
    1400 Jackson Street, Denver, Colorado
    80206 USA

Anthony L. Komaroff, MD
    Chief, Division of General Medicine
    Harvard Medical School, Brigham and
    Women's Hospital, 75 Francis Street,
    Boston, Massachusetts   02115 USA

Russell J.M. Lane, BSc, MD, MRCP
    Consultant Neurologist
    Regional Neurosciences Centre,
    Charing Cross Hospital, London
    W6 8RF, England

Luis Leon-Sotomayor, MD
    Doctors Clinic
    Internal Medicine
    6518 Memorial Drive
    Texas City, Texas   77591 USA

Paul H. Levine, MD
    Senior Clinical Investigator
    Viral Epidemiology Section,
    Environmental Epidemiology Branch,
    National Cancer Institute,
    National Institutes of Health,
    Building EPN, Room 434
    Bethesda, Maryland
    20892 USA

Andrew Lloyd, MD, MBBS, FRACP
    Visiting Fellow, Sydney, Australia
    Laboratory of Molecular Immunoregulation
    Building 560, Room #31-19
    National Cancer Institute
    Frederick, Maryland   21702-1 USA

Robert H. Loblay, MB, BS, FRACP, PhD
    Consultant Physician
    Director, Allergy Service,
    Department of Clinical Immunology,
    Royal Prince Alfred Hospital,
    Senior Lecturer, Clinical Immunology Research
    Centre, The University of Sydney, Sydney,
    N.S.W.   2006 Australia

Roger M. Loria, PhD
    Associate Professor

Department of Microbiology, Immunology
and Pathology, Medical College of Virginia,
Virginia Commonwealth University,
East 67th Street, MCV Station,
Richmond, Virginia   21298-0001 USA

Alberto Antonio Marinacci, MD
    515 Ocean Avenue
    Santa Monica, California
    90402 USA

W. John Martin, MD, PhD
    Professor of Pathology
    Director of Molecular Pathology,
    School of Medicine, University of Southern
    California, 1200 N. State Street, Los Angeles,
    California   90033 USA

Donatella Matteucci, BS
    Virology Section, Department of Biomedicine,
    University of Pisa
    Via S. Zeno 35-39   1-56127 Pisa, Italy

R.A. McCartney
    Enterovirus Reference Laboratory,
    Regional Virus Laboratory, Ruchill Hospital,
    G51 4TF   Glasgow, UK

David R. McCluskey, MD, FRCP
    Senior Lecturer
    Department of Medicine,
    Queen's University of Belfast, Grosvenor Road,
    Belfast, BT12 6BA Ireland

B. McLaughlin, MD
    Laboratory Services Branch,
    Ontario Ministry of Health, Box 9000
    Terminal A, Toronto, Ontario,
    M5W 1R5   Canada

Thomas McNamara, MD
    Professor of Radiological Sciences
    Chief of Cardiovascular Radiology
    UCLA
    10833 Leconte Avenue
    Los Angeles, California   90024 USA

Ismael Mena, MD
    Professor of Radiological Sciences
    UCLA School of Medicine, Director,
    Division of Nuclear Medicine,
    Harbor-UCLA Medical Center,
    1124 West Carson Street, Torrance, California
    90502-2064 USA

Harvey Moldofsky, MD
    Professor of Psychiatry and Medicine
    Western Division, Toronto Hospitals
    399 Bathurst Street, Toronto, Ontario
    Canada   M5T 2S8

James F. Mowbray, FRCP
  Professor of Immunopathology
  Department of Immunopathology,
  St. Mary's Hospital Medical School,
  Norfolk Place,
  London W2 1PG England

John Campbell Murdoch, MD, PhD, FRCGP,
  MRNZCGP
  General Practitioner, Mornington
  Health Centre/Elain Gurr Professor of
  General Practice
  Department of General Practice,
  Otago Medical School, University of Otago,
  P.O. Box 913, Dunedin, New Zealand

Karen A. Nackoul, PhD
  Memory and Neuropsychological Center,
  366 San Miguel, Suite 210, Newport Beach,
  California, University of California, Irvine,
  State Developmental Research Institute
  92717 USA

Newcastle Research Group, NCM Group
  New England House, Ridley Place
  Newcastle-Upon-Tyne, England   NE1 8JW

Brian E. Niven
  University of Otago, P.O. Box 913,
  Dunedin, New Zealand

P.J. Pacy, MD
  London School of Hygiene and
  Tropical Medicine, Keppel Street, London
  W6 8RF UK

J. Gordon Parish, MD
  Pear Tree Cottage
  Thorrington, Essex, England
  CO7 8EY

Gordon Parker, MD, PhD, FRANZCP
  Mood Disorders Unit, Prince Henry Hospital,
  Little Bay, N.S.W. 2036 Australia

Evan Patrick, MD
  Cardiologist
  1081 Carling Avenue, Suite 605
  Ottawa, Ontario Canada   K1Y 4G2

M. Pecht, PhD
  Department of Cell Biology,
  The Weizmann Institute of Science, Rehovot,
  Israel

Daniel L. Peterson, MD
  Suite 306, 865 Tahoe Boulevard, P.O. Box 7870,
  Incline Village, Nevada   89450 USA

Charles M. Poser, MD
  Lecturer on Neurology, Harvard Medical School/
  Senior Neurologist, Beth Israel Hospital
  330 Brookline Avenue, Boston, Massachusetts
  02215 USA

David C. Poskanzer, MD, MPH
  deceased

Deepak Prasher, MD
  Medical Research Council, Human Movement
  and Balance Unit, Section of Neuro-Otology,
  National Hospital Queen Square, London,
  W6 8RF UK

Jesus Prieto, MD
  Director of the Department of Medicine
  University Clinic, University of Navarra, 31080
  Pamplona, Spain

Hugh F. Pross, MD, PhD, FRCPC
  Professor of Microbiology and Immunology
  and Oncology
  Associate Dean of Undergraduate Medical
  Education
  Queen's University, Kingston, Ontario
  K7L 3N6   Canada

B. Rager-Zisman, PhD
  Department of Immunology and Virology,
  Ben-Gurion University, Beer-Sheva, Israel

A. Melvin Ramsay, MD
  deceased

Nancy L. Reichenbach, BS
  Temple University School of Medicine,
  Philadelphia, Pennsylvania   19140 USA

John Richardson, MB, BS
  Clinical Tutor
  Family Medicine, University of Newcastle
  upon Tyne, 22 Elmfield Road, Gosforth,
  Newcastle-Upon-Tyne NE3 4BA England

M. Riley, MD
  Department of Medicine, Queen's University
  and Royal Victoria Hospital, Belfast
  BT12 6BA Ireland

Henri Rubinstein, MD
  Neurology (EM6) Consultant
  Hopital St-Joseph, 11, rue Franklin,
  75116 Paris, France

I. Jon Russell, MD, PhD
  Associate Professor of Medicine
  Director, Brady-Green Clinical Research Center,
  The University of Texas Health Science Center
  at San Antonio, 7703 Floyd Curl Drive,
  San Antonio, Texas   78284-7874 USA

Index

Index of Photographs